W0227967

W. Hiddemann T. Büchner W. Plunkett
M. Keating B. Wörmann M. Andreeff (Eds.)

Acute Leukemias

Pharmacokinetics and Management
of Relapsed and Refractory Disease

With 246 Figures and 248 Tables

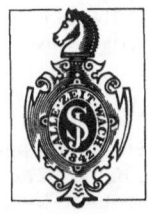

Springer-Verlag
Berlin Heidelberg GmbH

Prof. Dr. W. HIDDEMANN
Prof. Dr. T. BÜCHNER
Priv. Doz. Dr. B. WÖRMANN

University of Münster
Department of Internal Medicine
Albert-Schweitzer-Straße 33, D-4400 Münster,
Federal Republic of Germany

Prof. Dr. W. PLUNKETT
Prof. Dr. M. KEATING
Prof. Dr. M. ANDREEFF

M.D. Anderson Cancer Center
University of Texas
1515 Holocombe Boulevard
Houston, TX 77030, USA

ISBN 978-3-540-53949-0   ISBN 978-3-642-76591-9 (eBook)
DOI 10.1007/ 978-3-642-76591-9

27/3140/543210 – Printed on acid-free paper

Preface

Following the major breakthroughs in the treatment of acute leukemias in the seventies by the introduction of intensive combination regimens, therapeutic progress has slowed down and the impression of stagnation may even have occured. In contrast, the knowledge about the biology of leukemias is rapidly expanding and allows new insights into the pathophysiology of the disease. Further improvements also come from a better understanding of the pharmacokinetics and pharmacodynamics of cytostatic drugs and their mechanisms of action. Hence, novel treatment modalities can be developed on a more solid basis and rational. These achievements need to be complemented by effective eradiation of residual disease or its permanent control and new approaches have been derived from recent insights into the interaction between leukemic cells and the immune system as well as from new techniques allowing the sensitive detection of residual leukemic cells. Clinically, new therapeutic strategies are first explored in patients with advanced leukemias, which means with relapsed or refractory disease, before being incorporated into first-line treatment. These aspects deserve intensive and special efforts and frequent and thorough exchange of information. Hence, it was felt that a special series of symposia should be devoted to "Pharmacokinetics and Management of Relapsed and Refractory Disease" complementing the established meetings on "Prognostic Factors and Treatment Strategies" which will proceed in parallel. It was the aim of the international symposium "ACUTE LEUKEMIAS – Pharmacokinetics and Management of Relapsed and Refractory Disease" to provide an update of the present knowledge in this area and to stimulate further developments. As a sign for the closing distance between countries and the development of effective worldwide cooperation this symposium emerged from the joint efforts of the German AML Cooperative Group and the M.D. Anderson Cancer Center. International cooperation and effective exchange of information will lead to further improvements in biologic knowledge and therapy and will ultimately benefit patients with acute leukemias.

W. HIDDEMANN · T. BÜCHNER
W. PLUNKETT · M. KEATING
B. WÖRMANN · M. ANDREEFF

Table of Contents

Hematopoietic Growth Factors in Leukemia Therapy

Characterization of Complete Remission –
Molecular Biologic and Cytogenetic Approaches

X

Pharmacokinetics –
Preclinical Investigations and Therapeutic Implications

Post Remission Therapy

XVI

Idarubicin: New Aspects in the Treatment of Acute Leukemias

Novantrone: Current Status and Future Trends in the Treatment of Leukemias and Lymphomas

Authors and Institutions

AMADORI, S.
  Section of Hematology, Department of Human Biopathology,
  University La Sapienza, Via Benevento 6, 00161 Rome, Italy

ANDREEFF, M.
  University of Texas, MD Anderson Cancer Center,
  1515 Holcombe Blvd., Houston, TX 77030, USA

ARNOLD, R.
  Department of Internal Medicine III, University of Ulm,
  Robert-Koch-Str. 8, 7900 Ulm

AUL, C.
  Department of Internal Medicine, Hematology and Oncology
  Division, Heinrich Heine University, Moorenstr. 5,
  4000 Düsseldorf 1, FRG

BARTRAM, C.R.
  Section of Molecular Biology, Department of Pediatrics II,
  Prittwitzstr. 43, 7900 Ulm, FRG

BECK, W.T.
  Department of Biochemical and Clinical Pharmacology,
  St. Jude Children's Research Hospital, 332 N Lauderdale, Memphis,
  Tennessee 38101, USA

BEELEN, D.W.
  Department of Bone Marrow Transplantation,
  University Hospital Essen, Hufelandstr. 55, 4300 Essen 1, FRG

BERGMANN, L.
  Division of Hematology, Department of Internal Medicine,
  University Hospital, Theodor-Stern-Kai 7, 6000 Frankfurt am Main,
  FRG

BERMAN, E.
  Leukemia Service, Department of Medicine, Memorial Sloan
  Kettering Cancer Center, 1275 York Avenue, New York, NY 10021,
  USA

BIELACK, S.
  Department of Pediatric Hematology and Oncology,
  University of Hamburg, Martinistr. 52, 2000 Hamburg 20, FRG

BORSI, J.D.
2nd Department of Pediatrics, Semmelweis Medical School,
Budapest 1094 tuzolto u 7/9 Hungary

BÜCHNER, T.
Department of Hematology and Oncology, University of Münster,
Albert-Schweitzer-Str. 33, 4400 Münster, FRG

BUNJES D.
Department of Internal Medicine III, University of Ulm,
Robert-Koch-Str. 8, 7900 Ulm, FRG

CANNISTRA, S.A.
Division of Tumor Immunology, Dana Farber Cancer Institute,
44 Binney Street, Boston, Massachusetts, 02115, USA

CAPIZZI, R.L.
Comprehensive Cancer Center of Wake Forest University,
Bowman Gray School of Medicine, 300 S. Hawthorne Road,
Winston-Salem, NC 27103, USA

CARELLA, A.M.
Bone Marrow Transplantation Unit, Division of Hematology II,
Ospedale S. Martino, Via Acerbi 10/22, 16148, Genoa, Italy

CHYBICKA, A.
Department of Hematology and Oncology, Medical Academy,
ul. Bujwida 44 50-345 Wroclaw, Poland

CLIFT, R.A.
Fred Hutchinson Cancer Research Center, Veterans Administration
Medical Center and the University of Washington School of
Medicine, Seattle, USA

CREUTZIG, U.
Department of Pediatric Hematology and Oncology, University of
Münster, Albert-Schweitzer-Str. 33, 4400 Münster, FRG

DAENEN, S.
Department of Hematology, University of Groningen,
Oostersingel 59, 9713 EZ Groningen, The Netherlands

DEANE, M.
Department of Haematology, Royal Free Hospital School of
Medicine, London, UK

DRACH, J.
Department of Internal Medicine, University of Innsbruck,
Anichstr. 35, 6020 Innsbruck, Austria

EHNINGER, G.
Department of Internal Medicine, University of Tübingen,
Otfried-Müller-Str. 10, 7400 Tübingen, FRG

ENGERT, A.
  Department of Internal Medicine I, University of Köln,
  Josef Stelzmannstr., 5000 Köln 41, FRG

ERTTMANN, R.
  Department of Pediatric Hematology and Oncology,
  University of Hamburg, Martinistr. 52, 2000 Hamburg 20, FRG

ESTEY, E.
  Department of Hematology, University of Texas,
  M.D. Anderson Cancer Center, Houston, Texas, USA

FOA, R.
  Department of Biomedicine and Oncology,
  Section of Clinical Medicine, Via Genova 3, 10126 Torino, Italy

FRASSONI, F.
  Bone Marrow Transplantation Unit, Division of Hematology II,
  Ospedale S. Martino, Via Acerbi 10/22, 16148 Genoa, Italy

FREUND, M.
  Department of Hematology and Oncology, Hannover Medical
  School, Konstanty-Gutschow-Str. 8, 3000 Hannover 61, FRG

GANDHI, V.
  Department of Medical Oncology, Box 52, University of Texas,
  M.D. Anderson Cancer Center, 1515 Holcombe Boulevard,
  Houston, TX 77030, USA

GANSBACHER, B.
  Memorial Sloan Kettering Cancer Center, Box 402,
  1275 York Avenue, New York, N.Y. 10021, USA

GANSER, A.
  Department of Hematology, University of Frankfurt,
  Theodor-Stern-Kai 7, W-6000 Frankfurt 70, FRG

GARRITSEN, H.S.P.
  University of Twente, Department of Applied Physics,
  Cell Characterization Group, P.O. Box 217, 7500 AE Enschede,
  The Netherlands

GIESELER, F.
  Department of Internal Medicine, University of Würzburg,
  Klinikstr. 8, 8700 Würzburg, FRG

GLASS, B.
  Department of Internal Medicine II, University of Kiel,
  Chemnitzstr. 33, 2300 Kiel 1, FRG

GRIESINGER, F.
  Department of Hematology and Oncology, University of Münster,
  4400 Münster, FRG

GROOT, C.J. DE
Institute for Applied Radiobiology and Immunology TNO,
P.O. Box 5815, 2280 HV Rijswijk, The Netherlands

HAAS, R.
Department of Internal Medicine V, University of Heidelberg,
Hospitalstr. 3, 6900 Heidelberg, FRG

HAROUSSEAU, J.L.
Department of Hematology and Oncology, Hotel Dieu,
44035 Nantes Cedex, France

HEIL, G.
Department of Internal Medicine III, University of Ulm,
Robert-Koch-Str. 8, 7900 Ulm, FRG

HEINEMANN, V.
Department of Internal Medicine III, Klinikum Großhadern,
Marchioninistr. 15, 8000 München 70, FRG

HENSCHLER, R.
Department of Hematology and Oncology, University of Freiburg,
Medical Center, 7800 Freiburg, FRG

HIDDEMANN, W.
Department of Hematology and Oncology, University of Münster,
Albert-Schweitzer-Str. 33, 4400 Münster, FRG

HITTELMAN, W.N.
Department of Medical Oncology (Box 019), University of Texas,
M.D. Anderson Cancer Center, 1515 Holcombe Blvd., Houston,
Texas 77030, USA

HO, A.D.
Northeastern Ontario Regional Cancer Centre,
41 Ramsey Lake Road, Sudbury, Ontario P3E 5J2, Canada

HOLOWIECKI, J.
Department of Hematology, Silesian Medical Academy,
8 Reymonta, 40029 Katowice, Poland

HOVE, L. van
Department of Hematology, University Hospital of Leuven,
Herestraat 49, 3000 Leuven, Belgium

JANKA-SCHAUB, G.E.
Department of Pediatric Hematology and Oncology, University of
Hamburg, Martinistr. 54, 2000 Hamburg 20, FRG

JÜRGENS, H.
Department of Pediatric Hematology and Oncology,
Heinrich Heine University, Moorenstr. 5, 4000 Düsseldorf 1, FRG

KANTARJIAN, H.M.
M.D. Anderson Cancer Center, Department of Hematology, Box 61,
Houston, Texas 77030, USA

KASPERS, G.J.L.
Free University Hospital, Department of Pediatrics,
De Boelelaan 1117, 1081 HV Amsterdam, The Netherlands

KEATING, M.J.
University of Texas, MD Anderson Cancer Center,
1515 Holcombe Blvd., Houston, TX 77030, USA

KEMENA, A.
University of Texas, MD Anderson Cancer Center,
1515 Holcombe Boulevard, Houston, TX 77030, USA

KINGREEN, D.
Department of Hematology and Oncology, Klinikum Steglitz,
Hindenburgdamm 30, 1000 Berlin 45, FRG

KNUUTILA, S.
Department of Medical Genetics, University of Helsinki,
Haartmaninkatu 3, 00290 Helsinki, Finland

KOLB, H.J.
Department of Internal Medicine III, Klinikum Großhadern,
University of München, Marchioninistr. 15, 8000 München 70, FRG

KOLLER, E.
Ludwig-Boltzmann-Institute for Leukemia Research and
Hematology, Hanusch-Krankenhaus, Heinrich-Collin-Str. 30,
1140 Wien, Austria

KÖNEMANN, S.
Department of Hematology and Oncology, University of Münster,
Albert-Schweitzer-Str. 33, 4400 Münster, FRG

KÖPPLER, H.
Department of Hematology, University of Marburg, Baldingerstraße,
3550 Marburg, FRG

LAMBERTENGHI-DELILIERS, G.
Department of Medicine, University of Milan,
Via Francesco Sforza, 35, 21122 Milano, Italy

LEE, E.J.
University of Maryland Cancer Center, 22 S. Greene St., Baltimore,
MD 21201, USA

LINK, H.
Department of Hematology and Oncology, Hannover Medical
School, Konstanty-Gutschow-Str. 8, 3000 Hannover 61, FRG

LINKESCH, W.
Department of Internal Medicine II, University of Wien,
Garnisongasse 13, 1090 Wien, Austria

LISO, V.
Department of Hematology, University of Bari, Italy

LIST, A.F.
Arizona Cancer Center, 1515 North Campbell Avenue, Tucson,
AZ 85724, USA

MASCHMEYER, G.
Department of Hematology and Oncology, Evangelisches
Krankenhaus, Pattbergstr. 1–3, 4300 Essen 16 (Werden), FRG

MIRRO, J.
Department of Hematology and Oncology, St. Jude Children's
Research Hospital, P.O. Box 318, Memphis, TN 38101–0318, USA

MUNKER, R.
Department of Internal Medicine III, Klinikum Großhadern,
Marchioninistr. 15, 8000 München 70, FRG

MUUS, P.
Department of Hematology, University Hospital Nijmegen,
Nijmegen, The Netherlands

NOOTER, K.
Institute of Applied Radiobiology and Immunology TNO,
P.O. Box 5815, 2280 HV Rijswijk, The Netherlands

NOVOTNY, L.
Cancer Research Institute, Slovak Academy of Sciences,
Spitálska 21, 812 32 Bratislava, Czechoslovakia

OHNO, R.
Departmnet of Medicine, Nagoya University Branch Hospital,
1-1-20 Daiko-Minami, Higashiku, Nagoya 461, Japan

PIETERS, R.
Free University Hospital, Department of Pediatrics,
De Boelelaan 1117, 1081 HV Amsterdam, The Netherlands

PIETSCH, T.
Department of Pediatric Hematology and Oncology, Medical School
Hannover, Konstanty-Gutschow-Str. 8, 3000 Hannover 61, FRG

PIRKER, R.
Clinic for Internal Medicine I, Department of Oncology,
Währingergürtel 18–20, 1090 Wien, Austria

PLUNKETT, W.
Department of Medical Oncology, University of Texas,
M D Anderson Cancer Center, Houston, Texas 77030, USA

PRENTICE, H.G.
  Bone Marrow Transplant Programme,
  Royal Free Hospital School of Medicine, London, UK

RADTKE, H.
  Department of Internal Medicine I, University of Homburg,
  6650 Homburg, FRG

REIFFERS, J.
  Department of Hematology and Bone Marrow Transplant Unit,
  CHR Bordeaux, Hopital Haut-Leveque, 33604 Pessac, France

RITTER, J.
  Department of Pediatric Hematology and Oncology, University of
  Münster, Albert-Schweitzer-Str. 33, 4400 Münster, FRG

ROLLER, E.
  Department of Hematology, Oncology and Immunology,
  Robert-Bosch-Krankenhaus, Auerbachstr. 110, 7000 Stuttgart 50,
  FRG

ROWE, J.M.
  University of Rochester, Hematology Unit (JMR) and Cancer Center
  (JMB) Rochester, NY, USA

ROZMYSLOWICZ, T.
  Department of Internal Medicine, Institute of Hematology,
  Chocimska str. 5, 00-957 Warsaw, Poland

RUNDE, V.
  Department of Internal Medicine, Hematology and Oncology
  Division, Heinrich Heine University, Moorenstr. 5,
  4000 Düsseldorf 1, FRG

SCHÄFER, K.
  Department of Medicine V, Hematology and Oncology, Flurstr. 17,
  8500 Nürnberg 90, FRG

SCHLEYER, E.
  Department of Hematology and Oncology, University of Münster,
  Albert Schweitzer Str. 33, 4400 Münster, FRG

SCHMIDT, C.A.
  Department of Internal Medicine, Klinikum Rudolf Virchow,
  Spandauer Damm 130, 1000 Berlin, FRG

SCHWERDTFEGER, R.
  Department of Internal Medicine, KlinikumRudolf Virchow,
  Spandauer Damm 130, 1000 Berlin 19, FRG

SMITH, M.A.
  Department of Haematology, Royal United Hospital, Combe Park,
  Bath BA1 3NG, United Kingdom

TRIPPETT, T.
Memorial Sloan-Kettering Cancer Center, New York,
New York 1002, USA

UHAREK, L.
Department of Immunology, University of Kiel, Brunswiker Str. 4,
2300 Kiel, FRG

UNTERHALT, M.
Department of Hematology and Oncology, University of Münster,
Albert-Schweitzer-Str. 33, 4400 Münster, FRG

URASINSKI, T.
First Pediatric Department, Pomeranian Medical Academy,
ul. Unii Lubelskiej 1, 71-344 Szczecin, Poland

WEBER, E. (see KOLLER, E.)
Ludwig Boltzmann Institute for Leukemia Research and
Hematology, 1140 Wien, Austria

WEISBACH, V.
Department of Internal Medicine, Klinikum Rudolf Virchow,
Spandauer Damm 130, 1000 Berlin 19, FRG

WILEY, J.S.
Hematology Department, Austin Hospital, Heidelberg 3084,
Australia

WÖRMANN, B.
Department of Hematology and Oncology, University of Münster,
Albert-Schweitzer-Str. 33, 4400 Münster, FRG

ZINGSEM, J.
Department of Internal Medicine, Klinikum Rudolf Virchow,
1000 Berlin 19, FRG

ZURLUTTER, K.
Department of Hematology and Oncology, University of Münster,
Albert-Schweitzer-Str. 33, 4400 Münster, FRG

Drug Resistance in Leukemia

Multidrug Resistance and Its Circumvention in Acute Leukemia

A. F. List, C. M. Spier, and W. S. Dalton

Introduction

The use of intensive chemotherapy regimens produces complete remissions in up to 90 % of children with acute lymphocytic leukemia, and more than half of these patients are expected to be cured of their disease [1]. Among patients with acute myeloid leukemia (AML) and adults with acute lymphocytic leukemia, sustained complete remissions are achieved in only 20 %–40 % of cases [2, 3]. Remission rates in patients relapsing from a complete remission are substantially lower due to development of resistance to agents employed in primary therapy and other agents to which the patient has not been exposed. In experimental systems, resistance to multiple agents most often relates to expression of P-glycoprotein, or the multidrug resistance (MDR) phenotype. In this chapter we review the role of MDR in acute leukemia and current clinical trials at the Arizona Cancer Center aimed a-restoring chemosensitivity in these disorders.

Multidrug Resistance

Initial observations that tumor cell lines selected for resistance to a "natural product" antineoplastic may display cross-resistance to a variety of other agents was

first reported by Beidler and Riehm in 1970 [4]. Subsequent studies have shown that such resistance extends to many drugs that are dissimilar in structure and mechanism of action [5–7]. Multidrug-resistant cell lines accumulate and retain less drug than their drug-sensitive counterparts, which is believed to be the cellular basis for the MDR phenotype [8]. The observed changes in the cellular handling of such drugs is associated with expression of a 170-kDa membrane glycoprotein termed P-glycoprotein. P-glycoprotein traverses the plasma membrane in MDR cells and possesses ATP binding sites intracellularly, whereas carbohydrate moieties are restricted to the cell surface. Reduced drug retention by MDR cell lines is recognized to result from energy-dependent drug efflux that is mediated by P-glycoprotein. The gene encoding P-glycoprotein has been cloned, and is localized on the long arm of chromosome 7 [7q21.1] [9]. Gene transfection studies have provided convincing evidence that expression of P-glycoprotein is sufficient for expression of the MDR phenotype [10].

P-glycoprotein expression has been identified in a number of hematologic tumors, including leukemias, malignant lymphomas, and multiple myeloma. Various methodologies have been used to detect P-glycoprotein overexpression in tumor samples, including immunoblotting, immunocytochemistry, and RNA analysis. These assays allow for the correlation of P-glycoprotein expression and response to chemotherapy. If P-glycoprotein serves a functional role in conferring MDR in hematologic tumors, it may be possible to restore che-

Section of Hematology/Oncology, Department of Internal Medicine and Department of Pathology, University of Arizona College of Medicine, Tucson, Arizona, USA

mosensitivity by inactivating P-glycoprotein or utilizing drugs which are not affected by the MDR phenotype. Clinical studies using chemosensitizers to inhibit P-glycoprotein are just beginning; however, preliminary results are encouraging.

Acute Lymphoblastic Leukemia

The anthracyclines, vinca alkaloids, and the epipodophyllotoxins are integral components of induction regimens in acute lymphoblastic leukemia (ALL). Using conventional chemotherapy combinations, complete hematological remissions are achieved in 70%–90% of patients with adult or childhood acute lymphoblastic leukemia (ALL) [1, 3]. Although sustained remissions are more common in childhood, second remissions are achieved in a high percentage of relapsing patients. Not unexpectedly, expression of P-glycoprotein in ALL blasts is detected infrequently at initial diagnosis (Table 1). In childhood ALL in particular, studies by Goldstein et al. [11] and Rothenberg et al. [12] have noted overexpression of the *mdr1* gene transcript in fewer than 15% of cases at presentation or at relapse. Acquisition of the MDR phenotype, however, may be more frequent in adult ALL. Although the number of cases studied to date is small, Musto et al. [13] and others [14–17] have noted expression of the MDR phenotype in 50% or more cases of relapsing adult ALL. These observations are in keeping with the lower rate of successful reinduction in relapsed adult ALL that principally relates to drug-resistance failures.

The low prevalence of MDR detection in childhood ALL is in sharp contrast to observations in other lymphoid malignancies. Investigations at the Arizona Cancer Center [8, 18] and elsewhere have shown that while overexpression of P-glycoprotein is detected in fewer than 5% of patients with multiple myeloma at initial diagnosis, relapses following treatment with doxorubicin- or vincristine-containing regimens are commonly associated with elevated levels of P-glycoprotein. Similarly, immunohistochemical detection of P-glycoprotein using the C219 monoclonal antibody was found in over 75% of patients with non-Hodgkin's lymphoma relapsing after initial treatment with vincristine- and/or anthracycline-containing chemotherapy regimens [20]. The comparatively high frequency of expression of MDR in B-cell malignancies versus ALL may relate to inherent biological differences between these disorders. Capacity to express P-glycoprotein in normal tissues is linked to detoxification and/or secretory function and in tumors derived from such tissues, MDR expression is associated with mature or differentiated phenotypes [21, 22]. The higher frequency of MDR overexpression in relapsing B-cell malignancies may relate to intrinsic capacity for secretory function associated with a more differentiated phenotype.

Despite the low frequency of MDR detection in ALL, it may contribute to treatment failure in specific clinical and pathological subsets (Table 2). As noted

Table 1. Frequency of *mdr1* message or P-glycoprotein detection in acute lymphoblastic leukemia

Author	Pretreatment No. of cases	MDR+ (%)	Relapsed No. of cases	MDR+ (%)
Childhood				
Goldstein et al. [11]	9	1 (11)	20	3 (15)
Rothenberg et al. [12]	9	1 (11)	19	3 (16)
Adult				
Goldstein et al. [11]	15	2 (13)	0	0
Musto et al. [13]	20	2 (10)	12	7 (58)
Herweijer et al. [14]	8	4 (50)	1	1

Table 2. Acute lymphoblastic leukemia (ALL) variants associated with MDR

Disease subset	Reference
Relapsed adult ALL	[15]
Adult T-cell leukemia/lymphoma (ATL)	[23, 24]
T-cell ALL	[14, 15]
Haplodiploid ALL	[25]

earlier, adults with relapsing ALL have a lower remission rate with reinduction and may have a higher prevalence of MDR overexpression. Patients with the adult T-cell leukemia/lymphoma (ATL) syndrome in particular have a high prevalence of P-glycoprotein overexpression. Despite the use of intensive chemotherapy induction regimens in patients with ATL, remissions are generally of short duration and are associated with emergence of drug-refractory disease. Kuwazuru et al. [23], using immunoblotting with the C219 antibody, examined P-glycoprotein expression in specimens from 25 patients with the ATL syndrome. High levels of P-glycoprotein were detected in eight of 20 (40%) cases at presentation and each of six relapsed patients with drug-refractory disease. Interestingly, Herweijer et al. [14] and others [15] also noted a higher frequency of MDR overexpression in T-lineage ALL, implying that capacity for MDR expression may relate to lymphoblast lineage. Preliminary observations by Redner et al. [25] in the cytogenetically defined cohort of haplodiploid ALL indicate that the MDR phenotype may also contribute to treatment failure in this high-risk group.

Acute Myeloid Leukemia

The anthracyclines are the most active single agents in the treatment of AML, and remain an integral component of chemotherapy induction regimens [2]. Previous studies examining drug pharmacodynamics in AML have shown that cellular anthracycline concentration is an important determinant of response to therapy [26]. Anthracycline uptake by myeloblasts is influenced by a number of variables, including total leukemia burden [27] as well as duration of drug infusion [28, 29]. Accumulating evidence indicates that increased drug extrusion mediated by P-glycoprotein may underlie the heterogeneity in drug retention observed in AML samples. Accumulation of daunorubicin, as measured by cellular fluorescence, is enhanced by exposure to verapamil or other MDR antagonists in a subpopulation of blast cells in roughly 20% of previously untreated patients [31]. Indeed, intermediate or high levels of *mdr1* message or its glycoprotein product are detected in 10%–20% of cases of de novo AML (Table 3). Unlike ALL, AML appears to possess inherently greater potential for MDR expression following

Table 3. Multidrug resistance (MDR) expression in de novo AML

Author	Pretreatment No. of Cases	MDR⁺ (%)	Relapsed No. of Cases	MDR⁺ (%)
Goldstein et al. [11]	24	3 (13)	5	4
Sato et al. [32]	36	9 (25)	17	9 (53)
Nooter et al. [33]	6	1 (17)	10	6 (60)
Herweijer et al. [14]	7	1 (14)	10	8 (80)
Ito et al. [34]	10	1 (10)	14	2 (15)
Musto et al. [13]	12	1 (8)	8	6 (75)
Holmes et al. [35]	8	2 (25)	8	5 (62)

initial chemotherapy exposure. Although few patients have been studied serially for acquisition of MDR, P-glycoprotein or its message is demonstrable in more than 50 % of cases with relapsed or previously treated leukemia (Table 3).

Whether MDR expression in patients with previously untreated AML is related to recognized clinical or biologic parameters predictive of treatment outcome is not clear. To address this, we examined P-glycoprotein expression in clinically defined subsets of high-risk AML, myelodysplasia, and standard-risk de novo AML and its relation to karyotype and blast phenotype. Patients with treatment-related leukemia or AML preceded by an antecedent hematologic disorder have a characteristically high incidence of primary chemotherapy resistance and/or short-remission duration. P-glycoprotein expression in bone marrow specimens was determined by immunocytochemical staining with monoclonal antibodies directed against either the cytoplasmic domain (C219, JSB1) or a surface epitope (MRK-16) of P-glycoprotein, and performed in parallel with flow cytometry using the MRK-16 antibody [36]. The prevalence of P-glycoprotein expression in myelodysplastic syndromes was comparable to that observed in de novo AML (22 % versus 21 %) (Table 4). Antibody reactivity was restricted to blast forms and leukemic monocytes, but was otherwise absent from terminally differentiated blood cells. In contrast, acute leukemias preceded by a myelodysplastic syndrome and treatment-related hematologic disorders exhibit a comparatively high frequency of P-glycoprotein expression. The high incidence of

MDR expression in therapy-related hematologic disorders is not unexpected and may explain the observed refractoriness of these disorders to conventional induction therapy. Chemical-induced tumors in animal models often exhibit collateral resistance to a broad spectrum of naturally occurring antineoplastics associated with expression of the *mdr1* gene product [37, 38]. Interestingly, cytogenetic abnormalities affecting chromosomes 5 and 7 that characterize these high-risk AML subsets correspond to those linked in epidemiologic studies to occupational exposure to environmental toxins [39, 40]. Although MDR expression was not associated with specific chromosome abnormalities in our studies, we found a significant association between P-glycoprotein expression and stem cell (i.e., CD34) or monocytic phenotypes in the 74 cases studied ($P = 0.001$) [36]. The close association between MDR expression and specific cellular phenotypes in myeloid leukemia may reflect a normal physiologic function conserved in neoplastic counterparts. Whether the MDR product is expressed in normal hematopoietic stem cells remains unclear. Nonetheless, observations that MDR expression may be associated with an immature cell phenotype in myeloid leukemia represents a sharp deviation from observations in epithelial neoplasms.

Evidence that MDR contributes to treatment failure in AML, although quite strong, remains inconclusive. MDR expression in clinical cohorts associated with a high frequency of primary treatment failure such as relapsed AML, leukemic evolution from myelodysplasia, and treatment-

Table 4. Arizona Cancer Center studies of P-glycoprotein immunodetection in AML and myelodysplastic syndromes (MDS)[a]

Disease category	No. of cases	P-glycoprotein expression
De novo AML	19	4 (21 %)
MDS	32	7 (22 %)
MDS-AML	12	9 (75 %)
Treatment-related HD	11	9 (82 %)

MDS-AML, AML preceded by MDS; HD, hematologic disorders
[a] P-glycoprotein expression determined by flow cytometry (MRK-16) and immunocytochemistry (C219, JSB1, MRK-16)

related leukemia occurs with high frequency. Sato et al. [32] found a trend favoring a lower frequency of complete remission among patients whose leukemic cells contained moderate or high levels of the *mdr1* transcript (88% versus 58%). While this difference is not statistically significant, the number of patients requiring two courses of induction therapy to obtain remission was substantially higher in patients with high MDR expression ($P = 0.03$). Moreover, the median duration of remission for patients with low levels of MDR expression was over twice that observed in high expressors ($P = 0.003$), indicating that MDR may be an important determinant of outcome in patients receiving conventional anthracycline/cytarabine induction and consolidation therapy. It is important to note, however, that the predictive value of MDR studies as a determinant of outcome in AML may vary depending on the method of detection. The Cancer and Leukemia Group B (CALGB) found no relation between MRK-16 reactivity detected by flow cytometry and response or survival in 205 conventionally treated patients with de novo AML [41]. Recent reports describing a high incidence of epitope masking with MRK-16 [42] and failure to discriminate between monocyte and leukemia cell expression of P-glycoprotein may explain the conflicting results in the latter study. This issue is currently under investigation by the Southwest Oncology Group (SWOG) using multicolor flow cytometry to insure gating on antigenically defined blast populations. The relative merits of flow cytometric detection of MDR by two antibodies directed against surface epitopes will be compared to immunocytochemical and molecular methods and their prognostic value defined.

Clinical Circumvention of MDR

The observed associations between cellular anthracycline retention or MDR expression and treatment outcome in AML imply that treatment strategies to circumvent MDR may improve outcome in specific patient cohorts. Investigations at the Arizona Cancer Center in multiple myeloma and non-Hodgkin's lymphoma have shown that this can indeed be accomplished with agents that inhibit P-glycoprotein function, such as verapamil [43, 44]. Although responses can be restored in patients previously refractory to anthracyclines and/or vinca alkaloids, the dose of verapamil necessary for in vivo effectiveness is associated with inordinate cardiovascular toxicity. A number of other agents sharing the property of lipid solubility are potent inhibitors of P-glycoprotein and have immediate clinical applicability. Cyclosporine A in particular is an effective inhibitor of P-glycoprotein-mediated drug efflux at concentrations readily achieved in vivo in allograft transplantation [33, 45]. To test its safety and activity when administered in combination with chemotherapeutics as a resistance modifier, we initiated a phase I/II clinical trial at the Arizona Cancer Center in patients with high-risk AML. Eligible patients received a 5-day course of high-dose cytarabine (3 g/m^2) as a 3-h daily infusion, followed by a loading dose of cyclosporine and continuous infusion administered in conjunction with daunorubicin on days 6 through 8. Dose escalations of cyclosporine range from 1.0 to 16.0 mg/kg to reach projected whole blood levels of 1,000 to 2,000 ng/ml.

To date, 16 patients have been enrolled in the study and 14 are evaluable for toxicity and response. Diagnoses include relapsed or refractory AML [4], AML preceded by myelodysplasia [6], chronic myeloid leukemia in blast phase [1], treatment-related acute leukemia [2], and de novo AML with monosomy 7 [1]. Dose-limiting toxicities were observed in two of six patients treated at the highest dose level and included SWOG grade III renal and hepatic toxicity. Reversible hyperbilirubinemia occurred in four patients during cyclosporine administration. There was no apparent increase in myeloid toxicity, with the duration of neutropenia ranging from 19 to 25 days. Despite the inclusion of patients with only high-risk myeloid leukemia, preliminary results are encouraging. Complete remissions and/or restoration of chronic phase was achieved in ten of the 14 patients. There was one neutropenic death resulting from bacterial sepsis; however, an overall increased susceptibility to infection was not observed. Two additional patients achieved prolonged partial remissions. Because of the minimal toxicity observed in the initial phase of this study, the dose of daunorubicin will be escalated to 60 mg/m² per day to maximize anthracycline exposure. The potential clinical benefit of this approach is now being tested in a randomized fashion by the SWOG in patients with blast-phase chronic myelogenous leukemia.

Conclusions

Preliminary investigations in acute leukemia indicate that the MDR phenotype may contribute to treatment failure in high-risk subsets. Initial clinical trials suggest that strategies to inhibit P-glycoprotein function may restore anthracycline sensitivity in some patients. However, chemotherapy resistance in the major portion of patients with acute leukemia likely relates to multiple mechanisms. Additional studies delineating biologic features influencing MDR expression in acute leukemia and its relation to other mechanisms of resistance will provide needed insight concerning its cellular regulation and new approaches to clinical management.

References

1. Gaynon PS (1990) Primary treatment of childhood acute lymphoblastic leukemia of non-T-cell lineage (including infants). Hematol Oncol Clin North Am 4: 913–936
2. Champlin R, Gale RP (1987) Acute myelogenous leukemia: recent advances in therapy. Blood 69: 1551–1562
3. Champlin R, Gale RP (1989) Acute lymphoblastic leukemia in recent advances in biology and therapy. Blood 73: 2051–2066
4. Beidler JL, Riehm H (1970) Cellular resistance to actinomycin-D in Chinese hamster cells in vitro: cross-resistance, radioautographic, and cytogenetic studies. Cancer Res 30: 1174–1184
5. Beck WT (1987) The cell biology of multiple drug resistance. Biochem Pharmacol 36: 2879–2887
6. Endicott JA, Ling V (1989) The biochemistry of P-glycoprotein-mediated multidrug resistance. Annu Rev Biochem 58: 1137–1171
7. Pastan I, Gottesman M (1987) Multiple-drug resistance in human cancer. N Engl J Med 316: 1388–1393
8. Dalton WS, Grogan TM, Rybski JA, et al. (1989) Immunohistochemical detection and quantitation of P-glycoprotein in multiple drug-resistant human myeloma cells: association with level of drug resistance and drug accumulation. Blood 73: 747–752
9. Callen DF, Baker E, Simmers RN, Seshardri R, Roninson IB (1987). Localization of the human multiple drug resistance gene, mdr1, to 7q21.1. Hum Genet 77: 142–144
10. Gros P, Neriah YB, Croop JM, et al. (1986) Isolation in expression of a complementary DNA that confers multidrug resistance. Nature 23: 728–731
11. Goldstein LJ, Galsi H, Fojo A, et al. (1989) Expression of multidrug-resistant gene in human tumors. JNNCI 81: 116–124
12. Rothenberg ML, Mickley LA, Cole DE, Balis FM, Tsuruo T, Poplack DG, Fojo AT (1989) Expression of the mdr1/P-170 gene in patients with acute lymphoblastic leukemia. Blood 74: 1388–1395
13. Musto P, Melillo L, Lombardi G, Matera R, Di Giorgio G, Carotenuto M (1981) High risk of early resistant relapse for leukemic patients with presence of multidrug resistance associated P-glycoprotein positive cells in complete remission. Br J Haematol 77: 50–53
14. Herweijer H, Sonneveld P, Baas F, Nooter K (1990) Expression of mdr1 and mdr3 multidrug-resistance genes in human acute and chronic leukemias and association with stimulation of drug accumulation by cyclosporine. JNCI 82: 1133–1140
15. Berry JM, Brophy NA, Smith SD, Bergstrom SK, et al. (1988) Increased expression of the multidrug resistance gene mdr1 in human cancers. ASCO Proc 7: 51
16. Kato S, Ideguchi H, Muta K, Nishimura J, Nawata H (1990) Mechanisms involved in the development of Adriamycin resistance in human leukemias. Leuk Res 14: 567–573
17. Mattern J, Efferth T, Back M, Ho AD, Volm M (1989) Detection of P-glycoprotein in human leukemias using monoclonal antibodies. Blut 58: 215–217
18. Dalton WS, Grogan TM, Meltzer PS, et al. (1989) Drug-resistance in multiple myeloma in non-Hodgkin's lymphoma: detection of P-glycoprotein and potential circumvention by addition of verapamil to chemotherapy. J Clin Oncol 7: 415–424
19. Epstein J, Xiao H, Oba BK (1989) P-glycoprotein expression in plasma-cell myeloma is associated with resistance to VAD. Blood 74: 913–917

20. Miller TP, Grogan TM, Dalton WS, Spier CM, et al. (1991) P-glycoprotein expression in malignant lymphoma and reversal of clinical drug resistance with chemotherapy and high-dose verapamil. J Clin Oncol 9: 17–24
21. Kanamaru H, Kakehi Y, Yoshida O, Nakanishi S, Pastan J, Gottesman MM (1989) MDR1 RNA levels in human renal cell carcinomas: correlation with grade and prediction of reversal of doxorubicin resistance by quinidine in tumor explants. JNCI 81: 844–849
22. Bates SE, Mickley A, Chen YN, et al. (1989) Expression of drug resistance gene in human neuroblastoma cell lines: modulation by retinoic acid-induced differentiation. Mol Cell Biol 9: 4337–4344
23. Kuwazuru Y, Hanada S, Furukawa T, et al. (1990) Expression of P-glycoprotein in adult T-cell leukemia cells. Blood 76: 2065–2071
24. Kato S, Nishimura J, Muta K, Yufu Y, Nawata H, Ideguchi H (1990) Overexpression of P-glycoprotein in adult T-cell leukemia. Lancet 336: 573
25. Redner A, Hegewisch S, Haimi J, Stinherz P, Jhanwar S, Andreeff M (1990) A study of multidrug resistance and cell kinetics in a child with nearhaploid acute lymphoblastic leukemia. Leuk Res 14: 771–778
26. Kokenberg E, Sonneveld P, Delwel R, Sizoo W, Hagenbeek A, Lowenberg B (1988) In vivo uptake of daunorubicin by acute myeloid leukemia (AML) cells measured by flow cytometry. Leukemia 2: 511–517
27. Kokenberg E, Sonneveld P, Sizoo W, Hagenbeek A, Lowenberg B (1988) Cellular pharmacokinetics of daunorubicin: relationships with the response to treatment in patients with acute myeloid leukemia. J Clin Oncol 6: 802–812
28. Paul C, Tidefelt U, Liliemark J, Peterson C (1989) Increasing the accumulation of daunorubicin in human leukemia cells by prolonging the infusion time. Leuk Res 13: 191–196
29. Speth PAJ, Linssen PCM, Boezeman JBM, Wessels HMC, Haanen C (1987) Leukemic cell and plasma daunomycin concentrations after bolus injection and 72-hour infusion. Cancer Chemother Pharmacol 20: 311–315
30. Ross D, Ordonez J, Cuddy D, Wooten P, Lee E, Thompson B, Schiffer C (1989) Verapamil enhancement of daunorubicin uptake in subpopulations of blast cells from AML patients: relation to clinical outcome. ASCO Proc 8: 207
31. Maruyama Y, Murohashi I, Nara N, Aoki N (1989) Effects of verapamil on the cellular accumulation of daunorubicin in blast cells and on the chemosensitivity of leukemic blasts progenitors in acute myeloid leukemia. Br J Haematol 72: 357–362
32. Sato H, Preisler H, Day R, et al. (1990) Mrd1 transcript levels as an indication of resistant disease in acute myelogenous leukemia. Br J Haematol 75: 340–345
33. Nooter K, Sonneveld P, Oostrum R, Herweijer H, Hagenbeek T, Valerio D (1990) Overexpression of the mdr1 gene in blast cells from patients with acute myelocytic leukemia is associated with decreased anthracycline accumulation that can be restored by cyclosporine. Int J Cancer 45: 263–268
34. Ito Y, Tanimoto M, Kumazawa T, et al. (1989) Increased P-glycoprotein expression and multidrug-resistant gene (mdr1) amplification are infrequently found in fresh acute leukemia cells: sequential analysis of 15 cases at initial presentation in relapse stage. Cancer 63: 1534–1538
35. Holmes J, Jacobs A, Carter G, Janowska-Wieczorek A, Padua RA (1989) Multidrug resistance in haemapoietic cell lines, myelodysplastic syndromes and acute myeloblastic leukemia. Br J Haematol 72: 40–44
36. List AF, Spier CM, Cline A, Doll DC, Garewal H, Morgan R, Sandberg AA (1991) Expression of the multidrug resistance gene product (P-glycoprotein) in myelodysplasia is associated with a stem cell phenotype. Br J Haematol (to be published)
37. Fairchild CR, Ivy SP, Rushmore T, et al. (1987) Carcinogen-induced MDR overexpression is associated with xenobiotic resistance in rat premioplastic liver nodules in hepatocellular carcinomas. Proc Natl Acad Sci USA 84: 7705–7707
38. Keith WN, Mee PJ, Brown R (1990) Response of male skin tumors to doxorubicin is dependent on carcinogen exposure. Cancer Res 50: 6841–6847
39. Fourth International Workshop on Chromosomes and Leukemia (1984) Correlation of karyotype in occupational exposure to potential mutagenic/carcinogenic agents in acute nonlymphocytic leukemia. Cancer Genet Cytogenet 11: 326–331
40. Golomb HM, Alimena G, Rowley JD, et al. (1982) Correlation of occupation and karyotype in adults with acute nonlymphocytic leukemia. Blood 60: 404–411
41. Ball ED, Lawrence D, Malnar M, Ciminelli N, Mayer R, Wurster-Hill D, Davey FR, Bloomfield CD (1990) Correlation of CD34 in multidrug resistance P-170 with FAB and cytogenetics but not prognosis in acute myeloid leukemia. Blood 76 (Suppl 1): 252A
42. Cumber PM, Jacobs A, Hay T, Fisher J, Whittaker JA, Tsuruo T (1990) Expression of

the MDR gene (mdr1) and epitope masking in chronic lymphatic leukemia. Br J Haematol 76: 226–230

43. Durie BGM, Dalton WS (1988) Reversal of drug resistance in multiple myeloma with verapamil. Br J Haematol 68: 203–206

44. Dalton WS, Grogan TM, Meltzer PS, Scheper RJ, Durie BGM, Taylor CW, Miller TP, Salmon SE (1989) Drug-resistance in multiple myeloma and non-Hodgkin's lymphoma: detection of P-glycoprotein and potential circumvention by addition of verapamil to chemotherapy. J Clin Oncol 7: 415–424

45. Meador J, Sweet P, Stupecky M, et al. (1987) Enhancement by Cyclosporin-A of daunorubicin efficacy in Ehlich ascites carcinoma and murine hepatoma 129. Cancer Res 47: 6216–6219

The Role of DNA Topoisomerase II in Multidrug Resistance in Human Leukemia

W. T. Beck, T. Funabiki, and M. K. Danks

Introduction

Resistance to chemotherapy continues to be a major impediment and intellectual challenge to the cure of neoplastic diseases, and leukemias are no exception. Resistance of tumor cells to multiple "natural product" anticancer drugs, known as multidrug resistance (MDR), is now a well-documented phenomenon, and some excellent reviews have recently summarized its pharmacology and cell and molecular biology [1–5]. It is now clear that several types of natural product MDR exist experimentally: one is associated with P-glycoprotein (Pgp) over-expression (Pgp-MDR) [1–5], another with alterations in DNA topoisomerase II (at-MDR) (reviewed in [6]), and a third with features similar to Pgp-MDR but without Pgp overexpression [7, 8]. Although Pgp-MDR appears to have clinical correlates, we do not yet know about the clinical relevance of other forms of MDR. In this chapter, we focus on at-MDR.

Department of Biochemical and Clinical Pharmacology, St. Jude Children's Research Hospital, 332 N Lauderdale, Memphis, Tennessee 38101, USA

* The work reported in this paper is supported in part by research grant CA-30103 and Cancer Center Support (CORE) grant CA-21765, both from the National Cancer Institute, Bethesda, MD, and in part by American Lebanese Syrian Associated Charities

General Features of at-MDR

We and others have extensively characterized the biochemistry and pharmacology of the at-MDR phenotype over the past several years. Many of these studies have been summarized elsewhere [6, 9]. Briefly, while such resistant cells share overlapping cross-resistance profiles with cells expressing Pgp-MDR, "pure" at-MDR cells remain sensitive to vinca alkaloids [10], most likely because such cells do not express the *mdr1* gene or Pgp [11]. Further, modulators of Pgp-MDR, which bind to and interfere with the efflux function of Pgp, are without effect in at-MDR cells for the same reason. Fusion of at-MDR cells with drug-sensitive cells produced drug-sensitive hybrids, suggesting that at-MDR is expressed recessively [12], although other explanations are possible. Biochemically, these cells have either decreased amounts or activities of topoisomerase II (reviewed in [6]). The ability of topoisomerase II-acting drugs to form stable topoisomerase II-DNA "cleavable" complexes is decreased in the at-MDR cells, as is the catalytic activity of the enzyme [13]. In some cell lines, the amount of the enzyme is reduced [14, 15]. Moreover, we have shown that the enzyme from the at-MDR cells apparently binds ATP less well than its counterpart from the drug sensitive cells [16]. More recently, Fernandes et al. [17] showed that newly synthesized (nuclear matrix-bound) DNA was more susceptible to inhibition by VM-26 and m-AMSA, suggesting that matrix topoisomerase II was the most sensitive target of these drugs. In a subsequent study, we showed that the amount and activity of nuclear matrix topoisomerase II was decreased in at-MDR human leukemic cells [18]. Finally, Suttle et al. [19] have found a mutation in the topoisomerase II cDNA near the ATP binding fold. While many of these changes are associated with at-MDR, we do not yet know whether any of them actually cause the phenotype.

Is at-MDR Clinically Relevant?

Whether or not at-MDR is clinically relevant is the question that many of the studies of at-MDR are presently attempting to address. Several lines of reasoning suggest that tumor cells with an at-MDR phenotype will be found in patients. First, we know that neither the *mdr1* gene nor its product, Pgp, are expressed in all tumors from clinically drug-resistant patients [20]. Second, it is relatively easy to select at-MDR cell-lines experimentally [10]. Third, many of the drugs that are used to select for at-MDR in vitro – anthracyclines, epipodophyllotoxins, and aminoacridines – are used widely in the clinic. Accordingly, we suggest that tumor cells expressing the at-MDR phenotype will be found in patients' tumors. We are currently developing functional and molecular biological methods to test this hypothesis.

Functional Assays for at-MDR

We have exploited an assay that permits detection of topoisomerase II-DNA complexes in intact cells [21, 22]. An intact cell assay has several advantages. First, it can be used on clinical specimens, especially leukemia cells. Second, it can provide a functional assessment of the topoisomerase II in the cells. Third, by using an inhibitor of Pgp like verapamil, it may also be possible to assess the functional status of Pgp in the cells and consequently distinguish between cells expressing either at-MDR or Pgp-MDR. Such distinctions may allow us to determine whether these two forms of MDR are expressed in tumors and whether these phenotypes have relevance to the chemotherapeutic responsiveness of the patient.

Accordingly, we have modified an assay that quantitates drug-stimulated topoisomerase II-DNA complexes in intact tumor cells [21, 22]. Given that antitopoisomerase II drugs will "stimulate" the formation of such complexes [13], and given the fact that many antitopoisomerase II drugs such as epipodophyllotoxins and anthracyclines are substrates for Pgp, it is possible to distinguish between the two phenotypes by measuring the formation of complexes in the absence and presence of verapamil, an inhibitor of the efflux function of Pgp. Thus, as seen in Table 1, VM-26 will stimu-

Table 1. An intact cell assay for drug-stimulated DNA-protein complex formation distinguishes between cells that express Pgp-MDR and those that express at-MDR[a]

Cell line	^{3}H-DNA/^{14}C-protein, cpm precipitated		
	No drugs	30 µM VM-26	30 µM VM-26 + 10 µM verapamil
CEM	0.433	3.09	3.35
CEM/VLB$_{5K}$	0.380	1.26	3.08
CEM/VM-1	0.510	0.44	0.60

[a] Cells were incubated with ^{3}H-thymidine and ^{14}C-leucine for 18 h to label DNA and protein, respectively. Cells were then washed and incubated with VM-26 ± verapamil for another 30 min, after which they were washed again. DNA-protein complexes were precipitated with K$^+$-SDS and quantitated by liquid scintillation counting, as described by Trask et al. [21] and Zwelling et al. [22]. CEM/VLB$_{5K}$ overexpresses Pgp [23]; CEM/VM-1 does not overexpress Pgp [11] but does have altered topoisomerase II [13, 19].

late fewer complexes in cells expressing either Pgp-MDR or at-MDR, compared to drug-sensitive cells, but when Pgp-MDR cells are co-treated with VM-26 and verapamil, Pgp will be inhibited, intracellular drug levels will increase, and complex formation will be increased. However, in the at-MDR cells that express little or no Pgp [11], the effect of verapamil will be either attenuated or nonexistent.

DNA-Protein Complex Formation in Pediatric Acute Myeloid Leukemia Blasts

Whether this functional assay will correlate with clinical response remains to be determined. Shown in Fig. 1 are preliminary results of DNA-protein complex formation in acute myeloid leukemia (AML) blasts from four of our pediatric patients. We used two concentrations of VP-16, 3 μM and 30 μM, the former being a target level for free drug concentrations in the plasma. It appeared that the cells from patients 1 and 2 had an unresponsive topoisomerase II and no functional Pgp, as VP-16 produced no complexes and verapamil was without effect. However, we need independent verification that the cells actually accumulated drug. A VP-16 dose-response relationship

was seen in the cells from patient 4, and verapamil was able to permit more complexes to be formed, suggesting that these cells may have had a normal topoisomerase II but also may have expressed some Pgp. Finally, cells from patient 3 showed some response to VP-16 only in the presence of verapamil, suggesting that their topoisomerase II may be normal but that they express Pgp. We presently have no information on Pgp expression in these patients' cells, but intend to do immunohistochemical analysis with an anti-Pgp antibody. *NOTE ADDED IN PROOF: We have recently learned that only the cells from patient #2 highly expressed P-glycoprotein, as determined by immunohistochemical staining. Thus, other factors may be involved in the responsiveness of AML blasts in the intact cell assay shown in Fig. 1. These studies are ongoing.

Conclusions

Drug resistance continues to be a major obstacle to the cure of neoplastic diseases, including leukemias. Much is now known about the expression of *mdr1* or Pgp in patients' tumors. By contrast, little is known about the expression of topoisomer-

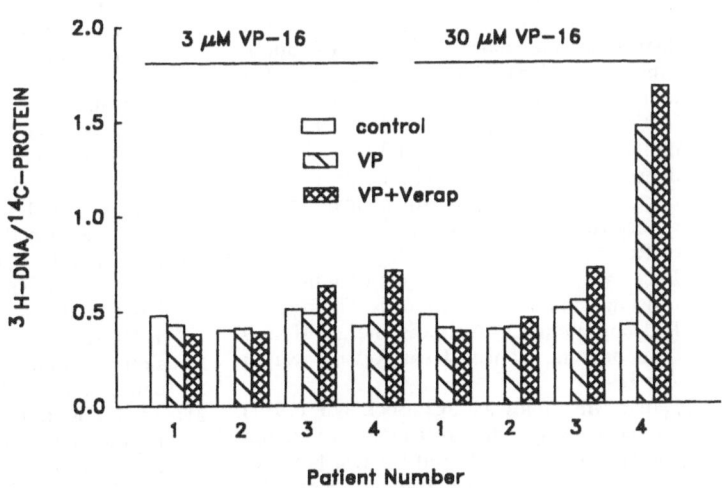

DNA−protein complex formation in AML blasts

Fig. 1. DNA-protein complex formation in acute myeloid leukemia (AML) blasts from four pediatric patients. (See footnote to Table 1 for details of the method.) The method for patients' blast cells differed from that for cell cultures in that the cells were incubated with VP-16 for 60 min at a higher number of cells/ml.

ase II in patients' tumors, so its clinical relevance remains obscure. The functional consequences of Pgp overexpression or altered topoisomerase II are implied by their presence in clinical specimens. It is our opinion that functional assays coupled with biochemical or molecular assays for markers of Pgp-MDR and at-MDR will be of considerable use in the diagnosis and treatment of tumors.

References

1. Beck WT (1987) The cell biology of multiple drug resistance. Biochem Pharmacol 36: 2879–2887
2. Moscow JA, Cowan KH (1988) Multidrug resistance. JNCI 80: 14–20
3. Endicott JA, Ling V (1989) The biochemistry of P-glycoprotein-mediated multidrug resistance. Annu Rev Biochem 58: 137–171
4. Van der Bliek AM, Borst P (1989) Multidrug resistance. Adv Cancer Res 52: 165–203
5. Roninson IB (1991) Molecular and cellular biology of multidrug resistance in tumor cells. Plenum, New York
6. Beck WT, Danks MK (1991) Multidrug resistance associated with alterations in topoisomerase II. In: Potmesil M, Kohn K (eds) DNA topoisomerases in cancer. Oxford University Press, New York pp. 260–275
7. Hindenburg AA, Gervasoni JE Jr, Krishna S, Stewart VJ, Rosado M, Lutzky J, Bhalla K, Baker MA, Taub RN (1989) Intracellular distribution and pharmacokinetics of daunorubicin in anthracycline-sensitive and -resistant HL-60 cells. Cancer Res 49:4607–4614
8. McGrath T, Center MS (1988) Mechanisms of multidrug resistance in HL60 cells: evidence that a surface membrane protein distinct from P-glycoprotein contributes to reduced cellular accumulation of drug. Cancer Res 48: 3959–3963
9. Beck WT (1990) Mechanisms of multidrug resistance in human tumor cells. The roles of P-glycoprotein, DNA topoisomerase II, and other factors. Cancer Treat Rev 17 (Suppl A): 11–20
10. Danks MK, Yalowich JC, Beck WT (1987) Atypical multiple drug resistance in a human leukemic cell line selected for resistance to teniposide (VM-26). Cancer Res 47: 1297–1301
11. Beck WT, Cirtain MC, Danks MK, Felsted RL, Safa AR, Wolverton JS, Suttle DP, Trent JM (1987) Pharmacological, molecular, and cytogenetic analysis of "atypical" multidrug-resistant human leukemia cells. Cancer Res 47: 5455–5460
12. Wolverton JS, Danks MK, Schmidt CA, Beck WT (1989) Genetic characterization of the multidrug-resistant phenotype of VM-26-resistant human leukemic cells. Cancer Res 49: 2422–2426
13. Danks MK, Schmidt CA, Suttle DP, Beck WT (1988) Altered catalytic activity of and DNA cleavage by DNA topoisomerase II from human leukemic cells selected for resistance to VM-26. Biochemistry 27: 8861–8869
14. Deffie AM, Batra JK, Goldenberg GJ (1989) Direct correlation between DNA topoisomerase II activity and cytotoxicity in adriamycin-sensitive and resistant P388 leukemia cell lines. Cancer Res 49: 58–62
15. Matsuo K, Kohno K, Takano H, Sato S, Kiue A, Kuwano M (1990) Reduction of drug accumulation and DNA topoisomerase II activity in acquired teniposide-resistant human cancer KB cell lines. Cancer Res 50: 5819–5824
16. Danks MK, Schmidt CA, Deneka DA, Beck WT (1989) Increased ATP requirement for activity of and complex formation by DNA topoisomerase II from human leukemic CCRF-CEM cells selected for resistance to teniposide. Cancer Commun 1: 101–109
17. Fernandes DJ, Smith-Nanni C, Paff MT, Neff T-A (1988) Effects of antileukemia agents on nuclear matrix-bound DNA replication in CCRF-CEM leukemia cells. Cancer Res 48: 1850–1855
18. Fernandes DJ, Danks MK, Beck WT (1990) Decreased nuclear matrix DNA topoisomerase II in human leukemia cells resistant to VM-26 and m-AMSA. Biochemistry 29: 4235–4241
19. Bugg BY, Danks MK, Beck WT Suttle DP (1991) Expression of a mutant DNA topoisomerase II in CCRF-CEM human leukemic cells selected for resistance to teniposide. Proc Natl Acad Sci USA 88: 7654–7658
20. Goldstein LJ, Galski H, Fojo A, Willingham M, Lai SL, Gazdar A, Pirker R, Green A, Crist W, Brodeur GM, Lieker M, Crossman J, Gottesman MM, Pastan I (1989) Expression of a multidrug resistance gene in human cancers. JNCI 81: 116–124
21. Trask DK, DiDonato JA, Muller MT (1984) Rapid detection and isolation of covalent DNA/protein complexes: application to topoisomerase I and II. EMBO J 3: 671–676
22. Zwelling LA, Hinds M, Chan D, Mayes J, Sie KL, Parker E, Silberman L, Radcliffe A, Beran M, Blick M (1989) Characterization of

an amsacrine-resistant line of human leukemia cells. J Biol Chem 264: 16411–16420

23. Qian X-d, Beck WT (1990) Binding of an optically pure photoaffinity analogue of verapamil, LU-49888, to P-glycoprotein from multidrug resistant human leukemic cell lines. Cancer Res 50: 1132–1137

Development of Sensitive Assays to Detect Antifolate Resistance in Leukemia Blasts

T. Trippett, J. T. Lin, Y. Elisseyeff, M. Wachter, S. Schlemmer, B. Schweitzer, and J. R. Bertino

Introduction

Despite the importance of drug resistance, both intrinsic and acquired following chemotherapy, relatively little is known of the mechanisms underlying resistance to chemotherapeutic agents in the clinic [1]. This lack of information is a result of the inherent difficulties in studying tumors from patients. Inadequate samples, tumor heterogeneity, and inability to obtain repetitive biopsies are some reasons for this paucity of information relative to the large amount of data regarding mechanisms of resistance to these drugs both at the phenotypic as well as the genetic level in experimental tumors.

We have chosen acute leukemia as the prototype disease, since malignant cells (blasts) can be obtained in relatively high purity with relative ease (blood, marrow) and repetitive sampling is possible. Acute lymphocytic leukemia (ALL) is an ideal disease to examine mechanisms of acquired methotrexate (MTX) resistance. MTX is probably the key drug in the curative regimens for this disease; however, despite a 90 %–100 % complete remission (CR) rate, most centers still report relapses in 30 %–40 % of patients [2]. Acute nonlymphocytic leukemia (ANLL) is an example of a human neoplasm that is intrinsically resistant to MTX; at the present time MTX is not used as part of treatment regimens for this disease. Study of ANLL thus allows an

understanding of mechanisms of intrinsic resistance to MTX.

Mechanisms of Acquired Resistance to MTX

MTX is an excellent model drug for the study of resistance. The major target for the drug is known (dihydrofolate reductase, DHFR), and cell lines have been developed with acquired resistance to the drug both from animal and human tumors that show one or more different mechanisms of resistance: decreased influx (decreased V_{MAX} or K_t), increased DHFR, altered DHFR that binds MTX less tightly than the wild-type enzyme, or decreased retention due to decreased polyglutamylation (reviewed in [3]).

Increased Levels of DHFR Via Gene Amplification as a Cause of MTX Resistance

Mouse, hamster, and human MTX-resistant cell lines with increased levels of DHFR activity have been described in recent years [3,5–10]. When these lines have been examined with appropriate cDNA probes, in almost all cases gene amplification has been found to accompany the increase in DHFR level, as well as a corresponding increase in the level of mRNA(s) for this enzyme. One exception to this generalization is a MTX-resistant cell line described by Dedhar et al. that was reported to have an elevated level of DHFR, but did not have an increase in mRNA or DHFR gene copies [4].

Memorial Sloan-Kettering Cancer Center, New York, USA

* Professor J. R. Bertino was supported by American Cancer Society Grant #BE-40F.

16

Following reports, indicating that gene amplification was a common mechanism of resistance observed in cell lines exposed to gradually increasing doses of MTX, four case reports appeared in the literature, one of which was from this laboratory, indicating that this event occurs in the clinic, albeit at low level, consistent with the expectation that a low level of amplification would be sufficient to cause clinical MTX resistance [11–14]. However, questions regarding the frequency with which this event occurs either in untreated or treated patients with malignancy, the stability of this type of resistance, or the influence of dose schedule on the frequency of resistance due to gene amplification, have not been adequately addressed.

Altered DHFR as a Mechanism for MTX Resistance

In experimental cell lines or in mouse tumors, alteration of DHFR as a cause of MTX resistance is less commonly observed than is impaired transport or an elevated DHFR [15]. In contrast to the relative infrequency of this mechanism of resistance in experimental human tumors, resistance to the antifolate, pyrimethamine, in falciparum malaria is almost always due to mutations in DHFR that lead to decreased binding of the drug to this enzyme (reviewed in [3]). It is of interest that in a recent study by Sirotnak (personal communication), three of 20 L1210 tumors propagated in vivo had an altered DHFR following development of MTX resistance. We have employed polymerase chain reaction (PCR) technology to amplify and sequence both cDNA and the individual exons of DHFR to determine the mutations in several of these altered cell lines (Table 1). Two of these altered enzymes have been expressed in high yield in E. coli and their characteristics studied [16, 17]. A gly-->trp mutation, which is found in the backbone of the DHFR molecule rather than in the active site, is currently under study.

It is now important to carefully examine human neoplams to determine if alterations in DHFR lead to intrinsic or acquired drug resistance. The possibility that inherent or natural resistance of ANLL to MTX is due to the presence of an altered form of DHFR in blasts of untreated patients has been suggested by the observations of Dedhar et al. [18]. This work, if confirmed, is of great potential importance for the understanding of natural and possibly acquired resistance to this drug.

In order to elucidate whether such point mutations play a role in the clinically resistant patient, we determined the nucleotide sequence of the DHFR gene of eight patients: six patients with ALL (four relapsed and two with ALL at primary diagnosis) and two patients with acute myelocytic leukemia (AML) at the time of the primary diagnosis. DHFR cDNA was amplified using PCR technology and sequenced. In all cases only wild-type sequence was found.

MTX Resistance Due to Impaired Transport

Decreased MTX uptake may be due to a reduced influx (decrease in V_{MAX} or altered K_t), or a decrease in retention (due to

Table 1. Altered mammalian DHFR enzymes from MTX resistant cells

Source	Decrease in MTX binding to DHFR	Mutation in coding sequence	Reference
3T6 (mouse)	270 fold	Leu 22→asp	[7]
CHL (hamster)	100 fold	Leu 22→phe	[8]
CHO (hamster)	100 fold	Leu 22→phe	[17]
HCT8 (human)	100 fold	Phe 31→ser	[16]
L1210 (mouse)	ND	Gly 15→trp	Unpublished

ND, not determined

decreased polyglutamylation). Decreased influx, like increased DHFR enzyme activity is a common mechanism of MTX resistance in experimental tumors [15]. Several groups are actively pursuing the molecular nature of this resistance by attempting to isolate the carrier for this active transport system (the reduced folate transport carrier) and to clone the gene or genes involved. Measurement of MTX uptake in patients with leukemia is difficult because of the number of cells required, issues related to quantitation (comparing subtypes of leukemia of varying cell size), and the requirement for untreated samples as well as samples after resistance develops. In addition to conventional uptake measurements, we have therefore explored the use of displacement assays in which cells are loaded with a fluorescent MTX compound [19–21], then displaced with either MTX or trimetrexate (TMTX); this latter drug does not require the reduced folate carrier for uptake. PT430, N^{α}-(4-amino-4-deoxy-N^{10}-methylpteroyl)-N^{ε}-(4'fluorescein thiocarbamyl)-L-lysine, synthesized in the laboratory of Andre Rosowsky at the Dana Farber Cancer Institute from fluorescein isothiocyanate and the lysine analogue of MTX, serves as an intracellular marker for transport of antifolate analogues across the membranes of blast cells. The compound is extremely lipophilic, allowing for rapid entry into cells and establishment of steady state concentrations in a period of 2 h. No evidence of cytotoxicity to cells is noted. The assay system uses competitors of DHFR, MTX, and TMTX to distinguish between cells that manifest transport defects and sensitive cells. The CCRF-CEM parent and transport defective cell lines were clearly distinguished with this assay system (Fig. 1a, b).

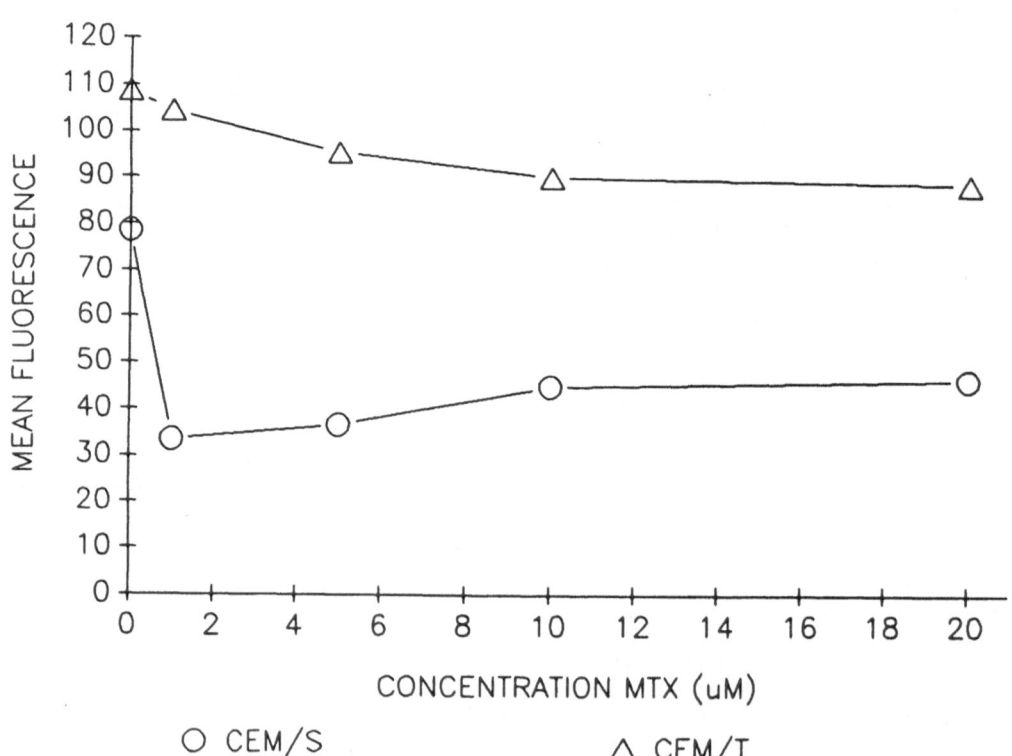

○ CEM/S   △ CEM/T

Fig. 1a. Displacement of the fluorescein analogue of MTX, PT430, in the CCRF-CEM parent cell line when incubated with an increasing concentration of MTX (2 h). Displacement is most notable at $3 \times 10^{-7} M$ MTX. Displacement of PT430 is absent in the CCRF-CEM transport resistant cell line (CEMT) when incubated with an increasing concentration of MTX

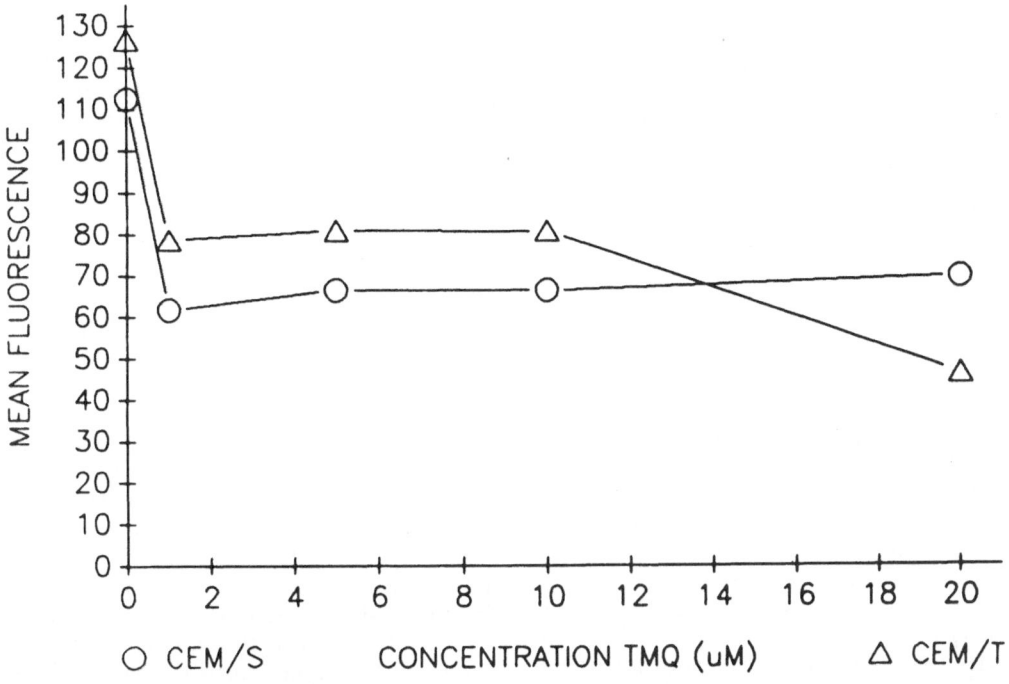

Fig. 1b. Displacement of PT430 in both the CCRF-CEM parent and transport resistant cell lines following incubation with an increasing concentration of TMTX. Displacement is most notable at 3×10^{-7} M TMTX

Resistance Due to Decreased MTX Polyglutamate Synthesis

Data from several laboratories have emphasized the importance of MTX polyglutamylation as a determinant of MTX cytotoxicity (reviewed in [3, 22]). Thus both intrinsic resistance to high pulse doses of MTX [23, 24] as well as acquired resistance may result from defective polyglutamate formation [25–27]. We recently examined the possibility that the dose schedule of MTX employed may influence the type of resistance obtained. CEM-CCRF cells were exposed to high pulse doses of MTX for 24 h (either 3 or 30 μM), and following regrowth, cells were repeatedly exposed to this drug in this same schedule. After 6–7 cycles of exposure, cell growth was no longer significantly affected by this dose of drug. The mechanism of resistance found in these cell lines (CCRF-CEM R 3/7 and CCRF-CEM R 30/6) was impaired polyglutamylation [27]. Of great interest was that relative sensitivity of these cell lines to

continuous exposure (for 72 h) of MTX was essentially unchanged. In collaboration with Dr. J. McGuire of Roswell Park, the MTX-resistant cell line was found to have an altered folylpolyglutamate synthetase enzyme (submitted for publication).

In pediatric patients with ALL, Whitehead and colleagues have recently shown that good prognosis is correlated with the ability of blast cells to accumulate MTX polyglutamates [28]. In a preliminary communication, it was reported that blast cells from patients with ANLL formed fewer polyglutamates than cells from patients with ALL [29]. Our studies extend these studies and underscore the importance of polyglutamylation in natural and acquired resistance to MTX.

Decreased MTX Polyglutamylation in ANLL Blasts as Compared to ALL Blasts

Patients with ANLL are considered to be naturally resistant to MTX, with clinical response rates of 15 % or less. To explore the reasons for this natural resistance, we examined several mechanisms known to produce MTX resistance in vitro, and compared these results with the results in a sensitive neoplasm, pediatric ALL. Comparing the two neoplasms, we found no significant difference in DHFR activity. The level of DHFR activity found in our ANLL samples was similar to the activity of 0.012 ± 0.018 µmol/h per mg protein found both in our previous studies and a recent report by Dedhar and colleagues [4]. Eighteen patients' samples were evaluated for formation of MTX polyglutamates. No significant differences were seen in the total amount of MTX plus polyglutamates between the two neoplasms, suggesting that transport resistance is not a common mechanism of intrinsic MTX resistance in ANLL.

However, although the total MTX plus polyglutamates was the same in ANLL and ALL, we found lower levels of long chain polyglutamates formed in ANLL cells than in ALL cells, although the amounts of long chain polyglutamates formed by ANLL blast cells were quite variable, and some ANLL patient samples formed as much MTX polyglutamates as the pediatric ALL blast cells. These long chain polyglutamates are the forms of MTX that are retained in cells after the withdrawal of external drug, and therefore are the forms that are most significant for cytotoxicity following a short term exposure to drug. This difference could be due to a decreased formation of MTX polyglutamates due to an altered folypolyglutamate synthetase (FPGS), a decreased amount or altered regulation of FPGS, or an increased catabolism of MTX polyglutamates. Further studies are underway to differentiate between these possibilities.

This study, together with our previous data, provides for the first time a plausible explanation for the intrinsic resistance of most ANLL patients to MTX treatment. In ANLL blasts, the lack of accumulation and retention of MTX because of poor polyglutamylation leads to rapid efflux of unbound drug as extracellular concentrations decrease, and DHFR levels in cells increase as a result of decreased DHFR degradation. As a consequence of both of these events, a higher concentration of DHFR is present in these cells, and as MTX dissociates from the enzyme, sufficient activity returns to allow enough tetrahydrofolate to be formed to allow the cells to resume DNA synthesis (see below).

MTX Polyglutamyate Formation in Adult Versus Childhood ALL

Sixteen adult and seven pediatric patient samples were evaluated for formation of MTX polyglutamates. Although there was a significant difference in the amount of total MTX plus MTX polyglutamates found in adult versus pediatric ALL blasts, most adult ALL blast cell samples were able to accumulate significant amounts of MTX plus polyglutamates, suggesting that transport resistance is not a common form of intrinsic MTX resistance in adults with ALL. Of interest is that about half of the adult ALL samples formed as many long chain (glu 3–6) polyglutamates as pediatric ALL blasts, whereas the remainder formed significantly less. The worse prognosis of adult patients with ALL may be related to the decreased ability of ALL blast cells from a significant proportion of these patients to accumulate MTX and form MTX polyglutamates. The patients studied are being followed prospectively to determine whether MTX polyglutamate formation correlates with prognosis.

„Induction" (Stabilization?) of DHFR after MTX Administration

Several years ago we reported that after treatment with MTX, the level of DHFR increases in leukemia cells and even in normal leukocytes and erythrocytes [30, 31]. The accumulated enzyme was found to be almost entirely bound to MTX, since activity at pH 5.9 was low or nondetectable, whereas there was good activity at pH 8.5, a pH at which MTX binds less tightly to DHFR [35]. When enzyme is freed from bound MTX by gel filtration at pH 9.0 in the presence of KCl, it has as much activity at pH 5.9 as at 8.5, consistent with the hypothesis that the accumulation of DHFR noted was due to complex formation between the enzyme and inhibitor in immature cells, where the rate of synthesis of this enzyme is rapid. As a consequence of decreased degradation of the enzyme due to inhibitor binding, a high concentration of the complex persists for the lifetime of the cell [30, 31]. This process was studied further in human lymphoblasts grown in vitro [32]. In the presence of MTX, at concentrations that retarded growth only slightly, DHFR increased markedly during logarithmic growth and persisted during plateau phase. Free reductase (assayed at pH 7.0) did not increase as compared to control cells. That the increased concentration of total reductase was due to decreased degradation of the enzyme was supported by experiments in which actinomycin D and cycloheximide were used [36]. However, it is also possible that an enhanced rate of expression of DHFR mRNA contributes to this increase.

As a consequence of these experiments, and later studies with ANLL patients [33], we suggested [34, 35] that the formation of the MTX-reductase complex allowed a large accumulation of this enzyme, and even a small amount of dissociation would lead to sufficient tetrahydrofolate synthesis to allow DNA synthesis to recover. We have now initiated studies to show that this phenomenon is linked with MTX polyglutamate formation and intrinsic resistance of ANLL to MTX.

Conclusions

The availability of new technology has now made it possible to begin to carefully investigate the basis of natural and acquired resistance to drugs. MTX is an important drug in the treatment of severe human malignancies, including ALL, and its mechanism of action is reasonably well established. It should be possible to further characterize the basis for natural and acquired resistance to this drug in acute leukemia, and based on this knowledge, to utilize this drug more effectively, as well as to develop alternative therapeutic opportunities.

References

1. Sobrero A, Bertino JR (1986) Clinical aspects of drug resistance. Cancer Surv 5: 93–107
2. Henderson ES, Lister TA (eds) (1990) Leukemia, 5th edn. Saunders, Philadelphia
3. Schweitzer BI, Dicker AP, Bertino JR (1990) Dihydrofolate reductase as a therapeutic target. FASEB J 4: 2441–2452
4. Dedhar S, Hartley D, Goldie JH (1985) Increased dihydrofolate reductase activity in methotrexate-resistant human promyelocytic leukemia (HL-60) cells. Biochem J 225: 609–617
5. Mini E, Srimatkandada S, Medina WD, Moroson BA, Carman MD, Bertino JR (1985) Molecular and karyological analysis of methotrexate-resistant and sensitive human leukemic CCRF-CEM cells. Cancer Res 45: 317–328
6. Srimatkandada S, Medina WD, Cashmore AR, Whyte W, Engel D, Moroson BA, Franco CT, Dube S, Bertino JR (1983) Amplification and organization of dihydrofolate reductase gene in human leukemic cell line K-562, resistant to methotrexate. Biochemistry 22: 5774–5781
7. Simonsen CC, Levinson AD (1983) Isolation and expression of an altered mouse dihydrofolate reductase cDNA. Proc Natl Acad Sci USA 80: 2495–2499
8. Melera PW, Davide JP, Hession CA, Scotto KW (1984) Phenotypic expression in E Coli and nucleotide sequence of two Chinese hamster lung cell cDNAs encoding different dihydrofolate reductases. Mol Cell Biol 4: 38–48
9. Kaufman RJ, Brown PC, Schimke RT (1979) Amplified dihydrofolate reductase genes in unstable methotrexate resistant cells are associated with double minute chromosomes. Proc Acad Sci USA 76: 5669–5673
10. Wolman SR, Craven ML, Grill SP, Domin BA, Cheng YC (1983) Quantitative correlation of homogeneously stained regions on chromosome 10 with dihydrofolate reductase enzyme in human cells. Proc Natl Acad Sci USA 80: 807–809
11. Horns RC, Dower WJ, Schimke RT (1984) Gene amplification in a leukemia patient treated with methotrexate. J Clin Oncol 2: 2–7
12. Carman MD, Schornagel JH, Rivest RS, Srimatkandada S, Portlock CS, Bertino JR (1984) Clinical resistance to methotrexate due to gene amplification. J Clin Oncol 2: 16–20
13. Curt GA, Carney DN, Cowan KH, Jolivet J, Bailey BD, Drake JC, Kao-Shan CS, Minna

JD, Chabner BA (1983) Unstable methotrexate resistance in human small cell cancer associated with double minute chromosomes. N Engl J Med 308: 199–202

14. Trent JM, Buick RN, Olson S, Horns RC Jr, Schimke RT (1984) Cytologic evidence for gene amplification in methotrexate-resistant cells obtained from a patient with ovarian adenocarcinoma. J Clin Oncol 2: 8–15
15. Sirotnak FM, Moccio DM, Kelleher LE, Goutas LJ (1981) Relative frequencey and kinetic properties of transport defective phenotypes among methotrexate-resistant L1210 clonal cells derived in vivo. Cancer Res 41: 4447–4452
16. Schweitzer BI, Srimatkandada S, Gritsman H, Sheridan R, Venkataraghavan RB, Bertino JR (1989) Probing the role of two hydrophobic active site residues in the human dihydrofolate reductase by site directed mutagenesis. J Biol Chem 264: 20786–20795
17. Dicker A, Volkenandt M, Schweitzer BI, Banerjee D, Bertino JR (1990) Identification and characterization of a mutation in the dihydrofolate reductase gene from the methotrexate resistant chinese hamster ovary cell line pro- 3 Mtx^{RIII}. J Biol Chem 265: 8317–8321
18. Dedhar S, Hartley D, Fitz-Gibbons D, Phillips G, Goldie JH (1985) Heterogeneity in the specific activity and methotrexate sensitivity of dihydrofolate reductase from blast cells of acute myelogenous leukemia patients. J Clin Oncol 3: 1545–1522
19. Assaraf YG, Molina A, Schimke RT (1989) Cross resistance to the lipid soluble antifolate trimetrexate in human carcinoma cells with the multidrug resistant phenotype. J N C I 81: 290–294
20. Assaraf YG, Schimke RT (1987) Identification of methotrexate transport deficiency in mammalian cells using fluoresceinated methotrexate and flow cytometry. Proc Natl Acad Sci USA 84: 7154–7158
21. Wright JE, Rosowsky A, Boeheim K, Cucchi CA, Frei E III (1987) Flow cytometric studies of methotrexate resistance in human squamous carcinoma cell cultures. Biochem Pharmacol 36: 1561–1564
22. Chabner BA, Allegra CJ, Curt GA, Clendenin NJ, Baram J, Koizumi A, Drake JC, Jolivet JJ (1985) Polyglutamylation of methotrexate. Is methotrexate a prodrug? Clin Invest Med 76: 907–912
23. Curt GA, Jolivet J, Bailey BD, et al. (1984) Synthesis and retention of methotrexate polyglutamates by human small cell lung cancer. Biochem Pharmacol 33: 1682–1686
24. Pizzorno G, Chang Y-M, McGuire JJ, Bertino JR (1989) Inherent resistance of human squamous carcinoma cell lines to methotrexate as a result of decreased polyglutamylation of this drug. Cancer Res 49: 5275–5280
25. Cowan KH, Jolivet J (1984) A methotrexate-resistant human breast cancer cell line with multiple defects, including diminished formation of methotrexate polyglutamates. J Biol Chem 259: 10798–10800
26. Rosowsky A, Wright JE, Cucchi CA, Lippke JA, Tantravahi R, Ervin TJ, Frei E III (1984) Phenotypic heterogeneity in cultured human head and neck squamous cell carcinoma lines with low level methotrexate resistance. Proc Natl Acad Sci USA 81: 2873–2877
27. Pizzorno G, Mini E, Coronnello M, McGuire JJ, Moroson BA, Cashmore AR, Lin JT, Mazzei T, Periti P, Bertino JR (1988) Impaired polyglutamylation of methotrexate as a cause of resistance in CCRF-CEM cells after short term, high-dose treatment with this drug. Cancer Res 48: 2149
28. Whitehead VM, Rosenblatt DS, Vuchich M-J, Shuster JJ, Witte A, Beaulieu D (1990) Accumulation of methotrexate and methotrexate polyglutamates in lymphoblasts at diagnosis of childhood acute lymphoblastic leukemia; a pilot prognostic factor analysis. Blood 76: 4433
29. Whitehead VM, Kalman TI, Rosenblatt DS, Vuchich M-J, Payment C (1988) Regulation of methotrexate polyglutamate (MTXPG) formation in human leukemic cells. Proc Am Assoc Cancer Res 29: 287
30. Bertino JR, Donohue DM, Simmons B, Gabrio BN, Silber R, Huennekens FM (1963) The "induction" of dihydrofolic reductase in leukocytes and erythrocytes of patients treated with amethopterin. J Clin Invest 42: 466
31. Bertino JR, Cashmore A, Fink M, Calabresi P, Lefkowitz E (1965) The "induction" of leukocyte and erythrocyte dihydrofolate reductase by methotrexate. II. Clinical and pharmacologic studies. Clin Pharmacol Ther 6: 763–770
32. Hillcoat BL, Swett V, Bertino JR (1967) Increase of dihydrofolate reductase activity in cultured mammalian cells after exposure to methotrexate. Proc Natl Acad Sci USA 58: 1632–1637
33. Bertino JR, Sawicki NL, Cashmore AR, Cadman E, Skeel RL (1977) Natural resistance to methotrexate in human acute nonlymphocytic leukemia. Cancer Treat Rep 61: 667–673
34. Bertino JR, Johns DG (1967) Folate antagonists. Annu Rev Med 18: 27–34

Sequential Analysis of P-Glycoprotein Expression in Childhood Acute Lymphoblastic Leukemia

D. Kingreen[1], C. Sperling[1], M. Notter[1], C. Schmidt[2], H. Diddens[3], H. Riehm[4], E. Thiel[1], and W.-D. Ludwig[1]

Introduction

Tumor-cell resistance to cytotoxic drugs is thought to be a major cause of failure in the chemotherapy of malignant tumors. One type identified as multidrug resistance (MDR) in experimental systems including human tumor cell lines was first described in 1970 in Chinese hamster lung and P388 leukemia cells [1]. Resistant tumor cells exhibit decreased sensitivity, not only to the initial drug used to promote resistance but also to a variety of structurally diverse molecules to which they have not been previously exposed (reviewed in [21]). At the molecular level, such resistant cells have been found to exhibit increased expression of P-glycoprotein (P-gp), a 170-kDa transmembrane glycoprotein encoded by the *MDR1* gene. The functionally relevant characteristic of MDR cells is a defective intracellular accumulation of cytotoxic drugs due to the overexpression of P-gp, which acts as an energy-dependent efflux pump for the transfer of cytotoxic drugs to the external medium.

Recent studies using various molecular techniques and immunocytochemical methods have indicated that several untreated human cancers including hematologic malignancies are associated with increased expression of the *MDR1* gene, suggesting that P-gp may be responsible for intrinsic drug resistance [3, 4]. Very few data, however, are as yet available on the expression of P-gp in acute lymphoblastic leukemia (ALL) [3, 5–13], and sequential analyses to determine the clinical relevance of the MDR phenotype have only been performed in one longitudinal study of a small number of patients with ALL [13].

The present study in a large series of children with ALL therefore applied monoclonal antibodies (mAbs) to different epitopes of the P-gp molecule for performing sequential analyses of P-gp expression at initial diagnosis and in relapse and for correlating the MDR phenotype with responsiveness to therapy.

Patients and Methods

This study included a total of 61 children with ALL, in 14 of whom P-gp expression was analyzed only at the time of initial diagnosis. Case control studies were conducted on leukemic cells (bone marrow and/or peripheral blood) of 47 patients at various phases of the disease: at diagnosis and first or further relapses ($n = 34$), at first and second or subsequent relapses ($n = 6$), and at diagnosis or relapse and blast persistence after induction therapy ($n = 7$).

The 61 patients (37 males and 24 females) ranged in age from 5 months to 14 years. All patients achieved complete remission after initial induction therapy. Thirty-two pa-

---

[1] Department of Hematology/Oncology, Klinikum Steglitz, Berlin, FRG
[2] Department of Internal Medicine, University Hospital R. Virchow, Berlin, FRG
[3] Medical Laser Center, Lübeck, FRG
[4] Department of Pediatrics, Hannover Medical School, Hannover, FRG
* Supported in part by Deutsche Krebshilfe e. V. and Deutsche Leukämie-Forschungshilfe.

23

tients had an early relapse (during front-line treatment or within the first 6 months thereafter) and 15 a late relapse. Treatment was carried out in accordance with the therapeutic protocols of the ALL-BFM 81, 83 and 86 studies [14].

Table 1 lists the properties of the three mAbs (C219, JSB-1, MRK16) used for detecting P-gp expression [15–17]. In view of the localization of the P-gp epitopes, the reactivity of C219 and JSB-1 was analyzed after fixation (acetone, 5 min, room temperature) by immunoperoxidase staining and that of MRK16 by both immunoperoxidase and the indirect immunofluorescence techniques, as previously described [18, 19]. Murine antibodies of the isotypes IgG1 and IgG2a were used as negative controls. The positive controls were two cell lines (CCRF and F4-6) whose characteristics are summarized in Table 2. The cell lines were maintained in RPMI 1640 medium (Gibco/BRL, Eggenstein, FRG) supplemented with 10 % fetal bovine serum (Gibco), 5 mM L-glutamine (Gibco), and 1 mM Napyruvate (Gibco).

Table 1. Characterization of monoclonal antibodies

	MRK16	C219	JSB-1
Reference	[17]	[16]	[15]
Immunogen (cell line)	K562	CHrA3	CHrC5
Specificity detection MDR cell lines	Human ovarian cancer	Syrian hamster Mouse Human CCRF	Human ovary (H134) Chinese hamster lung (DC3F) Human lung
Immunoprecipitation	Western blot analysis	Western blot analysis	Western blot analysis
Localization of the epitope	Extracellular	Intracellular	Intracellular
Isotype	IgG2a	IgG2a	IgG1
Source (of supply)	Tsuruo/Tokyo	Centocorps	Sanbio

Table 2. Characteristics of the MDR cell lines

	CCRF	F4-6
Species	Human	Mouse
Initial cell line	T-ALL (ATCC CLL 119) CCRF-CEM	Erythroleukemia (Friend virus) F4-6WT
Cytostatic used for selection	Actinomycin D	Pyromycin
Concentration reached	200 ng/ml	1 µg/l
Relative resistance (ID$_{50}$ res/ID$_{50}$ sens)	348-fold	125-fold
Resistant line	CCRF-DAC	F4-6ADM
Tested cross-resistance	Adriamycin, daunomycin, vincristine, vinblastine, VP16, VM26	Actinomycin D, daunomycin
Drugs to which sensitive	Bleomycin, cisplatin, MTX	Aclacinomycin
Method of detection of MDR/P-170	Northern blot analysis	Gene amplification Northern blot, APAAP
Supplier	Diddens/Lübeck	Ostertag/Hamburg

res, resistant; sens, sensitive; VP16, etoposide; VM26, teniposide; MTX, methotrexate; MDR, multidrug resistance; P-170, P-glycoprotein; APAAP, alkaline phosphatase-anti-alkaline phosphatase technique

Results

In cultured tumor cells, the mAbs JSB-1 and C219 yielded reliably reproducible results with a negative reaction in the drug-sensitive cells and clearly positive staining in the drug-resistant cell lines. The mAb MRK16 unspecifically stained both parental cells and their Actinomycin D- or Adriamycin-resistant derivatives and was therefore not used in the investigations of ALL specimens. P-gp-positive cells were found in three of 48 patients examined at the initial presentation; the percentage of leukemic cells showing the MDR phenotype in these cases ranged from 10% to 70%. These patients achieved complete remission. The case control studies yielded indications of scattered P-gp-positive leukemic blasts in 11 patients at different phases of their disease. The further clinical course of these patients is summarized in Table 3. Of the five patients disclosing P-gp-positive cells at the first relapse, three achieved a second complete remission, and one of three children analyzed during the second relapse responded to chemotherapy. In contrast to the findings in the leukemic cell lines, those in the ALL investigations did not reveal a uniform reaction pattern for the mAbs C219 and JSB-1 inasmuch as positive staining was largely only detected with the latter.

Discussion

Our present study indicates that increased P-gp expression occurred infrequently in leukemia cells from children with ALL. Only three of 48 patients (6%) disclosed P-gp-positive cells at initial presentation and 11 of 47 patients (23%) at the relapsed stage. No clear correlation was evident between the MDR phenotype and responsiveness to therapy.

Very few studies have as yet evaluated the incidence and clinical implications of increased P-gp expression in childhood ALL.

A recent study did not detect P-gp-positive cells in 28 untreated and 14 relapsed children with ALL and concluded that the MDR phenotype is not an important mechanism of drug resistance in childhood ALL [12]. In accordance with our observations, two other reports described a relatively low frequency of P-gp expression in initial and relapsed childhood ALL [7, 8].

There are some possible explanations for the absence or low incidence of P-gp expression in childhood ALL observed by us and others. Firstly, childhood ALL is considered to be a chemoresponsive malignancy with remissions achieved in more than 95% of patients at initial presentation [14]. Secondly, other mechanisms of cellular drug resistance or alterations of pharmacokine-

Table 3. Correlation between P-glycoprotein (P-170) expression and the clinical course

Patient	Time	Positive mAb	Further clinical course
1	4 rel	C219	Death 2 months after 4th rel
2	1 rel	C219/JSB-1	2nd rem, BMT, death 3 months after BMT
3	1 rel	JSB-1	No th, death after 7 weeks
4	1 rel	JSB-1	2nd rem, 2nd rel after 10 months, death 6 weeks after 2nd rel
5	2 rel	JSB-1	Death 2 months after 2nd rel
6	2 rel	JSB-1	Death 2 months after 2nd rel
7	1 rel	JSB-1	2nd rem, BMT, death 4 months after BMT
8	1 rel	JSB-1	2nd rem, 2nd rel after 10 months, death 2 months after 2nd rel
9	pers rel	JSB-1	Death in pers rel
10	2/3 rel	JSB-1	3rd rem, death 2 months after 3rd rel
11	1 rel	JSB-1	Unknown

rel, relapse; rem, remission; BMT, bone-marrow transplantation; th, therapy; pers rel, persistent relapse

tics may play a more important role in refractory childhood ALL patients [12]. Thirdly, studies evaluating the incidence of P-gp expression in childhood ALL were mainly performed in leukemia samples collected prior to the administration of chemotherapeutic induction regimens or salvage protocols and might therefore have failed to detect the induced MDR1 product [6].

In contrast to these findings in ALL, other recent studies have indicated a substantially higher incidence of increased *MDR-1* mRNA or P-gp expression both at diagnosis and relapse in myelodysplastic syndromes, acute myeloid leukemia, adult T-cell leukemia, and the blast crisis of chronic myeloid leukemia [13, 20–27]. Even more important for the clinical implications of the MDR phenotype were observations suggesting that the expression of P-gp and clinical refractoriness to chemotherapy are highly correlated in leukemic patients [23–27] and that the MDR phenotype can be reversed by various types of drugs including calcium-channel-blocking agents (e.g., verapamil), cyclosporin A and steroid antagonists (e.g., tamoxifen) [11, 28, 29]. These studies, however, mainly involved adult patients and demonstrated a more frequent overexpression of P-gp in patients with poor prognostic features such as a preceding myelodysplastic syndrome or acute myeloid leukemia following cytotoxic therapy for neoplastic disease or carcinogen exposure.

While molecular techniques – e.g., use of nucleic acid probes for Northern blot analysis as well as in situ hybridization or slot blot analysis to detect mRNA, and Western blotting to detect P-gp – are difficult and time-consuming [30]. Immunocytochemistry and immunofluorescence with mAbs make it fairly easy to analyze a large number of tumor cells for P-gp expression at the single-cell level. Some authors, however, have observed conflicting staining patterns when using different mAbs for detection of the MDR phenotype in tumor cell lines as well as in neoplastic human tissues [6, 31, 32]. Therefore, the reliability of mAbs for detection of P-gp must be checked thoroughly before interpreting the results of anti-P-gp mAbs in clinical specimens.

Comparison of the three mAbs used in this study against different epitopes of the P-gp molecule yielded some variability of reactions in leukemic cell lines and ALL samples. Although the staining pattern with JSB-1 paralleled that of C219 in drug-resistant cell lines, the two mAbs did not show a uniform reaction pattern with blasts in ALL. Positive staining results in ALL samples were mostly obtained only with JSB-1.

Other authors also reported a number of discrepancies such as weak staining with JSB-1 in the absence of *MDR-1* mRNA or diffuse positivity for C219 on neutrophils and some myeloid precursors [13, 21, 32]. It has therefore been proposed that a small panel of at least three anti-P-gp mAbs should be used and that a clinical specimen be considered P-gp-positive only if it reacts with all three mAbs [31]. Since MRK16 cross-reacts with molecules other than P-gp and nonspecifically reacts in both drug-sensitive parental cell lines and fresh acute leukemia cells, positive results obtained only with MRK16 probably cannot be considered as proof of the presence of P-gp [6, 31, 32].

Acknowledgements. We gratefully acknowledge the fruitful cooperation of participants in the ALL-BFM trials. We also wish to thank Dr. W. Ostertag for the drug-resistant cell line F4-6ADM, Dr. T. Tsuruo for the mAb MRK16, Ms. G. Gassner and Ms. B. Komischke for excellent technical assistance, and Mr. J. Weirowski for improving the English text.

References

1. Biedler JL, Riehm H (1970) Cellular resistance to actinomycin D in Chinese hamster cells in vitro: cross-resistance, radioautographic and cytogenetic studies. Cancer Res 30: 1174–1184
2. Van der Bliek AM, Borst P (1989) Multidrug resistance. Adv Cancer Res 52: 165–203
3. Goldstein LJ, Galski H, Fojo A, Willingham M, Lai SL, Gazdar A, Pirker R, Green A, Crist W, Brodeur GM, Lieber M, Cossman J, Gottesman MM, Pastan I (1989) Expression of a multidrug resistance gene in human cancers. JNCI 81: 116–124

4. Deuchars KL, Ling V (1989) P-glycoprotein and multidrug resistance in cancer chemotherapy. Semin Oncol 16: 156–165
5. Fojo AT, Ueda K, Slamon DJ, Poplack DG, Gottesman MM, Pastan I (1987) Expression of a multidrug-resistance gene in human tumors and tissues. Proc Natl Acad Sci USA 84: 265–269
6. Ito Y, Tanimoto M, Kumazawa T, Okumura M, Morishima Y, Ohno R, Saito H (1989) Increased P-glycoprotein expression and multidrug-resistant gene (mdr1) amplification are infrequently found in fresh acute leukemia cells. Cancer 63: 1534–1538
7. Rothenberg ML, Mickley LA, Cole DE, Balis FM, Tsuruo T, Poplack DG, Fojo AT (1989) Expression of the mdr-1/P-170 gene in patients with acute lymphoblastic leukemia. Blood 74: 1388–1395
8. Ubezio P, Limonta M, D'Incalci M, Damia G, Masera G, Giudici G, Wolverton JS, Beck WT (1989) Failure to detect the P-glycoprotein multidrug resistant phenotype in cases of resistant childhood acute lymphocytic leukaemia. Eur J Cancer Clin Oncol 25: 1895–1899
9. Mattern J, Efferth T, Bak M, Ho AD, Volm M (1989) Detection of P-glycoprotein in human leukemias using monoclonal antibodies. Blut 58: 215–217
10. Sugawara I, Kodo H, Ohkochi E, Hamada H, Tsuruo T, Mori S (1989) High-level expression of MRK 16 and MRK 20 murine monoclonal antibody-defined proteins (170,000–180,000 P-glycoprotein and 85,000 protein) in leukaemias and malignant lymphomas. Br J Cancer 60: 538–541
11. Redner A, Hegewisch S, Haimi J, Steinherz P, Jhanwar S, Andreeff M (1990) A study of multidrug resistance and cell kinetics in a child with near-haploid acute lymphoblastic leukemia. Leuk Res 14: 771–777
12. Pieters R, Hongo T, Loonen AH, Huismans DR, Broxterman HJ, Hählen K, Veerman AJP (1991) Drug resistance in children with relapsed acute lymphoblastic leukemia. In: Pieters R (ed) Drug resistance in childhood leukemia. Thesis, Amsterdam, p 79
13. Musto P, Melillo L, Lombardi G, Matera R, Di Giorgio G, Carotenuto M (1991) High risk of early resistant relapse for leukaemic patients with presence of multidrug resistance associated P-glycoprotein positive cells in complete remission. Br J Haematol 77: 50–53
14. Riehm H, Gadner H, Henze G, Kornhuber B, Lampert F, Niethammer D, Reiter A, Schellong G (1990) Results and significance of six randomized trials in four consecutive ALL-BFM studies. In: Büchner T, Schellong G, Hiddemann W, Ritter J (eds) Acute Leukemias II. Prognostic factors and treatment strategies. Springer, Berlin Heidelberg New York, pp 439–450 (Haematology and blood transfusion, vol 33)
15. Scheper RJ, Bulte JWM, Brakkee JGP, Quak JJ, van der Schoot E, Balm AJM, Meijer CJLM, Broxterman HJ, Kuiper CM, Lankelma J, Pinedo HM (1988) Monoclonal antibody JSB-1 detects a highly conserved epitope on the P-glycoprotein associated with multidrug-resistance. Int J Cancer 42: 389–394
16. Kartner N, Evernden-Porelle D, Bradley G, Ling V (1985) Detection of P-glycoprotein in multidrug-resistant cell lines by monoclonal antibodies. Nature 316: 820–823
17. Hamada H, Tsuruo T (1986) Functional role for the 170- to 180-kDa glycoprotein specific to drug-resistant tumor cells as revealed by monoclonal antibodies. Proc Natl Acad Sci USA 83: 7785–7789
18. Köller U, Stockinger H, Majdic O, Bettelheim P, Knapp W (1986) A rapid and simple immunoperoxidase staining procedure for blood and bone marrow samples. J Immunol Methods 86: 75–81
19. Ludwig WD, Bartram CR, Ritter J, Raghavachar A, Hiddemann W, Heil G, Harbott J, Seibt-Jung H, Teichmann JV, Riehm H (1988) Ambiguous phenotypes and genotypes in 16 children with acute leukemia as characterized by multiparameter analysis. Blood 71: 1518–1528
20. Ma DDF, Davey RA, Harman DH, Ibister JP, Scurr RD, Mackertich SM, Dowden G, Bell DR (1987) Detection of a multidrug resistant phenotype in acute non-lymphoblastic leukaemia. Lancet i: 135–137
21. Holmes J, Jacobs A, Carter G, Janowska-Wieczorek A, Padua RA (1989) Multidrug resistance in haemopoietic cell lines, myelodysplastic syndromes and acute myeloblastic leukaemia. Br J Haematol 72: 40–44
22. Sato H, Gottesman MM, Goldstein LJ, Pastan I, Block AM, Sandberg AA, Preisler HD (1990) Expression of the multidrug resistance gene in myeloid leukemias. Leuk Res 14: 11–22
23. Sato H, Preisler H, Day R, Raza A, Larson R, Browman G, Goldberg J, Vogler R, Grunwald H, Gottlieb A, Bennett J, Gottesman M, Pastan I (1990) MDR1 transcript levels as an indication of resistant disease in acute myelogenous leukaemia. Br J Haematol 75: 340–345
24. Kuwazuru Y, Yoshimura A, Hanada S, Utsunomiya A, Makino T, Ishibashi K, Kodama M, Iwahashi M, Arima T, Akiyama SI (1990) Expression of the multidrug transporter,

P-glycoprotein, in acute leukemia cells and correlation to clinical drug resistance. Cancer 66: 868–873

25. Kuwazuru Y, Yoshimura A, Hanada S, Ichikawa M, Saito T, Uozumi K, Utsunomiya A, Arima T, Akiyama SI (1990) Expression of the multidrug transporter, P-glycoprotein, in chronic myelogenous leukaemia cells in blast crisis. Br J Haematol 74: 24–29

26. Kuwazuru Y, Hanada S, Furukawa T, Yoshimura A, Sumizawa T, Utsunomiya A, Ishibashi K, Saito T, Uozumi K, Maruyama M, Ishizawa M, Arima T, Akiyama SI (1990) Expression of P-glycoprotein in adult T-cell leukemia cells. Blood 76: 2065–2071

27. Holmes JA, West RR, Whittaker JA, Jacobs A (1991) Correlation of MDR status with clinical outcome in patients with acute myeloblastic leukaemia. Br J Haematol 77: 130–131

28. Berman E, Adams M, Duigou-Osterndorf R, Godfrey L, Clarkson B, Andreeff M (1991) Effect of Tamoxifen on cell lines displaying the multidrug-resistant phenotype. Blood 77: 818–825

29. Sonneveld P, Nooter K (1990) Reversal of drug-resistance by cyclosporin-A in a patient with acute myelocytic leukaemia. Br J Haematol 75: 208–211

30. Rothenberg M, Ling V (1989) Multidrug resistance: molecular biology and clinical relevance. JNCI 81: 907–910

31. Van der Valk P, van Kalken CK, Ketelaars H, Broxterman HJ, Scheffer G, Kuiper CM, Tsuruo T, Lankelma J, Meijer CJLM, Pinedo HM, Scheper RJ (1990) Distribution of multi-drug resistance-associated P-glycoprotein in normal and neoplastic human tissues. Ann Oncol 1: 56–64

32. Wooten P, Cuddy D, Felsted P, Pan S, Ross D (1989) Comparison of anti-P-glycoprotein monoclonal antibodies MRK16, 265/F4 and C219 in the detection of multidrug resistant cells. Proc Am Assoc Cancer Res 30: 529

Expression of the *MDR1* Gene and Treatment Outcome in Acute Nonlymphocytic Leukemia

R. Pirker[1,2,3], J. Wallner[2], K. Geissler[1], P. Bettelheim[1], W. Linkesch[2], and K. Lechner[1]

Introduction

Drug resistance contributes to the poor prognosis of acute nonlymphocytic leukemia (ANLL) [1, 2]. In order to overcome drug resistance, knowledge of its exact nature is required.

Multidrug resistance is due to the expression of the *MDR1* gene and its protein product, P-glycoprotein [3]. This transmembrane protein functions as an energy-dependent drug efflux pump for anthracyclines and other hydrophobic natural compounds but does not affect alkylating agents and antimetabolites [3]. *MDR1* gene expression was detected in several normal human tissues [3] and in malignancies [4–7]. The observation of occasional expression of the *MDR1* gene in ANLL [4] led us to study the *MDR1* gene expression in de novo ANLL in a prospective manner and to assess its impact on treatment outcome. Our results, which have been described in detail elsewhere [6], are summarized in this report.

[1] First Medical Clinic and [2]Second Medical Clinic, University of Vienna, 1090 Vienna, Austria
[3] Clinic for Internal Medicine I, Department of Oncology, Währingergürtel 18–20, 1090 Vienna, Austria
* R. Pirker has been supported by the Austrian Science Foundation, Medizinisch-Wissenschaftlicher Fonds des Bürgermeisters der Bundeshauptstadt Wien, and Kommission Onkologie der Medizinischen Fakultät der Universität Wien.

Patients and Methods

Patients

From early 1988 to spring 1990, 50 consecutive patients (28 females, 22 males), aged 18–80 years (median 54), were studied. De novo ANLL was diagnosed according to standard criteria. Remission induction chemotherapy, described in detail elsewhere [6], was as follows: 39 patients received daunorubicin plus cytosine arabinoside (DA protocol), nine patients received these two drugs plus thioguanine (DAT chemotherapy) and two patients received high-dose cytosine arabinoside plus mitoxantrone (C-HAM chemotherpay). These protocols were equally distributed between *MDR1* RNA negative and positive patients [6]. Consolidation therapy consisted of either a DA protocol or C-HAM chemotherapy.

Leukemic Cells and Cell Lines

Blast cells were isolated from peripheral blood or bone marrow specimens as described [6]. Drug-sensitive KB-3-1 cells and multidrug-resistant KB-8-5 cells (provided by Dr. I. Pastan, National Cancer Institute, NIH, Bethesda, MD, USA) were grown as described [7].

Determination of MDR1 Gene Expression

MDR1 gene expression was determined at diagnosis prior to induction chemotherapy by measuring *MDR1* RNA levels of blast cells, using a slot blot technique as described by Pirker et al. [6] and Wallner et al. [7].

Hybridization was performed with a radiolabeled *MDR1* cDNA (probe 5A; provided by Dr. I. Pastan and Dr. M. Gottesman, address as above). The *MDR1* RNA signal in drug-sensitive KB-3-1 cells was negative, whereas an arbitrary value of 30 units was assigned to the *MDR1* RNA signal of 10 µg RNA from KB-8-5 cells [6, 7]. RNA loading was normalized to actin expression [6, 7].

Statistical Analysis

Durations of survival were estimated according to Kaplan-Meier. Comparison between *MDR1* RNA positive and negative patients was done with the log-rank test. Frequencies were tested by chi-square tests.

Results

In 50 previously untreated patients with de novo ANLL, *MDR1* RNA levels of blast cells were negative in 22 % and positive in 78 % (Table 1). Expression of the *MDR1* gene was termed positive when *MDR1* RNA was detected in peripheral and/or bone marrow blast cells. In most patients whose blasts were studied from both sources, there was no difference in *MDR1* gene expression between peripheral blasts and bone marrow blasts [6].

Age, white blood cells, percentage of blasts, lactate dehydrogenase and duration of observation were not different between *MDR1* RNA negative and positive patients [6].

The complete remission (CR) rate was 66 % for the whole study population (Table 1), but it was lower for patients with *MDR1* gene expression than for patients with undetectable expression (59 % vs 91 %; $p = 0.048$). The CR rates for patients with low, intermediate and high *MDR1* RNA levels were 75 %, 56 % and 53 %, respectively. Expression of the *MDR1* gene occurred in most patients refractory to chemotherapy and in all eight patients who expired within 4 weeks after treatment (Table 1).

At a median follow-up of 10 months, the durations of both overall survival and disease-free survival were significantly longer for the *MDR1* RNA negative patients than for the positive patients ($p = 0.044$ and 0.016, respectively) (Fig. 1).

Discussion

MDR1 gene expression, which was observed in 78 % of the untreated ANLL patients, was associated with lower CR rates, refractory disease, early death, and shorter duration of disease – free, as well as overall survival. These results indicate that drug-resistant cells are present already at

Table 1. *MDR1* RNA levels and outcome of induction chemotherapy

Status of patient	Number of patients (%)	Number of patients with CR (%)	ED	RD
MDR1 RNA negative	11 (22)	10 (91)	0	1
MDR1 RNA positive	39 (78)	23 (59)	8	8
Low levels (<2 U)	8 (16)	6 (75)	1	1
Intermediate levels (2–9 U)	16 (32)	9 (56)	4	3
High levels (> 9 U)	15 (30)	8 (53)	3	4
All	50 (100)	33 (66)	8	9

The CR rate of the *MDR1* negative patients was significantly higher than the CR rate of the positive group ($P = 0.048$)
CR, complete remission; ED, death within 4 weeks after treatment; RD, resistant disease; U, units

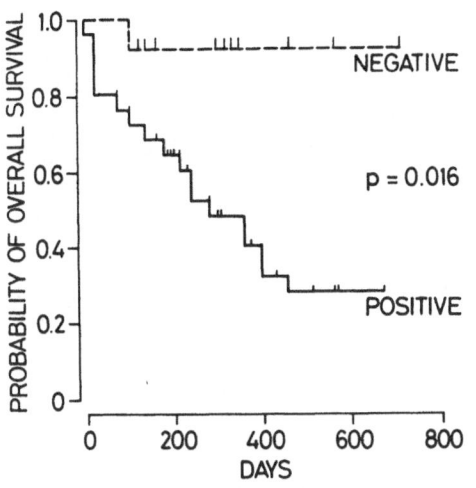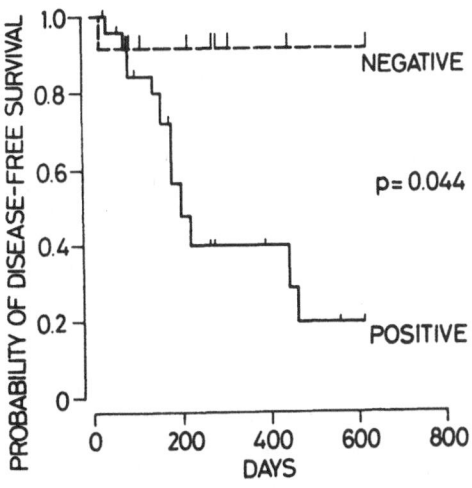

Fig. 1. *MDR1* RNA levels and survival. Durations of both disease-free survival and overall survival were estimated according to Kaplan-Meier

diagnosis and suggest that multidrug resistance is important for clinical drug resistance in ANLL. Other investigators also recently reported that expression of the *MDR1* gene (or P-glycoprotein) did occur in ANLL [8–10] and that this expression was associated with lower CR rates and shorter remission duration [8] as well as resistant disease [9].

Our findings could have impact on the current therapeutic strategies in ANLL. Since our results suggest that it is necessary to overcome multidrug resistance in order to improve the clinical outcome, clinical trials to overcome multidrug resistance by combining chemotherapy with reversing agents such as verapamil, verapamil analogues [11, 12] or cyclosporines [10] are warranted. Determination of *MDR1* gene expression should also be helpful for selecting patients for high-dose chemotherapy or early bone marrow transplantation. Finally, patients with undetectable *MDR1* RNA levels might be candidates for less aggressive treatment.

Summary

To prospectively assess the role of the *MDR1* gene expression in acute nonlymphocytic leukemia (ANLL), *MDR1* RNA levels of blast cells were determined at diagnosis and correlated with treatment outcome in 50 patients with de novo ANLL.

MDR1 RNA levels were negative in 22 % and positive in 78 % of the patients. The complete remission (CR) rate of induction chemotherapy was 66 % for the whole study population. However, the CR rate was 91 % for *MDR1* RNA negative patients and 59 % for *MDR1* RNA positive patients ($p = 0.048$). Kaplan-Meier curves revealed a decrease in duration of both disease-free survival and overall survival of patients with detectable *MDR1* gene expression as compared to the survival durations of *MDR1* RNA negative patients ($P = 0.044$ and $p = 0.016$, respectively). These data suggest that the *MDR1* gene is a clinically relevant drug-resistance gene in ANLL.

References

1. Wiernik PH (1989) Acute leukemias. In: DeVita VT Jr, Hellman S, Rosenberg SA (eds) Cancer: principles and practice of oncology. Lippincott, Philadelphia, pp 1809–1835
2. Hiddemann W, Büchner T (1990) Treatment strategies in acute myeloid leukemia (AML). Blut 60: 163–171
3. Pastan I, Gottesman MM (1987) Multiple-drug resistance in human cancer. N Engl J Med 316: 1388–1393
4. Goldstein LJ, Galski H, Fojo A, Willingham M, Lai S, Gazdar A, Pirker R, Green A,

Crist W, Brodeur GM, Lieber M, Cossman J, Gottesman MM, Pastan I (1989) Expression of a multidrug resistance gene in human cancers. J Natl cancer Inst 81: 116–124

5. Pirker R, Goldstein LJ, Ludwig H, Linkesch W, Lechner C, Gottesman MM, Pastan I (1989) Expression of a multidrug resistance gene in blast crisis of chronic myelogenous leukemia. Cancer Commun 1: 141–144

6. Pirker R, Wallner J, Geissler K, Linkesch W, Haas OA, Bettelheim P, Hopfner M, Scherrer R, Valent P, Havelec L, Ludwig H, Lechner K (1991) *MDR1* gene expression and treatment outcome in acute myeloid leukemia. J Natl Cancer Inst 83: 708–712

7. Wallner J, Depisch D, Hopfner M, Haider K, Spona J, Ludwig H, Pirker R (1991) *MDR1* gene expression and prognostic factors in primary breast carcinomas. Eur J Cancer In press

8. Sato H, Preisler H, Day R, Raza A, Larson R, Browman G, Goldberg J, Vogler R, Grunwald H, Gottlieb A, Bennett J, Gottes-man M, Pastan I (1990) *MDR1* transcript levels as an indication of resistant disease in acute myelogenous leukaemia. Br J Haematol 75: 340–345

9. Ma DDF, Davey RA, Harman DH, Isbister JP, Scurr RD, Mackertich SM, Dowden G, Bell DR (1987) Detection of a multidrug resistant phenotype in acute non-lymphoblastic leukaemia. Lancet i: 135–137

10. Sonneveld P, Nooter K (1990) Reversal of drug-resistance by cyclosporin-A in a patient with acute myelocytic leukaemia. Br J Haematol 75: 208–211

11. Pirker R, Keilhauer G, Raschack M, Lechner C, Ludwig H (1990) Reversal of multidrug resistance in human KB cell lines by structural analogs of verapamil. Int J Cancer 45: 916–919

12. Pirker R, FitzGerald DJP, Raschack M, Zimmermann F, Willingham MC, Pastan I (1989) Enhancement of the activity of immunotoxins by analogues of verapamil. Cancer Res 49: 4791–4795

Multidrug Resistance Proteins and their Functional Modulation in Human Leukemias as Analyzed by Flow Cytometry

L. Van Hove, K. Van Acker, and M. Boogaerts

Introduction

Resistance to chemotherapy is one of the major problems in the treatment of leukemia patients, and much effort has been put into elucidating the mechanisms. Several types of drug resistance have been identified with cell lines made highly resistant to different types of anticancer agents. One of the most important phenomena found is the multidrug resistance (MDR) phenotype [5]. MDR cells are resistant to a variety of naturally occurring drugs, like anthracyclines and vinca alkaloids. MDR is often associated with the presence of a 170 kDa transmembrane glycoprotein (P-glycoprotein), encoded by the human *mdr1* gene. P-glycoprotein functions as a rapid drug-efflux pump, resulting in a decreased, less toxic, intracellular drug accumulation. In humans a second highly homologous *mdr* gene has been identified, called *mdr3* [6]. A P-glycoprotein of the *mdr1* gene has been found to be active in human leukemias. Only one report suggests a functional drug-efflux pump to be active in some chronic B-cell lymphocytic leukemias, as a mdr 3 gene product [4].

Here we report on P-glycoprotein expression, as *mdr1* and *mdr3* gene products and intracellular drug accumulation in human leukemias and their MDR modulation by cyclosporin A.

Department of Hematology, University Hospital of Leuven, Leuven, Belgium.
* This work was supported by a cancer grant of the Fund for Medical Scientific Research (Belgium) (F.G.W.O. nr: 3.0019.91). L. Van Hove is Research Associate of the National Fund for Scientific Research (Belgium).

Materials and Methods

Patients

Of the 30 leukemia/lymphoma patients studied, 12 were untreated at the time of sample collection. Diagnosis was performed on the basis of the FAB and morphologic, immunologic and cytogenic (MIC) standard criteria [1, 2]. Treated patients always received at least one MDR-related drug e.g., vincristine, daunorubicin, or etoposide.

The leukemia cells were obtained from peripheral blood or bone marrow containing more than 30 % malignant cells. Blood was anticoagulated with ethylenediaminetetraacetate (EDTA), bone marrow with heparin. The erythrocytes were removed by hypotonic lysis.

Cell Lines

The drug-sensitive K-562 chronic myeloid leukemia cell line and its MDR variants K-562/VLB$_{20}$ and K-562/VLB$_{50}$, resistant to 20- and 50-ng/ml vinblastine, were used. Cells were grown in plastic flasks in Iscove's modified Dulbecco's medium (IMDM), supplemented with 10 % fetal calf serum at 37 °C in a humidified atmosphere of 5 % CO_2 in air. The resistant variants were obtained by growing the K-562 cells with increasing amounts of vinblastine.

33

Flow Cytometry

P-170 glycoprotein quantitation

Cells were fixed with methanol (70 %) for 8 min at $-20\,°C$, washed twice in phosphate-buffered saline (PBS), resuspended in 20 µl of fluorescein isothiocyanate (FITC)-conjugated C-219 monoclonal antibody (MoAb) (50 µg/ml) and incubated for 1 h at $4\,°C$, washed twice in PBS and analyzed with a FACScan flow cytometer (Becton Dickinson, Erembodegem, Belgium). A FITC-conjugated isotype-matched irrelevant mouse immunoglobulin (IgG2a) was always included as control. Staining with MRK-16, kindly provided by Dr. Tsuruo, Tokyo, Japan, was similar to that with C-219, except that fresh, unfixed cells were used. MRK-16 was diluted to 30 µg/ml in PBS containing 10 % human AB serum and, following secondary antibody reaction, the cells were fixed in 0.5 % paraformaldehyde. The proportion of cells expressing P-170 was calculated by determining the proportion of cells that had P-170-related (green) fluorescence above that of matching control (specific fluorescence). The level of P-170 expression was determined from the intensity of specific P-170-related fluorescence on a 10^4 fluorescence log scale and expressed as a P-170 ratio.

Drug Uptake Kinetic Studies

In vitro daunorubicin (DNR) uptake kinetics of leukemia cells were measured with a FACScan at 1 min intervals. The cells (5 × 10^5/ml in Hanks' medium with glucose, Ca and Mg ions, but without phenol red) were kept at $37\,°C$ in a reaction vessel surrounded by a thermostated water jacket. For each cell, forward light scatter, perpendicular light scatter, and DNR fluorescence (through a 585/42 nm long pass filter) data were stored. Data concerning 3000 cells at 25 selected time points, before and after the addition of DNR or MDR modifying agents, were collected. Dead cells and debris were excluded during the analysis. Dead cells were identified by staining with the nonvital dye propidium iodide. In the drug accumulation curves, the mean DNR fluorescence of the leukemic subpopulation (calculated at each of the 25 time points of data collection) is plotted versus the time after addition of the drug or its modifier.

Results

An example of P-150 flow cytometry (FCM) analysis is illustrated in Fig. 1 A, B. The vinblastine-resistant K-562/VLB$_{20}$ cell line showed 25-fold higher P-170 expression than its vinblastine-sensitive parent K-562. There was marked heterogeneity in P-170 expression on both the resistant and parent cells by immunocytochemical P-170 analysis (data not shown). The FCM reactivity patterns of these cell lines with the two MoAbs, C-219 and MRK-16, were remarkably similar ($r = 0.83$) and correlated directly with the level of drug resistance in tissue culture ($r = 0.94$, $r = 0.65$) and with the steady state (plateau) level of DNR accumulation in the cells ($r = 0.81$, $r = 0.99$). The proportion of P-170+ cells in blood and bone marrow of healthy adult donors was always lower than 1 %, with an intensity of specific P-170-related fluorescence (level of P-170 expression) smaller than 1.6 ± 0.53.

Heterogeneity in P-170 expression was also observed in clinical samples. In Fig 1 B a case of acute myeloid leukemia (AML) M1 with 100 % P-170+ myeloblasts and a high level of P-170-related fluorescence (P-170 ratio = 5.5:1) is shown. Increased P-170 expression was more frequently found with C-219 than with MRK-16. In Table 1, the obtained results on P-170 expression and DNR accumulation in clinical samples are summarized. Of 18 acute leukemias, seven (39 %) contained more than 30 % P-170+ blasts (see Table 1, cases 1, 2, 4, 5, 6, 7 and 8) and six (34 %) has a P-170 expression greater than 2.5. No correlation ($r = 0.13$) was found between these two parameters, although they pointed in the same direction. Half of the leukemias were treated and they were classified either as acute lymphoblastic leukemia (ALL) or AML. Both AMLs, postmyelodysplasia, showed a P-170 ratio of or greater than 3.0:1. Of 12 chronic hematologic disorders, three (25 %) had a P-170 ratio greater than 2.5:1 (one chronic lymphocytic leukemia

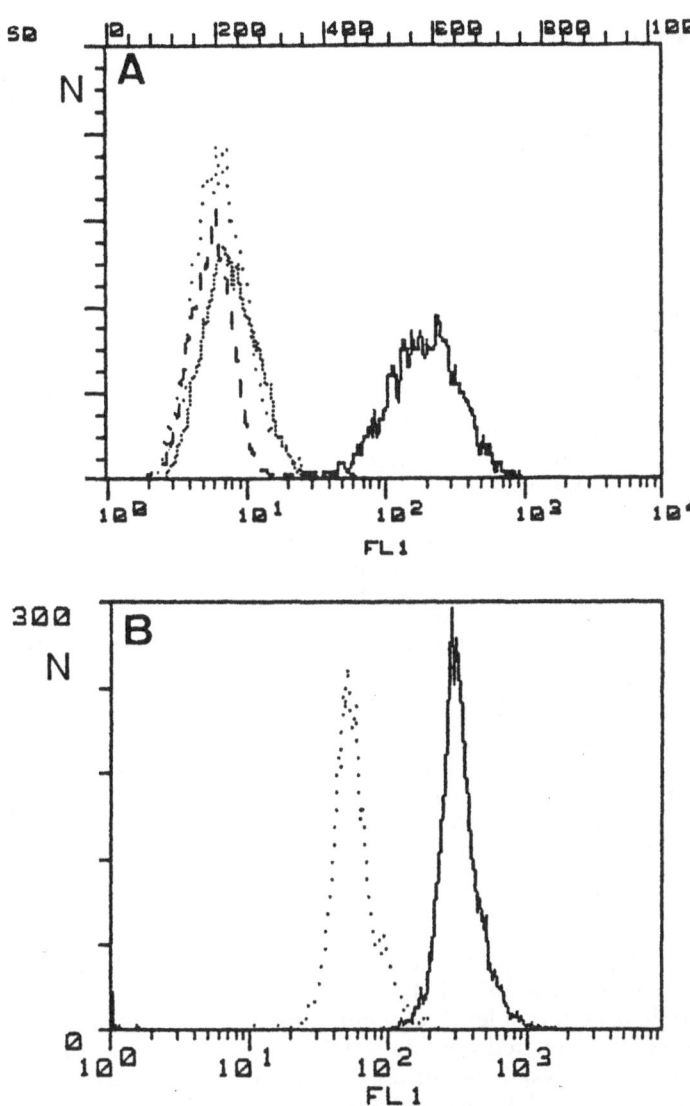

Fig. 1A, B. Overlay histograms of P-glycoprotein expression on K-562 cells (*A*) and on an AML M1 blood sample (*B*), analyzed with MoAb C-219. *A* K-562 parent cells with MoAb C-219 (– – –), K-562 parent cells with isotypic control (.   .   .), K-562/VLB$_{20}$ vinblastine-resistant cells with isotypic control (.....), and K-562/VLB$_{20}$ with MoAb C-219 (——); all cells expressed P-170 and a P-170 expression ratio of 25:1 is found. *B* AML M1 cells with isotypic control (...) and AML M1 cells with MoAb C-219 (——): all cells expressed P-170 and a P-170 ratio of 5.5:1 is found

(CLL), one chronic myeloid leukemia (CML) and one multiple myeloma; the last two were treated). Except for the CLL, these samples contained less than 50% malignant cells.

DNR accumulation kinetics by FCM were performed in 14 cases (see Table 1 for relevant cases). Lowered intracellular drug accumulation is related with the MDR phenotype and can be restored by MDR modifiers, like cyclosporin A. In order to have an idea of drug-accumulation-curves in MDR, DNR uptake was studied first in sensitive and vinblastine-resistant K-562

Table 1. Clinical and flow cytometric MDR data on leukemia/lymphoma patients

Cases	Class	Treatment	Response	P-170 glycoprotein		DNR accumulation kinetics	
				P-170+ cells (%)	P-170 ratio	DNR plateau	Cyclosporin A reversal (%)
1	Pre-pre-B ALL	ALL[b]	PD +	73	1.7	40	ND
2	Pre-pre-B ALL	ALL[a], VIM	RE	75	3.0	71	0
3	C-ALL	None		0	ND	39	ND
4	C-ALL	None		71	3.5	65	0
5	AML MO	None		36	2.7	70	6
6	AML M1	Hovon4	PD	100	5.5	ND	ND
7	AML M4	None		79	1.7	78	0
8	AML post-MDS	Ara-C, VP-16, Mitoxantrone	PD	46	3.0	ND	ND
9	B CLL	Chlorambucil, VIM, CEP	PD +	11	1.7	62	12
10	B CLL	Prednimustine	PD	7	2.4	67	20
11	Kahler	VAD	PD	–	1.2	60	ND
12	Kahler	VAD	PR	52	2.6	ND	ND

ALL, acute lymphoblastic leukemia; AML, acute myeloid leukemia; MDS, myelodysplastic syndrome; CLL chronic lymphocytic leukemia; DNR, daunorubicin; Ara-C, cytosine arabinoside; ALL[a]: scheme in adults consists of cyclophosphamide, vincristine, daunorubicin, asparaginase and prednisone, ALL[b]: scheme in children consists of the EORTC protocol nr. 58881 (vincristine, daunorubicin, ARA-C, ...), ND, no data; None, no treatment at diagnosis; CR, complete remission; PD, progressive disease; +, death; RE, first relapse; PR, partial response

cells (Fig. 2A) and on normal blood and bone marrow. K-562/VLB$_{50}$ cells, resistant to clinical relevant levels of vinblastine and DNR, accumulated only 25% DNR compared to the K-562 parent cells. Saline had no effect on DNR accumulation by these cells, whereas the addition of cyclosporin A to K-562/VLB$_{50}$ led to a complete restored accumulation profile (factor 5). No significant effect on K-562 parent cells was found. For normal blood and bone marrow cells, mean DNR accumulation values of 120 fluorescence intensity units (FIU) were found. Minor differences in DNR accumulation were observed between lymphocytes and neutrophils (98.3 FIU ± 4.4 and 143.5 ± 1.5). Addition of cyclosporin A increased DNR accumulation by a factor of 1.15 ± 0.05. Eight pathology cases were studied for cyclosporin A reversal of the MDR phenotype. Of the 14 cases studied, 13 (93%) showed a clear decreased DNR accumula-

tion. Five of them (36%) contained an increased proportion of P-170+ cells (cases 1, 2, 4, 5 and 7, Table 1) and three (21%) expressed also a higher level of P-170 (cases 2, 4 and 5). No correlation was found between P-170 expression and DNR accumulation in these clinical samples ($r = 0.07$). However, two pre-pre-B ALLs with progressive disease (cases 1 and 2, Table 1) and three leukemias at diagnosis (cases 4, 5 and 7) also showed an increased proportion of P-170+ cells as a reduced drug accumulation. Some leukemias, particularly B-CLL, and myelomas, expressed normal levels of P-170, but were deficient in DNR accumulation. In vitro addition of cyclosporin A, studied in eight cases, demonstrated an increased DNR accumulation effect in two CLLs (of about 12% and 20%). Both had been treated before and had progressive disease and no increased expression of P-170. One of them is shown in Fig. 2B.

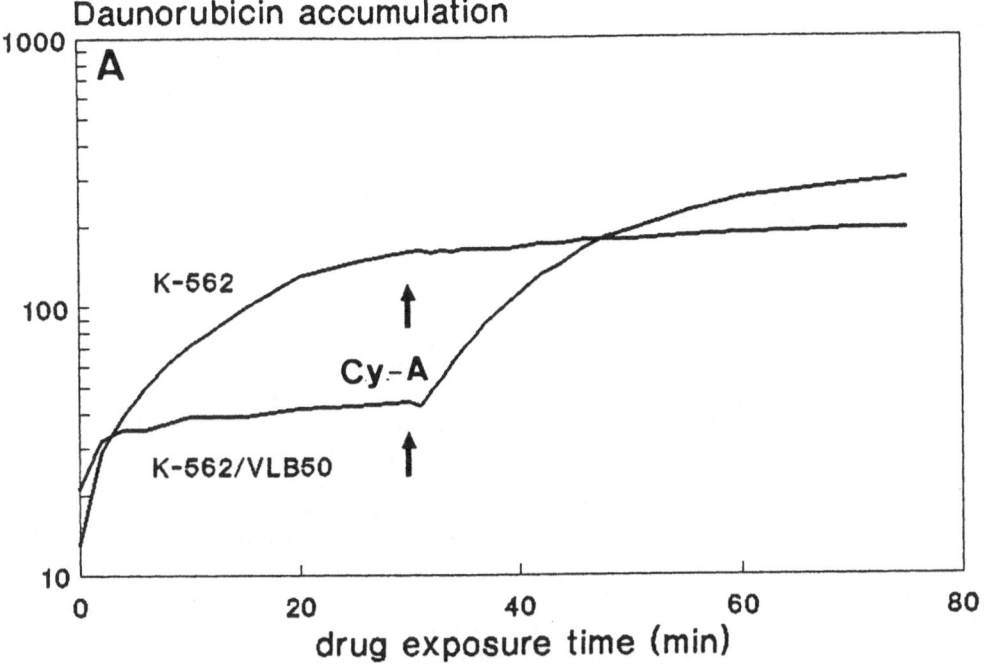

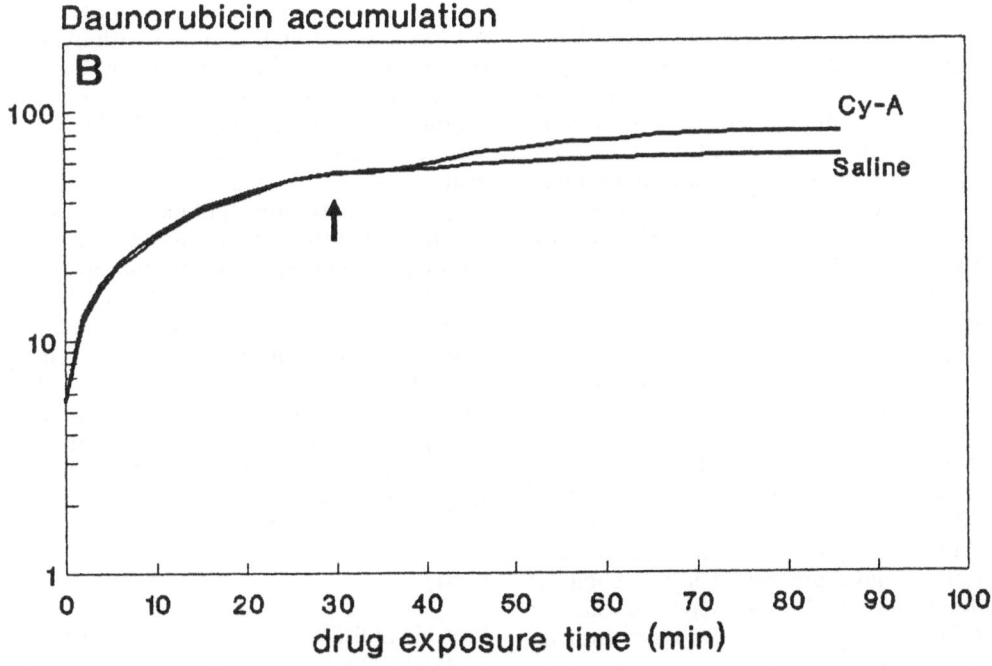

Fig. 2A, B. Daunorubicin (DNR) accumulation in vitro by the K-562 leukemic cells (*A*) and by the CLL cells (*B*) of a patient. Values are expressed as DNR fluorescence intensity in arbitrary units (Y-axis). *A* K-562 parent cells and K-562/VLB$_{50}$ vinblastine-resistant cells. *B* B-CLL cells from a blood sample. At t = 0, DNR was added to the cell suspension (final concentration 4 µM). Arrows indicate the time point of addition of cyclosporin A (Cy-A) (final concentration 3 µM)

Discussion

While the MDR phenotype is a well-established phenomenon in cell lines selected for resistance to high concentrations of certain drugs, it has not yet been recognized as a major mechanism for clinical drug resistance. Several problems have interfered with the assessment of the clinical relevance of MDR, including (a) the complexity of treatment protocols, (b) the difficulty in quantitating therapy responses, and (c) the lack of standardized methods for quantitating P-170 expression and drug accumulation in heterogeneous clinical samples. By FCM analysis of the MDR phenotype on leukemic cells of individual patients, a marked heterogeneity was found. Among the parameters examined, reduced DNR accumulation was most frequently observed (93 %), followed by an increased proportion of P-170+ cells (37 %), a raised level of P-170 expression (31 %) and the reversal of drug accumulation by cyclosporin A (4 %). The MDR phenotype differed from the resistant K-562 cell lines in that no correlation was found by orthogonal regression analysis between P-170 expression and drug accumulation for the clinical samples. These observations suggest the presence of different types of drug efflux pumps on acute leukemias, CLLs and myelomas. They can be visualized by a well-standardized DNR accumulation assay, but not by the MoAbs C-219 and MRK-16, directed against different epitopes on the P-170 glycoprotein, a *mdr1* gene product. Some of these P-170 negative efflux pumps might represent *mdr3* gene products, recently described by Herweijer et al. [4]. This is probably so for the CLLs with clinical evidence of drug resistance, since they accumulated only low amounts of DNR which was reversed by cyclosporin A. For the first time, we demonstrated that only P-170 glycoproteins can be visualized by the MoAbs C-219 and MRK-16, but not *mdr3* gene products or other types of drug efflux pumps. These observations indicate the necessity to incorporate a well-standardized DNR accumulation assay into the procedures for MDR phenotyping of individual leukemias and lymphomas. Standardization of FCM procedures for MDR analysis include negative controls, like isotypic irrelevant antibodies and the repetitive analysis of normal blood or bone marrow samples and positive controls that can consist of the analysis of drug-resistant cell lines, like our K-562/VLB variants. P-170 glycoprotein can best be visualized by the P-170 ratio, representing the P-170 expression level. Some leukemias with a low expression level, but a high proportion of P-170 weakly positive cells, might falsely explain the MDR phenotype as an increased expression of P-glycoprotein and hide, at the same time, some of the other efflux pumps. This might explain why no better correlation was found between P-170 glycoprotein expression, P-170+ cells and DNR accumulation in these clinical samples, which oppose our findings on the drug resistant K-562 cell lines and data published by other authors [3]. Therefore, we suggest, that observed P-170 overexpression should always be followed by further FCM analysis of the absolute numbers and proportion of P-170+ cells and by drug accumulation studies. If then an increased proportion of P-170+ cells is found together with overexpression of P-170 and reduced drug accumulation, the overexpression of a *mdr1* gene product is almost certain. Only by FCM can such combined observations be made as well in progressive leukemias as in newly diagnosed, untreated leukemias and lymphomas. Therefore, FCM may be useful in identifying patients prior to therapy who are likely to develop clinical MDR. Moreover, increased drug accumulation on addition of cyclosporin A, especially seen in progressive CLL patients, suggests the incorporation of MDR modifiers, like cyclosporin A, into the therapy protocols for leukemia and lymphoma with an MDR phenotype sensitive to MDR modifiers.

Summary

Typical multidrug resistance (MDR) in human cell lines is caused by overactivity of unidirectional transmembrane drug efflux pumps, encoded by the *mdr1* and *mdr3* genes. There is increasing evidence that overexpression of P-170 glycoproteins, as *mdr-1* gene products, play a crucial role in resistance to anticancer agents in several tumor types. However, only few data are available on other drug efflux pumps and drug resistance. Therefore, we studied tumor cell-associated expression of MDR with monoclonal antibodies (MoAbs) C-219 and MRK-16 and by intracellular accumulation of daunorubicin (DNR), using flow cytometry (FCM) on leukemias and lymphomas. By FCM analysis a marked heterogeneity was found in P-170 expression on the resistant cell lines and on 30 clinical samples. From the evaluated parameters, reduced DNR accumulation was most frequently seen (93%), followed by increased proportions of P-170+ cells (37%), a raised P-170 expression level (31%), and the reversal of DNR accumulation by cyclosporin A (4%). Findings were unlike those for the resistant cell lines; no correlation was found between P-170 expression and DNR accumulation. This indicates the necessity to incorporate standardized DNR accumulation asssays for the identification of drug efflux pumps different from the P-170 glycoproteins. Only the *mdr1* gene products can be identified by the MoAbs C-219 and MRK-16. P-170 negative efflux pumps can only be visualized by DNR accumulation studies, as proven by our study on five drug-resistant chronic lymphocytic leukemias (CLLs), which showed that only one had a minor overexpression of P-170, but that all showed a reduced DNR accumulation that could be increased by cyclosporin A. These observations were as well made in treated as newly diagnosed patients with acute leukemia (18), myelodysplasia (1), chronic myeloid leukemia (CML) (1), B-CLL (5) and multiple myelomas (5). The presence de novo of a high percentage of P-170+ cells with high P-170 expression and a reduced DNR accumulation, warrants systematic combined FCM analysis of P-170 expression prior to therapy to determine the implications for clinical therapy in acute and chronic leukemias and lymphomas expressing different types of drug efflux pumps, in particular, for response to treatment combinations of cytotoxic drugs plus agents that reverse MDR.

References

1. Bennett JM, Berger R, Catovsky D, Flandrin G, Foon A, Gralnick HG, Griffin JD, Hagemeijer A, Mecucci C, Minowada J, Milrelman F, Preud'homme JL, Sandberg A, Van den Berghe H (1988) Morphologic, immunologic and cytogenic (M.I.C.) working classification of the acute myeloid leukaemias. Br J Haematol 68: 487–494
2. Bennett JM, Catovsky D, Daniel M, Flandrin G, Galton DAG, Gralnick HR, Sultan C (1989) Proposals for the classification of chronic (mature) B and T lymphoid leukemias. J Clin Pathol 42: 567–584
3. Epstein J, Xiao H, Oba BK (1989) P-glycoprotein expression in plasma-cell myeloma is associated with resistance to VAD. Blood 74: 913–917
4. Herweijer H, Sonneveld P, Baas F, Nooter K (1990) Expression of mdr1 and mdr3 multidrug-resistance genes in human acute and chronic leukemias and association with stimulation of drug accumulation by cyclosporine. JNCI 82: 1133–1140
5. Ling V, Juranka PF, Endicott JA, Deuchars KL, Gerlach JH (1988) Multidrug resistance and P-glycoprotein expression. In: Woolley PVM, Tew KD (eds) Mechanisms of drug resistance in neoplastic cells. Academic, New York, pp 197–209, (Bristol-myers cancer symposia, vol 9)
6. Van Der Bliek AM, Kooiman PM, Schneider C, Borst P (1988) Sequence of mdr3 cDNA encoding a human P-glycoprotein. Gene 71: 401–411

Reversal of Multidrug Resistance with a New Calcium/Calmodulin Antagonist

E. Roller[1], B. Benz[1], M. Eichelbaum[1], V. Gekeler[2], K. Häußermann[1], B. Klumpp[1], and K. Schumacher[1]

Introduction

One of the major problems limiting optimal chemotherapy is the development of tumor cells with multidrug resistance (MDR) during treatment. These cells are cross-resistant to structurally different natural occurring drugs. One form of MDR is related to a reduction of drug accumulation in the resistant cells [7]. The drug efflux mechanism seems to be mediated by a 170 kDa plasma membrane glycoprotein which acts as an ATP-dependent drug efflux pump [4]. The MDR1 gene encodes for this protein, termed P-glycoprotein [2, 3].

Different classes of heterocyclic compounds were able to reverse the MDR phenotype in vitro [5, 6]. One group of these modulators belongs to calcium antagonists.

Niguldipine (B859-34), a dihydropyridine, is clinically used because of its antihypertensive effects [10]. The (−)isomer B859-35 has about 35- to 40-fold less effect on blood pressure [10]. Antiproliferative effect of B859-35 on small cell human lung tumor cells in vitro and for neuroendocrine lung tumors and nasa cavity tumors induced in hamsters in vivo has been demonstrated [11].

Material and Methods

Chemicals

B859-35, B859-34 and B8909-008 were gifts from Byk Gulden, Konstanz, FRG, while 3-(4,5-dimethylthiazol-2-yl)-2,5-diphenyl-tetrazolium bromide (MTT) and vincristine were purchased from Sigma Chemicals, Munich, FRG.

Cell Lines

The human lymphoblastoid cell line CCRF-CEM and its drug-resistant subline VCR 1000 were gifts from V. Gekeler, Tübingen, FRG.

Cytotoxicity Assays

The MTT assay was used to determine chemosensitivity [8].

Discussion

VCR 1000 cells are 1760-fold more resistant to vincristine than the parental cell line CCRF-CEM. They are also cross-resistant to daunomycin, adriamycin, and actinomycin D and show an increased expression of P170-glycoprotein as described by Gekeler et al. [2].

[1] Robert-Bosch Krankenhaus, Stuttgart, FRG
[2] Physiologisch-Chemisches Institut, Universität Tübingen, FRG
* Supported by the Robert Bosch Foundation, Stuttgart, FRG, and Byk Gulden, Konstanz, FRG.

Table 1. Effects of modulators on VCR 1000 cell growth without addition of cytostatica

	Growth inhibition[a] (%)		
μM	(−) Enantiomer	(+) Enantiomer	Metabolite
10	100 ± 0.0	100 ± 0.0	93 ± 6.5
5	97 ± 4.8	38 ± 2.5	56 ± 4.5
2	41 ± 8.3	9 ± 9.0	4 ± 4.7
1	17 ± 7.5	5 ± 4.5	9 ± 1.8
0.1	1 ± 0.5	2 ± 0.7	1 ± 0.3

[a] % growth inhibition determined with the MTT test; mean of five measurements ± SD

Table 2. Effects of modulators on CCRF-CEM cell growth without addition of cytostatica

	Growth inhibition[a] (%)		
μM	(−) Enantiomer	(+) Enantiomer	Metabolite
10	100 ± 0.0	100 ± 0.0	46 ± 10.5
5	35 ± 4.1	45 ± 3.5	16 ± 3.5
2	12 ± 6.4	19 ± 3.0	8 ± 3.0
1	5 ± 5.0	9 ± 8.5	11 ± 2.0
0.1	1 ± 1.0	2 ± 1.5	1 ± 0.0

[a] % growth inhibition determined with the MTT test; mean of five measurements ± SD

In Vitro Cytotoxicity Studies

Cytostatic activity of the modifiers was established using the MTT test. As shown in tables 1 and 2, each of the tested modifiers has an antiproliferative effect on VCR 1000 cells in concentrations ranging from 1 to 5 μM without addition of any cytostatica. A total cell kill was achieved for the (+) and (−) enantiomer at a concentration of 10 μM. For comparison we also tested the parental drug-sensitive cell line CCRF-CEM. At 2 μM and 5 μM, B859-35 growth of the resistant cells was inhibited by about 41% and 97% respectively, whereas the sensitive cells were inhibited by about 12% and 35%. For the tested (+) enantiomer there was less difference between the two cell lines, whereas the metabolite acted in a manner comparable to B859-35. The regulatory mechanism for neoplastic cell growth seems to be more sensitive for B859-35 in VCR 1000 than in CCRF-CEM cells. This proliferation inhibition is independent of blocking a calcium/calmodulin-dependent second messenger pathway, because B859-34 with higher affinity to calcium channels [1] is less active.

Effects of Modulators on Drug Sensitivity

In the presence of cytostatica (1 µg/ml VCR, a nontoxic concentration for VCR 1000 cells), an additive effect on cytotoxicity could be seen for all tested chemosensitizers (Table 3). The addition of B859-35 (1 μM) led to an enhancement of cytotoxicity (97%) compared to the untreated control. Cells were sensitive to the modifier per se, but the combination of cytostatica (VCR 1 µg/ml) in a suboptimal dose with the antagonist (B859-35, 1 μM) resulted in a sixfold higher cell-kill compared to B859-35 growth inhibitory effect alone. The mechanism of modulation seems to be related to the affinity of the modulators to P-glycoprotein [6]. The competitive inhibition of the drug

Table 3. Effects of modulators on VCR 1000 cell growth with addition of cytostatica

	Growth inhibition[a] (%)		
μM	(−) Enantiomer	(+) Enantiomer	Metabolite
10	100 ± 0.0	100 ± 0.0	100 ± 0.0
5	100 ± 0.0	100 ± 0.0	100 ± 0.0
2	99 ± 2.8	95 ± 1.1	89 ± 9.3
1	97 ± 3.1	41 ± 7.2	23 ± 6.8
0.1	21 ± 4.3	9 ± 1.5	8 ± 2.3

[a] % growth inhibition determined with the MTT test; 1 μg/ml vincristine was added to the medium; mean of five measurements ± SD

efflux pump leads to increasing intracellular concentration of the cytostatica [12].

Calcium channel blocking activity per se seems not to be necessary for the reversing potency. This fact has already been shown for the two enantiomers of verapamil [5, 9].

B859-35, with less effect on blood pressure, reduces tumor cell proliferation and potentiates the effect of suboptimal vincristine concentration in resistant cells expressing P-glycoprotein.

So we conclude that B859-35 should be tried as a new antitumor agent; furthermore, it seems to be a promising modulator of MDR.

human lymphoblastoid cell line CCRF-CEM and its multidrug-resistant subline VCR 1000 which expresses classical MDR phenotype including P-glycoprotein overexpression. We tested the compounds alone and in combination with vincristine for their cytotoxic effects. There were only slight differences in MDR reversing capacity and growth inhibitory effect between the isomers and the metabolite. At a noninhibitory concentration of vincristine for VCR 1000 cells addition of chemosensitizers in a nontoxic concentration led to a reversion of MDR independent of calcium-antagonistic activity.

Summary

Calcium antagonists are the most effective chemosensitizers of multidrug resistance (MDR) in experimental cancer chemotherapy. We tested a new calcium/calmodulin antagonist with 1,4 dihydropyridine structure for its MDR-reversing potency using the enantiomers (−)B859-35 [(−)-3-methyl-5- (3- (4,4-diphenyl-1-piperidinyl)-propyl) -1,4-dihydro-2,6-dimethyl-4- (3-nitro-phenyl) -pyridine-3,5-dicarboxylate-hydrochloride] and (+)B859-34 (Niguldipin-hydrochloride) and the common metabolite B8909-008 [3-methyl-5- (3-(4,4-diphenyl-1-piperidinyl) -propyl) -2,6-dimethyl-4- (3-nitrophenyl) -pyridine-3,5-dicarboxylate]. B859-35 is reported to have antitumor activity. For drug testing we used an in vitro system (MTT test) with the

References

1. Boer R, Grassegger A, Schudt C, Glossmann H (1989) (+)-Niguldipine binds with very high affinity to Ca2+ channels and to a subtype of a1-adrenoceptors. Eur J Pharmacol 172: 131–145
2. Gekeler V, Frese G, Diddens H, Probst H (1988) Expression of a P-glycoprotein gene is inducible in a multidrug-resistant human leukemia cell line. Biochem Biophys Res Commun 155: 754–760
3. Goldstein L, Galski H, Fojo A, Willingham S, et al. (1989) Expression of a multidrug resistance gene in human cancers. JNCI 81: 116–124
4. Gottesman MM, Pastan I (1988) The multidrug transporter, a double-edged sword. J Biol Chem 263: 12163–12166
5. Gruber A, Peterson C, Reizenstein P (1988) D-verapamil and L-verapamil are equally effective in increasing vincristine accumula-

tion in leukemic cells in vitro. Int J Cancer 41: 224–225

6. Kamiwatari M, Gagata U, Kikuche H, Yoshimura A, Sumizawa T, Shudo N, Sakoda R, Seto K, Akiyama S (1989) Correlation between reversing of multidrug resistance and inhibiting of 3H-Azidopine photolabeling of P-glycoprotein by newly synthesized dihydropyridine analogues in a human cell line. Cancer Res 49: 3190–3195

7. Kartner N, Ling V (1989) Multidrug resistance in cancer. Sci Am March: 44–51

8. Mosmann T (1983) Rapid colorimetric assay for cellular growth and survival: application to proliferation and cytotoxicity assays. J Immunol Methods 65: 55–63

9. Plumb JA, Milroy R, Kaye SB (1990) The activity of verapamil as a resistance modifier in vitro in drug resistance human tumour cell lines is not stereospecific. Biochem Pharmacol 39: 787–792

10. Sanders KH, Kolossa N, Beller K-D, Cettier B (1988) Acute and short term antihypertensive effects of niguldipine, a new long acting dihydropyrine in animals. Ann NY Acad Sci 522: 531

11. Schuller HM, Correa E, Orloff M, Reznik GK (1990) Successful chemotherapy of experimental neuroendocrine lung tumors in hamsters with an antagonist of Ca++/Calmodulin. Cancer Res 50: 1645–1649

12. Tsuruo T, Iida H, Tsukagoshi S, Sakurai Y (1982) Increased accumulation of vincristine and adriamycin in drug-resistant P388 tumor cells following incubation with calcium antagonists and calmodulin inhibitors. Cancer Res 42: 4730–4733

Characterization of Human Leukemic HL-60 Sublines as a Model for Primary and Secondary Resistance Against Cytostatics

F. Gieseler[1], F. Boege[1], R. Erttmann[2], H.-P. Tony[1], H. Biersack[1], B. Spohn[1], and M. Clark[1]

Introduction

Resistance against cytostatics is a major problem in the therapy of hematologic malignancies. The intracellular alterations can be studied *in vitro* and several molecular mechanisms affecting all cellular levels like altered membrane transport rates (P-glycoprotein) [1], "trapping" of cytostatics in vesicles [2], detoxification (glutathione-S-transferase) [3], and alteration of nuclear target proteins (topoisomerases) [4] have been described. A special problem is the exhibition of a multidrug-resistant (MDR) phenotype, resulting in resistance against a broad spectrum of substances from different classes.

Most of the studies on molecular mechanisms of cellular resistance have been done in cell lines which have been selected by, stepwise, increasing the concentration of cytostatics in the medium. Obviously, in these cells the overexpression of the *MDR1*-gene resulting in overexpression of P-glycoprotein is an important factor.

In this chapter we show that cells with primary resistance have molecular and biochemical characteristics different from those of selected cell lines which can be used as a model for secondary (induced) resistance. For these purposes, we compared the stem-cell line HL-60 with three multidrug-resistant sublines: HL-60R (primary resistance), HL-60ETO, and HL-60TENI (the last two selected against etoposide or teniposide).

Material and Methods

The following materials were used: fetal calf serum (Bethesda Research Laboratories, Karlsruhe, FRG); β-mercaptoethanol (Sigma Chemical, Deisenhofen, FRG); RPMI 1640 medium, penicillin/streptomycin (Seromed Biochrom KG, Berlin, FRG); pBR322 plasmid (Boehringer, Mannheim, FRG); HEPES (Roth KG, Karlsruhe, FRG); and HL-60 cells (American tissue culture collection #CCL240, Rockville, Maryland). Cells were grown in liquid culture (RPMI 1640 + 5% fetal calf serum, 1% penicillin strepomycin) in a humidified atmosphere containing 5% CO_2. Only cells in logarithmic growth phase (1–5 million cells/ml) were harvested. To determine cellular resistance to various cytostatics the half-lethal concentrations (LD_{50}) and the factor of resistance between two indicated cell lines is expressed as the LD_{50} quotient. Cell viability was evaluated by determining the cellular trypan blue exclusion rate after growing the cells for 48 h in the presence of various concentrations of the indicated substance and with or without verapamil (2 ng/ml; in this concentration viability of the cells was not affected by verapamil alone). The sublines HL-60ETO and HL-60TENI were selected by, stepwise, increasing the concentration of etoposide or teniposide in

[1] Medizinische Poliklinik, University of Würzburg, Würzburg, FRG
[2] Department of Pediatric Oncology, University of Hamburg, Hamburg, FRG
* Supported by DFG, SFB 172 (C9) and Sander Stiftung (90.038.01)

the medium over a period of 15 months. The subline HL-60R is a spontaneous mutation; the cells have not been selected against cytostatics. The assessment of topoisomerase II (topo II) activity was performed as described previously [5]. For topo II activation, 10 mM MgCl$_2$ and 2 mM ATP were freshly added. Activity was quantified from disappearance of supercoiled pBR322 substrate by densitometric scanning of photographic negatives. Surface marker analysis was done after staining with monoclonal antibodies using a FACscan (Becton Dickinson, Mountain View, California, USA). Ten thousand viable cells were analysed using forward/sidescatter gating. All antibodies are commercially available: CD33 phycorythrin (PE), HLA-DR fluorescein isothiocyanate (FITC), CD7-FITC, CD19-PE; Becton Dickinson, Heidelberg, FRG, CD13-FITC, CD2-PE, CD34-FITC; Dianova, Hamburg, FRG. For Partial purification of topoisomerases, 1 ml of crude nuclear extract from human promyelocytic HL-60 cells was adsorbed to 0.1 ml of hydroxyl apatite. The resin was washed and eluted with potassium phosphate (800 mM). Topo II activity was monitored by ATP-dependent pBR322 plasmid DNA relaxation, and protein content was measured with the Lowry procedure using bovine serum albumin as a standard. Anion exchange chromatography of nuclear extracts was carried out using an FPLC system (Pharmacia) [6]. Expression of the P-glycoprotein has been determined by cytochemistry using the following sandwich system: Cells, MDR1 polyclonal antibody (Oncogene Science Corp., N.Y. USA), Auroprobe TN goat antirabbit, and Intence SEM silver enhancer (Janson, Olen, Belgium).

Results

Surface Markers

For phenotypical characterization of HL-60 cells and sublines we used the following markers: CD33-PE, CD13-FITC, HLA-DR-FITC, CD7-FITC, CD2-PE, CD19-PE, and CD34-FITC. In Tab 1, the surface marker analysis of the used HL-60 lines is shown. All cell lines express the same markers; they do not differ in the state of differentiation and they are all subclones of promyelocytic HL-60 cells.

Sensitivity to Cytostatics

The following cytostatics and the influence of verapamil on sensitivity of the cells were tested: etoposide, teniposide, 4-(9-acridinylamino)methanesulfon-m-anisidide (mAMSA), daunoblastin, doxorubicin, mitoxantrone and vincristine. In Tab 2, the factor of resistance compared to HL-60 wild-type and the influence of verapamil are shown. In contrast to the stem cell line HL-60, the three sublines HL-60R, HL-60ETO, and HL-60TENI show a high resistance to a number of substances from different classes. The cell lines exhibit the following characteristics:

- High sensitivity against all cytostatics in the HL-60 stem cell-line
- MDR against a broad spectrum of substances in all sublines
- High reversibility of resistance (mostly more than 50 %) after addition of verapamil in the selected sublines HL-60ETO and HL-60TENI
- Low influence of verapamil on the resistance of HL-60R

Table 1. Surface maker analysis of HL-60 cell lines*

Cell Line	Monoclonal Antibodies						
	CD33	CD13	HLA-DR	CD7	CD2	CD19	CD34
HL-60	97	neg.	neg.	neg.	neg.	neg.	
	36						
HL-60R	100	71	neg.	neg.	neg.	neg.	neg.
HL-60ETO	98	40	neg.	neg.	neg.	neg.	neg.
HL-60TENI	100	73	neg.	neg.	neg.	neg.	neg.

* Percent positive cells

Table 2. Resistance of the cells against cytostatics*

Cell Line			Substance				
	eto	teni	mAMSA	dau	dox	mit	vic
HL-60	60/50	10/10	20/18	3/3	1/1	150/150	20/20
HL-60ETO	90/4	8/2	13/3	3/1	2/1	500/100	3/3
HL-60TENI	50/30	80/12	50/18	1/1	25/5	150/50	7/7

* Factor of resistance comparing LD50 of resistant strain to HL-60 wildtype without verapamil/with verapamil.

Table 3. Expression of P-glycoprotein*

Cell Line	Response to MDR1-Antibody			
	neg.	+	++	total pos.
HL-60	100	0	0	0
HL-R	100	0	0	0
HL-60ETO	6	91	3	94
HL-60TENI	3	86	11	97

* Percent cells

– Low resistance against vinca alkaloids in all sublines

Expression of P-Glycoprotein

In Tab 3, membrane expression of P-glyco-protein in the cells is shown. HL-60 cells as well as HL-60R cells have virtually no P-glycoprotein expressed. In the selected lines HL-60ETO and HL-60TENI, more than 90 % of the cells express P-glycopro-tein.

Characterization of Topoisomerases in the HL-60R Cells

By anion exchange chromatography we separated three active peaks with the fol-lowing characteristics: peak 1 (eluted at 50–100 mM) could be identified as topo I by p4-unknotting assay, negative immunos-taining using a topo II antibody and resis-tance to orthovanadate and topo II inhibi-tors (not shown); peaks 2 (eluted at 170 mM) and peak 3 (eluted at 200 mM) have been identified by the same methods to be isoforms of topo II. In Fig. 1, the pH-dependence of the isolated peaks revealed by changing the pH of the reaction buffer is shown: peak 1 (topo I) is active at pH 7.9, peak 2 (topo II) is active at pH 8.3, and peak 3 (topo II) is active at pH 7.9 and 9.0. Both peaks 2 and 3 contain the 170 and 180 kDa isoform as previously described [6].

In Fig. 2, the sensitivity of the peaks to mAMSA is shown. Peak 2, characterized as topo II, is as resistant to mAMSA as peak 1 (topo I); peak 3 is highly sensitive. This proves the existence of a resistant topo II isoform in the HL-60R cells.

Discussion

MDR cells with overexpression of the mem-brane-transport P-glycoprotein exhibit a high degree of resistance against lipophilic substances such as anthracyclines and vinca alkaloids [7, 8]. Apart from these cells an "AT (altered topoisomerase) pattern of resistance" has been described (9–11) fea-turing the following characteristics:
– High resistance against a broad spectrum of cytostatics

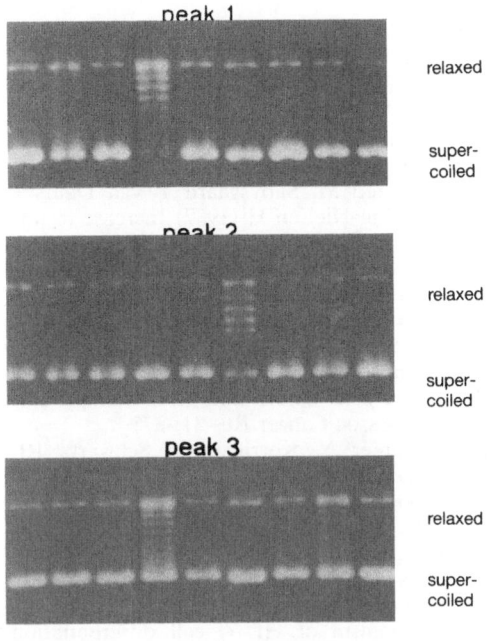

peak 1

relaxed

super-coiled

peak 2

relaxed

super-coiled

peak 3

relaxed

super-coiled

7.3 7.5 7.8 7.9 8.1 8.3 8.5 9.0 9.4

Fig. 1. pH profile of topoisomerase fractions revealed by anion exchange-chromatography from HL-60R cells. DNA relaxation activity of peak fractions was measured at the pH indicated

- Lower resistance against vinca alka-loids
- Weak modulation by verapamil
- Altered activity of topo II

The selected cell lines HL-60ETO and HL-60TENI, as well as the primary resistant line HL-60R, are resistant against cytostatics from several classes. Resistance of the lines HL-60ETO and HL-60TENI can be inhibited greatly by the addition of verapamil to the medium. Moreover, in contrast to the sensitive line, and in contrast to the MDR line HL-60R, these cells exhibit a high expression of P-glycoprotein in the membrane revealed by immunostaining. Also, topo II activity is altered in HL-60R cells, as these cells have a topo II isoform resistant against mAMSA. Obviously, in one cell several different topo II isoforms (probably due to posttranslational modifications) with different pH-activity peaks are active at the same time.

From these findings we conclude that overexpression of P-glycoprotein is an important molecular factor in selected cell lines which serve as a model for secondary resistance. In primary resistant cells addi-

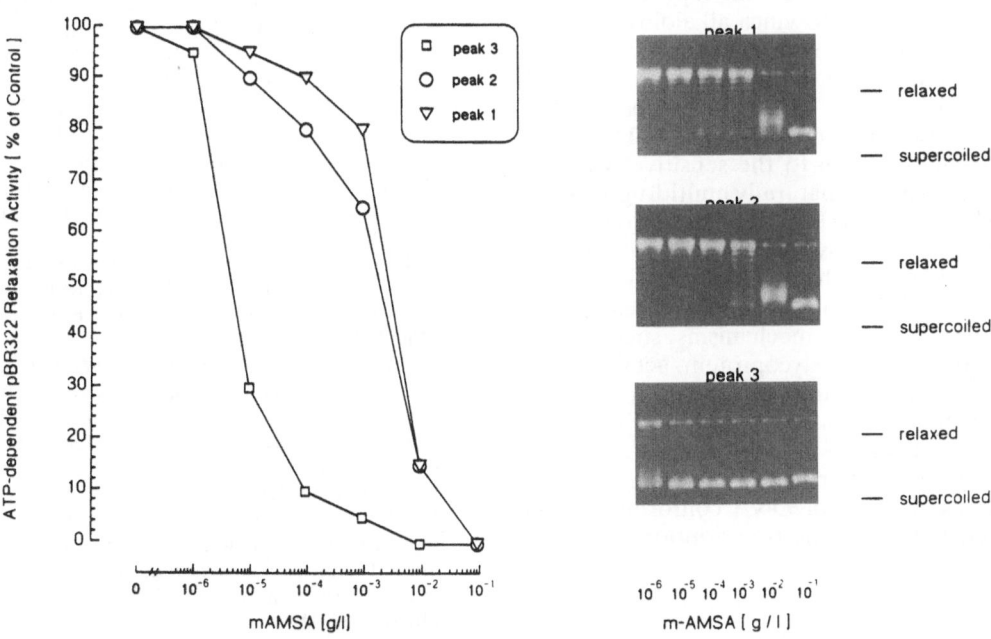

peak 1

— relaxed

— supercoiled

peak 2

— relaxed

— supercoiled

peak 3

— relaxed

— supercoiled

10^{-6} 10^{-5} 10^{-4} 10^{-3} 10^{-2} 10^{-1}

m-AMSA [g / l]

ATP-dependent pBR322 Relaxation Activity [% of Control]

□ peak 3
○ peak 2
▽ peak 1

mAMSA [g/l]

Fig. 2. *In vitro* inhibition of topoisomerase activity peaks revealed by anion exchange-chromatography from HL-60R cells by mAMSA at various concentrations. Controls without enzyme were run for each concentration of drug to exclude direct DNA effects (not shown)

47

tional factors, like alteration of topo II, are obviously more important. Consequently, it does not seem reasonable to treat primary resistant leukemias with drug modulators such as verapamil or derivates.

Summary

Several different molecular mechanisms of cellular resistance have been described, but alteration of topoisomerases seems to be one of the most important, as topoisomerase II (topo II) is the target enzyme for clinically important cytostatic drugs such as anthracyclines, epipodophyllotoxins, 4-(9-acridinyLamino)methanesulfon-m-anisidide (mAMSA) and mitoxantrone. These drugs act *via* inhibition of the enzyme after binding to the DNA ("cleavable complex"). Besides the "typical" resistance, caused by higher expression of P-glycoprotein, an "atypical" pattern of resistance has been described. These cells exhibit no amplification of P-glycoprotein and are not reversibel by P-glycoprotein-modulators, such as verapamil, an altered content or function of topo II, and a cross resistance to cytostatic drugs that interact with topo II, but with low resistance to vinca alkaloids.

To study these aspects, we selected HL-60 cell lines (human promyelocytic leukemia cells) against etoposide (labeled HL-60ETO) and teniposide (HL-60TENI) and compared them to the sensitive wild-type strain and to a naturally multidrug-resistant HL-60 strain (HL-60R). Alteration of topo II seems to play a major role in "primary" resistance. In the selected cells (which may be a model for "secondary" resistance), other molecular mechanisms, such as overexpression of P-glycoprotein, act synergistically. Modification of topo II results in a change of sensitivity to topo II inhibitors and a change of pH optima of the enzymes. This may affect DNA binding and has consequences for DNA conformation and regulation of gene transcription.

References

1. Kartner N, Everden-Porelle D, Bradley G, Ling V (1985) Detection of P-glycoprotein in multidrug-resistant cell lines by monoclonal antibodies. Nature 316: 820–826
2. Sehested M, Skovsgaard T, van Deurs B, Winther-Nielsen H (1987) Increase in nonspecific adsorptive endocytosis in anthracycline- and vinca-alcaloid resistant Ehrlich ascites tumor cell lines. JNCI 78: 171–175
3. Brophdy NA, Mc Fall P, Lewis AD, Smith SD. Sikic Bl (1990). Studies of drug resistant phenotypes and mechanisms in human leukemic cells before and after therapy. Proc Am Assoc Cancer Res 31: 375
4. Pommier Y, Kerrigan D, Schwartz RE, Swack JA. McCurdy A (1986) Altered DNA topoisomerase II activity in chinese hamster cells resistant to topoisomerase II inhibitors. Cancer Res 46: 3075–3081
5. Gieseler F, Boege F, Clark M (1990) Alteration of topoisomerase II action is a possible mechanism of HL-60 cell differentiation. Environ Health Perspect 88: 183–185
6. Boege F, Gieseler F, Biersack H, Clark M (to be published) Structural and functional heterogeneity of topoisomerase II in a multi-drug resistant HL-60 cell line revealed by anion-exchange chromatography and chromato-focussing. J Chromatogr
7. Beck W, Mueller T, Tanzer L (1979) Altered surface membrane glycoproteins in vinca alcaloid-resistant human leukemic lymphoblasts. Cancer Res 39: 2070–2075
8. Erttmann R, Gieseler F, Muenchmeyer M, Boetefuer A, Winkler K (1990) Atypical cross resistance against cytostatic drugs due to P-glycoprotein and reduced topoisomerase II activity in leukemic cells. Klin Padiatr 202: 294
9. Beck W, Danks M, Suttle D (1990) Multidrug resistance associated with alterations in topoisomerase II activity. J Cancer Res Clin Oncol (Suppl) 116: 1145
10. Erttmann R, Gieseler F, Wilms K, Winkler K (1990) Extended multidrug resistance in leukemic cells due to P-glycoprotein and altered topo-iosmerase II activity. Proc Am Soc Clin Oncol 9: 56
11. Boege F, Gieseler F, Biersack H, Clark M, Erttmann R (1990) Topo-isomerase II from multidrug-resistant leukemic cells exhibit altered enzyme activity and can not be inhibited by teniposid. J Cancer Res Clin Oncol 116: 418

Conserved Cytotoxic Activity of Aclacinomycin A in Multifactorial Multidrug Resistance

R. Erttmann[1], A. Boetefür[1], K. D. Erttmann[2], F. Gieseler[3], G. Looft[1], M. Münchmeyer[1], A. Reymann[4], and K. Winkler[1]

Introduction

Identification of anthracyclines which are able to overcome multidrug resistance would be a major step towards to improving antineoplastic chemotherapy.

Recently it has been shown [1] that 9-alkyl, morpholinyl anthracylines retain cytostatic activity in a multidrug resistant mouse mammary tumor cell line as well as in a multidrug resistant human small cell lung cancer cell line. It has been suggested that in these cell lines nonresponse to cytostatic drugs is due to the classical p-glycoprotein-related membrane transport resistance mechanism.

Another working group [2] has been able to show conserved cytotoxic activity of aclacinomycin A, which is also a 9-alkyl-substituted anthracycline (Fig. 1), in some multidrug-resistant human small cell cancer cell lines. Their in vitro model included different multidrug resistant cell lines,

which have been selected by cultivation under the pressure of daunorubicin. The daunorubicin-resistant cell lines obtained differed significantly in p-glycoprotein expression, which did not influence their sensitivity to aclacinomycin A. Therefore, it can be concluded that aclacinomycin A does overcome not only the classical type of p-glycoprotein mediated multidrug resistance but also other atypical mechanisms of multidrug resistance.

To prove this assumption we investigated the cytostatic activity of several anthracyclines including aclacinomycin A as a 9-alkyl-derivative in a doxorubicin-resistant mouse leukemia cell line. This cell line has been shown to have multifactorial resistance by at least two different molecular mechanisms: the classical p-glycoprotein

[1] Abteilung für Pädiatrische Hämatologie und Onkologie, Universitätskinderklinik, Hamburg
[2] Bernhard-Nocht-Institut für Tropenmedizin, Hamburg
[3] Medizinische Poliklinik, Universität Würzburg, Würzburg
[4] Abteilung für Allgemeine Pharmakologie, Pharmakologisches Institut der Universität, Hamburg
* Supported by Hamburger Krebsgesellschaft e.V., Fördergemeinschaft zur Erforschung und Heilung von Krebskrankheiten im Kindesalter e.V., Hamburg Deutsche Forschungsgemeinschaft, SFB 172, C9, Werner-Otto-Stiftung, Hamburg.

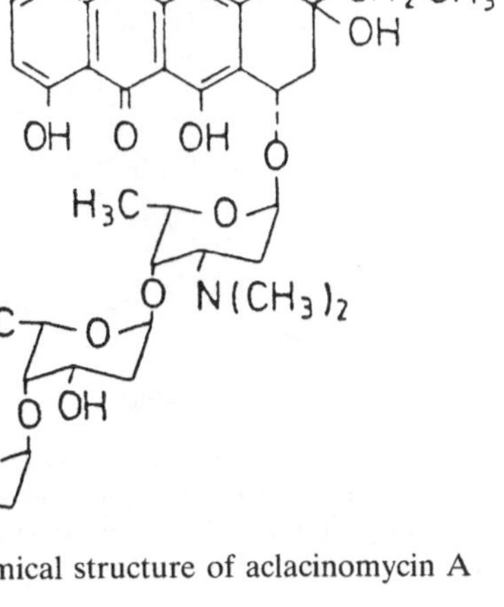

Fig. 1. Chemical structure of aclacinomycin A

mediated transport resistance as well as reduced DNA topoisomerase II activity. Despite the fact that this cell line shows a broad cross-resistance pattern to antineoplastic drugs of the antibiotic type its sensitivity to aclacinomycin A has been found to be nearly conserved.

Materials and Methods

A stable multidrug-resistant cell line (F4-6R) was selected by long-term exposure of the Friend mouse erythroleukemia cell line (F4-6) to increasing concentrations of doxorubicin. Both cell lines were propagated in suspension with Eagle's minimal essential medium (MEM alpha; Gibco Corp., Karlsruhe, FRG) supplemented with 10% fetal calf serum. The cells were collected in the late log phase of proliferation.

The sensitivity of the F4-6R cell, as well as of its parent line F4-6, to cytostatic substances was tested in the 48 h proliferation assay. Resistance factors of each cytostatic drug were determined as the ratio between the 50% inhibitory dosages (ED_{50}) for the F4-6R and the F4-6 cell lines.

Expression of p-glycoprotein was proven by immunogold cytochemistry using the Mdr1 polyclonal antibody (rabbit IgG; Oncogene Science Corp., Manhasset, NY, USA) with the following "sandwich system": Mdr1 polyclonal antibody – Auroprobe LM goat anti-rabbit – IntenSE M silver enhancer (Jansen Corp., Olen, Belgium). Moreover, the *MDR1* gene expression in both cell lines has been compared by Northern blotting using the pMDR cDNA probe related to the human *MDR1* gene as described by Chen et al. [3].

DNA topoisomerase II activity was measured after extraction from isolated nuclei of F4-6 and F4-6R cells by relaxation of 500 ng pBR322 plasmid DNA, as detailed by Gieseler et al. [4]. Aliquots of nucleic eluate were activated by 10 mM $MgCl_2$ and 2 mM ATP. After incubation at 37°C for 30 min the plasmid DNA was electrophoresed in 1% agarose gel. Topoisomerase II activity was quantified from disappearance of supercoiled pBR322.

Net uptake of anthracyclines into both cell lines was investigated by the silicone oil filtration method as well as by direct immunofluorescence microscopy as described in detail elsewhere [5, 6].

Results

The enhanced expression of *MDR1* gene in F4-6R cells in comparison to the parent line

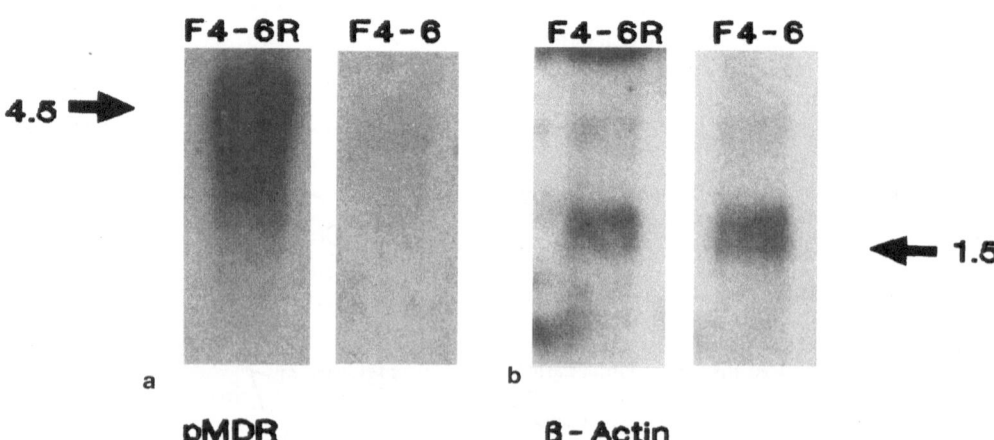

Fig. 2. a, b. Comparison of *MDR1* gene expression between F4-6R and F4-6 leukemia cells. Blot hybridization of mRNA (2 μg) from F4-6R and F4-6 cells is shown. *A* The Northern blot was hybridized with the pMDR1 0.7 kb probe. *B* As a control the same blot was rehybridized with a β-actin probe after removal of the pMDR1 probe

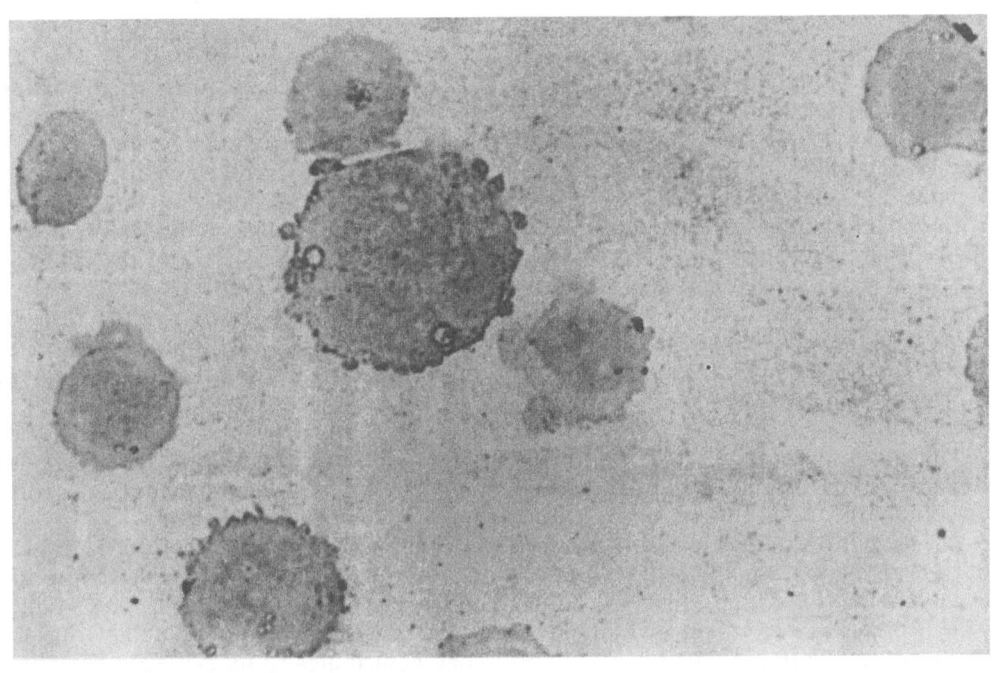

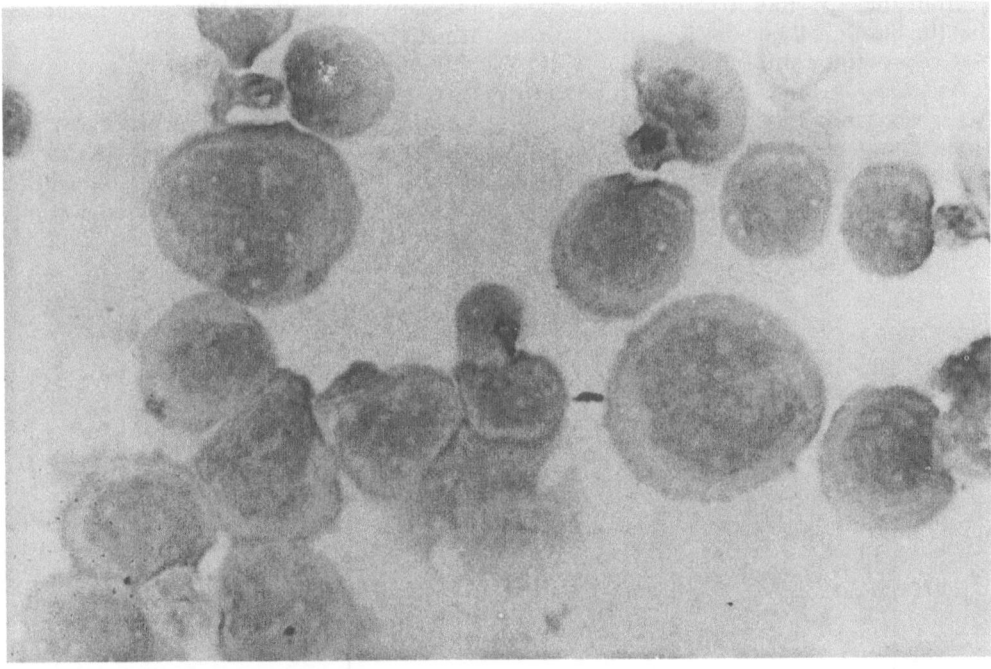

Fig. 3. Immunocytochemical detection of p-glycoprotein in F4-6R cells (lower part). Immunocytochemistry was performed with the immunogold method. The polyclonal IgG MDR1 antibody was used in the way described in the text

F4-6 was revealed by Northern blotting as well as by immunocytochemistry. In the Northern blot demonstrated in Fig. 2, the *MDR1*-related mRNA is compared in F4-6 and F4-6R cells showing overexpression in the resistant cell line. This corresponds well with the immunocytological detection of p-glycoprotein using the mdr1 antibody. As shown in Fig. 3, p-glycoprotein located in the membrane and in some vesicular structures of F4-6R cells could be found, whereas under the experimental conditions used, p-glycoprotein was undetectable in the parent cell line.

The p-glycoprotein-related multidrug-resistant (MDR) phenotype of the F4-6R cell line was found to be of functional relevance in terms of cellular anthracycline net accumulation. In Fig. 4 the reduced accumulation of daunorubicin in F4-6R cells compared to their wild-type is depicted. In additional drug release experiments (not demonstrated) the reduced net uptake of daunorubicin into F4-6R cells could be proven to be due to enhanced drug efflux.

From these results it can be concluded that the F4-6R cell line displays the classical p-glycoprotein-related MDR phenotype.

As shown in Table 1, the F4-6R cell line has a very broad spectrum of cross-resistance compared with that found in the classical MDR phenotype. The resistance spectrum of F4-6R includes such DNA-topoisomerase-II-related drugs as mitoxantrone and amsacrine. Therefore, we investi-gated the DNA topoisomerase II activity of F4-6R cells in comparison to the parent line. In Fig. 5 it is demonstrated that the turnover of supercoiled plasmid pBR322 DNA (in other words, the relaxation of the plasmid DNA) by nuclear extract of F4-6R cells is highly reduced compared with the nuclear relaxation activity of the wild-type cells (F4-6). This reflects reduced DNA topoisomerase II activity in the resistant cell line. As the DNA topoisomerase II in its active state during the generation of an enzyme-stabilized double strand break is the target for cytostatic drugs like anthra-cyclines, podophyllotoxins, and amsacrine, reduced activity of this enzyme confers drug resistance to these substances.

Therefore, it can be concluded that in addition to the classic p-glycoprotein-related phenotype the reduced DNA topoi-somerase II activity found in the F4-6R cell line contributes to its extended pattern of cross-resistance, as shown in Table 1. The F4-6R cell line has multifactorial resistance properties which consist of at least two molecular mechanisms: p-glycoprotein ex-pression and reduced DNA topoisomerase II activity.

In this context it should be mentioned that, as shown in Table 1, the 9-alkyl-substituted anthracycline aclacinomycin A is subjected only slightly to cross-resistance in the F4-6R model. In contrast to the other anthracyclines investigated the resistance factor of three does reflect grossly retained cytostatic activity.

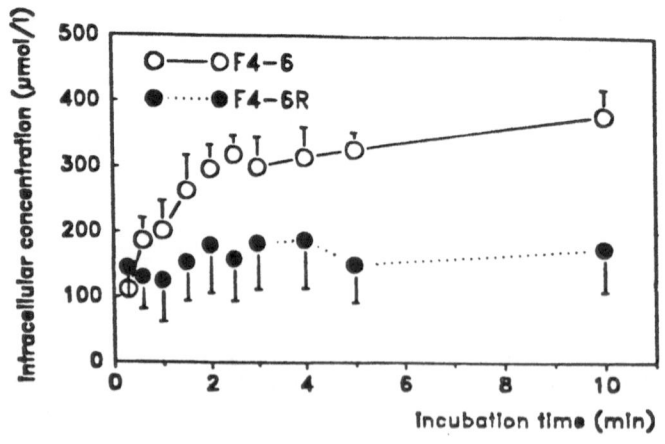

Fig. 4. Time dependence of daunorubicin uptake into F4-6 and F4-6R cells. The total cellular daunorubicin content (cytosolic and DNA-, RNA-, protein-bound) measured by the silicone oil filtration method is shown. The values are given as means ± SEM of seven to nine determinations from three cell passages

Table 1. Pleiotropic resistance of the F4-6R leukemic cell line

Cytostatic drug	Resistance factor
Doxorubicin	**51**
Daunorubicin	35
Idarubicin	12
Vincristine	19
Vepesid	17
Mitoxantrone	16
Amsacrine	11
Anthrapyrazole Cl-941	10
Aclarubicin	3

Resistance factor: ID_{50} F4-6R/ID_{50} F4-6

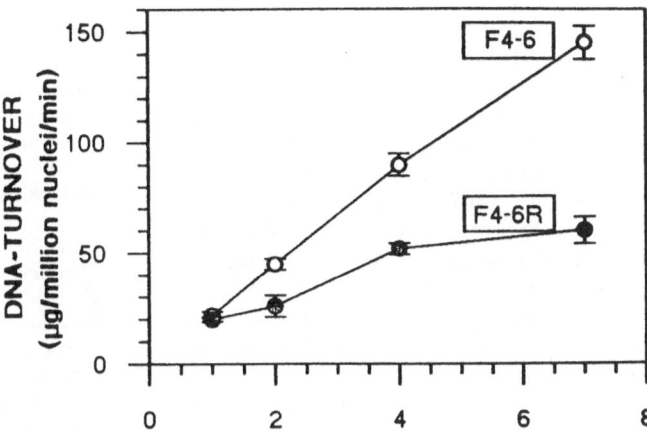

Fig. 5. DNA topoisomerase II activity in F4-6 and F4-6R cells. The median of three independent experiments ± SEM is shown. Topoisomerase II activity is achieved from nuclear extracts and has been quantified as relaxation effectivity of supercoiled DNA of the pBR322 plasmid. Incubation and activation were performed in the way described in the text

Discussion

The classical type of membrane-transport-dependent multidrug resistance and its relation to the drug eliminating properties of p-glycoprotein in resistant tumor cells are well described (see Weinstein et al. [1] for a comprehensive review). In acute myeloic leukemia and to a somewhat lesser extent acute lymphoblastic leukemia, expression of p-glycoprotein has been found before treatment and during advanced states of disease [8–13]. Therefore, a clinical role for p-glycoprotein in resistant acute leukemia can be assumed. At present prospective clinical trials asking this question are under way. In vitro it has been shown that the reduction of intracellular drug accumulation can be reversed by a lot of amphophilic drugs as for instance verapamil [14]. Therefore, pharmacological modulation of p-glycoprotein-related multidrug resistance may be possible.

Another way to circumvent pleiotropic membrane resistance would be the creation of cytostatic drugs with a favorable structure preventing p-glycoprotein-mediated membrane transport. Recently it has been shown by Coley et al. [1] that 9-alkyl, morpholinyl anthracyclines are able to overcome multidrug resistance of the membrane transport type. Similar results have been reported by Jensen et al. [2] for aclacinomycin A which is also a 9-alkyl-substituted anthracycline with a trisaccharide side chain in position 7. These authors found conserved cytostatic activity of aclacinomycin A in a p-glycoprotein-resistant small cell lung carcinoma subline selected by daunorubicin. In another daunorubicin-resistant cell line of the same parent strain no p-glycoprotein could be detected. In this model with atypical resistance aclacinomycin A also retained its cytostatic activity.

In our F4-6R mouse erythroleukemia cell line with multifactorial resistance selected by doxorubicin, aclacinomycin A nearly retains its cytotoxic activity, in contrast to daunorubicin and idarubicin. This result gives further evidence that the 9-alkyl-substitution of the anthracycline structure may provide protection against the p-glyco-protein efflux pumping system of multi-drug-resistant cells.

In addition, its special structure may improve the interaction of aclacinomycin A with altered DNA topoisomerase II to overcome atypical multidrug resistance. This question should be investigated further using atypically resistant p-glycoprotein negative cell lines with altered DNA topoisomerase II activity. Those models are described by several working groups [15, 16]. Whether the trisaccharide side chain of aclacinomycin A contributes to its favorable properties against different resistance mechanisms cannot be excluded and remains to be answered.

In conclusion, our in vitro data confirm the results of Coley et al. [1] that there is a correlation between 9-alkyl-substitution and cytotoxic activity of anthracyclines in p-glycoprotein-positive multidrug-resistant tumor cells. Moreover, it may be speculated, that the molecular structure of acla-rubicin A retains its cytotoxic activity against atypically multidrug resistant leukemic cells with altered DNA topoisomerase II activity.

Multifactorial drug resistance, as in our F4-6R model, reflects the main clinical problem of antileukemic therapy, because nearly all cytostatic drugs of the antibiotic type are included in the broad pleiotropic resistance pattern. The favorable structure activity relationship of aclacinomycin A in multidrug resistant leukemia cells found in vitro seems to correlate with its appreciable antileukemic activity in highly pretreated patients with acute myeloblastic leukemia [17–19].

References

1. Coley HM, Twentyman PR, Workman P (1990) 9-Alkyl, morpholinyl anthracyclines in the circumvention of multidrug resistance. Eur J Cancer 26: 665–667
2. Jensen PB, Vindelov L, Roed H, Demant EJF, Sehested M, Skovsgaard T, Hansen HH (1989) In vitro evaluation of the potential of aclarubicin in the treatment of small cell carcinoma of the lung (SCCL). Br J Cancer 60: 838–844
3. Chen C, Chin J, Ueda K, Clark DP, Pastan I, Gottesmann MM, Roninson IB (1986) Internal duplication and homology with bacterial transport proteins in the mdr1 (p-glycoprotein) gene from multidrug-resistant human cells. Cell 47: 381–389
4. Gieseler F, Boege F, Clark M (1990) Alteration of Topoisomerase II action is a possible mechanism of HL-60 cell differentiation. Environ Health Perspect 88: 183–185
5. Steinhoff A, Münchmeyer M, Looft G, Erttmann R (1989) Measurements of anthracycline accumulation in multidrug resistant and sensitive leukemia cells by fluorometry. Effect of verapamil and other membrane-transport modulating drugs. Naunyn Schmiedebergs Arch Pharmacol (Suppl) 339: R42
6. Reymann A, Edens L, Erb N, Erttmann R, Looft G, Woermann C (1989) Steady-state kinetics of anthracycline uptake in mouse Friend erythroleukemia cells. Naunyn Schmiedebergs Arch Pharmacol (Suppl) 340: R78
7. Weinstein RS, Kuszak JR, Kluskens LF, Coon JS (1990) P-glykoproteins in pathology: the multidrug resistance gene family in humans. Hum Pathol 21: 34–48
8. Ma DDF, Davey RA, Harman DH, Isbister JP, Scurr RD, Mackertich SM, Dowden G, Bell DR (1987) Detection of a multidrug resistant phenotype in acute non-lymphoblastic leukaemia. Lancet 135–137
9. Kemnitz J, Freund M, Dominis M, Cohnert TR, Uysal A, Georgii A (1989) Detection of cells with multidrug-resistant phenotype in myeloproliferative disorders before therapy. Hematol Pathol 3: 73–78
10. Holmes J, Jacobs A, Carter G, Janowska-Wieczorek A, Padua RA (1989) Multidrug resistance in haemopoietic cell lines, myelodysplastic syndromes and acute myeloblastic leukaemia. Br J Haematol 72: 40–44
11. Kuwazuru Y, Yoshimura A, Hanada S, Utsunomiya A, Makino T, Ishibashi K, Kodama M, Iwahashi M, Arima T, Akiyama S-Ig (1990) Expression of the multidrug trans-

porter, p-glycoprotein, in acute leukemia cells and correlation to clinical drug resistance. Cancer 66: 868–873

12. Rothenberg ML, Mickley LA, Cole DE, Balis FM, Tsuruo T, Poplack DG, Fojo A (1989) Expression of the mdr-1/p-170 gene in patients with acute lymphoblastic leukemia. Blood 74: 1388–1395

13. Noonan KE, Beck C, Holzmayer TA, Chin JE, Wunder JS, Andrulis IL, Gazdar AF, Willman CL, Griffith B, Von Hoff DD, Roninson I (1990) Quantitative analysis of MDR1 (multidrug resistance) gene expression in human tumors by polymerase chain reaction. Proc Natl Acad Sci USA 87: 7160–7164

14. Tsuruo T (1988) Mechanisms of multidrug resistance and implications for therapy. Jpn J Cancer Res 79: 285–296

15. Zijlstra JG, de Vries EGE, Mulder NH (1987) Multifactorial drug resistance in an adriamycin-resistant human small cell lung carcinoma cell line. Cancer Res 47: 1780–1784

16. Beck WT, Cirtain MC, Danks MK, Felsted RL, Safa AR, Wolverton Suttle DP, Trent JM (1987) Pharmacological, molecular and cytogenetic analysis of "atypical" multidrug-resistant human leukemic cells. Cancer Res 47: 5455–5460

17. Mathe G, Gil M-A, Delgado M, Bayssas M, Gouevia J, Ribaud R, Machover D, Misset J-L, de Vassal F, Schwarzenberg L, Jasmin C, Hayat M (1980) Phase II trial in acute leukemia and lymphosarcoma. In: Mathe G, Muggia FM (eds) Cancer chemo- and immunopharmacology I. Springer, Berlin Heidelberg New York, pp 217–222 (Recent results in cancer research, vol 74)

18. Pedersen-Bjeergard J, Brinker A, Ellegard J, et al. (1984) Aclarubicin in the treatment of acute non-lymphocytic leukemia refractory to treatment with daunorubicin and cytarabine: phase II trial. Cancer Treat Rep 68: 1233–1238

19. Mitrou PS, Kuse R, Anger H, et al. (1985) Aclarubicin (Aclacinomycin A) in the treatment of relapsing acute leukaemias. Eur J Cancer Clin Oncol 21: 919–923

Cytostatic Drug Resistance and Differentiation in Friend Erythroleukemia Cells

C. A. Schmidt[1], A. Schäfer[2], F. Lorenz[1], H. Oettle[1], F. F. Wilborn[1], D. Huhn[1], and W. Siegert[1]

Introduction

Cytostatic drug resistance is a common clinical problem in antitumor chemotherapy. To study mechanisms of drug resistance, in vitro model systems have been established. Frequently cross-resistance to other cytostatic drugs (i.e., chemically and structurally not related to the selective agent) was observed in these cell lines [1]. Multidrug resistance included medicaments often used in clinical therapy regimens such as vinca alkaloids or anthracyclines. Overexpression of a 170 kD glycoprotein was found to correlate with the multidrug-resistant phenotype [2, 3]. The gene encoding for the 170 kD glycoprotein, *mdr1*, has been cloned and sequenced [4, 5]. The multidrug-resistant phenotype could be transferred to drug-sensitive cells by transfection with *mdr1* cDNA [6, 7]. Resistant cells showed significant lower intracellular cytostatic drug levels, due to an activated drug efflux mechanism [8, 9]. *MDR* gene overexpression was detected in several leukemias and tumors and could be related to poor prognosis [10–13].

Beside the eradication of malignant cells by cytostatic drugs a new therapeutic approach – induction of differentiation – is presently being evaluated. It might be a valuable alternative in leukemia therapy and a way to circumvent multidrug resistance. To our knowledge, so far no data are available concerning cell differentiation and alterations in *mdr* gene expression. Friend erythroleukemia cells are a well known system for studying cell differentiation, since immature blast cells can be easily induced to differentiate to hemoglobin producing mature erythroid cells by adding dimethylsulfoxide (DMSO) [14, 15].

In this study we partially characterized a model system of drug sensitive Friend erythroleukemia cells and drug resistant subclones, using RNA dot blot analysis, immunocytochemistry, and fluorescence microscopy. This cell system will allow us to develop strategies for circumvention of drug resistance due to *mdr* gene overexpression and furthermore, to investigate *mdr* gene expression during terminal differentiation.

Material and Methods

Cell Lines

Friend erythroleukemia clone F4-6 [15] was grown in alpha medium without nucleosides, plus HEPES, pH. 7.2, supplemented with 10% fetal calf serum at 37 °C, 4% CO_2. These cells were kindly provided by Dr. W. Ostertag, H. Pette Inst. Exp. Virol., Hamburg, FRG. Doxorubicin-resistant cells (F4-6 ADM) were established by exposure of F4-6 wild-type (WT) cells to increasing Adriamycin concentrations. Finally, F4-6 ADM cells were still able to grow in the presence of 1 μg/ml Adriamycin.

[1] Freie Universität Berlin, Universitätsklinikum Rudolf Virchow, Abtlg Innere Medizin Spandauer Damm 130, Berlin, FRG
[2] Universität Hamburg, Abtlg Toxikologie Grindelallee 117, Hamburg, FRG

Induction of Differentiation

F4-6 WT and F4-6 ADM cells were grown for 5 days in alpha medium plus 10 % fetal calf serum in the presence of 1.5 % DMSO (210 mM) or varying concentrations of Adriamycin. Hemoglobin synthesis was determined by spectrophotometry methods [16].

RNA Dot Blot Analysis

Whole cellular RNA was prepared according to standard protocols [16]. A dilution of 10 µg, 3 µg, 1 µg and 0.3 µg RNA was blotted onto a nylon membrane (Hybond N, Amersham) for dot blot analysis. Filters were hybridized using the 1.3 kb ECORI ERI *mdr1* cDNA probe (kindly provided by Dr. M. M. Gottesman). To check equal loading of RNA, filters were washed and rehybridized using a β-actin probe (Clontech, Palo Alto, USA). Probes were labeled with ^{32}P dCTP using the Random Primed DNA Labelling Kit (Boehringer Mannheim, FRG). Hybridization and washing of filters were performed according to standard procedures [16]. Filters were exposed overnight to Kodak Xomat films at −70 °C.

To compare intracellular uptake of Adriamycin in F4-6 WT and F4-6 ADM cells, cell cultures were incubated for 4 h by adding the drug to the culture medium (final concentration 10 µM). Cells were washed twice. Intracellular accumulation and distribution of Adriamycin could be shown by fluorescence microscopy using the autofluorescence of this substance at 520 nm. Immunochemical determination of mdr1 protein was performed as described using an antibody against mdr protein (C-219, Centocor [15]). For negative controls, an unspecific myeloma immunoglobulin was used.

Results

As determined by trypan blue exclusion technique, only 2 % of F4-6 WT cells were viable after treatment with 15 ng/ml Adriamycin (doxorubicin) (Table 1). In contrast, 93 % of F4-6 ADM cells were growing after treatment with 250 ng/ml Adriamycin (Table 1); 54 % of F4-6 ADM cells survived a treatment of 1 µg/ml Adriamycin for 5 days.

Induction of differentiation was analyzed in F4-6 WT and F4-6 ADM cells. These cells could be induced to terminal differentiation by adding DMSO (final concentration 1.5 %) to the culture medium, as determined by hemoglobin (Hb) synthesis (228

Table 1. Induction of differentiation and inhibition of cell growth in F4-6 wild-type (WT) and doxorubicin-resistant (F4-6 ADM) cells

F4-6 WT cells	Control	DMSO concentration 1,5% (ng/ml)	Doxorubicin (ng/ml)			
			5	8	10	15
Hb (µg/10^8 cells)	29	228	46	47	56	46
vit. cells (% control)	100	51	80	52	18	2

F4-6 ADM cells	Control	DMSO concentration 1.5 %	Doxorubicin (ng/ml)		
			250	700	1000
Hb (µg/10^8 cells)	47	302	40	30	44
vit. cells (% control)	100	23	93	72	54

Hb, Hemoglobin; DMSO, dimethylsulfoxide

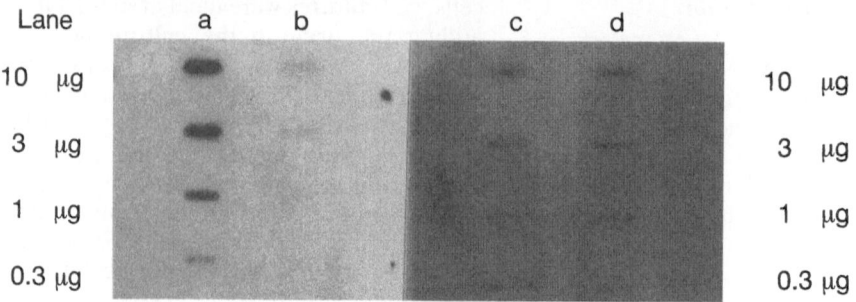

Fig. 1. Dot blot *mdr* gene expression in F4-6 WT cells. *Lane a*, F4-6 ADM cells; *lane b*, rehybridization of the filter with a β-actin probe; *lane c*, F4-6 WT cells; *lane d*, F4-6 ADM cells. For each cell line, 10 μg, 3 μg, 1 μg and 0.3 μg RNA were blotted. mdr1 and β-actin probes were labeled as described in material and me thods

μg Hb/10^8 cells in F4-6 WT and 302 μg Hb/10^8 cells in F4-6 ADM cells). Mean values of at least three independent experiments are given in Table 1. As shown in Table 1, Adriamycin has no capacity to induce differentiation in both subclones. Levels of *mdr* gene expression were determined by RNA dot blot analysis. As demonstrated in Fig. 1, high levels of *mdr* gene expression are present in F4-6 ADM cells, whereas no hybridization signal was observed in F4-6 WT cells. Equal loading of RNA was checked after washing the filter by reprobing with a β-actin probe.

As an assay for mdr glycoprotein function, Adriamycin uptake in F4-6 WT and F4-6 ADM cells was determined by using the autofluorescence of Adriamycin (not shown). Comparing fluorescence intensity in F4-6 WT and F4-6 ADM cells, resistant cells accumulated less of the cytostatic drug. Interestingly, different distribution patterns of Adriamycin were observed for both subclones. Whereas Adriamycin was detected predominantly in the cell nucleus of F4-6 WT cells, it was found mainly in the cytoplasm of F4-6 ADM cells. The expression of mdr protein was confirmed by immunocytochemical analysis using the monoclonal antibody C-219 (Centocor, not shown).

Discussion

We partially characterized F4-6 ADM cells, derived from F4-6 WT cells, by exposure to increasing Adriamycin concentrations. F4-6 ADM cells were still able to grow in the presence of 1 μg/ml Adriamycin in the medium, whereas only 2 % of F4-6 WT cells survived treatment with 2 ng/ml Adriamycin. Similar degrees of resistance have been described in other cell line systems [1]. F4-6 WT and F4-6 ADM cells could be induced to differentiation. By adding DMSO (final concentration 210 mM) hemoglobin synthesis could be detected in both subclones. To characterize mechanisms leading to drug resistance in F4-6 ADM cells, dot blot experiments were performed. High levels of *mdr* gene expression were detected in F4-6 ADM cells. Furthermore, immunocytochemical analysis revealed overexpression of mdr protein in these cells. Adriamycin uptake was significantly lower in F4-6 ADM compared to F4-6 WT cells as could be shown by fluorescence microscopy, exhibiting much less Adriamycin fluorescence in F4-6 ADM compared to F4-6 WT cells. Decreased intracellular drug accumulation has been described, when resistance was due to *mdr* gene overexpression [8–10]. Our data support the view that cytostatic drug resistance in F4-6 ADM cells is probably due to *mdr* gene overexpression. However, the possibility that other mechanisms contribute to Adriamycin resistance in F4-6 ADM cells cannot be excluded. Drug accumulation is one of the first steps in drug/cell interaction. Therefore, irrespective of whether other resistance mechanisms are present, these cells may be a suitable model system for studying multidrug resistance in mammal cells, and additionally will allow analysis of *mdr* gene expression during terminal differentiation.

References

1. McGrath T, Latoud C, Arnold ST, Safa A, Felsted R, Center M (1989) Mechanisms of multidrug resistance in HL 60 cells. Biochem Pharmacol 38: 3611–3619
2. Beck WT, Mueller TJ, Tanzer LR (1975) Altered surface membrane glycoproteins in Vinca alkaloid-resistant human leukemic lymphoblasts. Cancer Res 39: 2070–2076
3. Riordan JR, Deuchars K, Kartner N, Alon N, Trent J, Ling V (1985) Amplification of P-glycoprotein genes in multidrug-resistant mammalian cell lines. Nature 316: 817–819
4. Van der Bliek AM, Baas F, Van der Velde-Koerts T, Biedler JL, Myers MB, Ozols RF, Hamilton TC, Joenje H, Borst P (1988) Genes amplified and overexpressed in human multidrug resistant cell lines. Cancer Res 48: 5927–5932
5. Ueda K, Clark DP, Chen LJ, Roninson IB, Gottesman MM, Pastan I (1987) The human multidrug resistance (MDR1) gene: cDNA cloning and transcription initiation. J Biol Chem 262: 505–508
6. Ueda K, Cornwell MM, Pastan I, Roninson IB, Ling V, Riordan JR (1986) The mdr1 gene responsible for multidrug resistance, codes for P-glycoprotein. Biochem Biophys Res Commun 141: 956
7. Ueda K, Cardarelli C, Gottesman MM, Pastan I (1987) Expression of a full-length cDNA for the human "MDR1" gene confers resistance to colchicine, adriamycin, and vinblastine. Proc Natl Acad Sci USA 84: 3004–3008
8. Gros P, Neriah YB, Croop JM, Housman DE (1986) Isolation and expression of a complementary DNA that confers multidrug resistance. Nature 323: 728–731
9. Cornwell MM, Tsuruo T, Gottesman MM, Pastan I (1987) ATP-binding properties of P-glycoprotein from multidrug resistant KB cells. FASEB J 1: 51–54
10. Inaba M, Johnson RK (1987) Uptake and retention of adriamycin and daunorubicin by sensitive and anthracycline resistant sublines of P388 leukemia. Biochem Pharmacol 27: 2123–2130
11. Gros P, Croop J, Housman DE (1986) Mammalian multidrug resistance gene: complete cDNA sequence indicates strong homology to bacterial transport proteins. Cell 47: 371–380
12. Sato H, Preisler HD, Gottesman MM, Leukemia Intergroup (1988) Expression of the multidrug resistance gene (mdr) in the cells of patients with ANLL. Blood 72 (5/Suppl 1): 224a
13. Sato H, Gottesman MM, Goldstein LJ, Pastan I, Block AM, Sanberg AA, Preisler HD (1990) Expression of the multidrug resistance gene in myeloid leukemias. Leuk Res 44: 11–22
14. Steinheider G, Westendorf J, Marquardt H (1986) Induction of differentiation by the anthracycline antitumor antibiotics, Aclacinomycin A, Musettamycin and Marcellomycin. Leuk Res 10: 1233–1239
15. Ostertag W, Melderis H, Steinheider G, Kluge N, Dube SK (1972) Synthesis of mouse haemoglobin and globin mRNA in leukemic cell cultures. Nature N Biol 239: 231
16. Maniatis T, Fritsch EF, Sambrook J (1982) Molecular cloning. A laboratory manual. Cold Spring Harbor Laboratory Press, Cold Spring Harbor

On the Role of Aldehyde Dehydrogenase in a Cyclophosphamide-Resistant Variant of Brown Norway Rat Acute Myelocytic Leukemia*

C. J. de Groot[1], A. C. M. Martens[1], and A. Hagenbeek[1,2]

The development of resistance to chemo-therapeutic agents is still a major cause of treatment failure in cancer patients. The mechanisms by which drug resistance develops are poorly understood. Cyclophosphamide (CP) is widely used in the treatment of different hematological malignancies and in a variety of solid tumors. Furthermore, CP is incorporated in many conditioning regimens prior to bone marrow transplantation. Its in vitro active metabolite 4-hydroperoxycyclophosphamide is frequently used for purging purposes in case of autologous bone marrow transplantation for acute leukemia [1]. Obviously, given these clinical applications, studies on the mechanism(s) of CP resistance are highly relevant.

Brown Norway rat acute myelocytic leukemia (BNML) has been recognized as a realistic model for human acute myelocytic leukemia (AML), both for the development of new diagnostic tools as well as a preclinical model from which new clinical treatment strategies can be derived [2]. To investigate the biochemical mechanism(s) and ultimately the molecular basis of CP resistance, we have established a CP-resis-tant BNML line in vivo by repeated treatment of leukemic animals with CP [3].

CP first has to be activated in the liver to yield 4-hydroxy-CP/aldophosphamide, intermediates which by further metabolism yield the alkylating agent phosphoramide mustard (PM). Alternatively, activated CP can be inactivated to the nontoxic carboxy-phosphamide by the catalysis of aldehyde dehydrogenase (ALDH) or by the action of glutathione (GSH) or glutathione-dependent enzymes like, for instance, gluta-thione-S-transferases (GSTs), to 4-mercap-to-CP [4].

Some cell-lines resistant to CP have been shown to exhibit increased ALDH activity levels [5, 6]. To investigate whether increased detoxification of activated CP is involved in CP resistance of the BNML/CPR variant, we determined the ALDH enzyme activity levels in tissues of leukemic rats (Table 1). The cytosolic fraction of spleen and bone marrow of full-blown leukemic rats carrying CP-resistant cells revealed at least 6- to 7-fold higher ALDH activity levels than their CP-sensitive counterpart.

The cytosolic enzyme ALDH can specifically be inhibited by substances like disulfiram (DSF) [7]. Table 2 shows the in vivo data obtained after pretreatment of leukemic rats with DSF followed by CP treatment. A significant increase in the survival time of the CPR-carrying rats (reflected in an increase in log cell kill, LCK) was observed. Treatment with DSF alone hardly affected the survival time, while injection of CP alone resulted in 0.3–1.5 LCK, a range remaining within the limits of sensitivity of

[1] Institute of Applied Radiobiology and Immunology TNO, Rijswijk, The Netherlands
[2] Dept. Hemato-Oncology, The Dr. Daniel den Hoed Cancer Center, Rotterdam, The Netherlands
* These investigations were supported by the Dutch Cancer Society, the Josephine Nefkens Foundation, the Nijbakker-Morra Foundation, and ASTA-Werke A.G., Bielefeld, FRG.

Table 1. Aldehyde dehydrogenase (ALDH) enzyme activity levels in cytosolic tissue extracts of leukemic and nonleukemic rats

Source	ALDH activity (nmol min^{-1} mg protein^{-1}) Spleen	Bone marrow	Liver
Normal BN	0.13–0.36	<0.10	0.68
BNML/S (parent)	<0.10–0.38	<0.10	0.45
BNML/CPR	0.36–1.39	1.94	0.53

Table 2. Effect of pretreatment with disulfiram (DSF: ALDH inhibitor) on the antileukemic effect of cyclophosphamide (CP) in vivo

Group	DSF (mg/kg)	CP (mg/kg)	Number of rats	Cause of death Leukemia	Toxicity	LCK
BNML/CPR						
DSF + CP	50	100	8	6	2	5.3
	100	50	10	5	5	2.3
	100	100	18	6	1	4.3–6.5
DSF control	50	–	8	8	0	0.3
	100	–	18	18	0	0.1
CP control	–	100	24	24	0	0.3–1.5
BNML/S						
DSF + CP	50	100	8	4	4	5.1
	100	100	8	3	5	5.6
DSF control	50	–	8	8	0	0
	100	–	16	9	7	0
CP control	–	100	24	24	0	3.6–5.2

CP was injected i.p. in the dose indicated 4–4.5 h after DSF treatment. Note: 50 mg/kg CP alone has no cytotoxic effect on BNML/CPR cells.

the survival assay. However, pretreatment with DSF followed by CP did lead to a significant LCK, ranging from 4.3 to 6.5 in the case of BNML/CPR-carrying rats. In the groups receiving the highest dose of DSF and thereafter treated with CP – or even without, in the case of BNML/S cells – lethal toxicity within the first week after treatment hampered the evaluation of the in vivo experiments. The therapeutic effect of pretreatment with DSF of the rats carrying BNML/S cells was far less pronounced (Table 2).

Likewise, the effect on both cell lines of DSF treatment prior to incubation with mafosfamide, an in vitro active analogue of CP, was investigated (Table 3). In this par-

ticular experiment there was a considerable cytotoxic effect of mafosfamide (100 μM) incubation on the BNML/CPR cells (1.0 LCK, Table 3). Nevertheless, 15- to 150-fold differences in sensitivity to mafosfamide between the BNML/S and BNML/CPR cell lines were observed. As can be inferred from Table 3, preincubation of the BNML/CPR cells with the ALDH-inhibitor DSF led to a 20-fold increase in the cytotoxic effect of mafosfamide. Also in the case of the CP-sensitive cells a pronounced increase in cell kill was observed (3–5 LCK, Table 3). Since there is hardly any cytotoxic effect of incubation of the leukemia cells with DSF only, for the in vitro situation, as it was for in vivo, the conclusion can be drawn

Table 3. Effect of pretreatment with disulfiram (DSF) on the antileukemic effect of mafosfamide (MAFOS) in vitro

Group	MAFOS dose (μM)	LCK
BNML/CPR		
DSF + MAFOS	100	2.5
DSF control	–	0.2
MAFOS control	50	0
	100	1.0
	200	1.3
	500	2.7
BNML/S		
DSF + MAFOS	100	5–7[+a]
DSF control	–	0.4
MAFOS control	20	0.5
	50	2.2
	100	2.2

DSF incubation was for 60 min; mafosfamide incubation was for 30 min. Since there was no difference in rat survival time in the groups treated with DSF dissolved in ethanol or dimethylsulfoxide (DMSO) and its control groups, these data were pooled (4 × 5 rats/group). [a]In this incubation group, 2/9 rats did not develop leukemia, while 7/9 died of leukemia with a survival time corresponding with 1–100 surviving leukemic cells (indicated with a LCK of 5–7[+])

that by inhibition of ALDH with DSF, the CP- or mafosfamide-resistance of the BNML/CPR cells can be overcome.

Another more general detoxification mechanism of CP that has been reported to be implicated in resistance to CP and other alkylating agents, involves elevated GSH levels and increased GST activity [4, 8]. In case increased levels of ALDH are solely responsible for the CP resistance of the BNML/CPR cell line, it is to be expected that it has retained its sensitivity to PM, the alkylating product of CP metabolism [4]. Therefore, we investigated the sensitivity of the CP-resistant cell line to PM in comparison with the sensitive parent line, both in vivo and in vitro. By PM treatment in vivo up to a 4.2 LCK could be obtained with a dose of 120 mg/kg body weight in rats carrying the CPR cells, comparable to the 3.5 LCK obtained with the same dose in rats carrying the sensitive cell line (Fig. 1).

Incubation with PM in vitro of the CP-resistant and parent sensitive BNML cells, followed by injection into recipient animals showed similar results: an LCK of 2.2 for the BNML/CPR cells versus 3.0 for the

BNML/S cells at a PM concentration of 500 μM was observed (Fig. 2).

Depletion of GSH by treatment with buthionine sulfoximine (BSO), a specific inhibitor of GSH synthesis, can restore drug sensitivity in case elevated GSH levels or GST enzyme activity are involved in the mechanism of drug resistance [9]. To determine whether elevated GSH levels are involved, CP-resistant and -sensitive BNML cells were incubated in vitro for 6 h with BSO to deplete the intracellular GSH level, and subsequently incubated with PM. Only a marginal effect of BSO pretreatment on the cytotoxicity of PM for both cell lines was observed (data not shown). The comparable sensitivity of the BNML/S and the BNML/CPR cells to PM (Figs. 1, 2) and the fact that GSH depletion had no effect on the sensitivity of the CP resistant cells to PM, indicate that elevated GSH levels or increased GST activity plays no or only a minor role in the mechanism of CP resistance of the BNML/CPR cell line.

Both by conventional karyotyping and by flowkaryotyping the chromosomal aberrations of the BNML/S and the BNML/CPR

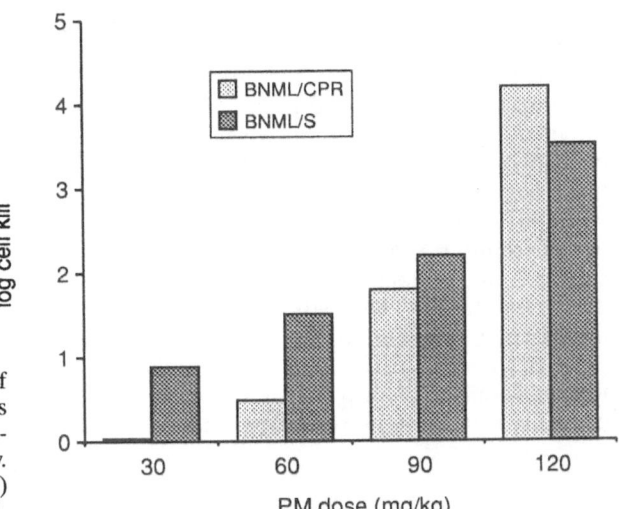

Fig. 1. Comparison of the response of the BNML/CPR and BNML/S cell lines to treatment with phosphoramide mustard (PM) in vivo. PM was injected i.v. on day 11 (60–120 mg/kg; 5 rats/group) or day 12 (30 or 60 mg/kg; $N = 16$ and 8, respectively)

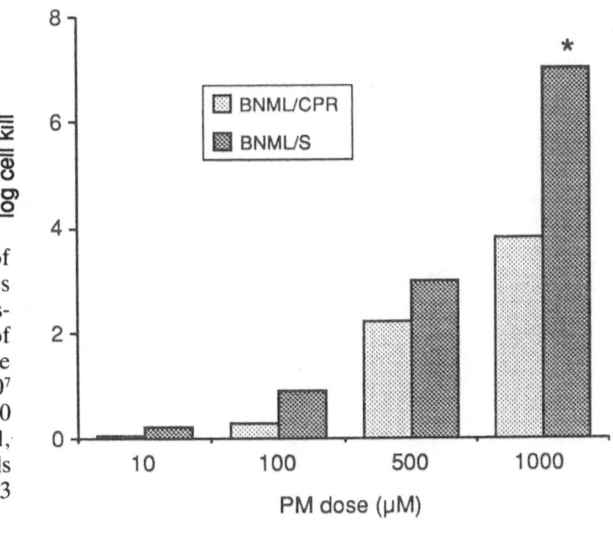

Fig. 2. Comparison of the response of the BNML/CPR and BNML/S cell lines to treatment with phosphoramide mustard (PM) in vitro. After incubation of the cells with PM (30 min, 37°C), the cells were washed and injected i.v. (10^7 cells/rat) into recipient animals (5–10 rats/group). Survival time was recorded, expressed as log cell kill. * No animals died of leukemia (observation period 63 days)

cells have been documented [10]. The CP-resistant variant is characterized by a specific $2p^+q^+$ marker chromosome, i.e., an elongation of the long arm of the $2p^+$ chromosome, which is one of the chromosomal aberrations characteristic for the BNML/S cell line [10]. By spot blot analysis of flow-sorted chromosomes of normal BN rat, and also CP-resistant and CP-sensitive BNML cells, we are currently establishing the chromosomal localization of the ALDH1 gene in these cells. Hopefully, this will tell us whether there is a direct causa-tive link between changed ALDH gene structure or localization, leading to the observed enhanced ALDH gene expression, and the extra chromosomal aberration, specific for the BNML/CPR cell line.

Summary

Brown Norway rat acute myelocytic leukemia (BNML) was made resistant in vivo to cyclophosphamide (CP) by repeated CP treatment of leukemic animals. The obtained BNML/CPR cell line was highly resistant to CP in vivo and to activated CP in vitro. In the spleen of BNML/CPR-carrying rats, the level of the CP-detoxifying enzyme aldehyde dehydrogenase (ALDH) was 6-fold higher, compared to non-resistant BNML spleen cells. Inhibition of ALDH by disulfiram led to reversal of CP resistance. These studies show that increased detoxification capacity can render cancer cells resistant to CP. Whether this mechanism of drug resistance occurs clinically can easily be tested in vitro.

References

1. Yeager AM, et al. (1986) Autologous bone marrow transplantation in patients with acute nonlymphocytic leukemia, using ex vivo marrow treatment with 4-hydroperoxy-cyclophosphamide. N Engl J Med 315: 141–147
2. Martens ACM, van Bekkum DW, Hagenbeek A (1990) The BN acute myelocytic leukemia (BNML) (A rat model for studying human acute myelocytic leukemia (AML)). Leukemia 4: 241–257
3. Martens ACM, de Groot CJ, Hagenbeek A (1991) Development and characterization of a cyclophosphamide resistant variant of the BNML rat medel for acute myelocytic leukemia (AML). Eur J Cancer (recently published =) Eur. J. Cancer 27: 161–166
4. Brock N (1989) Oxazaphosphorines cytostatics: past-present-future. Seventh Cain Memorial Award Lecture. Cancer Res 49: 1–7
5. Hilton J (1984) Role of aldehyde dehydrogenase in cyclophosphamide-resistant L1210 leukemia. Cancer Res 44: 5156–5160
6. Koelling TM, et al. (1990) Development and characterization of a cyclophosphamide-resistant subline of acute myeloid leukemia in the Lewis × Brown Norway hybrid rat. Blood 76: 1209–1213
7. Sladek NE, Landkamer GJ (1985) Restoration of sensitivity to oxazaphosphorines by inhibitors of aldehyde dehydrogenase activity in cultured oxazaphosphorine-resistant L1210 and cross-linking agent-resistant P388 cell lines. Cancer Res 45: 1549–1555
8. McGown AT, Fox BW (1986) A proposed mechanism of resistance to cyclophosphamide and phosphoramide mustard in a Yoshida cell line in vitro. Cancer Chemother Pharmacol 17: 223–226
9. Suzukake K, Petro BJ, Vistica DT (1982) Reduction in glutathione content of L-PAM resistant L1210 cells confers drug sensitivity. Biochem Pharmacol 31: 121–124
10. Arkesteijn GJA, et al. (1987) Bivariate flow karyotyping of acute myelocytic leukemia in the BNML rat model. Cytometry 8: 618–624

SAENTA-fluoresceins: New Flow Cytometry Reagents for Assessing Transport of Nucleoside Drugs in Acute Leukemia

J. S. Wiley[1], G. P. Jamieson[2], A. M. Brocklebank[2], M. B. Snook[1], W. H. Sawyer[2],
P. M. Dennington[1], J. McKendrick[1], R. K. Woodruff[1], and A. R. P. Paterson[3]

New strategies are needed to improve the outlook for patients with acute myeloid leukemia (AML). The use of granulocyte-macrophage colony stimulating factor (GM-CSF) given prior to and in combination with chemotherapy represents such a new approach and its safety and efficacy have been established [1, 2]. GM-CSF is a growth promoter of leukemic colony-forming cells in vitro [3, 4] and can render such cells more susceptible to the cytotoxic action of cytosine arabinoside (araC). When given in vivo to patients with AML, GM-CSF usually increases the proliferative activity of myeloblasts and in a small study is associated with a high remission rate to subsequent chemotherapy incorporating araC.

The basis for the increased sensitivity of cycling cells to nucleoside antimetabolites such as araC rests not only on the greater incorporation of araC into DNA but may also reflect differences in the accumulation of araC metabolites in cycling and quiescent cells. There is good evidence that araCTP is the active metabolite of araC and that this triphosphate reaches higher concentrations in proliferating cells in culture compared to quiescent cells such as peripheral blood lymphocytes [5, 6]. Our previous work has established that membrane transport of araC is rate-limiting for araCTP accumula-

tion when cells are exposed to araC plasma levels of $1 \mu M$ or less [5, 7] although at araC levels in excess of $10 \mu M$, the rate-limiting step for araCTP accumulation becomes deoxycytidine kinase [8]. It follows that proliferating cells must transport nucleosides such as araC at greater rates and this has been shown experimentally for peripheral blood lymphocytes which, after stimulation by the mitogen phytohemagglutinin, develop 30-fold greater transport capacity for araC [9]. Measurement of nucleoside transport site densities on a variety of fresh and cultured leukemic and lymphoid cells provides strong support for the concept that the expression of the transporter is greater on cycling cells than on quiescent cells. Cultured cell lines which are permanently committed to growth express 100 000–500 000 transporters per cell, which is 100-fold greater than values found on quiescent peripheral blood lymphocytes. Even in fresh clinical specimens of B-cell lymphomas, AMLs, and T-cell acute lymphoblastic leukemia (ALL) a linear relationship has been established between the number of transporter sites per cell and the proliferative fraction shown by percentage of S-phase cells [10, 11].

The measurements of nucleoside transporter density on fresh clinical samples of cells has proven value in predicting the effect of araC in T-cell ALL/lymphoblastic lymphoma [11]. Measurement of nucleoside transport sites in AML blasts before and after growth factor administration might also enable a rapid assessment of a subsequent response to araC chemotherapy. Nucleoside transport capacity is tradi-

Haematology Department and Ludwig Institute for Cancer Research, Austin Hospital, Heidelberg, Australia[1]
Russell-Grimwade School of Biochemistry, University of Melbourne, Australia[2] and
University of Alberta, Edmonton, Canada[3]

tionally assessed by ligand binding using nitrobenzylthioinosine (NBMPR), a high affinity and specific inhibitor of the equilibrative nucleoside transporter [12]. However, this technique, which employs a ^{3}H-labeled ligand, cannot identify subpopulations of cells with different transporter densities within a single sample.

A fluorescent ligand for the equilibrative nucleoside transporter would enable ligand-cell interactions to be analyzed by flow cytometry, a technique which can differentiate between subpopulations on the basis of light scatter and fluorescence intensity [13]. In addition, flow cytometry requires far fewer cells than are needed for analysis of ^{3}H-ligand binding. Although a fluorescent dansyl derivative of 6-thioguanosine has been synthesized and shown to bind to the equilibrative nucleoside transporter of human erythrocytes [14] this ligand had only moderate affinity (Kd 100–300 nM) as well as high nonspecific binding. We have reported the synthesis of a more suitable ligand formed by coupling fluorescein-5-isothiocyanate (FITC) to the amino group of $5'$-S-(2-aminoethyl)N^6-(4-nitrobenzyl)-$5'$-thioadenosine (SAENTA) to produce an analogue that binds tightly to the nucleoside transporter [15].

This fluorescent ligand is termed SAENTA-x_2-fluorescein where x_2 refers to the number of atoms in the linkage between fluorescein and SAENTA. This SAENTA-x_2-fluorescein ligand inhibited the influx of ^{3}H-nucleoside into cultured RC2a leukemic cells and moreover competed with ^{3}H-NBMPR for binding to the transporter in the same cell line. Thus SAENTA-x_2-fluorescein appears to interact with the same site on the transporter as NBMPR although the fluorescent ligand bound with a lower affinity (Kd 6.2 nM) than that found for NBMPR (Kd 0.2–1.0 nM). These estimates of the affinity of SAENTA-x_2-fluorescein for the transporter came from flow cytometry measurements on dilute cell suspensions equilibrated with a range of SAENTA-x_2-fluorescein concentrations. Such equilibration is rapid and complete within 10 min of mixing cells with ligand at room temperature. Histograms of cell-bound fluorescent were obtained at each concentration of SAENTA-x_2-fluorescein both in

the presence and absence of 1 μM NBMPR. This NBMPR-sensitive ligand binding (expressed as channels of fluorescence intensity) was plotted against the SAENTA-x_2-fluorescein concentration. Half maximal binding values obtained at low cell concentrations (10^5/ml) approximate the dissociation constant which for leukemic RC2a cells was 6.2 ± 1.0 nM ($n = 3$).

A potential drawback with SAENTA-x_2-fluorescein is its low fluorescence yield which was only 15 %–30 % of the values for FITC although the exact value depends on the solvent used for the measurement. A second SAENTA-based ligand for the transporter has been synthesized and has the structure shown in Fig. 1. This ligand has a longer spacer arm of eight atoms (x_8) between SAENTA and fluorescein and this results in a 60 % increase in fluorescence intensity. This ligand also gave extremely high specific binding to the nucleoside transporter of leukemic RC2a cells, as illustrated by the fluorescence histograms in Fig. 2. Incubation of cells with 1 μM NBMPR prior to addition of ligand reduced cell-associated fluorescence almost to the level of autofluorescence indicating very low nonspecific binding by this ligand.

Specific binding of SAENTA-fluorescein ligands can only be expressed in units of fluorescence intensity (i.e., channels of fluorescence on the flow cytometer). To allow comparison of measurements performed on different flow cytometers and on different days, a calibration is included with each run. Fluorescent standard beads containing known numbers of fluorescein molecules were analyzed under the same conditions as the leukemic cells. The fluorescence histograms are shown in Fig. 3 for beads containing 7000, 13000, 29000, and 62000 molecules of equivalent soluble fluorescein (MESF). Calibration curves of MESF against mean fluorescence channel number were constructed to enable specific binding of the SAENTA-fluoresceins to be expressed in units of MESF. Although SAENTA-x_8-fluorescein binds with 1:1 stoichiometry to the nucleoside transporter, SAENTA-x_8-fluorescein binding expressed in MESF does not simply equate with the number of nucleoside transporters due to differences in fluorescence quench-

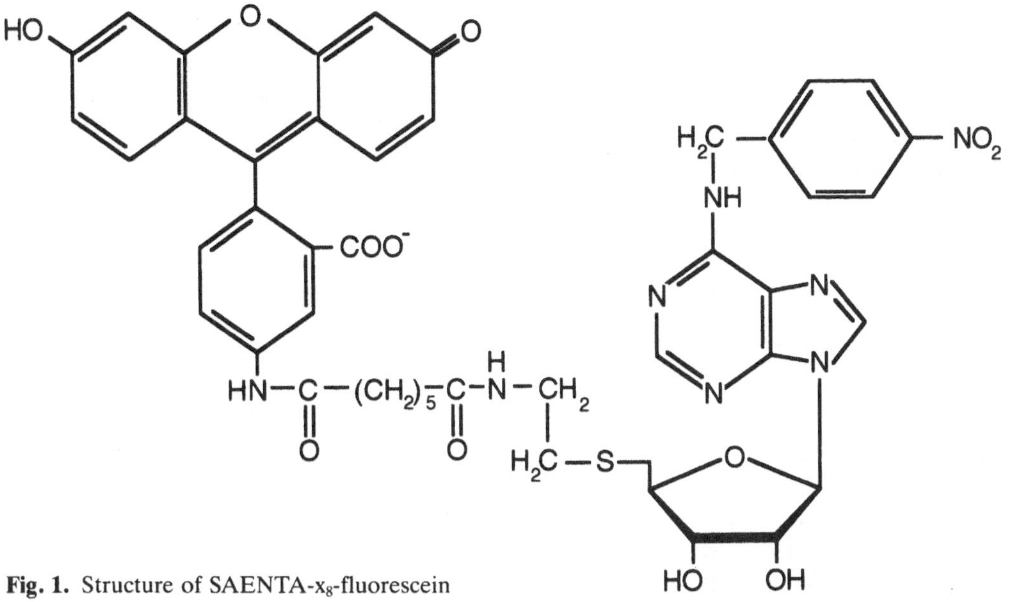

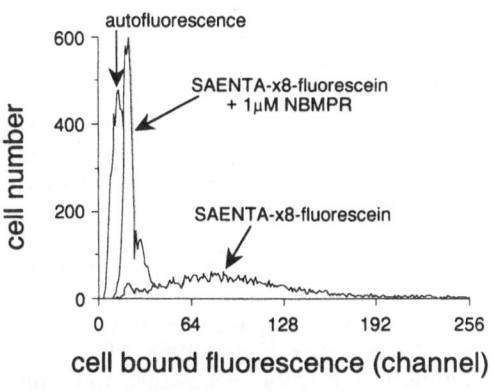

Fig. 1. Structure of SAENTA-x₈-fluorescein

Fig. 2. Fluorescence histograms of SAENTA-x₈-fluorescein binding and its inhibition by nitrobenzyilthioinosine (NBMPR). RC2a leukemic cells were preincubated with or without 1 μM NBMPR for 10 min at room temperature; 50 nM SAENTA-x₈-fluorescein was then added and the cells incubated for a further 15 min. Histograms of cell-bound fluorescence were obtained by flow cytometric analysis of cells. Excitation was at 488 nm and emission was collected between 515 nm and 550 nm. Integrated fluorescent signals generated from individual cells were assigned into 256 channel histograms. The autofluorescence histogram was obtained using untreated cells

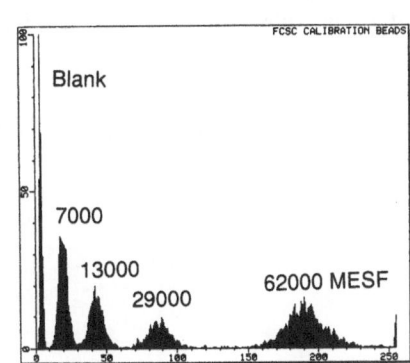

fluorescence (channel)

Fig. 3. Fluorescence histogram of a mixture of standard fluorescent microspheres containing known numbers of molecules of equivalent soluble fluorescein (MESF; Flow Cytometry Standards Corporation). Bead signals were compared to signals from SAENTA-x₈-fluorescein bound to leukemic cells under the same conditions and the same settings of the flow cytometer on each run

ing between the standard beads and the cell surface. By constructing nomograms of SAENTA-x_8-fluorescein binding (in MESF) against [^3H]NBMPR binding sites, the amount of cell-bound ligand (in MESF) can be translated to numbers of nucleoside transporters per cell.

The utility of the SAENTA-fluorescein probes has been assessed in a small clinical study of patients with relapsed or refractory AML given GM-CSF for 72 h before and then for 4 days after starting chemotherapy with araC plus daunorubicin. Bone marrow aspirates were taken at 0 and 72 h of GM-CSF administration and the mononuclear fraction analyzed for [^3H]thymidine labeling index, Ki-67 antigen expression, and density of nucleoside transport sites. The first patient (MZ) was diagnosed as having AML (FAB subtype M4) and failed initial induction therapy with araC plus daunorubicin (7 plus 3 regimen). Cytogenetics showed a monosomy 7, consistent with a myelodysplastic disorder [16] although there was no history of pre-existing cytopenias. The administration of GM-CSF subcutaneously, once daily at 5 µg/kg day produced a marked leukocytosis with total white cell count rising from 4 to 28 × 10^9/l after 72 h although subsequent chemotherapy controlled this rise (Fig. 4). The blast

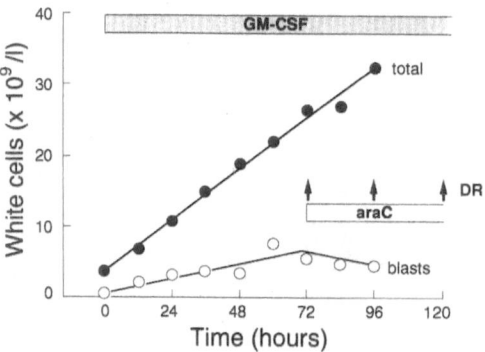

Fig. 4. Peripheral blood white cell counts of a patient with AML (MZ) receiving GM-CSF. Total white cell counts (0) and blast cell counts (0) are shown during the initial 96 h of GM-CSF therapy given s.c. at a dosage of 5 µg/kg day. After 72 h araC was given by continuous i.v. infusion at 100 mg/m^2 day for 7 days together with daunorubicin (DR) at 30 mg/m^2 per day for 3 days

count in the peripheral blood also rose with GM-CSF, as did the polymorphs, band forms, and monocytes. Large "monocytoid" cells appeared for the first time with diameters of 25–35 µm, folded or indented nuclei, 1–3 nucleoli, and faint granulation (Fig. 5). Although these cells appeared morphologically promonocytic, cytochemical staining with chloroacetate esterase positively identified them as giant dysplastic myelocytes and metamyelocytes. The appearance of abnormal giant forms of white cells following granulocyte colony-stimulating factor (G-CSF) therapy has been previously reported in patients recovering from cytotoxic chemotherapy induced neutropenia [17].

The bone marrow aspirates showed an increased percentage of blasts after GM-CSF pretreatment (from 37 % to 50 %) while [^3H]thymidine labeling index of bone marrow mononuclear fraction was likewise increased by the cytokine treatment from 8 % to 15 %. SAENTA-x_8-fluorescein binding to the blast subpopulation rose from 3070 to 6360 sites/cell after 48 h of GM-CSF pretreatment. In this patient only one colour (fluorescein) histograms were obtained on blast cells which were simply defined by their large size and lack of granularity on flow cytometry. This increase in nucleoside transport site expression is compatible with the increasing blast numbers and the rise in [^3H]thymidine labeling index, both of which indicate proliferation.

The second patient in (RV) presented with fever and swollen submandibular glands and was diagnosed as having AML (FAB subtype M4Eo) in 1988. He entered complete remission following araC plus daunorubicin combination chemotherapy and remission was maintained for 22 months. Neutropenia then developed and relapse was confirmed by a bone marrow showing 56 % blasts and 0.6 % eosinophils, including some with abnormal granulation (Table 1). Routine immunophenotyping confirmed that the blasts were CD34$^+$ and Ia$^+$. GM-CSF was administered for 72 h before commencing chemotherapy but the cytokine produced no increase in either the percentage of blasts in bone marrow or in absolute blast count in the peripheral blood

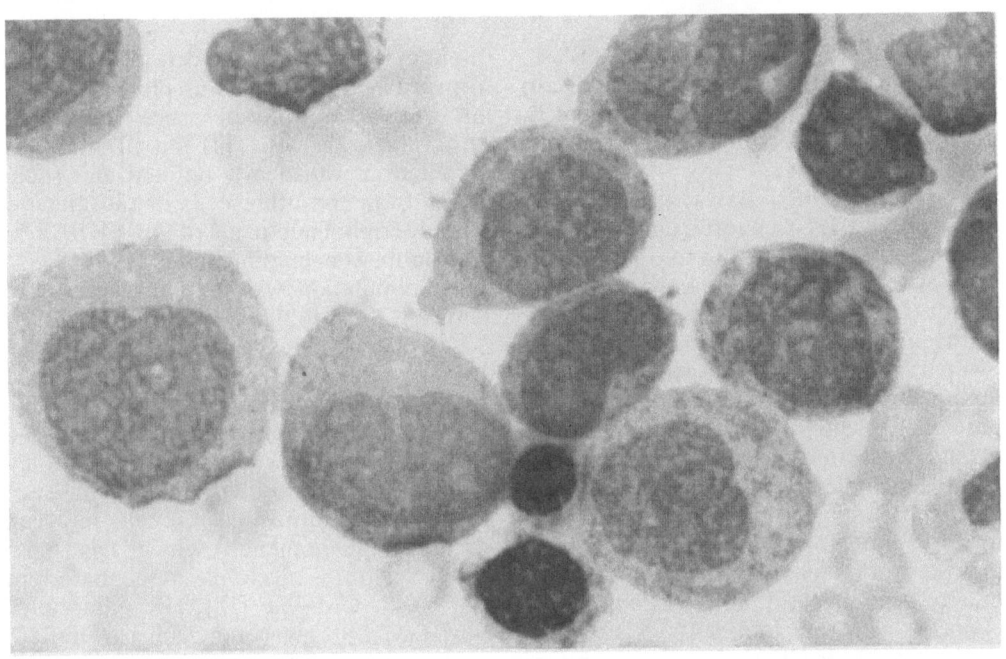

Fig. 5. Large atypical (dysplastic) myelocytes observed in the bone marrow of patient MZ 72 h after commencement of GM-CSF

Table 1. Effect of GM-CSF given in vivo on peripheral blood and bone marrow morphology, proliferation and nucleoside transporter expression on blasts

Duration of GM-CSF administration (5 µg/kg/day s.c.)

	0 h	72 h
PB	2.1	3.1
Total white cells		
PB blasts ($\times 10^9$/l)	0.37	0.34
Bone marrow % blasts	56	57
% eosinophils	0.6	2.8
% monocytes	0.8	0.2
Marrow mononuclears ^{3}H-thymidine LI	9.9	13.0
Ki-67 positive cells	36	46
SAENTA-x_8-fluorescein binding to CD34$^+$ cells (sites/cell)	5800	13 100

LI, labeling index; PB, peripheral blood

(Table 1). The parameters of proliferation in the marrow mononuclear fraction increased after the GM-CSF since [^{3}H]thymidine labeling index rose from 10 % to 13 % while K-67 positive cells also rose from 36 % to 46 % (Table 1). These measurements of proliferative activity, however, were not totally specific for the blast cell compartment since these cells made up only two-thirds of the marrow mononuclear sample. Residual normal myeloid precursors may have participated in the proliferative response to GM-CSF and elevated estimates of the percentage of S-phase cells in the sample. Binding of SAENTA-x_8-fluorescein was then measured specifically to the leukemic blast cell compartment by using one of the features of flow cytometry.

The flow cytometric assay usually measures SAENTA-x_8-fluorescein binding (green fluorescence) on discrete subpopulations of cells defined by forward angle light scatter (size) and side scatter (granularity). With leukemic bone marrow samples, these two parameters are not always sufficient to define the leukemic blast subpopulation, particularly when it comprises under 50 % of the nucleated cells. Flow cytometry allows leukemic blast subpopulations to be positively identified by measurement of a fourth parameter, red fluorescence from phycoerythrin labeled monoclonals against one of the myeloid antigens commonly expressed on myeloblasts, e.g., CD13, CD14, CD33, or CD34. Routine immunophenotyping of leukemic samples can be used to select the most appropriate antibody for this purpose. Figure 6 shows how phycoerythrin-labeled anti-CD34 can be used to define the myeloblast population in bone marrow. The two-dimensional histogram of forward scatter versus side scatter (left and panel, Fig. 6) shows a mixed population comprising blasts, lymphocytes,

monocytes, and nucleated red cells. When forward scatter (size) was plotted against intensity of red fluorescence (phycoerythrin-labeled anti-CD34) the CD34$^+$ blast population was clearly defined and separated from the other cells in the marrow sample (right hand panel of Fig. 6). SAENTA-fluorescein binding to this gated CD34$^+$ blast population was then measured and showed a 2.3-fold increase from 5800 to 13 100 sites/cell as a result of GM-CSF therapy (Table 1). Blast cell size estimated by forward angle light scatter on flow cytometry did not change so that the increase in SAENTA-x_8-fluorescein binding could not be attributed to a size increase but rather to recruitment of G_0 cells into cell cycle, a phenomenon which has been observed with myeloblasts incubated in vitro with GM-CSF [18]. The paradox of how GM-CSF given for 72 h can initiate proliferation in these myeloblasts without raising the percentage of blasts in the bone marrow is difficult to explain. Cell cycle kinetics are extremely sluggish in some patients with AML [19] and it is possible that while GM-CSF may rapidly recruit G_0 cells, in some patients progression through cell cycle to mitosis is far slower. Whatever the explanation, it is evident that SAENTA-fluorescein ligands for the nucleoside

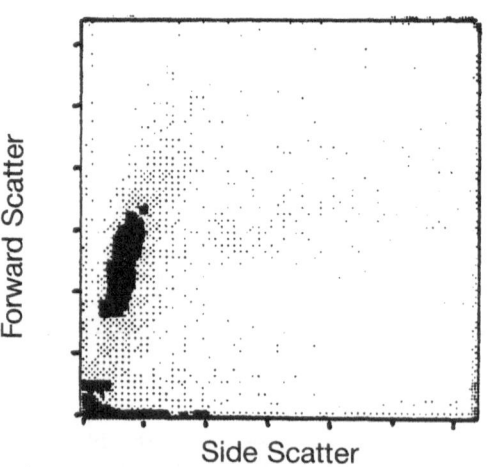 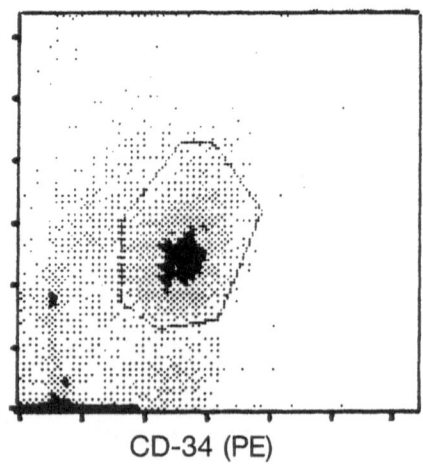

Fig. 6. Two-dimensional flow cytometric histograms of mononuclear cells in the bone marrow of patient RV with AML. The *left hand panel* is a two-dimensional histogram of forward scatter (size) against side scatter (granularity). These two parameters alone were insufficient to identify the blast cell population. The *right hand panel* plots forward scatter (size) against red fluorescence due to binding of phycoerythrin (PE)-labeled anti-CD34. A population of CD34-positive cells can be separated, and SAENTA-x_8-fluorescein binding to this gated population was measured

transporter offer a promising new tool to study the biology of leukemic cells which may help the clinician predict those patients who will be responsive to standard dose araC.

Acknowledgements. We thank Elaine Brigal for typing the manuscript and Dr. George Morstyn for helpful discussions. This work was supported in part by a grant from the Anti-Cancer Council of Victoria. The two patients described were part of a collaborative ongoing trial whose investigators included Dr. G. Begley, Dr. J. Bishop, Dr. J. Cebon, Dr. I. Cooper, Prof. R. Fox, Dr. W. Sheridan, Dr. G. Szer, Prof. M. van der Weyden, and Dr. M. Wolf.

References

1. Bettelheim P, Valent P, Andreeff M, Tafuri A, Haimi J, Gorischek C, Muhm M, Sillaber C, Haas O, Vieder L, Schulz G, Speiser W, Geissler K, Kier P, Hinterberger W, Lechner K (1991) RhGM-CSF in combination with standard induction chemotherapy in de novo acute myeloid leukemia. Blood 77: 700–711
2. Estey E, Kantarjian H, Keating M, Deisserath A, Gutterman J, Plunkett W (1990) Use· of GM-CSF prior to chemotherapy of AML: effects on circulating blast count, thymidine incorporation and ara-CTP formation. Blood 76: 142a
3. Griffin JD, Young D, Herrmann F, Wiper D, Wagner K, Sabbath KD (1986) Effects of recombinant human GM-CSF on proliferation of clonogenic cells in acute myeloblastic leukemia. Blood 67: 1448–1453
4. Asano Y, Shibuya T? Okamura S, Yamaga S, Otsuka T, Niho Y (1987) Effect of human recombinant granulocyte/macrophage colony-stimulating factor and native granulocyte colony-stimulating factor on clonogenic leukemic blast cells. Cancer Res 47: 5647–5648
5. Wiley JS, Taupin J, Jamieson GP, Snook M, Sawyer WH, Finch LR (1985) Cytosine arabinoside transport and metabolism in acute leukemias and T cell lymphoblastic lymphoma. J Clin Invest 75: 632–641
6. Jamieson GP, Snook MB, Bradley TR, Bertoncello I, Wiley JS (1989) Transport and metabolism of l-B-D-arabinofuranosylcytosine in human ovarian adenocarcinoma cells. Cancer Res 49: 309–313
7. Jamieson GP, Finch LR, Snook M, Wiley JS (1987) Degradation of l-B-D-arabinofurano-

8. White JC, Rathmell JP, Capizzi RL (1987) Membrane transport influences the rate of accumulation of cytosine arabinoside in human leukemia cells. J Clin Invest 79: 380–387
9. Smith CL, Pilarski LM, Egerton ML, Wiley JS (1989) Nucleoside transport and proliferative rate in human thymocytes and lymphocytes. Blood 74: 2038–2042
10. Wiley JS, Snook MB, Jamieson GP (1989) Nucleoside transport in acute leukemia and lymphoma: close relation to proliferative rate. Br J Haematol 71: 203–207
11. Wiley JS, Woodruff RK, Jamieson GP, Firkin FC, Sawyer WH (1987) Cytosine arabinoside in the treatment of T-cell acute lymphoblastic leukemia. Aust NZ J Med 17: 379–386
12. Gati WP, Paterson ARP (1989) Nucleoside transport. In: Agre P, Parker JC (eds) Red blood cell membranes. Dekker, New York, pp 635–661
13. Sklar LA (1987) Real-time spectroscopic analysis of ligand-receptor dynamics. Annu Rev Biophys Biophys Chem 16: 479–506
14. Shohami E, Koren R (1979) S-(N-Dansylaminoethyl)-6-mercaptoguanosine as a fluorescent probe for the uridine transport system in human erythrocytes. Biochem J 178: 271–277
15. Wiley JS, Brocklebank AM, Snook MB, Jamieson GP, Sawyer WH, Craik JD, Cass CE, Robins MJ, McAdam DP, Paterson ARP (1991) A new fluorescent probe for the equilibrative inhibitor-sensitive nucleoside transporter. 5-S-(2-Aminoethyl)-N^6-(4-nitrobenzyl)-5′-thioadenosine (SAENTA)-x$_2$-fluorescein. Biochem J 273: 667–672
16. Second MIC cooperative study group (1988) Morphologic, immunologic and cytogenetic (MIC) working classification of the myeloid leukemias. Br J Haematol 68: 487–494
17. Morstyn G, Campbell L, Souza LM, Alton NK, Keech J, Green M, Sheridan W, Metcalf D, Fox R (1988) Effect of granulocyte colony-stimulating factor on neutropenia induced by cytotoxic chemotherapy. Lancet *1*: 667–672
18. Tafuri A, Andreeff M (1990) Kinetic rationale for cytokine-induced recruitment of myeloblastic leukemia followed by cycle-specific chemotherapy in vitro. Leukemia 4: 826–834
19. Raza A, Maheshwari Y, Preisler HD (1987) Differences in cell cycle characteristics amongst patients with acute nonlymphocytic leukemia. Blood 69: 1647–1653

Hematopoietic Growth Factors in Leukemia Therapy

Human Stem Cell Factor: Biological Effects and Receptor Expression on Myeloid Leukemia Cells

T. Pietsch[1], U. Kyas[1], K. Zsebo[2], and K. Welte[1]

Introduction

Recently a novel hematopoietic growth has been identified and characterized that stimulates primitive mouse progenitor cells [13, 15]. This factor, termed stem cell factor (SCF), is a multipotent hematopoietic colony-stimulating factor (CSF) that acts after binding to its specific surface receptor, the protein encoded by the proto-oncogene c-*kit* [14, 12]. The cDNA for human SCF has been cloned, expressed in mammalian cells, and the recombinant factor purified to homogeneity [15, 6]. Whereas SCF for itself has only low capacity to induce colony formation in progenitor assays in vitro (CFU-GM, BFU-E, CFU-GEMM, and CFU-L) on normal bone marrow cells, it has strong synergistic activities with other factors. It synergizes with granulocyte CSF (G-CSF), granulocyte-macrophage CSF (GM-CSF), and interleukin-3 (IL-3) in myelopoiesis [8], with erythropoietin (EPO) in erythropoiesis [8], with IL-6 in megakaryopoiesis, with IL-7 in lymphopoiesis [9], and with IL-3 in mast cell growth [7]. The aim of this study was to investigate the mitogenic potential of SCF alone or in synergy with other factors and the pattern of its receptor expression on myeloid leukemia cells.

Materials and Methods

Cell Lines and Fresh Leukemic Cells

Most human myeloid leukemia cell lines were obtained from ATCC and DSM (Deutsche Sammlung für Mikroorganismen, Braunschweig, FRG). The GM-CSF-dependent cell line GM/SO was kindly provided by Dr. S. Oez, Universitätsklinikum Nürnberg, FRG [10]. The cell line GM-153 was provided by Dr. M. Freund, Medizinische Hochschule Hannover, FRG. The cell lines were cultured in RPMI 1640 (Gibco) with 10 % fetal calf serum (FCS; Gibco, Berlin, FRG) and 1 mM L-glutamine. Fresh leukemic cells were collected from two patients with acute promyelocytic (FAB M1) leukemia. Peripheral blasts (>95 % of leukocytes) were isolated by gradient centrifugation with Ficoll-Hypaque (Pharmacia, Freiburg, FRG) and depleted from aherent cells by plastic adherence for 1 h at 37 ° C. The purity of this preparation was checked by FACS analysis. All cultered cells and cell lines were tested and found free of mycoplasma contamination by DAPI staining and culture methods.

Human Recombinant Factors

Recombinant human SCF rhSCF and rhG-CSF were provided by Amgen, Thousand Oaks, California, USA, rhGM-CSF, rhIL-3, and rhEPO were from Behringwerke, Marburg, FRG, and M-CSF was from Alpha Therapeutics, Japan.

---

[1] Department of Pediatric Hematology and Oncology, Medical School Hannover, FRG
[2] Amgen, Thousand Oaks, California, USA

Antibodies

The monoclonal anti-*kit* antibody YB5.B8 [2] was kindly provided by Dr. L. Ashman, University of Adelaide, South Australia. This antibody was used in a 1:1000 dilution of ascitesfor FACS analysis.

^3H-Thymidine Incorporation Assays

The mitogenic activity of rhSCF alone or in combination with other CSFs (G-CSF, GM-CSF, M-CSF, IL-3, and EPO) was determined in a ^3H-thymidine incorporation assay. Myeloid leukemia cells in exponential growth phase were washed three times with complete medium (RPMI 1640, 10 % FCS, 1 m M L-glutamine) and then plated in a concentration of 5×10^4 cells/ml (cell lines) and 5×10^5 cells/ml (fresh leukemic blasts) in 96 well flatbottom microtiter plates (200 μl/well) containing various concentrations (0-500 ng/ml) of rhSCF alone or in combination with other CSFs. The other factors were used in concentrations known to be saturating (100 units/ml). After a culture period of 68 h at 37 ° C, 5 % CO_2, the cells were exposed to a 4 h pulse of 0.5 μ Ci ^3H-thymidine (25 Ci/mmol; Amersham). Finally, the cells were harvested on glass fiber strips and the incorporated radioactivity measured in a scintillation counter (Packard).

Binding Studies with ^{125}I-rhSCF, ^{125}I-rhG-CSF

rhSCF was radiolabeled by the lactoperoxidase/glucoseoxidase method using enzymobeads (Biorad) following the instructions of the manufacturer. Briefly, 10 μg of rhSCF was labeled by incubation with 1 mCi ^{125}I-Na (Amersham, Braunschweig, FRG) in the presence of enzymobeads to a specific activity of 10 μCi/μg. The rhG-CSF analogue Met-Lys-rhG-CSF (kindly provided by Dr. L. Souza, Amgen, Thousand Oaks, California, USA) was radioactively labeled according to the method described by Bolton and Hunter [4] using iodinated Bolton-Hunter reagent (Amersham). Free iodide was removed by passage through a desalting column (P6-DG; Biorad, Rich-mond, USA), equilibrated with phosphate-buffered solution (PBS), containing 0.02 % Tween 20 (Biorad) and 0.01 % NaN_3. Binding assays were performed on 4×10^6 leukemic blasts in a volume of 500 μl RPMI 1640 with 0.1 % gelatin with various concentrations of ^{125}I-rhSCF ranging between 100 and 30000 pmol/l. The incubation was performed at 37 ° C for 1 h. Identical incubations were also performed in the presence of 2.5 μmol/l unlabeled rhSCF. Aliquots of 125 # μl of the cell suspension were then layered onto silicon oil and centrifuged. The radioactivity in the pellet (bound) and the supernatant (free) was determined separately in a gamma-counter. The specific binding was calculated from the difference between the radioactivity bound in the absence and presence of unlabeled rhSCF. The dissociation constant and the number of binding sites per cell were determined using Scatchard analysis [11]. Fresh leukemic blasts were treated for 20 s with sodium citrate buffer (10 mmol/l, pH 4.0) and subsequently washed with RPMI 1640 prior to the binding assay in order to remove bound nSCF.

Flow Cytometry

Indirect immunofluorescence for staining with the anti-*kit* antibody YB5.B8 [2] was performed as described by Hadam [5] using commercial immunoglobulin (Gammonativ; Kabi, München, FRG) to competitively block Fc receptors and fluorescinated goat immunoglobulin F(ab')$_2$ fragments directed against mouse IgG and IgM (Dianova, Hamburg, Germany) as developing reagent. All incubations were carried out in PBS with 0.1 % bovine serum albumin and 0.02 % NaN_3. Flow cytometry was performed on a FACS 440 cell sorter (Becton-Dickinson, Heidelberg, FRG).

Results

Mitogenic Activity of rhSCF on Myeloid Leukemia Cells

We tested rhSCF on 21 myeloid leukemia cell lines and fresh leukemic blasts from two patients in proliferation assays. A significant proliaferative response to rhSCF was detected in four cell lines (GM-153, acute myeloid leukemia; GM/SO, chronic myeloid leukemia; HEL, erythroleukemia; and MO7$_e$, megakaryoblastic leukemia) and in one of the two fresh leukemias, both of promyelocytic (FAB M1) type (Table 1). Half maximal proliferation in response to rhSCF was found at concentrations of about 10 ng/ml (cell line MO7$_e$). Synergistic activity of rhSCF with other CSFs was detected in all SCF responsive cells. In MO7$_e$ cells, SCF showed synergistic activity with IL-3 and GM-CSF in inducing the proliferation. However, the proliferation of these cells in response to SCF alone was rather high (Table 2). In contrast to MO7$_e$

cells, GM/SO cells proliferated best in response to GM-CSF alone, or after stimulation with a combination of GM-CSF and SCF (Table 3). In these cells, SCF alone has only minor mitogenic activity. Interestingly, a synergistic activity of SCF was also found with EPO. The fresh leukemic blasts (M1, #1) responded only moderately to SCF and other single CSFs. Significant increases of

Table 1. Proliferative response of leukemia cells to stem cell factor (SCF)

Type of leukemia	Cell line	Proliferative response to rhSCF[a]
Acute myeloid	HL-60	–
	KG-1	–
	KG-1a	–
	RC-2A	–
	CTV-1	–
	OCI-AML-1	–
	OCI-AML-1a	–
	OCI-AML-2	–
	OCI-AML-3	–
	GM-153	+
	Fresh M1 (#1)	+
	Fresh M1 (#2)	–
Acute monocytic	THP-1	–
	ML-2	–
Monocytic	U-937	–
Chronic myeloid	GM/SO	+
	GDM-1	–
	TMM	–
Erythro-leukemia	KMOE	–
	K-562	–
	SPI-801	–
	HEL	+
Megakaryo-blastic	MO7$_e$	+

[a] Alone or in combination with G-CSF, GM-CSF, M-CSF, IL-3, or EPO.

Table 2. Proliferation (^3H-thymidine uptake) of MO7$_e$ cells in response to single or combined cytokines

Added factor	Stimulation index	
	Mean	Standard deviation
G-CSF	1.04	0.11
M-CSF	1.07	0.30
EPO	0.87	0.10
GM-CSF	45.07	2.65
IL-3	55.10	2.07
GM-CSF + IL-3	116.04	7.37
SCF	235.87	15.25
SCF + GM-CSF	251.25	10.94
SCF + IL-3	253.99	16.82
SCF + GM-CSF + IL-3	260.94	34.37

^3H-thymidine uptake in the absence of growth factors (spontaneous proliferation) was 288 ± 47 cpm.

Table 3. Proliferation (^3H-thymidine uptake) of chronic myeloid GM/SO cells

Added Factor	Stimulation Index	
	Mean	Standard deviation
G-CSF	1.24	0.29
M-CSF	1.12	0.12
EPO	4.97	0.88
GM-CSF	42.90	2.94
IL-3	1.80	0.13
SCF	7.72	0.83
SCF + GM-CSF	49.78	1.07
SCF + IL-3	8.07	0.23
SCF + EPO	13.14	0.25
SCF + GM-CSF + IL-3	56.27	7.43

[3] H-thymidine uptake in the absence of growth factors (spontaneous proliferation) was 3545 ± 906 cpm.

proliferation were found when SCF was combined with G-CSF, GM-CSF or IL-3 (Table 4). The strongest proliferative effect was seen with a combination of SCF, GM-CSF, IL-3, and G-CSF with stimulation indices up to 53.

Receptor Expression on Myeloid Leukemic Cells

The number of SCF binding sites on myeloid leukemia cells were determined using ^{125}I-radiolabeled rhSCF and subsequent Scatchard analysis. The number of binding sites for SCF on responding cells ranged between 2000 and 33 150 binding sites per cell (Table 5). The nonresponding line K-562 was used as control. In this cell line we were not able to detect binding sites for SCF. The cell lines with detectable binding sites also stained with the anti-kit oncoprotein antibody YB5.B8 (Table 5). The expression of SCF binding sites depended on the presence of cytokines in the culturue medium prior to the binding assay. MO7$_e$ cells demonstrated 33 150 binding sites when cultured with rhGM-CSF (100 U/ml for 3 days), but only 2000 when cultured in medium containing SCF (100 ng/ml).

Discussion

We were able to define a subset of myeloid leukemia cell lines and fresh leukemic blasts that have receptors for SCF and respond to this factor with proliferation. The ability to grow after stimulation with SCF seemed not to correlate with a distinct

Table 4. Proliferation (^3H-thymidine uptake) of fresh promyelocytic leukemia cells (#1)

Added Factor	Stimulation index	
	Mean	Standard deviation
G-CSF	3.64	1.42
M-CSF	2.26	0.35
GM-CSF	2.42	0.32
IL-3	9.51	1.17
GM-CSF + IL-3	6.91	0.23
SCF	12.51	1.00
SCF + GM-CSF	15.74	1.22
SCF + IL-3	25.57	2.05
SCF + GM-CSF + Il-3	27.37	0.95
SCF + G-CSF + GM-CSF + IL-3	53.51	2.65

^3H-thymidine uptake in the absence of growth factors (spontaneous proliferation) was 162 $\pm$ 74 cpm.

morphological type of myeloid leukemic cells. The responding cell lines had different FAB types. To exclude the possibility that myeloid leukemia cells are selected for responsiveness to SCF during long-term culture we have also tested freshly isolated blasts. One of the two blast preparations responded to SCF. The mitogenic activity of SCF on leukemic blasts seems to be important for the clinical behavior of myeloid leukemia cells in vivo. The expression of the antigen detected by the monoclonal antibody YB5.B8, which later turned out to be the SCF receptor, on myeloid leukemia cells defined a subset of acute nonlymphoblastic leukemia with poor prognosis [3]. Interestingly, in most leukemia cells, but not in the MO7$_e$ cell line, the response to SCF alone

Table 5. Stem cell factor binding sites on leukemia cells (Scatchard analysis)

Cell Line	Type	SCF binding sites per cell	Proliferative response to SCF	Staining with YB5.B8
K-562	Erythroleukemia	0	–	–
HEL	Erythroleukemia	3600	+	+
GM/SO	Chronic myeloid	29000	+	+
MO7$_e$	Megakaryoblastic			
(Cultured in rhSCF)		2000	+	+
(Cultured in rh GM-CSF)		33150	+	+

was rather moderate. This reflects the situation in normal bone marrow, where approximately 2 % of the mononucleated cells have SCF receptors [2]: the effects of SCF on normal bone marrow progenitor cells expressing receptors for SCF are barely detectable in progenitor cell assays like CFU-GM, BFU-E, or CFU-GEMM, if the factor is used alone. After combination of this factor with a lineage-restricted factor like EPO, GM-CSF, IL-3, or G-CSF synergistic effects are seen in respect to an increase of the number and size of colonies without a change in their cellular composition [8]. Hypotheses about the mechanisms of SCF action include that SCF helps quiescent normal stem cells to enter the cell cycle, and induce or increase the expression of specific receptors fo the other lineage-specific CSFs on the surface of the progenitor cell surface. We have evidence that this is also the case in the malignant counterpart of myelopoiesis, the myeloid leukemias. Preliminary studies on fresh promyelocytic blasts previously shown to express both G-CSF and SCF receptors showed an upregulation of G-CSF receptors when cultured for 24 h in the presence of 100 ng/ml SCF. Binding assays using ^{125}I-radiolabeled rhG-CSF showed an increase from 3000 to 4600 G-CSF binding sites. We have also evidence that the expression of SCF receptors is regulated by CSFs, because the receptor numbers for SCF vary depending on the presence of specific CSFs, as shown on the MO7$_e$ line (Table 5). When cultured in GM-CSF-containing medium, the cells expressed 33 150 receptors, with SCF only 2000. This corresponds to a higher proliferative response to SCF in cells cultured with GM-CSF (data not shown). The growth-promoting activity of SCF on leukemic blasts was most potent, when SCF factor was combined with one or more CSFs. This effect can also be explained by an upregulation of the specific receptors, so that the leukemic cells become more responsive to the corresponding factors. Because the expression of SCF receptors on myeloid leukemia cells defines a subset with poor prognosis, it is likely that this is due to the action of SCF. A role of SCF in lymphoblastic leukemia has also to be considered because SCF is known to synergize with IL-7 on normal lymphoblastic progenitor cells [9]. Agents like antibodies or soluble receptors may be able to block these actions and may be future therapeutic tools. On the other hand, SCF may be also a potent synchronizing agent to bring quiescent leukemic cells into cycle and increase the susceptibility of leukemic cells to chemotherapeutic agents [1]. Further studies are necessary to evaluate the potential clinical use of this factor or its antagonists.

Summary

A novel hematopoietic growth factor, the stem cell factor (SCF), for primitive hematopoietic progenitor cells has recently been purified and its gene has been cloned. In this study we tested the mitogenic activity of recombinant human (rh) SCF on myeloid leukemia cells as well as the expression of its receptor. We have investigated the proliferation of 21 myeloid leukemia cell lines as well as fresh myeloid leukemic blasts from two patients in a 72 h ^3H-thymidine uptake assay in the presence of various concentrations of rhSCF alone or in combination with saturating concentrations of G-CSF, GM-CSF, M-CSF, IL-3, or erythropoetin. Four out of 21 lines significantly responded to SCF, as well as leukemic cells from one patient with acute myeloid leukemia (FAB M1). The responding cell lines were of acute promyelocytic, chronic myeloid, megakaryoblastic and erythroleukemia origin. Synergistic activities of SCF were found with G-CSF, GM-CSF, erythropoetin, and IL-3. To determine the SCF binding sites on leukemic cells, we used ^{125}I-radiolabeled SCF in Scatchard analysis. The leukemic cells responding to SCF expressed between 2000 and 33 000 binding sites per cell. The SCF receptor expression is regulated by the presence or absence of hematopoietic growth factors. This study suggests that SCF may be an important factor for the growth of a subset of myeloid leukemia cells, either as a direct stimulus or as a synergistic factor for other cytokines.

Acknowledgements. We are indepted to A. Ohrdorf and P. Beenken for excellent technical assistance.

References

1. Andreeff M, Welte K (1989) Hematopoietic colony-stimulating factors. Semin Oncol 16: 211–229

2. Ashman LK, Cambereri AC, Cole SR, Gadd SJ (1989) Functional studies on a 150-kDA cell-surface antigen expressed by haemopoietic progenitor cells, mast cells and some AML cells, using mAb YB5.B8. In: Knapp W (ed) Leucocyte typing IV. Oxford University Press, pp 943–945

3. Ashman LK, Roberts MM, Gadd SJ. Cooper SJ, Juttner CA (1988) Expression of a 150kDa cell surface antigen identified with monoclonal antibody YB5.B8 is associated with poor prognosis in acute non-lymphoblastic leukemia. Leuk Res 12: 923–928

4. Bolton AE, Hunter WM (1973) The labelling of proteins to specific radioactivity by conjugates to a ^{125}I-containing acylating reagent. Biochem J 133: 529–539

5. Hadam MR (1985) Flow cytometry and surface marker phenotyping using monoclonal antibodies: a combined approach to precisely define the state of the immune system. In: Gillisen G, Theurer KE (eds) New aspects in physiological antitumor substances. Karger, Basel, pp 120–146

6. Martin F, Suggs S, Lu H, Langley K. Johnson M, Okino K, Morris C, McNiece I, Jacobson F, Johnson M, Parker V, Flores J, Patel A, Birkett N, Smith K, Fisher E, Erjavec H, Herrera C, Mendiaz E, Wypych J, Sachdev R, Pope JA, Zsebo K (1990) Primary structure and functional expression of rat and human stem cell factor DNAs. Cell 63: 203–211

7. Medlock E, Yung Y, McNiece I, Langley K, Mineo Daley C, Dubbell C, Mendiaz B, Sachdev R, Smith K, Zsebo K (1990) Role of stem cell factor (SCF) in the stimulation of the mast cell lineage. Blood 76 (Suppl 1): 155

8. McNiece IK, Langley KE, Zsebo MK (1991) Recombinant human stem cell factor synergizes with GM-CSF, G-CSF, IL-3 and Epo to stimulate human progenitor cells of the myeloid and erythroid lineages. Exp Hematol 19: 226–231

9. McNiece IK, Langley KE, Zsebo MK (to be published) The role of stem cell factor in B-cell differentiation: synergistic interactions with IL-7. J Immunol

10. Oez S, Tittelbach H, Fahsold R, Schaetzl R, Bührer C, Azpodien J, Kalden JR (1990) Establishment and characterization of a granulocyte-macrophage colony-stimulating factor-dependent human myeloid cell line. Blood 76: 578–582

11. Scatchard G (1949) The attraction of proteins for small molecules and ions. Ann NY Acad Sci 51: 660–672

12. Yarden Y, Kuang W-J, Yang-Feng T, Coussens L, Munemitsu S, Dull TJ, Chen E, Schlessinger J, Francke U, Ullrich A (1987) Human protooncogene c-kit: a new cell surface receptor tyrosine kinase for an unidentified ligand. EMBO J 6: 3341–3351

13. Zsebo K, Martin F, Suggs S, Wypych J, Lu H, McNiece I, Medlock E, Morris F, Sachdev R, Tung W, Birkett N, Smith K, Yuschenkoff V, Mendiaz E, Jacobson F, Langley K (1990) Biological characterization of a unique early acting hematopoietic growth factor. Exp Hematol 18(6): 703

14. Zsebo K, Williams D, Geissler E, Broudy V, Martin F, Atkins H, Hsu R-Y, Birkett N, Okino K, Murdock D, Jacobson F, Langley K, Smith K, Takeishi T, Cattanach B, Galli S, Suggs S (1990) Stem cell factor (SCF) is encoded at the *Sl* locus of the mouse and is the ligand for the c-*kit* tyrosine kinase receptor. Cell 63: 213–224

15. Zsebo K, Wypych J, MyNiece I, Lu H, Smith K, Karkare S, Sachdev R, Yuschenkoff V, Birkett N, Williams L, Satyagal V, Tung W, Bosselman B, Mendiaz E, Langley K (1990) Identification, purification, and biological characterization of hematopoietic stemm cell factor from buffalo rat liver conditioned medium. Cell 63: 195–201

Recombinant Human Granulocyte-Macrophage Colony-Stimulating Factor Following Chemotherapy in Patients with High-Risk AML

T. Büchner[1], W. Hiddemann[1], M. Koenigsmann[1], M. Zühlsdorf[1], B. Wörmann[1], A. Boeckmann[1], E. Aguion Freire[1], G. Innig[1], G. Maschmeyer[2], W.-D. Ludwig[3], M.-C. Sauerland[4], A. Heinecke[4], and G. Schulz[5]

Introduction

Despite great efforts in supportive care for patients with acute myeloid leukemia (AML), early death during the phase of induction treatment still remains an unsolved therapeutic problem. Multicenter trials [1–6] show early deaths in 17 %–32 % of patients at all ages and 27 %–52 % in those 60 years of age and older. In addition, intensive chemotherapy for relapsed and refractory AML produced up to 56 % complete remissions (CR) but also 29 % early deaths [7, 8] or probably more [9]. After postinduction intensification chemotherapy 5 %–20 % of patients died from toxicity [6]. Infections due to neutropenia were responsible for most of the early deaths during induction therapy [1–4] and represent the major dose-limiting toxicity. Thus, reducing the phase of critical neutropenia would allow more effective antileukemic chemotherapy.

Before this first study [10, 11] recombinant human granulocyte-macrophage colony-stimulating factor (GM-CSF) was not applied in AML. Under various other conditions GM-CSF has been proven to effectively stimulate granulopoiesis. In primates a dramatic rise of neutrophils was induced [12, 13] which similarly occurred in an animal with virus-induced pancytopenia [12]. After irradiation [14] or combined irradiation, cytostatic treatment, and autologous bone marrow transplantation [15, 16] the recovery of neutrophils was accelerated by GM-CSF. Given to humans, GM-CSF induced an increase of neutrophils in patients with AIDS [17] and in patients with aplastic anemia [18, 19]. The phase of therapy-induced critical neutropenia could be reduced after chemotherapy for sarcomas [20] and after chemotherapy followed by autologous bone marrow transplantation for breast cancers and malignant melanomas [21]. As preleukemic disorders, myelodysplastic syndromes have been treated now with GM-CSF [22–25] and showed an effective increase of neutrophil counts.

When considering GM-CSF as a part of treatment for AML its potential stimulatory effect on leukemic blasts has to be taken into account. In vitro leukemic blast growth in both colony assays and suspension cultures was stimulated in the presence of GM-CSF [26–32] in up to 97 % [28] of AMLs. In myelodysplastic syndromes some patients receiving GM-CSF responded with an increase of blasts and even a transformation into AML [23–25]. Thus, GM-CSF in AML was restricted in this first step to patients at high risk of early death due to early or multiple relapse or higher age. The clinical and hematological responses were evaluated in comparison with control groups not receiving GM-CSF and treated in phase II and III chemotherapy studies at the same institutions.

[1] Departments of Hematology/Oncology, University of Münster, [2] Evangelisches Krankenhaus Essen-Werden, FRG
[3] Free University Hospital, Steglitz, West Berlin, FRG
[4] Department of Biostatistics, University of Münster and [5] Behringwerke, AG Marburg, FRG

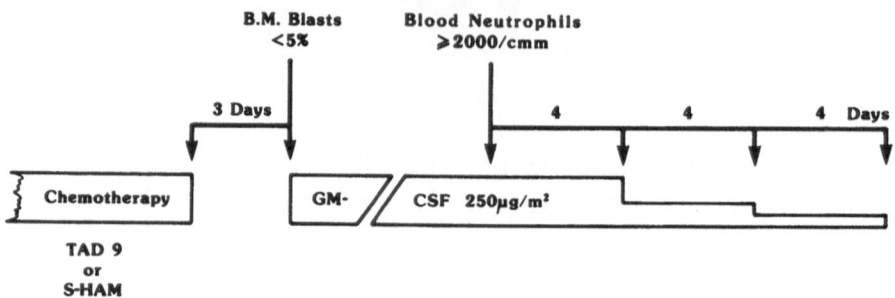

Fig. 1. Study design

Patients and Methods

Patients

The criteria for entering the GM-CSF study included (a) adult patients at all ages with early relapse occurring in the first 6 months of remission and with multiple relapse, and (b) patients 65 years of age and older with newly diagnosed AML or late relapse. Patients having had bone marrow transplantation before they relapsed and secondary leukemias were included in the GM-CSF study. A written informed consent was obtained from each patient. All investigations were performed after approval by the local ethical committee and in accordance with the Declaration of Helsinki. The historical control groups were treated at the same institutions and received the same chemotherapy.

Study Design

If the bone marrow 3 days after the end of chemotherapy was aplastic with less than 5 % blasts, GM-CSF 250 μg/m^2/day continuous i.v. infusion started on day 4. When a neutrophil count of 2000/mm^3 was achieved and maintained for 4 days the dose was reduced to 125 μg/m^2 for 4 days and to 50 μg/m^2 for another 4 days until the infusion was discontinued (Fig. 1).

Recombinant Human GM-CSF

Recombinant human GM-CSF was provided by Behringwerke AG Marburg, West

Germany. The recombinant protein was expressed in yeast and purified by Immunex Corporation (Seattle, WA, USA), as described by Cantrell et al. [33]. Sterility, general safety, and purity studies met Food and Drug Administration standards.

Chemotherapy

Early or multiple relapses were treated with sequential high-dose cytosine arabinoside (ara-C) and mitoxantrone (S-HAM) [34] combining high-dose ara-C randomly either 1 g/m^2 or 3 g/m^2 q 12 h by 3 h i.v. infusion on days 1, 2, 8, and 9, and mitoxantrone, 10 mg/m^2/day i.v. infusion on days 3, 4, 10, and 11. Only one course of S-HAM was given to each patient. Newly diagnosed AML and AML late relapses in the higher age group were treated with 9-day 6-thioguanine, ara-C and daunorubicin (TAD9) [4], containing 6-thioguanine, 100 mg/m^2 q 12 h orally on days 3–9; araC, both 100 mg/m^2/day continuous i.v. infusion on days 1 and 2 and q 12 h i.v. infusion over 30 min on days 3–8 and daunorubicin randomly either 30 or 60 mg/m^2/day i.v. injection on days 3–5. Patients with inadequate blast clearance received a second course of TAD9. After attaining CR, patients received one additional course of TAD9 for consolidation and monthly maintenance by 5-day courses of ara-C combined in rotation with daunorubicin or 6-thioguanine or cyclophosphamide for 3 years, as previously described [4]. No postremission chemotherapy was given to patients achieving CR after relapse.

Definitions of Outcome

CR was defined by a normocellular hematopoietic marrow with less than 5% leukemic cells and a peripheral blood with at least 1500 neutrophils/mm³ and 100 000 platelets/mm³. Remission duration was from achievement of CR until relapse. Adverse events were graded according to Eastern Cooperative Oncology Group (ECOG) criteria [35].

Laboratory Tests

Complete blood counts including white and red cell, reticulocyte, platelet and differential counts were done daily. Bone marrow aspirates and biopsies were obtained before and after chemotherapy and after GM-CSF when CR criteria in blood counts were achieved, or in case of persistent cytopenia. Bone marrow microscopy included quantification of cellularity, percentage of blasts and normal hematopoietic cells, and classification of leukemic cells according to FAB criteria [36]. DNA histograms from bone marrow cells were obtained by flow cytometry as previously described [37, 38]. DNA aneuploidy was defined by a clonal deviation of at least 5% of the cellular DNA content from admixed normal blood reference cells [39]. Colony forming progenitor cells in the bone marrow growing on methylcellulose were monitored using methods described by Rowley et al. [40]. Bone marrow aspirates were separated on Ficoll gradients and interphase cells were washed in Iscove's modified Dulbecco's medium (IMDM). Quadruplicate samples of 50 000 cells were seeded into 1.3% methylcellulose in IMDM, 30% fetal bovine serum, 50 μM beta-mercaptoethanol, 2 μM L-glutamine, 100 milliunits/ml penicillin and 100 µg/ml streptomycin. Parallel samples were grown with or without 100 units/ml GM-CSF (Behring) or with 5% phytohemagglutinin leukocyte-conditioned medium. After 14 days at 37 °C in a water-saturated atmosphere with 5% CO_2, colonies were scored under an inverted microscope (× 40). For verification of their morphology single colonies were picked from the plates, cytospun onto slides and Pappenheim stained. Leukemic colonies were identified morphologically and by their ability to grow in secondary plates.

Results

Therapeutic Response

Between September 1987 and December 1989, thirty six consecutive patients entered the GM-CSF study. Of these, 30 received GM-CSF and are listed in Table 1. GM-CSF was infused over a median of 18 (range 10–48) days. Of the patients receiving GM-CSF, 18 (60%) attained CR, three (10%) died in the first 6 weeks, seven (23%) died later in bone marrow hypoplasia with no blasts, and two patients (7%), in whom AML persisted, were classified as definite nonresponders. One of the nonresponders (patient 3) showed a 30% reinfiltration of his bone marrow 4 weeks after cessation of GM-CSF. The other nonresponder (patient 15) developed a marked leukemic regrowth under GM-CSF (as described later). Six patients remained untreated by GM-CSF due to persistent bone marrow blasts after two induction courses (two patients) or after one course (four patients) with contraindications against further chemotherapy. All six of these patients had newly diagnosed AML and were included in the calculation of response data in comparison with the controls. The control groups comprised 56 sequential patients treated by the identical chemotherapy at the same situations between 1985 and 1987 as parts of phase II and III studies of the AML Cooperative Group [4, 34]. Patient characteristics in the GM-CSF and control groups are compared in Table 2. Table 3 shows the response data for the whole GM-CSF group in comparison with the control group.

Adverse Events and Toxicity

After chemotherapy all patients in the GM-CSF and control groups exhibited grade 4 neutropenia and thrombocytopenia according to ECOG toxicity criteria [35]. Nonhematological adverse events are listed in Tables 4 and 5.

The overall frequency of weight gain not specified for different grades was higher in patients with GM-CSF than in the controls ($p = 0.007$) while edema, effusions, and higher grade weight gain did not differ significantly. The GM-CSF group showed a higher overall frequency including all grades of decrease in serum protein ($p = 0.023$), prothrombin ($p = 0.016$) and pseudocholinesterase levels ($p = 0.008$) with no significant difference in higher grade deficiencies in the three parameters. In the controls, elevation of serum transaminases was more frequent overall ($p = 0.0001$) and in lower grade elevations. Controls showed more frequent cardiac events ($p = 0.018$),

not significant within the different grades. There were more severe neurocortical events due to cerebral hemorrhage in the control groups. Infections overall were more frequent in patients after S-HAM chemotherapy in the control group ($p = 0.05$). There were no other differences in adverse events between TAD9 and S-HAM chemotherapy.

Hematologic Response

The recovery time to achieve 500 blood neutrophils/mm^3 and 20 000 platelets/mm^3 from start of GM-CSF is given in Table 6.

Table 1. Patient characteristics and therapeutic outcome

Patient	Age	Diagnosis		Special History	Outcome
1	65	AML (M1)	1st relapse		ED
2	44	AML (M4)	1st relapse		ED
3	61	AML (M2)	1st relapse	Tumor chemotherapy	AML regrowth, NR
4	54	AML (M5)	1st relapse		CR
5	75	AML (M2)	1st relapse		CR
6	64	AML (M2)	1st relapse		CR
7	61	AML (M4)	2nd relapse		CR
8	34	AML (M2)	2nd relapse	Auto BMT	CR
9	35	AML (M5)	2nd relapse	Allo BMT	NR (hypoplasia)
10	27	AML (M1)	2nd relapse	Auto BMT	ED
11	77	AML (M2)	1st relapse		CR
12	65	AML (M5)	De novo		ED
13	77	AML (M2)	De novo		CR
14	75	AML (M2)	De novo		CR
15	70	AML (M1)	De novo		AML regrowth, NR
16	84	AML (M6)	De novo		CR
17	75	AML (M3)	De novo		CR
18	66	AML (M2)	De novo		NR (hypoplasia)
19	83	AML (M2)	De novo		NR (hypoplasia)
20	68	AML (M1)	De novo		NR (hypoplasia)
21	72	AML (M4)	De novo		CR
22	69	AML (M5)	De novo		CR
23	68	AML (M1)	De novo		CR
24	65	AML (M4)	Secondary	Tumor chemotherapy	NR (hypoplasia)
25	78	AML (M5)	Secondary	MDS	AML regrowth, CR
26	75	AML (M5)	Secondary	MDS	ED
27	67	AML (M1)	De novo		CR
28	67	AML (M2)	De novo		CR
29	69	AML (M5)	De novo		CR
30	73	AML (M1)	De novo		NR (hypoplasia)

auto, autologous; allo, allogeneic; BMT, bone marrow transplant; ED, early death; MDS, myelodysplastic syndrome; NR, nonresponder; CR, complete remission

Table 2. Patient characteristics

	GM-CSF group	Controls	p^b
No. of patients	36[a]	56	
Age, median (range)	68 (27–84)	68 (19–80)	
FAB subtype			
M1	7 (19%)	10 (18%)	
M2	10 (28%)	19 (34%)	
M3	1 (3%)	1 (2%)	
M4	4 (11%)	10 (18%)	
M5	10 (28%)	10 (18%)	
M6	1 (3%)	3 (5%)	
M7	1 (3%)	0	
Hybrid AML/ALL	2 (5%)	1 (2%)	
Unknown	0	1 (2%)	
Newly diagnosed AML, age 65+	25	41	
Age, median (range)	70 (65–84)	70 (65–80)	
Prior tumor chemotherapy/radiotherapy	1	1	
AML after preleukemia	2	3	
Relapsed AML	11	15	
Age, median (range)	61 (27–77)	46 (19–65)	
Early 1st relapse (within 6 months)	6	2	0.038
Late 1st relapse	1	6	
2nd relapse	4	7	
Prior tumor chemotherapy/radiotherapy	1	1	
Prior BMT	3	0	
AML after preleukemia	0	3	
Hybrid AML/ALL	2	1	

[a] Including six patients not receiving GM-CSF with persistence of blasts in bone marrow after chemotherapy
[b] Fisher exact test
BMT, bone marrow transplant

Table 3. Therapeutic response to induction

No. of patients	GM-CSF group		Controls		p^b
	36[a]	(%)	56	(%)	
Complete remissions	18/36	(50)	18/56	(32)	0.09
In newly diagnosed AML	11/25	(44)	12/41	(29)	
In relapsed AML	7/11	(64)	6/15	(40)	
Early deaths (within 6 weeks)	5/36	(14)	22/56	(39)	0.009
In newly diagnosed AML	3/25	(12)	18/41	(44)	0.007
In relapsed AML	2/11	(18)	4/15	(27)	
Later hypoplastic deaths	7/36	(19)	7/56	(13)	
In newly diagnosed AML	6/25	(24)	6/41	(15)	
In relapsed AML	1/11	(9)	1/15	(7)	
Definite nonresponse	6/36	(17)	9/56	(16)	
In newly diagnosed AML	5/25	(20)	5/41	(12)	
In relapsed AML	1/11	(9)	4/15	(26)	

[a] Including six patients not receiving GM-CSF due to persistence of blasts in bone marrow after chemotherapy
[b] Chi-squared test

Table 4. Nonhematological adverse events exhibited by all patients in the GM-CSF and control groups following chemotherapy in high-risk AML. All grades (ECOG or accordingly)

	GM-CSF (%)	Controls (%)	p
Fever	100	98	
Documented infections	72	84	
Effusions	29	25	
Edema	16	13	
Weight gain	35	9	0.007
Cardiac	21	49	0.018
Serum-bilirubin elevation	48	65	
GOT/GPT elevation	24	77	0.0001
PCHE decrease	64	27	0.008
Protein decrease	92	68	0.023
Prothrombin time prolongation	88	60	0.016
Neurocortical	21	26	

GOT, aspartate aminotransferase; GPT, glutamine pyruvic transaminase; PCHE, pseudocholinesterase

Table 5. Nonhematological adverse events exhibited by all patients in the GM-CSG and control groups following chemotherapy in high-risk AML. Higher grades (ECOG or accordingly)

Grade		GM-CSF (%)	Controls (%)	p
Fever	3–4	28	38	
Weight gain	2–3	12	2	
Cardiac	4–5	14	21	
Serum-bilirubin elevation	3–4	40	40	
GOT/GPT elevation	3–4	4	10	
PCHE decrease	<750 U/l	16	4	
Protein decrease	<4.0 g/dl	8	2	
Prothrombin time prolongation	4	4	2	
Neurocortical	4	0	16	0.025

GOT, aspartate aminotransferase; GTP, glutamine pyruvine transaminase; PCHE, pseudocholinesterase; U, units

Neutrophil recovery time after GM-CSF is compared to that in the control group in Figs. 2 and 3 for the two chemotherapeutic regimens used. The medians are 10 vs 16 days ($p = 0.009$) after TAD9 and 15 vs 24 days ($p = 0.043$) after S-HAM. Median recovery time of platelets to 20 000/mm^3 after TAD9 was 15 days in the GM-CSF group and 11 days in the controls ($p = 0.28$). After S-HAM corresponding medians were 16 vs 20 days ($p = 0.64$). Platelet recovery time to 50 000 equally failed to show a significant effect of GM-CSF after TAD9 ($p = 0.75$) or S-HAM ($p = 0.55$). There was no difference in neutrophil or platelet recovery time according to the two different randomized doses of daunorubicin and ara-C. Table 6 also shows increases in blood eosinophils, monocytes and lymphocytes under GM-CSF. All multilineage responses were found to be rapidly reversible.

Response of Infections

After recovery of neutrophils under GM-CSF to at least 500 mm^3 temperature returned to normal within 2 days in 41 % of patients and within 7 days in 73 % of patients. Other signs of infections responded in two-thirds of the patients and

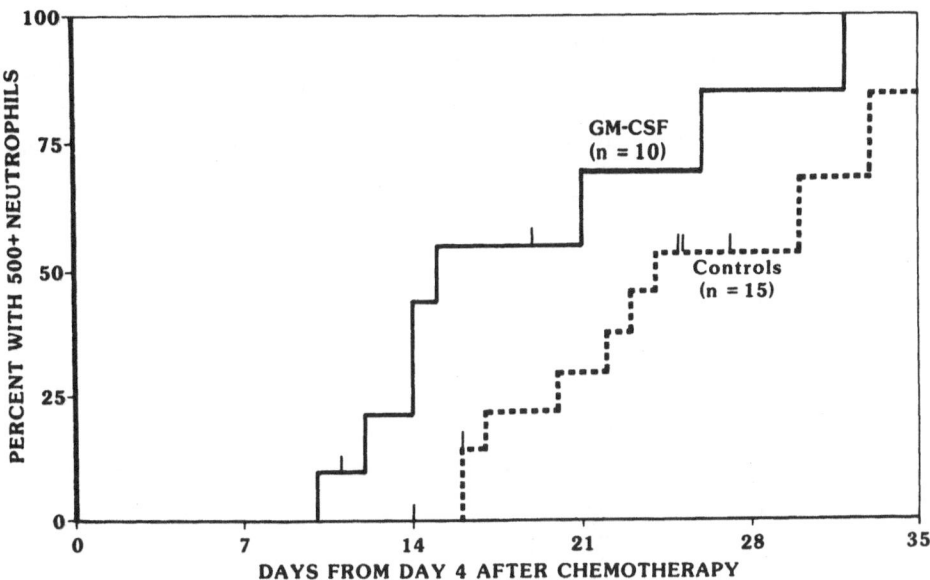

Fig. 2. Kaplan Meier test of blood neutrophil recovery time in patients receiving TAD9 chemotherapy (log-rank test, $p = 0.009$). *Thick marks* represent patients without neutrophil recovery at their last possible update

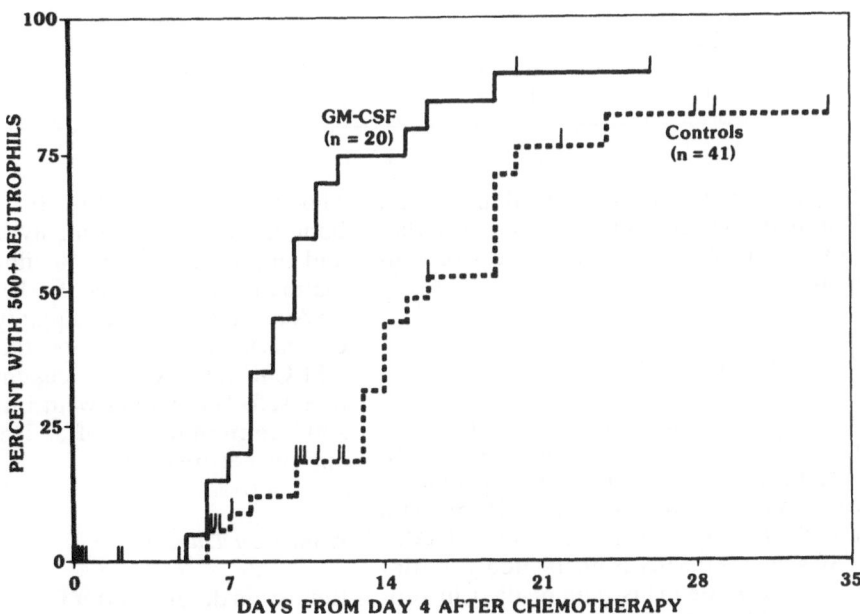

Fig. 3. Neutrophil recovery time in patients receiving S-HAM chemotherapy ($p = 0.043$). (See also Fig. 1)

Table 6. Response to GM-CSF in peripheral blood cells counts

Patient	Days from GM-CSF start to 500 neutrophils/mm³	Days from GM-CSF start to 20000 platelets/mm³	Response of other white blood cells (maximum counts/mm³)		
			Eosinophils	Monocytes	Lymphocytes
1	14	13			
2	21	29+			
3	14	2	1450		
4	11+	13+			
5	15	27			
6	12	16			
7	10	0	2725		
8	32	13			
9	26	90+			
10	19+	19+			
11	6		1600	2838	
12	5+	5+			
13	8	0			
14	7	5			
15	11	0		5694	
16	10	5			
17	9	51	1200	2682	3843
18	6	14+			
19	20+	20+			
20	26+	26+			
21	12	0		2544	
22	15	7		3315	
23	10	20	2065		
24	19	70	1176		
25	10	15			
26	11	13+			
27	8	8		4320	
28	16	17			
29	8	0		8160	
30	9	21+			

persisted longer in some fungal infections. This pattern of response was similar to that in the control group after recovery of neutrophils.

Leukemic Regrowth

Two patients under GM-CSF showed a marked regrowth of their blood blasts. In patient 15 this was associated with monocytosis. As shown in Fig. 4, monocytosis was rapidly reversible after cessation of GM-CSF whereas the blasts uneffectedly continued to increase. This patient died in progression of her AML. In patient 25 suffering from an AML M5 there was an increase of blood monocytes and promonocytes up to 11 600/mm³ under GM-CSF (Fig. 5). The bone marrow became highly hypercellular and infiltrated by 95% immature and mature monocytic cells. Pretherapeutically, no Auer rods, DNA aneuploidy or cytogenetic markers were present in this case. After GM-CSF cessation the leukemic regrowth reversed. The patient went into CR and is still free from relapse after 2 years without any further treatment.

Remission Duration

Remission duration after GM-CSF is shown in Figs. 6 and 7 and compared to that in the controls. Remission duration after GM-CSF in the patients treated for relapse

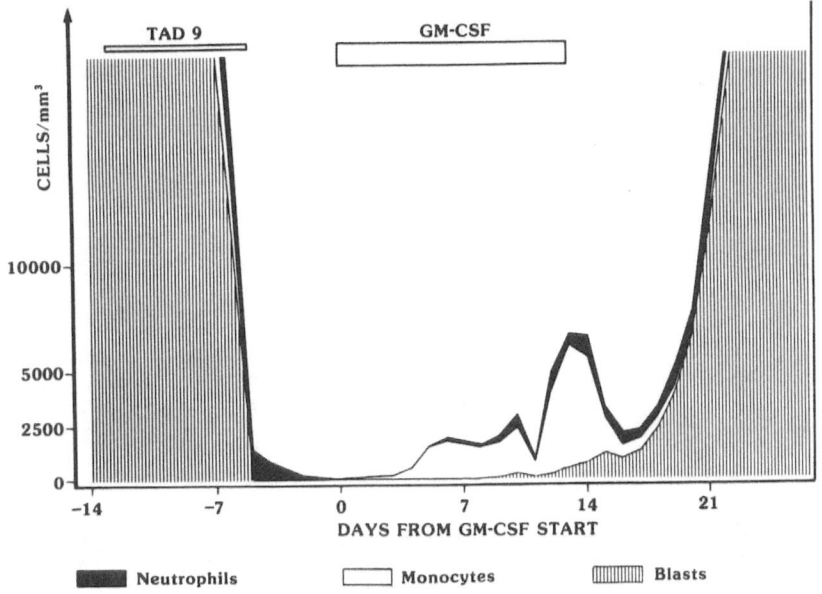

Fig. 4. Absolute counts of different white blood cells in patient 15 with AML M1 during TAD9 chemotherapy followed by GM-CSF. After cessation of GM-CSF, monocytosis is reversible while regrowth of leukemic blasts continues unaffectedly

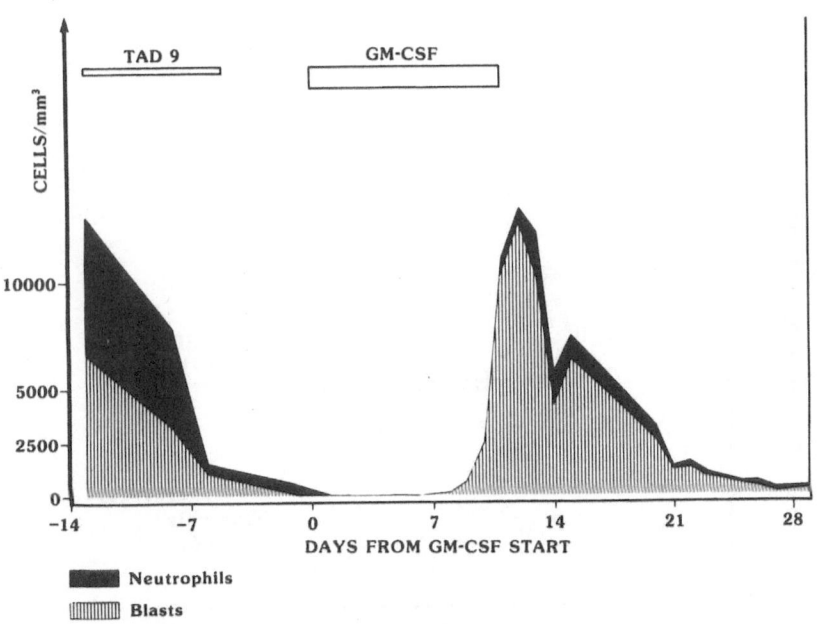

Fig. 5. Absolute counts of different white blood cells in patient 25 with AML M5 during TAD9 chemotherapy followed by GM-CSF. Leukemic regrowth is reversible after GM-CSF cessation

89

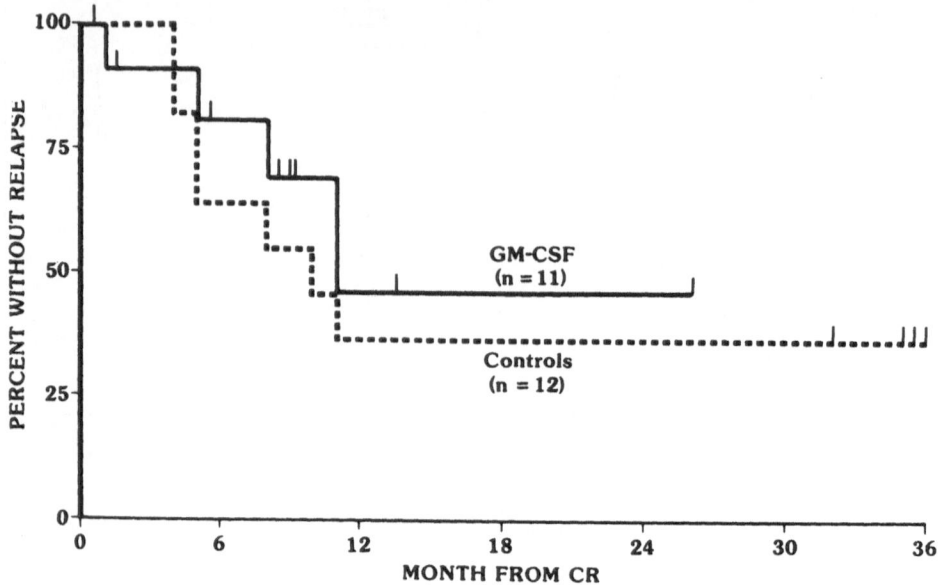

Fig. 6. Kaplan Meier test of remission duration in newly diagnosed AML. *Tick marks* represent patients in CR at last update

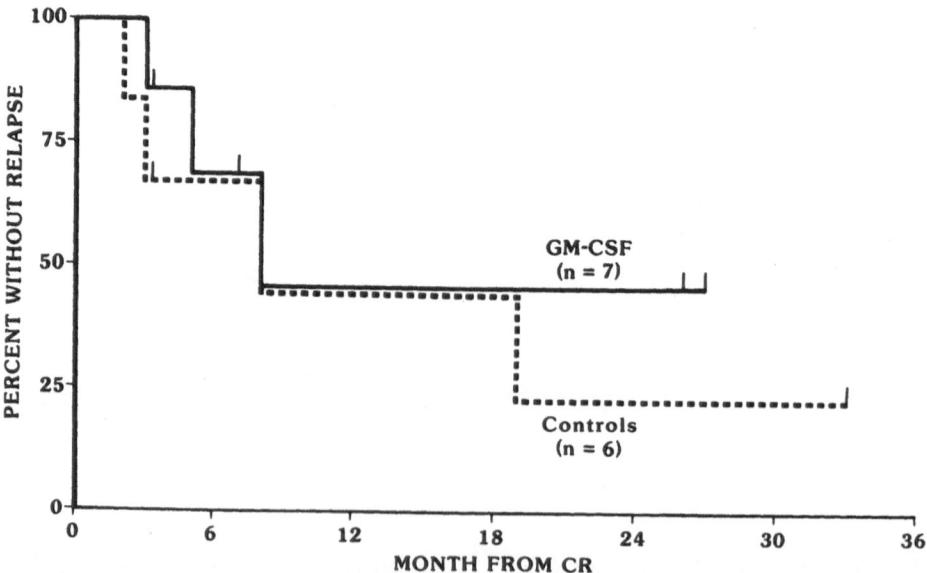

Fig. 7. Remission duration in patients treated for relapse (see also Fig. 6)

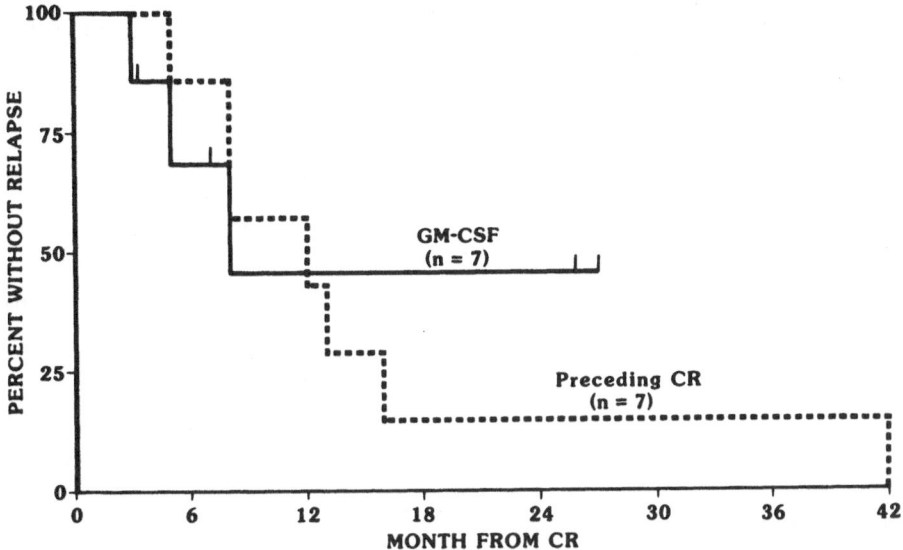

Fig. 8. Remission duration in patients treated for relapse, comparing remissions after GM-CSF to previous remissions in the same patient ($n = 7$). (See also Fig. 6)

compared to the duration of the preceding remissions shows no difference in the medians. In aptients 7 and 8 the duration of the new remissions is 27+ and 26+ months vs 8 and 13 months previously (Fig. 8).

DNA Aneuploidy

Cellular data on bone marrow DNA aneuploidy and leukemic colony growth are shown in Table 7. A hyperdiploid cell population was found in five out of 22 patients. It disappeared after chemotherapy in three out of four cases. It persisted and disappeared only after GM-CSF in one patient.

Leukemic Colony Growth

A pretherapeutic leukemic colony growth was found in 13/18 patients (Table 7). It was spontaneous in ten patients of whom six went into CR and one (patient 25) showed a leukemic regrowth. Leukemic colony growth was stimulated by GM-CSF in vitro in seven cases, six of whom went into CR, one after a reversible leukemic regrowth

(patient 25). A persistence of leukemic colony growth after chemotherapy was found in two out of 19 patients and was associated with nonresponse (patients 3 and 25).

Discussion

The results of this clinical study in patients with AML at high risk of early death provide good evidence that GM-CSF was of therapeutic benefit for the patients. This is reflected by the 60% CRs after GM-CSF with a comparatively low early death rate of 10%. The median age of responders was as high as 69 years ranging up to 84 years. Even when including the six patients with persistent blasts who did not receive growth factor the GM-CSF group compares favorably with the historical control group by its CR rate of 50% vs 32% and an early death rate of 14% vs 39%. This effect is more pronounced in newly diagnosed AMLs over the age of 65 years than in the relapses where the GM-CSF group, however, included three prior bone marrow transplantations and more early relapses.

91

Table 7. Bone marrow DNA aneuploidy and leukemic colony growth during course of treatment in patients receiving GM-CSF

Patient	DNA Index			CFU-L without/with GM-CSF in vitro		
	Before therapy	After Chemotherapy	After GM-CSF	Before therapy	After Chemotherapy	After GM-CSF
1	1.0	1.0		1/3 (× 3)		0/0
2						
3					10/4	
4	1.0			10/24 (× 2.4)	0/0	0/0
5	1.0					
6	1.0	1.0	1.0	67/70	0/0	
7	1.11	1.0	1.0	15/35 (× 2.3)		
8					0/0	
9	1.0			16/16	0/0	0/0
10					/0	
11	1.0	1.0	1.0			
12	1.0	1.0				
13	1.25	1.19	1.0	1/19 (× 19)	0/0	0/0
14					0/0	0/0
15	1.0	1.0		0/0	0/0	
16	1.0	1.0	1.0			
17	1.0	1.0	1.0	2/4 (× 2)	0/0	0/0
18	1.0		1.0	60/51	/0	0/0
19	1.0			7/7	/0	
20	1.0	1.0				
21				0/0		
22	1.0			14/4	0/0	0/0
23	1.18	1.0	1.0	0/1	0/0	0/0
24				0/1	0/1	
25	1.0	1.0	1.0	4/26 (× 6.5)	4/4	10/10
26	1.0	1.0	1.0	0/0	0/1	
27						
28	1.0			0/11 (× 11)	0/0	0/0
29	1.08	1.0		27/35	0/0	0/0
30	1.11					

CFU-L, leukemic colony forming units

The reduction in the early death rate mainly accounts for the improved response rate and is explained by a marked acceleration of the recovery from critical neutropenia. The median neutrophil recovery time was reduced by about 1 week after both the TAD9 and the more intensive S-HAM induction regimen. After recovery of neutrophils under GM-CSF to 500/mm^3, signs of documented infections or fever of unidentified origin reversed immediately or within a few days in most patients. We conclude that by reducing the phase of risk more patients survive their infections.

Estey et al. [41] recently reported that GM-CSF failed either to improve response rates or to accelerate neutrophil recovery in 12 patients with poor-prognosis newly diagnosed AML. This discrepancy in comparison to our results may be due to a lower daily dose of 120 µg/m^2 GM-CSF in the Houston study versus 250 µg/m^2 in our study. When using this higher dose but interrupting GM-CSF for 1 week in most patients the median neutrophil recovery time was reduced by 3.5 days when compared to controls, but differences in therapeutic outcome are not reported [45].

GM-CSF was generally well tolerated. The same adverse events occurring in the GM-CSF group, e.g., cardiac events, elevation of serum transaminases, and severe neurocortical events, were also observed in the controls, mostly at similar incidence or even more frequently. In the GM-CSF group the overall incidence of weight gain, hypoproteinemia, and prolongation of prothrombin time was increased but the difference was not significant for higher grade events. Together with the decrease of the pseudocholinesterase levels the three changes similarly reported by others [45] may reflect an impaired synthetic function of the liver. Those non-life-threatening events were reversible in part while GM-CSF was continued. Unlike others [45] we observed similar changes in the controls. Fever reactions were mostly explained as infectious and probably not GM-CSF-related [42]. No typical first-dose effect of GM-CSF as characterized by flushing, tachycardia, hypotension, musculoskeletal pain and dyspnea [43] was observed in our patients.

In addition to the response in neutrophil recovery 20% of patients showed an increase in blood eosinophils and monocytes under GM-CSF. All multilineage responses were found to be rapidly reversible after discontinuation of GM-CSF.

This study also provides data on the risk of stimulating the progress of AML by GM-CSF. We observed a marked leukemic regrowth under GM-CSF in two instances. In patient 15 the regrowth appeared to be unrelated to GM-CSF since it was unaffected in its kinetics by the cessation of infusion, while an additional monocytosis in this patient typically reversed rapidly. One could argue that GM-CSF in this case only triggered the regrowth by recruiting dormant leukemic stem cells into the cell cycle while not affecting proliferation. In the in vitro studies, however, an increase of colony numbers in the presence of GM-CSF occurred with an increase of colony size [27, 30] and a selective recruitment effect has not been reported. In patient 25 the leukemic regrowth was clearly related to GM-CSF, as indicated by its reversibility. In this AML M5 specific leukemic cell markers were not present. However, the selective increase of promonocytes and monocytes in blood up to 11 600/mm³ and the 95% infiltration and hypercellularity of the bone marrow by the corresponding type of cells

strongly suggest their leukemic nature. After cessation of GM-CSF and disappearance of her leukemic regrowth the 78-year-old patient has remained in continuous remission for now 2 years without further treatment.

These data suggest that there is only a low risk of activating minimal residual disease by GM-CSF leading to regrowth or early relapse. Indeed, remission duration after GM-CSF so far appears similar to that in the controls, and shows at least no increase in early relapses.

As shown in patient 13 a residual leukemic cell population marked by a DNA aneuploidy may persist after chemotherapy and disappear even after GM-CSF not followed by an early relapse. Furthermore, it is remarkable that two of seven responders treated for relapse have been achieving a remission duration after GM-CSF twice and three times that in the preceding remission (patients 7 and 8).

Confirming numerous data obtained from in vitro experiments [25–32] we found that in eight of 17 patients investigated leukemic colony growth (CFU-L) was stimulated by GM-CSF in vitro [44]. In the in vivo situation, however, only two patients developed a marked leukemic regrowth under the infusion of GM-CSF. Six patients went into CR with one early relapse and two long-term remissions. Thus, progenitor cells stimulated by GM-CSF in vitro may not be representative for the cells producing disease progression in the patient.

In conclusion, GM-CSF given in aplasia after chemotherapy to patients with AML at high risk of early death seems to improve their therapeutic outcome by accelerating the recovery of neutrophils. Adverse effects like stimulating disease progression are less important than expected from in vitro data. The data provide a basis for larger controlled trials that are highly warranted.

Summary

In order to reduce critical neutropenia after chemotherapy for AML, we gave recombinant human granulocyte-macrophage colony-stimulating factor (GM-CSF) to patients over the age of 65 years with newly diagnosed AML and to patients with early or second relapse. Chemotherapy was 9-day 6-thioguanine, ara-C, and daunorubicin (TAD9) in newly diagnosed AML and sequential high-dose ara-C and mitoxantrone (S-HAM) for relapse. In patients whose bone marrow was free from blasts a continuous i.v. infusion of GM-CSF , 250 μm/m^2 day, started on day 4 after chemotherapy. Of the 36 patients who entered the study, 30 received GM-CSF. For comparison, a historical control group of 56 patients was used. CR rate was 50 % (18/36) vs 32 % in controls ($p = .09$), and early death rate was 14 % vs 39 % ($p = .009$). Treatment with GM-CSF was not associated with major adverse events. Two patients showed a marked leukemic regrowth which was completely reversible in one patient and appeared GM-CSF-independent in the other patient. Remission duration seems not reduced after GM-CSF. Under GM-CSF the blood neutrophils recovered 6 and 9 days earlier in the TAD9 ($p = 0.009$) and S-HAM ($p = .043$) groups leading to a rapid clearance of infections in most patients. We conclude that GM-CSF was of therapeutic benefit to our patients which provides a basis for larger controlled trials.

References

1. Rai KR, Holland JF, Glidewell O, Weinberg V, Brunner K, Obrecht JP, Preisler HD, Nawabi IW, Prager D, Carey RW, Cooper MR, Haurani F, Hutchison JL, Silver RT, Falkson G, Wiernik P, Hoagland HC, Blumfield CD, James GW, Gottlieb A, Ramanan SV, Blom J, Nissen NI, Bank A, Allison RR, Kung F, Henry P, McIntyre OR, Kaan SK (1981) Treatment of acute myelocytic leukemia: a study by Cancer and Leukemia Group B. Blood 58: 1203
2. Yates J, Glidewell O, Wiernik P, Cooper MR, Steinberg D, Dosick H, Levi R, Hoagland C, Henry P, Gottlieb A, Cornell C, Behrenberg J, Hutchinson JL, Raich P, Nissen N, Allison RR, Frelick R, James GW, Falksohn G, Silver RT, Haurani F, Green M, Anderson E, Leone L, Holland JF (1982) Cytosine-arabinoside with daunorubicin or adriamycin for therapy of acute myelocytic leukemia: a CALGB-study. Blood 60: 454
3. Cassileth PA, Begg CB, Bennett JM, Bozdech M, Kahn SB, Weiler C, Glick JH (1984) A randomized study of the efficacy of consolidation therapy in adult acute nonlymphocytic leukemia. Blood 63: 843
4. Büchner T, Urbanitz D, Hiddemann W, Rühl H, Ludwig WD, Fischer J, Aul HC, Vaupel HA, Kruse R, Zeile G, Nowrousian MR, König HJ, Walter M, Wendt FC, Sodomann H, Hossfeld DK, von Paleske A, Loeffler H, Gassmann W, Hellriegel KP, Fülle HH, Lunscken C, Emmerich B, Pralle H, Pees HW, Pfreundschuh M, Bartels H, Koeppen HM, Schwerdtfeger R, Donhuijsen-Ant R, Mainzer K, Bartel B, Koeppler H, Zurborn KH, Ranft K, Thiel E, Heinecke A (1985) Intensified induction and consolidation with or without maintenance chemotherapy for acute myeloid leukemia (AML): two multicenter studies of the German AML Cooperative Group. J Clin Oncol 3: 1583
5. Rees JKH, Gray R (1987) Comparison of 1 + 5 DAT and 3 + 10 DAT followed by COAP or MAZE. Consolidation therapy in the treatment of acute myeloid leukemia: MRC ninth AML trial. Semin Oncol 14 (Suppl 1): 32
6. Preisler H, Davis RB, Kirshner J, Dupre Richards III F, Hoagland HC, Copel S, Levi AN, Carey R, Schulman P, Gottlieb AJ, McIntyre OR, Cancer and Leukemia Group B (1987) Comparison of three remission induction regimens and two post induction strategies for the treatment of acute non-lymphocytic leukemia: a Cancer and Leukemia Group B study. Blood 69: 1441
7. Hiddemann W, Kreutzmann H, Straif K, Ludwig WD, Mertelsmann R, Donhuijsen-Ant R, Lengfelder E, Arlin Z, Büchner T (1987) High-dose cytosine-arabinoside and mitoxantrone: a highly effective regimen in refractory acute myeloid leukemia. Blood 69: 744
8. Hiddemann W, Kreutzmann H, Straif K, Ludwig WD, Mertelsmann R, Planker M, Donhuijsen-Ant R, Lengfelder E, Arlin Z, Büchner T (1987) High-dose cytosine-arabinoside in combination with mitoxantrone for the treatment of refractory myeloid and lymphoblastic leukemia. Semin Oncol 14 (Suppl 1): 73
9. Capizzi RL, Powell BL (1987) Sequential high-dose Ara-C and asparaginas versus high-dose Ara-C alone in the treatment of patients with relapsed and refractory acute leukemias. Semin Oncol 14 (Suppl 1): 40
10. Büchner T, Hiddemann W, Zühlsdorf M, Königsmann M, Boeckmann A, van de Loo J, Schulz G (1988) Human recombinant granulocyte-macrophage colony-stimulating factor (GM-CSF) treatment of patients with

acute leukemias in aplasia and at high risk of early death. Behring Inst Mitt 83: 308

11. Büchner T, Hiddemann W, Königsmann M, Zühlsdorf M, Wörmann B, Boeckmann A, van de Loo J, Maschmeyer G, Wendt F, Schulz G (1988) Human recombinant granulocyte-macrophage colony-stimulating factor (GM-CSF) for acute leukemias in aplasia and at high risk of early death. Blood 72 (Suppl 1): 354

12. Donahue RE, Wang EA, Stone DK, Kamen R, Wong GG, Sehgal PK, Nathan DG, Clark SC (1986) Stimulation of haematopoiesis in primates by continuous infusion of recombinant human GM-CSF. Nature 321: 872

13. Mayer P, Lam C, Obenaus H, Liehe E, Besemer J (1987) Recombinant human GM-CSF induces leukocytosis and activates peripheral blood polymorph nuclear neutrophils in non-human primates. Blood 206

14. Monroy RL, Skelly RR, Taylor P, Dubois A, Donahue RE, MacVittey TJ (1988) Recovery from severe hematopoietic suppression using recombinant human granulocyte-macrophage colony-stimulating factor. Exp Hematol 16: 344

15. Nienhues AW, Donahue RE, Karlson SC, Agricola B, Antinoff N, Pierce JE Turner P, Anderson WF, Nahtan DG (1987) Recombinant human granulocyte-macrophage colony-stimulating factor (GM-CSF) shortens the period of neutropenia after autologous bone marrow transplantation on a primate model. J Clin Invest 80: 573

16. Monroy RL, Skelly RR, MacVittie TJ, Davies TA, Sauber JJ, Clark SC, Donahue RE (1987) The effect of recombinant GM-CSF on recovery of monkeys transplanted with autologous bone marrow. Blood 70: 1696

17. Groopmann JE, Mitsuyasu RT, DeLeo MJ, Oette DH, Golde DW (1987) Effect of recombinant human granulocyte-macrophage colony-stimulating factor on myelopoiesis in the acquired immunodeficiency syndrome. N Engl J Med 318: 593

18. Champlin RE, Nimer SD, Ireland P, Oette DH, Golde DW (1989) Treatment of refractory aplastic anemia with recombinant human granulocyte-macrophage colony-stimulating factor. Blood 73: 694

19. Vadhan-Raj SV, Büscher S, Broxmeyer HE, LeMaistre A, Lepe-Zuniga JL, Ventura G, Jeha S, Horowitz LJ, Trujillo JM, Gillis S, Hittelman WN, Gutterman JU (1988) Stimulation of myelopoiesis in patients with aplastic anemia by recombinant human granulocyte-macrophage colony-stimulating factor. N Engl J Med 319: 1628

20. Antman K, Griffin J, Elias A, Socinski M, Whitley M, Ryan L, Cannistra S, Oette D, Frei E, Schnipper L (1987) Use of rGM-CSF to ameliorate chemotherapy-induced myelosuppression in sarcoma patients. Blood 70 (Suppl 1): 373

21. Brandt SJ, Peters WP, Atwater SK, Kurtzberg J, Borowitz MJ, Jones RB, Shapaal EJ, Bast RC, Gilbert CJ, Oette DH (1988) Effect of recombinant human granulocyte-macrophage colony-stimulating factor on hematopoietic reconstitution after high-dose chemotherapy and autologous bone marrow transplantation. N Engl J Med 318: 869

22. Vadhan-Raj S, Keating M, LeMaistre A, Hittelmann W, McCredie K, Trujillo JM, Broxmeyer HE, Henney C, Gutterman JV (1987) Effects of recombinant human granulocyte-macrophage colony-stimulating factor in patients with myelodysplastic syndromes. N Engl J Med 317: 1545–1552

23. Hölzer D, Ganser A, Völkers B, Greher J, Walther F (1988) In vitro and in vivo action of recombinant human GM-CSF in patient with myelodysplastic syndromes. Blood Cells 14: 551

24. Ganser A, Völkers B, Groher J, Ottmann OG, Walther F, Becker R, Bergmann L, Schulz G, Hölzer D (1989) Recombinant human granulocyte-macrophage colony-stimulating factor in patients with myelodysplastic syndromes; a phase I/II trial. Blood 738 31

25. Herrmann FH, Lindemann A, Klein H, Lübbert M, Schulz G, Mertelsmann R (1989) Effect of recombinant human granulocyte-macrophage colony-stimulating factor in patients with myelodysplastic syndrome with excess blasts. Leukemia 3: 335

26. Griffin HD, Young D, Herrmann F, Wiper D, Wagner K, Sabbath KD (1986) Effects of recombinant human GM-CSF on proliferation of clonogenic cells in acute myeloblastic leukemia. Blood 67: 1448

27. Kelleher C, Miyauchi J, Wong G, Clark S, Minden MD, McCuloch EA (1987) Synergism between recombinant growth factors GM-CSF and G-CSF, acting on the blast cells of acute myeloblastic leukemia. Blood 69: 1489

28. Miyauchi J, Kelleher CA, Yang Y, Wong GC, Clark SC, Minden MD, Minken S, McCulloch EA (1987) The effect of three recombinant growth factors, IL-3, GM-CSF, and G-CSF, on the blast cells of acute myeloblasts leukemia maintained in short-term suspension culture. Blood 70: 657

29. Vellenga E, Ostapovicz D, O'Rurke B, Griffin B (1987) Effects of recombinant IL-3, GM-CSF, and G-CSF on proliferation of leukemic clonogenic cells in short-term and long-term cultures. Leukemia I: 584

30. Vellenga E, Young DC, Wagner K, Wiper D, Ostapovicz D, Griffin JD (1987) The effect of GM-CSF and G-CSF in promoting growth of clonogenic cells in acute myeloblastic leukemia. Blood 69: 1771

31. Murohashi I, Nagata K, Suzuki T, Maruyama Y, Nara N (1988) Effects of recombinant G-CSF and GM-CSF on the growth in methyl cellulose and suspension of the blast cells in acute myeloblastic leukemia. Leuk Res 12: 433

32. Young DC, Demetri DG, Ernst TJ, Cannistra SA, Griffin JD (1988) In vitro expression of colony-stimulating factor genes by human acute myeloblastic leukemia cells. Exp Hematol 16: 378

33. Cantrell MA, Anderson D, Cerretti DP, Price V, McKereghan K, Tushinski RJ, Mochizuki DY, Larsen A, Grabstein K, Gillis S, Cosman D (1985) Cloning, sequence, and expression of a human granulocyte/macrophage colony-stimulating factor. Proc Natl Acad Sci USA 82: 6250

34. Hiddemann W, Maschmeyer G, Pfreundschuh M, Ludwig WD, Büchner T (1987) High-dose cytosine arabinoside and mitoxantrone (HAM) for treatment of refractory acute leukemias: results of a multicenter study and preliminary data on a sequential application suggesting increased antileukemic efficacy. Blood 70 (Suppl 1): 778

35. Oken MM, Creech RH (1982) Toxicity and response criteria of the Eastern Cooperative Oncology Group. Am J Clin Oncol 5: 649

36. Bennett JM, Catovsky D, Daniel D, Flandrin G, Galton DAG, Gralnick HR, Sultan C (1976) Proposals for the classification of the acute leukemias. Br J Haematol 33: 451

37. Büchner T, Hiddemann W, Wörmann B, Kleinmeyer B, Schumann J, Göhde W, Ritter J, Müller KM, von Bassewitz DB, Rössner A, Grundmann E (1985) Differential pattern of DNA aneuploidy in human malignancies. Pathol Res Pract 179: 310

38. Hiddemann W, Wörmann B, Göhde W, Büchner T (1986) DNA aneuploidies in adult patients with acute myeloid leukemia: incidence and relation to patient characteristics and morphologic subtypes. Cancer 57: 2146

39. Hiddemann W, Schumann J, Andreeff M, Barlogie B, Herman CJ, Leif RC, Mayall BH, Sandberg AA (1984) Convention on nomenclature for DNA cytometry. Cancer Genet Cytogenet 13: 181

40. Rowley SD, Zühlsdorf M, Brayne HG, Colvin OM, Davis J, Jones RJ, Saral R, Sensenbrenner LL, Yeager A, Santos GW (1987) CFU-GM content of bone marrow graft correlates with time to hematological reconstitution following autologous bone marrow transplantation with 4-hydroxyperoxyclyclophosphamide-purged bone marrow. Blood 70: 271

41. Estey EH, Dixon D, Kantorjian HM, Keating MJ, McCredie K, Bodey GP, Kurzrock R, Talpaz M, Freireich EJ, Deisseroth AB, Gutterman JU (1998) Treatment of poor-prognosis, newly diagnosed acute myeloid leukemia with Ara-C and recombinant human granulocyte-macrophage colony stimulating factor. Blood 75: 1766

42. Peters WP, Shogan J, Shpall EJ, Jones RB, Kim CS (1988) Recombinant human granulocyte-macrophage colony-stimulating factor produces fever. Lancet I: 950

43. Lieschke GJ, Cebon J, Morstyn G (1969) Characterization of the clinical effects after the first dose of bacterially synthesized recombinant human granulocyte-macrophage colony-stimulating factor. Blood 74: 2634

44. Zühlsdorf M, Hiddemann W, Königsmann M, Wörmann B, Büchter U, Büchner T (1990) Different responsiveness of AML blasts to rhGM-CSF pre and post chemotherapy. Proc Am Assoc Cancer Res 31: 1159

45. Bettelheim P, Valent P, Andreeff M, Tafuri A, Haimi J, Gorischek C, Muhm M, Sillaber C, Haas O, Vieder L, Maurer D, Schulz G, Speiser W, Geissler K, Kier P, Hinterberger W, Lechner K (1991) Recombinant human granulocyte-macrophage colony-stimulating factor in combination with standard induction chemotherapy in de novo acute myeloid leukemia. Blood 77, 4: 700

Use of Granulocyte-Macrophage Colony-Stimulating Factor Prior to Chemotherapy of Newly Diagnosed AML

E. Estey, H. Kantarjian, S. O'Brien, M. Beran, K. McCredie, C. Koller, J. Schachner, and M. Keating

Introduction

A body of in vitro evidence suggests that use of granulocyte-macrophage colony-stimulating factor (GM-CSF) might increase the in vivo sensitivity of leukemic myeloblasts to daunorubicin-cytosine arabinoside (ara-C) chemotherapy [1–4]. If so, administration of GM-CSF prior to and during administration of daunorubicin/ara-C might overcome the resistance to therapy that is characteristic of acute myeloid leukemia (AML). This resistance is most obvious in patients with abnormalities of chromosomes 5, 7, (-5, -7, 5q-, 7q-) who frequently fail even to enter initial complete remission (CR), but it is also a major problem in patients with other aneuploidies (except INV(16), t (15; 17), or t (8; 21)), or with a normal karyotype or insufficient metaphases for analysis [5]. While the majority of these patients enter CR, their remissions rarely last more than 2 years.

In this study we administered GM-CSF to 58 patients with newly diagnosed AML (55 patients) or refractory anemia with excess of blasts (RAEB) or RAEB in transformation (RAEB-t) (three patients) prior to and during daunorubicin/ara-C chemotherapy. Our data fail to suggest that such use of GM-CSF decreases the early resistance rate in patients with those karyotypes associated with resistance as described above.

Department of Hematology, University of Texas M. D. Anderson Cancer Center, Houston, Texas

Patients and Methods

The median age of the 58 patients was 44 years (range 18–85). Patients with promyelocytic leukemia were ineligible. Only six of the patients had karyotypes associated with a high likelihood of entering CR (INV(16) or t(8; 21)). Twenty one patients had a normal karyotype; such is associated with an "average" probability of entering CR. The remaining 31 patients (53 %) had prognostically unfavorable karyotypes: ten patients had abnormalities of chromosomes 5 or 7 (-5, -7, 5q-, or 7q-), two patients had $+8$, ten had other aneuploidies, and nine had insufficient metaphases for analysis. Twenty five patients had a preleukemic phase, i.e., a documented abnormality in blood count for $\geq$ 1 month prior to diagnosis of AML. Only 28 patients (48 %) met Eastern Cooperative Ecology Group (ECOG) criteria [6] for entry to protocol for treatment of newly diagnosed AML: age < 65 years, de novo AML, no preleukemic phase, and adequate liver and kidney function.

Patients received GM-CSF (the recombinant human nonglycosylated product expressed in E. Coli and supplied by Schering-Plough Corp), 125 μg/m^2 by daily s.c. administration until the circulating blast count reached 50 000 or for 4 (later patients) – 7 (initial patients) days, whichever came first. Immediately thereafter patients began daunorubicin 45 mg/m^2 day for 3 days and ara-C 1.5 g/m^2 day by continuous infusion for 4 days (HDAC). GM-CSF continued until chemotherapy was completed. Patients who were not in

CR (a morphologically normal marrow with < 5% blasts, a platelet count > 100 000, and a neutrophil count > 1 000) after receiving two courses were changed to alternative treatments.

Results in patients receiving GM-CSF prior to chemotherapy were compared with those in patients receiving HDAC ± amsacrine (75 mg/m^2 day for 4 days) or mitoxantrone (7.5 mg/m^2 day for 4 days) but without GM-CSF during our two most recent trials in newly diagnosed AML. Since patients with acute promyelocytic leukemia (APL) were ineligible for the GM-CSF study, patients with APL given HDAC ± amsacrine or mitoxantrone were excluded from the comparisons. Expectations for attaining CR and for surviving the initial 28 days after beginning chemotherapy in each treatment group (historical or GM-CSF) were based on published logistic regression models relating probability of CR or 28 days survival following therapy with conventional dose ara-C (100 mg/m^2 day for 7 days by continuous infusion) + amsacrine (AMSAOAP) or Adriamycin (ADOAP) to various prognostic factors [7, 8].

Results

Of the 58 patients 31 entered CR (53%). Based on the predictive model mentioned above, 34 of the patients would have been expected to enter CR had they received ADOAP or AMSAOAP. Of the 27 patients who did not enter CR, 14 died (compared to an expected nine) within 28 days of beginning chemotherapy. The remaining 13 patients survived at least 29 days but failed to enter CR and were considered "resistant". Of these, 12 received two courses of therapy and none died in aplasia.

Table 1 compares results in patients given GM-CSF prior to daunorubicin + HDAC with those treated with similar chemotherapy (HDAC ± amsacrine or mitoxantrone) without GM-CSF. The number of deaths within 28 days of beginning chemotherapy divided by the number expected following ADOAP or AMSAOAP was between one and two, following either GM-CSF/daunorubicin + HDAC, HDAC alone, or amsacrine (or mitoxantrone)/HDAC. However, while the ratio of observed to expected CRs was 1.1:1 following the no GM-CSF regimes the ratio was 0.9:1 (31:34) following GM-CSF/daunorubicin + HDAC. This reflects a higher rate of resistance (defined above) in patients given GM-CSF prior to chemotherapy. This rate was 22% in the GM-CSF/daunorubicin + HDAC group, 14% in the amsacrine (or mitoxantrone) + HDAC group, and 13% in the HDAC group.

Table 2 examines the ratio of CR to resistant by cytogenetic group for patients receiving chemotherapy with or without preceding GM-CSF. Of the four patients with chromosome 5 or 7 abnormalities entering CR after GM-CSF/daunorubicin + HDAC, one relapsed within 4 months and entered a second CR after receiving daunorubicin + HDAC without GM-CSF, one died in CR 1 month after entering CR, and the other two remained in CR for < 2 months. Given this data and the data provided in Table 2 there seems to be no indication that GM-CSF will decrease the resistance rate in patients with prognostically "unfavorable" or "average" karyotypes.

Table 1. Comparison between GM-CSF + chemotherapy study and previous studies (chemotherapy, no GM-CSF)

	GM-CSF + daunorubicin + HDAC	Amsacrine (or mitoxantrone) + HDAC	HDAC
Patients	58	73	115
CR (CR expected)	31 (34)	55 (48)	73 (66)
Deaths within 28 days (expected)	14 (9)	8 (4)	27 (18)
Survived ≥ 29 days but no CR (resistant)	13	10	15

Table 2. The ratio of CR to resistant patients by cytogenetic group

Group	GM + daunorubicin + HDAC	HDAC or amsacrine + HDAC or mitoxantrone + HDAC
−5/−7	4:2	7:7
+8	0:1	7:0
Miscellaneous	8:2	25:4
Insufficient	1:2	12:2
Normal	13:5	46:7
Total	26:12	97:20

GM-CSF was in general well tolerated. The median time to attaining 1000 neutrophils in patients entering CR was 24 days after the start of chemotherapy in patients receiving GM-CSF/daunorubicin + HDAC vs 27 days in patients receiving amsacrine (or mitoxantrone) + HDAC and 26 days in patients receiving HDAC. The median time to a platelet count of 100 000 was 22, 24, and 23 days in the three groups respectively.

Discussion

Our results suggest that use of GM-CSF prior to and during daunorubicin + HDAC chemotherapy will not decrease the resistance rate in AML. Two important qualifying statements must be made. First, remission duration is as yet indeterminate in most patients; and second, the great majority of our patients had prognostically average or unfavorable karyotypes. It remains possible that the appropriate patients to receive GM-CSF prior to daunorubicin + HDAC are those with prognostically favorable karyotypes (INV(16) or t(8; 21)), i.e., those who are already relatively sensitive to chemotherapy but still have a relatively low cure rate. However, at least in patients with prognostically unfavorable or average karyotypes it can be calculated that given the resistance rate observed to date (12/38, Table 2) it is mathematically impossible to reduce the resistance rate from its historical 17 % (20/117, Table 2) to 10 %. Under these circumstances we have decided to close the study.

Summary

We gave 58 patients with newly diagnosed AML (55 patients) or RAEB or RAEB-t (three patients) GM-CSF 125 µg/m² until the circulating blast count reached 50 000 or for 4–7 days, whichever came first, followed by daunorubicin 45 mg/m² day × 3 and ara-C 1.5 g/m² day × 4 CI. (continuous infusion). GM-CSF continued until chemotherapy was completed. Of the 58 patients, 31 entered CR, 14 died within 28 days of beginning chemotherapy, and 13 survived > 29 days but never entered CR, being regarded as "resistant". Twelve of these 13 received two courses of chemotherapy and none died in aplasia. When the ratio of CR to resistant was compared in patients with prognostically unfavorable or prognostically average karyotypes receiving GM-CSF/daunorubicin + ara-C with the ratio in prognostically similar patients given similar chemotherapy without GM-CSF, there was no indication that use of GM-CSF was likely to decrease the resistant rate.

References

1. Cannistra SA, Groshek P, Griffin JD (1989) Granulocyte-macrophage colony-stimulating factor enhances the cytotoxic effects of cytosine arabinoside in acute myeloblastic leukemia and in the myeloid blast crisis of chronic myeloid leukemia. Leukemia 3: 328–334
2. Hiddemann W, Kiehl M, Schleyer E, Woermann B, Zuehlsdorf M, Buechner T (1989) Stimulating effect of GM-CSF and IL-3 on the metabolism and cytotoxic activity of cytosine arabinoside in leukemia blasts from patients with acute myeloid leukemia. Blood 74 (Suppl 1): 230a

3. Santini V, Noater K, Delwel R, Loewenberg B (1990) Susceptibility of acute myeloid leukemia cells from clinically resistant and sensitive patient to daunomycin: assessment in vitro after stimulation with colony stimulating factors. Leuk Res 14: 377–380

4. Tafuri A, Andreeff M (1990) Kinetic rationale for cytokine-induced recruitment of myeloblastic leukemia followed by cycle-specific chemotherapy in vitro. Leukemia 4: 826–835

5. Keating M, Cork A, Broach Y, Smith T, Walters R, McCredie K, Trujillo J, Freireich E (1987) Toward a clinically relevant cytogenetic classification of acute myelogenous leukemia. Leuk Res: 119–133

6. Cassileth PA, Harrington DP, Hines JD, Oken MM, Maza JJ, McGlave P, O'Connell MJ (1988) Maintenance chemotherapy prolongs remission duration in adult acute none lymphocytic leukemia. J Clin Oncol 6: 583–587

7. Keating M, Smith T, Kantarjian H, Cork A, Walters R, Trujillo J, McCredie K, Gehan E, Freireich E (1988) Cytogenetic pattern in acute myelogenous leukemia: a major reproducible determinant of outcome. Leukemia 2: 403–412

8. Estey E, Smith T, Keating M, McCredie K, Gehan E, Freireich E (1989) Prediction of survival during induction therapy in patients with newly diagnosed acute myelogenous leukemia. Leukemia 3: 257–263

G-CSF after Intensive Induction Chemotherapy in Refractory Acute Leukemia and Bone Marrow Transplantation in Myeloid Leukemia

R. Ohno[1], T. Masaoka[2], S. Asano[3], and F. Takaku[4]

Introduction

Acute leukemia has become a curable disease, although intensive therapy is required to obtain a cure [1, 2]. Therefore, a high degree of myelosuppression and resultant infectious complication are the major obstacles in its treatment.

Colony-stimulating factors (CSFs) are expected to be useful in the recovery from severe neutropenia after intensive therapy [3, 4]. However, clinical application of CSFs in leukemia has been controversial because they stimulate leukemia colonies as well as normal colonies in vitro [5, 6]. Additionally, there is some skepticism that CSFs may be ineffective when normal stem cells are severely damaged by highly intensive chemotherapy.

Therefore, in order to clarify these issues, we conducted a prospective randomized study of granulocyte CSF (G-CSF) after a remission induction therapy in refractory acute leukemia [7]. In addition, in order to assess a possible stimulation of myeloid leukemia cells by G-CSF, remission duration and diesease-free survival of patients with myeloid leukemia were analyzed in two double-blind controlled studies of G-CSF after bone marrow transplantation (BMT) [8, 9].

[1] Department of Medicine, Nagoya University Branch Hospital, Nagoya, Japan
[2] Department of Medicine, Osaka Adult Disease Center, Osaka, Japan
[3] Department of Medicine, Tokyo University Institute of Medical Science, Tokyo, Japan
[4] National Medical Center, Tokyo, Japan

Patinets and Methods

Adult patients with relapsed or refractory acute leukemia were entered from 41 institutions to the study after the remission induction therapy. In addition to acute myeloid leukemia (AML) or acute lymphoblastic leukemia (ALL), which had become refractory to conventional chemotherapy, chronic myeloid leukemia (CML) in blast crisis and acute leukemia derived from proven myelodysplastic syndromes (MDS) were regarded as refractory cases. Patients received one course of a response-oriented individualized induction therapy, which consisted of mitoxantrone, 5 mg/m² from day 1 to 3, etoposide, 80 mg/m² from day 1 to 5, and behenoyl cytosine arabinoside, 170 mg/m² daily for 8 to 12 days. Bone marrow aspiration was carned out on day 8, and if the marrow was not hypoplastic, additional mitoxantrone was given on day 8. Marrow aspiration was repeated on day 10 and occassionally on day 12, and additional mitoxantrone was given if the marrow was not hypoplastic. Therapy was stopped when marrows became severely hypoplastic. Then they were randomized according to age, type, and stage of leukemia.

Patients allocated to CSF received recombinant human G-CSF (rhG-CSF) (Kirin/Sankyo) 200 µg/m² daily by 30-min i.v. infusion, starting 2 days after the last day of induction therapy, until peripheral neutrophils exceeded 1500/mm³. Then the dose was tapered to 100 and 50 µg, and finally discontinued if neutrophils stayed over 1500/mm³. Care was taken to avoid unnecessary stimulation of neutrophil production, and not to give G-CSF when too many leukemia blasts remained in the bone marrow. In vitro assay of leukemia colony-forming units was encouraged.

In double-blind controlled studies of G-CSF after MBF, two studies were conducted using two kinds of rhG-CSFs; one produced in E. coli /Kirin/Sankyo) and the other in Chinese hamster cells (Chugai). In the Kirin/Sankyo study, 300 µg/m^2 G-CSF was given i.v. for 2 weeks from day 5 to 18 after BMT [8], and in Chugai's study, 5 µg/kg was given i.v. for 3 weeks (day 1–21) [9]. Among patients registered to these two studies, only patients with myeloid leukemia were analyzed.

Results and Discussion

After chemotherapy 108 patients were registered for the prospective randomized study. Eligibility and evaluability of each case were judged by an evaluation committee, before information on the randomization and the outcome of each case was disclosed. There were several reasons for the exclusion from further evaluation: one patient was erroneously registered twice;

one with CML in blast crisis did not receive the assigned G-CSF because his leukemia cells had responded to G-CSF in in vitro leukemia colony assay; two had hypercellular marrow; one received aclarubicin instead of mitoxantrone; one received four doses of therapeutic intrathecal methotrexate due to meningeal leukemia; and four were already in complete remission (CR) before the study.

Forty-eight patients in the G-CSF group and 50 in the control group were evaluable. There was no statistical difference in age, sex, type, and stage of leukemia. However, the G-CSF group was found to have been given slightly more antileukemia drugs in the induction therapy (Table 1).

Figure 1 shows the day when neutrophils recovered to over 500/mm^3. X-axis represents the day of recovery, and Y-axis represents the cumulative percentage of patients whose neutrophils exceeded 500. The neutrophil recovery was significantly faster in the G-CSF group. The median was 20 days for the G-CSF and 28 days for the control. The difference was significant even when they were compared in all registered patients including ten patients who had been excluded. The neutrophil recovery to

Table 1. Characteristics of patients

	G-CSF	Control	
Evaluable cases	48	50	
Age	39 ± 14	42 ± 13	ns
Sex			
Male	25	27	ns
Female	23	23	
Type			
AML	30	31	
ALL	12	15	ns
CML-BC	4	4	
MDS-AL	2	0	
Stage			
Primary refractory	9	8	
Relapsed	25	25	ns
Relapsed and refractory	12	13	
Untreated	2	2	
Drug dose (mg/m^2)			
Mitoxantrone	20.5 ± 6.0[a]	17.5 ± 4.5[a]	
Etoposide	448 ± 72[a]	408 ± 56[a]	
BHAC	1785 ± 442[a]	1581 ± 425[a]	

ns, not significant
[a]mean ± standard deviation, $p<0.05$

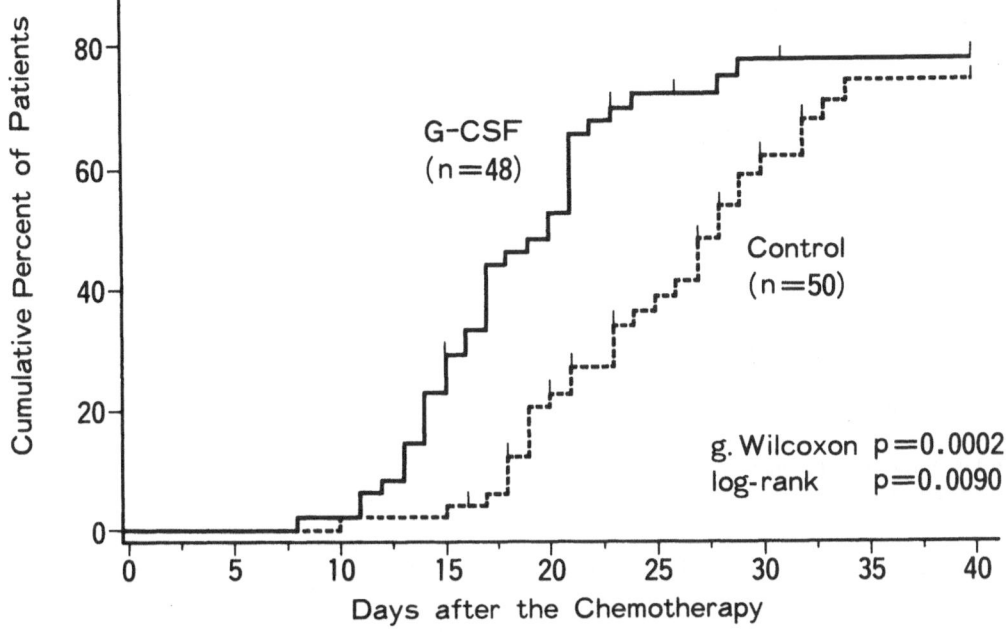

Fig. 1. Recovery of neutrophils to over 500/mm³ after induction therapy. X-axis represets the day after the end of chemotherapy, and Y-axis the cumulative percent age of patients whose neutrophil counts came to exceed 500/mm³

over 1000 neutrophils/mm³ was also significantly faster in the G-CSF. The median was 22 days for teh G-CSF and 34 days for the control.

No significant increase of lymphocytes, monocytes and eosinophils was noted. There was no difference in the recovery of platelets to over 100000/mm³ between the two groups. This indicated that the degree of myelosuppression was almost the same in spite of the fact that the G-CSF group received more drugs in the induction therapy.

Twenty-one of 48 patients in the G-CSF group and 17 of 50 in the control already had febrile episodes before the randomization (Table 2). Twenty-three of the remaining 27 in the G-CSF group and 32 of 33 in the control developed fever after the randomization. The total febrile days were fewer in the G-CSF, but not significantly. Mean days were 5.7±7.0 versus 6.5±4,4, and median days were 3 (range 0–31) versus 7 (0–14). Two patients in the G-CSF group had fever for 22 and 31 days without any documented infection, even after their neutrophils recovered to over 1000/mm³. If these two

patients were excluded, the mean febrile day of the former was 4.0±3.7, and the difference became significant ($p=0.0272$). Documented infections such as septicemia and pneumonia were significantly less frequent in the G-CSF group after the end of induction therapy. They were observed in five cases of the G-CSF and in 15 of the control (p=0.028) (Table 2).

The toxicities of G-CSF were mild. Only two patients complained of bone pain, and one nausea and vomiting. Abnormalities of blood chemistry included mild elevation of serum alkaline phosphatase (less than twice normal) in two patients and of serum GPT (less than twice normal) in one.

The regrowth of leukemia blasts was compared by examining the bone marrow 21 to 40 days after the end of induction therapy. As shown in Fig. 2, there was no difference between the two groups in the regrowth of blasts. In the G-CSF, the mean blasts were 56% before the chemotherapy and 11% after it, while in the control group, they were 44% before the chemotherapy and 14% after it. Regrowth rate was rather smaller in the G-CSF, but the difference was

Table 2. Febrile episodes and documented infections after the randomization

	G-CSF	Control
Afebrile before randomization	27	33
Became febrile	23	32
Stayed afebrile	4	1
Documented infections	5*	15*
Septicemia	3	6
Pneumonia	1	4
Septicemia + pneumonia	0	1
Perianal abscess	1	0
Cellulitis	0	1
Gingivitis/Pharyngitis	0	2
Cystitis	0	1
Fever of unknown origin	18	17
Total febrile days median (range) deviation	3 (0–31)	7 (0–14)
mean ± standard	5.7 ± 7.0	6.5 ± 4.4
	4.4 ± 3.7**	

*P=0.028 **P=0.0272 when two cases with fever for 22 and 31 days in spite of neutrophil recovery were omitted.

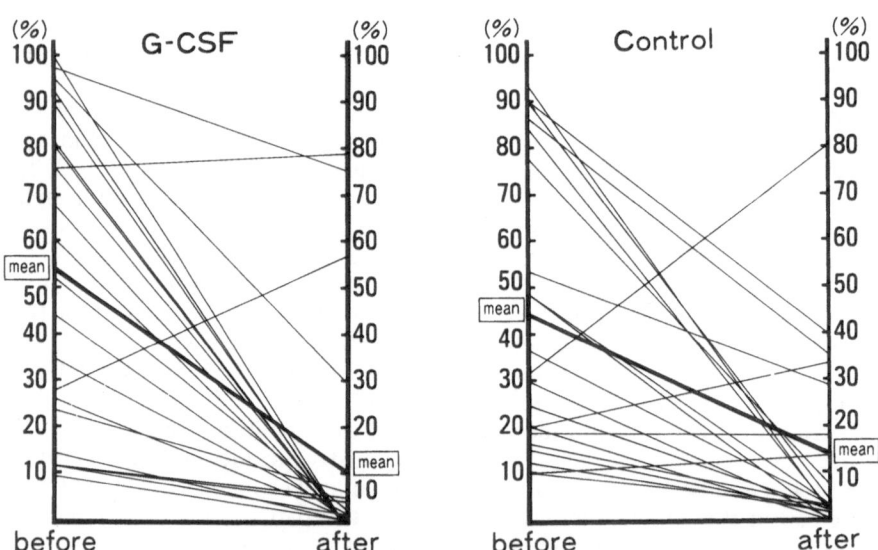

Fig. 2. Leukemia blasts in bone marrows before induction therapy and 21 to 40 days after the end of therapy. The highest values were chosen if there were multiple bone marrow samples in single patients

not significant. Since ALL cells are not stimulated by G-CSF, the regrowth of leukemia blasts was compared in the subgroups excluding ALL. However, there was alos no significant difference.

In the G-CSF group 50% of patients obtained CR, while 36% of the control achieved it (Table 3). Although the remission rate was higher in the G-CSF, the difference was not significant (p=0.162).

Table 3. Result of remission induction therapy

Group Type	No. of cases	No. of CR	%
G-CSF			
AML	30	17	(57)
ALL	12	7	(58)
CML-BC	4	0	(0)
MDS-AL	2	0	(0)
Total	48	24	(50)
Control			
AML	31	12	(39)
ALL	15	6	(40)
CML-BC	4	0	(0)
Total	50	18	(36)

CR, complete remission; AML, acute myeloid leukemia; ALL, acute lymphoblastic leukemia; CML, chronic myeloid leukemia; MDS, myelodysplastic syndrome

Since no CR was obtained in CML and myelodysplastic syndromes (MDS) in blast crisis, CR rates of AML and ALL were 57 % and 58 %, respectively, in the G-CSF, and 39 % and 40 % in the control. The remission rates in the G-CSF group were very good for relapsed or refractory acute leukemia.

Figure 3 shows the Kaplan-Meier curve of the remission duration in patients who had obtained remission at he median follow-up of 22 months. There was no difference between two groups ($p=0.8975$ by generalized Wilcoxon test). The curves are almost the same when only AML is analyzed. Since the G-CSF group had higher remission rate, and the relapse rates were almost the same, the G-CSF group tended to have better event-free survival ($p=0.1237$).

Although this randomized study after the intensive induction chemotherapy indicates that G-CSF is beneficial, and probably is used safely even in myeloid leukemia, we need more information to confirm this inportant issue.

There were two double-blind controlled studies in Japan in which different recombinant G-CSF from two companies were tested for their efficacy after BMT [8, 9]. Since these studies were not designed specifically to answer the above question, lymphoid and myeloid leukemia as well as aplastic anemia were included, and because the number of myeloid leukemias was not large enough to analyze the issue separately

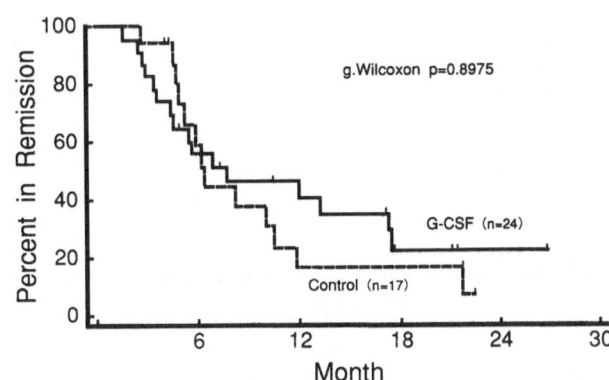

Fig. 3. Kaplan-Meier curve of probability in remission after chemotherapy

in each study, myeloid leukemias of both studies were analyzed together.

There were some differences in the two studies. Kirin's G-CSF is produced in *E.coli*, and Chugai's in Chinese hamster cells. Although the doses were almost equivalent, the administration schedules were slightly different; Kirin's G-CSF was given from day 5 to 18 [8], and Chugai's from day 1 to 21 [9]. However, from our previous experience with G-CSFs, the two sets of data are thought to be well comparable and able to be analyzed togehter.

A total of 129 patients were registered to the two studies, and 119 were evaluable, 56 of whom had myeloid leukemia. However, two patients in the placebo group in each study were given G-CSF due to infections after the 21-day observation period was over. Since the aim of the analysis was to see whether myeloid leukemia cells were stimulated by G-CSF in vivo, these four patients were included in the G-CSF group for further analysis.

Thus, there were 33 patients in the G-CSF group and 23 in the placebo group (Table 4). There were 16 AMLs in first remission, six AMLs in second or later

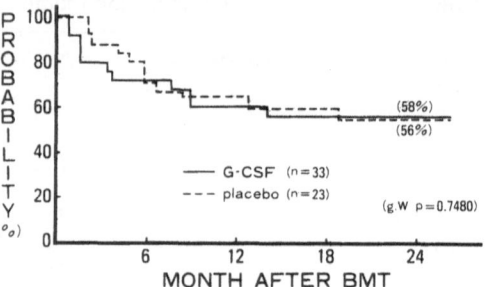

Fig. 4. Kaplan-Meier curve of probability in remission after bone marrow transplantation (BMT). Four patients in the placebo group who were later given G-CSF due to infectious episodes were included in the G-CSF group

remission, eight AMLs in relapse, 14 CMLs in chronic phase, ten CMLs in accelerated or blastic phase, and two MDSs. The age range of patients was 2–45 with a median of 30.

At the median follow-up of 23 months, there was no statistical difference in the remission duration ($P=0.8971$ by the generalized Wilcoxon test) (Fig. 4) and in the

Table 4. Two double-blind controlled studies of G-CSF in bone marrow transplantation (BMT) (myeloid leukemia only)

	G-CSF	Placebo	Total
Kirin/Sankyo study [8]	15 (2)	12	27
Chugai study [9]	18 (2)	11	27
AML			
First CR	10 (1)	6	16
Second or later CR	4	2	6
Relapse	5 (1)	3	8
CML			
Chronic phase	8	6	14
Accelerated phase	3 (2)	1	4
Blast crisis	2	4	6
MDS			
RAEB	1	0	1
REEB in T	0	1	1
Total	33 (4)	23	56

The number in parentheses indicates the number of patients in the placebo group who received G-CSF due to the delay of leukocyte recovery after the observation period was over, and who were thus included in the G-CSF group.
CR, complete remission; AML, acute myeloid leukemia; CML, chronic myeloid leukemia; MDS, myelodysplastic syndrome; RAEB, refractory anemia with excess of blasts

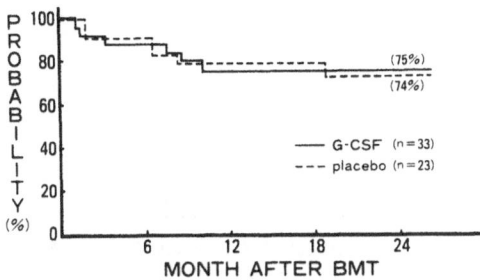

Fig. 5. Kaplan-Meier curve of diesease-free survival after bone marrow transplantation (BMT). Four patients in the placebo group who were later given G-CSF due to infectious episodes were included in the G-CSF group

disease-free survival ($P=0.7480$) (Fig. 5) between the groups which received either G-CSF or placebo after BMT. Since the prognosis of BMT is strongly influenced by the stage of disease at the time of transplantation, it is necessary to analyze the prognosis according to the stage. Therefore, AML in first CR, CML in chronic phase, and MDS in refractory anomia with excess of blasts (RAEB) were regarded as good risk, and others bad risk. However, there was no statistical difference in the disease-free survival either of good-risk patients ($P=0.4963$ by the generalized Wilcoxon test) or of poor-risk patients ($P=0.2811$).

In summary, the present prospective randomized studies in Japan revealed that G-CSF accelerated the neutrophil recovery significantly after intensive chemotherapy in leukemia, while causing no major toxicities. Documented infections were significantly less frequent in the G-CSF group. There was no evidence that G-CSF accelerated the regrowth of leukemia blasts after chemotherapy or BMT. Patients in the G-CSF group tended to have a higher remission rate. The incidence of leukemia relapse was not higher in the G-CSF group than in the control group after chemotherapy or BMT. However, when using CFSs in myeloid leukemia, great care must be taken not to give unnecessary stimulation to neutrophil production. Furthermore, the use of G-CSF should be limited to patients who are at high risk from life-threatening infections and who have minimal leukemia cells until the results of additional clinical studies become available.

Acknowledgement. We would like express our sincere gratitude to all participating physicians from 41 institutions in Japan for their cooperation in these multi-institutional studies. These studies are partly supported by Grants-in-Aid form the Japanese Ministry of Health and Welfare.

References

1. Gale RP, Foon KA (1987) Therapy of acute myelogenous leukemia. Semin Hematol 24: 40–54
2. Ohno R (1989) Recent progress in the treatment of acute leukemia. Acta Haematol Jpn 52: 1340–1344
3. Groopman JE, Molina J-M, Scadden DT (1989) Hematopoietic growth factors: biology and clinical applications. N Engl J Med 321: 1449–1459
4. Antman KS, Griffin JD, Elias A, et al. (1988) Effect of recombinant human granulocyte-macrophage colony-stimulating factor on chemotherapy-induced myelo suppression. N Engl J Med 319: 593–598
5. Souza LM, Boone TC, Gabrilove JL, et al. (1986) Recombinant human granulocyte colony-stimulating factor: effects on normal and leukemic myeloid cells. Science 232: 61–65
6. Inoue C, Hotta T, Murate T, Saito H (1990) Response of leukemic cells to the sequential combination of GM-CSF and G-CSF. Int J Cell Biol 8: 54–62
7. Ohno R, Tomonaga M, Kobayashi T, et al. (1990) Effect of granulocyte colony stimulating factor after intensive induction therapy in relapsed or refractory acute leukemia: a randomized controlled study. N Engl J Med 323: 871–877
8. Masaoka T, Moriyama Y, Kato S, et al. (1990) A double-blind controlled study of KRN 8601 (rhG-CSF) in patients received alogeneic bone marrow transplantation. Kyo-no-Ishoku 3: 233–239
9. Asano S, Masaoka T, Takaku F, Ogawa N (1990) Placebo controlled double blind controlled trial of recombinant human granulocyte colony-stimulating factor for bone marrow transplantation. Kyo-no-Ishoku 3: 317–321

Cytokinetic Resistance in Acute Leukemia: Recombinant Human Granulocyte Colony-Stimulating Factor, Granulocyte Macrophage Colony-Stimulating Factor, Interleukin-3 and Stem Cell Factor Effects In Vitro and Clinical Trials with Granulocyte Macrophage Colony-Stimulating Factor*

M. Andreeff[1], A. Tafuri[1, 3], P. Bettelheim[2], P. Valent[2], E. Estey[1], R. Lemoli[3], A. Goodacre[1], B. Clarkson[4], F. Mandelli[3], and A. Deisseroth[1]

Introduction

Human leukemia has been extensively investigated over the last 25 years regarding its cell kinetics, cytokine regulation, and molecular defects. It has been postulated that leukemic cells proliferate at variable rates, with DNA synthesis times as short as 6, cell cycle times as long as 200 h, and that cell kinetic parameters can be of prognostic importance [1–4]. In addition to the marked heterogeneity observed in cycling cells, seminal experiments conducted over 25 years ago demonstrated the presence of noncycling, quiescent leukemic cells [5]. It is believed that these cells are less sensitive to chemotherapy and thus constitute the residual cells which lead to clinical relapse at different time intervals after initial induction of remission. We have previously demonstrated that cell kinetic measure-

[1] University of Texas, M. D. Anderson Cancer Center, Houston, Texas, USA
[2] Department of Medicine, University of Vienna, Vienna, Austria
[3] Institue of Hematology, University of Roma "La Sapienza", Rome, Italy
[4] Memorial Sloan-Kettering Cancer Center, New York, New York, USA
* Supported in part by grants from NIH, CA 38980 and CA 05864. A. T. is supported in part by the Department of Human Biopathology, Hematology Section, University "La Sapienza", Rome, Italy. R. L. is supported by A.I.R.C. and the National Leukemia Association, Italy.

ments are correlated with remission incidence, remission duration, and survival in AML [6]. The most predictive parameter was found to be cellular RNA content, as determined by acridine orange flow cytometry. This cellular feature is asssociated with a quiescent state ("G_0"–low RNA content, and "G_1"–high RNA content). More refined measurements of genes expressed when cells enter the division cycle, including *Ki67, PCNA,* and c-*myc,* were also found to be useful in dissecting cell cycle kinetics, in particular, the important G_0-G_1 transition.

The advent of human recombinant growth regulatory molecules provides tools to effectively recruit cells into the cell cycle. We and others [7–13] have demonstrated that granulocyte colony-stimulating factor (G-CSF), granulocyte macrophage colony-stimulating factor (GM-CSF), and interleukin-3 (IL-3) can recruit leukemic cells. The mechanisms involved are poorly understood. Cellular receptor status, signal transduction, early response genes, degree of differentiation, and other cellular mechanisms may effect the ability of cytokines to recruit cells.

We now report that cytokine combinations containing IL-3 are significantly more effective in recruiting leukemic cells than G-CSF and GM-CSF, and that human cloned stem cell factor (SCF) may further enhance this effect. Studies previously conducted only in suspension culture systems have now been extended to clonogenic assays.

Our initial observation that recombinant human (rh) GM-CSF recruits leukemic cells into cycle in vitro provided the rationale for several clinical trials. Although cell kinetic data in patients are limited to date, we present here the cell cycle results of two clinical treatment regimens studied at the University of Vienna [14] and at the M. D. Anderson Cancer Center [15]. They demonstrate the induction of recruitment in vivo in some patients with rhGM-CSF. Future clinical trials will optimize this strategy by use of IL-3 and SCF.

Materials and Methods

Peripheral blood and bone marrow samples were obtained with informed consent, according to institutional policy, for both the in vitro and in vivo studies. Mononuclear cells were separated by Ficoll-Hypaque density gradient centrifugation (Pharmacia Fine Chemicals Co., Piscataway, N. J.). Samples used in the in vitro studies were suspended in fetal calf serum (FCS) and immediately cryopreserved using a mixture containing 5 % dimethylsulfoxide (DMSO) and 6 % hydroexythyl starch (HES) as described [16]. Cells were frozen at $-120 \,°C$ in a Revco Freezer (Revco Scientific, Inc., Asheville, N. C.). After rapid thawing, cells were suspended in Iscove's modified Dulbecco's medium (IMDM) (Gibco, Grand Island, NY) supplemented with 10 % FCS (Hyclone, Logan) and 60 U of deoxyribonuclease I (Cooper Biomedical, Malvern, PA) and incubated for 30 min on ice. Viable cells were recovered by Ficoll-Hypaque gradient and all samples contained more than 85 % blasts. Residual T cells were assessed by flow cytometry and were less than 2 % in all samples. Samples selected for these studies were chosen based on their known clonogenic efficiency.

Cytokines. rhIL-3 was kindly provided by Dr. S. Gillis (IMMUNEX, Seattle, WA) (20 ng/ml). rhG-CSF and rhGM-CSF was a gift from Dr. L. Souza (AMGEN, Thousand, Oaks, CA), both at a concentration of 500 U/ml. rhSCF was generously provided by Dr. K. Szebo (AMGEN, Thousand Oaks, CA) (200 ng/ml).

Culture Systems. Cells were suspended in IMDM supplemented by 10 % FCS, 1 % L-gluatime and 1 % penicillin-streptomycin (Gibco). Cell number was adjusted to a starting concentration of 0.5×10^6 cells/ml. Cells were cultured at 37 °C for 48 h in 5 % CO_2 with and without (control culture) two combinations of cytokines: IL-3 plus GM-CSF plus G-CSF and G-CSF plus GM-CSF. Cell number and viability were assessed by trypan blue exclusion. SCF was studied in serum-free medium (HL-1), in combination with G-CSF, GM-CSF, and IL-3. Read-out was on day 5.

Cell Kinetic Studies. Cell kinetics were analyzed after 48 h (or 5 d) of cytokine exposure using the acridine orange (AO) DNR/RNA technique, which allowes descrimination of cells in G_0, G_1, S, and G_2M as well as the mean RNA content per cell in each phase of the cell cycle as previously described [17]. Bromodeoxyuridine was used to label samples ex vivo for 60 min. Details have been described elsewhere [13]. Samples were measured in a FACScan flow cytometer (Becton Dickinson, Mountain View, CA). The software used included Consort 30, FACStar Research, Lysis, and Paint-a-gate (Becton Dickinson).

Clonogenic Assay. Culture medium for the leukemia-colony forming unit (CFU-L) assay consisted of 1 ml of IMDM supplemented with 24 % FCS, 0.8 % BSA, and 10^{-4} ml/l of Mercaptoethanol, methylcellulose at a final concentration of 1.32 %. MO-T cell line conditioned medium (kindly provided by Dr. Golde, UCLA, Los Angeles, CA) at 20 % v/v concentration was used as clonogenic stimulating activity. Irradiated autologous cells (1×10^5 cells at 3000 cGy) were added to the cultures. Colony growth was not observed in any culture when irradiated cells were cultured alone. Total number of cells plated was adjusted according to the previously studied clonogenic efficiency in order to generate about 100 colonies/ml of culture; 1×10^5 cells/ml were plated in the three experiments in which fresh samples were used. Quadruplicate cultures were incubated at 37 °C in a humidified atmosphere of 5 % CO_2. Plates

109

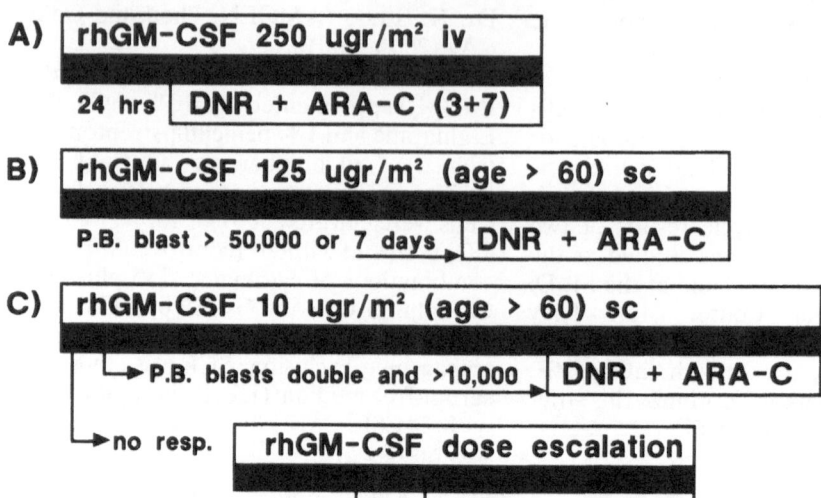

A)

rhGM-CSF 250 ugr/m² iv

| 24 hrs | DNR + ARA-C (3+7) |

B)

rhGM-CSF 125 ugr/m² (age > 60) sc

| P.B. blast > 50,000 or 7 days | DNR + ARA-C |

C)

rhGM-CSF 10 ugr/m² (age > 60) sc

→ P.B. blasts double and >10,000 | DNR + ARA-C

→ no resp. | rhGM-CSF dose escalation

→ DNR + ARA-C

Fig. 1. Treatment regimen combining GM-CSF and chemotherapy. *Regimen A*, University of Vienna; *Regimen B* and *C*, M. D. Anderson Cancer Center

were scored for colonies (greater than 20 cells) after 10 days of incubation.

Clinical Protocols. Patients were treated on three different protocols: Study A (Fig. 1) consisted of rhGM-CSF 250 ug/m² i.v. for 24 h, followed by daunorubicin and ara-C for 3 and 7 days, respectively. Details of this clinical trial are reported elsewhere [14]. Protocol B (Fig. 1) consisted of rhGM-CSF (125 ug/m² s. c.) given for up to 7 days or until the peripheral blast count exceeded 50000/μl (GM-CSF supplied by Schering-Plough Corp., nonglycosylated GM-CSF expressed in *E. coli*). Following GM-CSF, patients received daunorubicin 45 mg/m² daily X 3 days, and ara-C 1.5 g/m² daily by continuous infusion for 4 days. GM-CSF continued until chemotherapy was completed [15]. A third protocol (C, Fig. 1) used low dose GM-CSF (10 ug/m² s. c.) until the peripheral blast count exceeded 10000 or the peripheral blast count doubled. At that point, daunorubicin and ara-C were applied as above. The protocol also called for a GM-CSF dose escalation if no response was observed.

Statistical Analysis. Significance levels between different in vitro groups were determined by paired two-sided Student't t test. Linear regression analysis was also performed to investigate correlation between variables.

Results

In Vitro Stimulation with G-CSF, GM-CSF, IL-3 and SCF

Figure 2 shows the effects of G-CSF and GM-CSF in combination on AML cells in vitro. The upper panel compares changes in S phase and changes in CFU-L. In the majority of cases, no significant increase in S phase or CFU-L was observed, however in cases number 3 and 4, S phase increased significantly, and this was paralleled by increases in CFU-L. Cases 1 and 2 had only small S phase increases, although the increase in CFU-L was more pronounced. The lower panel shows the percentage of decrease of cells in G_0 as determined by DNA/RNA flow cytometry. Sample number 6 had the highest decrease, but decreases were also observed in samples 1, 3, and 4.

The enhanced cell kinetic effects of IL-3 can be seen in Fig. 3; the same samples were studied under identical conditions except for the addition of IL-3. It is apparent that 5/10 samples had significant increases in S phase and these increases were significantly higher than those observed with G and GM-CSF alone. Again, changes in S phase were paralleled by increases in CFU-L and in decreases in the percentage of cells in G_0.

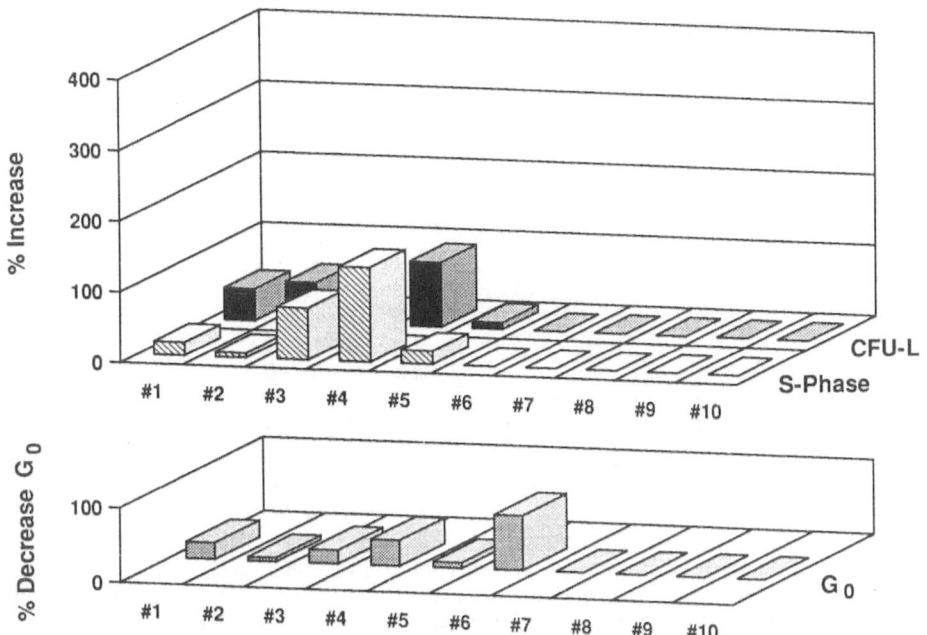

Fig. 2. Effects of rhG-CSF + GM-CSF in suspension culture and in clonogenic assays in vitro. Ten samples from patients with AML were analyzed by flow cytometry for percentage of cells in S phase and in G_0. Results were normalized to control samples and expressed as percent increase (S phase) and percent decrease (G_0 cells). Identical samples were studied by clonogenic assays (CFU-L) and changes are expressed as percent increase as compared to controls

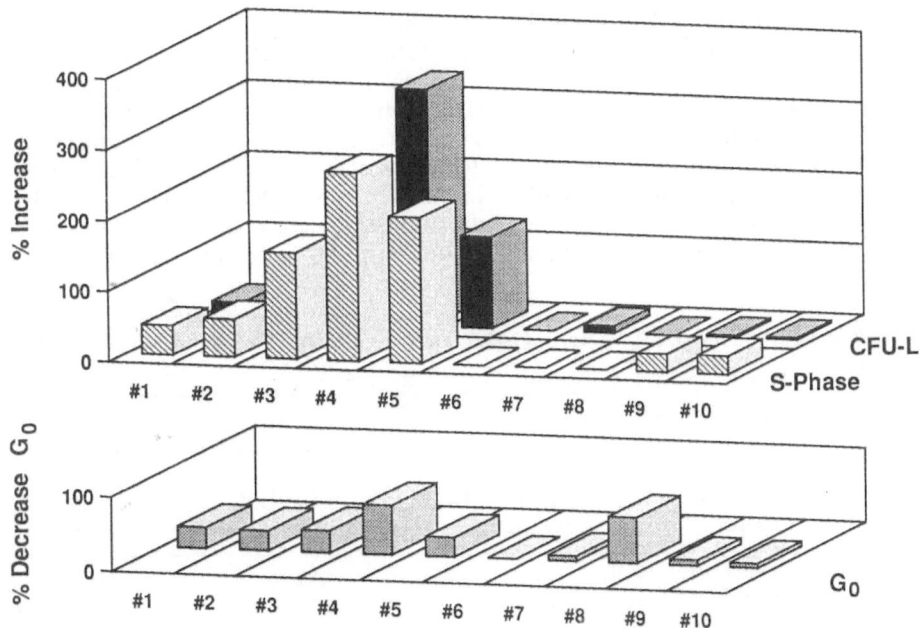

Fig. 3. Same samples as shown in Fig. 2: G-CSF + GM-CSF + IL-3 were used to stimulate proliferation (% change of cells in G_0 and in S phase) and clonogenicity (CFU-L). For further details, see Fig. 2

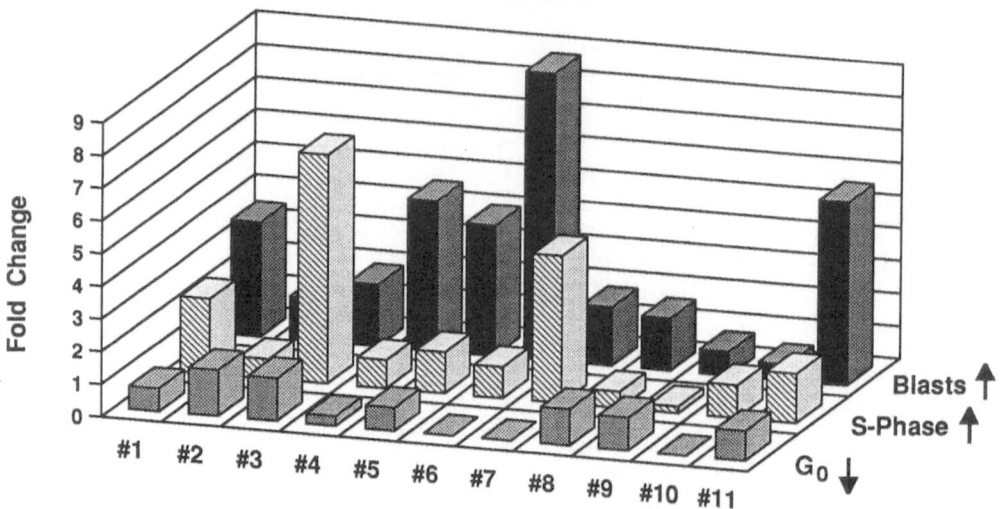

Fig. 4. Cell kinetic changes in AML patients treated with GM-CSF in vivo. Eleven patients were studied; results are expressed as change compared to pretreatment values. Increases are shown for cells in S phase and for the number of circulating blast cells. Changes shown for G_0 cells indicate decreases in the number of G_0 cells

Only case 8 had a decrease in G_0, which was not accompanied by increased clonogenicity or elevated S phase. One could postulate that cells were recruited from G_0 into G_1 but not into S phase, and that this did not result in an increased number of colony forming cells.

Comparison of Figs. 2 and 3 allows the conclusion that the addition of IL-3 results in more effective recruitment than that obtained with G- and GM-CSF combined. These experiments did not address the question whether IL-3 alone would result in

significantly increased clonogenicity and proliferation.

As shown in Table 1, the addition of SCF further enhances the proliferation induction observed by the combination of G-CSF, GM-CSF, and IL-3. These experiments were carried out in serum-free medium (HL1), and cell kinetic changes were measured after 5 days. It was apparent that the depletion of cells in G_0 was more significant when SCF was added ($p=0.01$), and that the number of cells in S increased from 9 % on day 0 to 12.3 % on day 5 in the presence

Table 1. Effect of stem cell factor (SCF), IL-3, G-CSF, and GM-CSF on AML Bone Marrow Cells in vitro

Cell Cycle	Day			P
	0 Bone Marrow Biopsy	5 G + GM + IL-3	5 G + GM + IL-3 + SCF	
G_0 (%)	67.5	59.4	38.7	0.01
G_1 (%)	24.5	15.4	22.2	n.s.
SG_2M (%)	9	12.3	24.2	0.01

Cells were grown in serum-free medium (HL-1). Changes in cell kinetics (G_0, G_1, SG_2M) were measured on day 0 and again after 5 days. Recruitment is evident by decrease of cells in G_0 and increase of cells in SG_2M. SCF significantly adds to the effects of G + GM + IL-3.

of G + GM + IL-3, and to 22.2% when SCF was added.

Cell Kinetic Changes in Patients Treated with GM-CSF

Table 2 summarizes patient characteristics for the 11 patients treated with GM-CSF and chemotherapy. Table 3 provides specifics of the doses of GM-CSF and the changes in the percentage of bone marrow cells in G_0 and in S phase, changes in peripheral blood blast numbers, and in the percentage of bone marrow blast cells. Columns labelled "pre-" and "start" reflect two pretreatment time points. In some of these patients, changes were observed with regard to the percentage of cells in G_0 and in S phase, which were unrelated to cytokine therapy. In other cases, significant changes are apparent only after cytokine therapy. Some of these changes may be related to sampling error, as only bone marrow aspirates were used in the kinetic studies of bone marrow leukemic cells. It is known that bone marrow biopsies provide more reliable material for this purpose.

Table 2. Characteristics of 11 patients treated with GM-CSF followed by chemotherapy

PATIENT	FAB	AGE	% BLASTS b.m.	RESP.
# 1	M1	25	86	CR
# 2	M5	46	79	CR
# 3	M4	66	84	CR
# 4	M1	60	94	Resist.
# 5	M2	62	50	Died
# 6	M1	49	73	CR
# 7	M2	21	34	CR
# 8	M2	33	74	CR
# 9	M2	38	36	Resist.
#10	n.c	50	29	Resist.
#11	M2	70	47	CR

Table 3. Details of clinical trials of GM-CSF and chemotherapy

#	Dose	%G_0(BM)			%S(BM)			PB blasts x 10^3			% BM blasts	
		Pre	Start	Post	Pre	Start	Post	Pre	Start	Post	Pre	Post
1	250 × 24h	75.6	86.9	60.1	4.4	3.8	8.7	/	0.2	0.7	86	92
2	250 × 24h	/	65.1	91.6	/	3.0	2.0	/	0.8	1.1	79	81
3	250 × 24h	/	57.7	74.6	/	1.3	9.1	/	12.7	24.2	84	95
4	250 × 24h	/	91.5	92.9	/	3.0	0.7	/	20.7	15.4	94	90
5	125 × 4d.	86.6	77.2	81.7	3.3	5.5	2.7	45.8	63.3	99.5	50	68
6	125 × 5d.	58.1	30.0	8.4	15.3	14.5	12.7	10.4	11.7	54.7	73	93
7	125 × 8d.	52.4	79.4	57.2	3.3	7.8	9.8	1.0	0.5	2.0	34	31
8	125 × 4d.	/	/	/	7.2	15.1	14.3	7.2	4.7	41.7	74	49
9	125 × 8d.	/	/	/	4.2	7.5	7.7	3.8	15.4	9.1	36	70
10	125 × 7d.	76.7	61.4	54.3	7.2	6.7	10.2	1.4	3.2	18.1	29	21
11	10–20 × 22d.	/	/	/	8.5	3.1	14.0	5.5	5.5	10.1	47	62

Dose of GM-CSF given in μm/m² X time of in vivo therapy. Cell kinetics is given as percentage of cells in G_0 and S Phase, as measured by DNA/RNA flow cytometry in bone marrow cells. PB blasts X 10^3 indicates circulating leukemic blast cells. Percentage of bone marrow blast cells is given before and after GM-CSF. "Pre-" and "Start" signify two pretreatment time points.

Table 4. Ex vivo BUdR incubation for 1 h of AML samples, before and after treatment with GM-CSF. Four of seven patients have significant increases in S Phase cell

Case #	Sample	Pre	Post
1	B.M.	2.3 %	5.9 %
	P.B.	0.3 %	2.0 %
2	B.M.	1 %	2.5 %
3	B.M.	5.5 %	20.1 %
	P.B.	3.4 %	17.9 %
4	B.M.	1.2 %	1.4 %
8	B.M.	15.1 %	14.3 %
9	B.M.	7.5 %	7.7 %
11	B.M.	3.1 %	14.1 %

S-phase ↑ 4/7

Changes in S phase cells were also studied using ex vivo BUdR labelling as shown in Table 4. This technique is considered superior to DNA measurement alone, and it is obvious that a significant increase in S phase cells was observed in 4/7 patients.

The kinetic changes are summarized in Table 5: 33 % of patients had a significant decrease in G_0 cells and 36 % had an increase in S phase cells of more than 50 %. In one quarter of patients, decreases in G_0 were accompanied by increases in S phase cells. The majority of patients had changes in peripheral blasts, and four out of 11 patients had changes in bone marrow blasts. The higher number of peripheral blasts was not always correlated to cell kinetic changes.

Table 5. Summary of cell kinetic changes in patients treated with GM-CSF and chemotherapy (for details, see text)

Kinetic changes	Patient number	% of cases
GO ↓ >25 %	1, 6, 7	33
S phase ↑ >25 %	1, 3, 7, 10, 11	45
↑ >50 %	1, 3, 10, 11	36
GO ↓ + S ↑	1, 7	25
PB Blasts ↑ >25 %	1, 2, 3, 5, 6, 7, 8, 10, 11	81
↑ >50 %	1, 3, 5, 6, 8, 10, 11	63
BM Blasts ↑ >25 %	5, 6, 9, 11	36

Discussion

Cytokinetic manipulations of acute myeloid leukemia have been attempted for many years, since ara-C and anthracyclins were found to act in a cell cycle specific manner. Cytosine arabinoside, the backbone of AML therapy to date, is specifically effective against cells in S phase. Topoisomerase II inhibitors, such as daunomycin, idarubicin, and etoposide, require increased levels of the enzyme Topo II to be effective. Cells in G_0 express only very low levels to Topo II, and increases in Topo II when cells enter G_1 have been demonstrated [18]. Cytokine-induced recruitment would therefore modulate the target cells in a way that would render them more susceptible to chemotherapy.

Another mechanism of enhanced drug action was recently described by Wiley [19, 20]. Cells incubated with GM-CSF significantly increased their nucleoside-transporter concentration and increased ara-C cytotoxicity was observed. This effect appeared to be unrelated to changes in the proliferative compartment of the leukemic cell population.

Previous studies from our and other groups have demonstrated a recruiting effect of G-CSF, GM-CSF, and IL-3 [21–25]. We have extended our initial observations, which were obtained in short-term suspension culture systems, to include clonogenic assays and results indicate that changes observed in suspension cultures parallel those observed in clonogenic assays. This may be related to the relatively small number of samples investigated. Nevertheless, a short term suspension culture assay for 48 h with subsequent flow cytometric measurement of cell cycle parameters (e. g., DNA/RNA, Ki67, PCNA) may be a useful tool in predicting in vivo response of individual patients to cytokines. Our studies demonstrate that the combination of G- plus GM-CSF is far inferior to combinations containing IL-3: the number of samples showing recruitment and the degree of recruitment observed increased significantly. This observation provides rationale for a clinical trial with IL-3 prior to chemotherapy in patients with AML, which will begin shortly at the M. D. Anderson Cancer

Center. The additional recruitment obtained with SCF provides rationale for future trials.

The limited recruitment by GM-CSF observed in vitro was also demonstrated in our in vivo studies. Although different clinical trials are combined in this analysis, it is apparent that only some patients demonstrated significant recruitment in vivo induced by GM-CSF. This may be related to the absence of GM-CSF receptors, and future studies of GM-CSF receptors will investigate whether the absence of receptors predicts for the absence of kinetic responses.

Our studies also demonstrate that increases in peripheral blast counts are not paralleled in all cases by cell kinetic recruitment. All cases with recruitment showed a concommitent increase in circulating blasts, but the reverse was not true. This may be related to the down regulation of adhesion molecules on myeloblasts by GM-CSF.

We hope that the in vitro observations and the initial clinical trials will become starting points for a new period of leukemia therapy: manipulations of drug dosage and scheduling have probably reached a plateau at the present time, and we propose, therefore, to modulate cellular features in order to render leukemic cells more sensitive to chemotherapy.

Many open questions remain. These include the selective stimulation of leukemic versus normal progenitor cells. This question will be answered by a combination of cell kinetic and fluorescence in situ hybridization studies. Furthermore, the induction of differentiation by cytokines was recently observed in patients with AML and may diminish the subsequent efficacy of chemotherapy [26]. Timing of cytokine treatment will therefore play a major role in the planned studies, and these issues require careful clinical investigation.

Summary

Previous studies have demonstrated that hematopoietic growth factors can enhance cytotoxicity of cell cycle therapeutic agents in acute myeloblastic leukemia (AML). We and others have previously reported that recombinant human G-CSF, GM-CSF, and IL-3 recruit leukemic cells into the cell cycle and that recruitment is associated with increased cell killing by cytosine arabinoside (ara-C) and daunorubicin (DNR). We now report detailed cytokinetic and clonogenic analysis of ten AML samples and compare the effects of G-CSF and GM-CSF with those of G-CSF, GM-CSF, and IL-3 combined. Cytokinetic analysis includes determination of quiescent G_0 cells and of cells in G_1 and S phase. Increased clonogenic growth of leukemic colonies (CFU-L) in methylcellulose was observed by the combination of G-CSF, GM-CSF, and IL-3 in 4/10 samples studied. Flow cytometric analysis of cell cycle kinetis was indicative of recruitment in 5/10 samples. Importantly, the IL-3 containing combination was significantly more effective than the combination of G-CSF and GM-CSF. rhSCF was found to further enhance recruitment in serum free medium.

Results in 11 AML patients treated with rhGM-CSF indicate induced recruitment in vivo: the doses used were 125 and 250 µg/m² s. c. for 1–8 days or 25 µg/m² for 3–22 days. Five of 10 patients treated with high dose GM-CSF showed either a decrease in G_0 cells or an increase in S cells, or both. An increase in circulating blasts was seen in 7/10 patients. All patients with cell kinetic changes also had increases in circulating blast cells.

The in vitro experiments would predict a significantly increased efficacy for IL-3 alone or in combination with other cytokines in the recruitment of leukemic cells.

References

1. Paietta E, Mittermayer K, Schwarzmeier J (1980) Proliferation kinetics and cycline AMP as prognostic factors in adult acute leukemia. Cancer 46: 102–108
2. Raza A, Maheshwari Y, Preisler HD (1987) Differences in cell cycle characteristics among patients with acute nonlymphocytic leukemia. Blood 69: 1647
3. Andreeff M (1986) Cell kinetics of leukemia. Sem Hematol 23: 300
4. Andreeff M, Gaynor J, Chapman D, Little C, Gee T, Clarkson BD (1987) Prognostic fac-

tors in acute lymphoblastic leukemia in adults: the Memorial Hospital experience. In: Buechner T, Shellong G, Hiddemann W, Urbanitz D, Ritter W (eds) Haematology and blood transfusions. Springer, Heidelberg New York, p 111

5. Clarkson BD, Fried J, Strife A, Sakai Y, Ota K, Ohkita T (1970) Studies of cellular proliferation in human leukemia. III Behavior of leukemic cells in three adults with acute leukemia given continuous infusion of 3H-Thymidine for 8 or 10 days. Cancer 25: 1327

6. Andreeff M, Assing G, Cirrincione C (1984) Prognostic value of DNA/RNA flow cytometry in myeloblastic and lymphoblastic leukemia in adults: RNA content and S-phase predict remission duration and survival in multivariate analysis. Ann NY Acad Sci 467: 387

7. Vellenga E, Ostapovica D, O'Rourke B, Griffin JD (1987) Effects of recombinant Il-3, GM-CSF, and G-CSF on proliferation of leukemic clonogenic cells in short-term and long-term cultures. Leukemia 1: 584

8. Strife A, Lambek C, Wisniewski D, Gulati S, Gasson JC, Golde DW, Welte K, Gabrilove JL, Clarkson B (1987) Activities of four purified growth factors on highly enriched human hematopoietic progenitor cells. Blood 69: 1508

9. Kelleher C,, Miyauchi J, Wong G, Clark S, Minden MD, McCulloch EA (1987) Synergism between recombinant growth factors, GM-CSF and G-CSF, acting on the blast cells of acute myeloblastic leukemia. Blood 69: 1948

10. Lista P, Porcu P, Avanzi GC, Pegoraro L (1988) Inteleukin-3 enhances the cytotoxic activity of 1-beta-d-arabinofuranosylcytosine (ara-c) n acute myeloblastic leukemia (AML) cells. British Journal of Haematology 69: 121

11. Cannistra SA, Groshek P, Griffin JD (1989) Granulocyte-macrophage colony-stimulating factor enhances the cytotoxic effects of cytosine arabinoside in acute myeloblastic leukemia and in the myeloid blast crisis phase of chronic myeloid leukemia. Leukemia 3: 328

12. Miyauchi J, Kelleher CA, Wang C, Minkin S, McCulloch EA (1989) Growth factors influence the sensitivity of leukemic stem cells to cytosine arabinoside in culture. Blood 73: 1272

13. Tafuri A, Andreeff M (1990) Kinetic rationale for cytosine-induced recruitment of myeloblastic leukemia followed by cycle-specific chemotherapy in vitro. Leukemia 12: 826

14. Bettelheim P, Valent P, Andreeff M, Tafuri A, Haimi J, Gorischek C, Muhm M, Sillaber C, Haas O, Vieder L, Maurer D, Schulz G, Speiser W, Geissler K, Kier P, Hinterberger W, Lechner K (1991) Recombinant human granulocyte-macrophage colony-stimulating factor in combination with standard induction chemotherapy in de novo acute myeloid leukemia. Blood 77: 700

15. Estey E, Kantarjian H, O'Brien S, Beran M, McCredie K, Koller C, Schachner J, Keating M (1991) Use of GM-CSF prior to chemotherapy of newly-diagnosed AML. In: Acute leukemias. Pharmacokinetics and management of relapsed and refractory disease. Hiddemann W, Buechner T, Keating M, Plunkett W, Andreeff M (eds)

16. Lemoli RM, Gulati SC, Strife A, Lambek C, Perez A, Clarkson BD (1991) Proliferative response of human acute myeloid leukemia cells and normal marrow enriched progenitors cells to human recombinant growth factors IL3, GM-CSF and G-CSF alone and in combination. Leukemia (in press)

17. Andreeff M, Darzynkiewicz Z, Sharpless TK, Clarkson BD, Melamed MR (1980) Discrimination of human leukemia subtypes by flow cytometric analysis of cellular DNA and RNA. Blood 55: 282

18. Estey E, Adlakha RC, Hittelman WN, Zwelling LA (1987) Cell cycle stage-dependent variations in drug-induced topoisomerase II-mediated DNA cleavage and cytotoxicity. Biochemistry 26: 4338–4344

19. Wiley JS, Brocklebank AM, Snook MA, Jamieson GP, Sawyer WH, Craik JD, Cass CE, Robins MJ, McAdam DP, Paterson RP (1991) A new fluorescent probe for the equilibrative inhibitor-sensitive nucleoside transporter. Biochem J 273: 667–672

20. Wiley JS, Jamieson GP, Brocklebank AM, Snook MB, Sawjer WH, Paterson ARP (1991) Saenta-fluorescein: new flow cytometry reagent for the nucleoside transporter of leukemic cells. Ann Hematol 62: A7–A7

21. Lista P, Brizzi MF, Rossi M, Resegotti L, Clark SC, Pegoraro L (1990) Different sensitivity of normal and leukaemic progenitor cells to ARA-C and IL-3 combined. Br J Haematol 76: 21

22. Tafuri A, Hegewisch S, Souza L, Andreeff M (1988) Stimulation of leukemic blast cells in vitro bu colony stimulating factors (G-CSF, GM-CSF) ad interleukin-3 (IL-3): evidence of recruitment and increased cell killing with cytosine arabinoside (ara-C). Blood 72: 105 a

23. Tafuri A, Andreeff M (1990) Cell kinetic modulation of hematological malignancies

116

by cytokines: recruitment therapy to overcome cytokinetic resistance. In: Mertelsmann R, Herrmann F (eds) Hematopoietic growth factors in clinical application. Dekker, New York, pp 381–399

24. Cannistra SA, DiCarlo J, Groshek P, Kanakura Y, Berg D, Mayer RJ, Griffin JD (1991) Simultaneous administration of granulocyte-macrophage colony-stimulating factor and cytosine arabinoside for the treatment of relapsed acute myeloid leukemia. Leukemia 3: 230–238

25. Wang YF, Kelleher CA, Minkin S, McCulloch EA (1991) Effects of rGM-CSF on the cisplatin sensitivity of the blast cells of acute myeloblastic leukemia. Leukemia 3: 239–248

26. Wormann B, Terstappen LW, Safford M, Konemann S, Piechotka K, Rottmann R, Hiddeman W, Buechner T (1991) In vivo effects of GM-CSF on leukemic blasts in acute myeloid leukemia. Proc ASCO, #749

Simultaneous Administration of Granulocyte-Macrophage Colony-Stimulating Factor and Cytosine Arabinoside for the Treatment of High-Risk Myeloid Leukemia*

S. A. Cannistra, J. DiCarlo, P. Groshek, Y. Kanakura, D. Berg, R. Stone, R. J. Mayer, and J. D. Griffin

Introduction

Patients with refractory or relapsed acute myeloid leukemia (AML) are often treated with regimens containing high-dose cytosine arabinoside (ARA-C), resulting in complete response rates of approximately 30% to 50%, with a median remission duration of approximately 4 months [1]. Likewise, patients with the myeloid blast crisis of chronic myeloid leukemia (CML) are often treated with high dose ARA-C, with re-establishment of a short-lived stable phase in only about 20% of cases [2]. An important reason for treatment failure in these high-risk patients is likely to be pharmacologic resistance to ARA-C, which may be due to multiple mechanisms including decreased intracellular levels of deoxycytidine kinase and decreased intracellular uptake of ARA-C. Since ARA-C is a cell-cycle-specific drug, another potential mechanism of resistance may be related to the observation that a large fraction of leukemic clonogenic cells is not in S phase at the time of ARA-C exposure [3]. We have attempted to overcome kinetic resistance to ARA-C in vitro by recruiting leukemic cells into S phase through the use of recombi-

nant human granulocyte-macrophage colony-stimulating factor (rhGM-CSF), a humoral factor which supports the in vitro proliferation of clonogenic cells from the majority of patients with AML [4]. We have previously shown in tissue culture that this agent is able to effectively increase the fraction of leukemic clonogenic cells in S phase, and that this effect is associated with a significant increase in ARA-C-mediated cytotoxicity [5]. Since rhGM-CSF is biologically active and well-tolerated when administered to patients with normal bone marrow function [6–8], we chose to study the in vivo kinetic and therapeutic effects of combined rhGM-CSF and high dose ARA-C treatment in a population of high risk patients with myeloid leukemia. We now report the results of this treatment strategy in six patients with relapsed or refractory AML, and in two patients with the myeloid blast crisis of CML.

Materials and Methods

Patient Selection

High-risk myeloid leukemia patients eligible for this study have been previously defined [9]. Briefly, patients appropriate for this study include (a) those with AML which is refractory to two courses of standard induction chemotherapy (3 days of daunorubicin and 7 days of ARA-C, followed by 2 days of daunorubicin and 5 days of ARA-C if bone marrow blasts persist by day 14), (b) those with AML which has relapsed within 1 year of achieving com-

The Divisions of Tumor Immunology and Medical Oncology, Dana-Farber Cancer Institute, Harvard Medical School, Boston, Massachusetts, USA
* Supported in part by Public Health Service Grants No CA 36167, CA 42802, and CA 34183, Biomedical Research Support Grant No SO7RR05526-26, and by the U.S. Cancer Research Council.

plete remission, or (c) those with the myeloid blast crisis of CML as defined by the development of at least 30 % bone marrow myeloblasts (as determined by morphology and surface marker analysis) in the setting of Philadelphia chromosome-positive CML. Other criteria necessary for enrollment include: peripheral blast count $\leq$ 75 000/mm/³, no evidence of leukostasis or clotting diathesis, no evidence of severe systemic infection, $\geq$ 30 % bone marrow blasts, no prior history of cerebellar dysfunction, no history of neurologic toxicity to ARA-C; normal renal and hepatic function, age greater than 18 years, Eastern Cooperative Ecology Group (ECOG) performance status 0-2, and written informed consent. The study was approved by the Scientific Review Committee and the Human Protection Committee of the Dana-Farber Cancer Institute.

Study Design

This was an open labeled, nonrandomized phase I clinical study in which all patients received an 18 h "priming" period of recombinant human rhGM-CSF as described below, followed by the institution of high dose ARA-C therapy. rhGM-CSF was administered throughout the duration of ARA-C therapy, after which both drugs were discontinued. rhGM-CSF was administered intravenously at a dose of either 0.45 μg/kg h (CHO-derived material) or 0.21 μg/kg h (E. Coli-derived material) as a continuous infusion through a central venous catheter. As stated below, the first six patients received CHO-derived GM-CSF, after which the product was switched to E. Coli-derived material in order to accommodate a policy change on the part of the supplier. ARA-C was initially administered intravenously over 3 h at a dose of 3 g/m², every 12 h for a total of six doses. After treating patient 1, the protocol was modified by reducing the ARA-C dose to 2 g/m² for a total of eight doses in order to reduce the risk of ARA-C-mediated neurotoxicity. The protocol called for stopping rhGM-CSF prematurely if leukemic exacerbation occurred during treatment, defined as the development of leukostasis or a peripheral

blast count of greater than 150 000/mm³. Standard supportive measures including broad spectrum antibiotic administration for the treatment of fever in the setting of neutropenia were provided.

rhGM-CSF

rhGM-CSF was provided by two sources. For the first six patients, the rhGM-SCF was supplied by Sandoz Pharmaceuticals (Basel, Switzerland) and was purified from media conditioned by transfected CHO cells, with a specific activity of 5.4×10^6 units/mg glycoprotein (8.0×10^6 units/mg aglycoprotein). For the last two patients, rhGM-CSF was provided by Schering-Plough and was purified from media conditioned by transfected E. coli.

Laboratory Studies

Sources of Human Cells

Bone marrow was aspirated into heparinized syringes immediately prior to and 18 h after the institution of rhGM-CSF therapy. The mononuclear fraction was separated by Ficoll-Hypaque density gradient centrifugation and used for the study of cell cycle kinetics and GM-CSF receptor occupancy as described below. All mononuclear cell specimens from the three patients studied in this report contained between 68 % and 90 % blast forms, the remainder of cells being promyelocytes, myelocytes, metamyelocytes, bands, and monocytes.

Cell Cycle Analysis

Three separate techniques were used to evaluate the cell cycle status of leukemic blasts in this study. The S phase fraction of leukemic blasts was determined by (a) in vitro incorporation of bromodeoxyuridine (BrdU) as assessed by fluorescence microscopy, (b) DNA histogram analysis with propidium iodide (PI) as assessed by flow cytometry, and (c) thymidine suicide analysis of leukemic clonogenic cells. The details of these techniques have been previously reported [9].

Binding of Iodinated rhGM-CSF to Leukemic Myeloblasts

The procedure for the binding of rhGM-CSF to myeloid cells was performed as previously described [10]. rhGM-CSF was iodinated by the Bolton-Hunter reagent, with a maximum binding capacity of approximately 80 % and a specific activity of 50–100 µCi/µg protein as determined by self-displacement analysis. Equilibrium binding was determined to occur after 1.5 h of incubation at 37 °C in the presence of sodium azide (0.02 % w/v). Receptor number was determined by Scatchard analysis using mean data from duplicate samples at each concentration of iodinated rhGM-CSF [10]. The standard error of the mean for duplicate samples was ≤ 15 %.

Analysis of GM-CSF Receptor Occupancy in Leukemic Myeloblasts

We have previously shown that acid treatment of myeloid cells (phosphate-buffered solution, (PBS) pH 3.0 for 2 min at 4 °C) removes approximately 80 % prebound rhGM-CSF while completely preserving receptor integrity, permitting an assessment of the degree of receptor occupancy by comparing the results of Scatchard analysis of cells treated with or without acid. The details of this technique have been previously reported [10].

Measurement of rhGM-CSF Plasma Levels

An enzyme-linked immunoabsorbant assay (ELISA) was used to determine rhGM-CSF levels prior to an 18 h after the start of rhGM-CSF therapy. The details of this technique have been reported [9]. The lower limit of detection of this assay is approximately 100 pg/ml rhGM-CSF.

Statistical Analysis

Significance levels for comparison between treatment groups were determined using the two-sided Student's t test for unpaired samples.

Results

Clinical Characteristics

The characteristics of the eight patients with high-risk myeloid leukemia who were enrolled in this study are shown in Table 1. Of note is that AML patients 1, 3, and 4 had disease refractory to standard therapy, and AML patients 2, 5, and 6 had disease which relapsed after achievement of complete remission. Patient 2 was entered onto protocol therapy after his fifth AML relapse (after having received multiple courses of high dose ARA-C). Patient 7 presented with the myeloid blast crisis of CML and received initial treatment with hydroxyurea in order to acheive white count control prior to study entry. Patient 8 had a previous history of CML which had progressed to myeloid blast crisis 5 years before study entry. At that time, he was successfully induced into a second stable phase with high dose ARA-C alone. Five years later he was entered into the current study at the time of his second myeloid blast crisis.

Effects of In Vivo rhGM-CSF Administration on the Fraction of Leukemic Cells in S Phase

Each patient received a priming period of continuous infusion rhGM-CSF for 18 h prior to the institution of ARA-C therapy, permitting assessment of the S phase fraction of leukemic cells prior to and after 18 h of treatment. Kinetic studies were performed on bone marrow blasts for each patient at 0 h and 18 h. As shown in Table 2, six of seven evaluable patients demonstrated a significant rise in the percentage of bone marrow blasts in S phase after 18 h of rhGM-CSF therapy as assessed by BrdU analysis. No increment in the S phase fraction was observed for patient 8. In contrast, no significant change was observed in the DNA histogram obtained after staining with PI in most patients, with the exception of patient 2, who demonstrated a borderline significant increase in the leukemic S phase fraction after 18 h (Table 2). The insensitivity of the PI technique most likely relates to the fact that

Table 1. Patient Characteristics

Patient	Age/sex	Dx (FAB)	First line Rx[a]	Outcome of first line Rx	Second line Rx at relapse	Outcome of second line Rx	% BM blasts at study entry	WBC at entry (% blasts)[b]
1	64/F	AML(M2)	3+7	CRX3mo	HiDAC	persistent Dz	52	9.1 (57)
2	59/M	AML(M4E)	3+7	CRX2y	HiDAC	CRX4mo	76	0.8 (9)
3	43/M	AML(M1)	3+7/2+5	persistent Dz	none[c]	NA	30	10.3 (1)
4	17/M	AML(M1)	3+7/2+5	persistent Dz	HiDAC	persistent Dz	65	8.7 (36)
5	19/F	AML(M1)	3+7/2+5/HiDAC	CRX3mo	none[c]	NA	83	1.7 (12)
6	20/F	AML(M1)	3+7/2+5/HiDAC	CRX7mo	none[c]	NA	38	6.0 (21)
7	24/M	CML MBC	hydroxyurea	WBC control	NA	NA	31	12.9 (26)
8	32/M	CML MBC	HiDAC	SP X 5 y	hydroxyurea	WBC control	48	16.4 (48)

Dx, diagnosis; AML, acute myeloid leukemia; CML MBC, chronic myeloid leukemia in myeloid blast crisis; CR, complete remission; mo, month; y, years; WBC, white blood count; SP, stable phase; Rx, treatment; BM, bone marrow; Dz, disease; HiDAC, high dose ARA-C; NA, not applicable
[a] 3+7=3 days of daunorubicin (45 mg/m² day) and 7 days of ARA-C (200 mg/m²/day); 2+5=2 days of daunorubicin and 5 days of ARA-C; Hi-DAC=2–3 g ARA-C/m²/day × 6–8 doses.
[b] Value expressed as WBC/mm³ × 10⁻³.
[c] no second-line treatment was administered prior to study entry.

121

Table 2. Effects of GM-CSF on the S phase fraction of leukemic blasts in vivo

Patient	Time (h)	%S phase (BrdU)[a]	%S phase (PI)[b]
1	0	23[c]	9.7[d]
		$p = 0.009$[e]	$p = $ NS
	18	36	8.0
2	0	10	5
		$p = 0.04$	$p = 0.05$
	18	15	9
3	0	34	17
		$p = 0.04$	$p = $ NS
	18	44	20
4	0	ND	4
			$p = $ NS
	18	ND	6
5	0	35	12
		$p = 0.04$	$p = $ NS
	18	42	14
6	0	7	15
		$p = 0.001$	$p = $ NS
	18	15	14
7	0	9	15
		$p = 0.02$	$p = $ NS
	18	14	14
8	0	18	16
		$p = $ NS	$p = $ NS
	18	19	10

NS, not significant; ND, not determined

[a] The fraction of blasts incorporating bromodeoxyuridine (BrdU) was assessed by fluorescence microscopy as previously described [9].

[b] DNA histogram analysis was performed on a flow cytometer after staining nuclei with propidium iodide (PI) as previously described [9].

[c] Represents the mean S phase value of quadruplicate determinations (100 cells counted per determination). Standard error of the mean was less than 15% in each case.

[d] Represents the mean S phase value of duplicate determinations as assessed by analysis of the DNA histogram by the PARA-1 computer modeling program [9]. Standard error of the mean was less than 15% in each case.

[e] P values were determined by using the two-sided Student's t-test for unpaired samples.

cells in early S phase may initially contain a DNA content which is close to that of cells in G_0/G_1, although these cells would be expected to be actively incorporating BrdU during this time period. In addition to studying whole populations of leukemic mononuclear cells by the BrdU and PI techniques, the kinetics of clonogenic cells from patient 1 and 8 were studied by the thymidine suicide technique [9]. The fraction of leukemic clonogenic cells in S phase at 0 h and 18 h in patient 1 was 33% and 55%, respectively ($p = 0.008$), whereas corresponding values for patient 8 were 44% and 53%, respectively ($p = $ not significant). Due to insufficient numbers of peripheral blood leukemic cells, kinetic assessment of circulating blasts was possible only in patient 1, whose peripheral blood contained 90% blasts after Ficoll-Hypaque density centrifugation. The peripheral blasts of this patient demonstrated an increase in the fraction of S phase from 3% $\pm$ 1% at 0 h to 6.7% $\pm$ 2% at 18 h ($p = 0.02$) as assessed by BrdU analysis.

Effects of rhGM-CSF Therapy on GM-CSF Receptor Expression in Leukemic Blasts

In order to evaluate the effects of in vivo rhGM-CSF administration on GM-CSF receptor expression in AML, Scatchard analysis was performed on leukemic blasts from patients 1, 2, 4, and 8 at 0 h and 18 h. Immediately prior to Scatchard analysis, the cells were treated with or without acid in order to remove previously bound rhGM-CSF and to thereby obtain an assessment of GM-CSF receptor occupancy both before and during rhGM-CSF therapy. Specific in vitro binding was demonstrated in all four patients tested (range: 45–126 receptors per cell, Table 3). Prior to the start of rhGM-CSF therapy, there was no difference in receptor density with or without acid treatment, suggesting that the GM-CSF receptor of leukemic blasts was not initially occupied by ligand in vivo. However, patients 1 and 2 demonstrated a decrease in rhGM-CSF binding at 18 h which was reversible upon acid treatment, suggesting that sufficient quantities of administered

Table 3. Effects of GM-CSF on GM-CSF receptor expression in leukemic myeloblasts

Patient	1		2		4		8	
Time (h)	0	18	0	18	0	18	0	18
Receptor								
Media	45[a]	16	117	78	120	126	92	87
Acid	39[b]	40	110	103	116	118	85	78
% occupancy[c]	0	60	0	24	0	0	0	0
% downregulation:[d]	0		6		0		8	

[a] Receptor number per blast cell as determined by Scatchard analysis [10].

[b] Acid treatment (PBS pH 3.0 for 2 min at 4°C) was used to remove prebound GM-CSF prior to performing Scatchard analysis in order to assess receptor occupancy as previously described [10].

[c] % occupancy = 100 X [receptor (time=18,acid) – receptor(time=18,media)]/[receptor-(time=18,acid)].

[d] % down-regulation=100 X [receptor(time=0,acid) – receptor(time=18,acid)]/[receptor-(time=0,acid)].

rhGM-CSF were binding to blasts in vivo and that significant receptor down-regulation had not occurred at 18 h (60% and 24% receptor occupancy, for patients 1 and 2, respectively, Table 3). In contrast, no evidence for significant receptor occupancy was observed for either patients 4 or 8 at 18 h. Since patient 4 demonstrated an increment in the S phase fraction after 18 h of GM-CSF therapy (Table 2), the absence of significant receptor occupancy suggests that our acid wash technique may be insensitive at detecting low levels of in vivo binding which may still be biologically relevant.

Alternatively, it is possible that the increase in the S-phase fraction is not directly mediated by GM-CSF administration in this patient. In contrast, the absence of receptor occupancy in patient 8 correlates well with the lack of S-phase increment after 18 h of GM-CSF therapy (Table 2).

The lack of significant receptor down-regulation after 18 h of GM-CSF exposure (Table 3) suggests that tachyphylaxis to the proliferative effects of this growth factor might not occur. Therefore, in order to determine whether leukemic cells obtained before and during rhGM-CSF therapy would be equally responsive to this growth factor in vitro, a dose-response curve of day 7 leukemic cluster formation as a function of rhGM-CSF concentration was obtained for patient 1. No difference was observed in the dose-response curves for leukemic blasts obtained at 0 h or 18 h over a rhGM-CSF concentration range of 0–25 ng/ml (data not shown).

Measurement of rhGM-CSF Levels During Treatment

Patients 1–4 had daily determinations of rhGM-CSF plasma levels by the ELISA technique, both prior to and during the infusion of rhGM-CSF. No patient had detectable rhGM-CSF levels prior to the institution of rhGM-CSF therapy. Steady state levels of rhGM-CSF were observed at 18 h of infusion, with the values for patients 1, 2, 3, and 4 being 7.9, 8.4, 12.0, and 9.0 ng/ml, respectively. These levels have been previously shown to provide a sufficient stimulus for the in vitro growth of leukemic clonogenic cells in agar culture [4]. Patient 2 required evaluation of cerebrospinal fluid obtained through a previously placed Ommaya reservoir to rule out the possibility of central nervous relapse. A sample of this cerebrospinal fluid revealed no measurable rhGM-CSF after 18 h of therapy. The half life of GM-CSF was determined in patient 4 to be bisphasic, with an initial $t_{1/2}$ of 2.5 h and a second $t_{1/2}$ of 4 h.

Hematologic Response During rhGM-CSF/ARA-C Therapy

GM-CSF administration resulted in a >2-fold increase in circulating blasts in five of the eight patients studied (range 1.3 to ten-fold, Table 4). No patient developed leukostasis or required GM-CSF discontinuation due to a blast count in excess of 150 000/mm^3. The total white count uniformly decreased after treatment day 2 in all patients despite continuation of GM-CSF during ARA-C administration. Patients 7 and 8 developed a first-dose reaction characterized by subacute onset of dyspnea, hypoxia (arterial PO$_2$ in the 50-60 mmHg range), flushing, and mild diaphoresis during the initial 4 h of GM-CSF administration, associated with the development of profound neutropenia (<500/mm^3). Electrocardiography and chest radiographs were normal in both patients. The patients were treated with intravenous hydration, supplemental oxygen, and temporary discontinuation of GM-CSF. Symptoms, hypoxia, and neutropenia, resolved within 6 h, after which GM-CSF was resumed without recurrence of the first dose reaction in either patient.

Toxicity of rhGM-CSF/ARA-C Therapy

The side effects of rhGM-CSF/ARA-C therapy are shown in Table 4. Of the five patients evaluable for duration of neutropenia, the median duration of < 500 neutrophils/mm^3 was 19 days (range 14–28, Table 4). Fever as high as 39.3 °C P.O. during GM-CSF/ARA-C administration was a frequent side effect, occurring in seven out of eight patients and resolving after drug discontinuation except in patient 8, who experienced coexistent Hickman line infection with Staphylococcus aureus on day 4. Patient 1 developed dysarthria and dysmetria consistent with ARA-C cerebellar neurotoxicity approximately 24 h after discontinuation of ARA-C. This progressed to include stupor and grand mal seizures by day 10. The ARA-C dose was decreased to 2 g/m^2 per dose, eight total doses, for subsequent patients. Although no other patient experienced CNS toxicity directly attributable to GM-CSF/ARA-C, patient 3 developed nystagmus felt to be consistent with the effect of phenothiazine, and patient 4 developed bilateral seventh nerve palsies due to leukemic meningitis. From a cardiac standpoint, patient 1 developed chest pain shortly after GM-CSF discontinuation and was found to have a pericardial friction rub. The ECG was consistent with pericarditis, assumed to be related to GM-CSF administration, and she was treated symptomatically. No other patient developed a GM-CSF-induced cardiac complication, although patient 6 experienced self-limited sinus tachycardia (heart rate $\approx$ 110–120/min) on day 14 probably due to a malpositioned Hickman catheter, and patient 8 developed reversible hypotension on day 4 due to S. aureus Hickman line sepsis. Two out of eight patients developed a first dose reaction as noted above. During the first week of treatment, three of eight patients developed transient, mild renal dysfunction manifested by increases in the serum creatinine in the 2 mg/dl range, and five out of eight developed reversible increases in liver function tests (Table 4).

Response to rhGM-CSF/ara-C Therapy

All patients experienced initial clearing of peripheral blood blasts by day 5 of therapy. Three of eight patients achieved a satisfactory response to GM-CSF/ARA-C therapy (38 %). Specifically, a complete remission was reestablished in AML patients 2 and 6, and return of stable phase disease was achieved in CML patient 7. Patient 2 remained in remission for 4 months (approximately the same duration as his previous remission), after which he relapsed and subsequently died of disease refractory to VP-16 and mitoxantrone. Patient 6 underwent an ex vivo purged autologous marrow transplant three weeks after recovery from GM-CSF/ARA-C therapy and was without evidence of relapse 5 months after transplant. Patient 7 recovered > 500/mm^3 neutrophils on day 19 with a subsequent bone marrow consistent with stable phase disease. After approximately 3 months, during which he has remained in stable phase, he is currently undergoing a partially

Table 4. Outcome of patients treated with GM-CSF/ARA-C

Patient	Blasts[c]	Hematologic S phase[d]	Neutropenia[e]	first dose Reaction[a]	Fever[b]	CNS	Cardiac	Renal	Hepatic	Response
1	1.3	1.6	+8	None	+	+[f]	+[g]	+[h]	+[i]	Persistent dz
2	3.5	1.5	28	None	+	None	None	+	+	CRX4mo
3	10.0	1.3	15	None	None	+[j]	None	None	+	Persistent dz
4	2.3	No change	14	None	+	+[k]	None	None	None	Persistent dz
5	3.7	1.2	+13	None	+	None	None	None	None	Persistent dz
6	1.5	2.1	19	+[m]	+	None	+[l]	None	None	CR, transplant
7	1.3	1.6	19	+[m]	+	None	None	None	+	Stable phase
8	3.2	No change	+20	None	+	None	+[n]	+	+	Persistent dz

a As described in text.

b Defined as P.O. temperature above 100.8 °F (approximately 38.2 °C) occurring during GM-CSF/ARA-C administration.

c Ratio of maximum level of circulating blasts during GM-CSF administration to baseline value prior to treatment.

d Ratio of S phase fraction at 18 h to S phase fraction prior to treatment (see Table 2).

e Duration of neutropenia expressed in days. Plus sign indicates that patient was not fully evaluable due to being withdrawn from study (due to persistent disease) prior to bone marrow recovery.

f Developed severe, irreversible ARA-C neurotoxicity on day 5.

g Developed pericarditis on day 5.

h Transient increased creatinine during first week of GM-CSF/ARA-C therapy.

i Transient increased bilirubin during first week of GM-CSF/ARA-C therapy.

j Developed bilateral seventh nerve palsies in the setting of positive CSF cytology on day 15.

k Developed nystagmus on days 2–4 consistent with phenothiazine effect.

l Sinus tachycardia on day 14 probably due to malpositioned Hickman catheter.

m Developed within the first 4 h of GM-CSF administration and associated with profound, reversible neutropenia.

n Hypotension on day 4 due to Staphylococcus aureus Hickman line sepsis and associated anterior chest wall cellulitis.

mismatched allogeneic bone marrow transplant.

Patients 1, 3, 4, 5, and 8 did not achieve either a complete remission or resumption of stable phase disease after GM-CSF/ARA-C treatment. Patient 1 died on day 13 of hemodynamic compromise related to pericardial tamponade. At autopsy, the pericardium was filled with hemorrhagic fluid and a fibrinous pericarditis was observed. There was no evidence of inflammatory or leukemic cell infiltration on histologic review. The brain showed evidence of cerebellar degeneration and Purkinje cell loss consistent with ARA-C neurotoxicity. Post-mortem bone marrow examination revealed hypocellularity with residual leukemic blasts. Patients 3, 4, and 5 have subsequently died of complications related to active disease. Patient 8 remains alive 3 months after failure of GM-CSF/ARA-C treatment and is currently undergoing ablative therapy with VP-16, cytoxan, and daunorubicin followed by reinfusion of previously collected peripheral blood stem cells.

Discussion

The treatment of patients with relapsed/refractory AML or CML myeloid blast crisis remains a difficult clinical problem. High-dose ARA-C-containing regimens offer the most effective therapy for these patients, producing short-lived complete response rates of between 20% and 50% [1, 2]. Although pharmacologic resistance to ARA-C undoubtedly represents a major obstacle in the treatment of these patients, kinetic resistance due to the presence of a quiescent population of leukemic blasts that are not actively proliferating may also play an important role in treatment failure. It is known that a significant fraction of leukemic cells is not actively synthesizing DNA at the time of therapy. For example, it has been shown that generally less than 50% of leukemic clonogenic cells are in S phase by using either thymidine or ARA-C suicide techniques [3], which suggests that strategies designed to increase the fraction of clonogenic cells in S phase may enhance the degree of ARA-C-mediated cytotoxici-

ty. In this regard, we have previously demonstrated that in vitro treatment of leukemic blasts with rhGM-CSF for 24 h provides an effective stimulus for the recruitment of myeloid leukemic blasts into S phase, and that this effect is associated with a significant increase in cell killing by ARA-C [5]. These results have also been confirmed by other investigators, who have suggested that GM-CSF is capable of both enhancing the leukemic S phase fraction and mobilizing leukemic blasts from the G_0 to G_1 phases of the cell cycle [11].

Although in vitro studies have demonstrated that GM-CSF may enhance ARA-C-mediated killing of leukemic myeloblasts, it is possible that this effect might not result in a significant clinical benefit. For instance, myeloid leukemic cells may already be exposed to a maximal proliferative stimulus in vivo which may or may not be related to endogenous rhGM-CSF secretion. Several other hematopoietic growth factors are known to stimulate myeloid leukemic cell growth, including IL-3 and G-CSF, and it is possible that these factors may be partly or wholly responsible for in vivo leukemic cell proliferation [4]. Therefore, the present clinical trial was designed to investigate whether exogenously administered rhGM-CSF could increase leukemic cell proliferation above baseline levels, and whether this treatment approach resulted in acceptable toxicity in high risk myeloid leukemia patients. The data presented in this study suggest that rhGM-CSF is capable of enhancing the S phase fraction of leukemic myeloblasts over a relatively short "priming" period of 18 h, and that this effect is often associated with a rise in the level of circulating blasts (Table 4). The toxicity profile of this regimen appears to be acceptable in this small series, with no patient experiencing leukostasis and with tolerable durations of neutropenia. Although the study design does not allow an assessment of the efficacy of this regimen when compared to ARA-C alone, a 38% response rate in this high risk patient population is encouraging. Although the small numbers of patients preclude a meaningful analysis of the relationship between kinetic response and outcome, it is interesting to note that three out of four patients who experienced a $\geq$ 1.6-fold increment in the leukemic S phase fraction during GM-CSF treatment entered either complete remission or stable phase disease (Table 4).

The use of fluorescence microscopy to detect BrdU incorporation by leukemic blasts may offer several advantages over standard DNA histogram analysis using PI. First, the technique may be applied to bone marrow samples with low cell numbers which may not otherwise be amenable to flow cytometric analysis. Also, the technique allows assessment of nuclear morphology and thereby reduces the possibility of including nonleukemic cells in the analysis. This is important in view of the fact that each of our leukemic samples contained a small fraction of other myeloid cells such as metamyelocytes, bands, and monocytes, which could be readily distinguished from blasts on the basis of nuclear shape. Because it is impossible to discriminate between the nuclear morphology of blasts, promyelocytes, and myelocytes by fluorescent microscopy, it is possible that contamination of the leukemic samples by these more mature myeloid cell types could have partially contributed to the increase in S phase observed with GM-CSF. Nevertheless, data obtained from the $_3$H-thymidine suicide technique in patient 1 suggest that the observed increase in the S phase fraction involves the leukemic clonogenic cell population. Finally, the BrdU technique allows more sensitive detection of cells in early S phase, before they have synthesized enough DNA to be detectable by DNA histogram analysis with PI (Table 2) [12].

In this study, we have also shown that it is possible to achieve biologically relevant concentrations of GM-CSF in plasma, associated with significant rhGM-CSF binding to bone marrow leukemic blasts in some patients. Importantly, there was no evidence of significant GM-CSF receptor down-regulation over an 18 h period in four out of four patients tested (Table 3). The absence of significant receptor down-regulation in leukemic myeloblasts by GM-CSF in vivo is in agreement with our previous in vitro observations [13] and suggests that tachyphylaxis to the proliferative effects of this factor might not occur. This conclusion is also supported by the observation that

the sensitivity of leukemic blasts to the proliferative effects of rhGM-CSF in vitro was unchanged after rhGM-CSF exposure in patient 1. Our data are also in agreement with those of Broxmeyer et al, who found no evidence of progenitor cell resistance to rhGM-CSF in patients with the myeloproliferative syndrome treated with rhGM-CSF for up to 2 weeks [14].

It is possible that the simultaneous administration of rhGM-CSF and ARA-C may result in undesirable side effects such as exacerbation of leukemia, or prolonged durations of neutropenia due to co-stimulation of normal bone marrow myeloid progenitor cells by rhGM-CSF. No patient experienced leukemic exacerbation during the administration of rhGM-CSF/ARA-C therapy, although all patients experienced a transient increase in the absolute numbers of circulating blasts (Table 4). Although this increase was asymptomatic, all of our patients began therapy with relatively low numbers of circulating blasts (Table 1). Therefore, it is still possible that treatment of patients with initially high levels of circulating blasts may result in the development of leukostasis. None of our evaluable patients experienced durations of neutropenia that were unexpected for such a heavily pretreated population receiving high dose ARA-C. The possibility of prolinged duration of neutropenia with combined rhGM-CSF/ARA-C therapy is based upon the known ability of this growth factor to stimulate multipotent, committed progenitor cells (i.e., CFU-GEMM), potentially increasing ARA-C-mediated cytotoxicity of normal bone marrow precursors. Although we cannot rule out a significant effect of combined rhGM-CSF/ARA-C therapy on bone marrow recovery in view of the small number of patients studied thus far, the fact that rhGM-CSF is a relatively poor stimulator of the earliest pluripotent stem cell which can be identified in vitro (i.e., CFU-BLAST) suggests that this effect may not be clinically significant [15].

Pericarditis is a rare complication of rhGM-CSF therapy, usually when this factor is administered at doses higher than that used in the present study [16]. Whether synergistic pericardial toxicity exists between rhGM-CSF and ARA-C is unknown at present, although it is becoming increasingly clear that receptors for rhGM-CSF are not restricted to the hematopoietic lineage [17]. In view of the observed pericardial toxicity of rhGM-CSF/ARA-C therapy in patient 1, the expression of GM-CSF receptors by pericardial mesothelium deserves further study. In addition, patient 1 developed severe ARA-C-associated neurotoxicity, raising the possibility that rhGM-CSF may have altered the permeability of the blood-brain barrier, resulting in elevated levels of ARA-C in the CNS. Although levels of rhGM-CSF or ARA-C were not evaluated in the cerebrospinal fluid of patient 1, there was no detectable rhGM-CSF in the cerebrospinal fluid of patient 2 after 18 h of therapy, suggesting that rhGM-CSF itself does not cross the blood-brain barrier. Since ARA-C neurotoxicity is observed in approximately 15 %–20 % of patients above the age of 50 [18], it is also possible that the neurologic toxicity observed in patient 1 is solely related to ARA-C.

Our study is in agreement with the experience of Muhm et al, who also documented in vivo recruitment of leukemic blasts into the cell cycle after a 24–48 h pretreatment of AML patients with rhGM-CSF [19]. However, it is also possible that some of the changes observed in the leukemic S phase fraction in our study may be due to variability in cell cycle kinetics over time in this patient population, rather than induction of leukemic cell proliferation by rhGM-CSF. Since there is no information regarding serial cell cycle kinetic measurements over an 18 h period in patients with AML, this issue would be best addressed as part of a future clinical trial designed to investigate the cell cycle kinetics of patients randomized to receive either placebo or GM-CSF treatment prior to chemotherapy administration. Furthermore, since our study was designed to assess the biological effects and toxicity of rhGM-CSF/ARA-C therapy in high-risk patients with myeloid leukemia, it is impossible at the present time to precisely evaluate the effectiveness of this strategy on clinical outcome. Nevertheless, the results of this trial suggest that cell-cycle recruitment of myeloid leukemic cells in an attempt to improve the effectiveness of S-phase specific drugs is feasible through the use of recombinant hematopoietic growth factors such as rhGM-CSF. Further clinical investigation of the use of GM-CSF as a cell-cycle recruiting agent in patients with high-risk myeloid leukemia who are not already pharmacologically resistant to ARA-C are warranted.

Summary

High dose cytosine arabinoside (ARA-C) is often used in the treatment of patients with relapsed or refractory acute myeloid leukemia (AML), or those with the myeloid blast crisis of chronic myeloid leukemia (CML). This therapy typically results in short-lived complete response rates of 20 %–50 %. We have previously shown that entry of myeloid leukemic cells into S phase can be accelerated in vitro through the use of recombinant human granulocyte-macrophage colony stimulating factor (rhGM-CSF), resulting in enhancement of ARA-C-mediated cytotoxicity. In order to evaluate the in vivo biological and clinical effects of this strategy in patients with high-risk myeloid leukemia, we have treated six patients with either refractory or relapsed AML, and two patients with CML myeloid blast crisis, with a continuous infusion of rhGM-CSF for 18 h, followed by the institution of high dose ARA-C therapy. Recombinant GM-CSF was continued throughout the 4-day duration of ARA-C treatment and was stopped after the last dose of ARA-C was administered. Prior to therapy, four out of four patients tested had no detectable levels of circulating rhGM-CSF. There was no evidence of GM-CSF receptor occupancy (pretherapy) in leukemic myeloblasts of 4/4 patients tested. After 18 h of rhGM-CSF therapy, four out of four evaluable patients had biologically active levels of circulating rhGM-CSF (7.9–12.0 ng/ml). A significant rise in the S phase fraction of leukemic myeloblasts was observed at 18 h of rhGM-CSF treatment in five of six patients evaluated by BrdU incorporation. Five out of eight patients showed a > two-fold rise in the peripheral blast count during rhGM-CSF/ARA-C administration, followed by profound, but clinically tolerable, myelosuppression. No patient developed clinical evidence of leukostasis during GM-CSF therapy. The median duration of neutropenia ($< 500/mm^3$) was 19 days. There were three out of eight clinical responses (38 %). Two out of six patients with AML experienced complete morphologic remission, with one patient subsequently receiving a purged autologous transplant three weeks later, and the other patient relapsing after a remission duration of 4 months. One of two patients with CML myeloid blast crisis reentered a second stable phase. These results suggest that exogenously administered rhGM-CSF is capable of rapidly mobilizing leukemic cells into S phase in vivo and theoretically should be useful in overcoming kinetic resistance to ARA-C.

References

1. Mayer RJ (1987) Current chemotherapeutic treatment approaches to the management of previously untreated adults with de novo acute myelogenous leukemia. Semin Oncol 14: 384–396
2. Iacoboni SJ, Plunkett W, Kantarjian HM, Estey E, Keating MJ, McCredie KB, Freireich EJ (1986) High dose cytosine arabinoside: treatment and cellular pharmacology of chronic myelogenous leukemia blast crisis. J Clin Oncol 4: 1079–1088
3. Minden MD, Till JE, McCulloch EA (1978) Proliferative state of blast cell progenitors in acute myeloblastic leukemia (AML). Blood 52: 592–600
4. Vellenga E, Ostapovicz D, O'Rourke B, Griffin JD (1987) Effects of recombinant IL-3, GM-CSF, and G-CSF on proliferation of leukemic clonogenic cells in short-term and long-term cultures. Leukemia 1: 584–589
5. Cannistra SA, Groshek P, Griffin JD (1989) Granulocyte-macrophage colony-stimulating factor enhances the cytotoxic effects of cytosine arabinoside in acute myeloblastic leukemia and in the myeloid blast crisis phase of chronic myeloid leukemia. Leukemia 3: 328–334
6. Devereux S, Linch DC, Costa DC, Spittle MF, Jelliffe AM (1987) Transient leucopenia induced by granulocyte-macrophage colony-stimulating factor. Lancet 1: 1523–1524
7. Socinski MA, Cannistra SA, Sullivan R, Elias A, Antman K, Schnipper L, Griffin JD (1988) Granulocyte-macrophage colony-stimulating factor induces the expression of the CD11b surface adhesion molecule on human granulocytes in vivo. Blood 72: 691–697
8. Socinski MA, Cannistra SA, Elias A, Antman KH, Schnipper L, Griffin JD (1988) Granulocyte-macrophage colony stimulating factor expands the circulating haemopoietic progenitor cell compartment in man. Lancet 1: 1194–1198
9. Cannistra SA, DiCarlo J, Groshek P, Kanakura Y, Berg D, Mayer RJ, Griffin JD (1991) Simultaneous administration of granulocyte macrophage colony stimulating factor and cytosine arabinoside for the treatment of relapsed acute myeloid leukemia. Leukemia 5: 230–238
10. Cannistra SA, Groshek P, Garlick R, Miller J, Griffin JD (1990) Regulation of surface expression of the granylocyte/macrophage colony-stimulating factor receptor in normal human myeloid cells. Proc Natl Acad Sci USA 87: 93–97
11. Andreeff M, Tafuri A, Hegewisch-Becker S (1990) Colony-stimulating factors (G-CSF, GM-CSF, IL-3, and BCGF) recruit myeloblastic and lymphoblastic leukemia cells and enhance the cytotoxic effects of cytosine-arabinoside. Hamatol Bluttransfus 33: 747–762
12. Dolbeare F, Gratzner H, Pallavicini MG, Gray JW (1983) Flow cytometric measurement of total DNA content and incorporated bromodeoxyuridine. Proc Natl Acad Sci USA 80: 5573–5577.
13. Cannistra SA, Koenigsmann M, DiCarlo J, Groshek P, Griffin JD (1990) Differentiation-associated expression of two functionally distinct classes of GM-CSF receptor by human myeloid cells. J Biol Chem 265: 12656–12663
14. Broxmeyer HE, Cooper S, Williams DE, Hangoc G, Gutterman JU, Vadhan-Raj S (1988) Growth characteristics of marrow hematopoietic progenitor/precursor cells from patients on a phase I clinical trial with purified recombinant human granulocyte-macrophage colony-stimulating factor. Exp Hematol 16: 594–602
15. Leary AG, Yang YY, Clark SC, Gasson JC, Golde DW, Ogawa M (1987) Recombinant gibbon interleukin 3 supports formation of multilineage colonies and blast cell colonies in cuture: comparison with recombinant human granulocyte-macrophage colony-stimulating factor. Blood 70: 1343–1348
16. Lieschke GH, Maher D, Cebon J, O'Connor M, Green M, Sheridan W, Boyd A, Rallings M, Bonnem E, Metcalf D, Burgess AW, McGrath K, Fox RM, Morstyn G (1989)

Effects of bacterially synthesized recombinant human granulocyte-macrophage colony-stimulating factor in patients with advanced malignancy. Ann Intern Med 110: 357–364

17. Bussolino F, Wang JM, Defilippi P, Turrini F, Sanavio F, Edgell CJS, Aglietta M, Arese P, Mantovani A (1989) Granulocyte- and granulocyte-macrophage-colony stimulating factors induce human endothelial cells to migrate and proliferate. Nature 337: 471–473

18. Herzig RH, Hines JD, Herzig GP, Wolff SN, Cassileth PA, Lazarus HM, Adelstein DJ, Brown RA, Coccia PF, Strandjord S, Mazza JJ, Fay J, Phillips GL (1987) Cerebellar toxicity with high-dose cytosine arabinoside. J Clin Oncol 5: 927–932

19. Muhm M, Andreeff M, Geissler K, Gorischek C, Haas O, Haimi J, Hinterberger W, Schulz G, Speiser W, Sunder-Plassmann G, Valent P, Lechner K, Bettelheim P (1989) RhGM-CSF in combination with chemotherapy – a new strategy in the therapy of acute myeloid leukemia. Blood 74: 117a

Modulation of Cytotoxicity and Differentiation-Inducing Potential of Cytosine Arabinoside in Myeloid Leukemia Cells by Hematopoietic Cytokines*

R. Henschler, M. A. Brach, T. Licht, R. Mertelsmann, and F. Herrmann

Introduction

Cytosine arabinoside (ara-C) has been used extensively in the treatment of acute myelogenous leukemia (AML) for many years (see [4] for review). Besides the conventional low-dose regimen worked out by Frei et al. [16], high dose regimens [29] as well as combinations of ara-C with anthracycline derivatives [30] have further expanded and improved today's therapeutic repertoire for remission induction of AML. Despite considerable success in improving complete remission (CR) rates using new ara-C-based treatment modalities, we still face appallingly high relapse rates. Further improvement of AML induction therapy is thus mandatory.

The advent of recombinant hematopoietic growth factors and their clinical use gave us a powerful tool to mediate specific signals to selected cells resulting in either proliferation or differentiation of the respective set of cells. Accelerating the recovery of normal hemopoiesis after chemotherapy is now becoming the major field of the clinical use of colony stimulating factors (CSFs). However, a growing number of

investigations has been performed on leukemic cells themselves as targets of pharmacotherapy with hematopoietic growth factors. On the basis of the capability of CSFs to recruit leukemic blasts into cell cycle, it has been speculated that the proportion of leukemic cells responsive to the S-phase specific drug ara-C, and thus the efficacy of ara-C, may be substantially augmented when CSFs are given in conjunction with or prior to ara-C.

After a brief introduction into basic principles of the mode of action of CSFs and ara-C on leukemic cells, this chapter focuses on in vitro studies aimed at elucidating possible mechanisms of synergistic interactions between CSFs and ara-C, and at giving rationales for the design of experimental therapeutic regimens using combinations of CSFs and ara-C. We report that besides recruiting leukemic blasts into cell cycle, CSFs may function by altering intracellular ara-C metabolism as well as by promoting terminal differentiation of blast cells. In addition to the more early acting growth factors interleukin-3 (IL-3) and granulocyte-macrophage colony-stimulating factor (GM-CSF), consideration will be given to the potential use of other factors such as macrophage colony-stimulating factor (M-CSF) and leukemia inhibitory factor (LIF) in conjunction with ara-C; possible further strategies in the search for alternative molecular events influenced by CSFs that might alter the action of chemotherapeutic agents will also be considered. Finally, a short summary of experimental therapeutic regimes currently underway will include first clinical results.

* Supported by the Mildred Scheel Stiftung (MAB) and the Deutsche Forschungsgemeinschaft (FH, TL and RH).

Department of Hematology and Oncology, University of Freiburg
Medical Center, Freiburg, FRG

Mode of Action of ara-C on Leukemic Cells

Ara-C is converted intracellularly into its major metabolite and active form, the deoxyribonucleotide analogue ara-CTP [21]. Incorporation of ara-CTP into DNA will lead to alterations in DNA structure, slowing down of DNA elongation and, eventually, chain termination [12, 54]; ara-C was also found to inhibit DNA polymerase by competing with dCTP [17]. The latter effect is mediated by misincorporated 3'-ara-CMP residues [41].

Resistance to ara-C is common; two different kinds of mechanisms have been identified. On a pharmacological basis resistance may occur by an increase of the intracellular dCTP pool and thus a decrease in the intracellular ara-CTP:dCTP ratio. Other mechanisms of pharmacological resistance include decreased cellular retention of ara-CTP or loss of DNA polymerase binding affinity for Ara-CTP. To overcome pharmacological resistance of ara-C, the drug may be given as a bolus every 12 h [31], or, more effective and less toxic, by continuous i.v. infusion [45].

A different mechanism of resistance to ara-C is due to increasing proportions of leukemic cells that remain in G_0 and do not enter S phase, thus escaping action of the drug. As continuous infusion of ara-C alone is often insufficient to overcome resistance, it seems convincing that CSFs might be used to recruit quiescent leukemic cells into cell cycle in order to make them more susceptible to the action of ara-C. The basic questions for this concept are: to which growth factors are leukemic cells receptive, and how do they react?

Mode of Action of CSFs on Leukemic Cells

Fresh primary AML samples as well as various permanent myeloid leukemia cell lines have been studied concerning their reactivity to a range of CSFs and other growth factors in either semisolid medium or suspension culture [27] (for review). We and others have shown previously that leukemic progenitor cells are responsive in

particular to GM-CSF [23, 25]. In one-half to two-thirds of AML samples, GM-CSF and IL-3 support clonogenic leukemia growth in vitro. G-CSF in this context is only rarely active, whereas application of M-CSF will almost exclusively result in differentiation rather than proliferation [50, 14, 43, 39, 40]. Leukemic cell lines such as HL-60 (promyelocytic) and U937 (monoblastic) are induced by these CSFs to differentiate [48, 8, 36]. Whereas clonogenic survival is lost in some cell lines (e.g., U937), others display undiminished self-renewal (e.g., HL-60). In our experiments both KG-1 myeloblasts and primary AML cells were recruited into S phase most effectively by IL-3, and to a lesser degree also by GM-CSF or G-CSF (Fig. 1, panel A).

Combined Action of ara-C and CSFs on Leukemic Cells

Several groups have confirmed that AML blasts stimulated to proliferate by GM-CSF undergo enhanced cell killing by subsequent exposure to ara-C as compared to untreated cells [40, 32, 9]. Cannistra et al. [9] extended these findings to myeloid blast crisis of CML. Concomitantly, the effect of ara-C to suppress self-renewal of leukemic blasts was enhanced by pretreatment of the cells with GM-CSF. Moreover, Bhalla et al. [3] found that GM-CSF enhances the effects of ara-C by interfering with ara-C metabolism resulting in increased intracellular ara-CTP/dCTP ratios in both normal and leukemic cells.

As IL-3 is even more effective than GM-CSF in stimulating proliferation of AML blasts, [34], regimes combining IL-3 and ara-C can be expected to be more powerful than GM-CSF/ara-C combinations [5, 37]. When we exposed KG-1 myeloblasts or AML samples representing FAB subtypes M1, M2, M4 and M5 in suspension culture to either ara-C alone, or ara-C in the presence of IL-3, the number of leukemia cells surviving the clonal cultures was reduced by 83 % (low-dose ara-C) and 94 % (high-dose ara-C) by a combination of IL-3 and ara-C, as compared to reductions in cell numbers of 49 % and 74 % with ara-C alone

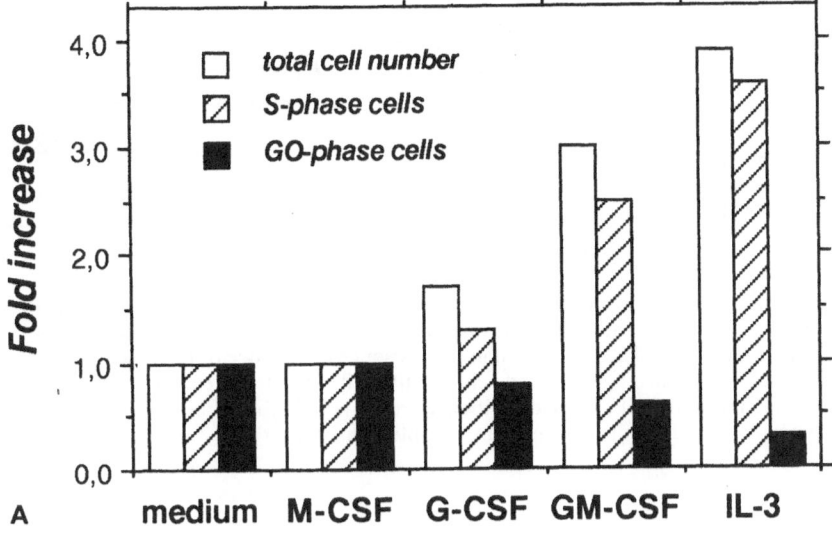

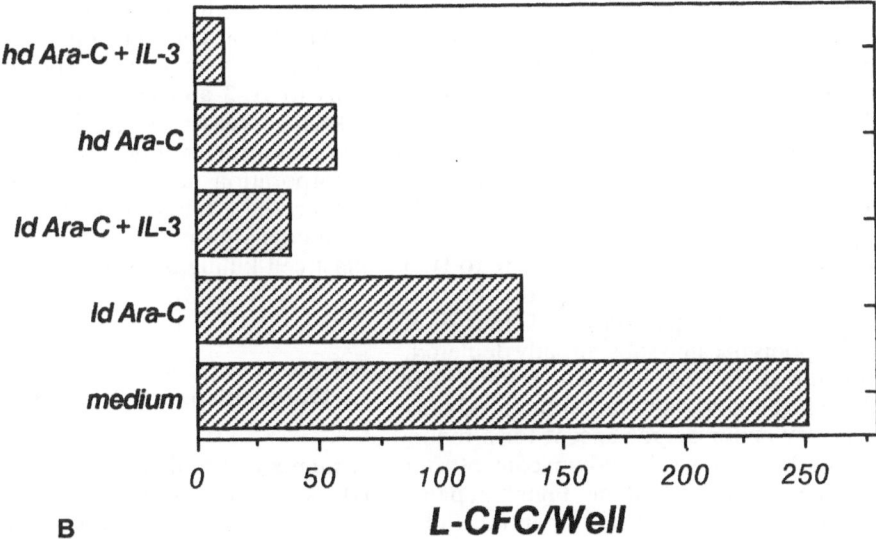

Fig. 1. A Effect of various CSFs on total cell number, number of cells in S phase and number of cells in G_0 phase of the cell cycle. Freshly sampled AML cells depleted of T lymphocytes and adherent cells (>95% pure blast cells by morphology) were exposed either to M-CSF (1000 Units/ml), G-CSF, GM-CSF or IL-3 (20 ng/ml each) for a period of 36 h. Proportions of cells in S phase and G_0 phase were determined by DNA histogram analysis and measurements of DNA/RNA content. Results represent mean values of nine independent experiments with blasts from different donors. I.B. Effect of IL-3 on ara-C-mediated cytotoxicity in clonogenic AML cells. Myeloid leukemia cells (cell line KG-1 or purified blasts from four patients with AML) were cultured for 24 h in the presence or absence of IL-3 (20 ng/ml) with or without ara-C at low (10^{-7} M) or high (10^{-3} M) doses. After several washings cells were recultured in soft agar. After 6 days numbers of blast colonies were enumerated. Reduction of colony growth was 41%–59% (low-dose ara-C), 64%–79% (high-dose ara-C), 71%–87% (low dose ara-C +IL−3), 94%–98% (high dose ara-C + IL-3). The results shown represent means of all experiments

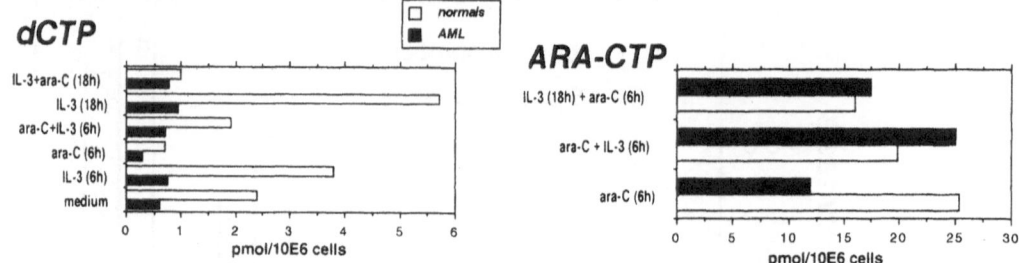

Fig. 2. Effect of IL-3 on dCTP and ara-CTP accumulation in normal and leukemic (*AML*) bone marrow cells treated with ara-C. Normal density bone marrow cells (*open bars*) and AML blasts (*solid bars*) were incubated at 10^6 cells/ml in the presence or absence of IL-3 (20 ng/ml) or ara-C (10^{-3} M) as indicated. Neutralized periodated acid soluble cell extracts were analyzed for intracellular dCTP and ara-CTP levels by HPLC as described previously [3]. Values are expressed as pmol/10^6 cells and represent the means of four separate samples for each group

(Fig. 1, panel B). Similar experiments using GM-, G- and M-CSF instead of IL-3 revealed that IL-3 was by far the most active CSF in enhancing ara-C cytotoxicity against leukemic cells. The increasing proportions of cells recruited into S phase by CSF treatment were in parallel to the percentage of dead cells after ara-C treatment. We also studied the effect of rhIL-3 on ara-C metabolism. As shown in Fig. 2 (left panel), normal low density bone marrow cells (open bars) exhibit strong increases in intracellular dCTP levels after exposure to IL-3 compared to the medium control (bottom experiment). If exposed to ara-C plus IL-3, dCTP pools became substantially depleted. In contrast, in leukemic cells intracellular dCTP levels generally were influenced only to a very minor degree except for a reduction by ca. 50 % of the medium control after treatment with ara-C alone. Figure 2, panel B, shows the effects of IL-3 on intracellular ara-CTP levels in ara-C treated cells. Whereas in normal cells levels of ara-CTP were lowered by a combination of ara-C and IL-3 compared to application of ara-C alone (open bars), again leukemic cells behaved differently and showed increased intracellular ara-CTP levels. Overall, in leukemic cells the ratio of intracellular ara-CTP/dCTP was unchanged after treatment with IL-3/ara-C compared to ara-C alone, which is in striking contrast to the effects in normal cells. These data suggest that unlike the effects of GM-CSF, those of IL-3 on

ara-C metabolism are of minor importance.

In another series of experiments, we investigated the incorporation of ^{3}H-ara-C into leukemic cells. The upper panel of Fig. 3 shows that sequential exposure of AML cells to IL-3 and ara-C results in a 2- to 3-fold increase in ara-C incorporation, whereas after simultaneous exposure ara-C incorporation rather decreased. Taken together, these findings indicate that there is strong synergism of IL-3 and ara-C on AML blast cell killing in vitro.

Effects of ara-C and CSFs
on Differentiation of Leukemic Cells

A number of leukemic cell lines including HL-60 promyelocytes, K562 erythroleukemia cells, ML-1 myelomonocytic leukemia cells, and U937 monoblasts undergo maturation when treated with sublethal (low dose) ara-C [22, 52, 47, 11]. This is commonly associated with decreased steady state c-myc mRNA levels and increased expression of the *c-fos* gene [42]. More recent work revealed that ara-C also activates the differentiation-associated transcription of *c-jun* and *junB* in these cells [13, 44, 33, 24]. Although in the case of KG-1 cells and of primary AML blasts ara-C failed to induce terminal differentiation, molecular changes consistent with early

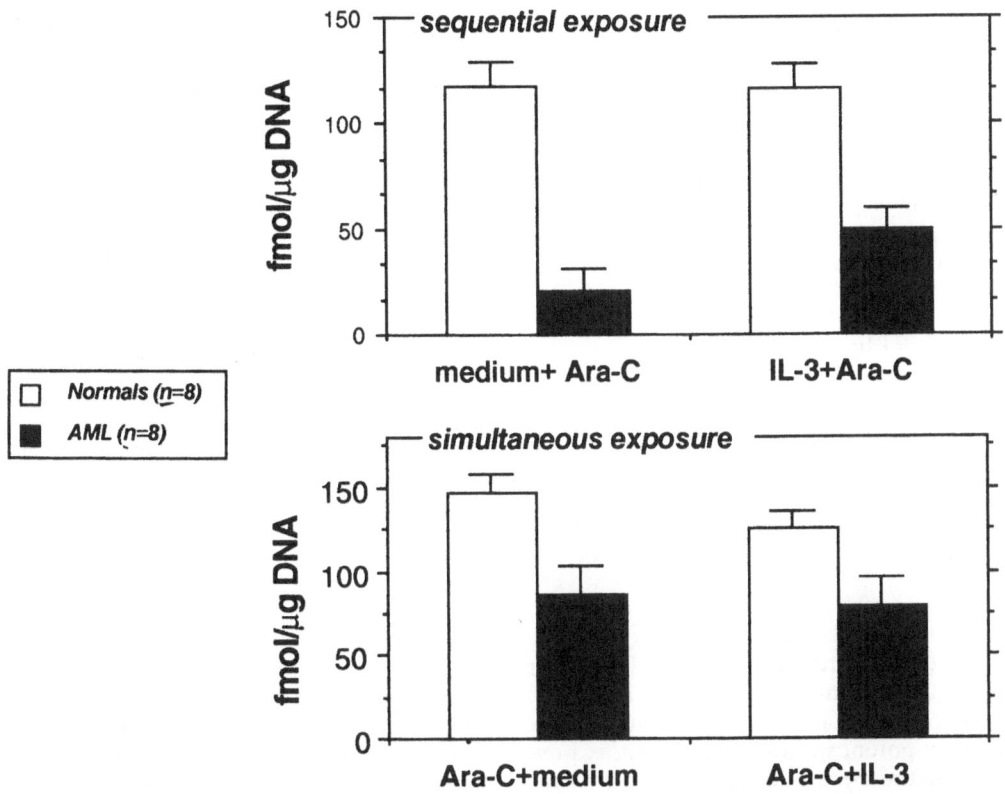

Fig. 3. Effect of IL-3 on ^{3}H-ara-C DNA incorporation into normal and leukemic bone marrow cells. *Upper panel*, Normal low density bone marrow cells (*open columns*) and AML blasts (*solid columns*) were cultured at 10^6 cells/ml in experiments in which a 12 h treatment with IL-3 (20 ng/ml) (or medium) was preceded by a 6 h pulse with ^{3}H-ara-C (10 μM). Incorporation of ^{3}H-ara-C into DNA was quantitated by scintillation counting as described by Bhalla et al. [3]. *Lower panel*, Analogue experiments in which IL-3 and ara-C were both present for the whole culture period of 18 h. Values are expressed as fmol/μg DNA and represent the means of three separate sample ± standard errors for each group

events in differentiation were accomplished [5, 33, 24].

A different strategy in designing synergistic combinations of ara-C and cytokines is to make use of the differentiation-inducing potential of a number of cytokines in an attempt to support ara-C-mediated maturation of leukemic cells, thus bringing down the self-renewing capacity of leukemic blasts. To this end, although GM-CSF by itself is able to induce differentiation in monoblastic U937 cells [8], there are no convincing data that GM-CSF or G-CSF in combination with ara-C have any synergistic effects on differentiation of leukemia cells. In our studies using combined IL-3/ara-C treatment of leukemic myeloid cells, no evidence for features indicating generation of a more mature phenotype was seen, e.g., expression of differentiation markers such as c-*fms* or myeloperoxidase gene expression, or expression of maturation-associated surface antigens [5]. An important candidate cytokine for this concept is the leukemia inhibitory factor (LIF). LIF exhibits growth inhibitory effects on primary AML cells, most likely due to prolongation of the generation time of leukemic stem cells [51]. LIF was also found to suppress clonogenicity of HL-60 and U937 cells in synergy with GM-CSF and G-CSF [38].

The effects of a study from our group [6] investigating a combined treatment of KG-

Table 1. Effect of recombinant human IL-3 and leukemia inhibitory favour (LIF) on ara-C-induced proto-oncogene expression in the myeloblast KG-1 cell line and the monoblast U937 cell line

	KG-1			U937		
	c-*fos*	c-*jun*	c-*fms*	c-*fos*	c-*jun*	c-*fms*
Treatment						
ara-C	+	+	−	+	+	−
IL-3	+	−	−	−	−	−
ara-C + IL-3	+	+	−	+	+	−
LIF	−	−	−	+	−	−
ara-C + LIF	+	+	−	+	+	+

KG-1 or U937 cells were cultured in the presence or absence of ara-C (10^{-7} *M*), rhIL-3 (20 ng/ml), rhLIF (100 units/ml), or combinations of ara-C, IL-3, or LIF. After the culture period indicated below, RNA was extracted and hybridized with cDNAs specific for the c-*fos*, c-*jun*, and c-*fms* oncogenes. Hybridization of c-*fos* mRNA was performed after 2 h of culture and of c-*jun* after 6 h of culture; c-*fms* transcripts were detected 12 h after initiation of cultures.

1 and U937 cells with ara-C and two different cytokines are pointed out in Table 1. In KG-1 cells, combinations of LIF and ara-C and combinations of IL-3 and ara-C were equally potent in inducing mRNA expression of the c-*fos* and c-*jun* genes that are associated with early differentiation. In U937 cells, however, LIF but not IL-3 induced c-*fos* gene expression. More terminal differentiation, as assessed by expression of the c-*fms* gene, was only achieved with LIF/ara-C, but not with IL-3/ara-C. CD14 surface antigen expression (as determined by MOl antibody) and the capacity of the cells to reduce nitroblue tetrazolium (NBT) were synergistically increased by simultaneous administration of LIF and ara-C (Fig. 4). These findings suggest that low-dose ara-C can be effectively combined with cytokines in an effort to overcome the block in differentiation of AML blasts. It appears mandatory to investigate other growth factors such as M-CSF and IL-6 in this context.

Alterations by CSFs of other Molecular Events that Influence Cytotoxicity of Cytostatic Drugs

Up to now, only very limited attention has been paid to mechanisms by which CSFs will either augment or diminish the action of chemotherapeutic drugs. One of the mechanisms of chemoresistance that has been under most profound investigation is the multiple drug resistance (*MDR*) gene family. A series of still partly preliminary experiments in our group has monitored the expression of P-glycoprotein, the product of the *MDR1* gene, under the influence of CSFs such as the ones used in combinations with ara-C mentioned above. In experiments with vindesine (VDS)-sensitive solid tumor cells (pleural mesothelioma cell line PXF 1118) expression of P-glycoprotein was almost completely suppressed when cells were treated with IL-3 in combination with VDS, whereas P-glycoprotein was induced in a high percentage of these cells when they were treated with VDS alone (Fig. 5). To what extent characteristics of PXF 1118 cell growth and differentiation were also affected and whether expression of other *MDR* genes is altered in the presence of IL-3 remains to be elucidated. Ongoing experiments including leukemic cells investigate the ability of other cytokines to bring about alterations in the induction of chemoresistance in vitro. The observation that CSFs may profoundly influence the ability of tumor cells to acquire chemoresistance may bring entirely new and innovative aspects into therapy with CSFs. The hope is that benefit will result for certain patients who may be kept from developing chemor-

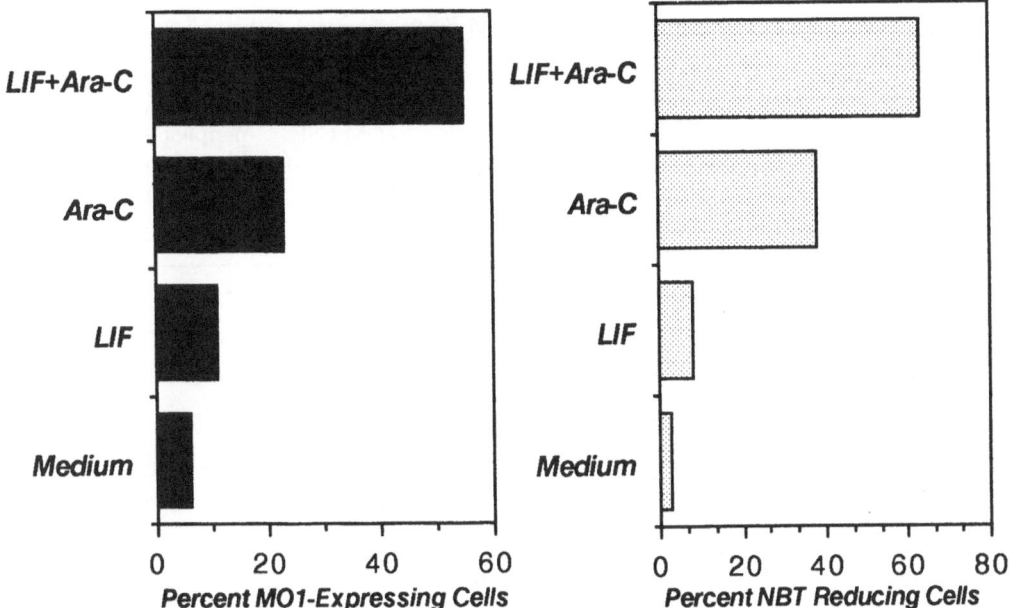

Fig. 4. Effect of leukemia inhibitory factor (*LIF*) on differentiation of U937 cells in the presence of ara-C. U937 cells grown in suspension culture at 10^6 cells/ml were treated with either medium alone, LIF (100 units/ml), ara-C (10^{-7} *M*), or LIF and ara-C at the same time. After 36 h, cells were washed and assayed for their ability to bind an anti-MOl fluorescein labeled antibody by FACS analysis or for their ability to reduce the nitroblue tetrazolium reagent (*NBT*). Results represent the mean values of three independent experiments

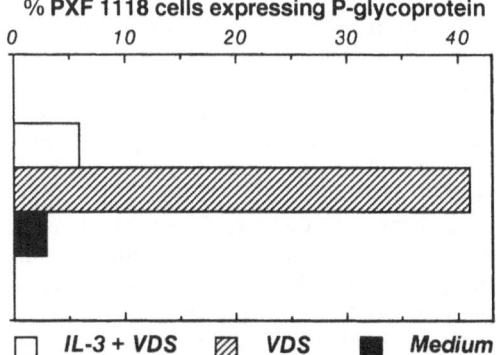

Fig. 5. Effect of IL-3 on P-glycoprotein expression in PXF 1118 pleural mesothelioma cells. Initially vindesine (VDS)-sensitive PXF 1118 cells, grown to confluence in plastic flasks, were treated with medium only, IL-3 (20 ng/ml), VDS (0.01 µg/ml) or a combination of IL-3 and VDS for 21 days. P-glycoprotein was assayed by immunostaining with MRK16 monoclonal antibody. Values represent percentages of enumerations of three separate experiments

esistance by receiving CSF therapy. Extended and more fundamental research in vitro as well as in vivo will be needed to give us the amount of insight into these phenomena that is necessary before patients can profit from it.

Clinical use of CSFs in Combination with ara-C

Although several trials using ara-C in combination with CSFs have been undertaken, only sparse and very preliminary data are yet available concerning clinical outcomes. Data of a first series of studies combining ara-C and GM-CSF in AML therapy are summarized in Table 2 [15, 46, 7, 35]. These regimens were all designed to recruit "dormant" leukemic stem cells to reenter cell cycle and enter S phase and thereby become sensitive to ara-C. Forty-six patients have so far entered the trials. During the prechemo-

Table 2. Clinical experience with rhGM-CSF-based cycle recruitment therapy utilizing an ara-C-containing regimen

Reference	No. of patients	Diagnosis	Chemotherapy	GM-CSF schedule	Onset of GM-CSF therapy relative to chemotherapy (day)	Increase in peripheral blast counts (n)	Cell kinetic changes (n)[a]
Estey et al.	18	de novo AML	ara-C Daunorubicin	125 µg/ m²/d s.c.	−8	13	5
Tafuri et al.	10	AML	ara-C Daunorubicin	125–250 µg/ m²/d s.c. or c.i.v.	−2	7	7
Burke et al.	8	relapsed AML	ara-C Daunorubicin VP-16	1–5 µg/kg/ d s.c. or c.i.v.	−3	8	8
Lacombe et al.	10	relapsed AML	ARA-C m-AMSA	3 µg/kg/d, 4 h infusion	−2	6	3

c.i.v., continuous intrachenous infusion; m-AMSA, amsacrine
[a] cell kinetic measures include: ^{3}H-thymidine uptake, ara-CTP formation, bromodeoxyuridine and propidium iodide staining, and measurement of DNA/RNA content.

therapy period, GM-CSF raised both peripheral neutrophil and blast counts. The number of blasts in S phase and blast uptake of bromodeoxyuridine and ^{3}H-thymidine all underwent substantial increases. No evidence was reported suggesting uncontrolled recruitment of leukemia growth or prolongation of postchemotherapy bone marrow aplasia. Interestingly, Tafuri et al. [46] reported that only patients who had GM-CSF-related cell kinetic changes experienced CR, whereas patients who had no cell kinetic changes did not. More data have to be awaited to further assess the effectiveness of these regimes. Based on the first experiences using GM-CSF and ara-C, trials with combinations of IL-3 and Ara-C in AML are now planned. Since it has been demonstrated that certain solid tumor cells also proliferate in vitro upon stimulation with CSFs [2], it seems promising to include these types of malignancies in this sort of study as well.

Besides recruiting tumor cells into cell cycle, CSFs have also been used in clinical trials for assisting ara-C in induction of differentiation. Although no in vitro data are currently available to show that GM-

CSF and ara-C cooperate in inducing terminal differentiation, patients with myelodysplastic syndrome (MDS) respond in vivo to either agent with improvements in blood counts [53, 49, 1, 19, 26]. Cheson et al. [10] have questioned the use of ara-C as a differentiation-inducing treatment modality for MDS. The use of GM-CSF in MDS is presently under critical reevaluation since responses have been limited mainly to the myeloid series and usually disappear upon withdrawal of the growth factor [28]. A study started very recently by Ganser et al. [18], using GM-CSF/ara-C in patients with advanced MDS, reported an increase in peripheral neutrophil counts in all nine patients who had so far entered the trial, and increased platelet counts in six of them. Eight patients had achieved a reduction in bone marrow blasts and an improved bone marrow maturation index (ratio of postmitotic to mitotic bone marrow cells). RFLP analysis of some of these patients documented stimulation of nonclonal hemopoiesis, suggesting that differentiation of the malignant cell population was induced in vivo by GM-CSF/ara-C [20].

Conclusion

In conclusion, in vitro data on synergism of hematopoietic growth factors and inhibitors of DNA synthesis revealed promising results. According to the qualities enabling each hematopoietic growth factor to induce its individual profile of proliferative and differentiative cellular events in tumor cells, further in vitro studies will have to explore a wider experimental basis that will provide the experience to elaborate and optimize the therapeutic use of a direct synergy between chemotherapeutic substances and CSFs.

References

1. Antin JH, Smith BR, Holmes W, et al. (1988) Phase I/II study of recombinant human granulocyte-macrophage colony-stimulating factor in aplastic anemia and myelodysplastic syndrome. Blood 72: 705–713
2. Berdel WE, Danhauser-Riedl S, Doll M, Herrmann F (1990) Effect of hematopoietic growth factors on the growth of nonhematopoietic tumor cell lines. In: Mertelsmann R, Herrmann F (eds) Hematopoietic growth factors in clinical applications. Dekker, New York, pp 339–362
3. Bhalla K, Birkhofer M, Arlin Z, et al. (1988) Effect of recombinant GM-CSF on metabolism of cytosine arabinoside in normal and leukemic bone marrow cells. Leukemia 2: 810–813
4. Bolewell B, Cassileth P, Gale R (1988) High dose cytoarabine: a review. Leukemia 2: 253–260
5. Brach M, Klein H, Platzer E, et al. (1990a) Effect of interleukin-3 on cytosine arabinoside-mediated cytotoxicity of leukemic myeloblasts. Exp Hematol 18: 748–753
6. Brach M, Riedel D, Mertelsmann R, Herrmann F (1990b) Synergistic effect of recombinant human leukemia inhibitory factor (LIF) and 1-β-D-arabinofuranosylcytosine on protooncogene expression and induction of differentiation in human U937 cells. Leukemia 4: 646–649
7. Burke PJ, Wendel KA, Nichols PD, et al. (1990) A phase I trial of GM-CSF and humoral stimulating activity as biomodulators of timed sequential therapy of AML. Blood 76 (Suppl 1): 1023a
8. Cannistra SA, Rambaldi A, Spriggs DR, et al. (1987) Human granulocyte-macrophage colony-stimulating factor induces expression of the tumor necrosis factor gene by the U937 cell line and by normal human monocytes. J Clin Invest 79: 1720–1728
9. Cannistra SA, Groshek P, Griffin JD (1989) Granulocyte-macrophage colony-stimulating factor enhances the cytotoxic effects of cytosine-arabinoside in acute myeloblastic leukemia and in the myeloid blast crisis phase of chronic myeloid leukemia. Leukemia 3: 328–332
10. Cheson BD, Jasperse DM, Simon R, Friedman MA (1986) A critical appraisal of low dose cytosine arabinoside in patients with acute non-lymphocytic leukemia and myelodysplastic syndromes. J Clin Oncol 4: 1857–1864
11. Chomienne C, Balitrand N, Abita J (1983) Effect of 1-β-D arabino-furanosylcytosine on differentiation of U937 cells. ICTS Med Sci 11: 731–732
12. Chu M, Fischer G (1968) The incorporation of ³H-cytosine arabinoside and its effect on murine leukemic cells. Biochem Pharmacol 17: 753–767
13. Datta R, Kharbanda S, Kufe D (1990) Regulation of junB expression by 1-β-D arabinofuranosycytosine in human myeloid leukemia cells. Mol Pharmacol 38: 435–439
14. Delwel R, Salem M, Pellens C, et al. (1988) Growth regulation of human acute myeloid leukemia: effect of five recombinant hematopoietic growth factors in a serum-free culture system. Blood 72: 1944–1950
15. Estey E, Kantarjian H, Keating M, et al. (1990) Use of GM-CSF prior to chemotherapy of AML: effect on circulating blast count, thymidine incorporation and ara-CTP formation. Blood 76 (Suppl 1): 558a
16. Frei E, Bickers JN, Hewlett JS, et al. (1969) Dose schedule and antitumor studies of arabinosylcytosine. Cancer Res 29: 1325–1332
17. Furth J, Cohen S (1971) Inhibition of mammalian DNA polymerase by the 5′-triphosphate of 1-β-D arabonofuranosyladenine. Cancer Res 28: 2061–2067
18. Ganser A, Hoelzer D (1990a) GM-CSF/ara-C in myelodysplastic syndrome. In: Mertelsmann R, Herrmann F (eds) Hematopoietic growth factors in clinical applications. Dekker, New York, pp 255–277
19. Ganser A, Völkers B, Greher J, et al. (1989) Recombinant human granulocyte-macrophage colony-stimulating factor in patients with myelodysplastic syndromes: phase I/II trial. Blood 73: 31–37
20. Ganser A, Bartram CR, Ottmann OG, et al. (1990b) Stimulation of nonclonal hematopoiesis in patients with hematological disord-

ers by recombinant GM-CSF or interleukin-3. Blood 76 (Suppl 1): 568a

21. Graham F, Whitmore G (1970) Studies in mouse L-cells on the incorporation of 1-β-D arabinofuranosyl 5'-triphosphate. Cancer Res 30: 2636–2644

22. Griffin JD, Munroe D, Major P, Kufe D (1982) Induction of differentiation of human myeloid leukemia cells by inhibitors of DNA synthesis. Exp Hematol 10: 776–783

23. Griffin JD, Young D, Herrmann F, et al. (1986) Effects of recombinant human GM-CSF on proliferation of clonogenic cells in acute myeloblastic leukemia. Blood 66: 1448–1453

24. Henschler R, Brennscheidt U, Mertelsmann R, Herrmann F (1991) Induction of c-jun expression in the myeloid leukemia cell line KG-1 by 1-β-D-arabinofuranosylcytosine. Mol Pharmacol 39: in press

25. Herrmann F, Oster W, Lindemann A, et al. (1987) Leukemic colony-forming cells in acute myeloblastic leukemia: maturation hierarchy and growth conditions. Haematol Blood Transfus 31: 185–195

26. Herrmann F, Lindemann A, Klein H, et al. (1989) Effect of recombinant human granulocyte-macrophage colony-stimulating factor in patients with myelodysplastic syndrome with excess blasts. Leukemia 3: 335–338

27. Herrmann F, Vellenga E (1990) The role of colony-stimulating factors in acute leukemia. J Cancer Res Clin Oncol 116: 175–282

28. Herrmann F, Ganser A, Lindemann A, et al. (1991) Clinical use of recombinant hematopoietic growth factors (GM-CSF, IL-3, EPO) in patients with MDS. Biotechnol Ther: in press

29. Herzig RH, Wolff SN, Lazarus HM, et al. (1983) High dose cytosine arabinoside therapy for refractory leukemia. Blood 62: 361–369

30. Herzig RH, Lazarus HM, Wolff SN, et al. (1985) High dose cytosine arabinoside therapy with and without anthracycline antibiotics for remission reinduction of acute non-lymphocytic leukemia. J Clin Oncol 3: 997–999

31. Hiddemann W, Kreuzmann H, Straif K, et al. (1987) High dose cytosine arabinoside in combination with mitoxantrone for the treatment of refractory acute myeloid or lymphoblastic leukemia. Semin Oncol 14 (Suppl 1): 74–77

32. Karp JE, Burke JE, Donehover RC (1990) Effect of rh GM-CSF on intracellular ara-C pharmacology in vitro in acute myelogenous leukemia: comparability with drug-induced humoral stimulatory activity. Leukemia 4: 553–556

33. Kharbanda S, Sherman ML, Kufe D (1990) Transcriptional regulation of c-jun gene expression by arabinofuranoxylcytosine in human KG-1 acute myelogenous leukemia cells. J Clin Invest 86: 1517–1523

34. Kobayashi M, Van Leeuwen BH, Elsbury S, et al. (1989) Interleukin-3 is significantly more effective than other colony-stimulating factors in long-term maintenance of human bone marrow-derived colony-forming cells in vitro. Blood 72: 1298–1303

35. Lacombe F, Dumain P, Puntous M, et al. (1990) Clinical and biological results in AML patients treated with GM-CSF and intensive chemotherapy. Blood 76 (Suppl 1): 1157a

36. Lindemann A, Riedel D, Oster W, et al. (1988) Recombinant human granulocyte-macrophage colony-stimulating factor induces secretion of autoinhibitory monokines by U937 cells. Eur J Immunol 18, 369–374

37. Lista P, Brizzi MF, Rossi M, et al. (1990) Different sensitivity of normal and leukemic progenitor cells to ara-C and IL-3 combined treatment. Br J Haematol 76: 21–26

38. Maekawa T, Metcalf D (1989) Clonal suppression of HL60 and U037 cells by recombinant human leukemia inhibitory factor in combination with GM-CSF. Leukemia 3: 270–276

39. Miyauchi J, Kelleher CA, Yang YC, et al. (1987) The effects of three recombinant growth factors, IL-3, GM-CSF, G-CSF, on the blast cells of acute myeloblastic leukemia maintained in short-term suspension culture. Blood 70: 657–663

40. Miyauchi J, Kelleher CA, Wang C, et al. (1989) Growth factors influence the sensitivity of leukemic stem cells to cytosine arabinoside in culture. Blood 73: 1272–1277

41. Mikita T, Beardsley GP (1988) Functional consequences of the arabinosylcytosine structural lesion in DNA. Biochemistry 27: 4698–4705

42. Pinto A, Attadia V, Rosati R, et al. (1988) Differentiation of human leukemic cell lines and fresh leukemia cells by low-dose ara-C: monitoring by expression of c-myc and c-fos oncogenes. Med Oncol Tumor Pharmacol 5: 91–97

43. Sealand S, Caux C, Favre C, et al. (1988) Effect of recombinant human interleukin-3 in CD 34 enriched normal hematopoietic progenitors and on myeloblastic leukemia cells. Blood 72: 1580–1588

44. Sherman M, Stone R, Datta R, et al. (1990) Transcriptional and posttranscriptional regulation of c-jun expression during induction of

monocytic differentiation. J Biol Chem 265: 3320–3323

45. Spriggs DR, Robbins G, Artur K, et al. (1988) Prolonged high dose ara-C in leukemia. Leukemia 2: 304–306

46. Tafuri A, Estey E, Valent P, et al. (1990) Cell kinetic effects in vivo of rh GM-CSF as preinduction treatment in acute myeloblastic leukemia. Blood 76 (Suppl 1): 663a

47. Takeo K, Mioawada J, Bloch A (1982) Kinetics of appearance of differentiation-associated chracteristics of ML-1, a line of human myeloblastic leukemia cells after treatment with 12-0-tetradecanoyl-phorbol-13-acetate, dimethyl sulfoxide, or 1-β-D arabinofuranoxylcytosine. Cancer Res 42: 5152–5157

48. Tomonaga M, Golde DW, Gasson JC (1986) Biosynthetic (recombinant) human GM-CSF effects on normal bone marrow and leukemic cell lines. Blood 67: 31–36

49. Vadhan-Raj S, Keating M, Maistre A, et al. (1987) Effect of recombinant human granulocyte-macrophage colony-stimulating factor in patients with myelodysplastic syndromes. N Engl J Med 317: 1545–1552

50. Vellenga E, Ostapovicz D, O'Rourke B, Griffin JD (1987) Effect of rh IL-3, GM-CSF and G-CSF on proliferation of leukemic clonogenic cells in short term and long term culture. Leukemia 1: 548–560

51. Wang C, Lishner M, Minden MD, McCulloch EA (1990) The effect of leukemia inhibitory factor (LIF) on the blast stem cells of acute myeloblastic leukemia. Leukemia 4: 548–552

52. Watanabe T, Mitchell T, Sariban E, et al. (1985) Effects of phorbolester and 1-β-D arabinofuranoxylcytosine on induction of K562 erythroleukemia cell differentiation. Mol Pharmacol 27: 683–688

53. Wisch JS, Griffin JD, Kufe DW (1983) Response of preleukemic syndromes to continuous infusion of low-dose cytarabine. N Engl J Med 309: 1599–1602

54. Zahn R, Mueller W, Foster W, et al. (1972) Action of 1-β-D arabinofuranosylcytosine on mammalian tumor cells. I: Incorporation into DNA. Eur J Cancer 8: 391–396

The Effect of Growth Factors on the Sensitivity of CFU-GM and CFU-Blasts to Cytosine Arabinoside

M.A. Smith and J.G. Smith

Introduction

With the recent advent of recombinant human (rh) cytokines, interest has focused on their possible use in association with cell cycle specific cytotoxic agents in the treatment of haematological malignancy. We have evaluated the effect of haemopoietic growth factors (rh interleukin-3, IL-3; rh granolocyte-macrofhage colony-stunulaling factor, GM-CSF; and CM 5637) on normal and blast cell progenitors with a view to increasing the cytotoxic effect of cytosine arabinoside (Ara-C). This study incorporates an investigation of the relative sensitivity of normal myelodysplastic syndromes (MDS) and acute myeloid leukaemia (AML) marrow precursors to Ara-C in vitro. We investigate the possibility of modifying the susceptibility of these cells to Ara-C by pre-incubating them in liquid culture with growth factors prior to clonogenic culture with the drug.

Materials and Methods

Patient Groups

Marrow was aspirated from the posterior iliac crests of patients with MDS ($n=5$) and AML ($n=5$), and individuals with B 12/folate deficiency whose haemopoiesis could normalised in vitro ($n=18$). This latter group comprised the "normal" control marrows.

CFU-GM/Blast Culture

Light density marrow cells (LDMCs) (sp. gr.<0.077), were T-cell-depleted using complement-mediated cytolysis of CD4 and CD8 populations by a previously described method [1]. T-cell-depleted LDMCs were either cultured immediately (day 0), or subjected to pre-incubation periods of 6, 24, 48 or 72 h. This liquid culture was performed in Biorich (a serum-free complete medium) alone or with the inclusion of rhIL-3 (5#ng/ml), rhGM-CSF (100# units/ml) or CM 5637 (10 % v/v).

A pre-incubation time of 48 h was established as optimal during preliminary experiments so this was the period of time selected for assays involving pre-treatment with growth factors. Semi-solid culture was performed in triplicate using 5×10^4 cells/0.5 ml well in Dulbeccos medium (supplemented), 20 % foetal calf serum, 0.8 % methylcellulose and GM-CSF (100# units/ml). Colonies were enumerated on day 12 and in some instances were evaluated morphologically by Wright's staining and by alkaline phosphatase-anti-alkaline phosphatase (APAAP), technology using MPO 7, a monoclonal antibody which recogniges the myeloid lineage.

Statistical Analysis

Analysis of significance was performed using a two-sample paired t test.

Department of Haematology, Royal United Hospital, Combe Park, Bath, England.

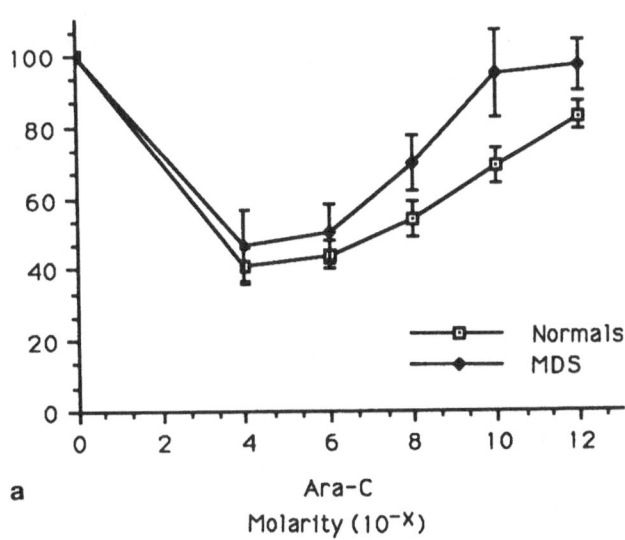

% SURVIVAL

a

Ara-C
Molarlty (10^{-x})

% SURVIVAL

Fig. 1 a, b. The effect of Ara-C (10^{-4} # M to 10^{-12} # M) on marrow progenitors from normal subjects ($n=18$) and patients with MDS ($n=5$) (a) and those with AML ($n=5$) (b) n. Numbers of surviving colonies are expressed as a percentage of control (no Ara-C) and are presented as mean values ± 1 standard error

b

Ara-C
Molarlty (10^{-x})

Results

Figure 1 demonstrates that Ara-C across a dose range is always detrimental to normal, MDS and AML colony formation. The responses of MDS and normal marrows were similar and consistent while AML marrow exhibited variable sensitivity to the drug. This may suggest variability in the length of cell cycle of AML progenitors

from different patients. Table 1 indicates that the optimum pre-incubation time should not exceed 48 h as CFU-GM survival is impaired beyond this point. Pre-incubation with growth factors appears to confer greater CFU-GM survival potential than with Biorich alone.

Figure 2 demonstrates the effect of pre-incubation of normal MDS and AML progenitors for 48 h with growth factors on

Table 1. The effects of liquid phase pre-incubation of LDMCs for 6, 24, 48 or 72 h with Biorich, CM 5637, GM-CSF, or IL-3 on subsequent CFU-GM colony survival in semi-solid culture. Numbers of surviving colonies are presented as a percentage of data obtained from cultures set up at time 0 with no pre-incubation

		CM5637	GM-CSF	IL-3
(h)	(%)	(%)	(%)	(%)
0	100	100	100	100
6	97±3	99±1	100±1	101±2
24	92±4	98±6	93±4	94±4
48	62±4	97±2	92±4	93±4
72	38±12	15±15	68±4	77±7
	$n=7$	$n=2$	$n=5$	$n=5$

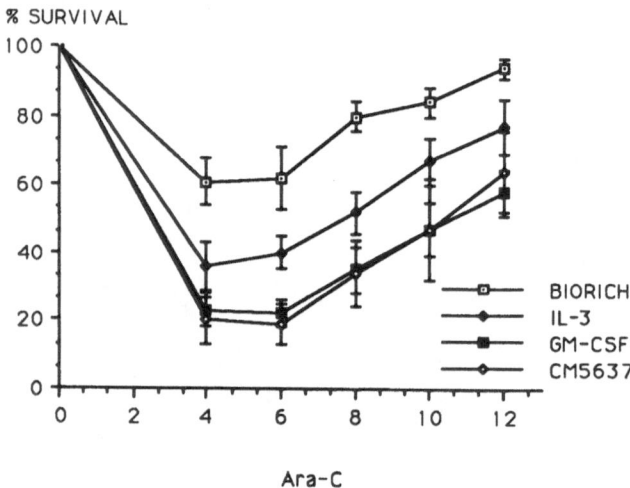

a

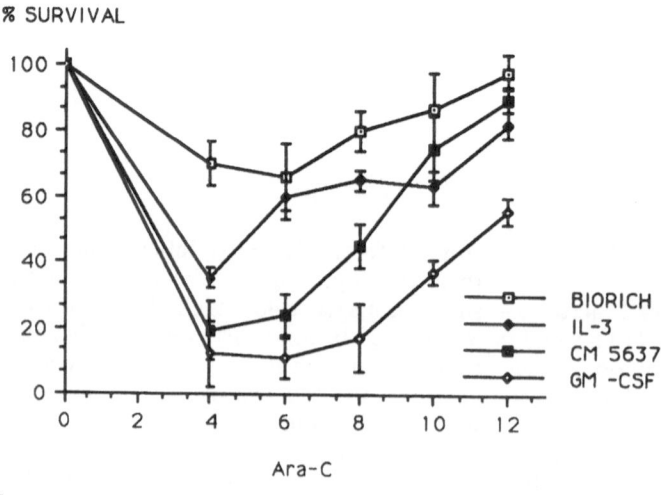

b

Fig. 2 a,b. Marrow sensitivity to Ara-C in semi solid culture after 48 h pre-incubation in liquid culture with growth factors. *a* Normal, $n=18$; *b* MDS, n = 5

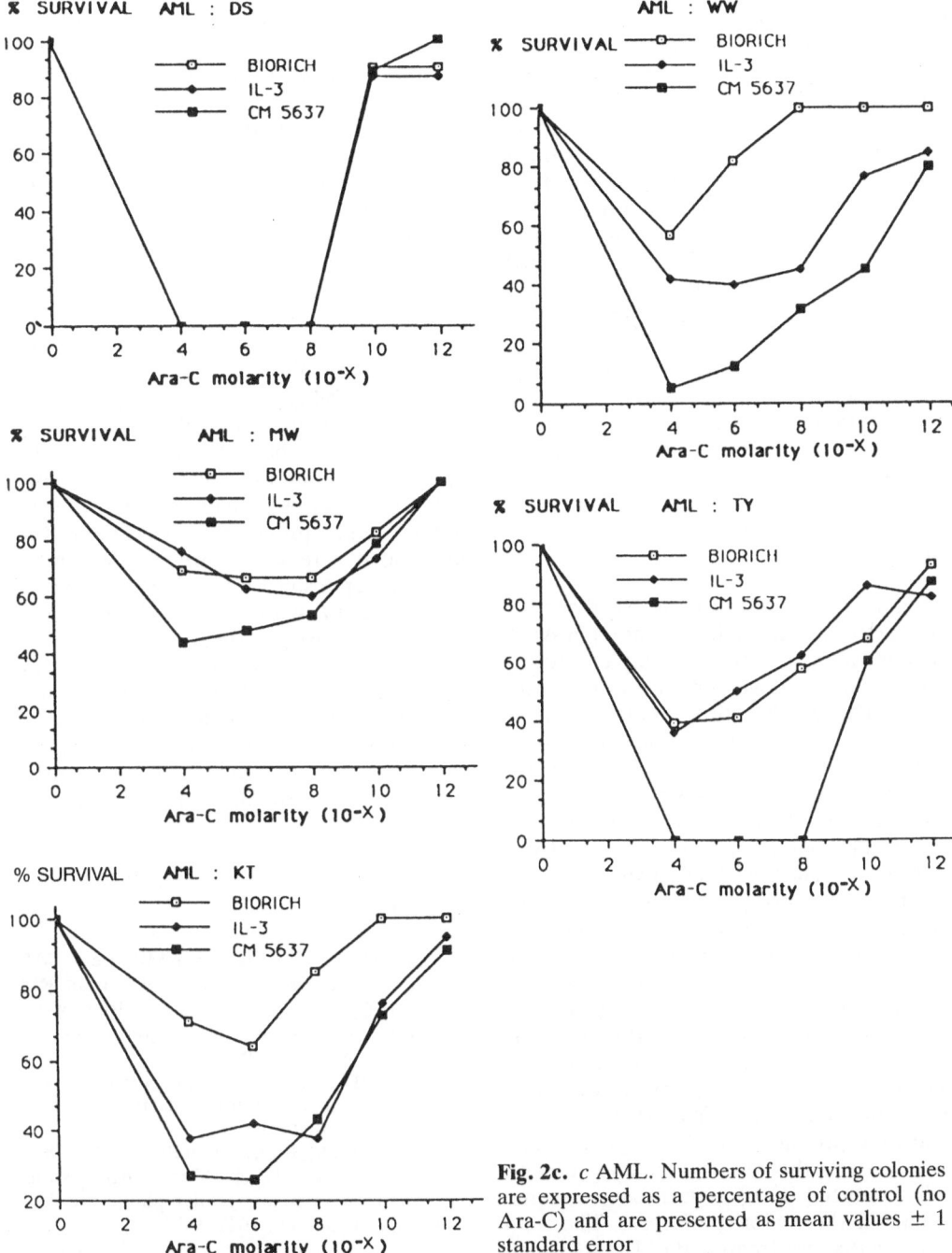

Fig. 2c. *c* AML. Numbers of surviving colonies are expressed as a percentage of control (no Ara-C) and are presented as mean values ± 1 standard error

their subsequent sensitivity to Ara-C. Compared with day 0 data (Fig. 1), pre incubation of normal and MDS LDMCs with GM-CSF and CM 5637 significantly improved the cytotoxic effect of Ara-C, while IL-3 did so to a lesser but still significantn

extent. All data indicate that the optimal cytotoxic effect occurred between Ara-C concentrations of 10^{-4} # M (equivalent to 100 # mg/^{2}) and 10^{-6} M. Biorich induced significant resistance to Ara-C in normal and MDS marrows. Figure 2 (c) illustrates the variable response of AML marrows to Ara-C following the pre-treatment manoeuvre. In patient DS, whose marrow was relatively sensitive to Ara-C on day 0, pre-incubation does not improve cytotoxicity. There was a slight but significant increase in effect ($p<0.05$) in marrow from patient MW after pre-incubation with CM 5637, but not with IL-3. Marrow from patients KT, WW and TY showed much improved susceptibility to Ara-C after 48 h in the presence of CM 5637 ($p<0.01$, 0.01 and 0.025 respectively). IL-3 caused a less dramatic but still significant ($p<0.02$ and 0.05) increase in cell toxicity in KT and WW, but not in TY. In patients KT and WW pre-incubation in Biorich alone promoted resistance to Ara-C.

Discussion

Problems associated with the use of chemotherapeutic agents in the treatment of AML include failure to obtain complete remission and/or the development of drug resistance. The proliferating compartment in AML is small [2] with the majority of blast cells remaining in G_o [3]. Using specific growth factors it is possible to induce proliferation of AML blasts [4, 5], thus potentially increasing blast cell sensitivity to cell-cycle specific drugs such as Ara-C.

Ara-C is considered nowadays as the mainstay of chemotherapy for patients with AML. It is also an important agent in higher grades of MDS. Thus marrow from patients within these disease categories was included in this study. Since the cytotoxic effect of Ara-C is S-phase-dependent, the increased cytotoxicity observed in normal, MDS and four out of five AML marrows following pre-incubation with growth factors suggests that this manoeuvre successfully induced DNA synthesis to some extent in the majority of cases. The data indicate that pre-treatment of LDMCs with GM-CSF and CM 5637 greatly improved the cytotoxic index of Ara-C, with IL-3 doing so to a lesser but still significant extent. Conversely, pre-incubation without growth factors appeared to confer resistance to Ara-C, possibly as a result of clonogenic cells entering G_0.

The fact that GM-CSF and IL-3 bind to common or closely related membrane receptors on AML and normal precursor cells [6], would be in accordance with our observation that both blast cells and CFU-GM progenitors are rendered more susceptible to Ara-C after pre-treatment with these growth factors. As a consequence, pre-treatment of patients with cytokines prior to the use of cytotoxic agents should be approached with caution due to the risk of prolonged pancytopenia resulting from increased destruction of normal haemopoietic stem cells.

The variability in degree and pattern of response to in vitro Ara-C demonstrated by AML marrows has also been noted by others [7]. This may be due to heterogeneity in cell cycle status or in maturation stage of the leukaemic progenitor cells. Due to the intrinsic differences between AML marrows in response to Ara-C with or without pre-treatment with growth factors, our observations would suggest that in vitro assessment of response to such therapeutic combinations should be seriously considered. Further research is required to define those therapeutic options which will maximise blast cell cytolysis whilst minimising damage to the normal stem-cell compartment.

References

1. Smith JG, Seenan AK, Smith MA, Lesko MJ, Lucie NP, Robertson MRI and Rowan RM (1985) Cyclical neutropenia and T-lymphocyte mediated stimulation of granulopoiesis. Br J Haematol 60: 481–489
2. Griffin JD and Lowenberg B (1986) Clonogenic cells in acute myeloblastic leukemia. Blood 68: 1185–1195
3. Raza A, Maheshwari Y and Preisler H (1987) Differences in cell cycle characteristics among patients with acute nonlymphoblastic leukaemia. Blood 69: 1647–1653
4. Lista P, Brizzi MF, Avanzi GC, Veglia F, Resegotti L and Pegorano L (1988) induction of proliferation of acute myeloblastic leukaemia (AML) cells with haemopoietic growth factors. Leuk Res 12: 441–447
5. Delwel R, Dorssers L, Touw I, Wagermaker G and Lowenberg B (1987) Human recombinant multilineage colony stimulating factor (Interleukin 3): stimulator of acute myelocytic

leukaemia progenitor cells in vitro. Blood 70: 333–336

6. Budel LM, Elbaz O, Hoogerbrugge H, Delwel R, Mahmoud L, Lowenberg B and Touw IP (1990) Common binding structure for granulocyte macrophage colony-stimulating factor and Interleukin 3 on human acute myeloid leukaemia cells and monocytes. Blood 75: 1439–1445

7. Misago M, Chiba S, Kikuchi M, Tsukada J, Sato T, Oda S and Eto S (1990) Usefulness of neutral red uptake method for investigation of the effects of recombinant growth factors on leukaemic blasts in proliferation. Leuk Res 14: 559–565

Proliferation – Inducing Effects of Recombinant Human Interleukin-7 and Interleukin-3 in B-Lineage Acute Lymphoblastic Leukemia

A. Ganser[2], M. Eder[2], O.G. Ottmann[2], T.E. Hansen-Hagge[2], C.R. Bartram[2], S. Gillis[3], and D. Hoelzer[1]

Introduction

Acute lymphoblastic leukemia (ALL) is a clonal disorder characterized by derangements of self-renewal and differentiation of lymphoid precursor cells in the bone marrow. Corresponding to the inconsistent stimulatory effects of the recombinant hematopoietic growth factors studied to date on B-lineage ALL blasts in vitro [1], a reproducible culture assay that supports proliferation and maturation of ALL blasts has not yet been reported.

Recently, a new cytokine has been defined by its stimulatory effects on DNA synthesis in murine pre-B cells from Whithlock-Witte culture [2]. This stromal-cell-derived cytokine, termed interleukin-7 (IL-7), has been purified and molecularly cloned and the recombinant murine and human proteins are now available [3, 4]. Since IL-7 also stimulates murine pre-B cells from bone marrow [5], murine thymocytes, and (as comitogen) mature T-cells [6], and induces proliferation of human T-cells [7], we investigated (a) whether or not IL7 could stimulate DNA synthesis in B-lineage

ALL blasts in suspension culture, and (b) the capacity of IL-7 to induce blast cell maturation in vitro.

Materials and Methods

Low density peripheral blood ($n=10$) or bone marrow ($n=4$) cells were separated by Ficoll-Hypaque density centrifugation and were classified as precursor-B-ALL(cALL) ($n=10$; HLA-DR+/CD10+/CD19+/sIg-) or B-ALL ($n=4$; HLA-DR+/CD10- or CD10+/CD19+/sIg+) [8]. All samples were depleted of adherent cells before incubation with OKT4, OKT8, and OKM1 and rabbit complement in order to eliminate mature myeloid and T-lymphoid cells. Cells were cultured in Iscove's modified Dulbecco's medium (IMDM), 20% fetal calf serum (FCS), 1% L-glutamine and 1% penicillin/streptomycin supplemented by IL-7 (50 units/ml, Immunex) or IL-3 (50 ng/ml, Behring Werke, Marburg and incubated in 96 well plates at $1–2.5 \times 10^5$ cells/well (quadruplicate values). After 7 days of liquid culture, samples were pulsed with ^3H-thymidine (1 µCi/well) for 4 h and harvested on nitrocellulose filters. Thymidine uptake was defined by liquid scintillation counting. Cells of responsive samples were further characterized by four parameter flow cytometry using a panel of monoclonal antibodies (moAb) and by immunogenotyping in order to monitor individual leukemic cell populations prior to and after suspension culture. All moABs were from Becton-Dickinson (anti-CAL-LA CD10, Leu 12 CD19, Leu 16 CD20,

[1] Department of Hematology, University of Frankfurt, Frankfurt, FRG
[2] Department of Pediatrics II, Molecular Biology Section, University of Ulm, Ulm, FRG
[3] Immunex Corporation, Seattle, Washington, USA

* This work was supported by grants Ga 333/1–3 and Ba 770/2–3 from the Deutsche Forschungsgemeinschaft and by a grant from the Deutsche Krebshilfe.

anti-kappa, anti-lambda, anti-HLA-DR, Leu M9 CD33, and anti-HPCA 1 CD34), Coulter Clone (My 7 CD13), and Medac (goat-anti-mouse IgG for indirect immuno-fluorescence staining). After culture one sample was incubated with Leu 12 and propidium iodide (PI) in order to examine viability and CD19 expression in different cell populations characterized by their light scatter properties.

Southern blot analysis was performed in the way described by Rhagavachar et al. [9]. *Eco*RI and *Hind*III digests were hybridized to a 2.4 kb Sau3a JH probe and *Bam*HI and *Hind* III digests to a 1.3 kb *Eco*RI Cμ probe, as well as a Ck probe to demonstrate Ig gene rearrangements. To analyse configuration of T-cell receptor genes *Eco*RI, *Bam*HI and *Hind*III digests were hybridized to a TCRβ probe and to a TCRγ probe, and *Hind*III and *Bgl*II digested DNA was hybridized to the TCRδ probe Js_{S16}.

Results and Discussion

The stimulation indices (SI), as defined as cpm of the sample/cpm of control, are given in Table 1. With an arbitrary cut-off of an SI value > 5, four out of ten cases of presursor-B-ALL (cALL) (samples 5, 7, 8, and 9) and one out of four cases of B-ALL (sample 14)

were stimulated by IL-7. IL-3 stimulated DNA synthesis in five out of nine cALL and three out of four B-ALL samples. In the cALL samples responsive to IL-7, IL–7 was more potent than IL-3 in two cases (samples 8 and 9), whereas IL-3 was more effective than IL-7 in all examined B-All samples.

To further define the nature of prolifer-ating cells and the maturation stage of the leukemic blasts, samples 6, 8, 9, and 14 were analyzed by fluorescence activated cell sorter (FACS) and Southern blot ana-lysis prior to and after liquid culture. Table 2 summarizes the results of immunopheno-typing, and Fig. 1 presents the analysis of sample 14. Analysis gates were fitted to light scatter properties of PI negative cells in order to gate preferentially viable cells after liquid culture. Case 6 which was Ph-positive revealed a marked increase in the percentage of CD33 and CD13 positive cells at day 7, suggesting that nonlymphoid cell populations preferantially proliferated during suspension culture. In sample 8 a decrease of CD34 and CD19 expression and of the percentage of CD10/CD19 double positive cells was detectable, while the percentage of CD20 positive cells was unchanged. Case 9 revealed a decrease in CD34 positive cells, but CD19 expression was unchanged and CD10/CD34 double positive cells were detectable after 7 days of

Table 1. Stimulation indices (SI) of ALL blasts stimulated by IL-7 and IL-3

Sample	Diagnosis	IL-7 (50 U/ml)	IL-3 (50 ng/ml)
1	cALL	1.5	1.5
2	cALL	2.6	nd
3	cALL	3.3	0.6
4	cALL Ph	1.3	1.8
5	cALL	5.1	6.7
6	cALL Ph	2.3	6.8
7	cALL	15.8	25.5
8	cALL	5.9	1.5
9	cALL	53.6	37.1
10	cALL	3,4	45.1
11	B-ALL	1.8	3.5
12	B-ALL	2.6	9.2
13	B-ALL	1.5	15.6
14	B-ALL	8.9	18.3

U, unit; Ph, Philadelphia positive
Mean SI of quadruplicate cultures (cpm of sample/cpm of control). cpm of control were < 850 in all examined cases.

Table 2. Surface marker analysis prior to and after suspension culture of ALL samples

Sample[a]	Antigen	Day 0	Day 7
6 cALL	CD34	11	54
	CD33	3	43
	CD13	<1	75
8 cALL	CD34	24	9
	CD19	69	45
	CD20	36	41
	CD10/CD19	69	37
9 cALL	CD34	96	75
	CD19	68	64
	CD20	6	4
	CD10/CD19	63	47
	CD10/CD34	92	42
14 B-ALL	CD34	<1	<1
	CD19	14	57
	CD20	72	82
	sIg kappa	36	<1

% positive cells

[a] samples 8, 9 and 14 were stimulated by IL-7 (50 units/ml), and sample 6 by IL-7 (50 units/ml) combined with IL3 (50 ng/ml)

liquid culture suggesting proliferative potential of B-lineage-restricted cells. A net increase of CD19 positive cells (data not shown) combined with the lack of surface bound Ig-kappa light chains was found in case 14 suggesting proliferation of B-lineage-restricted cells during the culture period. The lack of surface bound Ig-kappa light chains and the consistent pattern of Ig recombination prior to and after liquid culture (see below) suggest that leukemic transformation occurred at a maturation level preceding B-cell stage. Maturation induction, e.g., expression of surface-bound Ig after liquid culture was not detectable in any of the examined cases.

As indicated in Table 3, the immunogenotype corresponded to the immunophenotype of the examined cases. In order to monitor individual leukemic cell populations defined by specific molecular genetic markers, cells were analysed prior to and after liquid culture. In cases 9 and 14, IL-7 and IL-3 induced almost exclusively proliferation of the leukemic cell clone as indicated by the consistent pattern of the Ig recombination pattern prior to and after liquid culture. In samples 6 and 8, nonleu-

Table 3. Immunogenotype of ALL samples

Sample	Phenotype	Rearrangement	Proliferative population[a]
6	cALL Ph	IgH, TCRδ	Nonleukemic
8	cALL	IgH, TCRγ, TCRδ	Nonleukemic
9	cALL	IgH, TCRγ, TCRδ	Leukemic
14	B-ALL	IgH, Ig	Leukemic

[a] Proliferation of the leukemic cell clone was concluded from the consistent pattern of Ig recombination observed prior to and after liquid culture

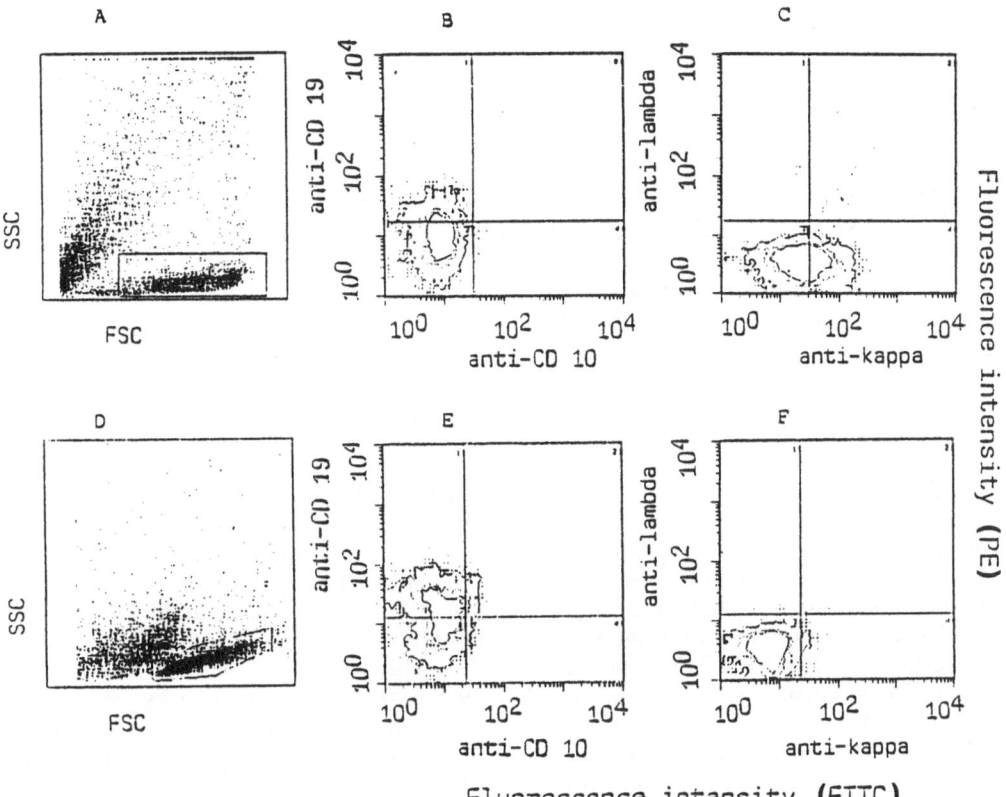

Fig. 1.
Scatter profile of sample 14 (B-ALL) before (A, B, C) and after (D, E, F) in vitro culture with II3+IL-7+IL-6 for seven days. Only the more immature, kappa-negative B-cells persisted in culture.

kemic cell proliferation associated with the generation of CD33 and CD13 positive cells (case 6) and detection of BFU-E and CFU-GM (case 8, data not shown) was observed after liquid culture when cultures were stimulated by IL-7 or IL-3. The detection of nonleukemic cells generated during suspension culture with IL-7 or IL-3 therefore underlines the necessity to exactly define the nature of proliferating cells in responsive samples.

We conclude that IL-7 and IL-3 can stimulate proliferation of leukemic cells in a subset of B-lineage restricted ALL without evidence of concurrent maturation induction. However, additional growth factors which could be provided by stromal cells are required to improve the in vitro culture of ALL blasts.

Acknowledgements. We gratefully appreciate the excellent technical assistance of P. Reutzel, P. Sauer, S. Ströcker-Pels, C. Tell, and U. Mehr.

References

1. Touw, et al. (1989) Leukemia 3: 356–362
2. Namen, et al. (1988) J Exp Med 167: 988–1002
3. Namen, et al. (1988) Nature 333: 571–573
4. Goodwin, et al. (1989) Proc Natl Acad Sci USA 86: 302–306
5. Lee, et al. (1989) J Immunol 142: 3875–3883
6. Henney. (1989) Immunol Today 10: 170–173
7. Armitage, et al. (1990) J Immunol 144: 938–941
8. Thiel, et al. (1987) Hamatol Bluttransfus 30: 95–103
9. Rhagavachar, et al. (1986) Blood 68: 658–662

Interleukin-1 Production by Mononuclear Cells and Natural Killer Cell Activity in Children with Acute Lymphoblastic Leukemia

A. Chybicka[1], J. Boguslawska-Jaworska[1], W. Budzyński[2], Cz. Radzikowski[2], and W. Jaworski[3]

Introduction

Interleukin 1 (IL-1) plays a major role in the response to infection, in inflammation, and in every immunological challenge. Over the past 10 years a variety of additional activities, especially of purified IL-1 on various target cells in vitro, has been reported [1]. As shown by Shirakawa et al. [2], IL-1 enhances also natural killer (NK) cell cytotoxic effect and proliferation. Expression of IL-2 receptors on NK cell surface can be regulated by IL-1 [3]. [4] Although IL-1 acts directly on many immunocompetent cells its role in malignant diseases has not yet been extensively explored [5]. We have previously reported apparent deficiency of IL-1 production by mononuclear cells of children with acute lymphoblastic leukemia (ALL) during the whole period of cytostatic therapy [6].

The of the current investigation was to discover whether a relationship exists between NK cell function and the IL-1 decreased level in children with ALL before any treatment, during and after completing chemotherapy, and in disease-free children (during the period 1–24 months).

Material and Methods

Our patient population included 60 children with ALL aged from 1 to 15 years (median 6 years) treated in the Department of Hematology and Oncology, Medical Academy, Wroclaw during the period 1988–1991. Nineteen healthy children in the same age group served as controls for IL-1 level examinations and 12 for NK cell count and cytotoxic activity in vitro studies. The ALL children were treated according to BFM protocols [6].

The initial characteristics of ALL children are presented in Table 1.

Heparinized vein blood samples were drawn from children at different stages of their disease: at the time of diagnosis, during therapy (from induction through consolidation to supportive remission therapy), and after completing the course of therapy.

Mononuclear cells were isolated on Lymphoprep (Nesco) gradient. Mononuclear cells for determination of NK cell numbers were incubated for 30 min with fluorescein conjugated with monoclonal antibody (CD_{16}) from Becton-Dickinson. After three subsequent washes slide preparations were made and examined using a fluorescent microscope. For cytotoxic in vitro assay a conventional ^{51}Cr release method was used [7]. Briefly, 0.5 # × # 10^4 K-562 erythroleukemic cells radiolabeled with ^{51}Cr were added in 0.1 ml volume to serial dilutions of peripheral blood on microplates (Plastomed). Triplicate cultures were maintained at 37° C in a humidified atmosphere con-

[1] Department of Hematology and Oncology, Medical Academy, Wroclaw
[2] Department of Tumor Immunology, Institute of Immunology and Experimental Therapy Polish Academy of Science, Wroclaw
[3] Department of Children Surgery, Medical Academy, Wroclaw
* This work was supported by grant of Polish Academy of Science No C.P.B.P 0601.

Table 1. The initial characteristics of ALL children

	n	%	n	%
Total	60		19	
Sex				
Girls	22	36.6	8	42.1
Boys	38	63.3	11	57.9
Age (years)				
< 2	4	6.6	–	–
2–10	44	73.3	14	73.6
> 10	12	20	5	26.3
Risk groups				
Low	15	25	3	15.7
Middle	38	63.3	12	63.1
High	7	11.6	4	21
Duration of observation				
Range	1–34 months			
Median	18 months			

taining 5% CO_2 in air for 4 h. After incubation, the supernatants were removed and measured in a gamma scintillation counter. The percentage of cytotoxity was calculated according to the formula:

$$\frac{\text{experimental cpm.} - \text{SR cpm}}{\text{MR cpm} - \text{SR cpm}} \times 100,$$

where SR indicates spontaneous release of ^{51}Cr and MR indicates maximal release of ^{51}Cr. # Lytic units (LU), defined as the number of effector cells required to lyse 1000 target cells (LU (20%/10^6 cells) were calculated according to a computer method described by Pross [8]. The method of IL-1 level determination described by Zimecki and Wieczorek [9] was used. It is based on IL-1 dependent reduction of the number of thymocytes forming autologous rosettes. Mononuclear cells were counted, resuspended in Eagle medium containing 10% fetal calf serum (FCS) and placed in an incubator at a concentration of 2×10^6 cells/ml; after 24 h of incubation the supernatants were removed. The thymocytes, in number 10^7 cells/1.8 ml of RPMI, supple-

mented by 10% FCS and antibiotics, were incubated with 0.2 ml of supernatant, at various dilutions for 24 h in CO_2 incubator.

The Rosette Assay

The cells were resuspended in a concentration of 3×10^6 cells/ml in Eagle medium supplemented by 10% mouse serum/preabsorbed with syngeneic erythrocytes. To 0.1 ml of the cell suspension 0.1 ml of 12% syngeneic erythrocytes was added, and mixed and centrifuged for 5 min at 200 g at 4 °C. After 24 h incubation at 4 °C, 0.5 ml of Hank's medium and 0.1 ml of 0.1% acridine orange solution were added; the cells were then gently resuspended and kept in an ice bath. The percentage of autologous rossettes formed by thymocytes from 2 months CBA mice were counted and the number varied from 28%–33%. Control samples consisted of referential r-IL-1 dilution. All the results were expressed in units of IL-1. One unit of IL-1 inhibited 50% of rossette formation.

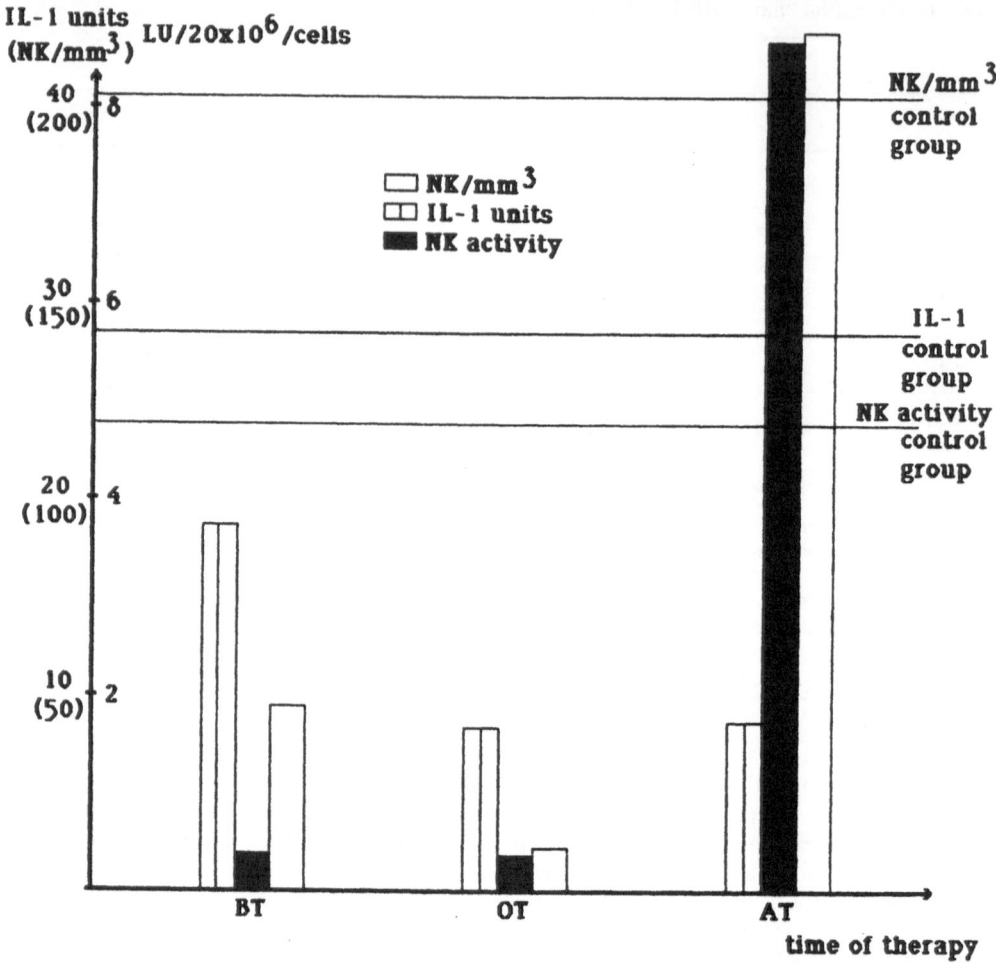

Fig. 1. Interleukin-1 (IL-1) production, natural killer (NK) cell number, and activity in children with ALL during cytostatic therapy (median values). *BT*, before treatment; *OT*, on cytostatic treatment; *AT*, after treatment

Results

The interleukin-1 production by cells from leukemic patients before chemotherapy ranged from 4 to 64 units, the median value being 18.4 units. This value was lower than that of the control group (2–64 units median 28 units).

Before initiation of treatment analysis revealed a significant decrease in NK cell count as compared with the control group value (median 48/mm³ versus 202/mm³). Similarly, the NK cells' cytotoxic activity was lower than that of the control group (median 0.48 LU versus 4.9 LU).

The striking decrease in IL-1 production was observed during the whole period of chemotherapy as compared to the control group (median 8 U versus 28 U). After a prednisone pretreatment phase the median value was 0 U, and after intensive multidrug induction the median value was 4 units; during remission maintenance therapy this value was 8 U (data not shown). At the same time the decrease in NK cell number to the median value of 15.9//mm³ was observed. The median value of NK cells' cytotoxic activity (0.58 LU) analysed during chemotherapy was similar to that found before treatment was started.

154

Table 2. Interleukin-1 (IL-1) production and (natural killer) (NK) cell activity in children with ALL treated according to BFM protocols. $p = 0.05$ - IL production results; m, median

Examination performed	Il-1 production units	Mononuclear cells/mm³	NK activity, lytic units	NK/mm³
Before treatment $n=10$ (IL-1) $n=8$ (NK)	x, 28.7 δ, 20.7 m, 18.4	x, 6233 δ, 8304 m, 3600	x, 1.75 δ, 2.9 m, 0.48	x, 76 δ, 60.2 m, 48
During cytostatic therapy from (induction therapy to supplement remedial treatment) $n = 46$ (IL-1) $n = 8$ (NK)	x, 10.4 δ, 11.5 m, 8	x, 995 δ. 598 m, 830	x 0.8 δ, 0.6 m, 0.58	x 38 δ, 64 m, 15
After treatment $n=10$ (IL-1) $n= 8$ (NK)	x, 14.1 δ, 17.1 m, 8.3	x, 1891 χ, 1013 m,2100	x, 28.62 χ, 29 m, 11.58	x, 303 δ, 139 m, 399
Control group $n=19$ (IL-1) $n=12$ (NK cells)	x, 29.42 δ, 13.5 m, 28	x, 2300 δ, 200 m, 2000	x, 7.27 δ, 5.3 m, 4.9	x, 181.78 δ, 150 m, 202

Il production results, $p=0.05$ NK cells activity n.s.

The examinations performed in children after therapy revealed an increase in IL-1 production (median 8.3 units without reaching the initial value. In the same period the increased value of NK cell numbers (median 399/mm³) and NK activity (median 11.58 LU) was observed.

Concluding Remarks

A number of reports have shown reduced NK activity in patients with hematologic malignancies [7, 13, 14]. In the present study we have investigated the NK activity in children with ALL before, during, and after cessation of chemotherapy. # The NK activity in children before and during treatment was found to be depressed as compared to the control group (0.48 LU and 0.58 LU versus 4.9 LU respectively). Similarly the number of NK cells/mm³ in leukemic children was severely decreased in comparison with control values. The reason for down-regulation of NK activity in untreated cancer patients is still not completely elucidated al though there are many data implicating the role of suppressor cells, prostaglandins, exhaustion of lytic function, inhibition of IL-2 production, etc [11]. After cessation of chemotherapy both NK cell activity and numbers were found to be highly elevated. It has been demonstrated in others reports [13, 14] that NK activity after completion of chemotherapy was to some extent comparable to the control values. In our studies including small numbers of patients (eight) it seems that high lytic activity and the number of NK cells could be explained by concomitant infection with hepatitis B virus recorded in some of the children.

Our studies showed that the level of IL-1 production in leukemic children before treatment was lower than that of the control group (18.4 U versus 28 U). This level remained lowered in children during cytotoxic treatment and may have been influenced by cytostatic drugs. However, after cessation of chemotherapy there was still a decreased level of IL-1 [15]. This low level of IL-1 in children before and during treatment corellated well with down-regulation of NK cell activity. Perhaps IL-1 can be regarded as one of the factors responsible for NK activity in children with ALL. The studies of Shirakava et al. [2] showed that incubation of large granular lymphocytes (LGL) with IL-1 enhances the induction of IL-2 receptors on them in a doese-dependent manner. Data obtained by Lange et al. [12] indicated that IL-1 exerted additive effect to IL-2 in generation of lytic activity of phagocyte-depleted non-adherent low density mononucleear cells in in vitro culture. However, the role level of IL-1 after successful chemotherapy needs futher study and observation.

References

1. Fibbe E, Schaafsma MR, Falkenburg FJ, Willmze R (1989) The biological activities of interleukin 1. Blut 59: 177
2. Shirakawa F, Tanaka Y, Eto S, Suzuki H, Yodo Y, Yamashita U, (1986) Effect of interleukin 1 on the expression of interleukin 2 receptor (TAC antigen) on human natural killer cells and natural killer-like cell line (YT cells). J Immunol 137: 551
3. Kataoka Y, Todo S, Morioka Y, Sugie K, Nakamura Y, Yodoi J, Imashuku S (1990) Impaired natural killer activity and expression of interleukin 2 receptor antigen in familial erythophagocytic lymphohistiocytosis. Cancer 65: 1937
4. Peppoloni S, Bossu P, Boraschi D, Tagliabue A (1989) A short synthetic peptide fragment of human interleukin 1β increases both human and murine natural killer activity. Nat Immun Cell Growth Regul 8:10–19
5. Herman JA, Kew MC, Rabson AR (1984) Defective interleukin-1 production by monocytes from patients with malignant diseases: interferon increasas IL-1 production. Cancer Immunol Immunother 16: 182–185
6. Chybicka A, Boguslawska-Jaworska J (1990) Interleukin 1 production in childhood acute lymphoblastic leukemia during chemo- and radiotherapy according to BFM (Berlin-Frankfurt-Munster) protocol. In: Büchner T et al. Acute leukemias II. Berlin Heidelberg New York 33: 72 (Hematology and blood transfusion)
7. Frydecka I (1985) Natural killer cell activity during the course of disease in patients with Hodgkin's disease. Cancer 56: 2799
8. Pross HF, Maroun JA (1984) The standardisation of NK cell assays for use in studies of biological response modifiers. J Immunol Methods 68: 235
9. Zimecki M, Wieczorek Z (1987) IL-1 decreases the level of thymocytes forming rosettes with autologous erythrocytes, a new method of determination of Il-1 activity. Arch Immunol Ther Exp (Warsz) 355: 371
10. Migliorati G, Cannarile L, D'Adamio L, Herberman RB, Riccardi C (1987) Interleukin 1 auguments the interleukin 2 dependent generation of natural killer cells from bone marrow precursor. Nat Immun Cell Growth Regul 6: 306
11. Pross HF, Baines M (1987) Alterations in natural killer cell activity in tumor-bearing hosts. In: Herberman RB, et al. (eds) Immune responses to metastases. CRC Press, Boca Raton, p 57
12. Lange A, Flad HD, Jack A, Ulmer AJ (1986) Effect of human recombinant interleukin 2 on natural killing of low density percoll fraction cells. Immunol Lett 12: 243–250
13. Douer D, Shaked N, Ramot B (1987) Normal natural killer activity in Hodgkin's disease patients in remission. Clin exp Immunol 69: 660–667
14. Mehta BA, Satam MN, Advani H, Nadkarin JJ (1989) In vitro modulation of natural killer cell activity in non-Hodgkin's lymphoma patients after therapy. Cancer Immunol Immunother 28: 148–152
15. Tanaka Y (1981) Natural killer NK activity in children with acute lymphoblastic leukemia. Hiroshima J Med Sci 30: 127

Lymphokine Combination Vectors:
A New Tool for Tumor Vaccination in Leukemias/Lymphomas

B. Gansbacher and E. Gilboa

Introduction

Previously, we have shown that CMS5, a fibrosarcoma, could be induced to secrete lymphokines into the immediate surroundings of the tumor cells following transduction with the interleukin-2 (IL-2) or mouse interferon gamma (IFN-gamma) gene, resulting in a potent antitumor immune response [1, 2]. To explore this system in detail an appropriate animal model, analogous to human tumors which are essentially nonimmunogenic, is required. Since CMS5 is immunogenic and generates a cellular immune response it is not by itself ideal for this purpose. On the other hand, the murine B cell lymphoma 38C13, produced in a C3H/eB mouse depleted of T-cells is weakly immunogenic and expresses an idiotype which essentially constitutes a tumor specific marker. This idiotype has been studied in detail and used in immunotherapeutic models to induce antitumor respones [3–5]. While both humoral and cellular immune responses are important in vivo for resistance to tumor growth, in the 38C13 system the cellular antitumor immune response has been quite suboptimal [6]. We will use these genetically modified malignant B-lymphocytes, which we have transduced with lymphokine genes using retroviral

Department of Hematology/Lymphoma and Molecular Biology, Memorial Sloan Ketterin Cancer Center, New York, USA
* This work was supported in part by funds from the Schultz Foundation (B.G.) and the Kleberg Foundation (E.G.).

gene transfer, to generate specific cytotoxic T-cells in vitro and a cellular antitumor response in vivo. Our findings in the CMS5 system provide a rationale for the hypothesis that lymphokine gene transfer may be successful in enhancing the host's antitumor response to 38C13.

Results

Generation of Tumor Cell lines Expressing IL-2 or Interferon Gamma

Figure 1a, b shows the retroviral vector constructs that were used to introduce and express the human IL-2 and IFN-gamma genes into tumor cells. The retroviral vectors used in this study were derived from Moloney murine leukemia virus (MLV) and are based on the high titer N2 retroviral vector, which also contains the bacterial neomycin resistance (neo) selectable gene [7]. Vector DNA was converted to corresponding virus using established procedures. Briefly, vector DNA was transfected into a packaging cell line, and neomycin-resistant colonies were selected with G418. Drug-resistant colonies were isolated and expanded to cell lines, and virus-containing cell-free supernatant was used to infect 38C13 cells. G418-resistant colonies were isolated and expanded to cell lines for further analysis. However, prior to infection it was necessary to assess the intrinsic G418 resistance of the 38C13 cells. These cells (quantity: 1×10^5/ml) were placed in 0.25, 0.5, 0.75, and 1.0 mg/ml of G418 in complete medium (RPMI 1640 medium

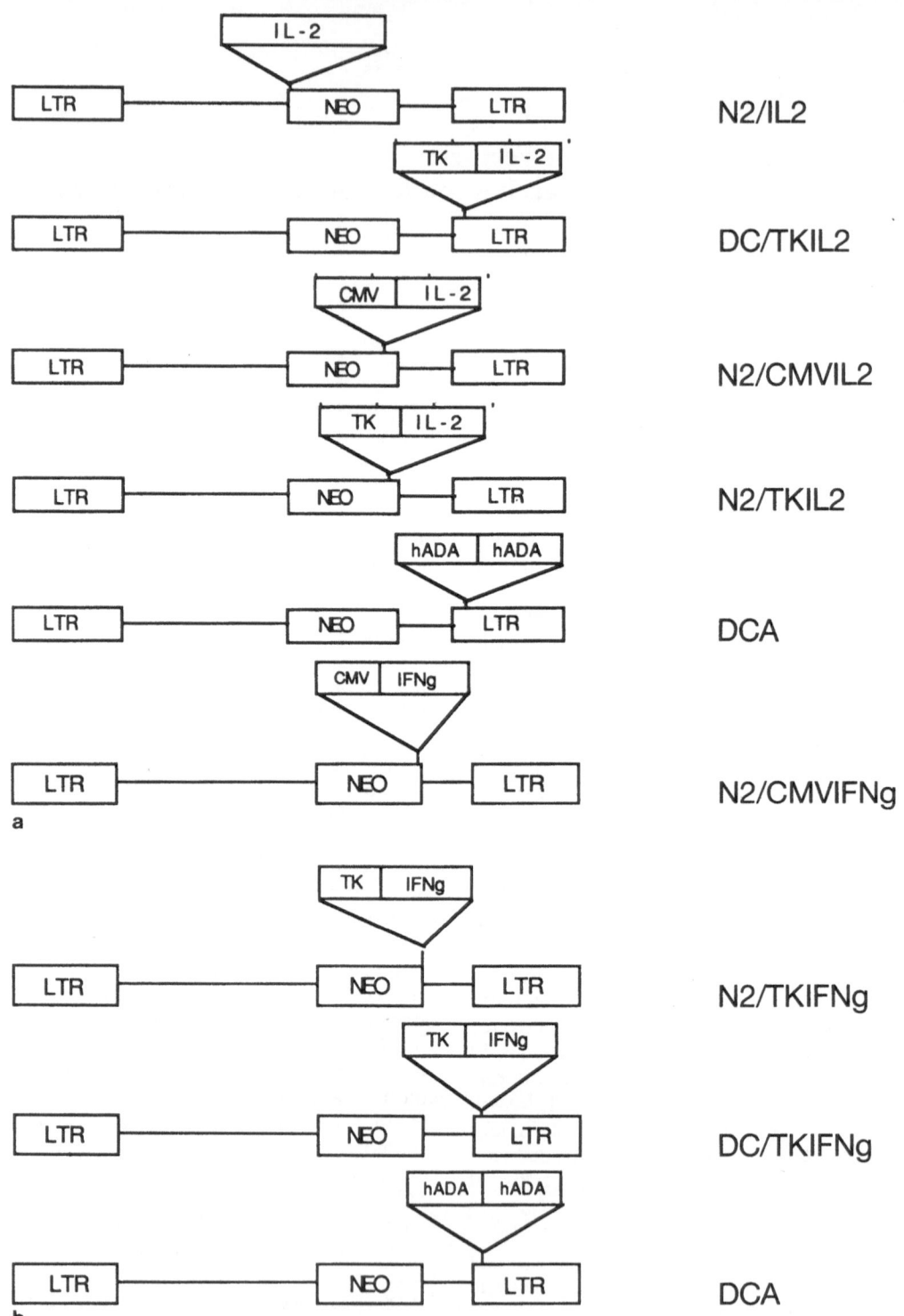

Fig. 1a, b. Structure of the retroviral vectors containing the human IL-2 (*a*) or the mouse IFN-gamma (IFNg) gene (*b*) (for additional details see [1] and [2])

supplemented with 10% fetal calf serum (FCS), 2 μ8 mM glutamine, 100 units/ml penicillin, 100 μ9 ug/ml streptomycin, and 5×10^{-5} M 2-ME). Cells were checked for viability with trypan blue and resuspended in new G418-containing medium every 2 days. At a G418 concentration of 0.5 mg/ml, 100% of uninfected cells were dead by day 10 and this G418 concentration was chosen for all further infections. Once we knew the G418 concentration required for selection, the cells were infected with four IL-2, two IFN-gamma and one adenosine deaminase (ADA) recombinant virus, since it was not possible to predict which construct would work best in these cells. The ADA virus, deoxycorticosterone acetate (DCA), serves as our negative control. The amphotrophic viruses, N2/IL-2, DC/TKIL-2, N2/CMVIL-2, N2/TKIL-2, DC/IFN-gamma, N2/CMVIFN-gamma, and DCA (Fig. 1 a, b), were used to avoid interference from endogenous ecotropic viruses in 38C13 cells. For infection, 38C13 cells were resuspended at 1×10^5 cells/ml, centrifuged, and resuspended in 1-ml virus-containing complete medium containing 8 mg/ml of polybrene. Polybrene is believed to facilitate virus adhesion to the cell surface. One sample of cells, to serve as an uninfected control, was resuspended in complete medium containing no virus and another was used in a mock infection with medium containing 8 mg/ml of polybrene, but no virus. After overnight incubation, the cells were resuspended in fresh complete medium for 48 h to allow cell proliferation which is important if viral integration is to occur. The uninfected control did not get any G418 and served in this way as a control for normal cell viability and proliferation. All other samples were grown in medium containing 0.5 mg/ml G418. The mock infected cells were used as the indicator of the G418 effect. Since virus integration is stable, once all mock infected 38C13 cells had died in the G418-containing medium the virus infected cells could be expanded in complete medium without G418. Appropriate integration of the provirus into the cell genome was assessed by Southern blot analysis using the restriction

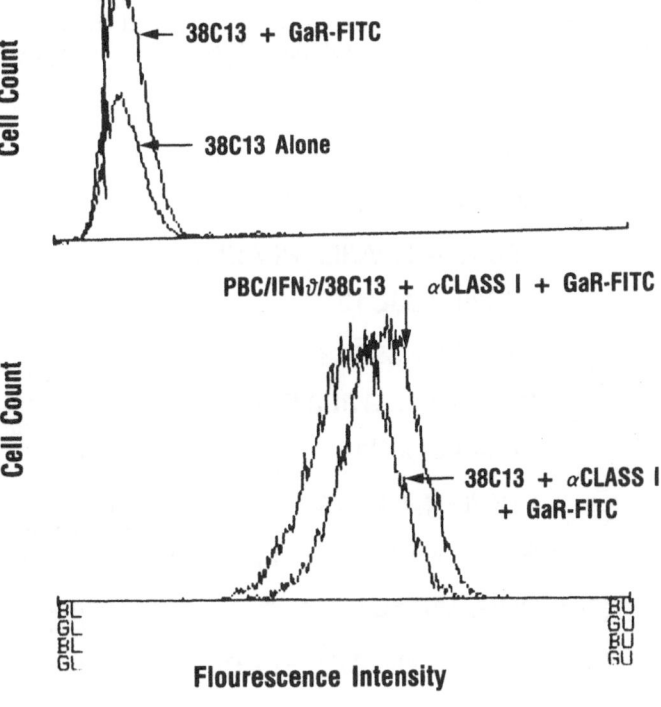

Fig. 2. Southern blot analysis of the structure of the proviral DNA in 38C13 cells infected with the cytokine – carrying vectors. The proviral DNA was excised from the host genome by digestion with *KpnI* which cuts once in the viral LTRs. As a size control, the appropriate cytokine-containing plasmid which was digested with the same enzyme was used. Of note is that the IL-2 and the IFN-gamma cDNAs are of similar size; consequently only one plasmid was used as a size marker. Hybridization was performed with a neospecific probe

enzyme *KpnI* which cuts in both viral LTRs and therefore excises the provirus from the host genome. This is done to exclude rearrangements and to ensure appropriate integration of the provirus into the host DNA. DNA from uninfected 38C13 cells served as the negative control. To check for the expected band in the infected 38C13 cell DNA we ran the appropriate vector-containing plasmid which was used to generate the recombinant virus side-by-side with the test samples on an agarose gel. Following transfer, hybridization was performed using the neomycin probe, since that gene is located between the proviral LTRs and normally is not present in mammalian cells (Fig. 2).

Expression of the IL-2 gene in 38C13 cells transduced with the retroviral vectors was determined by measuring the secretion of the corresponding cytokine into the cell supernatant using an appropriate bioassay, and confirmed by an enzyme-linked immunoabsorbant assay (ELISA) test. Clonal isolates of 38C13 cells were found to vary in their ability to express and secrete the IL-2 and IFN-gamma gene products depending on the retroviral vector used. Secretion of human IL-2 or mouse IFN-gamma from 38C13 cells had no discernible effect on cell morphology or on growth rate in culture when compared to parental 38C13 cells

transduced with the control DCA vector (data not shown). These results underscore the importance of retroviral vector design and choice of expression system, and provide an opportunity to test the effects of varying the level of cytokine production on the biological system under study.

MHC Class I Expression of Cytokine Producing 38C13 Cells

Studies have shown that treatment of highly tumorigenic cells with IFN-gamma led to a significant decrease in their tumorigenicity, presumably due to the induction of MHC class I gene expression [8]. In order to see whether a similar mechanism could account for the observed antitumor effect of IFN-gamma-producing 38C13 cells, quantitative analysis of MHC class I gene expression on the cell surface of parental 38C13 and cytokine-producing counterparts was performed by indirect immunofluoresence staining and analysis using a fluorescence-activated cell sorter (FACS). The results of such an experiment (Fig. 3) showed that even though parental 38C13 cells, as well as IL-2-producing cells, already express high levels of MHC class I molecules on the surface, MHC class I expression in 38C13 cells transduced with PBC/IFN-gamma

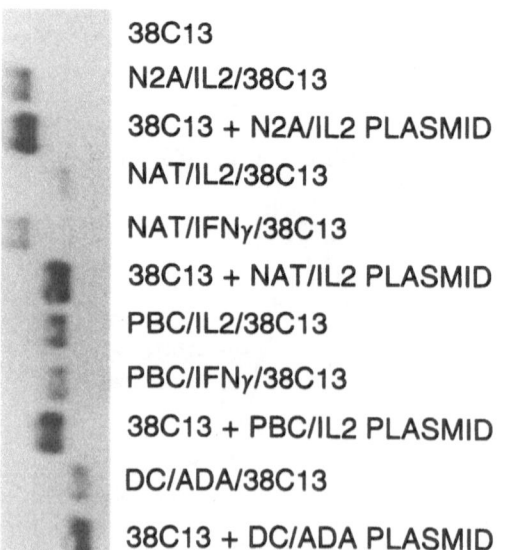

38C13

N2A/IL2/38C13

38C13 + N2A/IL2 PLASMID

NAT/IL2/38C13

NAT/IFNγ/38C13

38C13 + NAT/IL2 PLASMID

PBC/IL2/38C13

PBC/IFNγ/38C13

38C13 + PBC/IL2 PLASMID

DC/ADA/38C13

38C13 + DC/ADA PLASMID

Fig. 3. MHC class I expression on parental and cytokine-secreting 38C13 cells. Live cells were labeled with an MHC class I monomorphic monoclonal antibody (ATCC.TIB 126) followed by fluorescein isothicyocyanate-conjugated affinity-purified goat anti-rat IgG (GaR-FITC), and analyzed with an Epics V fluorescence-activated cell sorter (FACS) (Coulter Electronics, Inc.). As a control, µ8 specific antibody was omitted from reaction with 38C13 cells. Of note is that 38C13 cells infected with the IL-2-carrying vector did not show any upregulation of class I expression

(identical to N2/CMV/IFN-gamma) was upregulated above this background.

Discussion

When CMS5 cells were transduced with the IL-2 or IFN-gamma gene, delivery of these lymphokines to the tumor site had a dramatic effect on the outcome of the antitumor response against a normally lethal tumor, supporting our starting hypothesis. We showed that local secretion of IL-2 or IFN-gamma abrogated the tumorigenicity of the cytokine producing CMS5 cells and induced a long-term protective immune response against a subsequent tumor graft [1, 2]. Expression of MHC class I antigen increased 10 to 30-fold on the cell surface of IFN-gamma, but not IL-2 producing cells, which may explain their increased immunogenicity. In vitro analysis of spleen-derived cytotoxic T-cell activity against CMS5 cells indicated that IL-2 or IFN-gamma producing tumor cells prevented the establishment of tumor specific immunosuppression and were also capable of circumventing an existing state of immunosuppression [1, 2]. By choosing a tumor cell-line such as 38C13 with a well defined tumor antigen, it should be possible to extend these results so that they may be more relevant to the human setting. In addition, it should enable us to dissect the antitumor response in detail, permitting us to understand the underlying mechanism and optimize its potential application.

38C13 tumor cells express complement receptors, FcR, surface Ig and Ia. Most relevant to our work, extensive studies have shown the idiotype expressed by these cells can be used as a target for immunotherapy. Immunization with the idiotype hase led to tumor rejection, although the response was weak and could be overcome by increasing the tumor cell number used in the challenge. Because of the weakness of the response, anti-idiotypic therapy has been shown to benefit from the addition of IL-2 [5], IFN [4], and cytoxan [9], curing in some cases even mice which had established tumors. Unfortunately, idiotypic variants of 38C13 have been observed by immunoselection with anti-idiotype monoclonal antibody (MAb). Sequencing of the V region of the heavy and light chain has shown that the idiotypic heterogeneity which allowed the tumor to escape the immunotherapy arose as a consequence of alternative light chain rearrangements rather than point mutations [3]. Our system should enable a response even against these mutants by generating heterogeneous T-cell lines which are specific for a multitude of peptides expressed by this idiotype.

Our data demonstrate that retroviral vectors can be used to introduce the IL-2 or IFN-gamma gene into leukemia/lymphoma cells. With the exception of NAT/IFN-gamma/38C13 (identical to DC/IFN-gamma/38C13) in lane 5 (Fig. 3) all proviruses are of the appropriate size and not rearranged. The IFN-gamma secreting 38C13 cells showed upregulation of MHC class I expression and the 38C13 cells infected with the IL-2-containing vector secreted significant amounts of recombinant IL-2. Since IL-2 exerts its biological effect on the lymphocyte effector populations while IFN-gamma does so on the tumor cell population, lymphokine combination vectors have been constructed. We are now in the process of converting these vectors to hybrid viruses. In all further experiments those vectors will be used as well. The objective of these future studies will be to investigate whether the local secretion of cytokines, IL-2 and IFN-gamma, from the genetically modified 38C13 cells will induce a cellular anti-idiotypic immune response in vivo and thereby decrease or abolish their tumorigenicity. Like antigen vaccination approaches, this strategy would prevent clonal expansion of tumor cells carrying this specific idiotypee. These experiments are now underway.

References

1. Gansbacher B, Zier K, Daniels B, Cronin K, Bannerji R, Gilboa E (1990) IL-2 gene transfer into tumor cells abrogates tumorigenicity and induces protective immunity. J Exp Med 172: 1217
2. Gansbacher B, Bannerji B, Zier K, Daniels B, Cronin K, Gilboa E (1990) Retroviral vector

mediated IFN-gamma gene transfer into tumor cells generates a potent and long lasting anti-tumor response. Cancer Res 50: 7820

3. Carrol WI, Starnes CO, Levy R, Levy S (1988) Alternative Vk gene rearrangements in a murine B cell lymphoma. J Exp Med 168: 1607

4. Basham, TY, Race ER, Campbell MJ, Reid TR, Levy R, Merigan TC (1988) Synergistic antitumor activity with IFN and monoclonal anti-idiotype for murine B cell lymphoma. J Immunol 141: 2855

5. Bernstein N, Starnes CO, Levy R (1988) Specific enhancement of the therapeutic effect of anti-idiotypic antibodies on a murine B cell lymphoma by IL-2. J Immunol 140: 2839

6. Campbell MJ, Esserman L, Byars NE, Allison AC, Levy R (1990) Idiotype vaccination against murine B cell lymphoma. Humoral and cellular requirements for the full expression of antitumor immunity. J Immunol 145: 1029

7. Armentano D, Yu S-F, Kantoff PW, von Ruden T, Anderson WF, Gilboa E (1987) Effect of internal viral sequences on the utility of retroviral vectors. J Virol 61: 1647–1650

8. Hammerling, GJ, Klar D, Pulm W, Momburg F, Moldenhauer G (1987) The influence of major histocompatibility complex class I antigens on tumor growth and metastasis. Biochim Biophys Acta 907: 245–259

9. Campell MJ, Eserman L, Levy R (1988) Immunotherapy of established murine B cell lymphoma. Combination of idiotype immunization and cylophosphamide. J Immunol 141: 3227

Regulation of Erythropoietin Production in Patients with Myelodysplastic Syndromes

C. Aul, A. Heyll, V. Runde, M. Arning, and W. Schneider

Introduction

Preleukemic syndromes or myelodysplastic syndromes (MDS) comprise a heterogeneous group of acquired bone marrow disorders, probably resulting from malignant transformation of a multipotent hematopoietic stem cell [1, 2]. In the elderly they are rather common diseases. Analysis of our own data referring to the population of Düsseldorf (Germany) yields an age-specific incidence rate of about 25/100 per year in people over the age of 70 [3]. Hallmarks of MDS include ineffective hematopoiesis, hypercellular bone marrow, and peripheral blood cytopenias [4]. In the majority of cases the etiology remains unkown.

Although MDS appears to arise from a multipotent stem cell, the initial hematological picture is dominated by abnormalities of the erythroid lineage, including hyperplasia and prominent dysplastic features. These early phases of the disease are almost always associated with anemia, whereas the peripheral granulocyte and platelet counts may be normal or even increased [5, 6]. With progression of MDS, granulopoietic cells gradually replace erythropoiesis and the bone marrow displays increasingly malignant features. Interestingly, a similar sequence of proliferation and maturation defects of hematopoietic cells has been observed during experimental induction of leukemia in animals [7]. The mechanism by which MDS evolves from an erythroid to a myeloid phenotype has not been clarified, but it may reflect an altered response of medullary precursor cells to hematopoietic growth factors or other cytokines. To study the role of erythropoietic growth factors in preleukemia, we determined the serum concentrations of erythropoietin (Epo) in 46 patients with primary or secondary MDS.

Patients and Methods

Patients

Forty-four patients (22 male, 22 female) with primary MDS and two patients (both female) with secondary (radiotherapy-induced) MDS were examined. Their median age was 68 years (range 7–88). The criteria proposed by Bennett et al. [8] constituted the basis for morphological classification of MDS. Diagnoses were refractory anemia (RA) in four, RA with ring sideroblasts (RARS) in nine, RA with excess of blasts (RAEB) in nine, RAEB in transformation (RAEB/T) in nine, and chronic myelomonocytic leukemia (CMML) in 12 cases. Three additional patients were studied after evolution of MDS to overt leukemia (MDS/AML). Of the 46 patients, 39 were anemic (median hemoglobin concentration 9.3 g/dl; range 5.7–14.6 g/dl) and 22 had leuko- and/or thrombocytopenia. In all cases examined, serum creatinine levels were within the normal range ($\leq$ 1.2 mg/dl). Before enter-

Department of Internal Medicine, Hematology and Oncology Division, Heinrich Heine University, Düsseldorf, FRG

ing the study, none of the patients had received red blood cell transfusions or any other therapy for MDS. Infections, hemorrhages or other malignant diseases which may have interfered with the Epo measurement were not present at the time of investigation.

Hematological Methods

Standard methods were used for measurement of hemoglobin concentration, red cell indices, reticulocyte count, serum ferritin and lactate dehydrogenase (LDH). Bone marrow smears were routinely stained with Pappenheim, Prussian blue and periodic acid Schiff (PAS). To determine the percentage of erythroid cells, at least 500 nucleated bone marrow cells were examined. We further tried to assess the degree of dyserythropoiesis by using the following criteria. Marked dysplasia was defined by the presence of gross morphological abnormalities (multinuclearity, giant forms, karyorrhexis, nuclear budding, megaloblastic transformation, and positive PAS reaction) in more than 80 % of the erythroblasts. Mild dyserythropoiesis was defined by the presence of nuclear cytoplasmic asynchrony or subtle megaloblastic changes in less than 30 % of the erythroblasts. Intermediate cases were classified as having moderate dyserythropoiesis.

Epo Measurement

Serum Epo levels were measured by a competitive binding disequilibrium radioimmunoassay (Epo-Trac ^{125}I RIA, Incstar, Minnesota, USA). Using this assay, the normal range of immunoreactive Epo in 21 healthy adults (age range 21–84 years) was 15.3 ± 8.7 mU/ml (mean ± SD). Serum samples were kept frozen at $-20\,°C$ until measurement.

Results

Estimates of serum Epo for the whole group of MDS patients ranged from 12 to 4530 mU/ml. Compared with normal adults, 39 (85 %) out of 46 patients had increased serum Epo values. We observed a considerable variation of Epo titers in all morphological categories, and although patients with RA and CMML tended to have the lowest levels, no clear-cut correlation between Eop activity and FAB subtype was noticed. In accordance with these findings, the measured Epo levels were not significantly related to the medullary blast cell count.

Figure 1 illustrates the relationship between serum Epo activity and hemoglobin concentration. Although both parameters were found to be inversely correlated ($r = -0.35$; $p = 0.02$), Epo titers differed markedly between patients at comparable degrees of anemia. For example, in five patients with a hemoglobin concentration of 7 g/dl, the measured Epo levels ranged from 61 to 4530 mU/ml. We further identified four anemic patients (hemoglobin concentration 8.3–11.1 g/dl) with unexpectedly low Epo levels (12–24 mU/ml) as well as rare cases without anemia in whom Epo titers were significantly increased. As shown in Fig. 2, we also noted a significant relationship between circulating Epo levels and the mean corpuscular volume (MCV) of the erythrocytes ($r=0.38$; $p=0.01$).

Besides the degree of anemia, the proliferative activity of the erythroid marrow may be an important factor influencing the serum Epo concentrations. In our study, however, no clear relation between red cell mass and Epo activity was found (Fig. 3). On the other hand, we observed striking differences in Epo titers when patients were analysed according to their degree of medullary dyserythropoiesis (Fig. 4). Patients with mild qualitative changes of erythroblasts had significantly lower serum Epo levels (median, 33 mU/ml) than those presenting with moderate or svere dyserythropoiesis (212 and 913 mU/ml, respectively) ($p<0.005$). Other parameters investigated in this study (e.g., reticulocyte count, LDH, ferritin, and percentage of ringed sideroblasts) were not found to be correlated with the Epo response.

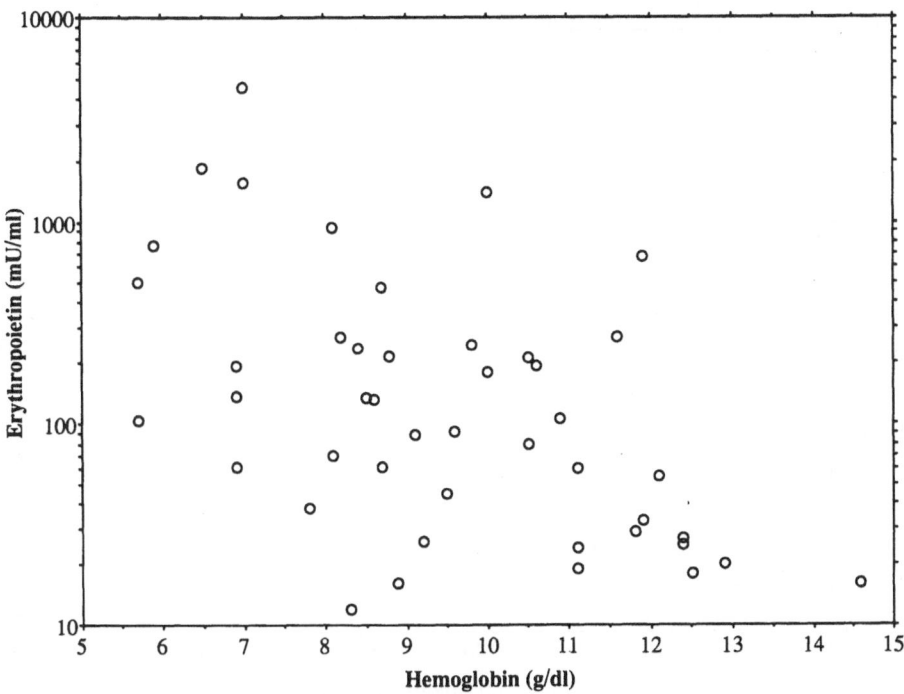

Fig. 1. Relationship between serum erythropoietin and hemoglobin concentrations in 46 patients with MDS ($r = -0.35$; $p=0.02$).

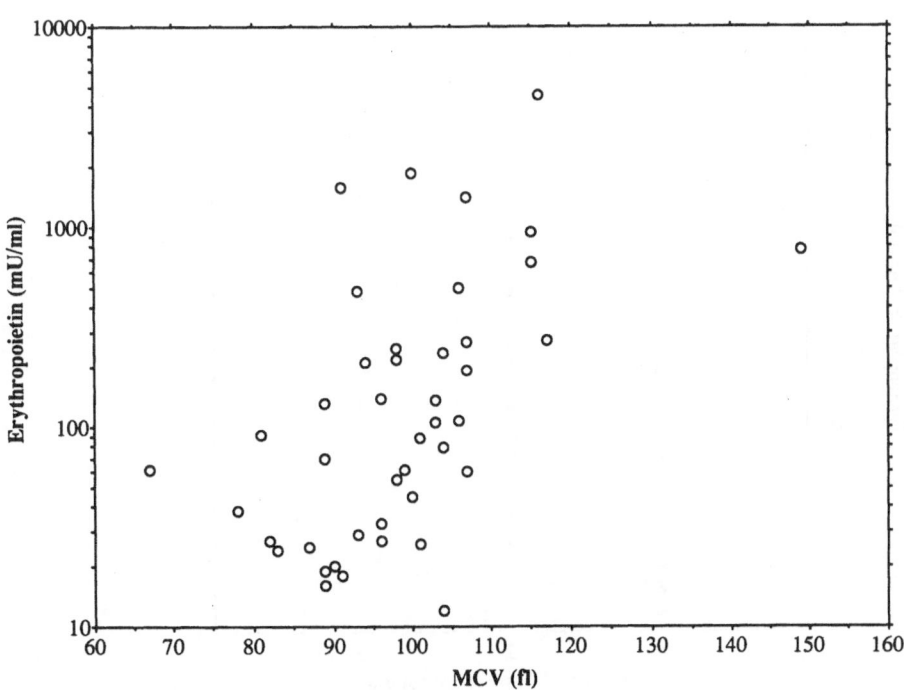

Fig. 2. Relationship between erythropoietin concentrations and mean corpuscular volume (MCV) of red blood cells ($r=0.38$; $p=0.01$).

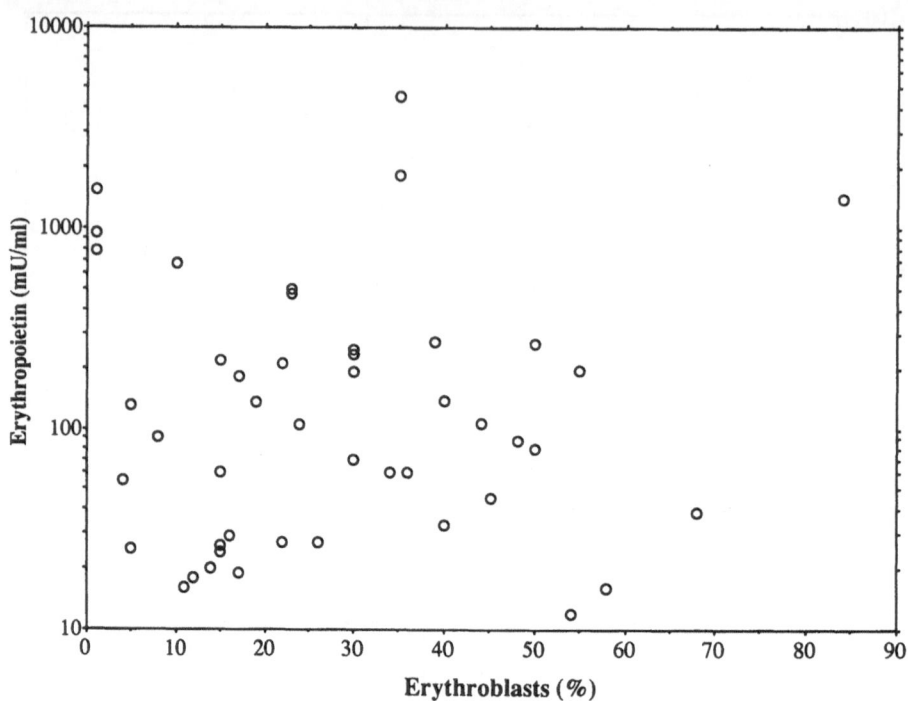

Fig. 3. Relationship between erythropoietin activity and percentage of bone marrow erythroblasts.

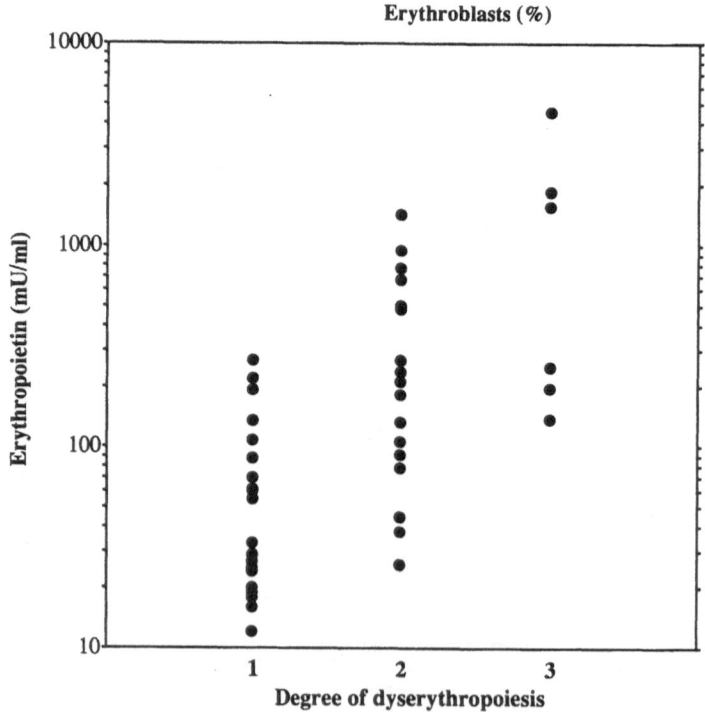

Fig. 4. Serum erythropoietin concentrations by degree of medullary dyserythropoiesis (*1*, mild; *2*, moderate; *3*, severe).

Discussion

Ineffective erythropoiesis with reduced production of erythrocytes is an early feature of MDS. The precise cause underlying the disturbed red cell proliferation and maturation in the bone marrow is presently unknown. It has been suggested that altered production of, and marrow cell response to, growth regulatory factors contribute to pathogenetic mechanisms in these disorders [9]. By measuring the serum levels of immunoreactive Epo in a large group of nontransfused patients, we tried to obtain more information on erythropoietic control mechanisms in MDS.

Although some cases were identified which had relatively low Epo levels for their degree of anemia, the majority of patients exhibited increased hormone concentrations, excluding an endogenous Epo deficiency as the cause of the anemia. Increased Epo production has been described in a variety of anemic disorders [10, 11] and represents a physiological renal response to decreased oxygen supply. In contrast to other types of nonrenal anemia, however, we found only a weak correlation between serum Epo and hemoglobin concentrations in our MDS patients. Similar data have recently been reported by Jacobs et al. [12], whereas other authors found a much closer relationship between Epo production and severity of anemia in MDS [13].

From their study, Jacobs et al. [12] concluded that different rates of Epo utilization by medullary erythroid cells account for the wide range of Epo titers in MDS. They found that circulating Epo levels were inversely correlated with the amount of erythropoiesis in the bone marrow. Patients with marked erythroid hypoplasia were shown to have particularly high Epo titers. These observations, however, could not be confirmed in our study. Based on our own data, we suppose that qualitative rather than quantitative changes of erythropoiesis have an important influence on the individual Epo response in MDS. Abnormally high Epo values were encountered only in patients with severe dyserythropoiesis, whereas patients with mild dysplastic features produced much lower amounts of Epo. It may be assumed that the degree of dyserythropoiesis reflects, at least in part, functional impairment of erythroid progenitor cells. Abnormal erythroid precursors may lose their sensitivity to Epo, either by altered receptor expression or disturbed function of the signal transduction pathway. As demonstrated by in vitro culture systems, erythroid colony growth in patients with MDS is often decreased and requires high concentrations of exogenous Epo [14]. In view of these findings, it is tempting to speculate that the marked elevations of Epo found in some MDS patients represent a compensatory mechanism, directed to overcoming the functional defect of aberrant target cells in the bone marrow.

References

1. Raskind WH, Tirumali N, Jacobson R, Singer J, Fialkow PJ (1984) Evidence for a multistep pathogenesis of a myelodysplastic syndrome. Blood 63: 1318–1323
2. Janssen JWG, Buschle M, Layton M, Drexler HG, Lyons J, Van Den Berghe H, Heimpel H, Kubanek B, Kleihauer E, Mufti GJ, Bartram CR (1989) Clonal analysis of myelodysplastic syndromes: evidence of multipotent stem cell origin. Blood 73: 248–254
3. Aul C, Schneider W (1990) Epidemiological and aetiological aspects of myelodysplastic syndromes: analysis of 441 cases (Abstract). Blut 61: 189
4. Aul C, Fischer JT, Schneider W (1984) Diagnostik der myelodysplastischen Syndrome („Präleukämien"). Dtsch Med Wochenschr 109: 506–510
5. Gattermann N, Aul C, Schneider W (1990) Two types of acquired idiopathic sideroblastic anaemia (AISA). Br J Haematol 74: 45–52
6. Bunn HF (1986) 5q- and disordered haematopoiesis. Clin Haematol 15: 1023–1035
7. Fritz TE, Tolle DV, Seed TM (1985) The preleukemic syndrome in radiation-induced myelogenous leukemia and related myeloproliferative disorders. In: Bagby GC (ed) The preleukemic syndrome (hemopoietic dysplasia). CRC Press, Boca Raton, pp 87–100
8. Bennett JM, Catovsky D, Daniel MT, Flandrin G, Galton DAG, Gralnick HR, Sultan C (1982) Proposals for the classification of the myelodysplastic syndromes. Br J Haematol 51: 189–199

9. Greenberg PL (1983) The smoldering myeloid leukemic states: clinical and biological features. Blood 61: 1035–1044
10. Erslev AJ, Wilson J, Caro J (1987) Erythropoietin titers in anemic, nonuremic patients. J Lab Clin Med 109: 429–433
11. De Klerk G, Rosengarten PCJ, Vet RJWM, Goudsmit R (1981) Serum erythropoietin (ESF) titers in anemia. Blood 58: 1164–1170
12. Jacobs A, Janowska-Wieczorek A, Caro J, Bowen DT, Lewis T (1989) Circulating erythropoietin in patients with myelodysplastic syndromes. Br J Haematol 73: 36–39
13. Vadhan-Raj S, Hittelman WN, Lepe-Zuniga J, Gutterman JU, Broxmeyer HE (1990) Regulation of endogenous erythropoietin levels in anemia associated with myelodysplastic syndromes (Correspondence). Blood 75: 1749–1750
14. Aoki I, Higashi K, Homori M, Chikazawa H, Ishikawa K (1990) Responsiveness of bone marow erythropoietic stem cells (CFU-E and BFU-E) to recombinant human erythropoietin (rh-Ep) in vitro in aplastic anemia and myelodysplastic syndrome. Am J Hematol 35: 6–12

Characterization of Complete Remission – Molecular Biologic and Cytogenetic Approaches

Detection of Minimal Residual Disease in Acute Lymphoblastic Leukemia Patients by Polymerase Chain Reactions

C. R. Bartram[1], S. Yokota[1], A. Biondi[2], J. W. G. Janssen[1], and T. E. Hansen-Hagge[1]

Introduction

Significant progress has been achieved in the treatment of acute lymphoblastic leukemia (ALL) by the introduction of modern chemotherapeutic strategies [1]. However, disease relapse following successful remission induction still poses a major clinical challenge. The quantity and kinetic behavior of residual leukemic cells remains largely enigmatic due to the limitation of most currently available techniques to identify less than 1 %–5 % neoplastic cells in the population being examined [2]. The use of double-color immunofluorescence has markedly improved the sensitivity with which persisting disease can be detected in distinct leukemias characterized by phenotypic features that are extremely rare or absent on normal hematopoietic counterparts [3]. More recently the development of polymerase chain reaction (PCR) strategies has opened a new era in the analysis of minimal residual disease by allowing the identification of neoplastic cells at a 10^{-4} to 10^{-6} level [4]. In the following we will summarize our experience with the application of PCR techniques in monitoring ALL patients during the course of the disease.

Preparation of Clonospecific $TCR\delta$ Probes

Leukemia cell clones of virtually all ALL patients exhibit a unique pattern of immunoglobulin (Ig) and/or T-cell receptor (TCR) gene rearrangements. Based on the individual immunogenotype different PCR-methods have been proposed for the evaluation of therapeutic efficacy [5–7]. An approach initiated in our laboratory takes advantage of the observation that the vast majority of ALLs show a $TCR\delta$ gene recombination and are characterized by a preferential involvement of distinct $TCR\delta$ elements depending on the immunological phenotype [5, 8, 9]. In our series of immunogenotype analyses performed in approximately 500 ALL patients enrolled in the German multicenter ALL trials BFM (children) and BMFT (adults), a $TCR\delta$ rearrangement and/or deletion was demonstrated in 97 % of T-ALL and 88 % of cALL cases. Due to the limited repertoire of germline elements, specific patterns of recombinations can be identified by Southern blot analysis (Fig. 1). Along this line we established a prevalance of $V\delta_1 DJ\delta_1$ (29 %), $V\delta_2 DJ\delta_1$ (11 %), and $D\delta_2 J\delta_1$ (19 %) recombinations in T-ALL, while a predominance of $V\delta_2 D\delta_3$ (52 %) and $D\delta_2 D\delta_3$ (16 %) rearrangements was observed in cALL patients. Proceeding from this restricted pattern of $TCR\delta$ recombinations on one hand and the enormous junctional diversity due to imprecise joining and extensive insertion of N-region nucleotides on the other hand, we have amplified and isolated $TCR\delta$ junctional regions of ALL

[1] Section of Molecular Biology, Department of Pediatrics II, Prittwitzstr. 43, University of Ulm, 7900 Ulm, FRG
[2] Department of Pediatrics, Ospedale S. Gerado (Monza), University of Milan, Italy

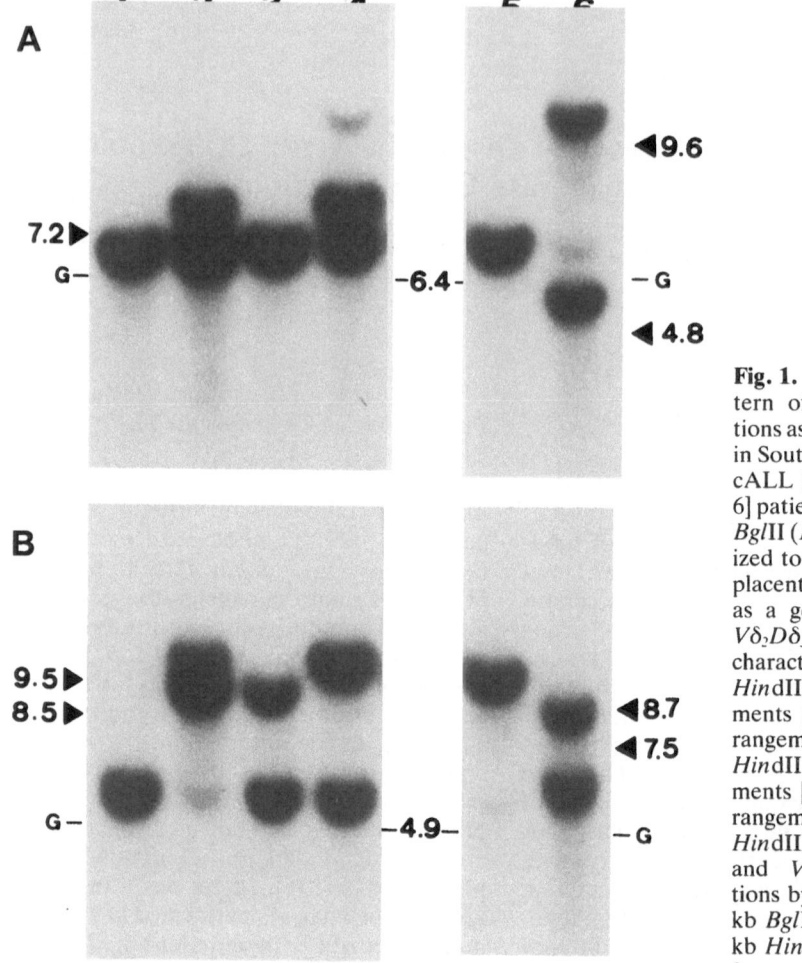

Fig. 1. Representative pattern of *TCRδ* recombinations as frequently observed in Southern blot analyses of cALL [2–4] and T-ALL [5, 6] patients. *Hin*dIII (*A*) and *Bgl*II (*B*) digests are hybridized to a *Jδ₁* probe; human placenta DNA is included as a germline control [1]. *Vδ₂Dδ₃* recombinations are characterized by 7.2 kb *Hin*dIII/9.5 kb *Bgl*II fragments [2, 4], *Dδ₂Dδ₃* rearrangements by 6.4 kb *Hin*dIII/8.5 kb *Bgl*II fragments [2, 3], *Vδ₂DJδ₁* rearrangements by 6.4 kb *Hin*dIII/8.7 kb *Bgl*II [5], and *Vδ₁DJδ₁* recombinations by 9.6 kb *Hin*dIII/7.5 kb *Bgl*II fragments [6]; 4.8 kb *Hin*III and 4.9 kb BglII fragments indicate a *Dδ₂Jδ₁* recombination [6]

patients characterized by either *Vδ₁DJδ₁* (T-ALL) or *Vδ₂Dδ₃* (cALL) recombinations and consecutively used them as clonospecific probes [5, 8–10]. It appears to be a particular advantage of this approach that it does not require sequence analyses of the junctional regions and synthesis of leukemia-specific oligonucleotide probes.

Thus far we have attempted to isolate clonospecific probes from 60 ALL patients and succeeded in 58 cases (Table 1). In two cALLs we did not obtain a distinct DNA fragment after the second PCR round but rather a smear of amplification products; both leukemias were therefore excluded from further analysis. The detection limit of

each clonospecific probe was individually determined by at least two independent dilution and amplification series. In the majority of cases leukemia DNA could be detected when representing as little as 0.001 % of total DNA (Table 2, Fig. 1). Probes derived from two T-ALLs exhibited a relatively low sensitivity of $10^{-2/-3}$. Sequence analyses of respective *Vδ₁DJδ₁* junctions revealed that this limitation was due to deletions of *Vδ₁* coding sequences represented in the 5' oligomer primer. Another *TCRδ* probe showed a considerable degree of nonspecific background signal and was therefore skipped in further investigations (Table 1).

Table 1. Preparation and application of clonospecific $TCR\delta$ probes in 60 ALL patients

1. *Isolation of probes*
   - Successful preparation in 58 cases
   - Failure in 2 cases (smears instead of distinct amplification products)

2. *Monitoring of residual leukemia*
   - Successful application in 54 cases
   - Restricted value of probe in 4 cases:
     a) Limited specificity indicated by cross-hybridization with normal blood cell DNA (1 cALL)
     b) Detection limit of only $10^{-2/-3}$ (2 T-ALL)
     c) Continuing recombination at the $TCR\delta$ locus represented in the clonospecific probe (1 cALL)

Table 2. Detection limits of 57 clonospecific $TCR\delta$ probes

ALL cells	$10^{-2/-3}$	$10^{-3/-4}$	10^{-4}	10^{-5}	10^{-6}
No. of cases	2	3	19	26	7

Table 3. Polymerase chain reaction analysis of 47 ALL patients using clonospecific $TCR\delta$ probes

Therapeutic Phase	Months after Diagnosis	No. of samples[a]	PCR status Positive	Negative
Consolidation	1–3	4	2	2
	4–6	10	8	2
Maintenance	7–12	15	4	11
	13–18	5	3	2
	19–24	10	2	8
Termination	>24	32	1	31

[a] Evaluation of 76 BM samples obtained from 47 ALL patients in complete remission

We next used the 57 suitable clonospecific probes to analyze bone marrow (BM) or peripheral blood (PB) samples obtained from the respective 47 pediatric and 10 adult ALL patients. This study included 35 cALL and 22 T-ALL cases.

Detection of Residual Leukemia in Continuing Complete Remission

In a first series of experiments we investigated 47 ALL patients in continuing complete clinical and hematological remission. From many patients multiple follow-up samples were available (Table 3). Southern blot analyses of respective specimens failed to detect the $TCR\delta$ gene rearrangement initially characterizing the leukemias. One interesting result of this study is the observation that the bone marrow of most cases analyzed during the phase of consolidation therapy following remission induction exhibited residual leukemia. The level of neoplastic cells varied between 10^{-2} and 10^{-4}. In all instances, where both PB and BM specimens of a patient were available for PCR analyses, PB samples contained significantly less residual cells, if any. The findings obtained in 30 BM samples taken during maintenance therapy appear even more remarkable. Thus a considerable

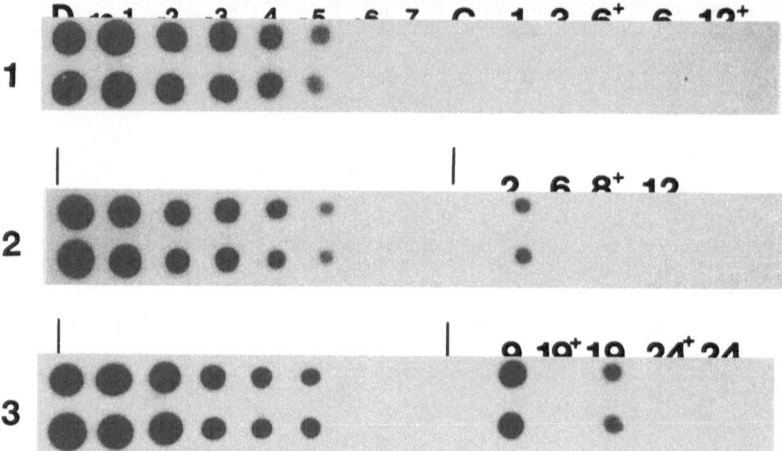

Fig. 2. Detection of minimal residual disease in three ALL patients by PCR technology. DNAs of leukemia cells at diagnosis (*D*) were diluted into peripheral blood cell DNA of three healthy individuals (*C*) at 10^{-1} to 10^{-7} and established a detection limit of approximately 10^{-5} leukemic cells in all cases. Bone marrow or peripheral blood (+) DNA samples obtained during the patients' complete clinical-hematological remission were also included (*numbers* indicate months after diagnosis). Upon amplification, the corresponding DNA fractions (20 ng) were spotted onto nylon filters and hybridized to the clonospecific probes. Note considerable differences in the elimination of residual leukemia among the three patients

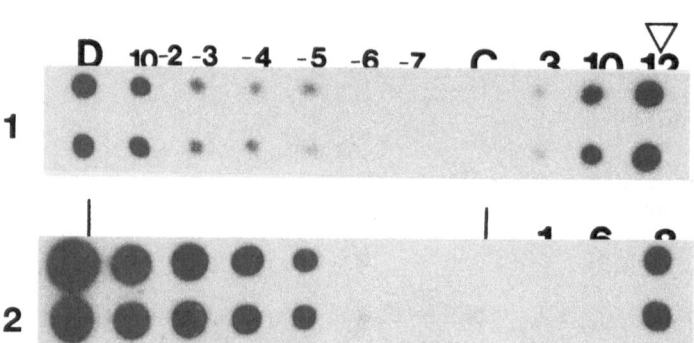

Fig. 3. Reemerging leukemic cells detected by PCR analyses prior to clinical relapse in bone marrow DNA of two cALL patients. While in case 1 a steady increase of the neoplastic cell population indicates a relapse several months before clinical manifestation (*arrowhead*), leukemia cells become detectable again 8 months after starting therapy in case 2, i.e., only 3 weeks prior to clinical relapse

number of patients show remaining blasts up to 19 months after diagnosis at frequencies of 10^{-3} to 10^{-6}. However, longitudinal analysis disclosed marked individual differences in the intervals between achievement of clinical remission and disappearance of residual disease below the detection limit of PCR (Fig. 2). It is noteworthy that these dynamic disparities in the reduction of residual leukemia did not correlate with known risk factors [9]. Thus some patients at standard risk showed persistence of leukemic cells for more than 1 year, while patients at an elevated risk became PCR negative in less than 6 months. These data also illustrate the limited value of a single PCR analysis as prognostic parameter. More relevant appears the proliferation capacity of a residual subclone as indicated in serial studies. A steady, yet prolonged decline of neoplastic cells (Fig. 2, case 3) may be associated with a favorable course, while a continuous increase of blasts (Fig. 3, case 1) may indicate an imminent clinical relapse.

Monitoring of leukemia patients by PCR might therefore identify novel components of the individual response to chemotherapy. The fact that only 1 of the 32 BM samples obtained from 22 patients 6–41 months after termination of treatment did exhibit residual leukemia (Table 3) makes us confident that PCR analysis is not inappropriately sensitive, but rather constitutes a valuable tool for the identification of clinically relevant leukemia cell populations. Similar results have recently been reported by two other groups in eight and five ALL patients, respectively [11, 12].

Serial PCR Analysis in Relapsed Patients

In order to elucidate further the prognostic value of longitudinal PCR analyses after successful remission induction we also studied 32 BM samples obtained from 10 ALL patients who eventually experienced a clinical relapse. In all but one case identical $TCR\delta$ rearrangements were observed in leukemia cells at initial diagnosis and relapse. In one T-ALL patient PCR analysis failed to detect leukemia relapse due to continuing recombination at the $TCR\delta$ locus represented in the clonospecific probe (Fig. 4). The frequency of secondary alterations at rearranged $TCR\delta$ genes during the course of the disease is currently not known, but might occur in less than 10% of cases according to our preliminary data. This proportion could be regarded as relatively low, since clonal variations at, e.g.,

rearranged IgH loci have been observed in 30% of ALL patients [13], a major problem for PCR strategies based on the analysis of specifically rearranged Ig loci. However, continuing rearrangements affecting clonospecific probes constitute a significant limitation of any PCR technique used for the monitoring of residual leukemia (Table 1).

A heterogeneous pattern of PCR results was obtained in the other nine cases. In five patients reemerging and/or constantly increasing numbers of residual blasts preceded the clinical manifestation by 5–12 months (Fig. 3, case 1). In two cases only remission samples taken 12 and 15 months prior to relapse were available and revealed a negative PCR status. More relevant in this context, however, appears the fact that PCR analyses in two cALL patients failed to identify residual neoplastic cells in multiple BM specimens obtained up to 2 and 3 months before relapse, respectively. Leukemia cells eventually became detectable 3 and 6 weeks prior to clinical manifestation in these cases (Fig. 3, case 2). One might speculate that the focal nature of residual disease has interfered with an earlier demonstration of an impending relapse in the latter patients [14].

Rearrangements of BCR-ABL in ALL Patients

As an alternative approach to monitoring minimal residual disease we have used another genetic marker, which appears particularly suitable in adult cALL patients, the $BCR\text{-}ABL$ oncogene [15]. In a recent

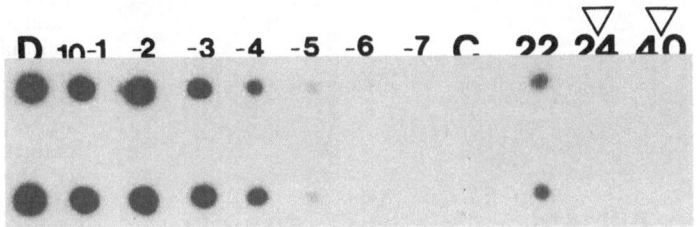

Fig. 4. Failure to detect leukemia relapse by PCR analysis due to continuing recombination at the $TCR\delta$ locus. Note that the initial leukemia cell clone is still detectable 22 months after starting therapy, but not 2 months later at first and consecutively at second relapse (*arrowheads*)

study including more than 300 ALLs, a *BCR-ABL* rearrangement, the molecular equivalent of the Philadelphia translocation, was observed in 55 % of adult cALL patients in contrast to only 6 % of children with cALL [16]. Thus far we have analyzed eight BCR/ABL-positive patients (six adults, two children) who achieved a complete clinical and hematological remission following polychemotherapy. Twelve BM samples obtained 4–12 months after initial diagnosis were available for PCR analysis and showed residual leukemia in all but one patient (Fig. 5). In three leukemias concurrent studies with clonospecific *TCRδ* probes were performed. The respective data matched in each case. Both methods may therefore be used to confirm and complement results mutually.

Prospect

In the nearer future a considerable number of hematopoietic neoplasias will become accessible to PCR analysis. A case in point is the growing list of malignancies with a known molecular basis of associated chromosomal defects. Monitoring of leukemia patients by PCR techniques will certainly be useful in elucidating the biology of neoplastic cell populations after therapeutic interventions and might ultimately offer a tool for the evaluation of a patient's individual demand for maintenance therapy and thus define a rationale for case-adapted treatment modifications. However, the value of PCR in clinical settings is far from being settled. Prospective analyses of the remission status using the PCR approaches discussed above have therefore been initiated in the German multicenter ALL trials. Additional methods, e.g., double-color immunofluorescence and PCR studies on rearranged *TCRγ* and *IgH* loci are also available. Since all techniques bear relevant limitations and specific advantages, the combined use of several approaches will be required to evaluate this issue and to balance interpretations derived from individual methods.

Acknowledgements. We thank Drs. H. Heimpel, D. Hoelzer, E. Kleihauer, W. D. Ludwig, G. Masera, and H. Riehm for continuous support and gratefully acknowledge the fruitful cooperation with the participants of the Multicenter ALL Trials for Children, BFM (Germany, Italy) and Adults, BMFT (Germany). The study was supported by grants from the Deutsche Forschungsgemeinschaft, Deutsche Krebshilfe, and Förderkreis für tumor- und leukämiekranke Kinder Ulm. S. Yokota was a recipient of a fellowship from the Alexander-von-Humboldt-Stiftung.

References

1. Champlin R, Gale RP (1989) Acute lymphoblastic leukemia: recent advantages in biology and therapy. Blood 73: 2051–2066

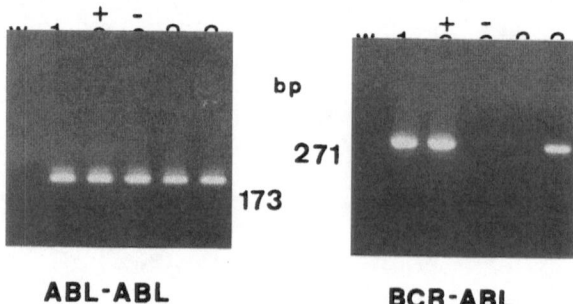

Fig. 5. Polymerase chain reaction analysis of three cALL patients in complete remission. Leukemia cells exhibited an m-*bcr* breakpoint at initial diagnosis. Following the generation of cDNA from RNA samples of bone marrow cells, two equal volumes were amplified by use of oligomers detecting either normal ABL-ABL (173 bp) or rearranged BCR-ABL (271 bp) fragments. A water sample (*w*) is included as a negative control for both reactions; a Ph-positive CML (M-*bcr* breakpoint) sample (C−) and a specimen obtained from patient 2 at initial diagnosis (C+) are included as negative and positive cellular controls, respectively. Samples were run on 2.5 % agarose gels and visualized by ethidium bromide staining. Patients 1 and 3 exhibit residual leukemic cells

2. Hagenbeek A, Löwenberg B (eds) (1986) Minimal residual disease in acute leukemia. Nijhoff, Dordrecht
3. Campana D, Coustan-Smith E, Janossy G (1990) The immunologic detection of residual disease in acute leukemia. Blood 76: 163–171
4. Saiki RK, Gelfand DH, Stoffel S, Scharf SJ, Higuchi R, Horn GT, Mullis KB, Erlich HA (1988) Primer-directed enzymatic amplification of DNA with a thermostable DNA polymerase. Science 239: 487–491
5. Hansen-Hagge TE, Yokota S, Bartram CR (1989) Detection of minimal residual disease in acute lymphoblastic leukemia by in vitro amplification of rearranged T-cell receptor δ chain sequences. Blood 74: 1762–1767
6. D'Auriol L, MacIntyre E, Galibert F, Sigaux F (1989) In vitro amplification of T cell γ gene rearrangements: a new tool for the assessment of minimal residual disease in acute lymphoblastic leukemias. Leukemia 3: 155–158
7. Yamada M, Hudson S, Tournay O, Bittenbender S, Shane SS, Lange B, Tsujimoto Y, Caton AJ, Rovera G (1989) Detection of minimal disease in hematopoietic malignancies of the B-cell lineage by using third-complementarity-determining region (CDR-III) specific probes. Proc Natl Acad Sci USA 86: 5123–5127
8. Yokota S, Hansen-Hagge TE, Bartram CR (1991) T-cell receptor δ gene recombination in common acute lymphoblastic leukemia: preferential usage of $V\delta_2$ and frequent involvement of the $J\alpha$ cluster. Blood 77: 141–148
9. Yokota S, Hansen-Hagge TE, Ludwig WD, Reiter A, Raghavachar A, Kleihauer E, Bartram CR (1991) The use of polymerase chain reactions to monitor minimal residual disease in acute lymphoblastic leukemia patients. Blood 77: 331–339
10. Campana D, Yokota S, Coustan-Smith E, Hansen-Hagge TE, Janossy G, Bartram CR (1990) The detection of residual acute lymphoblastic leukemia cells with immunologic methods and polymerase chain reaction: a comparative study. Leukemia 4: 609–614
11. Yamada M, Wasserman R, Lange B, Reichard BA, Womer RB, Rovera G (1990) Minimal residual disease in childhood B-lineage lymphoblastic leukemia. Persistence of leukemic cells during the first 18 months of treatment. N Engl J Med 323: 488–495
12. Macintyre EA, d'Auriol L, Duparc N, Leverger G, Galibert F, Sigaux F (1990) Use of oligonucleotide probes directed against T cell antigen receptor gamma delta variable(diversity)-joining junctional sequences as a general method for detecting minimal residual disease in acute lymphoblastic leukemias. J Clin Invest 86: 2125–2135
13. Raghavachar A, Thiel E, Bartram CR (1987) Analyses of phenotype and genotype in acute lymphoblastic leukemias at first presentation and in relapse. Blood 70: 1079–1083
14. Martens ACM, Schultz FW, Hagenbeek A (1987) Nonhomogenous distribution of leukemia in the bone marrow during minimal residual disease. Blood 70: 1073–1078
15. Kurzrock R, Gutterman JU, Talpaz M (1988) The molecular genetics of Philadelphia chromosome-positive leukemias. N Engl J Med 319: 990–998
16. Maurer J, Janssen JWG, Thiel E, van Denderen J, Ludwig WD, Aydemir Ü, Heinze B, Fonatsch C, Harbott J, Reiter A, Riehm H, Hoelzer D, Bartram CR (1991) Detection of chimeric BCR-ABL genes in acute lymphoblastic leukaemia by polymerase chain reaction: frequency and clinical relevance. Lancet 337: 1055–1058

Detection of Minimal Residual Disease in B-Lineage Leukemia by Immunoglobulin Gene Fingerprinting*

M. Deane[1], A. V. Hoffbrand[1], H. G. Prentice[1], and J. D. Norton[1,2]

Introduction

Immunoglobulin and/or T-cell-receptor gene rearrangement occur in the vast majority of lymphoid malignancies and can be readily detected by molecular genetic approaches [1, 2]. Since an identical immunoglobulin or T-cell-receptor gene rearrangement occurs in all members of a single clone, detection of such rearrangements provides a useful marker of clonality. Until recently, the standard means of demonstrating these clonal gene rearrangements has been analysis of the gene structure by Southern hybridisation. The advent of the polymerase chain reaction (PCR) technology has prompted several groups to develop PCR-based strategies as an alternative rapid and simple means of demonstrating lymphoid clonality [3–6]. These methods can be used to detect clonal populations at a sensitivity comparable to that of Southern blotting (1 %–5 %) [7]. This level of sensitivity, though useful in assessing clonality, is not sufficient to monitor residual disease following treatment. Several groups have therefore developed highly sensitive methods of detecting clonal populations by initially characterising the clonal rearrangement of interest and generating clonespecific primers of probes which can then be used in subsequent PCR and/or hybridisa-tion steps [8–12]. Though two groups have applied such approaches in detection and quantitation of residual disease in acute lymphoblastic leukemia (ALL) [13, 14], the widespread application of such methods is limited by their laborious and complex technology. Because of the paucity of clinical studies applying these sensitive methods, the frequency of occurrence and clinical relevance of very low levels of residual leukemia detected by molecular methods in remission is not known. However, immunophenotypic studies analysing leukemia-specific combination of surface markers, expressed in over 30 % of cases of B-lineage ALL, suggest that detection of residual disease at levels of 0.01 % or more is predictive of relapse, although absence of such findings cannot exclude this [15]. The immunoglobulin heavy chain (IgH) gene fingerprinting method is a technically simple PCR-based method which allows discrimination of clonal B-cell populations on the basis of size of their clonal IgH gene rearrangements and has a level of sensitivity comparable to that of surface marker analysis (0.01 %–0.1 %) [16]. Since the majority of cases of B-lineage ALL are amenable to analysis using this approach, it could potentially provide a means of selecting a group of patients with a high probability of relapse, thereby enabling the effect of therapeutic intervention to be evaluated.

We have analysed serial bone marrow samples from 11 cases of B-lineage ALL using the IgH gene fingerprinting method. Our results suggest that detection of residual disease by this approach may be pre-

---

[1] Department of Haematology, Royal Free Hospital School of Medicine, London, UK
[2] Present address: Paterson Institute for Cancer Research, Christie Hospital, Manchester, UK
* This work was funded by the UK MRC.

dictive of relapse in a high proportion of patients.

Materials and Methods

Clinical Material. Cases of ALL were diagnosed according to standard morphological and immunophenotypic criteria [17]. Cases in this study were selected on the basis of availability of follow-up material. Patients L5, L8, L9, L13 and L15 were under 16 years of age at the time of diagnosis. Normal bone marrow was used as a control in all experiments.

Extraction of DNA. DNA was extracted from Ficoll-gradient-separated mononuclear cell fractions of bone marrow or from material recovered from stored bone marrow slides as described previously [16]. Serial follow-up material from individual patients was prepared on separate occasions to reduce the likelihood of cross-contamination.

Polymerase Chain Reaction Gene Amplification of DNA. DNA amplification using a panel of variable region (V_H) family-specific PCR primers together with a single joining region (J_H) primer for *IgH* gene fingerprinting was performed as described previously [15]. The J_H region primer was 5′ end-labelled with [γ³²P]ATP prior to addition to the PCR mix. The reaction mix was irradiated for 15 min with a UV lamp (254 nm) and transilluminator (302 nm, UVP Inc., California) to degrade potential contaminants in the reagents prior to addition of test DNA [18]. Normal bone marrow DNA was always analysed in parallel with test DNAs as a control. Twenty-five cycles of amplification were performed under conditions adapted for each primer set in order to reduce background amplification products to a minimum as described previously [16]. Labelled, amplified DNA was extracted using phenol chloroform, precipitated in ethanol, washed, dried and redissolved in 10 mM Tris-HCl, 2 mM EDTA and analysed on a denaturing 6 M urea 6 % polyacrylamide DNA sequencing gel. Initially, DNA samples from each patient were screened for the presence of clonal V_H family-specific rearrangements by ethidium bromide-stained gel analysis of an aliquot

of the PCR reaction as described previously [4]. Subsequent fingerprinting experiments on serial DNA samples were done using the V_H primer set appropriate for the clonal *IgH* rearrangement at disease presentation.

Results

IgH VDJ gene rearrangements can be detected in the majority of cases of B-lineage ALL (>90 %) using a panel of V_H family-specific primers together with a single J_H primer [16]. High-resolution gel electrophoresis of the radiolabelled amplification products generates an *IgH* gene fingerprint. A ladder of products within a size range determined by the relative positions of the 5′ and 3′ primers is generated from the VDJ rearrangements in polyclonal B cells and against this background a clonal rearrangement can be seen as a single more intense product (see Figs. 1–3). Sequential bone marrow samples from 11 cases of B-lineage ALL were examined in this study, all of which had one or more clonal *IgH* gene rearrangement demonstrable by the fingerprinting method at disease presentation or relapse. The details of the patients examined and the overall results of the analysis are shown in Table 1.

Analysis of Patients Who Relapsed

Six of the 11 patients relapsed and in 5 of these cases (L6, L9, L108, L110) the presence of a residual clone was demonstrated by fingerprinting during morphological remission. In some cases, positive PCR fingerprinting results during remission were obtained several months or years prior to relapse (see Table 1). The fingerprinting profiles of three of these cases are illustrated in Fig. 1. In the case of L13, two dominant products are seen (Fig. 1, December 1986) during induction treatment for second relapse, representing clonal *IgH VDJ* rearrangements involving members of the same V_H family, as well as a faint background of amplified *IgH* gene rearrangements from accompanying polyclonal B cells. This polyclonal profile which

Table 1. Morphological and PCR analysis of clinical samples

Patient No. and diagnosis	Disease status	Sample date	PCR results	% blasts		Patient No. and diagnosis	Disease status	Sample date	PCR results	% blasts
L6 cALL	First relapse	20/1/86	15	+		L109 cALL	Presentation	26/7/88	90	+
	Remission	23/4/86	< 5	+			Persisting disease	17/8/88	30	+
	Second relapse	13/8/86	8	+			Persisting disease	7/9/88	60	+
	Remission	2/11/86	< 5	+			Persisting disease	10/10/88	35	+
	Third relapse	2/87	80	ND			Persisting disease	11/10/88	80	+
L9 cALL	Second relapse	12/11/86	77	+		L9 pre-B ALL	Presentation	29/9/88	70	+
	Remission	14/1/87	< 5	+			Persisting disease	12/10/88	9	+
	Remission	30/1/87	< 5	+			Remission	24/1/89	< 5	+
	Remission	30/6/87	< 5	+		L15 cALL	Presentation	30/6/89	90	+
	Remission	30/9/87	< 5	+			Remission	30/10/90	< 5	+
	Third relapse	2/88	30	+		L5 cALL	Presentation	26/1/87	90	+
L13 cALL	Second relapse	2/12/86	6	+			Remission	25/2/87	< 5	−
	Remission	7/7/87	< 5	+			Remission	18/5/87	< 5	−
	Third relapse	15/2/88	90	+			Remission	10/6/87	< 5	−
L108 cALL	First remission	3/5/85	< 5	+			Remission	13/7/87	< 5	−
	First relapse	28/2/89	80	+			Remission	19/5/88	< 5	−
L110 Null ALL	Presentation	22/10/87	20	+			Remission	1/91	ND	ND
	Persisting disease	19/11/87	20	+		L41 cALL	Presentation	3/4/86	94	+
	Remission	12/5/88	< 5	+			Remission	24/6/86	< 5	+
	First relapse	3/11/89	96	+			Remission	9/2/87	< 5	+
	First relapse	4/1/90	50	+			Remission	27/3/87	< 5	−
L8 cALL	First relapse	9/12/85	93	+			Remission	16/2/88	< 5	−
	Remission	20/1/86	< 5	−			Remission	1/91	ND	ND
	Remission	7/5/86	< 5	−						
	Remission	30/9/86	< 5	−						
	Second relapse	24/2/87	90	+						

ᵃ ND, not determined

appears as a ladder of products representing *IgH* gene rearrangements of random size can be clearly seen in the normal bone marrow DNA (Fig. 1C) amplified in parallel. Seven months later, during morphological remission, one of the original two clonal rearrangements is still clearly visible against a polyclonal background. The patient relapsed 7 months later and the fingerprinting profile at this time (Fig. 1, February 1988) shows the presence of clonal rearrangements identical to those seen on the first examination. In the case of L108, two identical clonal products are seen during first remission and at relapse 4 years later (see Fig. 1). Since the fingerprinting method is not quantitative, the intensity of the clonal products does not give an indication of the size of that clone. Similarly, in the case of L110 (Fig. 1), two dominant products of identical sizes are seen at presentation (October 1987, November 1987), during morphological remission (May 1988) and at first relapse (November 1989, January 1990). In one of the six cases (L8), the fingerprinting profile was normal during remission though the patient subsequently relapsed (Fig. 2). The fingerprinting profile was identical in both first and second relapse in L8, showing several distinct clonal rearrangements involving the same V_H family on each occasion. These results suggest that residual disease was present during remission at a lower level than could be detected by the fingerprinting method.

Analysis of Patients Remaining in Clinical Remission

Two patients, L139 and L15, showed evidence of residual disease during remission

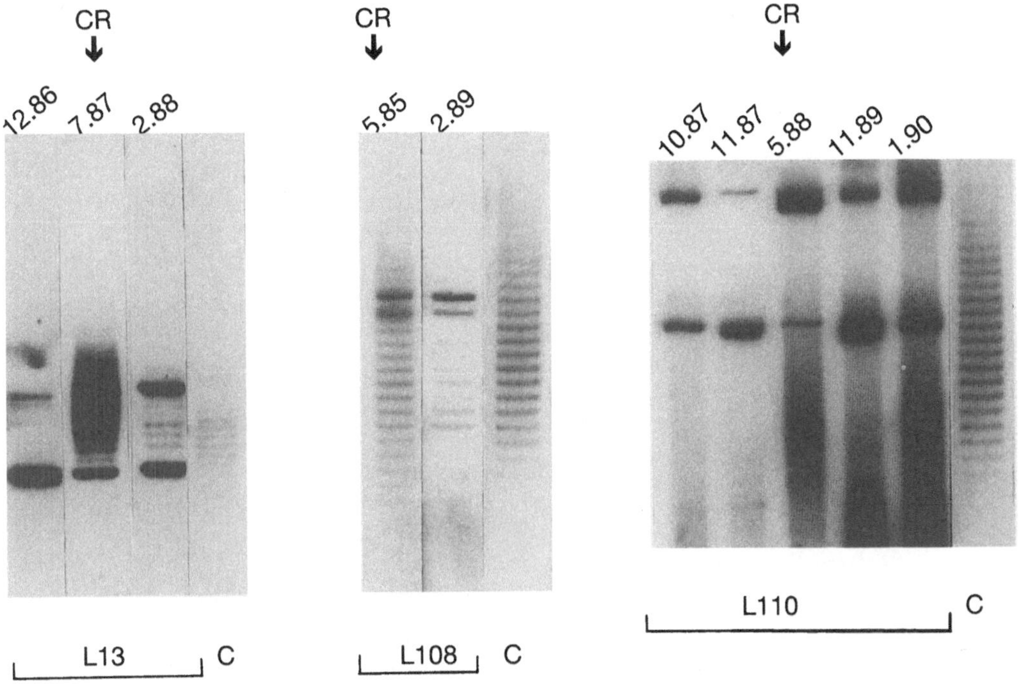

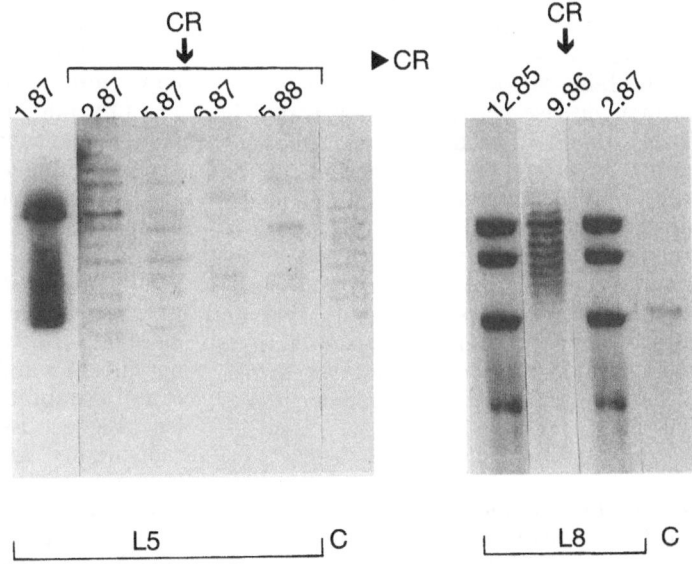

Fig. 1. Analysis of *IgH* gene rearrangements in leukemic DNA by *IgH* gene fingerprinting. Genomic DNA was PCR amplified using ^{32}P-labelled J_H primer in combination with a panel of primers specific for each of the six V_H families. The amplified DNA was electrophoresed on a denaturing sequencing gel to generate an *IgH* gene fingerprint. Fingerprinting lanes displaying dominant clonal PCR-amplified fragments are from overnight direct autoradiographic exposures. Otherwise, all exposures were for 1–2 weeks with intensifying screens. Normal bone marrow (*C*) was amplified in parallel with each leukemia as a control

Fig. 2. Analysis of *IgH* gene rearrangements in leukemic DNA by *IgH* gene fingerprinting. As Fig. 1

181

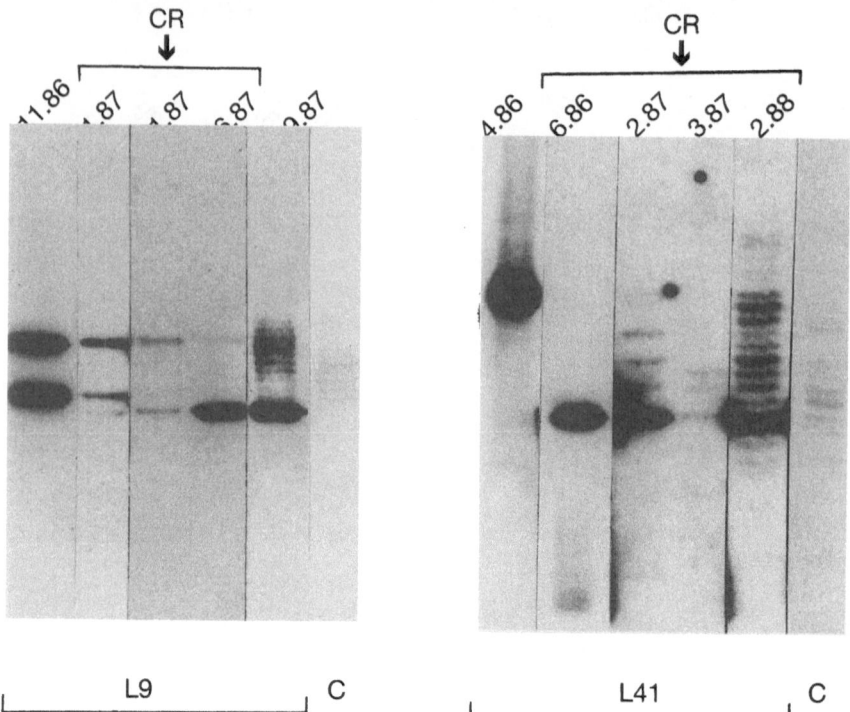

Fig. 3. Analysis of *IgH* gene rearrangements in leukemic DNA by *IgH* gene fingerprinting. As Fig. 1

and remain in remission 27 and 19 months respectively after presentation (Table 1). These patients are currently being followed up. Patients L5 and L41 have both been in remission for 4 years and are likely to be cured (Table 1). In the case of L5 (Fig. 2), residual disease was not demonstrated in serial examinations during and following treatment over a 16-month period. In the case of L41, however, a clonal rearrangement (distinct from that a presentation) could be demonstrated 2 months after presentation (Fig. 3, April 1986 and June 1986). The patient subsequently had an autologous bone marrow transplantation, and subsequent fingerprint analysis over a 12-month period gave negative results (Fig. 3).

Detection of Clonal Instability and Oligoclonality

Since the fingerprinting method employs a series of V_H family-specific primers and clonal rearrangements are discriminated on the basis of size, it provides a means of simultaneously monitoring coexisting clonal populations. The importance of being able to monitor more than a single dominant clone is illustrated in several of the cases examined. Of the 11 patients examined, 3 had more than two dominant *IgH* gene rearrangements, involving 1 or more V_H family, demonstrable by fingerprinting (data not shown). An example is seen in the case of L8 in Fig. 2 where the fingerprint profile at presentation shows three *IgH* gene rearrangements of similar intensity involving the same V_H family. Two of the patients, L9 and L41, showed evidence of clonal instability during the disease course (see Fig. 3). L9 had two dominant rearrangements at second relapse. During induction treatment (January 1987) a third rearrangement is seen and this rearrangement dominated during the subsequent examinations (January 1987, June 1987) and predominated at relapse (September 1987). These findings suggest the presence of at least two B-cells clones in L9. In the case of L41, a single dominant product is demonstrated at disease presentation (Fig. 3, April 1986). However, a new rearrangement is seen in the subsequent examination (June 1986), which also involves the same V_H family. Sequence analysis of these two products shows that they are independent rearrangements involving distinct D and J regions (data not shown). These results again suggest the presence of at least two clonal B-cell populations.

Discussion

The IgH gene fingerprinting method employing a panel of V_H family-specific primers as applied in this study allows the detection of the IgH gene rearrangement in the majority of cases of B-lineage ALL (>90%) [16]. Moreover, the reliability of detection of IgH gene rearrangement by this PCR approach appears to be superior to alternative PCR methods which employ a consensus 3' V_H primer [5, 6, 10–12]. As a result of variable deletion of V_H primer target sequence during V-DJ recombination, together with somatic mutation (in the context of more mature B-cell malignancies), these latter methods do not detect a significant minority of IgH VDJ alleles [19, 20]. Clonal evolution is recognised to be a frequent event in ALL [7, 20, 21]. Similarly oligoclonality has been observed in 10%–30% of cases of B-lineage ALL [7, 22, 23] and analysis using more sensitive PCR-based methods suggests that this may occur in a much higher proportion of cases (unpublished observations). Both oligoclonality and clonal evolution have important implications for the design of strategies for the detection of minimal residual disease, and suggest that the use of probes or primers specific to a single clone may not be adequate in many cases. Since the IgH gene fingerprinting method effectively scans the entire repertoire of IgH VDJ rearrangements, it provides advantages in those cases displaying clonal instability, as is illustrated in some of the cases in this study.

Although the fingerprinting approach is less sensitive than some of the more sophisticated PCR-based methods, the results from this study suggest that detection of residual disease at levels of 0.01% or more is predictive of relapse in many cases of B-lineage ALL. Similar findings have recently been reported based on immunophenotypic studies [15]. We found that five of the six patients who relapsed in our study had residual leukemic cells in remission at a level detectable by IgH gene fingerprinting. In the sixth case, the patient relapsed with the same clone as was seen at disease presentation, though this clone was not demonstrated by fingerprinting during remission. It is worth noting that, in most of the cases who relapsed, residual disease could be demonstrated by fingerprinting several months to years prior to relapse. Two patients who had residual clonal rearrangements demonstrable in remission have not relapsed and clearly need careful monitoring to determine the significance of this finding.

The availability of a widely applicable method to monitor residual disease in the majority of cases of B-lineage ALL is an important adjunct to immunophenotypic methods which have been particularly useful in monitoring T-lineage ALL [15]. Clearly, larger studies are needed to fully establish the biological significance of various levels of residual disease. The possibility of selecting a sizeable group of patients at high risk of relapse would allow assessment of the effect of tailored therapeutic regimens.

Acknowledgements. We would like to thank Professor George Janossy, Department of Immunology, for providing the immunophenotyping data, some of the clinical specimens, and for helpful discussions.

References

1. Arnold A, Cossman J, Bakshi A, Jaffe ES, Waldmann TA, Korsmeyer SJ (1985) Immunoglobulin gene rearrangement as unique clonal markers in human lymphoid neoplasms. N Engl J Med 309: 1593–1599
2. Korsmeyer SJ, Arnold A, Bakshi A, Ravetch JV, Siebenlist U, Hieter PA, Sharron SO, Lebien TW, Kersey JA, Poplack DG, Leder P, Waldman TA (1983) Immunoglobulin gene rearrangement and cell surface

antigen expression in acute lymphocytic leukemia of T and B cell precursor origins. J Clin Invest 71: 301–313

3. Deane M, Norton JD (1990) Detection of immunoglobulin gene rearrangement in B lymphoid malignancies by polymerase chain reaction gene amplification. Br J Haematol 74: 251–256

4. Deane M, Norton JD (1990) Immunoglobulin heavy chain variable region family usage is independent of tumour cell phenotype in human B lineage leukaemias. Eur J Immunol 20: 2209–2217

5. McCarthy KP, Sloane JP, Wiedemann LM (1990) Rapid method for distinguishing clonal from polyclonal B cell populations in surgical biopsy specimens. J Clin Pathol 43: 429–432

6. Trainor KJ, Brisco MJ, Story CJ, Morley AA (1990) Monoclonality in B-lymphoproliferative disorders detected at the DNA level. Blood 75: 2220–2222

7. Wright JJ, Poplack DG, Bakshi A, Reaman G, Cole D, Jensen JP, Korsmeyer SJ (1987) Gene rearrangements as markers of clonal variation and minimal residual disease in acute lymphoblastic leukemia. J Clin Oncol 5: 735–741

8. D'Auriol L, Macintyre E, Galibert F, Sigaux F (1989) In vitro amplification of T cell γ gene rearrangements: a new tool for the assessment of minimal residual disease in acute lymphoblastic leukaemias. Leukemia 3: 155–158

9. Hansen-Hagge TE, Yokota S, Bartram CR (1989) Detection of minimal residual disease in acute lymphoblastic leukaemia by in vitro amplification of rearrnged T-cell receptor delta chain sequences. Blood 74: 1762–1767

10. Yamada M, Hudson S, Tournay O, Bittenbeider S, Shane SS, Lange B, Tsujimoto Y, Caton AJ, Rovera G (1989) Detection of minimal disease in hemopoietic malignancies of B-cell lineage by using third-complementarity-determining region (CDR-III)-specific probes. Proc Natl Acad Sci USA 86: 5123–5127

11. Jonsson OG, Kitchens RL, Scott FC, Smith RG (1990) Detection of minimal residual disease in acute lymphoblastic leukemia using immunoglobulin hypervariable region specific oligonucleotide probes. Blood 76: 2072–2079

12. Brisco MJ, Tan LW, Orsborn AM, Morley AA (1990) Development of a highly sensitive assay, based on the polymerase chain reaction, for rare B-lymphocyte clones in a polyclonal population. Br J Haematol 75: 163–167

13. Yamada M, Wasserman R, Lange B, Reichard BA, Womer RB, Rovera G (1990) Minimal residual disease in childhood B-lineage lymphoblastic leukemia. N Engl J Med 323: 448–455

14. Yokota S, Hansen-Hagge TE, Ludwig W-D, Reiter A, Raghavachar A, Kleihauer E, Bartram CR (1991) Use of polymerase chain reactions to monitor minimal residual disease in acute lymphoblastic leukemia patients. Blood 77: 331–339

15. Campana D, Coustan-Smith E, Janossy G (1990) The immunological detection of minimal residual disease in acute leukemia. Blood 76: 163–171

16. Deane M, Norton JD (1991) Immunoglobulin gene 'fingerprinting': an approach to analysis of B lymphoid clonality in lymphoproliferative disorders. Br J Haematol 77: 274–281

17. Campana D, Janossy G (1986) Leukemia diagnosis and testing of complement fixing antibodies for bone marrow purging in ALL. Blood 68: 1264–1271

18. Sarkar G, Sommer SS (1990) Shedding light on PCR contamination. Nature 343: 27

19. Deane M, McCarthy KP, Wiedemann LM, Norton JD (1991) An improved method for detection of B lymphoid clonality by polymelase chain reaction. Leukemia 5: 726–730

20. Deane M, Norton JD (1991) Detection of immunoglobulin gene rearrangement in B cell neoplasias by polymerase chain reaction gene amplification. Leukemia Lymphoma, 5: 9–22

21. Raghavachar A, Thiel E, Bartram CR (1987) Analyses of phenotype and genotype in acute lymphoblastic leukemias at first presentation and in relapse. Blood 70: 1079–1083

22. Bird J, Galili N, Link M, Stites D, Sklar J (1988) Continuing rearrangement but absence of somatic hypermutation in immunoglobulin genes of human B cell precursor leukemia. J Exp Med 168: 229–245

23. Kitchingman GR, Mirro J, Stass S, Rovigatti U, Melvin SL, Williams DL, Raimondi SC, Murphy SB (1986) Biological and prognostic significance of the presence of more than two μ heavy-chain genes in childhood acute lymphoblastic leukemia of B precursor origin. Blood 67: 698–703

Probing the Pathophysiology of Leukemic Response by Premature Chromosome Condensation*

W. N. Hittelman and R. Vyas

Introduction

The myeloid leukemic process is generally thought to involve a series of genetic changes in a hematopoietic progenitor or stem cell that results in a dysregulation of proliferation and maturation of myeloid elements. The clinical manifestation of this process is the impaired production of mature myeloid elements and platelets culminating in an increased risk for fatal infection and hemorrhage. Remission induction is generally thought to decrease the tumor burden by cytotoxic mechanisms and allow restoration of normal hematopoiesis. While it is useful to think of leukemic response in such terms, there is increasing evidence to suggest that other processes might be involved such as induced maturation of leukemic elements and modulation of the factors elicited by leukemic elements that impact normal hematopoiesis.

Premature Chromosome Condensation: Predicting Relapse in Acute Leukemia

In early studies, our laboratory was interested in examining the levels of chromosome damage induced in the bone marrow cells of patients with acute myeloid leuke-

mia receiving chemotherapy. Since most of the bone marrow cells are not in mitosis, we utilized the technique of premature chromosome condensation to directly visualize the chromosomes of interphase cells. With this technique, factors from tissue culture cells in mitosis, when fused with the interphase cells of interest, act on the interphase component to break down the nuclear membrane and induce the interphase chromatin to prematurely condense into discrete chromosomal units called prematurely condensed chromosome (PCC) [1]. The morphology of the PCC reflects the stage of the cell in the cell cycle at the time of fusion. The morphology of the PCC is also useful in determining the substage of each cell within each cell cycle phase (i.e., early verses late) [2]. In particular, early G1 phase cells gave rise to highly condensed G1 PCC whereas late G1 phase cells gave rise to highly elongated G1 PCC. Of interest, it was also found that when normal cells come to rest in G1 under conditions of nutrient starvation or crowded conditions, their G1 PCC have the morphology of cells in early G1 phase. In contrast, when transformed cells are similarly growth arrested, their G1 PCC suggest that they arrest in late G1 phase. Thus the morphology of the G1 PCC suggests an altered mode of cell cycle regulation in transformed cells.

A similar pattern of G1 PCC morphologies is also observed in bone marrow populations. Cells derived from normal bone marrow exhibit G1 PCC predominantly in early G1 phase, whereas bone marrow cells from individuals with active acute leukemia exhibit relatively higher fractions of cells in

[1] Department of Medical Oncology, University of Texas MD Anderson Cancer Center, 1515 Holcombe Blvd., Houston, TX 77030, USA
* This work was supported in part by CA-27931 and CA-45746 from the National Institutes of Health.

late G1 phase, despite similar frequencies of actively cycling cells in S and G2 phases [3, 4]. When patients are treated with remission induction therapy and obtain complete remission, the fraction of cells in late G1 phase returns to lower levels. However, by serially following patients during complete remission, it was found that the fraction of cells in late G1 phase returned to high levels, usually 2–3 months prior to any clinical or morphological evidence of relapse [5, 6].

This last observation was difficult to understand. In the period just prior to relapse, the maturing hematopoietic elements were morphologically normal, yet their underlying chromatin phenotype was that of a malignant cell. Two alternate hypotheses might explain this apparent contradiction. First, the leukemic elements might have already returned, but, under the conditions of low tumor burden, they might still be capable of maturation. Alternatively, in the period just before clinically evident relapse, the leukemic cells might be increasing in number and at the same time eliciting factors which might allow normal maturing cells to pass from early G1 phase to late G1 phase (e.g., a growth factor).

With regard to the first possibility, there has been increasing evidence to suggest that leukemic elements are susceptible to maturation induction when treated in vitro with a variety of agents including dimethyl sulfoxide (DMSO), phorbol esters, HMBA, retinoids, and even some commonly used cytotoxic agents [7, 8]. Thus, it might be possible that one component of response in patients undergoing therapy for acute leukemia might be induced maturation of the leukemic elements. However, the test of this hypothesis is difficult since the maturing cells cease cell division and cannot be analyzed by conventional cytogenetic techniques to distinguish cells derived from the normal or abnormal clone. We have therefore again utilized the technique of premature chromosome condensation to address this issue since this technique allows direct visualization of the interphase chromosomes of nondividing mature cells. Moreover, the PCC can be enumerated and banded by conventional methods to detect cells with abnormal karyotypes [9].

Detecting Maturation of Abnormal Myeloid Elements

Our laboratory has utilized this technique to examine the pathophysiology of response in a number of treatment situations. For example, after treatment of acute myeloblastic leukemia (AML) patients with low-dose cytosine arabinoside, we have been able to demonstrate the presence of the abnormal clone in the mature granulocyte fraction, suggesting that induced maturation of the leukemic elements might be a component of clinical response [10]. Similar findings have also been found in a number of clinical situations where induced maturation was the goal of the treatment (e.g., HMBA treatment of patients with myelodysplasia and AML, mithramycin treatment of patients with accelerated chronic myeloblastic leukemia (CML)). Evidence for maturation of the abnormal clone has also been garnered using the PCC technique in patients undergoing high-dose cytotoxic treatment [11]. For example, three patients with cytogenetic abnormalities were recently studied who all received high-dose cytosine arabinoside followed by recombinant human granulocyte-macrophage colony-stimulating factor. At the time of complete remission, the mature peripheral blood granulocytes were enriched and analyzed by the PCC technique. In two of the patients, the granulocytes were shown to be derived from the normal residual hematopoietic elements. In contrast, the granulocytes from the third patient were shown to be predominantly derived from the cytogenetically abnormal (trisomy 8) clone [12]. Thus, in this third patient, while morphological and functional clinical complete remission was obtained, myeloid hematopoiesis was still dominated by the abnormal clone that was now capable of apparently normal maturation. This might suggest that, in some cases, the leukemic elements might be capable of induced maturation with the proper stimulation.

Probing the Mechanism of Response to All-*Trans*-Retinoic Acid

Recently, several clinical trials have reported the clinical utility of *trans*-retinoic acid in the treatment of acute promyelocytic leukemia (APL) [13, 14]. These trials were based on the in vitro findings that retinoic acid can induce the maturation of promyelocytic leukemia cells [15, 16]. More recently, it was also found that the cytogenetic abnormality most commonly observed in APL, i.e., a translocation of chromosomes 15 and 17, involves a break in the nuclear retinoic acid receptor α gene located on chromosome 17, and this results in the production of an abnormal transcription product [17, 18]. When APL patients were treated with *trans*-retinoic acid in the clinic, complete remission was found to be induced in greater than 75 % of these patients. Moreover, these remissions occurred without an interceding hypoplastic phase, suggesting that the mechanism of response might be different from that of conventional cytotoxic therapy. Thus it was of interest to determine if induced maturation of the leukemic elements was the predominant mode of action of all-*trans*-retinoic acid.

To better understand the pathophysiology of response in APL, we have utilized the technique of premature chromosome condensation to determine the karyotype of the maturing cells after treatment with *trans*-retinoic acid (TRA). The patients were treated at either Albert Einstein Cancer Center, New York (Dr. Peter H. Wiernik and colleagues) or Memorial Sloan-Kettering Cancer Center, New York (Dr. Raymond P. Warrell, Jr., and colleagues) and blood specimens were then sent to the MD Anderson Cancer Center. To facilitate the determination of the karyotype of the blood cells, a "chromosome painting" technique was used whereby the PCCs were hybridized with the biotinylated chromosome 17-specific DNA probe, and the hybridized chromosome 17 product was visualized by an immunocytochemical reaction with an avidin intermediate [19, 20]. When a diploid PCC is probed in this fashion, two normal chromosome 17 hybridizations are observed. When a PCC containing the 15; 17 translocation products is present, one normal and two translocated chromosome 17 products are easily visualized as three distinct staining regions. In case where other cytogenetic markers distinguished the abnormal clone, either G- or C-banding was utilized.

The first case was a patient with APL in relapse after conventional treatment and who had already responded to TRA when the blood sample was obtained. At this time the PCC technique showed that the mature granulocytes were completely derived from the diploid elements rather than from the abnormal clone. Upon relapse, however, cells with t(15; 17) made up the immature blast fraction.

The second patient studied was a patient with a promyelocytic blast crisis CML. While the patient did not exhibit the typical t(15; 17), the abnormal clone was characterized by karyotype of 48, XY, +17, +der (1), t(1; ?) (p13; ?), t(9; 22) (q34; q11). Upon treatment with TRA the white count decreased, the enlarged spleen became unpalpable, and the patient appeared to revert back to a chronic phase situation. Peripheral blood from this patient was examined by the PCC technique on day 60 of treatment at a time when no blasts were apparent in the blood. Approximately 30 % of the cells with low density (<1.077) contained 48 chromosomes with most of the remaining cells showing 46 chromosomes. Analysis of the cells with 48 chromosomes per cell demonstrated the abnormal chromosome 1 derivative. It was likely that these PCCs were derived from rather large cells exhibiting an intermediate myeloid morphology (i.e., nuclear hypersegmentation, with six to eight lobes) and which occurred with a similar frequency in the light density population. In contrast, the higher density cells representing the mature granulocyte forms yielded PCCs with 46 chromosomes per cell. Thus it appeared that the abnormal clone became capable of partial maturation after *trans*-retinoic acid treatment, and normal elements then became capable of growth and maturation.

To obtain a better idea of the progression of events during response of patients with APL to *trans*-retinoic acid, we are now studying patients sequentially during treatment. As illustrated in the next patient, a recurrent theme appears to be occurring. Early during treatment, there was morphological evidence of a partial maturation process and these partially maturing cells were derived predominantly from the abnormal clone (i.e., contain the t(15; 17)). However, the rise of fully maturing populations of granulocytes with time was accompanied by the increasing frequency of cells exhibiting a diploid karyotype. These results suggest that the pathophysiology of response in APL to *trans*-retinoic acid is somewhat unique. It appears that there is an induction of a partial maturation of the abnormal elements, and this process releases the inhibitory effect of the leukemic population and normal hematopoiesis is restored. During conventional cytotoxic treatment, is is generally thought that the inhibitory effect of the leukemic elements is removed when the bone marrow becomes hypoplastic. In the case of treatment with *trans*-retinoic acid, it appears that there is a downregulation of leukemic inhibitory activity without a substantial decrease in the leukemic burden.

Conclusion

In summary, it is apparent that the pathophysiology of response of patients with acute leukemia is different in different therapeutic situations. In some cases, response to therapy apparently occurs through a mechanism of cytotoxic elimination of the leukemic bulk followed by restoration of hematopoiesis predominated by the residual normal elements. In some cases, however, the leukemic clone can be induced to mature and remission is characterized by a reregulation of the maturation capacity of the abnormal clone. And in cases such as that found after treatment of patients with APL with *trans*-retinoic acid, remission is achieved by a partial induced maturation of the abnormal clone followed by a restoration of the growth and maturation capacity of the normal elements. The technique of premature chromosome condensation is a useful tool with which to dissect out the pathophysiology of res-

ponse, and it will serve as a useful intermediate marker to determine when specific regulatory events are taking place. This will facilitate the study of the molecular and biochemical factors which regulate normal and leukemic hematopoiesis.

Acknowledgements. The authors thank Drs. Saroj Vadhan Raj and Jordon Gutterman for their support.

References

1. Johnson RT, Rao PN (1970) Mammalian cell fusion: induction of premature chromosome condensation in interphase nuclei. Nature 226: 717–722
2. Hittelman WN, Rao PN (1978) Mapping of G1 phase by the structural morphology of the prematurely condensed chromosomes. J Cell Physiol 95: 333–342
3. Hittelman WN, Rao PN (1978) Predicting response or progression of human leukemia by premature chromosome condensation of bone marrow cells. Cancer Res 38: 416–423
4. Hittelman WN, Broussard LC, McCredie K (1979) Premature chromosome condensation studies in human leukemia: 1. Pretreatment characteristics. Blood 54: 1001–1014
5. Hittelman WN, Broussard LC, Dosik G, McCredie KB (1980) Predicting relapse of human leukemia by means of premature chromosome condensation. N Engl J Med 303: 479–484
6. Hittelman WN, Menegaz SD, McCredie KB, Keating MJ (1984) Premature chromosome condensation studies in human leukemia. 5. Prediction of early relapse. Blood 64: 1067–1073
7. Hozumi M (1983) Fundamentals of chemotherapy of myeloid leukemia by induction of leukemia cell differentiation. Adv Cancer Res 38: 121–169
8. Sachs L (1987) Cell differentiation and bypassing of genetic defects in the suppression of malignancy. Cancer Res 47: 1981–1986
9. Hittelman WN, Petkovic I, Agbor P (1988) Improvements in the premature chromosome condensation technique for cytogenetic analysis. Cancer Genet Cytogenet 30: 301–312
10. Beran M, Hittelman WN, Andersson BS, McCredie KB (1986) Induction of differentiation in human myeloid leukemia cells with cytosine arabinoside. Leuk Res 10: 1033–1039

11. Hittelman WN, Agbor P, Petkovic I, Andersson B, Kantarjian H, Walters R, Koller C, Beran M (1988) Detection of leukemic clone maturation in vivo by premature chromosome condensation. Blood 72: 1950–1960

12. Tigaud J-D, Estey E, Gutterman JU, Hittelman WN (1988) Proliferation and maturation of diploid and aneuploid elements after treatment of AML with cytarabine (AraC) followed by recombinant human granulocyte-macrophage colony stimulating factor (rh GM-CSF). Blood 72: 150a

13. Huang ME, Ye VC, Chen SR, Chai JR, Lu JX, Zhoa L, Gu LJ, Wang ZY (1988) Use of all-*trans* retinoic acid in the treatment of acute promyelocytic leukemia. Blood 72: 567–572

14. Castaigne S, Chomienne C, Daniel MT, Ballerini P, Bengen R, Fenaux P, Degos L (1990) All-*trans* retinoic acid as a differentiation therapy for acute promyelocytic leukemia. I. Clinical Results. Blood 76: 1704–1709

15. Breitman TR, Selonick SE, Collins SJ (1980) Induction of differentiation of the human promyelocytic leukemia cell line (HL-60) by retinoic acid. Proc Natl Acad Sci USA 77: 2936–2940

16. Breitman T, Collins SJ, Keene B (1981) Terminal differentiation of human promyelocytic leukemia cells in primary culture in response to retinoic acid. Blood 57: 1000–1004

17. De The H, Chomienne C, Lanotte M, Degos L, deJean A (1990) The t(15; 17) translocation of acute promyelocytic leukemia fuses the retinoic acid receptor alpha gene to a novel transcribed locus. Nature 347: 558–561

18. Miller WH Jr, Warrell RP, Frankel SR, Jakubowski A, Gabrilove JL, Muindi J, Dmitrovsky E (1990) Novel retinoic acid receptor-alpha transcripts in acute promyelocytic leukemia responsive to all-trans-retinoic acid. J Natl Cancer Inst 82: 1932–1933

19. Pinkel D, Straume T, Gray JW (1986) Cytogenetic analysis using quantitative, high sensitivity, fluorescence hybridization. Proc Natl Acad Sci USA 83: 2934–2938

20. Zwelling LA, Mayes J, Deisseroth K, Hinds M, Grant G, Pathak S, Ledley FD, Vyas R, Hittelman W (1990) A restriction fragment length polymorphism for human topoisomerase II: Possible relationship to drug-resistance. Cancer Commun 2: 357–361

Combination of In Situ Hybridization Cytogenetics and Immunologic Cell Identification in Diagnosing Minimal Residual Disease

S. Knuutila, M. Wessman, and M. Tiainen

Introduction

In leukemias about 60 %–80 % of patients have a clonal chromosome abnormality [8]. It is generally believed that healthy bone marrow is free from clonal chromosome aberrations. Thus chromosome aberrations are considered to be some of the best cancer-specific markers. Furthermore, there are a large number of aberrations in leukemias that are closely associated with certain morphological, immunological, or clinical subtypes of leukemia [19].

In principle any clonal abnormality observed can be used to follow up the leukemic disease and to detect minimal residual disease. In practice, however, conventional chromosome study has not proved sensitive enough to find residual cells. Supposing that the proportion of residual cells is similar among mitotic and interphase cells, one would have to analyze hundreds of metaphases before there is a statistical probability of finding a cell with the abnormal karyotype. This is not feasible in routine work and, furthermore, there is the possibility that residual cells do not undergo mitoses at the same rate as normal cells.

In situ hybridization (ISH) with chromosome-specific probes has made possible the chromosome analysis of interphase cells [4, 5, 13, 14, 16, 17]. We have combined in situ hybridization with another technique known as MAC (morphology antibody chromosomes) [11, 18, 20] that allows the study of the cell morphology, immunophenotype, and chromosomes of the same interphase or mitotic cell. This article describes the combination technique, MAC-ISH, and its application for the detection of minimal residual cells.

Methods

Morphology Antibody Chromosome Methodology

The procedure for MAC preparations has been described in detail elsewhere [11]. For slide preparation, 10^5 cells are suspended in a mixture of 1 ml incubation medium and 1 ml of a hypotonic solution. We use a hypotonic solution containing 50 mmol/l glycerol, 5 mmol/l KCl, 10 mmol/l NaCl, 0.8 mmol/l MgCl, 1 mmol/l CaCl$_2$, and 10 mmol/l sucrose (pH 7.0) After 5 min the suspension is divided into 12 cytocentrifuge chambers (Cytospin, Shandon Elliot, Runcorn, UK) and centrifuged at 400 g for 5 min. After air drying overnight, the slides are ready for analytical procedures.

For morphological cell classification we use Giemsa, Sudan black, and α-naphtyl acetate/esterase (ANAE), and for immunocytochemical classification immunofluorescence, immunoperoxidase, or alkaline phosphatase antialkaline phosphatase (APAAP). These MAC preparation techniques have also been described elsewhere [11].

Department of Medical Genetics, University of Helsinki, Haartmaninkatu 3, 00290 Helsinki, Finland

In Situ Hybridization and Chromosome In Situ Suppression Hybridization

The hybridizations are carried out with a biotin-labeled, chromosome-specific alpha satellite DNA probe or human chromosome-specific library DNA probes obtained from the American Type Culture Collection. The probes are labeled by nick translation using biotin-11-dUTP (Bethesda Research Laboratories) or biotin-16-dUTP (Boehringer Mannheim) according to the instructions of the supplier. Hybridizations are performed using a modification of methods described earlier [9, 10, 13, 16, 20].

Morphology antibody chromosome preparations are destained by incubation in methanol/acetic acid fixative for 1 h at room temperature and air dried. Then the preparations are treated with pepsin (0.01–0.1 mg/ml) to remove the cytoplasm. The hybridization mixture consists of 0.001–0.004 µg/µl biotinylated chromosome-specific alpha satellite DNA or 0.1 µg/µl biotinylated chromosome-specific library DNA, 50 %–65 % formamide, 10 % (w/v) dextran sulfate, 2 × SSC, and 0.5 µg/µl herring sperm DNA. When chromosome-specific library DNA probes are used, 0.2 µg/µl human genomic DNA is added to the hybridization mixture. Denaturation of the probes and the cells is performed at 70°–75 °C for 3–5 min. The slides are incubated in a moist chamber at 37°–42 °C for 12–16 h. After posthybridization washes the signals of alpha satellite probes are detected by immunocytochemical methods [3] and the signals of chromosome library probes by fluorescence methods [13, 16].

Advantages and Limitations of MAC-ISH Methodology for Minimal Residual Disease

The in situ hybridization techniques can be considered sensitive and reliable methods in the study of minimal residual cells (Table 1). No cell culture is needed; mitotic cells are not necessary. Nevertheless, dividing cells can be used to confirm results, especially with chromosome library probes that do not always give clear hybridization signals on interphase cells. With MAC metaphase the signals can be reliably interpreted. Mitotic cells also yield information about the proliferation kinetics of residual cells.

One cytospin preparation contains up to 10^4 cells. These cells can be scored in 2–3 h. It is likely that this procedure will be automated in the future. As the technique allows immunological cell classification, in

Table 1. Morphology antibody chromosome in situ hybridization in minimal residual disease

Advantages Practical/fast	Various types of preparations can be used
	No special equipment needed
	No radioactive chemicals needed
	Probes easily available[a]
Reliable	Cancer-specific markers (i.e., clonal chromosome abnormalities and/or monoclonal antibodies) are used
	Low number of false-positive signals
	No cell culture needed, specimen closely resembles the situation in vivo[a]
Sensitive/quantitative	Up to 10^5 cells can be scored in a reasonable time
	Analysis can be focused on certain cell lineages (e.g., immunoglobulin light-chain clonality in B-cell leukemias)
Qualitative	Origin (cell lineage) of residual cells
Limitations	A suitable chromosome aberration needed: polyploidies, trisomies, some translocations, and some inversions can be studied. Monosomies and deletions cannot be studied because of the high frequency of false-negative cells

cases where the immunocytochemical analysis reveals a single immunophenotype among all neoplastic cells (e.g., in B-cell leukemias there is often immunoglobulin light-chain clonality), one is able to concentrate on such immunophenotypically clonal cells. In other cases (such as the myeloid leukemias or myelodysplastic syndromes) where several cell lineages are involved, it is possible to trace the immunophenotypic origin of each residual cell, which is essential if in the future residual cells will be destroyed using target-specific treatments.

An example of the usefulness of the MAC-ISH method comes from our study of 12 trisomy in a patient with chronic lymphocytic leukemia [15]. In this patient with lambda light-chain clonality, the frequency of kappa-positive cells was less than 1% of all cells for analysis. However, we had no difficulty in finding 200 kappa-positive cells. None of these cells had three hybridization signals, whereas 87% of the clonal cells contained trisomy 12 (Fig. 1). Even though the above example does not concern minimal residual disease directly, it does illustrate the potential of the technique in studying the normality/abnormality of cell lineages representing a small minority of all cells. The above study also showed that, when the 12-specific repetitive probe was used, no false-positive signals were detected in the controls.

Another example of the sensitivity of the technique is derived from MAC-ISH study with Y-specific probe of minimal residual male host cells after bone marrow transplantation from female donors [21]. This study showed that Y-specific signals were detected in two of the three patients, both in clinical remission in 6 and 7 cells out of 1000 cells analyzed. The presence of host cells has been confirmed in a later study (Wessman et al. in preparation). Interestingly, in one patient a fragment of a blood vessel could be demonstrated on the basis of cell morphology (M. Wessman et al., in preparation). All these cells contained the Y chromosome. Thus the technique revealed a contamination associated with bone marrow aspiration. This means that other sensitive techniques that do not reveal cell morphology/immunophenotype (e.g., polymerase chain reaction with Y-specific primers) do not provide reliable detection of minimal residual male host cells.

In addition to classification according to cell lineage, the MAC-ISH technique allows quantitation of residual cells, a feature which other techniques lack. Residual cell counts can be used for evaluating the clinical importance of residual cells and for monitoring efficacy of the treatment(s).

The main limitation of the MAC-ISH technique lies in the requirement of a suitable chromosome aberration for follow-up. Abnormalities that can be used are polyploidies, trisomies, and partial trisomies. There are reports that some structural abnormalities can also be studied by ISH [2, 6].

In interphase cells repetitive probes give less ambiguous signals than do chromosome library probes. The signals of the latter are often uninterpretable in a large number of cells because of overlapping. Unspecific hybridization of some repetitive probes (e.g., for acrocentric chromosomes) may be a problem in interphase cells but not to the same extent in mitotic cells, where chromosomes can be recognized morphologically.

In interphase cytogenetic studies of leukemias, several chromosome-specific repetitive probes, such as those for chromosomes 1, 7, 8, 9, 12, and Y, have been used [1, 12, 15, 21]. Apart from ourselves, no other investigators have used these probes in immunologically and morphologically classified cells. We have also adapted chromosome library probes to MAC preparations (Tiainen et al., in preparation).

Because hybridization rate hardly ever approaches 100% and because the interpretation of the number of signals is not reliable for every cell especially when library probes are used, the MAC-ISH technique cannot be used for the detection of minimal residual cells with chromosome monosomy or deletion.

Use of MAC-ISH in Minimal Residual Disease

The MAC-ISH technique should not be used alone but in combination with stand-

ard chromosome banding analysis. G-band-
ing at the time of diagnosis provides the
basis for choosing a probe or probe combination for follow-up of the disease. Before
adoption, the probe(s) chosen will be tested
on a specimen obtained at the time of
diagnosis. Standard immunophenotyping
should also be performed at the time of
diagnosis to enable one to pick the right
antibodies for efficient detection of neoplastic cells (e.g., kappa/lambda light-chain
clonality in B-cell diseases). In cases where
immunophenotyping can not be expected
to yield additional information, however,

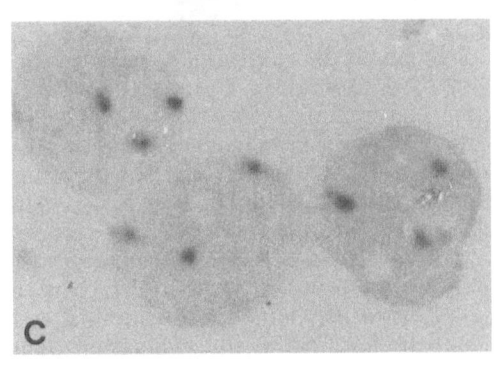

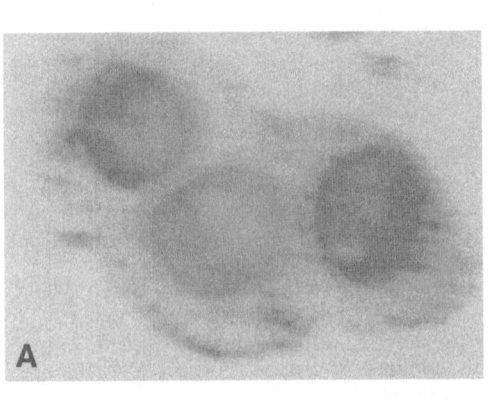

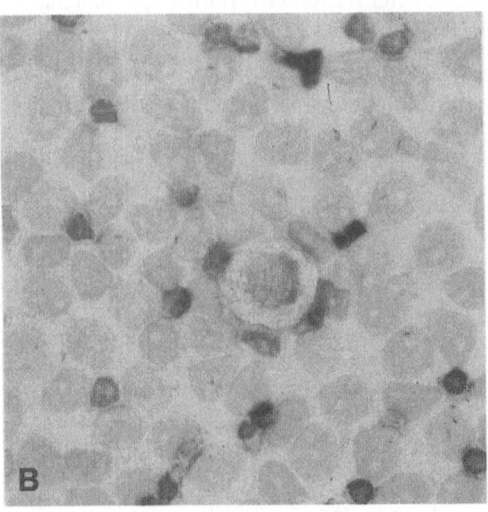

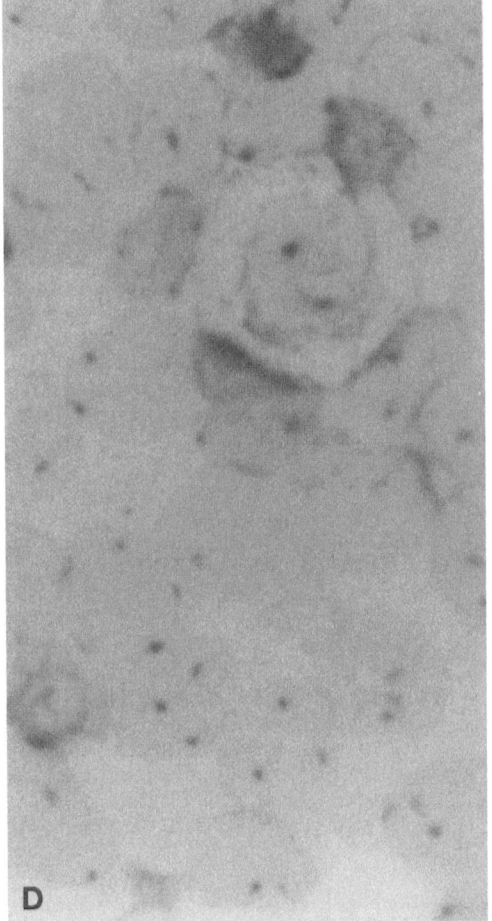

Fig. 1A–D. A cytospin preparation stained by immunoperoxidase technique from a patient with
chronic lymphocytic leukemia. Three lambda (**A**) positive cells and one kappa (**B**) positive cell after
immunoperoxidase staining. In situ hybridization with chromosome 12-specific alpha satellite DNA
probe *pSP12-1* (Greig et al. [7]) demonstrates that the lambda-positive cells contain trisomy 12 (**C**),
whereas the kappa-positive cell shows two in situ hybridization spots (**D**). Most of the kappa-negative
cells have trisomy 12

ISH should be performed primarily on standard chromosome preparations, skipping the immunocytochemistry stage (1–2 days). Without immunocytochemistry, ISH takes 1–1½ days to perform. Today routine investigations of leukemia patients at our laboratory include both standard cytogenetic analysis and MAC-ISH. The future will tell the real value of the MAC-ISH methodology in the detection of minimal residual disease and in the evaluation of its clinical significance.

Acknowledgements. This work was supported in part by grants from the Finnish Cancer Society, Sigrid Juselius Foundation, and Helsinki University.

References

1. Anastasi J, Le Beau MM, Vardiman JW, Westbrook CA (1990) Detection of numerical chromosomal abnormalities neoplastic hematopoietic cells by in situ hybridization with a chromosome-specific probe. Am J Pathol 136: 131–139
2. Arnoldus EPJ, Wiegant J, Noordermeer IA, Wessels JW, Beverstock GC, Grosveld GC, van der Ploeg M, Raap AK (1990) Detection of the Philadelphia chromosome in interphase nuclei. Cytogenet Cell Genet 54: 108–111
3. Burns J, Chan VTW, Jonasson JA, Fleming KA, Taylor S, McGee JOD (1985) Sensitive system for visualising biotinylated DNA probes hybridised in situ: rapid sex determination of intact cells. J Clin Pathol 38: 1085–1092
4. Cremer T, Landegent J, Brückner A, Scholl HP, Schardin M, Hager HD, Devilee P, Pearson P (1986) Detection of chromosome aberrations in the human interphase nucleus by visualization of specific target DNAs with radioactive and non-radioactive in situ hybridization techniques: diagnosis of trisomy 18 with probe L1.84. Hum Genet 74: 346–352
5. Cremer T, Lichter P, Borden J, Ward DC, Manuelidis L (1988) Detection of chromosome aberrations in metaphase and interphase tumor cells by in situ hybridization using chromosome-specific library probes. Hum Genet 80: 235–246
6. Dauwerse JG, Kievits T, Beverstock GC, van der Keur D, Smit E, Wessels HW, Hagemeijer A, Pearson PL, Ommen G-JB, Breuning MH (1990) Rapid detection of chromosome 16 inversion in acute nonlymphocytic leukemia, subtype M4: regional localization of the breakpoint in 16p. Cytogenet Cell Genet 53: 126–128
7. Greig GM, Parikh S, George J, Powers VE, Willard HF (1991) Molecular cytogenetics of alpha satellite DNA chromosome 12: fluorescence in situ hybridization and description of DNA and array length polymorphisms. Cytogenet Cell Genet 56: 144–148
8. Heim S, Mitelman F (1987) Cancer cytogenetics. Liss, New York
9. Hopman AHN, Ramaekers FCS, Raap AK, Beck JLM, Devilee P, van der Ploeg M, Voojis GP (1988) In situ hybridization as a tool to study numerical chromosome aberrations in solid bladder tumor. Histochemistry 89: 307–316
10. Hopman AHN, Poddighe PJ, Smeets AWGB, Moesker O, Beck JLM, Vooijs P, Ramaekers FCS (1989) Detection of numerical chromosome aberrations in bladder cancer by in situ hybridization. Am J Pathol 135: 1105
11. Knuutila S, Teerenhovi L (1989) Immunophenotyping of aneuploid cells. Cancer Genet Cytogenet 41: 1–17
12. Kolluri RV, Manuelidis L, Cremer T, Sait S, Gezer S, Raza A (1990) Detection of monosomy 7 in interphase cells of patients with myeloid disorders. Am J Hematol 33: 117–122
13. Lichter P, Cremer T, Borden J, Manuelidis L, Ward DC (1988) Delineation of individual human chromosomes in metaphase and interphase cells by in situ suppression hybridization using recombinant DNA libraries. Hum Genet 80: 224–234
14. Lichter P, Cremer T, Chang Tang CJ, Watkins PC, Manuelidis L, Ward DC (1988) Rapid detection of chromosome 21 aberrations by in situ hybridization. Proc Natl Acad Sci USA 85: 9664–9668
15. Perez Losada A, Wessman M, Tiainen M, Hopman AHN, Willard HF, Solé F, Caballin MR, Woessner S, Knuutila S (1991) Trisomy 12 in chronic lymphocytic leukemia – an interphase cytogenetic study. Blood 78: 775–779
16. Pinkel D, Landegent J, Collins C, Fusco J, Segraves R, Lucas J, Gray JW (1988) Fluorescence in situ hybridization with human chromosome specific libraries: detection of trisomy 21 and translocations of chromosome 4. Proc Natl Acad Sci USA 85: 9138–9142
17. Rappold GA, Cremer T, Hager HD, Davies KE, Müller CR, Yang T (1984) Sex chromosome positions in human interphase nuclei as studied by in situ hybridization with chromo-

some specific DNA probes. Hum Genet 67: 317

18. Teerenhovi L, Knuutila S, Ekblom M, Borgström GH, Tallman JK, Andersson L, de la Chapelle A (1984) A method for simultaneous study of the karyotype, morphology, and immunologic phenotype of mitotic cells in hematologic malignancies. Blood 64: 1116–1122

19. Trent JM, Kaneko Y, Mitelman F (1989) Report of the committee on structural chromosome changes in neoplasia. Cytogenet Cell Genet 51: 533–562

20. Wessman M, Knuutila S (1988) A method for the determination of cell morphology, immunologic phenotype and numerical chromosomal abnormalities on the same mitotic interphase cancer cell. Genet (Life Sci Adv) 7: 127–130

21. Wessman M, Ruutu T, Volin L, Knuutila S (1989) In situ hybridization using a Y-specific probe – a sensitive method for distinguishing residual male recipient cells from female donor cells in bone marrow transplantation. Bone Marrow Transplan 4: 283–286

Detection of Residual Leukemic Cells in AML

B. Wörmann[1], S. Könemann[1], A. Humpe[1], M. Safford[2], K. Zurlutter[1], K. Schreiber[1], K. Piechotka[1], Th. Büchner[1], W. Hiddemann[1], and L. W. M. M. Terstappen[2]

Introduction

Sixty to seventy percent of adult patients with newly diagnosed AML can achieve a complete remission (CR) through intensive chemotherapy [1–6]. However, the majority of these patients will suffer relapse within 2 years. With the exception of age, secondary leukemias, and a small group of cytogenetically defined AML, no universally accepted prognostic marker has been identified which would allow early treatment stratification. Thus AML treatment is highly uniform, consisting of intensive induction chemotherapy, followed by consolidating postremission therapy with or without bone marrow transplantation. The "gold standard" for the diagnosis of AML and therapy monitoring is the light microscopic evaluation of cytology and cytochemistry. Its sensitivity for the detection of residual leukemic cells is 5%.

In the past 5 years several cell biological markers and appropriate methods with high sensitivity have been described, which might be helpful in the detection of residual leukemic cells in AML. We have applied several of these techniques in bone marrow aspirates of patients with newly diagnosed disease as part of a prospective study. The methods and initial results will be discussed in the following chapters.

Methods for the Detection of Residual Leukemic Cells

Immunophenotyping by Multiparameter Flow Cytometry

The generation of murine monoclonal antibodies against myeloid leukemic cell lines and myeloid leukemic blasts from patients raised high hopes for improvements in the diagnosis and classification of AML [7–12]. However, it soon became obvious, that all leukemia-associated antigens were also present on the surface of normal myeloid progenitor cells. Thus the use of monoclonal antibodies for the detection of leukemic cells is limited by the incidence of normal committed progenitor cells within the bone marrow sample. A further limitation is the high heterogeneity of AML. No single antigen has been described with an incidence of >75% in AML [12]. The maturation of hematopoietic progenitor cells to mature effector cells is characterized by the sequential acquisition and the loss of cell surface antigens [13]. Using a combination of two or three monoclonal antibodies the maturation pathway of normal cells of myeloid, monocytoid, erythroid, and lymphocytic lineage has been established based on the analysis of normal bone marrow aspirates [14–16]. Delwel et al. [17], Terstappen et al. [18], and Campana et al. [19] have applied fluorescence-optical methods, in order to distinguish normal and leukemic myeloid progenitor cells. The characteristic feature of leukemic cells is the aberrant (asynchronous) expression of cell surface antigens. The technical require-

[1] University of Münster, Department of Internal Medicine A, University of Münster, Albert-Schweitzer Str. 33, 4400 Münster, FRG
[2] Becton Dickinson Immunocytometry Systems, San José, CA, USA

ments are met by automated flow cytometers equipped with argon lasers. Cells can first be characterized using their light catter profile. The combination of forward light scatter and orthogonal light scatter makes possible the separation of granulocytes, monocytes, lymphocytes, myelocytes, promyelocytes, erythrocytes, erythroid progenitors, and blast cells [20, 21]. Using simultaneous staining of cells with three monoclonal antibodies conjugated to three fluorescent dyes, the cell surface antigen expression can be analyzed within each subpopulation. A sensitivity of 0.1 % can be achieved for the detection of cells with the leukemic phenotype within otherwise normal bone marrow aspirates. The combination of the in vitro culture technique for clonogenic leukemic blasts and the aberrant antigen expression of B-lineage antigens on myeloid cells has also been described as a useful marker for detection of residual leukemic cells in AML [22].

In April 1989 we started a collaborative study for the multidimensional analysis of leukemic blasts in patients with newly diagnosed AML. Bone marrow aspirates were analyzed before therapy, after the first course of induction chemotherapy, at achievement of hematological CR, before consolidation therapy, before maintenance therapy, and in relapse. Monoclonal antibodies were used against CD2 [23], 3, 4, 7, 8, 11b, 11c, 13, 14, 15, 16, 33, 34, 38, 45, and HLA-DR. The antibodies were either directly conjugated to the fluorochromes fluoresceinisothiocyanite (FITC) or phycoerythrin (PE), or they were biotinylated. The latter conjugates were visualized using the tandem dye Duochrome (Becton Dickinson).

In the first series of 60 patients, 59 showed aberrant antigen expression which enabled the leukemic cells to be identified [24]. The patterns of aberrant antigen expression are as follows:
1. Expression of lymphoid antigens on myeloid cells
2. Asynchronous expression of stage-specific myeloid antigens
3. Overexpression of myeloid-lineage-associated antigens
4. Lack of myeloid-lineage-associated antigens.

The clinical course of 42 patients was followed. Residual leukemic cells were detected in the bone marrow aspirates of 39/42 patients after one cycle of TAD9 and in 20/27 patients in hematological and microscopic CR. One clinical course is shown in Fig. 1. The patient's leukemic cells were characterized by the expression of a lymphoid-associated antigen on the myeloid leukemic blasts. After double-induction chemotherapy he achieved a hematological remission, the bone marrow aspirate showing no significant infiltration of resi-

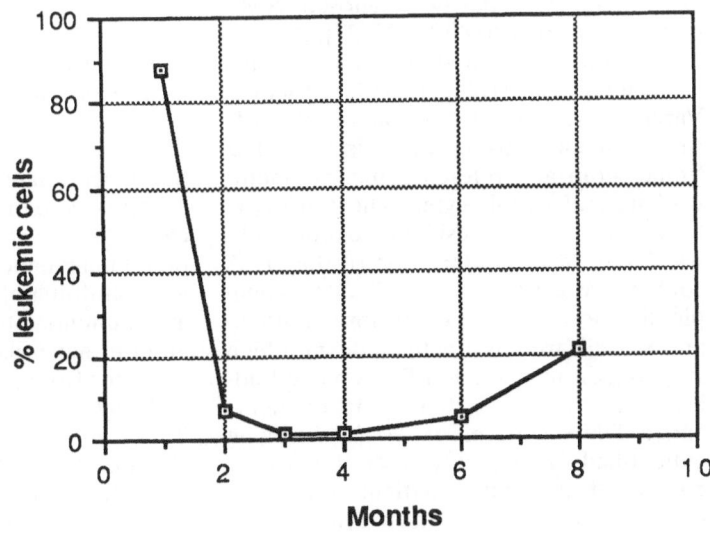

Fig. 1. Detection of leukemic cells by multiparameter flow cytometry. Leukemic cells were characterized by aberrant antigen expression using antibodies against myeloid- and lymphoid-lineage-associated antigens. The relative number of leukemic cells is shown on the y-axis. The patient entered hematological CR at 2 months and had overt relapse at 10 months. Multiparameter flow cytometry detected persistent leukemic cells throughout the whole period and a significant increase at 8 months after initial diagnosis

dual leukemic cells. However, multiparameter flow cytometry revealed a persistent population of cells with the leukemic phenotype. This population was consistently detected at unchanged frequency after consolidation chemotherapy (4 months) and during maintenance chemotherapy (6 months). At 8 months, the incidence of leukemic cells increased significantly. However, the microscopic evaluation of the bone marrow aspirate by an independent hematocytologist confirmed a percentage of <5% leukemic cells. Clinical relapse occurred at 10 months. The median observation time in this patient group is too short for a definitive evaluation of the clinical significance of persistent cells with the leukemic phenotype. Preliminary analysis shows a high incidence of early relapses in patients with residual leukemic cells after consolidation therapy.

DNA Aneuploidy

The detection of aneuploidies by automated quantitative DNA analysis is highly specific for malignant cells. Comparative studies using flow cytometry and cytogenetics have shown a good correlation of DNA aneuploidies and numerical chromosomal aberrations [25]. This analysis is fast and allows measurement of >10000 cells within 5–10 min. The incidence of DNA aneuploidies in the bone marrow aspirates of patients with newly diagnosed AML ranges from 20% to 40% [25–27]. A prospective study in our laboratory has revealed an incidence of 41.2% (54/131 patients). Variations from the DNA content of ≥5% were detectable using an optimized electronic setup and reference measurements with normal lymphocytes. The sensitivity for the detection of residual leukemic cells was 1%–5% if the deviation of the DNA content was ≥15%. Cells with DNA aneuploidies closer to the $G_{0/1}$ of normal mononuclear cells were not detectable with high sensitivity. The median of DNA aneuploidies in our study was 1.10. Only five patients had a DNA content of ≥1.15 and one patient had a hypoploidy of <0.9. Thus the number of informative patients for detection of residual cells by flow cytometry is relatively low. If a significant deviation of the cellular DNA content is present, this marker presents a simple, fast, and reliable method for the identification of leukemic cells.

Chromosomal Breakpoints

Acute myeloid leukemia is a very heterogenous disease. This is also reflected in the wide range of cytogenetic abnormalities associated with this disease [28]. Some entities are now well defined by a clonal chromosomal abnormality, a typical cytological and immunophenotypic pattern, and a characteristic clinical course. These well-characterized subgroups include the acute promyelocytic leukemia (FAB M3) with t(15; 17) [29–31]; the t(6; 9) in AML M2 [32]; the AML M4Eo with inv16 [33, 34]; the AML M2 with t(8; 21) [35]; and the AML M5a with translocation or deletion of 11q23 [36]. In some cases the molecular biological analyses have defined the genetic breakpoint at the DNA and RNA level, thus enabling polymerase chain reaction (PCR) techniques analogous to the procedures used in chronic myeloid leukemia to be applied [37, 38]. This method combines a highly specific marker such as the DNA/RNA sequence of a chromosomal breakpoint and a highly sensitive method such as PCR. The group of informative patients is still small.

Immunoglobulin and T-Cell Receptor Gene Rearrangements

Gene rearrangements can be detected by Southern analysis and by PCR. These analyses were first used for the detection of clone-specific gene rearrangements in lymphoid malignancies using the physiological gene shuffling of the T-cell receptor (TCR) and immunoglobulin (Ig) gene loci. Several authors have also analyzed bone marrow aspirates from patients with bonified AML and have detected rearrangements of the TCRγ and δ chains and/or the Ig heavy chain in up to 10% [39–42]. A correlation of TCR and Ig gene rearrangements with expression of terminal deoxynucleotidyl transferase (TdT) has been described [43]. Southern analysis has a sensitivity of 1%–5% for the detection of clonal rearrangements. A physiological mechanism of diversity generation in *TCR* and *Ig* genes is the insertion of additional nucleotides at the genetic breakpoints. These randomly inserted bases constitute a highly specific marker for one respective lymphoid cell clone and have been used for the detection of minimal residual disease by PCR at the DNA level [44–46]. A sensitivity of 0.001% for the identification of clonal lymphoid cells can be achieved. In a prospective study of 93 patients with newly diagnosed AML at our institution, only 2 patients had a *TCRδ* and one patient had an *IgH* gene rearrangement, which could be exploited by PCR. Both patients with *TCRδ* gene rearrangements failed to achieve a CR.

X-Linked Restriction Fragment Length Polymorphism

Another useful marker for the determination of clonality is the analysis of restriction fragment length polymorphism (RFLPs) based on the random inactivation of X chromosomal genes [47]. This method can only be applied in women. The incidence of informative patients for RFLPs of the phosphoglycerine kinase gene and the hypoxanthine-guanine phosphoribosyl transferase gene is about 20%–25% [48]. Using the recently described *M27β* probe, the percentage of informative female patients can be raised to 90% [49]. The sensitivity of this analysis by the Southern technique is 1%–5%.

Oncogene Point Mutations

The most extensively studied point mutations are those of the *ras* genes. They occur in well-defined regions of the N-*ras* genes at codons 12, 13, and 61 [50–52]. Using a set of appropriate oligonucleotides, these point mutations can be detected in 20%–25% of patients with AML. They are not leukemia-specific, but are found in a wide variety of malignant and premalignant conditions,

including myelodysplastic syndromes [53]. Most probably they constitute one event in a multistep concept of malignant transformation. The level of sensitivity for the detection of cells with point mutations within a population of cells in germline configuration is 2%–5%. Specificity and sensitivity categorize *ras* oncogene point mutations as a useful marker of clonality.

Oncogene Transcription

Overexpression of protooncogenes has been observed in a variety of hematological malignancies. In patients with AML, abnormally high levels of c-*myc* protein and persistence of a high c-*myc* transcription rate have been related to poor prognosis [54, 55]. Evinger-Hodges et al. have analyzed the c-*myc* transcription in patients in morphological remission using a rapid and sensitive in situ hybridization technique [56]. They reported a shorter remission duration in patients with abnormally high levels and proposed this method as a sensitive marker for minimal residual disease. As part of our prospective study, we have also analyzed bone marrow aspirates and peripheral blood samples of 25 patients with newly diagnosed AML. Twenty-two patients were treated with TAD, three patients with cytosine arabinoside low-dose (ara-C) and idarubicine. Cells were prepared and hybridized as previously described [56]. Elevated transcript levels were found in 21 of the 25 patients. All patients showed a rapid decrease in the transcription level during the first 3 days of chemotherapy. No significant differences in the initial c-*myc* levels or its decrease were observed in the 11 patients who entered CR, compared with the patients without adequate blast clearance after induction chemotherapy. Persistent cells with high c-*myc* transcription were found in 6/11 patients in CR. However, control bone marrow aspirates from three of four patients with acute lymphoblastic leukemia (ALL) in regeneration after high-dose chemotherapy with ara-C plus mitoxantrone also revealed the presence of cells with overexpression of c-*myc* transcription. These observations suggest that "abnormally" high transcription levels of c-*myc* may also occur physiologically in regenerating bone marrow.

Discussion

In the past 5 years several methods have been developed for the detection of leukemia-associated markers. The sensitivity ranges from 0.001 % for PCR-based markers to 5 % for markers of clonality. Figure 2 shows a schematic graph of residual leukemic cells in AML. A significant reduction of the relative number of leukemic cells can be achieved in the majority of patients, resulting in the recovery of normal hematopoiesis and hematological CR. Our data using multiparameter flow cytometry suggest that the relative percentage of residual leukemic cells in the majority of these patients is in the range of 0.1 %–10 % [57]. Some patients have an even higher number of leukemic cells consistent with the concept of clonal remission. A small number of patients will not have detectable leukemic cells by flow cytometry, but will ultimately relapse. More sensitive methods using amplification of leukemia-associated gene sequences by PCR can identify those patients.

The vast majority of studies for minimal residual disease in AML use only one method to detect leukemic cells. The widespread use of the different methods now allows prospective studies comparing the different markers and their predictive value for the patient's prognosis. Based on the results, a clinical trial on treatment of early relapse can be conceived.

Summary

Sixty to seventy percent of patients with newly diagnosed acute myeloblastic leukemia (AML) can achieve a complete remission (CR) after intensive chemotherapy, but only 20 %–30 % can be potentially cured. In the absence of widely accepted prognostic markers for early treatment stratification, the therapy of AML is highly standardized and uniform. One approach

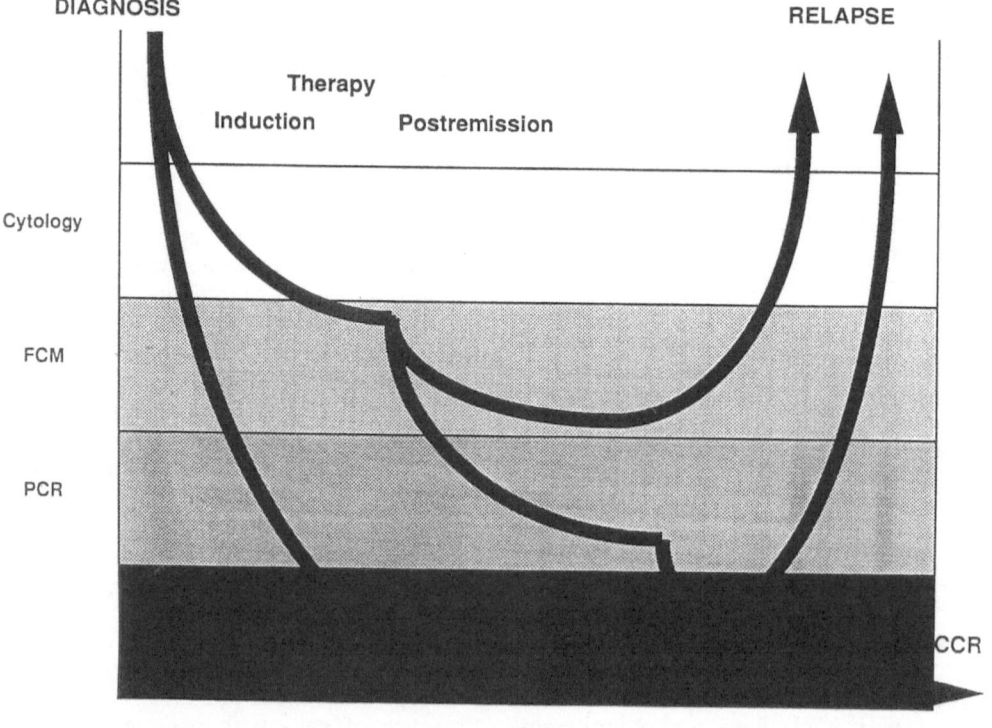

Fig. 2. Schematic diagram of residual leukemic cells in AML

for risk-adapted postremission therapy is the identification of residual leukemic cells in the bone marrow aspirates of AML patients in CR. Several leukemia-associated markers have been proposed (prevalence in brackets) including clonal chromosomal translocations (50 %), DNA aneuploidies (35 %), gene rearrangements (1 %–10 %), aberrant oncogene transcription (60 %), aberrant surface antigen expression (95 %), oncogene point mutations (20 %–25 %), and restriction fragment length polymorphisms (80 %–90 % of female patients). Strengths and weaknesses of the different markers and methods are discussed.

In April 1989 we started a prospective study on residual leukemic cells in AML. Using multiparameter flow cytometry for immunophenotyping, the leukemic cells were identified in 59/60 patients with newly diagnosed AML based on aberrant antigen expression. Residual leukemic cells were detected in the bone marrow aspirates of 39/42 patients after one cycle of TAD9 and in 20/27 patients in hematological and microscopic CR. The aim of the study was the evaluation of the prognostic significance of residual cells with the leukemic phenotype in CR and comparison of different markers.

The clinical value of the detection of persistent leukemic cells has not been established, nor has the value of the different methods been compared in prospective studies. With the use of currently available methods strategies for a more individualized chemotherapy can be developed.

References

1. Rai KR, Holland JF, Gliedewell OJ et al. (1981) Treatment of acute myelocytic leukemia: a study by Cancer and Leukemia Group B. Blood 58: 1203–1212
2. Büchner T, Urbanitz D, Hiddemann W et al. (1985) Intensified induction and consodilation with or without maintenance chemotherapy for acute myeloid leukemia (AML) (1985). Two multicenter studies of the German AML Cooperative Group. J Clin Oncol 3: 1583–1589
3. Preisler H, Davis RB, Kirshner J et al. (1987) Comparison of three remission induction regimens and two post-induction strategies for the treatment of acute nonlymphocytic leukemia: a Cancer and Leukemia Group B Study. Blood 69: 1441–1449
4. Cassileth PA, Harrington DP, Hines JD, Oken MM, Mazza JJ, McGlave P, Bennett JM, O'Connell MJ (1988) Maintenance chemotherapy prolongs remission duration in adult acute nonlymphocytic leukemia. J Clin Oncol 6: 583
5. Kurrle E, Ehninger G, Fackler-Schwalbe E, Freund M et al. (1990) Consolidation therapy with high-dose arabinoside: experiences of a prospective study in acute myeloid leukemia. In: Büchner T, Schellong G, Hiddemann W, Ritter J (eds) Acute leukemias II. Springer, Berlin Heidelberg New York, pp 254–260
6. Büchner T, Hiddemann W, Blasius S et al. (1990) Adult AML: the role of chemotherapy intensity and duration. Two studies of the AMLCG. In: Büchner T, Schellong G, Hiddemann W, Ritter J (eds) Acute leukemias II. Springer, Berlin Heidelberg New York, pp 261–266
7. Martens AC, Hagenbeck A (1985) Detection of minimal disease in acute leukemia using flow cytometry: studies in a rat model for human acute leukemia. Cytometry 6: 342–347
8. Foon KA, Gale RP, Todd RF 3d (1986) Recent advances in the immunologic classification of leukemia. Semin Hematol 23: 257–283
9. Neame PB, Soamboonsrup P, Browman GP, Meyer RM, Benger A, Wilson WE, Walker IR, Saeed N, McBride JA (1986) Classifying acute leukemia by immunophenotyping: a combined FAB-immunologic classification of AML. Blood 68: 1355–1362
10. Griffin JD, Davis R, Nelson DA, Davis FR, Mayer RJ, Schiffer C, McIntyre OR, Bloomfield CD (1986) Use of surface marker analysis to predict outcome of adult acute myeloblastic leukemia. Blood 68: 1232–1241
11. White DL, Ashman LK, Dart GW, Zola H, Toogood IR, Kimber RJ (1987) The expression of mature myeloid cell differentiation markers in acute leukemia. Pathology 19: 137–142
12. Drexler HG (1987) Classification of acute myeloid leukemias – a comparison of FAB and immunophenotyping. Leukemia 1: 697–705
13. Terstappen LWMM, Safford M, Loken MR (1990) Flow cytometric analysis of human bone marrow. III. Neutrophil maturation. Leukemia 4: 657–663
14. Loken MR, Shah VO, Dattilio KL, Civin CI

(1987) Flow cytometric analysis of human bone marrow: I. Normal erythroid development. Blood 69: 255–263

15. Loken MR, Shah VO, Dattilio KL, Civin CI (1987) Flow cytometric analysis of human bone marrow: II. Normal B lymphocyte development. Blood 70: 1316–1324

16. LeBien TW, Wörmann B, Villablanca JG, Law CL, Steinberg LM, Shah VO, Loken MR (1990) Multiparameter flow cytometric analysis of human fetal bone marrow B cells. Leukemia 4: 354–358

17. Delwel R, van Gurp R, Bot F, Touw I, Löwenberg B (1988) Phenotyping of acute myelocytic leukemia (AML) progenitors: an approach for tracing minimal numbers of AML cells among normal bone marrow. Leukemia 2: 814

18. Terstappen LWMM, Loken MR (1990) Myeloid cell differentiation in normal bone marrow and acute myeloid leukemia assessed by multi-dimensional flow cytometry. Anal Cell Pathol 2: 229–240

19. Campana D, Coustan-Smith E, Janossy G (1990) The immunologic detection of minimal residual disease in acute leukemia. Blood 76: 163–171

20. Brunsting A, Mullaney PF (1972) Light scattering from coated spheres: model for biological cells. Appl Optics 11: 675–680

21. Salzman GC, Growell JM, Martin JC (1975) Cell classification by laser light scattering: identification and separation of unstained leukocytes. Acta Cytol 19: 374–377

22. Gerhartz HH, Schmertzer H (1990) Detection of minimal residual disease in acute myeloid leukemia. Leukemia 14: 508–516

23. Knapp W, Dörken B, Gilks WR, Rieber EP, Schmidt RE, Stein H, von dem Borne AEGK (eds) (1989) Leukocyte Typing IV. White Cell differentiation Antigens. Oxford University Press, New York

24. Terstappen LWMM, Safford M, Könemann S, Loken MR, Zurlutter K, Büchner T, Hiddemann W, Wörmann B (1991) Flow cytometric characterization of acute myeloid leukemia. II. Extreme heterogeneity at diagnosis. Leukemia (in press)

25. Barlogie B, Hittelman W, Spitzer G, Hart JS, Trujillo JM, Smallwood L, Drewinko B (1977) Correlation of DNA distribution abnormalities with cytogenetic findings in human adult leukemia and lymphoma. Cancer Res 37: 4400–4407

26. Andreeff M, Redner A, Thongprasert S, Eagle B, Steinherz P, Miller D, Melamed MR (1985) Multiparameter flow cytometry for determination of ploidy, proliferation and differentiation in acute leukemia: treatment effects and prognostic value. In: Büchner T,

Bloomfield CD, Hiddemann W, Hossfeld DK, Schumann J (eds) Tumor aneuploidy. Springer, Berlin Heidelberg New York, pp 81–105

27. Hiddemann W, Wörmann B, Göhde W, Büchner T (1986) DNA aneuploidies in adult patients with acute myeloid leukemia (1986) Incidence and relation to patient characteristics and morphologic subtypes. Cancer 57: 2146–2152

28. Arthur DC, Berger R, Golomb HM, Swansbury GJ, Reeves BR, Alimena G, van den Berghe H, Bloomfield CD, de la Chapelle A, Dewalt GW, Garson OM, Hagemeijer A, Kaneko Y, Mitelman F, Pierre KV, Ruutu T, Sakurai M, Lawler SD, Rowley JD (1989) The clinical significance of karyotype in acute myelogenous leukemia. Cancer Genet Cytogenet 40: 203

29. Borrow J, Goddard AD, Sheer D, Solomon E (1990) Molecular analysis of acute promyelocytic leukemia breakpoint cluster region on chromosome 17. Science 249: 1577–1580

30. de Thé H, Chomienne C, Lanotte M, Degos L, Dejean A (1990) The t(15; 17) translocation of acute promyelocytic leukaemia fuses the retinoic receptor alpha gene to a novel transcribed locus. Nature 347: 558–561

31. Biondi A, Longo L, Rambaldi A, Pandolfi PP, Mencarelli A, LoCoco F, Diverio D, Pegoraro L, Avanzi G, Donti E, Zangrilli D, Alcalay M, Barbui T, Masera G, Grignani F, Pelicci PG (1990) Molecular analysis of the t(15; 17) in acute promyelocytic leukemia: rearrangements and aberrant expression of the retinoic acid receptor alpha (RAR alpha) gene. Blood [Suppl] 76: 227 (abstract 898)

32. Von Lindern M, Poustka A, Lerach H, Grosveld G (1990) The (6; 9) chromosome translocation, associated with a specific subtype of acute nonlymphocytic leukemia, leads to aberrant transcription of a target gene on 9q34. Mol Cell Biol 10: 4016–4026

33. Arthur DC, Bloomfield CD (1983) Partial deletion of the long arm of chromosome 16 and bone marrow eosinophilia in acute nonlymphocytic leukemia: a new association. Blood 61: 994

34. LeBeau MM (1983) Association of an inversion of chromosome 16 with abnormal marrow eosinophils in acute myelomonocytic leukemia. A unique cytogenetic-clinicopathological association. N Engl J Med 309: 630

35. Rowley JD, Testa JR (1982) Chromosome abnormalities in malignant hematologic diseases. Adv Cancer Res 36: 103

36. Yunis JJ (1981) All patients with acute nonlymphocytic leukemia may have a chro-

mosome defect. N Engl J Med 305: 135

37. Lee MS, Chang KS, Freireich EJ, Kantarjian HM, Talpaz M, Truhillo JM, Stass SA (1988) Detection of minimal residual *bcr/abl* transcripts by a modified polymerase chain reaction. Blood 72: 893–897

38. Kawasaki ES, Clark SS, Coyne MY, Smith SD, Champlin R, Witte ON, McCormick F (1988) Diagnosis of chronic myeloid and acute lymphocytic leukemias by detection of leukemia-specific mRNA sequences amplified in vitro. Proc Natl Acad Sci USA 85: 5698

39. Cheng GY, Minden MD, Toyonaga B, Tak WM, McCulloch EA (1986) T-cell receptor and immunoglobulin gene rearrangements in acute myeloblastic leukemia. J Exp Med 163: 414

40. Rovigatti UY, Mirro J, Kitchingman G, Dahl G, Ochs J, Murphy S, Stass S (1986) Heavy chain immunoglobulin gene rearrangement in acute nonlymphocytic leukemia. Blood 63: 1023

41. Greenberg JM, Quertermous T, Seidman JG, Kersey JH (1986) Human T cell gamma chain rearrangement in acute lymphoid and nonlymphoid leukemia. Comparison with the T cell receptor beta chain gene. J Immunol 137: 2043

42. Oster W, König K, Ludwig WD, Ganser A, Lindemann A, Mertelsmann R, Herrmann F (1988) Incidence of lineage promiscuity in acute myeloblastic leukemia: diagnostic implications of immunoglobulin and T-cell receptor gene rearrangement analysis and immunological phenotyping. Leuk Res 12: 887–895

43. Foa R, Casorati G, Giubellino MG, Basso G, Schiro R, Pizzolo G, Lauria F, LeFrance MP, Rabbitts TH, Migone N (1987) Rearrangements of immunoglobulin and T-cell receptor beta and gamma genes are associated with terminal deoxynucleotidyl transferase expression in acute myeloid leukemia. J Exp Med 165: 879

44. Hansen-Hagge TE, Yokota S, Bartram CR (1989) Detection of minimal residual disease in acute lymphoblastic leukemia by an in vitro amplification of rearranged T-cell receptor delta chain sequences. Blood 74: 1762

45. Yamada M, Hudson S, Tomay O, Rovera G (1989) Detection of minimal disease in hematopoietic malignancies of the B-cell lineage by using third-complementary-determining region (CDR-III) specific probes. Proc Natl Acad Sci USA 86: 5123–5127

46. Yamada M, Wasserman R, Lange B, Reichard BA, Womer RB, Rovera G (1990) Minimal residual disease in childhood B-lineage lymphoblastic leukemia – persistence of leukemic cells during the first 18 months of treatment. N Engl J Med 323: 448–455

47. Vogelstein B, Fearon ER, Hamilton SR, Feinberg AP (1985) Use of restriction fragment length polymorphisms to determine the clonal origin of human tumors. Science 27: 642

48. Bartram CR, Ludwig WD, Hiddemann W, Lyons J, Buschle M, Ritter J, Harbott J, Fröhlich A, Janssen JW (1989) Acute myeloid leukemia: analysis of *ras* gene mutations and clonality defined by polymorphic X-linked loci. Leukemia 3: 247–256

49. Abrahamson G, Fraser NJ, Boyd J, Craig I, Wainscoat JS (1990) A highly informative X-chromosome probe, *M27 beta,* can be used for the determination of tumour clonality. Br J Haematol 74: 371–372

50. Hirai H, Tanaka S, Azuma M, Anraku Y, Kobayashi Y, Fujisawa M, Okabe T, Takaku F (1985) Transforming genes in human leukemia cells. Blood 66: 1371–1378

51. Bos JL, Toksoz D, Marshall CJ, deVries MV, Veeneman GH, van der Erb AJ, van Boom JH, Janssen JWG, Steenvoorden AC (1985) Amino acid substitutions at codon 13 of the N-*ras* oncogene in human acute myeloid leukemia. Nature 315: 726–730

52. Gambke C, Hall A, Moroni C (1985) Activation of an N-*ras* gene in acute myeloblastic leukemia through somatic mutation in the first exon. Proc Natl Acad Sci USA 82: 8798–8882

53. Janssen JWG, Steenvoorden ACM, Lyons J, Anger B, Böhlke JU, Bos JL, Seliger H, Bartram CR (1987) *Ras* gene mutations in acute and chronic myelocytic leukemias, chronic myeloproliferative disorders, and myelodysplastic syndromes. Proc Natl Acad Sci USA 84: 9228

54. Preisler HD, Raza A (1987) Proto-oncogene transcript levels and acute nonlymphocytic leukemia. Semin Oncol 14: 207

55. Preisler HD, Sato H, Yang P, Wilson M, Kaufman C, Watt R (1988) Assessment of c-*myc* expression in individual leukemic cells. Leuk Res 12: 507–516

56. Evinger-Hodges MJ, Spinolo JA, Spencer V, Vieto P, Dicke KA (1989) Detection of minimal residual disease in acute myelogenous leukemia by RNA-in situ hybridization. Bone Marrow Transplant 4 [Suppl 1]: 13–15

57. Wörmann B, Könemann S, Safford M, Loken MR, Zurlutter K, Büchner T, Hiddemann W, Terstappen LWMM (1991) Selective elimination of leukemic subpopulations in acute myeloid leukemia through induction chemotherapy. To be published

Detection of Residual Leukemic Cells in the Majority of AML Patients After the Administration of TAD9

K. Zurlutter[1], S. Könemann[1], M. Safford[2], K. Schreiber[1], Th. Büchner[1], W. Hiddemann[1], B. Wörmann[1], and L. W. M. M. Terstappen[2]

Introduction

The maturation and differentiation pathway of normal bone marrow cells can be followed by monoclonal antibodies. Using five-dimensional flow cytometry (forward and side scatter, and three immunofluorescence signals) normal cell maturation is characterized by gradual changes of light-scattering properties and by gradual loss or acquisition of specific cell surface antigens [1–4]. Leukemic blasts can be distinguished from normal bone marrow cells by aberrant expression of surface antigens, e.g., abnormal quantitative expression and coexpression of cell surface antigens not occurring during normal maturation [5–7].

In an ongoing prospective study (begin: 4/89), the bone marrow aspirates of 54 patients with de novo acute myeloid leukemia (AML) were examined by using monoclonal antibodies and flow cytometry before and after induction chemotherapy. The reduction of the leukemic cell load by the first induction chemotherapy reflects the sensitivity of the blasts to the cytostatic agents and has been previously described as an indicator of prognosis. We analyzed leukemic populations before chemotherapy according to their degree of maturation and the relative proportion of leukemic cells. We investigated the modification of leukemic populations under the influence of one

[1] Department of Internal Medicine A, Albert-Schweitzer Str. 33, 4400 Münster, FRG
[2] Becton Dickinson Immunocytometry Systems, 2350 Qume Drive, San José, CA 95131, USA

cycle of TAD9 (thioguanine, cytosine arabinoside, daunorubicin).

Material and Methods

Bone marrow aspirates were obtained from patients with newly diagnosed acute myeloid leukemia (AML). Patient data are summarized in Table 1. For lysis of erythrocytes, a volume of bone marrow was diluted with 14 volumes of lysis solution. This mixture was incubated for 15 min at a temperature of 37 °C and centrifuged at 400 $\times g$ for 10 min. The pellet was resuspended with RPMI 1640 and the solution was centrifuged again at 400 $\times g$ for 10 min. This washing step was repeated twice. After this procedure the pellet was resuspended with RPMI 1640 for a final concentration of 2 $\times$ 10^5–1×10^6. Then the cells were incubated for 20 min with 15 µl pretitered monoclonal antibody in six combinations of three antibodies and in two combinations of two antibodies on ice at 4 °C. The fluorochromes FITC (fluoresceinisothiocyanite), PE (phycoerythrin), and Duochrome (Becton Dickinson, San José, CA, United States) were used. Antibodies were directed against the following antigens: CD (cluster designation) 2 (Leu5b), CD7 (Leu9), CD11b (Leu15), CD11c (LeuM5), CD13 (LeuM7), CD14 (LeuM3), CD15 (L16), CD15 (LeuM1), CD16 (Leu11a), CD19 (Leu12), CD20 (Leu16), CD22 (Leu14), CD33 (LeuM9), CD34 (HPCA-1), CD38 (Leu17), CD41 (IIIa), CD45 (HLe-1), and HLA-DR (HLA-DR). The antibodies were

Table 1. Patient characteristics

Number		54						
Age	Median:	61.5 years						
	<60 years:	25						
	>60 years:	29						
Sex	M:	32						
	F:	22						
FAB	M1	M2	M3	M4	M5	M6	M7	AUL
	6	11	4	13	12	5	1	2

Therapy outcome						
ED		NR		PR	CR	CCR
7		14		2	17	14

CCR: 7+ to 19+ months

Table 2. Maturation data

Subpopulation	Patient (n)	No maturation	Maturation	Both
1	11	8	3	–
2	25	3	4	18
3	15	1	1	13
4	2	–	–	2
5	1	–	–	1
	54	12	8	34

generously provided by Becton Dickinson Immunocytometry Systems (BDIS).

After each staining step the cells were washed with 2 ml phosphate-buffered saline (PBS) and centrifuged at 1200 × g for 2 min. Finally the antibody-labeled cells were fixed in 1% PFA (paraformaldehyde) in PBS. The samples were analyzed on a FACScan (BDIS).

Results

Subpopulations

The bone marrow aspirates of 54 patients with de novo AML were classified according to the number of leukemic subpopulations and the degree of maturation before therapy. Maturation was defined as a degree of differentiation analogous to normal myeloid cell development. Data of these subpopulations are shown in Table 2. We analyzed the changes in the phenotypes and the incidence of these subpopulations through TAD9 chemotherapy. Detailed analysis before and after administration of TAD9 revealed five different patterns:
1. Loss of all populations
2. No change
3. Appearance of new populations
4. Loss of populations but persistence of at least one population
5. Combinations of categories 3 and 4

The results of the respective patterns are listed in Table 3.

Immunophenotypic Changes After Administration of TAD9

As described in Table 2, 43 of 54 patients (80%) patients had more than one subpopulation. In 34 patients (63%) we found less and more mature subpopulations. Only 20

205

Table 3. Immunophenotypic changes after administration of TAD9

	Category				
	1	2	3	4	5
Patients ($n = 39$)	3	18	1	12	5

Table 4. Correlation of residual disease after administration of TAD9 and therapy outcome

% leukemic cells	Therapy outcome			
	NR	PR	CR	CCR
0 %–5 %	–	–	4	7
>5 % <25 %	2	1	5	2
>25 % <50 %	4	–	2	1
>50 %	6	–	1	–
Total	12	1	12	1

NR, no remission; PR, partial remission; CR, complete remission; CCR, continuous complete remission

patients (37 %) had only one type of sub-population. After administration of TAD9 (Table 3) only 3/39 patients (7 %) lost all of their leukemic cells. In 18/39 patients (46 %) there was no change, one new population appeared in 1/39 patients (3 %), and we found the loss of at least one population in 12/39 patients (31 %). In 5/39 (13 %) cases the changes can be described as a combination of categories 3 and 4.

Residual Blasts After Administration of TAD9 and Therapy Outcome

We correlated the percentage of residual blasts with therapy outcome. Data are shown in Table 4. All patients with less than 5 % residual leukemic cells by FCM reached a complete remission. This result was independent of the second induction course, which was randomized for TAD9 or high-dose cytosine arabinoside (ara-C) and mitoxantrone. Of the 17 patients with less than 50 % residual blasts, 10 achieved a complete remission after the second induction course, while 6 did not respond and 1 achieved a partial remission. One patient had more than 50 % residual leukemic cells on day 16. This patient suffered from systemic fungal infection after the first induc-

tion course and did not receive further chemotherapy for 4 weeks. After that period he had another bone marrow aspirate taken which showed a blast count of less than 5 % by light microscopy. The complete remission lasted 3 months.

Discussion

Only 10 %–20 % of all adult patients with newly diagnosed acute myeloid leukemia will have an event-free survival of more than 5 years. Attempts for improvements of these results include introduction of new treatment concepts, use of new drugs or better use of "old" drugs, and preselection of patient according to risk group. Prognostic factors include age, secondary leukemia, and cytogenetically defined subgroups. Widespread application of the latter marker is hampered by the time-consuming technique. One approach for the identification of high-risk groups is the quantification of residual leukemic cells after the first treatment course. In the vast majority of therapy protocols, the first part of the induction therapy includes ara-C and anthracyclines, which are the most efficient drugs in AML treatment. Quantification can be done by light microscopy or by use of

206

other methods, which are able to distinguish leukemic cells from normal myeloid progenitor cells. Multiparameter flow cytometry using combinations of monoclonal antibodies has proven to be such a method and we have started a prospective study to determine the value of detecting residual leukemic cells during and after intensive chemotherapy.

In this part of the study we have analyzed the significance of residual cells 7 days after TAD9 treatment. All patients with less than 5% leukemic cells at this time point achieved a complete remission, while in the group with more than 50% leukemic cells only one patient achieved CR. The detailed analysis of the leukemic cells showed a wide variability. Some subpopulations disappeared completely below the level of detectability by flow cytometry, while others revealed an antigenic shift. In one bone marrow aspirate, a previously unrecognized subpopulation was detected. It was probably masked by other dominating subpopulations at initial diagnosis.

The results suggest that multiparameter flow cytometry offers a method for objective calculation of residual leukemic cells after chemotherapy. It measures the in vivo sensitivity of AML blasts to cytostatic agents and might provide a reliable technique for early treatment stratification.

References

1. Loken MR, Shah VO, Dattillo KL, Civin CI (1987) Flow cytometric analysis of human bone marrow: I. Normal erythroid development. Blood 69: 255–263
2. Loken MR, Shah VO, Dattillo KL, Civin CI (1987) Flow cytometric analysis of human bone marrow: II. Normal B lymphocyte development. Blood 70: 1316–1324
3. LeBien TW, Wörmann B, Villablanca JG, Law CL, Steinberg LM, Shah VO, Loken MR (1990) Multiparameter flow cytometric analysis of human fetal bone marrow B cells. Leukemia 4: 354–358
4. Terstappen LWMM, Safford M, Loken MR (1990) Flow cytometric analysis of human bone marrow. III. Neutrophil maturation. Leukemia 4: 657–663
5. Delwel R, van Gurp R, Bot F, Touw I, Löwenberg B (1988) Phenotyping of acute myelocytic leukemia (AML) progenitors: an approach for tracing minimal numbers of AML cells among normal bone marrow. Leukemia 2: 814–820
6. Campana D, Coustan-Smith E, Janossy G (1990) The immunologic detection of minimal residual disease in acute leukemia. Blood 76: 163–171
7. Terstappen L et al. (1990) Myeloid cell differentiation in normal bone marrow and acute myeloid leukemia assessed by multidimensional flow cytometry. Anal Cell Pathol 2: 229

Flow Cytometric Characterization of Therapy-Resistant Leukemic Subpopulations in Relapse

S. Könemann[1], K. Zurlutter[1], M. Safford[2], K. Schreiber[1], Th. Büchner[1], W. Hiddemann[1], B. Wörmann[1], and L. W. M. M. Terstappen[2]

Introduction

Diagnosis and monitoring of acute myeloid leukemia (AML) is conventionally performed using light microscopy on Pappenheim- and cytochemically stained cells. The sensitivity of this technique is 5 % for the detection of leukemic cells. Recently, more sensitive methods have been developed for the detection of minimal residual disease, including the identification of leukemic cells by flow cytometry using the aberrant expression of cell surface antigens. The main advantage of this technique is its representative cell analysis (30 000 examined cells or more) and the high percentage of informative patients [1]. In the present study, we have characterized leukemic cells by using multiparameter flow cytometry at diagnosis, during chemotherapy, and in relapse. For studies on residual leukemic cells two aspects are important:

1. Are the residual leukemic blasts responsible for relapse?
2. Is there a selection of malignant cells caused by chemotherapy?

Material and Methods

This prospective study contains 83 patients. A unique patient number (MS...) was assigned to each patient. All patients were

treated at the Department of Internal Medicine A at the University of Münster according to the protocol of the German AML Cooperative group [2], with the exception of three patients who were given palliative chemotherapy only. Bone marrow aspirates were obtained before therapy (A) and at different time points of therapy evaluation, i.e., after induction therapy (B), in complete remission (C), before consolidation (D), and before or after maintenance therapy (E, F). Eight patients were also immunophenotyped in relapse. Their characteristics are given in Table 1.

For flow cytometric analysis the nonnucleated erythroid cells were lysed in hypotonic NH_4Cl solution, centrifuged, and washed three times in RPMI 1640. For immunological staining, 1×10^6 cells were resuspended in 1 ml phosphate-buffered saline (PBS) containing 1 % bovine serum albumin and incubated with 20 1 fluorescence-labeled monoclonal antibodies for 20 min. Antibodies against the following antigens were used: CD3 (Leu4), CD4 (Leu3), CD7 (Leu9), CD8 (Leu2), CD11b (Leu15), CD11c (Leu M5), CD13 (Leu M7), CD14 (Leu M3), CD15 (L16 and Leu M1), CD16 (Leu16), CD33 (Leu M9), CD34 (HPCA-1), CD38 (Leu17), CD45 (Hle-1), and HLA DR [3], LDS was added to identify nucleated cells. All monoclonal antibodies were labeled directly or indirectly with three different fluorochromes fluoresceinisothiocyanite (FITC), phycoerythrin (PE), and DUOchrome or PerCP). After staining, cells were fixed in paraformaldehyde (PFA 1 %) and analyzed on a

[1] Department of Internal Medicine A, University of Münster, 4400 Münster, FRG
[2] Becton Dickinson Immunocytometry Systems, San José, CA 95131, USA

flow cytometer (FACScan, Becton Dickinson Immunocytometry Systems, BDIS using Paint A Gate Software (BDIS).

Results

Multiparameter Flow Cytometric Analysis of Leukemic Blasts Before Chemotherapy

At diagnosis leukemic blasts were characterized according to the following four groups of aberrations [1].

Coexpression of Myeloid-Lineage and Lymphoid-Lineage-Associated Antigens

Figure 1 shows the antigenic profile of patient MS6. Two leukemic subpopulations were detected, the dominating leukemic population coexpressing the T-lymphoid marker CD7 and the myeloid lineage-associated antigen CD13 (black dots). The normal T lymphocytes, which are only CD7 positive, are printed gray. The mature neutrophils express CD7 unphysiologically.

Two leukemic populations were further distinguished by their expression of CD14 (not shown).

Asynchronous Expression of Immature and Mature Antigens

Figure 2 shows the initial antigenic profile of patient MS74. Two leukemic populations were detected. The dominating leukemic population is CD34+ (dim to intermediate), CD38+, and CD15 (L16)-. This population is printed in black and gray dots. The second smaller population (black dots) expresses CD34, CD38, and CD15 (L16). The latter population is an example of the unphysiological coexpression of the stem cell-associated antigen CD34 and an antigen (CD15) that is normally expressed on mature neutrophils.

Overexpression of Antigens

The majority of leukemic blasts of patient MS33 are characterized by their unphysiologically high expression of CD34 (black

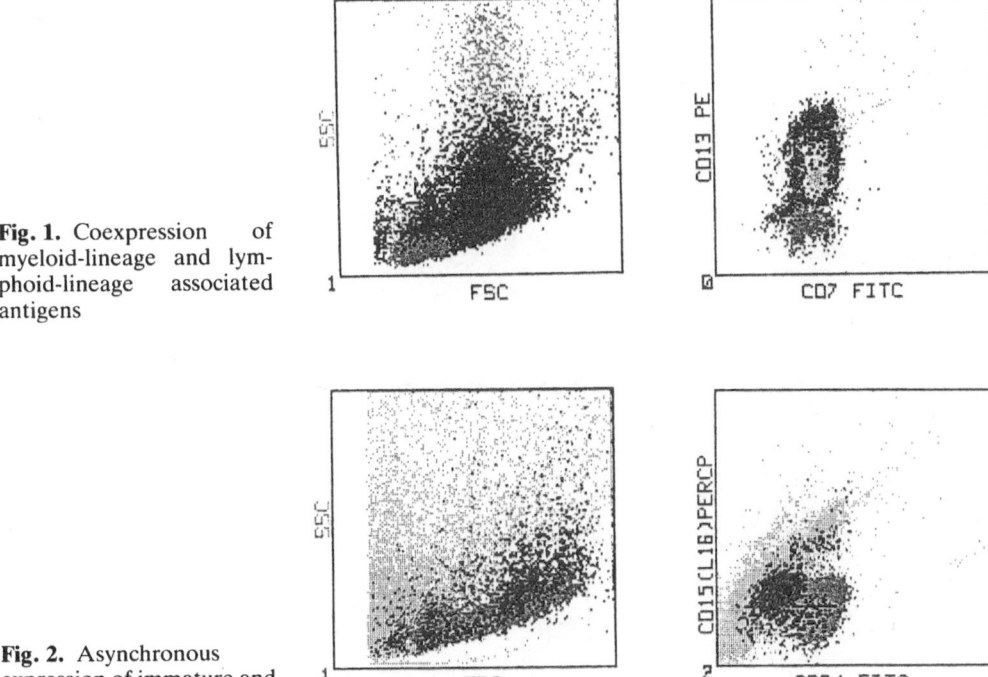

Fig. 1. Coexpression of myeloid-lineage and lymphoid-lineage associated antigens

Fig. 2. Asynchronous expression of immature and mature antigens

209

dots, Fig. 3). These cells lack CD33 and CD15 (Leu M1), compatible with immature cells in the normal maturation pathway. The second leukemic population is weakly positive for CD34 and coexpresses CD33. This population shows a partial maturation, visible by the acquisition of CD15 (Leu M1).

Unphysiological Absence of Antigens

The only leukemic population of patient MS17 (FAB M3) is colored black in Fig. 4. Based on the light scatter profile, these cells can be identified as promyelocytes. In normal bone marrow, cells of this stage of maturation are positive for CD33, CD11b, CD11c, and CD15. The leukemic blasts of this patient, however, lack CD11c. The few mature neutrophils also lack CD11c. In addition, the leukemic cells are HLA DR-. Data on the detection of subpopulations in the eight patients, who were also analyzed in relapse, are listed in Table 1.

Comparison of Immunophenotypic Features of Leukemic Blasts Before Chemotherapy and in Relapse

The antigenic profile of the leukemic blasts in relapse was compared with their initial phenotype at diagnosis. Three different types were distinguished:

Reidentification of Initially Present Leukemic Subpopulations

No Change in the Immunophenotype. All initially present leukemic subpopulations of four patients (MS8, MS60, MS74, MS76) were reidentified at relapse. The immunophenotypic profile of the leukemic cells was nearly unchanged. Figure 5 shows two leukemic populations (patient MS76), characterized by CD7, CD14, and HLA-DR, which can clearly be detected at diagnosis and at relapse. One initially present subpopulation is HLA-DR+, CD7+, and CD14− (marked X). The same subpopulation can be identified at relapse. The second leukemic subpopulation coexpressing

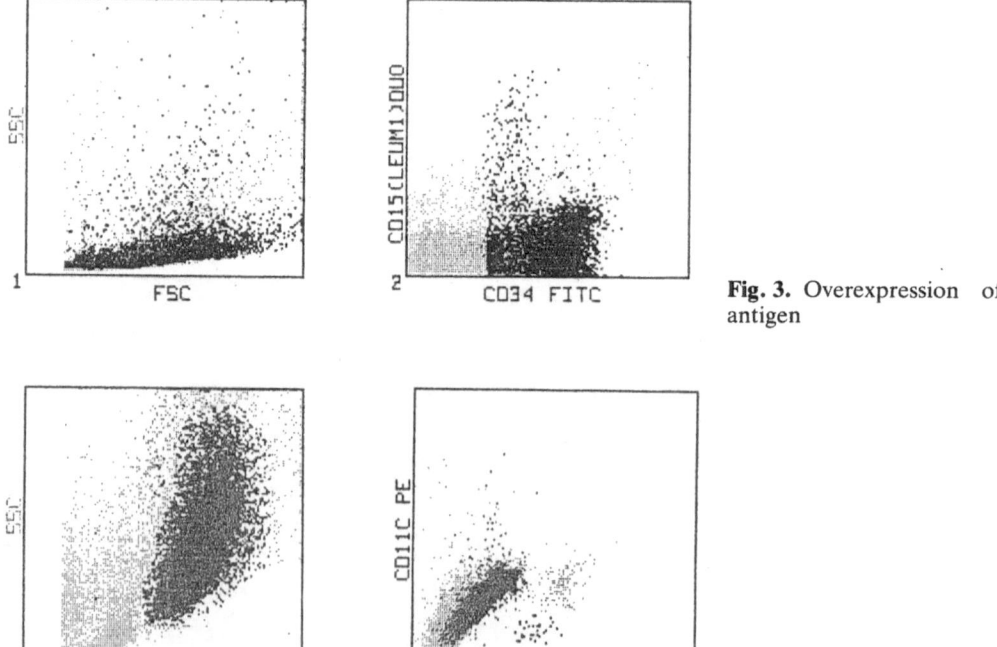

Fig. 3. Overexpression of antigen

Fig. 4. Unphysiological absence of antigens

Table 1. Patient characteristics and number of leukemic subpopulations at diagnosis

UPN	3	8	14	51	60	74	76	88
Sex	m	f	m	m	f	m	f	m
Age	68	27	36	57	66	66	37	24
CR duration (in months)	8	6	14	10	3	5	4	1
Subpopulations	3	1	3	2	2	2	2	3

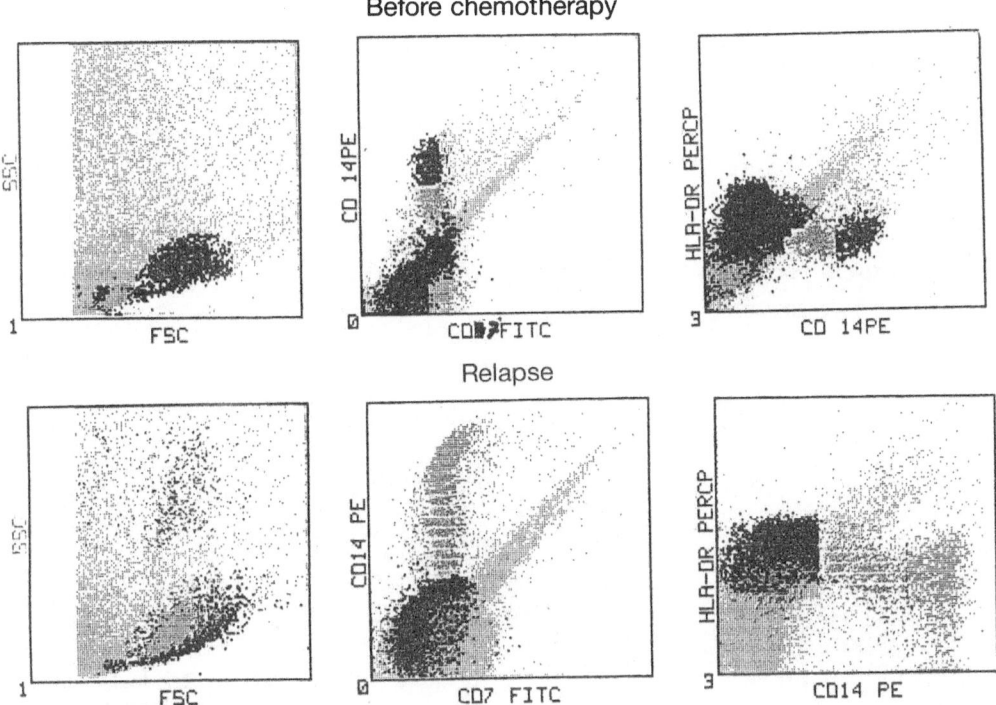

Fig. 5. Reidentification of leukemic subpopulations

CD14 (marked O) is also present in relapse.

Elimination of Subpopulations. In three cases (MS14, MS51, MS88) the number of initially present populations was reduced to only one population in relapse. In these cases the only relapse population was similar to one of the initially present leukemic subpopulations. In two of these patients the antigen density changed between initial diagnosis and relapse.

Identification of "New" Populations at Time of Relapse

The majority of leukemic blasts of patient MS3 were CD33 positive and partially CD34 positive at relapse. Compared with the immunophenotype of the three initially present populations, it became obvious that this population was not detectable at diagnosis.

211

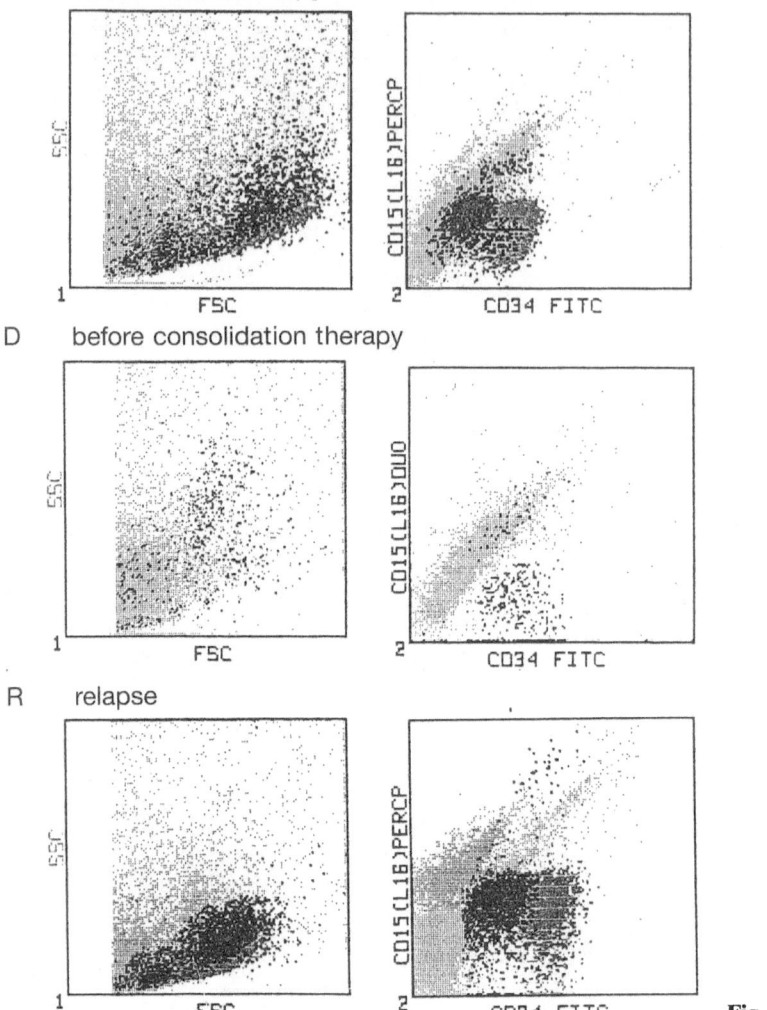

A   before chemotherapy

D   before consolidation therapy

R   relapse

Fig. 6. Residual leukemic blasts causing relapse

Identification of Residual Leukemic Cells During Chemotherapy

In seven of eight patients (exception: patient MS3) residual leukemic cells were identified during chemotherapy which had a similar antigenic profile to the leukemic blasts at relapse. An example is given in Fig. 6. Initially two leukemic subpopulations were detected (patient MS74). One population was double positive for CD34 and CD38 but negative for CD15 (L16). This population was detectable before consolidation therapy and in relapse. The second leukemic population coexpressed CD34 and CD15 (L16) and additionally expressed CD38 strongly. This population was also present before consolidation therapy and in relapse.

Discussion

Eighty-three consecutive adult patients with newly diagnosed AML were included in this prospective study on (minimal) residual disease. Goals were the identification of leukemic cells prior to chemotherapy, the detection and characterization of residual leukemic cells during chemotherapy, and finally the reidentification of leukemic cells in relapse. The majority of patients were treated according to the AML protocol of the German Cooperative group, with double induction therapy, maintenance, and consolidation therapy. Three patients were treated with low-dose ara-C and idarubicin only. Twelve patients have relapsed so far, and eight were immunophenotyped in relapse, and at several time points in bone marrow aplasia and in complete remission. Using multiparameter flow cytometry, the majority of patients had two or three leukemic subpopulations at diagnosis. In four of the eight patients all initially present populations were detectable during chemotherapy and in relapse. In three cases chemotherapy caused the elimination of one or more initially present subpopulations. The relapse population was also seen in complete remission. A shift of antigen density of residual leukemic cells was observed. In one patient a previously undetected subpopulation of leukemic cells appeared in relapse. These data suggest that it is possible to determine a combination of informative antibodies at diagnosis and use if for the monitoring of residual cells. Some subpopulations seem to be more malignant, i.e., resistant to chemotherapy and with higher proliferative capacity than others, thus explaining their sole reappearance in relapse. The observation of a previously undetected subpopulation in relapse could be due to antigenic shifts after chemotherapy, to genetic instability, or to selective elimination of other dominating subpopulations through induction and consolidation therapy. At present, we have no convincing experimental evidence for any of these hypotheses. The chemotherapy-resistant, relapse-causing cells were also detectable in complete remission, supporting the use of multiparameter flow cytometry for monitoring of residual disease. This could be the basis for a more individualized chemotherapy in the extremely heterogeneous AML which could be better able to meet the problem of chemotherapy-resistance.

Summary

In a prospective study on patients with newly diagnosed acute myeloid leukemia (AML), several leukemic subpopulations were identified and characterized prior to chemotherapy using multiparameter flow cytometry. In seven of eight patients the relapse population was identical to at least one of the initially present leukemic subpopulations. In some relapse populations a shift in the antigen density of residual leukemic blasts was observed. In one of eight patients the relapse population was different from the initially present leukemic subpopulations but was identified with the selected combination of antibodies.

References

1. Büchner T, Urbanitz D, Hiddemann W et al. (1985) Intensified induction and consolidation with or without maintenance chemotherapy for acute myeloid leukemia (AML). Two multicenter studies of the German AML Cooperative Group. J Clin Oncol 3: 1583–1589
2. Terstappen LWMM, Safford M, Könemann S, Loken MR, Zurlutter K, Büchner T, Hiddemann W, Wörmann B (1991) Flow cytometric characterization of acute myeloid leukemia. II. Extreme heterogeneity at diagnosis. Leukemia (in press)
3. Knapp W, Dörken B, Gilks WR, Rieber EP, Schmidt RE, Stein H, von dem Borne AEGK (eds) (1989) Leucocyte typing IV. White cell differentiation antigens. Oxford University Press, New York

Chronic Myelogenous Leukemia in Blastic Phase: A Model of Heterogeneity and Resistance in Acute Leukemia

H. M. Kantarjian[1], M. Talpaz[2], M. Wetzler[2], S. O'Brien[1], E. Estey[1], W. Plunkett[1], W. Zhang[1], M. J. Keating[1], and A. Deisseroth[1]

The heterogeneity and resistance of chronic myelogenous leukemia in blastic phase (CML-BP) are attributed to: (1) the involvement of the earliest progenitor cell by the disease process and (2) the acquisition of multiple mutational events during the evolution from the chronic to the blastic phase.

The heterogeneity of CML-BP is expressed at the morphologic, cytogenetic, and molecular levels, and in the mechanisms of blastic transformation. CML-BP is the most frustrating and resistant form of acute leukemia, and has the worst prognosis. The unique characteristics of the disease and the recent therapeutic trends will be reviewed.

Morphologic Heterogeneity of CML-BP

The capacity of CML to evolve from a very primitive stem cells is exhibited by the wide spectrum of morphologies seen during blastic transformation. In a review of 247 patients studied in CML-BP, 129 (52%) showed a myeloid, 62 (25%) an undifferentiated, and 56 (23%) a lymphoid blastic morphology. When a subset of patients with "undifferentiated" blasts were further analyzed by immunophenotyping and electron microscopic studies, most (80%) expressed myeloid markers on their blasts. This suggested that the undifferentiated blastic phase was more similar to the myeloid rather than the lymphoid blastic phase. This was supported by the patterns of survival and response to acute lymphoid leukemia (ALL) treatment. The median survivals of patients with myeloid and undifferentiated CML-BP were 3 and 4 months respectively, compared with 9 months for those with lymphoid CML-BP (Fig. 1; $p < 0.01$). Response to frontline CML-BP therapy was also significantly better in those with lymphoid morphology (Table 1). A subset of 51 patients were treated with the vincristine, doxorubicin, and dexamethasone (VAD) regimen, also used in ALL. Of 38 patients with lymphoid blastic phase, 17 (45%) achieved a complete remission (CR) and 3 (8%) a partial response (PR) for an overall response rate of 53%. This compared with only one PR (8%) among 13 patients with undifferentiated blastic phase treated with VAD. Thus, the morphologic heterogeneity in CML-BP is associated with significant therapeutic and prognostic differences.

In other studies where more detailed analyses were performed (electron microscopy and platelet peroxidase staining, heterologous antibodies against factor VIII, monoclonal antibodies against glycoprotein IIb/IIIa, glycophorin antibody), less than 10% of patients were found to have megakaryocytic or erythroid blastic transformation.

[1] Departments of Hematology and [2]Clinical Immunology and Biological Therapy, MD Anderson Cancer Center, 1515 Holcombe Blrd., Houston, Texas 77030, USA
Dr. Kantarjian is a Scholar of the Leukemia Society of America.

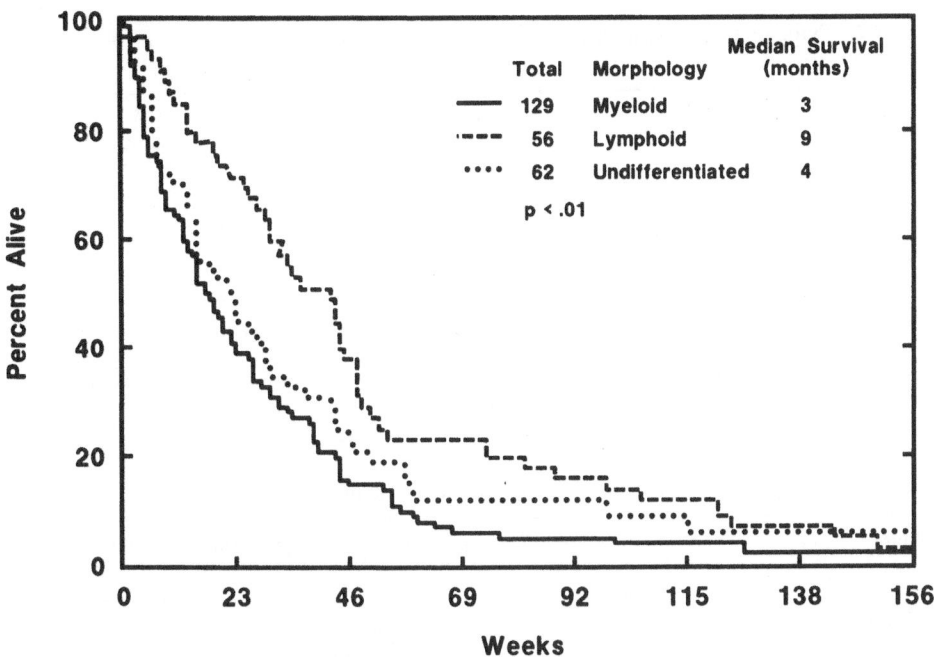

Fig. 1. Survival of patients with chronic myelogenous leukemia in blastic phase according to the blast morphology

Table 1. Response to first therapy in chronic myelogenous leukemia in blastic phase by blast morphology and therapy

Characteristic	No. treated	No. CR	(%)	
A. *Morphology*				
Myeloid	116	18	(16)	
Undifferentiated	52	5	(10)	$p < 0.01$
Lymphoid	52	29	(56)	
B. *VAD therapy*				
Lymphoid	38	17	(45)	$p < 0.01$
Undifferentiated	13	0	(0)	

CR, complete response; VAD, vincristine, doxorubicin, and dexamethasone

Cytogenetic Heterogeneity of CML-BP

Cytogenetic abnormalities in malignancy serve as useful "fingerprints" to investigate the abnormal molecular events in a particular tumor. Such strategies have been fruitful in chronic phase CML [Philadelphia chromosome (Ph) and *bcr/abl* oncogene], Burkitt's lymphoma (translocations between chromosome 8 and 14, 2, or 22, and the *myc* oncogene), and other cancers. The evolution of CML into the blastic phase is associated with frequent nonrandom chromosomal changes. A double Ph, trisomy 8, and isochromosome 17 abnormality are found alone or in various combinations in 73% of patients with chromosomal abnormalities in addition to Ph [1] (Table 2). Despite these cytogenetic "fingerprints," the molecular abnormalities are not well clarified, as will be discussed below (Table 3). Patients who develop additional

Table 2. Cytogenetic abnormalities in chronic myelogenous leukemia in blastic phase (192 patients)

Karyotype	No. patients (%)
Philadelphia chromosome only	78 (41)
Additional abnormalities	114 (59)
– Double Philadelphia	49 (26)
– Trisomy 8	49 (26)
– Isochromosome 17	34 (18)
– Any combination of the above	83 (43)
– Other changes	31 (16)

[a] Eighty-three of 114 patients (73 %) with additional abnormalities had changes involving a double Philadelphia, trisomy 8, or isochromosome 17

Table 3. Pathophysiology of chronic myelogenous leukemia

Phase	Cytogenetic fingerprint	Possible molecular abnormality
Chronic	Philadelphia chromosome	*bcr/abl*
Accelerated	Double Philadelphia	*bcr/abl*
Blastic	Trisomy 8	*myc*
	Isochromosome 17	p53
		G-CSF
		IL1
Monocytic transformation		*ras* mutations
Chronic myelomonocytic leukemia, juvenile chronic myelogenous leukemia		GM-CSF, IL6

chromosomal abnormalities in CML-BP have lower CR rates and shorter survival compared with those who do not [1].

Molecular and Pathophysiologic Heterogeneity of CML-BP

The presence of a double Ph and trisomy 8 led to the investigation of whether the *bcr/abl* or *myc* oncogene expressions were altered in CML-BP. Elevated *bcr/abl* levels were observed in a subset of patients with CML-BP [2, 3]. Increased *myc* expression was also found in CML-BP, but was similar when immature cells from blastic and chronic phase were compared.

The isochromosome 17 abnormality led to studies of mutations or rearrangements of p53, a suppressor gene localized to the short arm of chromosome 17. This could explain the loss of chronic phase control and

disease acceleration. In three studies, a low incidence (3 %) of p53 mutation or rearrangement was found in chronic phase; this increased slightly (up to 20 %–25 %) with disease transformation in some studies [4–6] (Table 4). Zhang et al. [7] have shown that the nuclear levels of p53 were elevated in blastic phase compared with chronic phase CML, this being due to prolongation of the p53 half-life from 20 min to more than 3 h.

Wetzler et al. [9] reported the constitutive expression of IL-1β to be elevated in patients with accelerated or blastic phase CML, as well as in those with clinical resistance to α-interferon while in chronic phase (Table 5). They hypothesized that autocrine and paracrine IL-1β production may be responsible for CML transformation and resistance.

Juvenile CML and chronic myelomonocytic leukemia may be pathophysiologically

Table 4. Rearrangement or point mutations in p53 in chronic myelogenous leukemia

Study (reference)	No. analyzed	No. with p53 abnormality (%)
A. *Chronic phase*		
Kelman et al. (4)	39	1 (3)
Bar-Eli et al. (5)	34	1 (3)
Mashal et al. (6)	39	1 (3)
B. *Accelerated-blastic phase*		
Kelman et al. (4)	14	4 (29)
Bar-Eli et al. (5)	34 (blastic)	6 (24)
	4 (accelerated)	1 (25)
Mashal et al. (6)	29	1 (3)

Table 5. Constitutive expression of Il-1β in interferon-resistant chronic phase and in transformed phases of chronic myelogenous leukemia

CML phase	No. positiv/total (%)	
	IL-1 mRNA	IL-1 protein
Chronic		
– Interferon sensitive	4/14 (29)	3/13 (23)
– Interferon resistant	12/18 (67)	12/16 (75)
Accelerated-blastic	7/14 (50)	10/13 (77)

Table 6. *Ras* mutations in chronic myelogenous and myelomonocytic leukemia

Disease (reference)	No. patients	No. with *ras* mutations (%)
Ph-positive CML (11)		
– Chronic	29	0 (0)
– Blastic	22	2 (9)
Ph-negative CML (12)	6	0 (0)
Chronic myelomonocytic leukemia	16	11 (69)
– Padua et al. (13)		
– Ginsberg et al. (12)	30	17 (57)

related to production of granulocyte-macrophase colony stimulation factor (GM-CSF) and interleukin-6 [9, 10]. Our group has also found that mutations in the *ras* oncogene are rare in Ph-positive CML, but are frequent in chronic myelomonocytic leukemia (Table 6) [11, 12]. This suggested a role for *ras* oncogene mutations in monocytic disease evolution. The presence of *ras* oncogene mutation may also be related to patient survival: in 30 patients with CMML analyzed, the median survival was 35 months among 13 patients with no *ras* mutations, and 11 months among 17 patients with *ras* mutations [12].

Therapeutic Heterogeneity and Resistance in CML-BP

Three therapeutic concepts have been investigated in CML-BP: (1) marrow ablative therapy followed by allogeneic or autologous stem cell transplantation, (2) intensive chemotherapy to induce marrow hypoplasia and regrowth of normal or chronic phase CML cells, and (3) differentiation therapy.

Marrow Ablative Therapy

Allogeneic bone marrow transplantation (BMT) is the only curative modality in CML-BP, although the results of therapy are significantly worse than those achieved in chronic phase. Long-term disease-free survival (DFS) is reported in 10%–15% of patients treated [14, 15]. The realistic DFS rate is less, considering that many patients in CML-BP with available donors cannot be transplanted due to poor performance status, infections, or organ dysfunction. Most failures following allogeneic BMT were due to inadequate eradication of the CML-BP clones, which have become resistant to proven myeloblastic regimens. The relapse rate following allogeneic BMT is 50%–90% in CML-BP compared with 5%–30% in chronic phase (Table 7).

The results of autologous BMT in CML-BP are disappointing (Table 7). Using autologous stem cells collected in chronic phase for marrow repopulation, a second chronic phase is achieved in 50%–60% of patients. The median duration of second chronic phase is short, however, ranging from 3 to 6 months [16, 17]. Improvement in prognosis may be achieved with: (1) better marrow ablative regimens, (2) the use of double autologous BMT, (3) post-BMT maintenance therapy (α-interferon, interleukin-2), or (4) infusion of "purged" stem cells (enrichment of normal stem cells by in vivo therapy or in vitro manipulation).

Intensive Chemotherapy

This approach has so far yielded disappointing results. At our institution, we have conducted a series of studies with high-dose cytosine arabinoside (ara-C) alone, in com-

Table 7. Bone marrow transplantation results in CML-BP

Study (reference)	No. patients	Survival percentage at 4 years	Leukemia relapse (%)
I. *Allogeneic*			
Thomas et al. [14]	42	14	80
Goldman et al. [15]	22	14	40
International BMT registry	54	16	45
II. *Autologous*		Percentage achieving second chronic phase	Median survival (months)
Haines et al. [16]	51	94	6
Reiffers et al. [17]	45	76	4.5
Compiled studies	38	29 to 60	4 to 7

Table 8. High-dose cytosine arabinoside (HD ara-C) containing regimens in CML-BP

Study (reference)	Regimen	No. patients	Percentage CR	Median survival (weeks)
Iacoboni et al. [18]	HD ara-C	22	23	16
Kantarjian et al. [19]	Mitoxantrone + HD ara-C	27	27	14
MDACC (unpublished)	Daunorubicin + HD ara-C + GM-CSF	20	25	15

bination with mitoxantrone, and in combination with daunorubicin and GM-CSF. The CR rates were modest and were not improved by the addition of anthracyclines [18, 19]. GM-CSF as supportive therapy following intensive chemotherapy did not shorten the duration of myelosuppression, or reduce the overall incidence of febrile episodes (Table 8). Other intensive chemotherapy programs which have been previously reviewed have also produced poor results [1].

Differentiation Therapy

Differentiation therapy is an interesting concept hich proposes to induce the maturation of CML-BP blasts and reinstitution of a chronic phase. Differentiating agents investigated have included: (1) low-dose ara-C, (2) mithramycin and hydroxyurea, (3) homoharringtonine, and (4) tiazofurin. Retinoids are other potentially useful agents. Therapy with low-dose ara-C was associated with a low response rate, which was probably attributable to the myelosuppression rather than differentiation properties of ara-C [20].

Mithramycin, and inhibitor of RNA synthesis, induces in vitro differentiation of blasts and reduction in *abl* and *myc* expression in CML blast cells. Koller and Miller treated patients with CML blastic phase

with low doses of mithramycin (1 mg/m² intravenously two to three times weekly) and hydroxyurea and observed responses in six of nine patients treated, all responders exhibiting a myeloid blast cell morphology [21]. A subsequent update of a larger series, using remission criteria of acute leukemia, resulted in 2 partial remissions among 6 patients with myeloid blastic phase (33 %) but no responses in 15 patients with undifferentiated blastic phase [22]. Similar low response rates were observed in two other studies, with only 1 complete response obtained among 16 patients (6 %) with CML blastic phase [23, 24].

Homoharringtonine is a plant alkaloid which was reported to have antileukemic activity in acute myelogenous leukemia, but was associated with significant cardiovascular toxicity. A lower dose schedule of 2.5 mg/m² daily for 14–21 days lessened the cardiovascular toxicity. In vitro studies showed homoharringtonine to be able to differentiate the HL-60 leukemic cell line. This led to our present study using homoharringtonine at a low-dose prolonged-exposure schedule in CML-BP. While the results are preliminary, only one of the first eight patients (12.5 %) treated achieved an objective remission.

Tiazofurin, a nucleoside analog, is metabolized to thiazole-4-carboxamide adenine dinucleotide (TAD), which inhibits the activity of the inosine monophosphate

Table 9. Therapy of CML-BP with differentiating agents

Study (reference)	Therapy	No. patients	No. responses	(%)
DiRaimondo et al. [20]	Low-dose ara-C	7	1	(14)
Koller and Miller [21]	Mithramycin + hydroxyurea	Myeloid, 6	6	(100)
		Other, 3	1	(33)
Koller et al. [22]	Mithramycin + hydroxyurea	Myeloid, 6	2	(33)
		Undifferentiated, 15	0	(0)
Trumper et al. [23]	Mithramycin + hydroxyurea	9	1	(11)
Antimi et al. [24]	Mithramycin + hydroxyurea	7	0	(0)
Tricot et al. [25]	Tiazofurin	9	4 CR + 3 hematologic improvement	(78)
MDACC (unpublished)	Tiazofurin	5	0	(0)

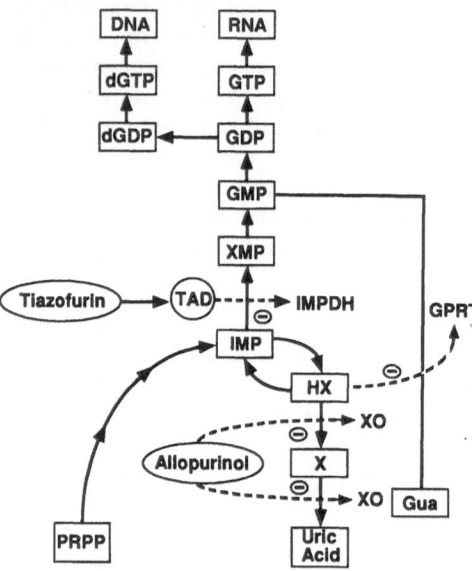

Fig. 2. Mechanisms of actions of tiazofurin and allopurinol (Adapted from Tricot et al. [25])

dehydrogenase enzyme (IMPD), thus reducing the formation of guanine triphosphase (GTP) pools, interfering with DNA and RNA synthesis, and leading to cell death (25) (Fig. 2). TAD is accumulated 20-fold more in leukemic compared with normal cells. IMPD enzymatic activity is also higher in leukemic cells. Based on this rationale, a biochemically directed clinical trial was conducted by Tricot et al. [25] which delivered tiazofurin at 2200 mg/m² daily for 15 days, the dose being adjusted by increments of 1100 mg/m² daily to achieve a suppression of IMPD levels below 10%, and of GTP pools below 20%. The daily dose of allopurinol is also adjusted to keep hypoxanthine levels between 40 and 80 μM, to prevent GTP formation through the salvage pathway. In their recent update [25], four of nine patients treated achieved CR, and three others had a hematologic improvement. Most patients achieved the biochemical targets, which also correlated with patient response. A similar study initiated at our institution did not produce objective responses in the first five patients treated. This may be due to differences in population characteristics, since only one of our five patients achieved the biochemical targets at the highest dose level allowed in this study (4400 mg/m² daily). Clearly further investigation of this interesting compound is warranted to define its antitumor activity and optimal schedule.

Retinoids are an interesting group of differentiating agents which have demonstrated significant activity in premalignant and malignant conditions including at least one form of leukemia, acute promyelocytic leukemia. Studies investigating the differentiation potential of some retinoids (particularly all-*trans* retinoid acid) in various CML phases are presently underway.

References

1. Kantarjian HM, Keating MJ, Talpaz M, Walters RS, Smith TL, Cork A, McCredie KB, Freireich EJ (1987) Chronic myelogenous leukemia in blast crisis: an analysis of 242 patients. Am J Med 83: 445–454
2. Collins SJ (1986) Breakpoints on chromosomes 9 and 22 in Philadelphia chromosome-positive chronic myelogenous leukemia (CML). Amplification of rearranged *c-abl* oncogenes in CML blast crisis. J Clin Invest 78: 1392–1396
3. Andrews DF III, Collins SJ (1987) Heterogeneity in expression of the *bcr-abl* fusion transcript in CML blast crisis. Leukemia 1: 718–724
4. Kelman Z, Prokocimer M, Peller S, Kahn Y, Rechavi G, Manor Y, Cohen A, Rotter V (1989) Rearrangements in the p53 gene in Philadelphia chromosome positive chronic myelogenous leukemia. Blood 74: 2318–2324
5. Bar-Eli M, Ahuja H, Foti A, Sun X-Z, Cline MJ (1989) The P53 gene in blast crisis, other hematologic malignancies and solid tumors. Blood 74 [Suppl 1] 465
6. Mashal R, Shtalrid M, Talpaz M, Kantarjian H, Smith L, Beran M, Cork A, Trujillo J, Gutterman J, Deisseroth A (1990) Rearrangement and expression of *p53* in the chronic phase and blastic crisis of chronic myelogenous leukemia. Blood 75: 180–189
7. Zhang W, Del Giglio A, Kantarjian H, Talpaz M, Deisseroth A (1991) Nuclear p53 protein increases from normal levels inc hronic phase CML to high levels in peripheral blood cells of most blast crisis CML patients. Soc Clin Oncol (to be published)
8. Wetzler M, Kurzrock R, Estrov Z, Shtalrid M, Troutman K, Kantarjian H, Gutterman JU, Talpaz M (1990) Constitutive expression of interleukin-1 beta correlates with interfe-

ron-alpha resistance in chronic myelogenous leukemia. Blood 76 [Suppl 1]: 335a

9. Everson MP, Brown CB, Lilly MB (1980) Interleukin-6 and granulocyte-macrophage colony-stimulating factor are candidate growth factors for chronic myelomonocytic leukemia cells. Blood 74: 1472–1476

10. Gualtieri RJ, Emanuel PD, Zuckerman KS, Martin G, Clark SC,Shadduck RK, Dracker RA, Akabutu J, Nitschke R, Hetherington ML, Dickerman JD, Hakami N, Castleberry RP (1989) Granulocyte-macrophage colony-stimulating factor is an endogenous regulator of cell proliferation in juvenile chronic myelogenous leukemia. Blood 74: 2360–2367

11. LeMaistre A, Lee MS, Talpaz M, Kantarjian HM, Freireich EJ, Deisseroth AB, Trujillo JM, Stass SA (1980) *RAS* oncogene mutations are rare late stage events in chronic myelogenous leukemia. Blood 73: 889

12. Hirsch-Ginsberg C, LeMaistre AC, Kantarjian H, Talpaz M, Cork A, Freireich EJ, Trujillo JM, Lee M-S, Stass SA (1990) *RAS* mutations are rare events in Philadelphia chromosome-negative/*bcr* gene rearrangement-negative chronic myelogenous leukemia, but are prevalent in chronic myelomonocytic leukemia. Blood 76: 1214–1219

13. Padua RA, Carter G, Hughes D, Gow J, Farr C, Oscier D, McCormick F, Jacobs A (1988) *RAS* mutations in myelodysplasia detected by amplification, oligonucleotide hybridization, and transformation. Leukemia 2: 503–510

14. Thomas ED, Clift RA, Fefer A, Appelbaum FR et al. (1986) Marrow transplantation for the treatment of chronic myelogenous leukemia. Ann Intern Med 104: 155–163

15. Goldman JM, Apperley JF, Jones L, Marcus R et al. (1986) Bone marrow transplantation for patients with chronic myeloid leukemia. N Engl J Med 314: 202–207

16. Haines LD, Goldman JM, Worsley AM, McCarthy DM et al. (1984) Chemotherapy and autografting for chronic granulocytic leukaemia in transformation: probably pro-

longation of survival for some patients. Br J Haematol 58: 711–721

17. Reiffers J, Gorin N, Michallet M, Maraninchi D, Herve P (1986) Autografting for chronic granulocytic leukemia in transformation. J Natl Cancer Inst 76: 1307–1310

18. Iacoboni SJ, Plunkett WK, Kantarjian H, Estey E, Keating MJ, McCredie KB, Freireich EJ (1986) High dose cytosine arabinoside: treatment and cellular pharmacology of chronic myelogenous leukemia blast crisis. J Clin Oncol 4: 1079–1088

19. Kantarjian H, Walters R, Keating M, Talpaz M, Andersson B, Beran M, Mcredie K, Freireich E (1988) Treatment of the blastic phase of chronic myelogenous leukemia with mitoxantrone and high-dose cytosine arabinoside. Cancer 62: 672–676

20. DiRaimondo F, Milone G, Guglielmo P, Cacciola E, Giustoliso R (1985) Treatment of CML blast crisis with low dose ara-C. Br J Haematol 60: 773–774

21. Koller CA, Miller DM (1986) Preliminary observations on the therapy of the myeloid blast phase of chronic granulocytic leukemia with plicamycin and hydroxyurea. N Engl J Med 315 (23): 1433–1438

22. Koller C, Keating M, Walters R et al. (1988) Mithramycin and hydroxyurea in chronic myelogenous leukemia and other hematologic malignancies. Blood 72 [Suppl 1]: 209a

23. Trumper L, Lie JVD, Goudsmit R, Ho AD, Hunstein W (1988) Therapy of the myeloid blast phase of chronic granulocytic leukemia with plicamycin and hydroxyurea: a retrospective analysis. 22nd Congress of ISH, Milan, SYM-TU-6-6, 1988

24. Antimi M, Poeta GD, Cianciulli P, Scimo MT et al. (1988) Plicamycin and hydroxyurea in the treatment of blast phase and accelerated phase of the Ph' chronic myelogenous leukemia. 22nd Congress of ISH, Milan, OP-TU-6-6, 1988

25. Tricot G, Jayaram HN, Weber G, Hoffman R (1990) Tiazofurin: biological effects and clinical uses. Int J Cell Cloning 8: 161–170

Myelomonocyte Differentiation Antigens in the Diagnosis of Acute Nonlymphocytic Leukemia: the Relevance of CDw65 Antigen as a Screening Marker and the Prognostic Significance of CD15 Expression*

J. Holowiecki, D. Lutz, V. Callea, M. Brugiatelli, F. Kelenyi, B. Stella-Holowiecka, S. Krzemien, and K. Jagoda

Immunological phenotyping of acute lymphoblastic leukemia (ALL) correlates with clinical findings and has contributed to the understanding of the pathophysiology of lymphoid malignancies. On the contrary, the role of cell markers in acute nonlymphoblastic leukemia (ANLL) has only recently acquired relevance. The detection by monoclonal antibodies (MoAbs) of some myelomonocyte differentiation antigens such as CD11b, 13, 14, 15, 33, and CDw65 has proved useful for the recognition of poorly differentiated leukemias which otherwise would have remained unclassifiable or could have been misdiagnosed as ALL [1–5]. There is also evidence of the prognostic significance of immunophenotyping of ANLL. Our group proved CD15 expression to be a positive prognostic index for a higher CR rate and for surival [6, 7] and this has been recently confirmed by Campos and coworkers [2]. Although there are more than 20 well-defined cluster-designated (CD) myelomonocyte antigens, only a small number react with early myeloid cells and are potentially useful as first-line screening reagents of myelomono-

cyte line-derived leukemias. Most authors recommend a combination including CD13 and CD33 [1, 2, 4, 8, 9] and evidence for the usefulness of CDw65 [3, 5, 10, 11] is omitted. We report herewith the comparative analysis of the diagnostic significance of the most important myelomonocyte antigens. The main objectives of this study were: (1) selection of a single marker useful as a screening reagent in ANLL (also for automated analysis) and (2) selection of an optimal combination of two to three markers.

Materials and Methods

Two hundred and fourteen adults with de novo ANLL were classified according to FAB morphocytochemical criteria and immunophenotyped using a panel of monoclonal antibodies detecting CDw65 (Vim2, BMA-0210), CD13 (My7), CD33 (My9), CD14 (Vim 13), CD11b (Vim12), CD15 (VimD5), IaDr, CD41, glycophorin A, CD34 (in some cases), and lymphocyte antigens CD1, 2, 3, 7, 10, 19/24. The MoAbs of the Vi series were kindly donated by W. Knapp. Reactivity of cells was tested in indirect immunofluorescence using FITC-labeled goat F(ab)2 antibodies against mouse IgG + IgM (Grubb) as a secondary reagent [6]. A positive result was determined when at least 20 % of leukemia cells revealed a given antigen.

* This paper was written on behalf of the International Society for Chemoimmunotherapy Cooperative Group, Vienna, Katowice, Reggio, Calabria, Pecs

Results

A comparison of the proportion of patients exhibiting positivity for the main myelo-monocyte antigens in the whole group and in particular FAB subgroups is shown in Fig. 1. The most prevalent markers in the whole group were CDw65, CD33, and CD13, which were found in 92.1%, 76.6%, and 69.6% of patients, respectively. It was of interest to note that the expression of these markers was strong even in the M1-FAB subgroup. On the contrary, CD15 was exhibited mainly in more mature FAB subtypes whereas CD14 and to a lesser extent CD11b were restricted to M4-M5. The next analyses therefore concerned initially all the CDw65, CD33, and CD13 antigens, which appeared to be the best candidates for a screening marker.

The results obtained using CDw65, -33, and -13 as a single marker and in various combinations are compared in Fig. 2, which demonstrates that CDw65 enables a significantly higher proportion of ANLL to be detected than the remaining antigens used a single markers ($p < 0.001$) and gives equivalent results to those obtained with combi-nations of two markers ($p > 0.01$). The combination of CDw65 with either CD13 or CD33 is significantly more effective (both 95.8% of positive cases) than the commonly recommended pairs of CD13 + CD33 (86.9%, $p < 0.01$). The triple combination including CDw65 + CD13 + CD33 identifying 97.7% of ANLL cases was significantly more effective than each of the single markers ($p < 0.001$) and the CD13 + CD33 combination ($p < 0.01$) but not CDw65 + CD13 or CDw65 + CD33. The reactivity of leukemic cells with these three antigens in particular FAB subgroups is presented in Fig. 3, clearly demonstrating the prevalence of CDw65. A separate analysis of cases which were nonreactive with pairs of MoAbs detecting CD13 + CDw65, CD13 + CD33, and CD33 + CDw65 shows the potential diagnostic usefulness of other myelomonocyte antigens in these patients, again confirming the lowest efficacy of the CD13 + CD33 combination, demonstrating that in patients negative for these markers relatively frequently the expression of the following antigens is noted: CD14, CD11b, CD15, or CDw65 (Fig. 4). In addition this analysis suggests that the CDw65 + CD13

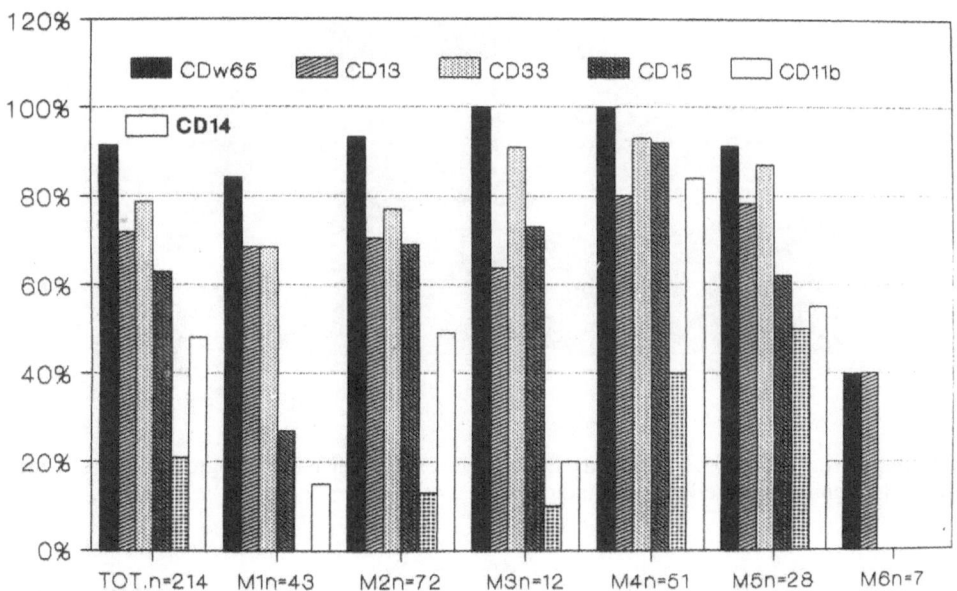

Fig. 1. Comparison of myelomonocyte antigen expression in ANLL. Percentage of positive cases in FAB subgroups

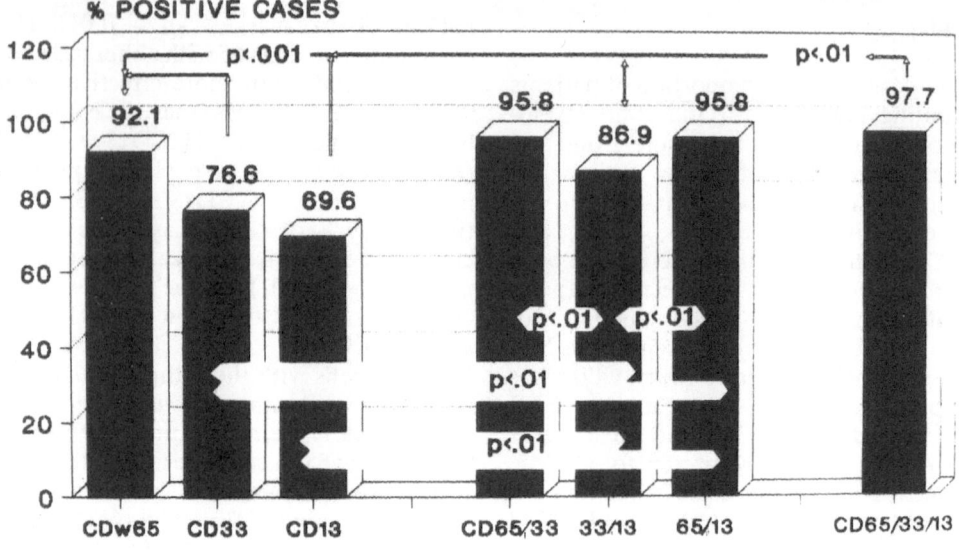

Fig. 2. Comparison of CDw65 (Vim2), CD13 (My7), and CD33 (My9) expression in 214 ANLL patients (percentage of positive cases). *First column*, single markers; *second column*, one of two markers present; *third column*, one of three markers present. Significant differences are indicated

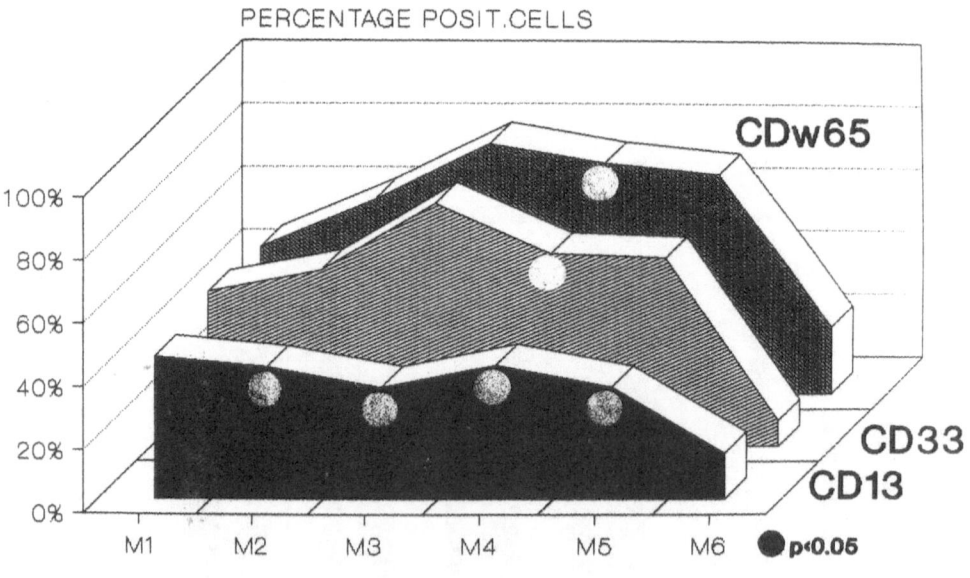

Fig. 3. Comparison of CDw65, CD13, and CD33 antigen expression in FAB subgroups (percentage of positive cells, significant differences are indicated)

combination is more effective if compared to the CDw65 + CD33 pairs. The superiority of this combination is also supported by the analysis of the results obtained in particular FAB subgroups (Table 1). In a separate study (to be published) we proved that CDw65 is suitable for tests on fixed cells using the APAAP method and the

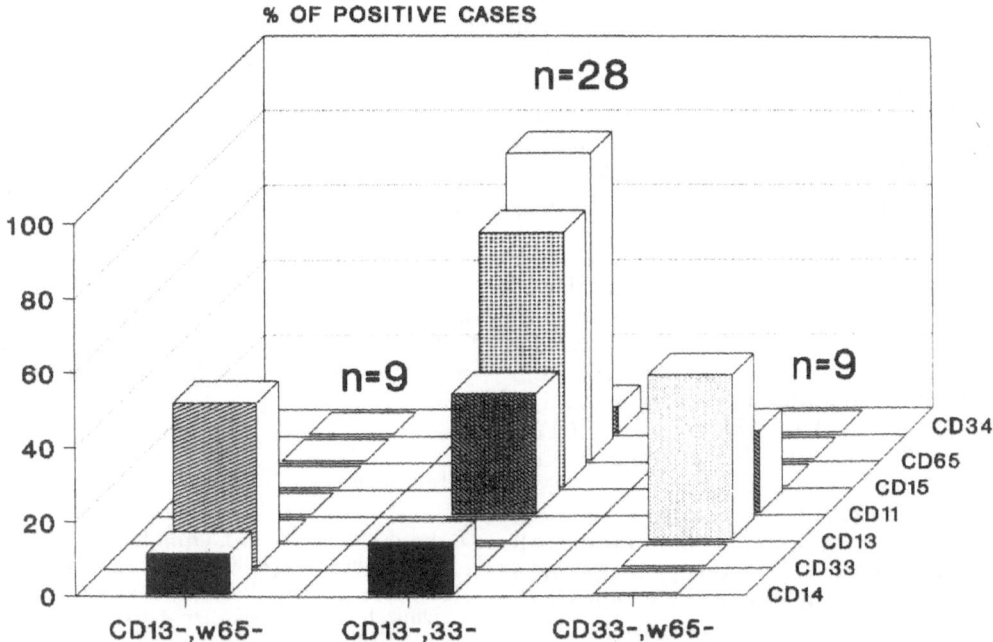

Fig. 4. Expression of different myelomonocyte markers in subgroups of ANLL patients nonreactive with pairs of basic markers: CD13 + CDw65, CD13 + CD33, and CD33 + CDw65

Table 1. Proportion of undetected cases with different pairs of MoAbs in FAB subgroups; n (%)

CD13 / CD33	CD13 / CDw65	CD33 / CDw65
M1: 6 (15.7%)	1 (2.6%)	3 (7.8%)
M2: 11 (17.7%)	4 (6.4%)	2 (3.2%)
M3: 0	0	0
M4: 2 (4.7%)	0	0
M5: 2 (8.6%)	0	1 (4.3%)
M6: 3 (60%)	2 (40%)	3 (60%)

results correlate well with the fluorescence analysis (correlation index = 0.65, $p < 0.01$).

Discussion

This study, which has been concerned with finding screening markers for ANLL, suggests that the CDw65 antigen is of great value both as a single marker and in combination with other cell differentiation antigens. It was significantly more frequently expressed in ANLL when compared to the commonly recommended antigens CD13 and CD33. CDw65 was present in 92% of the cases studied, its combination with CD13 or CD33 raising the positivity up to 96% ($p > 0.01$) and the use of all three markers further improved the result to 98% ($p < 0.01$). From a practical point of view it is important that CDw65 is strongly expressed on blastic cells of different FAB subtypes (Figs. 1, 2) and gives equivalent results to those obtained with a combination of two antigens including the commonly recommended CD13 + CD33 pair. Most of the studies comparing myelomonocyte antigen expression in ANLL concern only selected markers [3, 4, 8, 9, 10] and only few reports [3, 11] deal with a wide panel of antigens. The results presented in these papers are in the main in agreement with ours. Knapp and coworkers [10], comparing CDw65 (Vim2) and CD13 (MCS2), found their expression in 91 % and 80 % of ANLL cases respectively. Van der Schoot et al. [11] also reported high CDw65 expression (81 %), whereas reactivity with CD13 (54 %) and CD33 (34 %) was relatively low. Drexler [3] has calculated from data in the literature the following positivity rates: CDw65, 76 %; CD13 (MCS2/My7), 86 %/82 %; and CD33 (My9), 80 %. The discrepancies are mainly concerned with CD13, which is expresed first in the cytoplasm and later on the cell membrane [8]. The reactivity is therefore much higher with immunoenzymatic staining and is relatively strong in subtypes without maturation ([3] and Fig. 2). The results appear also to be dependent upon the MoAb used; MCS2 giving rather higher positivity than My7 [3, 8]. Our results and the data of others [3, 11] confirm the usefulness of CDw65 for the identification of ANLL without maturation. There is also evidence indicating its efficacy in clarifying the nature of undifferentiated leukemia [5]. It is to be tressed, however, that none of the applied markers is able to detect every case of ANLL because of the great heterogeneity of leukemia. In consequence the myelomonocytic markers may be exhibited in some ALL cases: CD13 in 5 %–11 %, CD33 in 5 %–10.8 %, and CD65 in 5 % [1, 3, 10]. CD34 is a nonlineage immaturity marker of practical use but present both in 51 % of ANLL and in up to 30 % of ALL cases [2, 11]. Thus, at present in some cases only a complex analysis including multimarker studies, ultrastructural cytochemistry [9]. MoAbs against myeloperoxidase [11], and molecular analysis may help clarify the cellular origin of leukemia. In spite of these restrictions our observations and the cited data by others clearly indicate that CDw65 is a good marker of ANLL blasts, displaying a strong expression in different FAB subtypes and suitable for both immunoenzymatic and fluorescence studies. In conclusion, CDw65 seems to be at present the best single screening marker of ANLL blasts useful for traditional and automated analysis of leukemic cells.

Concerning the prognostic significance of myelomonocyte marker expression, our studies did not confirm the prognostic significance of CDw65. In contrast a long follow-up of 424 de novo patients with ANLL confirms our earlier reports [6, 7] indicating that the expression of CD15 antigen is an independent positive prognostic factor for achieving CR (logistic regression; $p = 0.03$) and for survival (Cox models, $p = 0.001$).

References

1. Bradstock KF, Kirk J, Grimsley PG, Kabral A, Hughes WG (1989) Unusual immunophenotypes in acute leukemias: incidence and clinical correlations. Br J Haematol 72: 512–518
2. Campos L, Guyotat D, Archimbaud E, Devaux Y, Treille D, Larese A, Maupas J, Gentilhomme O, Ehrsam A, Fiere D (1989) Surface marker expression in adult acute myeloid leukaemia: correlations with initial characteristics, morphology and response to therapy. Br J Haematol 72: 161–166
3. Drexler HG (1987) Classification of acute myeloid leukemias – a comparison of FAB and immunophenotyping. Leukemia 1 (10): 697–705
4. Lo Coco F, Pasqualetti D, Lopez M, Panzini E, Gentile A, Latagliata R, Monarca B, De Rossi G (1989) Immunophenotyping of acute myeloid leukaemia: relevance of analysing different lineage-associated markers. Blut 58: 235–240
5. San Miguel JF, Gonzales M, Canizo MC, Anta JP, Zola H, Borrasca AL (1986) Surface marker analysis in acute myeloid leukaemia and correlation with FAB classification. Br J Haematol 64: 547–560
6. Holowiecki J, Lutz D, Krzemien S, Stella-Holowiecka B, Graf K, Kelenyi G, Schranz V, Callea V, Brugiatelli M, Neri A, Magyarlaki T, Ihle R, Jagoda K, Rudzka E (1986) CD-15 antigen detected by the VIM-D5 monoclonal antibody for prediction of ability to achieve complete remission in acute nonlymphocytic leukemia. Acta Haematol 76: 16–19
7. Holowiecki J, Lutz D, Callea V, Brugiatelli M, Krzemien S, Stela-Holowiecka B, Neri A, Ihle R, Schranz V, Graf E, Kelenyi G, Jagoda K, Zintl F, Reves T, Kardos G,

Barceanu S (1989) Expression of cell differentiation antigens as a prognostic factor in acute leukemia. In: Neth R, Gallo RC, Greaves MF, Gaedicke G, Ritter J (eds) Modern trends in human leukemia VIII. Springer, Berlin Heidelberg New York, pp 104–108

8. Pombo de Oliveira MS, Matutes E, Rani S, Morilla R, Catovsky D (1986) Early expression of MCS2 (CD13) in the cytoplasm of blast cells from acute myeloid leukaemia. Acta Haematol 80: 61–64

9. Matutes E, Pombo de Oliveira M, Foroni L, Morilla R, Catovsky D (1988) The role of ultrastructural cytochemistry and monoclonal antibodies in clarifying the nature of undifferentiated cells in acute leukaemia. Br J Haematol 69: 205–211

10. Knapp W, Majdic O, Stockinger H, Bettelheim P, Liszka K, Koller U, Peschel C (1984) Monoclonal antibodies to human myelomonocyte differentiation antigens in the diagnosis of acute myeloid leukemia. Med Oncol Tumor Pharmacother 1 (4): 257–326

11. Van der Schoot CE, von dem Borne AEGK, Tetteroo PAT (1987) Characterisation of myeloid leukemia by monoclonal antibodies, with an emphasis on antibodies against myeloperoxidase. Hemato-Oncology and Hemato-Immunology: Proceedings of the 2nd International Conference, Catania, 1986. Acta Haematol 78 [Suppl 1]: 32–40

Surveillance of Acute Leukemia by Multiparameter Flow Cytometry

J. Drach, H. Glassl, and C. Gattringer

Introduction

The standard definition of remission in acute leukemia is the presence of less than 5 % bone marrow blasts. However, even a much lower number of leukemic cells, referred to as "minimal residual disease" (MRD), may be associated with immediate relapse. Detection of MRD by means of immunocytological criteria is mainly hampered by the fact that no truly leukemic-specific antigen has been identified as yet. Thus, it is difficult to distinguish reliably between normal and leukemic blast cells, in particular when signs of bone marrow regeneration are present. In this study we attempted to overcome these obstacles by use of maker combinations and flow cytometric multiparameter analysis. We tried to explore to what extent acute leukemias could be monitored by this strategy and whether this approach is sensitive enough to predict relapse at an early stage.

Materials and Methods

Patients and Cells

So far, 60 patients with de novo acute leukemia have been investigated. Eleven patients had acute lymphoblastic leukemia (ALL) (2-T-ALL, 9 B-lineage ALL as identified by immunological criteria), and 49

Division of Hematology and Oncology, Department of Internal Medicine, University of Innsbruck, Anichstraße 35, 6020 Innsbruck, Austria

had acute myeloid leukemia (AML) which could be classified according to FAB criteria as follows: 20 AML M1, 18 AML M2, 1 AML M3, 3 AML M4, 6 AML M5, and 1 AML M6. In addition, three patients with T-ALL were studied during follow-up examinations. Peripheral blood and bone marrow samples were obtained at the time of diagnosis and routine follow-up studies. Mononuclear cells were separated by density centrifugation over Ficoll-Paque (Lymphoprep) and washed in phosphate-buffered saline (PBS).

Antibodies

The following monoclonal antibodies were employed in this study: Leu-1 (CD5), Leu-2 (CD8), Leu-3 (CD4), Leu-4 (CD3), Leu-5 (CD2), Leu-9 (CD7), Leu-12 (CD19), Leu-14 (CD22), Leu-M3 (CD14), Leu-M1 (CD15), la (HLA-DR), cALLA (CD10), all obtained from Becton Dickinson (Mountain View, CA); T6 (CD1), J5 (CD10), Mo-1 (CD11b), My-7 (CD13), My-9 (CD33), My-4 (CD14), purchased from Coulter Immunology (Hialeh, FL); and IOM-34 (CD34), IOP-41 (CD41), and anti-lycophorin-A obtained from Immunotech. A TdT Immunofluorescence kit (including a polyclonal rabbit anti-TdT serum) was purchased from Supertechs.

Immunofluorescence

Double-color immunofluorescence studies of surface antigens were performed using

228

PE- and FITC-labeled monoclonal antibodies: The antibodies were added at saturation concentration to 10^6 cells and incubated for 30 min at 4 °C. After two washes with PBS, cells were analyzed on a FACStar flow cytometer (Becton Dickinson). Nucelar TdT was detected according to a recently described method [1].

DNA Analysis

Simultaneous determination of surface markers and nuclear DNA content was carried out as described recently [2]: Briefly, cells were incubated with a FITC-labeled monoclonal antibody, then fixed with saponin (0.5 % in PBS; Sigma), and counterstained with propidium iodide (50 μg/ml PBS, Sigma) afterwards.

Results

Experimental Design

In this study, we tried to document aberrant and/or asynchronous antigenic features of leukemic cells which are not expressed on their nonmalignant counterparts. Thus, two-color immunofluorescence tests were carried out, and cells were analyzed by flow cytometry. In addition, we tested leukemic cells for DNA aneuploidy which – if present – is unequivocally associated with the leukemic stem line (see Fig. 1).

Detection of Leukemia-Associated Phenotypes at Diagnosis

Cells of 60 patients with de novo acute leukemia were immunophenotyped using a large panel of monoclonal antibodies (see "Materials and methods"). Aberrant/asynchronous antigen expression was detected in 24/60 patients (40 %); an example is given in Fig. 2. In 40 patients analysis of nuclear DNA content was performed; leukemic cells of 10 patients (25 %) showed a DNA-aneuploid stem line. Taken together, leukemmia-associated phenotypes were detected in 32 cases (53,3 %). The leukemia-associated phenotypes are summarized in Tables 1 and 2.

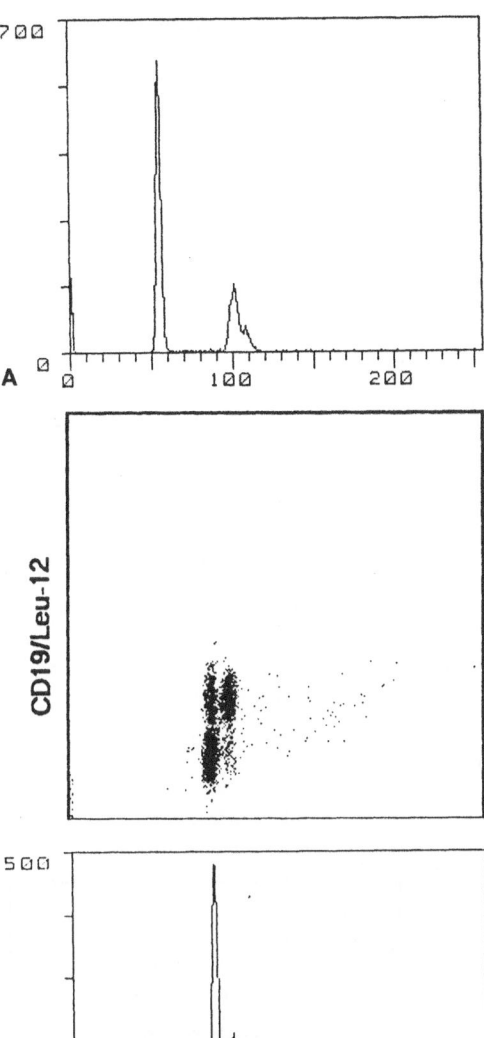

Fig. 1 A, B. DNA aneuploidy in acute leukemia. *A* Common ALL with DNA hypoploidy (DNA index = 0.54); *B* Common ALL with DNA hyperploidy (DNA index = 1.12). Peripheral blood with 30 % lymphoblasts; note CD19-positive DNA-hyperploid cells

Leukemia-Associated Phenotypes During Follow-up Studies

Bone marrow cells from eight patients with leukemia-associated phenotypes were

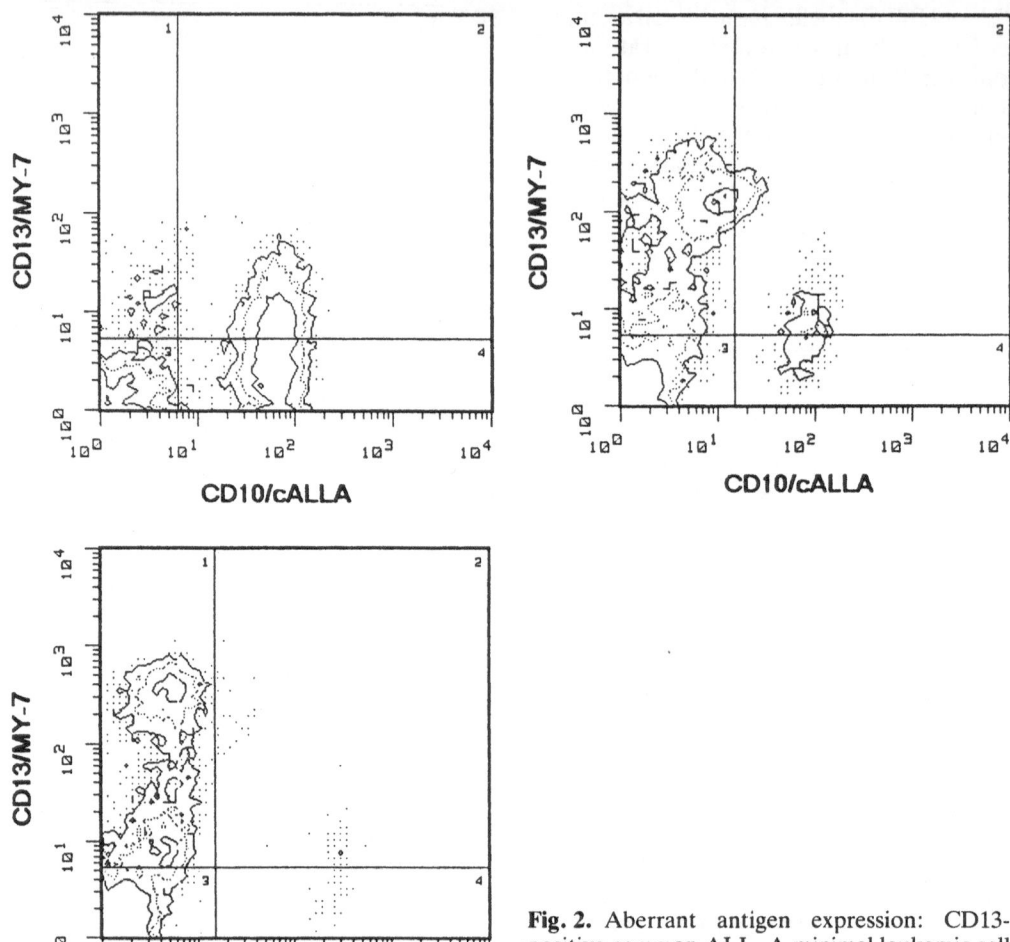

Fig. 2. Aberrant antigen expression: CD13-positive common ALL. A minimal leukemic cell population (CD10+/CD13+) could be demonstrated after induction chemotherapy. Relapse of the cALL was diagnosed 6 weeks later

Table 1. Leukemia-associated phenotypes in ALL

T-ALL ($n = 2$)	TdT + CD5	2
B-lineage ALL ($n = 9$)	CD13+	2
	CD11B+	1
	CD7+/CD14+	1
	DNA aneuploidy	5

studied during follow-up examinations. All patients were in full morphological remission. In three, a minimal leukemic blast cell population was identified by multiparameter flow cytometry (see Fig. 2). Two of these patients hadd a morphological and clinical relapse 4 and 6 weeks later, respectively; no clinical data on the third patient are available at the moment.

In five patients, no bone marrow cells with leukemia-associated phenotypes were detectable even when analyzing up to 10^5

Table 2. Leukemia-associated phenotypes in AML (n = 49)

CD7+	5
CD7+/TdT+	1
TdT+	2
CD5+/TdT+	1
CD2+	1
CD34+/CD13+/CD33-	4
CD34+/CD33+/HLA-DR-	2
CD14: MY-4+/Leu-M3-	3
DNA aneuploidy	5

cells. Four patients are still in remission (median 24 weeks later, range 20–38 weeks) and one patient succumbed due to interstitial pneumonia during chemotherapy-induced aplasia. Table 3 summarizes these follow-up studies.

Study of Peripheral Blood Samples

When no leukemia-associated marker is present, discrimination of small leukemic cell populations from normal hematopoietic cells is impossible. We thus tried to explore whether examination of peripheral blood samples for immature cells (CD34+/CD33+, CD34+/CD13+, TdT+/CD19+) provides valuable information about residual leukemic blast cells. We studied peripheral blood cells from five patients with ALL recovering from intensive chemotherapy, and myeloid progenitor cells (CD34+/CD33+, CD34+/CD13+) were detected in all of them (0.1% – 10%

Table 3. Leukemia-associated phenotypes during follow-up studies

Diagnosis (leukemia-associated feature) Time of follow-up	Results at follow-up	Status (time after follow-up studies)
1 T-ALL (CD5+/TdT+) 24 weeks after diagnosis	CD5 + TdT: 0	CR (36 weeks)
2 T-ALL (CD5+/TdT+) 32 weeks after diagnosis	CD5 + TdT: 0	CR (24 weeks)
3 T-ALL (CD5+/TdT+) 52 weeks after diagnosis	CD5 + TdT: 0	CR (24 weeks)
4 cALL (CD13+) 8 weeks after diagnosis	CD10 + CD13: 0.6%	Relapse (6 weeks)
5 cALL (DNA hypoploidy) 8/16/24 weeks after diagnosis	CD10 + DNA: 0	CR (8 weeks)
6 cALL (DNA hyperploidy) 8 weeks after diagnosis	CD10 + DNA: 0	Lethal infection
7 AML (CD7+) 8 weeks after diagnosis	CD7 + CD13: 0.8%	Relapse (4 weeks)
8 pre-pre B-ALL (TdT+/CD19+/CD10-/CD22+/CD34+) 8 weeks after diagnosis	CD 34 + CD22: 0.5%	Now under chemotherapy

of mononuclear cells). The study on lymphoid progenitor cells in peripheral blood samples is still under progress.

Discussion

A significant percentage of patients with acute leukemia still fail treatment and succumb to their disease. Such failure is presumably due to residual leukemic cells that resist standard therapy. Therefore, sensitive and specific assays are needed to improve the detection of MRD and to direct the development of strategies for prevention of disease recurrence. Double-color immunofluorescence [1, 3] and molecular biological methods including polymerase chain reaction (PCR) [4, 5] are currently the most important techniques used for the identification of rare leukemic cells. In this study we used double-color immunofluorescence analysis and multiparameter flow cytometry to characterize phenotypic features that are absent in normal hematopoietic cells (leukemia-associated phenotypes). These marker combinations as defined by aberrant Tasynchronous antigen expression and DNA aneuploidy were detectable in 53,3 % of patients with adult acute leukemia. Flow cytometric analysis of leukemia-associated marker combinations is a sensitive tool for monitoring acute leukemias: At least 0.1 % of leukemic cells can be reliably detected by this method, which was also verified by dilution experiments [1, 3, unpublished results]. At this moment only few data on follow-up studies of our patients are available; however, these first results are promising with respect to the identification of patients at high risk of immediate relapse. This is in accordance with data published recently [3].

We further wanted to elucidate the possibilities of peripheral blood studies in cases when no leukemia-associated feature is present. However, staining for myeloid precursor cells (CD34+/CD33+, CD34+/CD13+) is not suited for peripheral blood monitoring of AML since immature myeloid cells can be detected in elevated numbers in peripheral blood samples during various states of bone marrow regeneration. Whether detection of peripheral TdT-positive lymphoblasts (TdT+/CD19+, TdT+/CD10+) may contribute to surveillance of ALL remains to be shown [6]. Since the presented method turned out to be sensitive, specific, and rapid, the proposed strategies of bone marrow examination appear to become a clinically useful approach for the detection of MRD in acute leukemia. It is envisaged that the combined use of different methods (especially flow cytometry and PCR-based studies) will extend our knowledge about residual leukemia and tell us how to deal with it in the clinical situation.

References

1. Drach J, Gattringer C, Huber H (1991) Combined flow cytometric assessment of cell surface antigens and nuclear TdT for the detection of minimal residual disease in acute leukemia. Br J Haematol 77: 37–42
2. Drach J, Gattringer C, Huber H (1991) Expression of the neural cell adhesion molecule (CD56) by human myeloma cells. Clin Exp Immunol 83: 418–411
3. Campana D, Coustan-Smith E, Janossy G (1990) The immunologic detection of residual disease in acute leukemia. Blood 76: 163–171
4. Yamada M, Wassermann R, Lange B, Reichard BA, Womer RB, Rovera G (1990) Minimal residual disease in childhood B-lineage lymphoblastic leukemia. N. Engl J Med 323: 448–455
5. Yokota S, Hansen-Hagge TE, Ludwig WD, Reiter A, Raghavachar A, Kleihauer E, Bartram CR (1991) Use of polymerase chain reactions to monitor minimal residual disease in acute lymphoblastic leukemia patients. Blood 77: 331–339
6. Smith RG, Kitchens RL (1989) Phenotypic heterogeneity of TdT positive cells in the blood and bone marrow: implications for surveillance of residual leukemia. Blood 74: 312–319

Bone Marrow Blast Count at Day 28 as the Single Most Important Prognostic Factor in Childhood Acute Lymphoblastic Leukemia*

G. E. Janka-Schaub[1], H. Stuehrk[1], B. Kortuem[1], U. Graubner[2], R. J. Haas[2], U. Goebel[3], H. Juergens[3], H. J. Spaar[4], and K. Winkler[1] for the COALL Study Group

Introduction

Intensification of therapy and risk-adapted treatment have increased the cure rates for childhood acute lymphocytic leukemia (ALL) to 60%–70% [1–5]. Among the prognostic parameters the initial white blood count (WBC) has been considered to be the most important factor in several studies [4, 6, 7]. Other predictors for relapse include age, sex, immunological subtype, and structural chromosomal changes [4, 7–9]. Also in earlier reports it was suggested that the rapidity of lymphoblast cytoreduction during the first 1–2 weeks of treatment correlates with the probability of disease-free survival (DFS) [4, 10, 11]. In the present study the prognostic value of the percentage of lymphoblasts in the bone marrow at day 28 was evaluated.

* Supported by the Hamburger Landesverband für Krebsbekämpfung
[1] Children's Hospital, University of Hamburg Department of Hematology and Oncology, Martinistr. 54, 2000 Hamburg 20
[2] Children's Hospital, University of Munich Department of Hematology and Oncology, Lindwurmstr. 4, 8000 München 2
[3] Children's Hospital, University of Düsseldorf Department of Hematology and Oncology, Moorenstr. 5, 4000 Düsseldorf
[4] Prof. Hess Kinderklinik, St. Juergensstr., 2800 Bremen 1

Patients and Treatment

In a cooperative multicenter treatment study for childhood ALL (COALL-85), 305 patients age 3 months to 18 years were entered between January 1985 and April 1989. After the first six infants the study was closed for this age group because of a high relapse rate. One hundred and sixty-nine high-risk patients (WBC≥ 25/nl, T/null-ALL, age ≥ 10 years) were randomized to receive intensive chemotherapy with rapid or slow rotation of 6 different drug combinations with 12 cytostatic agents. The treatment program has been reported in detail elsewhere [12]. One hundred and thirty-six low-risk patients received four-drug induction therapy followed by three courses of medium high-dose methotrexate (0.5 g/m² 24 h infusion; leukovorin rescue at 48 h) together with cytoarabine i.v. and 6-mercaptopurine p.o. [13]. All patients with a WBC above 5/nl had cranial irradiation and comcomitant intrathecal methotrexate. Maintenance therapy for low- and high-risk patients consisted of oral 6-mercaptopurine daily and methotrexate weekly until 2 years from diagnosis. In all patients a bone marrow examination was done at day 28 or a couple of days later if the WBC was still below 1/nl. Study participants were asked to submit slides to the study center for evaluation. Two hundred to 500 nucleated cells were counted by 2 independent investigators (G. J., H. St.).

Definitions

Complete remission (CR) was defined as a lymphoblast count of less than 5% with evidence of recovery of normal hematopoiesis. Patients without CR at day 28 had another bone marrow aspirate at day 42 after the next drug combination or at the latest at day 56 after the following treatment cycle. Relapse was defined as more than 25% lymphoblasts in the bone marrow or more than 5/μl cells in the CSF with unequivocal lymphoblasts. Definition of late response or nonresponse is shown in Table 1.

Probability of event-free survival (EFS) was estimated by the life-table method [14] and differences between the curves were calculated by log-rank test. As events, nonresponse at day 56 and relapse or death in CR were counted. Patients receiving a bone marrow transplant were censored at the time of transplantation. The six infants were included in the analysis. The Cox regression model for life-table data was used in the multivariate analysis [15].

Results

Complete remission at day 28 was achieved in 289/305 (94.8%) patients. One low-risk patient died of infection during the first 4 weeks of treatment and 15 patients (1 low-risk, 14 high-risk) failed to enter CR by day 28. Six of these 15 patients had a blast count >25% (32%–78%), 5 had a blast count of 10%–18%, and 4 of 6%–9%. The initial characteristics of the poor response group compared to the remission group are shown in Table 2. Chromosome studies were successful in only seven patients; five were normal, one showed a translocation 4;11 and one a 5 q⁻. In relapse one child was found to have a transloction 9;22. Twelve patients (late responders) were in CR at day 42 (six out of nine with a bone marrow aspirate at day 42) or day 56. The three patients who did not achieve CR by day 56 (nonresponders) subsequently went into short-lived remission.

The clinical outcome of late and nonresponders is shown in Table 3. All patients with a day 28 bone marrow blast count of

Table 1. Definition of late and nonresponse

Late responder	(12/305)
No remission	day 28
Remission	day 56[a]
Nonresponder	(3/305)
No remission	day 28
No remission	day 56

a Most already in CR day 42

Table 2. Initial characteristics of late and non responders compared to the remission group

	Late/non-responder	Remission group
Boys	9/15	166 (57%)
Age <1> 10 years	2+8/15	4+60 (22%)
WBC >100/nl	7/15	36 (12%)
Liver/spleen >5 cm	6/15	59 (20%)
T/NULL-ALL	6+2/15	47+10 (20%)
Initial CNS disease	2/15	6 (2.1%)
Mediastinal mass	4/15	26 (9%)

Table 3. Clinical outcome of late and nonresponders

Blasts day 28	Number of patients	Relapse	BMT
5%–10%	4	2	0
>10%	11	9	2

BMT, bone marrow transplant

10% or more were either nonresponders or suffered an early relapse between 4 and 19 months except two patients who were transplanted in first remission. Two of the four patients with a blast count between 5% and 10% also relapsed and two are still in CR at 44 and 48 months. The site of relapse was the bone marrow in ten and the CNS in one patient.

Probability of EFS in the poor response group was 0.15 vs. 0.71 in the remission group (Fig. 1). All events in the poor response group were due to relapses; in the remission group three low-risk and three high-risk patients were lost due to infec-

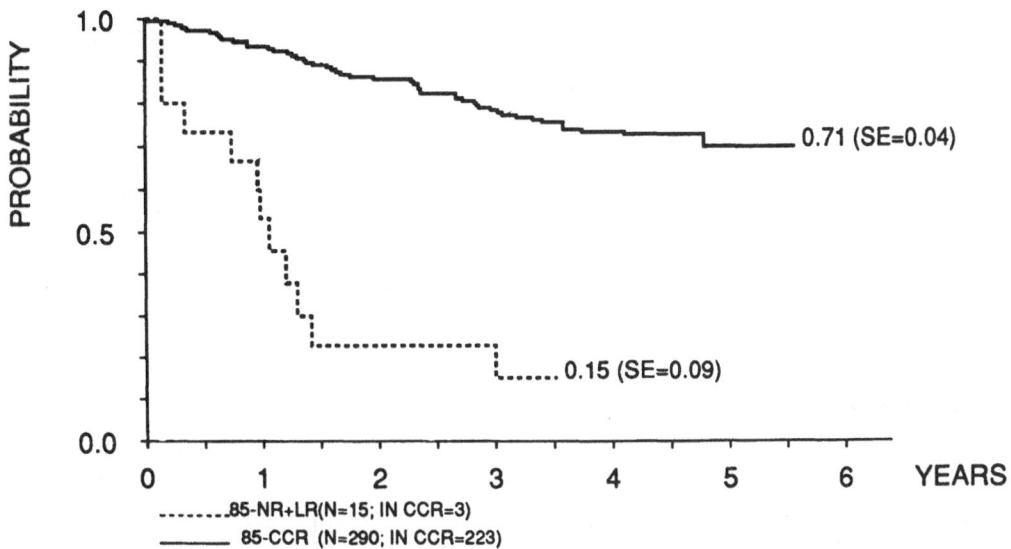

Fig. 1. Probability of event-free survical *(EFS)* in late *(LR)* and nonresponders *(NR)* compared to the remission group *(CCR)* in COALL-85

Table 4. Treatment results for all patients according to different prognostic factors

Risk factor	Event-free survival
Low-risk vs high-risk	0.65 vs. 0.70
WBC < vs. > 100/nl	0.69 vs. 0.65
AGE < vs. > 10 years	0.70 vs. 0.61
T/NULL-ALL vs. c-ALL	0.70 vs. 0.66
Slow vs. rapid rot	0.72 vs. 0.69
Late/nonresponse vs. remission group	0.15 vs. 0.71

tions. There was no statistically significant difference in EFS between low- and high-risk patients, WBC below and above 100/nl, age below and above 10 years, immunological subtype T/null-ALL and common-ALL, or slow and rapid rotation arm (Table 4). By multivariate analysis only late and nonresponse was a significant prognostic factor in high-risk patients above 1 year of age.

Discussion

In the present study 5.2 % of all patients did not achieve remission after 4 weeks of induction therapy. Although most were in remission 2–4 weeks later, the EFS was extremely poor in spite of continued intensive chemotherapy. Nearly all late and nonresponders had adverse prognostic characteristics, i. e., high WBC, very young or old aged, and T-cell leukemia. However, the high relapse rate cannot be attributed to these factors since in this study they were of no prognostic significance except age below 1 year (6/6 relapses). Even patients with a WBC above 100/nl had an EFS of 0.65; this shows that treatment itself is a very important prognostic factor. Other authors have reported than early response to initial chemotherapy as determined during the first 1–2 weeks of treatment has a great impact on DFS. In the ALL-BFM 83 study the reduction of peripheral lymphoblasts was measured after 1 week with only prednisolone therapy [16]. As in our study poor responders were often over 10 years of age, had T-or null-cell leukemia and a high WBC. EFS in the prednisone poor response group was 0.43 compared to 0.75 in the responding patients. The Boston group tested early response to therapy by calculating the absolute leukemic infiltrate at day 5 by bone marrow aspirate and biopsy (11). Children who had less than 50%

cytoreduction had a much higher relapse rate than patients having a greater than 50% cell kill by day 5. Jacquillat et al. reported that children requiring only one to two doses of vincristine and daunomycin to achieve CR had a better prognosis (10). The day 14 bone marrow was also examined in the protocol 160 series of the Children's Cancer Study Group and found to be a highly significant predictor of DFS by univariate and multivariate analysis. Whereas patients with CR on day 14 had a DFS above 60% it dropped below 50% in patients with a blast count of 5%–25% and below 30% if the blast count was above 25% [17].

Evaluation of the bone marrow at a later time should increase the accuracy of prediction of relapse. This is confirmed by our study in which 11/13 patients without remission at day 28 and no transplant suffered a relapse in spite of continuing intensive multiagent chemotherapy. Sallan et al. reported relapses in only 8/22 children not achieving remission at day 30; however, the median observation in this study was only 26 months [2]. It is important to emphasize that most poor responders are missed if a bone marrow aspirate is done later than 4–5 weeks. Also it is intersting that poor responders were found in a nearly even proportion in high-risk patients receiving 4 weeks induction therapy with vincristine, daunomycin, and prednisolone (slow rotation) or 2 weeks of these drugs followed by cyclophosphamide, high-dose methotrexate, and asparaginase (rapid rotation) [12]. It seems that poor response is not a matter of resistance to one drug or one drug combination but that it is rather a general biological characteristic of the disease.

Acknowledgement The authors thank Mrs C. Kirstein for excellent documentation of the COALL studies and for preparation of the manuscript.

References

1. Riehm H, Gadner H, Welte K (1977) Die West-Berliner Studie zur Behandlung der akuten lymphoblastischen Leukämie des Kindes. Klin Paediatr 189: 89–102
2. Sallan SE, Camitta BM, Cassady JR, Nathan DG, Frei E III (1978) Intermittent combination chemotherapy with adriamycin for childhood acute lymphoblastic leukemia: clinical results. Blood 51: 425–433
3. Henze G, Langermann HJ, Gadner H, Schellong K, Welte H, Riehm H (1981) Ergebnisse der Studie BFM 76/79 zur Behandlung der akuten lymphoblastischen Leukämie bei Kindern und Jugendlichen. Klin Paediatr 193: 28–40
4. Miller DR, Sandford L, Albo V, Sather H, Karon M, Hammond D (1983) Prognostic factors and therapy in acute lymphoblastic leukemmia of childhood: CCG-141. A report from Childrens Cancer Study Group. Cancer 51: 1041–1049
5. Graubner UB, Haas RJ, Janka G, Gaedicke G, Kohne E, Rieber EP (1985) Münchner Studie zur Behandlung der akuten lymphoblastischen Leukämie im Kindesalter (ALL 77-02). Klin Paediatr 197: 207–214
6. Henze G, Langermann HJ, Kaufmann U, Ludwig R, Schellong G, Stollmann B, Riehm H (1981) Thymic involvement and initial white blood count in childhood acute lymphoblastic leukemia. Am J Pediatr Hematol Oncol 3: 369–376
7. Crist W, Boyett J. Pullen J, van Eys J, Vietti T (1986) Clinical and biologic features predict poor prognosis in acute lymphoid leukemias in children and adolescents: Pediatric Oncology Group Review. Med Pediatr Oncol 14: 135–139
8. Ludwig WD, Teichmann JV, Sperling C, Komischke B, Ritter J, Reiter A, Odenwald E, Sauter S, Riehm H (1990) Inzidenz, klinische Merkmale und prognostische Bedeutung immunologischer Subtypen der akuten lymphoblastischen Leukämie (ALL) im Kindesalter: Erfahrungen und Therapiestudien ALL-BFM 83 und 86. Klin Paediatr 202: 243–252
9. Pui CH, Raimondi SC, Dodge RK, Rivera GK, Fuchs LAH, Abromowitch M, Look AT, Furman WL, Crist WM, Williams DL (1989) Prognostic importance of structural chromosomal abnormalities in children with hyperdiploid (>50 chromosomes) acute lymphoblastic leukemia. Blood 73: 1963–1967
10. Jacquillat C, Weil M, Gemon MF, Auclerc G, Loisel JP, Delobel J, Flandrin G, Schaison G, Izrael V, Bussel A, Drech C, Weisgerber C, Rain D, Tanzer J, Najean Y, Seligmann M, Boiron M, Bernard J (1973) Combination therapy in 130 patients with acute lymphoblastic leukemia (protocol 06 LA 66-Paris). Cancer Res 33: 3278–3284
11. Frei E III, Sallan SE (1978) Acute lymphoblastic leukemia: treatment. Cancer 42: 828–838

12. Janka-Schaub GE, Winkler K, Goebel U, Graubner U, Gutjahr P, Haas RJ, Juergens H, Spaar J for the COALL Study group. Rapidly rotating combination chemotherapy in childhood acute lymphoblastic leukemia: preliminary results of a randomized comparison with conventional treatment. Leukemia 2 [Suppl]: 73S–78S

13. Janka GE, Winkler K, Juergens H, Goebel U, Gutjahr P, Spaar JH Für die Mitglieder der COALL-Studien (1986) Akute lymphoblastische Leukämie im Kindesalter: die COALL-Studien. Klin Paediatr 198: 171–177

14. Kaplan EL, Meier P (1958) Nonparametric estimation from incomplete observations. J Am Stat Assoc 53: 457–481

15. Cox DR (1972) Regression models and life tables. J R Stat Soc (B) 34: 187–220

16. Riehm H, Reiter A, Schrappe M, Berthold F, Dopfer R, Gerein V, Ludwig R, Ritter J, Stollmann B, Henze G (1986) Die Corticosteroid-abhängige Dezimierung der Leukämiezellzahl im Blut als Prognosefaktor bei der akuten lymphoblastischen Leukämie im Kindesalter (Therapiestudie ALL-BFM 83). Klin Paediatr 199: 151–160

17. Miller DR, Coccia PF, Bleyer WA, Lukens JN, Siegel SE, Sather HN, Hammond GD (1989) Early response to induction therapy as a predictor of disease-free survival and late recurrence of childhood acute lymphoblastic leukemia: a report from the Childrens Cancer Study Group. J Clin Oncol 7: 1805–1815

GM-CSF, CD14, and C-fms Genes in 12 Patients with 5q Abnormalities

E. Weber, H. Karlic, O. Krieger, R. Grill, and D. Lutz

Introduction

Aberrations of the long arm of chromosome 5 (5q) are recurrent chromosomal anomalies in (secondary) acute myeloid leukemia (AML) and myelodysplastic syndrome (MDS) [1]. Common clinical features of these patients are poor response to cytostatic therapy and shorter survival time in comparison to patients with other cytogenetic abnormalities. In a recent evaluation of AML and MDS patients a critical region consisting of bands 5q23-32 was identified. These findings led to the hypothesis that the genes encoding for growth factors and growth factor receptors (e.g., *GM-CSF, M-CSF, IL3, CSF-1-rec. = CD14*) located within this region play an important role in the pathogenesis of these diseases [2]. Several authors described loss of heterozygosity of these genes [3–6], and Cheng et al. [7] detected structural alterations of the *GM-CSF* gene in two cases of AML that could not be found in remission.

We investigated 12 patients with a 5q-aberration and the human cell line HL60 using three different DNA probes *(GM-CSF, CD14)* to confirm the studies about gene loss in these diseases. On the other hand, we wanted to know more about

Ludwig Boltzmann Institute for Hematology and Leukemia Research and 3rd Medical Department, Hanusch Hospital, Heinrich Collinstr. 30, 1140 Vienna, Austria
* This work was supported by the Fond zur Förderung der wissenschaftlichen Forschung, Austria.

aberrant fragments and their use as clonal markers.

Patients

Clinical, cytogenetic features and molecular genetic results are summarized in Table 1. We investigated bone marrow and peripheral blood samples from 12 patients, six males and six females, with 5q-abnormality. Six patients had AML, four MDS, and two chronic myeloid leukemia. Five patients had a translocation involving chromosome 5, 2 × t(3;5), 1 × t(5;7), t(5;17), t(2;5); five patients had a 5q deletion, three out of five a complex karyotype aberration, and two patients monosomy 5.

Cytogenetic Methods

Bone marrow and peripheral blood samples were cultured by standard methods. Chromosomal preparations were stained with a three-stain fluorescence technique [8] and analyzed according to the International System of Human Cytogenetic Nomenclature [9].

Southern Blot Analysis

DNA was extracted by a modified method of Miller [10] from bone marrow and/or peripheral blood cells separated by a Percoll gradient. The DNA was digested with three restriction enzymes *(BamHI, EcoRI, HindIII)*, and the Southern blot was per-

Table 1. Cytogenetic and molecular biological results

Case	Initials	Age (years)	Sex	Diagnosis	Karyotype (partial)	Molecular biology GM-CSF	c-fms	CD14
1	W. M.	65	m	AML(M2)	t(3;5)	* (E 12.5)	*	N
2	W. H.	35	m	AML(M2)	t(3;5)	*	*	*
3	E. J.	72	m	CMML	t(5;17)	* (E 7, B 4)	*	*
4	K. A.	43	f	AML(M2)	t(2;5)	*	N	*
5	S. F.	37	m	CML-BC	t(5;7)	* (E7, B2.6, H16)	*	*
6	P. F.	68	f	RA/M4	5q-	*	*	*
7	N. H.	86	f	RA	5q-	* (mult.ab)	N	*
8	R. A.	82	f	CML	5q-(complex)	*	*	*
9	S. J.	81	m	AML	5q-(complex)	* (E7, B2.6, H20)	*	*
10	W. M.	85	f	RAEBT	5q-(complex)	*	*	*
11	B. K.	59	m	RAEB	Mono 5	*	*	*
12	H. R.	82	f	AML	Mono 5	*(E, H)	nd	nd

* loss of heterozygosity; N, normal; restriction enzymes: E, EcoRI; B, BamHI; H, HindIII

formed as previously described. Southern hybridization was carried out with a nonradioactive method with the following DNA probes: a 5.2-kb HindIII genomic subclone of the GM-CSF gene [3], a CD14 C-DNA probe, a Sst-Xho fragment kindly provided by Goyert et al. [11], and a genomic 0.9-kb probe of the fifth exon of c-fms (Amersham). Hemizygosity was detected by Southern blotting with a c-sis probe (1 kb Pst-BamHI fagment, Amersham) as a control.

Results

We found loss of heterozygosity of the GM-CSF gene in all investigated cases and the cell line HL-60. Six patients and the cell line showed structural alterations= aberrant bands. Cytogenetic anomaly in three out of five cases was a translocation involving chromosome 5, two had a 5q-, and one case a monosomy 5 within a complex karyotype. In the Soutern blot with the c-fms probe we could not detect aberrant fragments in all investigated samples. In the double hybridization c-fms with c-sis, 9/11 patients and the HL-60 cell line had only 1 allele. Two patients, one RA/5q- and one M2/t(2;5), had both c-fms alleles. With the CD14 DNA probe we could not detect any aberrant bands. Ten out of 11 analysed cases were hemizygous, and only 1 patient M2/t(3;5) was heterozygous.

Discussion

Our studies confirm reports about allele loss of 5q-located genes in hematological malignancies [3–6]. In a recent paper,

Cheng et al. described aberrant fragments in AML patients that could not be detected in remission. Blast cells of these patients had a larger mRNA [7].

We demonstrated structural abnormalities of the *GM-CSF* gene in 6/12 patients with 5q abnormalities. The aberrant fragments may be the result of multistep interstitial deletion as it is proposed for the HL-60 cell line [12]. The evidence of aberrant bands could also be used as a clonal marker for detection of residual disease in remission. As yet we have not had the opportunity to investigate DNA from these patients in remission; therefore we cannot confirm their use as clonal markers. The relevance of these findings may lie in the increasing importance of gene loss (tumor suppressor genes). Interestingly, familiar polyposis, an inherited cancer, has also been mapped to 5q and is associated with allele loss [13]. It is not yet clear whether the GM-CSF gene polymorphisms and the hemizygosity of 5q-located genes may be simply considered as clonal markers or if potential candidates for tumor suppressor genes are also deleted within this region. Further molecular studies will have to explain the importance of gene loss in 5q-abnormalities.

References

1. Nimer SD, Golde DW (1987) The 5q- abnormality. Blood 70: 1705
2. Le Beau MM, Albain KS, Larson R, Vardiman JW, Davies EM, Blough RR, Golomb HM,, Rowley JD (1986) Clinical and cytogenetic correlations in 63 patients with therapy related myelodysplastic syndromes and acute nonlymphocytic leukemia: further evidence for characteristic abnormalities of chromosome no.5 and 7. J Clin Oncol 4: 325
3. Huebner K, Isobe M, Croce CM, Golde DW, Kaufmann SE, Gasson JC (1985) The human gene encoding GM-CSF is at 5q21-q32, the chromosome region deleted in the 5q- anomaly. Science 230: 1282
4. Le Beau MM, Pettenati MJ, Lemons RS, Diaz MO, Westbrook CA, Larson RA, Sherr CJ, Rowley JD (1986) Assignment of the *GM-CSF, CSF-1,* and *fms* genes to human chromosome 5 provides evidence for linkage of a family of genes regulating hematopoiesis and for their involvement in the deletion (5q) in myeloid disorders. Cold Spring Harb Symp Quant Biol 51: 899
5. Pettenati MJ, Le Beau MM, Lemons RS, Shima EA, Kawasaki ES, Larson RA, Sherr CJ, Diaz MO, Rowley JD (1987) Assignment of CSF-1 to 5q33.1: evidence for a clustering of genes regulating hematopoiesis and for their involvement in the deletion of the long arm of chromosome 5 in myeloid disorders. Proc Natl Acad Sci USA 84: 2970
6. Nienhuis AW, Bunn HF, Turner PH, Gopal TV,, Nash WG, O'Brien SJ, Sherr CJ (1985) Expression of the human c-*fms* proto-oncogene in hematopoietic cells and its deletion in the 5q- syndrome. Cell 42: 421
7. Cheng GYM, Kelleher CA, Miyauchi J, Wong G, Clark SC, McCulloch EA, Minden MD (1988) Structure and expression of genes of GM-CSF and G-CSF in blast cells from patients with acute myeloblastic leukemia. Blood 71: 204–208
8. Schweizer D (1981) Counterstain enhanced chromosome banding. Hum Genet 57: 307
9. Harden DG, Klinger HP (eds) (1985) ISCN: An international system for human cytogenetic nomenclature. Birth defects Original article series, 21/1. March of Dimes Birth Defect Foundation, New York
10. Miller SA, Dykes DD, Polesky HF (1988) A simple salting out procedure for extracting DNA from human uncleated cells Nucleic Acids Res 61 (3): 1215
11. Goyert SM, Ferrero E, Rettio WJ, Yenamandra AK, Obata F, Le Beau MM (1988) The CD14 monocyte differentiation antigen maps to a region encoding growth factors and receptors. Science 239: 497
12. Nagarajan L, Lange B, Cannizzaro L,, Finan J, Nowell PC, Huebner K (1990) Molecular anatomy of a 5q interstitial deletion. Blood 75: 82
13. Bodmer NF, Bailly CJ, Bodmer J, Bussey HVR, Ellis A, Gorman P, Lucibello FC, Murday VA, Rider SH, Scambler P, Sheer D, Solomon E, Spurr NK (1987) Localisation of the gene for familial adenomatous polyposis on chromosome 5 (1987) Nature 328, 614

Characterization of the Predominant T-Cell Receptor Delta (TCRδ) Rearrangements in Non-T, Non-B ALL

F. Griesinger[1, 2], E. R. Grümayer[1], B. Van Ness[3], and J. H. Kersey[1]

Introduction

The gene that encodes the T-cell-receptor delta chain *(TCRδ)* has recently been identified [1, 2]. The gene product is expressed as a *TRCγ/δ* heterodimer on a minority of T lymphocytes in peripheral blood and thymus. The genomic repertoire of rearranging regions of *TCRδ* is rather limited [3–11]. We and others have shown limited diversity of *TCRδ* rearrangements by Southern blotting in common non-T, non-B lymphoid precursor ALL (LP-ALL) [3–6]. The purpose of the current study was: (1) the characterization and determination of the nucleotide sequence of the predominant *TCRδ* rearrangements in LP-ALL and (2) the evaluation of mechanisms that are functional in the diversification of the junctional sequences of the *TCRδ* gene in LP-ALL.

Materials and Methods

Southern blotting using *Vδ* (kindly provided by M. S. Krangel, Boston), *Jδ1* (kindly provided by T. H. Rabbitts, Cambridge), and *Dδ1/2* (kindly provided by M. D. Minden, Toronto) gene probes was carried out in 35 CD10+/- CD19+ CD24+/-

non-T, non-B lymphoid precursor ALL or leukemic cell lines, as described previously [3]. Monoallelic *Vδ2-(D)-Dδ3* and *Dδ2-Dδ3* rearrangements of 14 leukemias and 3 leukemic cell lines were amplified by the polymerase chain reaction (PCR) with primers 1 and 2 or 1 and 3, respectively as indicated in Fig. 1. For amplification and detection of inversional rearrangements, primers 4, 5, and 6 were used (the sequences of the primers will be provided upon request). The nucleotide sequence of amplification products was determined by the Sanger dideoxynucleotide sequencing method using internal primers and single-strand amplification products generated by asymmetrical PCR. Briefly, double-stranded amplification products were purified by three rounds of centricon microconcentrator (Amicon) centrifugation. A quantity of 1%–5% of the amplification products was asymmetrically amplified using amplification primers at concentration ratios of 1:50 to 1:100. Amplification products were purified by three rounds of centricon microconcentrator centrifugation and subsequently sequenced with a T7-polymerase-based sequencing kit.

Results

Our own and others' previous analysis of *TCRδ* rearrangements in lymphoid precursor ALLs (LP-ALLs) showed a frequency of 65%–90% of *TCRδ* rearrangements ([3, 7, 8]; C. R. Bartram, this volume) and that the predominant rearrangements, i.e., >90% of all rearranged alleles, represent

[1] Departments of Laboratory Medicine and Pathology, and Pediatrics, University of Minnesota, Minneapolis, Minnesota 55455, USA
[2] Present address: Department of Hematology, University of Münster, Münster, FRG
[3] Institute of Human Genetics and Department of Biochemistry, University of Minnesota, Minneapolis, Minnesota 55455, USA

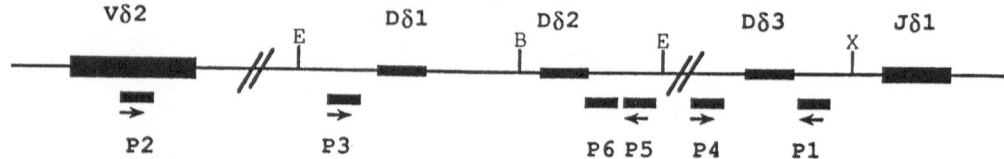

Fig. 1. Map of the *TCRδ* gene locus indicating the position and orientation of amplification primers P1-5 and primer P6 used for the detection of inversional arrangements

incomplete *Vδ2 – Dδ3* and *Dδ2-Dδ3* (Fig. 2, [6]). The junctional sequences of the PCR products derived from *Vδ2-Dδ3* rearrangements are shown in Table 1. The following pattern emerged for the *Vδ2* rearrangements. All recombinations represented "coding joints" [12, 13] between *Vδ2* and *Dδ3*. Extensive insertions of N-nucleotides with a bias toward addition of C/G (41 of 69 bases) over A/T (28 of 69 bases) were found in most of the joints. Diversity elements in addition to *Dδ3* were involved in only two rearrangements (cases 4 and 11), where at least four nucleotides were found to be identical to published sequences of *Dδ1* or *Dδ2* [11]. Twenty of 32 coding region borders were trimmed and up to 19 nucleotides (Nalm 16) of the *Vδ2* region were deleted. In 9 of 13 instances where the coding region borders remained intact P-mononucleotides (6 instances) or -dinucleotides (3 instances) were observed [14, 15].

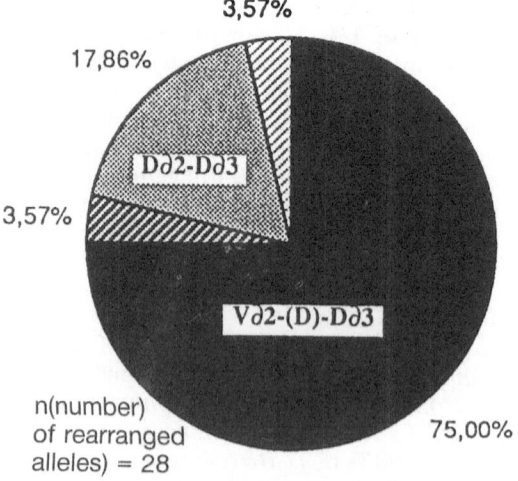

Fig. 2. Distribution of *TCRδ* rearrangements in non-T, non-B LP-ALL

The junctional sequences of three *Dδ2-Dδ3* rearrangements (Table 2) revealed a great degree of heterogeneity. Two samples (#12 and 13) showed coding joints between *Dδ2* and *Dδ3*, most likely as a result of a deletional rearrangement (Fig. 3A). The same principles of junctional diversification as in the *Vδ2-(D)-Dδ3* rearrangements, with the exception of insertion of further diversity elements, were observed in the *Dδ2-Dδ3* joins. The *Dδ2-Dδ3* rearrangement in Nalm 16 was unusual in that it involved joining of the 3' border of *Dδ2* and the 3' heptamer of *Dδ3*, the latter having the four most proximal nucleotides missing. In leukemic sample 14, the PCR product of P1 and P3 primers revealed an unexpected signal joint between the 5' signal sequence of *Dδ2* and the 3' signal sequence of *Dδ3* (Table 2). This leads to a circular excision product representing a coding join in which Dδ3 is located 5' of *Dδ2* and a chromosomal signal join which was amplified in this leukemia, as illustrated in Fig. 3B. One nucleotide (counting from the coding border) of the *Dδ2* heptamer was mutated from G to C. Four non-germline-encoded N-nucleotides were inserted in this signal joint. In the event that, prior to recombination, an inversion of the transcriptional orientation of one of the diversity elements has occurred, such a rearrangement will lead to a chromosomal *Dδ3-Dδ2* coding in which *Dδ3* is located 5' of *Dδ2*, as indicated in Fig. 3C (inverted arrangement of diversity elements). Therefore, we analyzed 62 previously published productive *Vδ1-D-D-Jδ1* and *Vδ2-D-D-Jδ1* rearrangements in nonleukemic T lymphocytes [9, 11, 16, 17]. We found evidence that the junctional regions of five of these rearrangements may be acccounted for by inverted arrangements of diversity elements (Table 3). This

Table 1. Vδ2-(D)-Dδ3 rearrangements in LP-ALL

Germline	Vδ2 GGT CTT ACT ACT CCT GTG ACA CC	P	N	Dδ1 GAA ATA GT	P	N	Dδ2 CCT TCC TAC	N	P	Dδ3 / Dδ33 ACT GGG GGA TAC G
	GGT CTT ACT ACT CCT GTG ACA CC			GAA ATA GT			CCT TCC TAC			ACT GGG GGA TAC G
KOPN-1	GGT CTT ACT ACT CCT GTG AC							TTG CGC	T	ACT GGG GGA TAC G
Nalm 16	GGT CTT A							TCG A	GT	G GGA TAC G
IE8		G	TT	ATA G				GG		ACT GGG GGA TAC G
1	GGT CTT ACT ACT CCT GTG AC							GCC ATA CCC CA	T	ACT GGG GGA TAC G
2	GGT CTT ACT ACT CCT GTG A							CCA AAG G	GT	ACT GGG GGA TAC G
3	GGT CTT ACT ACT CCT GTG							AAC C		ACT GGG GGA TAC G
4	GGT CTT ACT ACT CCT GTG ACA CC							GA		CT GGG GGA TAC G
5	GGT CTT ACT ACT CCT GTG G							CCC TCG GGA C	T	ACT GGG GGA TAC G
6	GGT CTT ACT ACT CCT GTG G	GG						TCC CCC T		CT GGG GGA TAC G
7	GGT CTT ACT ACT CCT GTG ACA CC	G						GG		ACT GGG GGA TAC G
8	GGT CTT CT ACT CCT GTG ACA CC							A	T	CT GGG GGA TAC G
9	GGT CTT ACT ACT CCT GTG ACA CC							GAG GGA TT		ACT GGG GGA TAC G
10	GGT CTT ACT ACT CCT GTG ACA C							CT		ACT GGG GGA TAC G
11	GGT CTT ACT ACT CCT GTG GT		TTC				CC T			CT GGG GGA TAC G

Table 2. Dδ2-Dδ3 rearrangements in LP-ALL

Germline	Dδ2 CCT TCC TAC	12 bp spacer act gat gtg	Heptamer ttt cat tgt g	P	N	P	Dδ3 ACT GGG GGA TAC G	Heptamer cac agt g	23 bp spacer cta caa aac..
	CCT TCC TAC	act gat gtg	ttt cat tgt g				ACT GGG GGA TAC G	cac agt g	cta caa aac..
Coding joint									
12	CCT TCC TA	act gat gtg	ttt cat tgt g		GGA GCG AAA AAG G	G	ACT GGG GGA TAC G		
13	CCT TCC TAC	act gat gtg	ttt cat tgt g		GAC	G	ACT GGG GGA TAC G		
Nalm 16	CCT TCC T	act gat gtg	ttt cat tgt g	GT			ACT GGG GGA TAC G		
Signal joint									
14		act gat gtg	ttt cat tct g		aac c			cac agt g	cta caa aac..

243

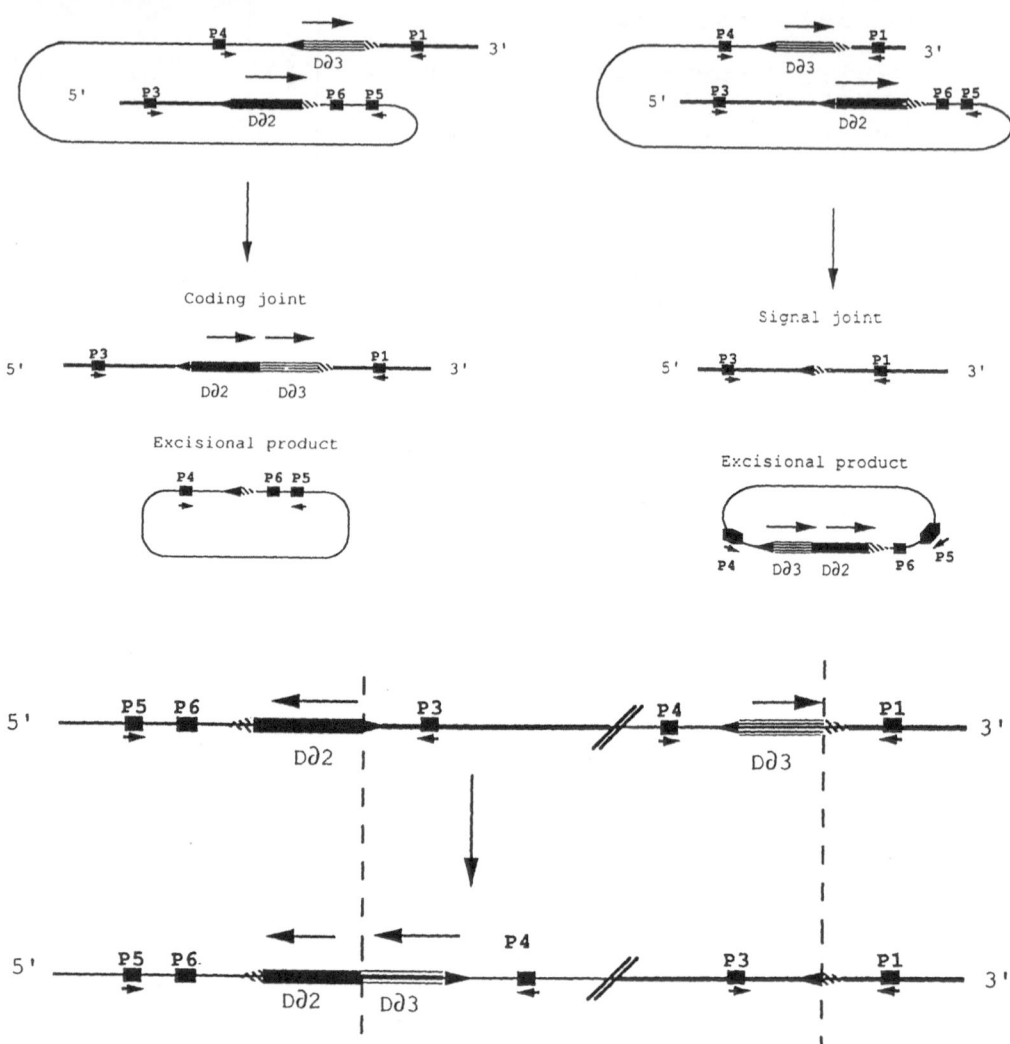

Fig. 3A. Deletional rearrangement in leukemic samples 12, 13 and NALM 16. **B** Deletional rearrangement in leukemic sample 14. **C** Dδ3–Dδ2 rearrangement subsequent to an inversional rearrangement

mechanism may considerably increase the junctional diversity of *TCRδ* joins, which encode the third complementarity-determining region which most likely interacts with the antigen detected by the T-cell antigen receptor [18].

Discussion

In the present paper, we provide direct evidence that the two predominant *TCRδ* rearrangements in LP-ALL are Vδ2-(D)-

Dδ3 or *Dδ2-Dδ3* joints, which is consistent with their immature stage of differentiation and maturation. These findings are in agreement with our previous hypothesis that the cell which undergoes malignant transformation in non-T, non-B LP-ALL may represent a lineage uncommitted precursor cell, which retains the capacity to undergo both immunoglobulin and T-cell receptor rearrangements [5, 6, 7]. It is of interest that all rearrangements (with the exception of the *Dδ2-Dδ3* rearrangement in Nalm 16 and sample 14) are potentially translatable if further joining events to joining and/or variable regions occur.

Our studies show that the rearrangements are incomplete joining events and, in the present configuration, will not give rise to a functional protein. They are similar to incomplete DJ_H or DJ_β rearrangements, observed as cross-lineage rearrangements in T- or B-lineage cells, respectively [19, 20, 21]. It has to be emphasized that cross-lineage rearrangements seem to occur also in nonleukemic immature lymphoid cells. Born and colleagues [19] showed that, in thymocytes, IgH rearrangements frequently occurred after $TCR\beta$ and γ had been functionally rearranged. Interestingly, these rearrangements were biased toward utilization of the most 3' diversity element D_{Q52}. Thus, the incomplete $TCR\delta$ rearrangements are similar to D_{Q52}-J_H rearrangements which are characteristically observed in immature B lymphocytes [21–25]. It has been suggested that the preferential utilization of proximal rearranging regions is due to increased accessibility of these regions to the recombinase [25, 26]. Whether only chromosomal proximity or other factors result in the preferential usage of these regions remains to be determined.

The insertion of N- and P-nucleotides and of further diversity elements in some instances, and trimming of the rearranging regions, led to highly diversified junctional regions specific for each leukemic clone. Thus, it may be possible to use $TCR\delta$ rearrangements for the detection of residual leukemic disease using PCR technology in the most frequent type of acute lymphoblastic leukemia. Due to the conserved rearranging genomic sequences of the $V\delta2$-(D)-$D\delta3$ joint, a set of "framework" oligonucleotides can be used to amplify the respective leukemic clone-specific junctional region. This amplification product could subsequently serve as a "signature" probe for the detection of leukemic minimal disease ([27, 28]; C. R. Bartram, this volume). However, it is clear that these methods may not be applicable in all cases of LP-ALL. In the majority of cases (9/11), the junctional region contains only one N-region. In 6 out of 11 cases, less than five N-nucleotides were inserted. In those

cases, the junctional diversity of the $TCR\delta$ rearrangement may not be sufficient to create a probe which would discriminate between residual leukemic and nonleukemic cells with the same rearrangement. Although not detectable by Southern analysis of fetal bone marrow cells or sorted $CD10^+SmIgM^-$ fetal bone marrow cells [29], $V\delta2$-(D)-$D\delta3$ can be readily detected by PCR in adult bone marrow, peripheral blood, and fetal hematopoietic organs (E. R. Grümayer, F. Griesinger and J. H. Kersey, unpublished results). We conclude that the detection of leukemic clone specific $TCR\delta$ rearrangements by PCR may be applicable for the detection of minimal residual leukemic disease in selected cases of LP-ALL.

The $D\delta2$-$D\delta3$ rearrangements display a great deal of heterogeneity. Two cases of $D\delta2$-$D\delta3$ excisional rearrangements (Fig. 3A), which result in coding joints, were observed (samples 12, 13). The rearrangement in Nalm 16 was unusual, in that it involved the joining of $D\delta2$ and the 3' heptamer of $D\delta3$. The sequence of rearrangement in sample #14 proved to be a signal joint between the 5' heptamer of $D\delta2$ and the 3' heptamer of $D\delta3$ which leads to an inverted arrangement of diversity elements in the circular excision product. If, however, the orientation of one of the two diversity elements had been changed prior to the rearrangement, the signal joint observed in leukemia 14 would represent the reciprocal joint of an inversional $D\delta3$-$D\delta2$ rearrangement remaining in the chromosome (Fig. 3C). It is noteworthy that such a rearrangement leaves the 5' signal sequence of $D\delta3$ and the 3' signal sequence of $D\delta2$ intact, thus allowing further rearrangements to variable and joining regions. Such a mechanism would introduce a considerably higher degree of diversity in the junctional regions of V-D-D-$J\delta$ rearrangements.

While there is a very restricted genomic repertoire of the $TCR\delta$ gene, diversification of CDR3, the paratope of the T-cell receptor, depends on the junctional region [44]. Therefore, we have searched for evidence of possible inversions of $D\delta1$, $D\delta2$, or $D\delta3$ in published productive human V-D-D-J $TCR\delta$ rearrangements (Table 3, modified

Table 3. Sequences of productive Vδ1-Jδ1 and Vδ2-Jδ1 rearrangements in nonleukemic T lymphocytes according to references cited in Results. The sequences are shown so as to demonstrate possible inversions of diversity elements

	Vδ1	P	N	Dδ1 GAAATAGT	N	P	Dδ2 CCTTCCTAC	N	Dδ3 ACTGGGGATACG	N	Dδ2 CCTTCCTAC	N	P	Jδ1 ACACCGATAAA
Germline	...TTGGGGAACT			GAAATAGT			CCTTCCTAC	TAGAAAGGAA	ACTGGGGATACG		CCTTCCTAC	AT		ACACCGATAAA
IDP2	...TTG	G	CTGTACGGG	GAAA	AC		TCCT		TGGGGGATACG	CGGTCT	TTCC			CCGATAAA
PBL L1A	...TTGGGGAA	G	TCCCAACCTCCCT	GAAA					ACTGGGGATACG	CAGGA	TCCT			ACACCGATAAA
Germline									D delta 1 GAAATAGT		D delta 2 CCTTCCTAC			
PBL C 1	...TTGGGGAAC		CCGGCTC				CCTAC	AG	TGGGGG	TGGGGTCGTGGG	ATAG	GTGG		A
Germline (Vδ2)	...TGTGACACC													
N1B.D9	...TGTGACACC	G	T						TGGG	TTTA	CTTCCT	C	GT	ACACCGATAAA
N1B.D12	...TGTGACACC	G	CT			GT			ACTGGGGGAT		CCTTC		GT	ACACCGATAAA

from [45, 46]). The junctional sequences 3' of Dδ3 of IDP2, PBL L1a, N1B.D9, and N1B.D12 contain the sequences TTCC, TCCT, CTTCCT, and CCTTC, respectively. As shown in Table 3, these nucleotides may be derived directly from a Dδ2 element. This conclusion seems to be almost certain in the two latter clones, where six and five nucleotides are identical to the published sequence of Dδ2. Similarly, the junctional sequence 3' of Dδ3 of PBL C1 contains the sequence ATAG which may be derived from Dδ1. If these nucleotides 3' of Dδ3 are encoded by D elements, no nucleotides possibly derived from the respective diversity elements would be expected 5' of Dδ3. This is clearly the case in PBL L1a, PBL C1, N1B.D9, and N1B.D12 where no Dδ2 or Dδ1 sequences can be found 5' of Dδ3 (Table 3). Thus, these results strongly suggest that normal, nonleukemic mature T lymphocytes increase their junctional diversity by inverting the arrangement of D elements in productive Vδ1-D-D-Jδ1 and Vδ2-D-D-Jδ1 rearrangements. We propose that this may represent a novel mechanism for the creation of diversity which is most likely unique to the TCRδ gene, since only this gene uses more than one diversity element for recombination.

Acknowledgement. We would like to thank Dr. J. M. Greenberg for invaluable discussion, and P. Medberry for excellent technical assistance.

Summary

The current study was designed to determine the nucleotide sequence of two distinct TCRδ rearrangements which are observed in >90% of all rearranged alleles, i.e., in 50%–60% of all non-T, non-B common lymphoid precursor acute lymphocytic leukemia (LP-ALL). Cloning of the genomic rearrangements was performed with the polymerase chain reaction (PCR) using oligonucleotide primers complementary to intronic sequences 3' of Dδ3, 5' of Dδ1, and to Vδ2, respectively. Nucleotide sequences determined by the Sanger dideoxynucleotide method of single-stranded amplification products revealed: (1) The most frequent rearrangement in

LP-ALL is an incomplete *Vδ2-(D)-Dδ3*
coding joint; (2) the second most frequent
rearrangement is an incomplete *Dδ2-Dδ3*
coding joint in the majority of cases; and (3)
the remarkable diversity of the rearrangements created by insertion of N- and P-
nucleotides and in some cases extensive
trimming of the rearranging regions demonstrate the clonal specificity and potential for
detection of residual leukemic disease.
However, in some cases, the number of
nucleotide differences may not be sufficient
for the discrimination of leukemic and
nonleukemic cells carrying *Vδ2-(D)-Dδ3*
rearrangements. A novel inversional rearrangement was demonstrated in one case.
This novel joint potentially increases the
degree of diversity of the junctional region
which encodes the antigen-binding domain
of *TCRδ*.

References

1. Hata S, Brenner MB, Krangel MS (1987)
   Science 238: 678
2. Band H, Hochstenbach F, McLean J, Krangel MS, Brenner MB (1987) Science 238:
   682
3. Griesinger F, Greenberg JM, Kersey JH
   (1989) J Clin Invest 84: 506
4. Griesinger F, Grümayer ER, Kersey JH
   (1989) Blood 74 [Suppl I]: 245a
5. Griesinger F, Kersey JH (1989) International
   Congress of Immunology, Berlin. Fischer,
   Stuttgart, p 36 (abstract 9–11)
6. Biondi A, di Celle PF, Rossi V, Casorati G,
   Matullo G, Giudici G, Foa R, Migone N
   (1990) Blood 75: 1834
7. Loiseau P, Gugliemi P, Le Paslier D, MacIntyre E, Gessain A, Bories J-C, Flandrin G,
   Chen Z, Sigaux F (1989) J Immunol 142:
   3305
8. Hara J, Benedict SH, Champagne E, Takihara Y, Mak TW, Minden M, Gelfand EW
   (1988) J Clin Invest 82: 1974
9. Hata S, Clabby M, Devlin P, Spits H, de Vries
   JE, Krangel MS (1989) J Exp Med 169: 41
10. Takihara V, Reimann J, Michalopoulos E,
    Ciccone E, Moretta L, Mak TW (1989) J Exp
    Med 169: 393
11. Loh EY, Swirla S, Serafini AT, Phillips JH,
    Lanier LL (1988) Proc Natl Acad Sci USA
    85: 9714
12. Lewis S, Gellert M (1989) Cell 59: 585–588
13. Lieber MR, Hesse JE, Mizuuchi K, Gellert
    M (1988) Proc Natl Acad Sci USA 85:
    8588
14. Lafaille JJ, DeCloux A, Bonneville M, Taka-
    gaki Y, Tonegawa S (1989) Cell 59: 859
15. McCormack WT, Tjoelker LW, Carlson LM,
    Petryniak B, Barth CF, Humphries EH,
    Thompson CB (1989) Cell 56: 785
16. Hata S, Satyanarayana K, Devlin P, Band H,
    McLean J, Strominger JL, Brenner MB,
    Krangel MS (1988) Science 240: 1541
17. Tamura N, Horoyd KJ, Banks T, Kirby M,
    Okayama H, Crystal RG (1990) J Exp Med
    172: 169
18. Davis MM, Bjorkman PJ (1988) T cell antig-
    en receptor genes and T-cell recognition.
    Nature 334: 395
19. Born W, White J, Kappler J, Marrack P (1988)
    Rearrangement of IgH genes in normal thy-
    mocyte development. J Immunol 140: 3228
20. Mitzutani S, Ford AM, Wiedemann LM,
    Chan LC, Furley AJW, Greaves MF, Mol-
    gaard HV (1986) EMBO J 5: 3467
21. Yancopoulos GD, Desiderio SV, Paskind M,
    Kearney JF, Baltimore D, Alt FW (1984)
    Nature 311: 727
22. Alt FW, Yancopoulos GD, Blackwell TK,
    Wood C, Thomas E, Boss M, Coffman R,
    Rosenberg N, Tonegawa S, Baltiore D (1984)
    EMBO J 3: 1209
23. Ravetch JC, Siebenlist V, Korsmeyer S, Wald-
    mann TA, Leder P (1981) Cell 27: 583
24. Nickerson KG, Berman J, Glickman E,
    Chess L, Alt FW (1989) J Exp Med 169:
    1391
25. Schroeder HW, Hillson JL, Perlmutter R
    (1987) Science 238: 791
26. Schlissel MS, Baltimore D (1989) Cell 58:
    1001
27. Hansen-Hagge TE, Yokota S, Bartram CR
    (1989) Blood 74: 1762
28. D'Auriol L, MacIntyre E, Galibert F, Sigaux
    F (1989) Leukemia 3: 155
29. LeBien TW, Elstrom RL, Moseley M, Ker-
    sey JH, Griesinger F (1990) Blood 76:
    1196

247

Diagnosis of Both c-ALL and Sarcoidosis in the Same Patient

K. Schäfer, H. Wandt, and W. M. Gallmeier

Introduction

The simultaneous manifestation of systemic sarcoidosis and a malignant disorder, especially a malignant lymphoma, is a rare phenomen on [1]. While some argue for a common pathogenesis in the simultaneous occurrence of the two disorders [2], others believe that the steroid treatment in sarcoidosis is responsible for the development of a malignant lymphoma in these cases [3, 4]. But this would not account for the predominance of Hodgkin's disease as opposed to other lymphomas in the reported cases [5]. Brinker [6] called it a "sarcoidosis-lymphoma syndrome," whereby the observed number of lymphoproliferative diseases appears to be about 5.5 times the expected number. This syndrome is characterized by late onset of systemic sarcoidosis (median age, 41 years), a chronic form of disease, and the sarcoidosis preceding the diagnosis of lymphoma by an average of 24 months.

It is difficult to distinguish between the simultaneous manifestation of systemic sarcoidosis and a malignant disorder and the so-called sarcoid-like reaction, which can be seen in lymph nodes, draining a carcinoma, in the tumor itself, or even in distant tissues. Such a reaction, which is histologically identical to that occurring in systemic sarcoidosis, occurs in 19 % of Hodgkin's disease and in 7 % of non-Hodgkin's lymphomas [7–10]. Three criteria are discussed in the literature, which argue for the simultaneous manifestation of the two diseases [11]. First, each diagnosis should be confirmed separately by biopsies from unrelated anatomical regions. Second, each disorder should be characterized by appropriate clinical, radiological, and biochemical features. Third, the sarcoidosis should remit or remain stable, while the malignant lesion progresses; this seems to be an unrealistic criterion, since sarcoidosis may also progress.

Furthermore, it seems useful to determine the angiotensin-converting-enzyme (ACE) level, because the ACE level is high in sarcoidosis and low in malignant lymphomas and leukemias. There was also no elevation of ACE in one patient with local noncaseating epithelioid granuloma and Hodgkin's disease [12]. There are some theories concerning the pathogenesis of the simultaneous occurrence of the two diseases, for example, a common viral origin [6, 13], or the high mitotic activity of lymphocytes in sarcoidosis [6].

There are case reports describing the occurrence of sarcoidosis in cases of Hodgkin's disease non-Hodgkin's lymphoma (NHL), acute myeloid leukemia (AML), and chronic myeloid leukemia (CML) [6, 14]. But there is just one report concerning the simultaneous manifestation of sarcoidosis and acute lymphoblastic leukemia [15]. Therefore, our case report seems to be worth mentioning. It contributes to the differential problems of interpreting pulmonary infiltration in cases of leukemia.

Fifth Medical Clinic, Institute for Hematology and Oncology, Flurstr. 17, W-8500 Nürnberg 90, FRG

Case Report

A 32-year-old man was well until 2 months before admission, when a dry cough, hoarseness, and a low-grade fever occurred for some days. These symptoms reappeared 4 weeks later, and for 2 weeks before admission a permanent dry cough, low-grade fever, and night sweat persisted. In the chest X-ray a diffuse fine reticular infiltration was seen and the patient was referred to hospital. On clinical examination, the only abnormalities were a tachypnea of 25/min, a palpable lymph node in the left supraclavicular region (1×1 cm), and a palpable spleen 4 cm below the left rib margin. The only abnormal laboratory parameters except blood count were moderately elevated serum glutamat-pyrovat pyruvic transaminase (SGPT) lactate dehydrogenase (LDH), γ-glutamyltransferase (γ-GT), and alkaline phosphatase (AP). The blood cell count showed a mild anemia with an Hb of 10.5 g/dl. The leukocyte count was in the normal range, but in the differential count 7 % lymphatic blasts were seen.

Ten days later, when the blasts had increased to 48 %, a bone marrow aspirate resulted in sicca-punction and the biopsy showed a dense infiltration of lymphatic blasts. On cytochemical examination the blasts were negative for periodic acid Schiff (PAS), peroxidase, esterase, and acid phosphatase. Immunocytologically the blasts were positive for CD10, CD19, CD20, CD24, HLA-DR, and Tdt (by flow cytometry). Because of the diffuse fine reticular infiltration of the middle parts of the lung, a bronchoscopic examination was done, which showed a normal appearance of the bronchi, but histologically there was an infiltration with non-caseating epitheloid-cell granulomas, giant cells of the Langhans type, and surrounding lymphocytes. In the bronchoalveolar lavage (BAL) a lymphocytic alveolitis, with 17 % lymphatic cells (64 % T4 cells, 24 T8 cells), was seen. The ACE level was 36 U/l (normal <30 U/l). A toxoplasmosis complement fixation test (KBR) 1:40 and a toxoplasmosis indivect fluorescent antibody (IF) with 1:1024 were indicative of an acute infection. An open lung biopsy was done to distinguish precisely between a sarcoidosis, a toxoplasmosis of the lung, and an infiltration with lymphatic blasts. This examination again showed a picture of sarcoidosis; no trophozoites or lymphatic blasts were seen.

Because of a rapid progressive thrombocytopenia no other invasive diagnostic study, such as a liver biopsy, was done. Summarizing all the diagnostic procedures, three diagnoses were made:

1. c-ALL
2. Systemic sarcoidosis stage III
3. Acute toxoplasmosis [organ involvement other than the lung and brain (CT scan) was not proved].

We started combination chemotherapy according to the protocol for ALL in adults (BMFT), first without steroids, because of the toxoplasmosis infection. The antibiotic treatment for toxoplasmosis consisted of

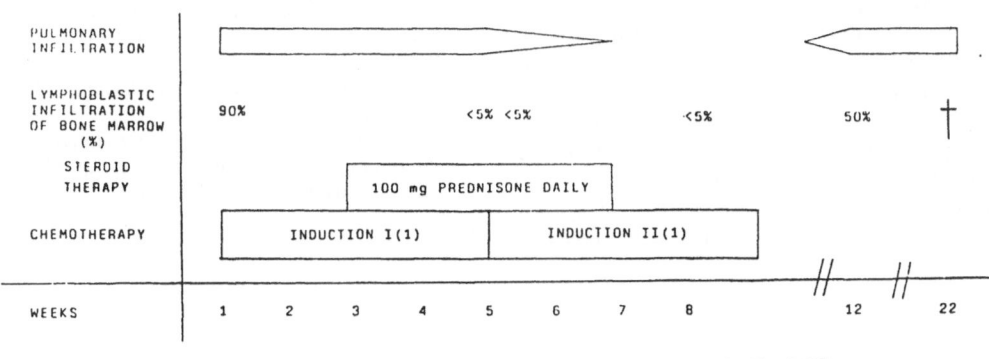

(1) TREATMENT ACCORDING TO THE PROTOCOL FOR ALL IN ADULTS (BMFT)

Fig. 1. Pattern of pulmonary infiltration

pyrimethamine and sulfadiazine. After 2 weeks of chemotherapy, we started steroids at a dose of 100 mg prednisone daily and after 2 weeks of this treatment no pulmonary infiltration was seen. Antibiotic treatment was terminated after 8 weeks, when the IgM titer of toxoplasmosis was negative and the IgG titer retrograde. After 8 weeks of induction treatment, there was a complete remission of the ALL in bone marrow. On termination of the steroid therapy the pulmonary infiltration reappeared in the same manner 4 weeks later. Four weeks later the end of induction therapy, a relapse of the ALL with a dense infiltration of bone marrow occurred. The blasts were cytochemically and immuncytologically identical to the blasts of ALL origin. Two different reinduction regimens with high-dose ara-C, etoposide (VePesid), and amsacrine failed to produce a second remission of the ALL and the patient died 3 months after the relapse. The pulmonary infiltration showed the same pattern as in the beginning of his illness (Fig. 1).

Summary

We think that our patient had systemic sarcoidosis and ALL at the same time. He met three criteria, which are discussed in the literature as signs of the simultaneous manifestation of sarcoidosis and a malignant disorder.

First, histological diagnosis of the two diseases was made from two different anatomical sites, above all, there was no sign of lymphoblastic infiltration of pulmonary tissue in both lung biopsies. Second, the ACE level was elevated. Third, the pulmonary infiltration showed a rapid regression when steroid therapy was started and reappeared when steroid therapy was ceased. The ALL was in complete remission at that time. In the following month the extent of the pulmonary infiltration was stable, although there was a relapse and progression of the ALL.

References

1. James DG, Sharma OP (1985) Overlap syndromes with sarcoidosis. Postgrad Med J 61: 769–771
2. Brinker H, Wilbeck E (1974) The incidence of malignant tumors in patients with respiratory sarcoidosis. Br J Cancer 29: 247–251
3. Romer FK (1980) Sarcoidosis and cancer – a critical view. In: Jones Williams W, Davies BH (eds) Eighth international conference on sarcoidosis and other granulomatous diseases. Alpha Omega, Cardiff, pp 201–205
4. Romer FK (1982) Sarcoidosis and cancer. N Engl J Med 306: 1490 (letter)
5. Mc Inerney PD (1986) Sarcoidosis and lymphoma: is there an association? Postgrad Med J 62: 809–810 (letter)
6. Brinker H (1986) The sarcoidosis-lymphoma syndrome. Br J Cancer 54: 467–473
7. Brinker H (1986) Sarcoid reactions in malignant tumors. Cancer Treat Rev 13: 147–153
8. Heymer B (1980) Sarcoid-like granulomatous reactions against malignancies. In: Grundmann E (ed) Metastatic tumor growth. Fischer, Stuttgart, pp 167–172
9. Goldfarb BL, Cohen SS (1970) Coexisting disseminated sarcoidosis and Hodgkin's diseases. JAMA 211: 1525–1528
10. Brinker H (1972) Sarcoid reactions and sarcoidosis in Hodgkin's disease and other malignant lymphomata. Br J Cancer 26: 120–128
11. Brennan NJ, Towers RP, Fenelly JJ, Fitzgerald MX (1983) Sarcoidosis and lymphoma in the same patient. Postgrad Med J 59: 581–585
12. Romer FK, Emmertsen K (1980) Serum angiotensin-converting enzyme in malignant lymphomas, leukemia and multiple lymphoma. Br J Cancer 42: 314–318
13. Blayney DW, Rohatgi PK, Hines W et al (1983) Sarcoidosis and the human-T-cell leukemia-lymphoma virus. Ann Intern Med 99: 409 (letter)
14. Reich JM (1985) Acute myeloblastic leukemia and sarcoidosis. Cancer 55: 360–369
15. Harousseau IL, Schaison G, Cauberrere I, Tricot G (1980) Leucemie algue lymphoblastique. Nouv Presse Med 9: 1310

Pharmacokinetics – Preclinical Investigations and Therapeutic Implications

Pharmacologically Guided Leukemia Therapy*

W. Plunkett, V. Gandhi, H. Kantarjian, and M. J. Keating

Hypotheses relevant to the pharmacokinetics and pharmacodynamics of anticancer drugs in human leukemias during therapy provide the focus for this review. The postulates presented are offered as approaches to investigations that experience suggests are likely to be useful to the overall goal of improving the treatment of leukemia and extending patient survival. It is important to conduct these investigations because the answers to the questions posed by these postulates will aid our understanding of clinical activity of the therapeutic agents. It is possible to propose these approaches because of the accessibility of leukemia to investigators and the sensitivity of the analytical procedures to be employed.

Biochemical Modulation

The influence of one drug, either directly or at a distance, on the metabolism and action of another drug is referred to as biochemical modulation. Nucleoside analogues must be phosphorylated to the respective triphosphates to elicit biological activity. Deoxycytidine kinase (dCyd kinase) catalyzes the initial and generally rate-limiting step in the phosphorylation of several drugs used or under development in leukemia: arabinosylcytosine (ara-C), fludarabine (F-ara-A),

Departments of Medical Oncology and Hematology, University of Texas MD Anderson Cancer Center, 1515 Holcombe Boulevard, Houston, Texas 77030 USA
* Supported by grant CA32839 from the National Cancer Institute, DHHS.

2-chloro-2'-deoxyadenosine (CldAdo), 2'-deoxy-5-azacytidine, arabinosyl-5-azacytosine, deoxycoformycin, 2', 2'-difluoro-deoxycytidine (dFdC). Therefore, additional investigations of the regulation of dCyd kinase are required to understand its role in nucleoside metabolism and to optimize the design of clinical protocols for combination chemotherapy using these analogues. We can expect that the recent molecular cloning and expression of the human enzyme will provide reagents that will greatly enhance present efforts to understand the activity and regulation of this enzyme [1].

In vitro assays of dCyd kinase demonstrated that its activity is subject to inhibitory feedback regulation by dCTP [2]. dCTP is of additional significance to the action of ara-C and dFdC because the respective 5'-triphosphates, ara-CTP [3] and dFdCTP [4], compete with dCTP in the inhibition of DNA polymerase and for incorporation into DNA. We sought to define the regulation of dCyd kinase in terms of the concentration of physiological ribo- and deoxynucleotides present in intact cells, to understand the inhibitory role of ara-CTP previously described in cell free extracts, and to identify the role of F-ara-ATP on the activity of this enzyme [5–7]. The regulated nature of dCyd kinase is not maintained in cell extracts which have traditionally been used to quantitate enzyme activity [5].

Because F-ara-A 5'-triphosphate (F-ara-ATP) inhibits ribonucleotide reductase [8] and therefore dNTP levels, we hypothesized that the activity of dCyd kinase could be modulated in cells treated with F-ara-A

253

[6, 7]. Ara-C was used at saturating concentrations as a clinically relevant alternative substrate for dCyd kinase because dCyd would raise cellular dCTP levels and inhibit the enzyme. The rate of ara-CTP accumulation was maximal in K562 cells with 10 μM ara-C (35 μM/h). However, cells preloaded with F-ara-ATP exhibited a three fold increase in the rate of ara-CTP accumulation, a modulation that resulted in cellular ara-CTP levels of >400 μM after 5 h. This stimulation was proportional to the cellular concentration of F-ara-ATP, achieving a maximal effect between 75 and 100 μM.

To analyze whether the stimulation of ara-CTP accumulation is cell cycle specific, exponentially growing K562 cells were fractionated into G_1-, S-, and G_2+M phase-enriched subpopulations by centrifugal elutriation. The rates of ara-CTP accumulation after incubation with F-ara-A were similar among these three phases, indicating that the stimulation of ara-C metabolism occurs in all phases of cell cycle [9]. Consistent with this, stimulation of ara-CTP synthesis was also observed when lymphocytes isolated from patients with chronic lymphocytic leukemia were studied before and after fludarabine phosphate therapy [10]. A strong relationship was observed between the cellular concentration of F-ara-ATP at the beginning of the ara-C incubation and the subsequent potentiation of ara-CTP accumulation. These studies strongly suggest that a protocol designed to administer fludarabine phosphate prior to ara-C infusion will augment ara-CTP accumulation by leukemia cells by biochemical modulation of dCyd kinase.

Biological Modulation

Although ara-C is the most effective agent in the treatment of myelogenous leukemia, the scope of its activity is limited by the fact that it is a cell cycle-specific drug. As such, it kills only those cells that are synthesizing DNA when cellular ara-CTP concentrations are at toxic levels. The portion of the leukemic population with self-renewal capacity that is cycling is high on a percentage basis [11, 12]. However, if only 1 % of the initial leukemic burden with progenitor capacity were quiescent, this might constitute 10^6–10^8 cells. This kinetically insensitive population could escape ara-C action and eventually expand to cause a relapse. One approach to such kinetic resistance is to stimulate this population into cycle prior to ara-C therapy.

Several recombinant human growth factors now available for clinical evaluation are capable of stimulating leukemic cell proliferation in vitro. In particular, GM-CSF increased the S phase fraction and induced proliferation of clonogenic leukemia cells in vitro from patients with AML and CML blast crisis [13]. Consistent with this, GM-CSF-treated myeloblasts showed increased sensitivity to ara-C [14]. In vitro incubation with GM-CSF did not affect ara-CTP accumulation in myeloblasts, but decreased it in normal marrow mononuclear cells [15], suggesting a pharmacologic basic for selectivity. We have demonstrated that after 3 days of clinical treatment with GM-CSF (125 μg/m² per day x 7 days, preceding ara-C/daunorubicin chemotherapy), the accumulation of myeloblasts in blood of patients with untreated AML was increased as was the ability of myeloblasts to accumulate ara-CTP ex vivo [16].

Nevertheless, in vitro studies are limited in their ability to reproduce actual concentrations, the pharmacokinetics of drugs and bilogics experienced by target cells in vivo, the lack of physical and chemical interactions among cells, and the consequences of the physical disruption of tissue architecture. These factors compromise our ability to determine actual effect of GM-CSF on ara-CTP metabolism. Therefore, we have designed a protocol for higher-risk patients specifically to determine ara-CTP pharmacokinetics in circulating blasts before and after GM-CSF administration. In this treatment, patients receive ara-C (1 g/m² over 2 h) and the pharmacology of ara-CTP in circulating leukemia cells is studied. GM-CSF (125 μg/m²) is administered daily for 3 days, followed by another dose of ara-C. The area under the accumulation and elimination curves of ara-CTP in circulating myeloblasts before and after GM-CSF administration is then compared. Results seen after the first three patients studied have not supported the hypothesis that

GM-CSF would augment ara-CTP metabolism. Nevertheless, it will be important to determine whether clonogenic cells are sensitized to ara-C by GM-CSF treatment. Together, these studies should provide an indication of the pharmacodynamic impact of GM-CSF on leukemic cell growth.

Pharmacologic Determinants of Response

A major tenet in clinical pharmacology is that a knowledge of the pharmacokinetics of the active drug species and its pharmacodynamic actions in the target cell will be valuable in understanding the effects of the drug, in predicting clinical outcome, and for optimizing drug administration for populations or individuals. Cancer chemotherapists have rarely had the opportunity to evaluate these parameters because of the necessity for invasive measures to approach tumors responsive to therapy and, to a lesser extent, the lack of sensitive assays for appropriate drug metabolites. Ara-C is a notable exception in that relatively noninvasive procedures are required to obtain leukemia cells for pharmacokinetic sampling, and its 5'-triphosphate ara-CTP is readily quantitated after extraction from leukemia cells. Investigations of the pharmacologic determinants of response of acute leukemia to ara-C therapy have resulted in new knowledge with respect to correlations between these parameters and clinical response, evaluation of hypotheses designed to optimize both intermittent and continuous infusion dose rates, and for the design of combination protocols [17].

Difluorodeoxycytidine is a new nucleoside antimetabolite that differs from deoxycytidine and ara-C by the presence of geminal fluorines at the 2' position of the carbohydrate moiety [18]. Its metabolism is qualitatively similar to ara-C, and its action is characterized by a specific inhibition of DNA synthesis, which is dependent upon the cellular accumulation of dFdC nucleotides. dCyd kinase is also required for phosphorylation of dFdC to the monophosphate. The 5'-triphosphate dFdCTP is the major nucleotide derivative of dFdC; its cellular concentration appears to be in a constant ratio with the mono- and diphosphates. dFdCTP is incorporated into DNA, although its molecular pattern of inhibition appears to differ from that of ara-C and F-ara-A [4]. dFdC 5'-diphosphate inhibits ribonucleotide reductase and decreases cellular deoxynucleotide pools in a concentration-dependent manner [19, 20]. The decrease in cellular dCTP may lead to self-potentiation of dFdC metabolism by modulation of dCyd kinase activity and of its competition for incorporation into DNA.

Clinically, we have demonstrated other parallels of dFdC with ara-C. Our phase I trial of dFdC in patients with solid tumors indicated that accumulation of dFdCTP by mononuclear cells is saturated by dose rates (225–350 mg/m^2 per 30 min) that achieve 15–20 μM dFdC in plasma [20].

Saturation kinetics had previously been demonstrated for the formation of ara-CTP in circulating leukemia cells during high-dose ara-C therapy [21]. We therefore postulate that understanding the relationship of the dFdC concentration in plasma to the rate of dFdCTP accumulation by leukemia cells will be an important factor for designing the dFdC dose schedule. Similarly, knowledge of the pharmacodynamics of this treatment on DNA synthesis and cellular deoxynucleotides will be critical to understanding the action of dFdC.

Programmed Cell Death

It is now recognized that the death of numerous cell and tissue types in response to diverse stimuli is characterized by a distinct pattern called apoptosis, or programmed cell death (PCD) [22]. This is distinguished from necrosis on both morphologic and biochemical grounds. The hallmarks of PCD include distinctive morphologic changes in nucleus and cytoplasm along with cleavage of chromatin at regularly spaced sites. During PCD, the selective action of an endogenous endonuclease produces double-strand DNA cleavage at integer multiples of about 190 base pairs [23]. This endogenous degradation of chromatin is apparently induced by a Ca^{2+}/Mg^{2+}-dependent endonuclease that cuts the DNA in exposed linker regions between nucleosomes. This activity, detected as characteristic structured DNA banding ladders by gel analysis, is an early event in PCD that occurs within a few hours of the appropriate stimulus, preceding the loss of dye exclusion capabilities.

Programmed cell death occurs in lymphoid cells following deprivation of growth factors, after addition of physiologic regulatory hormones (e. g., glucocorticoids), in response to attacks by cytotoxic T lymphocytes and natural killer cells, and after exposure to radiation. Recent results demonstrate DNA fragmentation to nucleosomal multimers in cells treated with topoisomerase-active drugs [24], cisplatin [25], and ara-C [26].

Recently, remarkable clinical activity has been demonstrated for fludarabine phosphate in chronic lymphocytic leukemia [27] and for 2-chlorodeoxyadenosine in hairy cell leukemia [28] and chronic lymphocytic leukemia [29], but it has been difficult to discern mechanisms by which these ostensibly cell cycle-active drugs act in indolent lymphocytic diseases. F-ara-A and CldAdo are nucleoside analogues that inhibit ribonucleotide reductase and are incorporated into DNA. There are, however, indications that these drugs may activate a PCD response in quiescent lymphoid cells. Thus, quiescent lymphocytes treated with CldAdo show an increase in ADP ribosylation accompanied by decreases in cellular NAD+ and ATP [30]. These activities are associated with DNA strand breaks detected by alkaline elution and by gel electrophoresis. Thus, promising leads have been developed that should be pursued in the lymphocytes of patients treated with fludarabine and CldAdo.

References

1. Chottiner EG, Shewach DS, Datta NS et al. (1991) Cloning and expression of human deoxycytidine kinase cDNA. Proc Natl Acad Sci USA 88: 1531–1535
2. Kim M-Y, Ives DH (1989) Human deoxycytidine kinase: kinetic mechanism and end product regulation. Biochemistry 28: 9043–9047
3. Furth JJ, Cohen SS (1968) Inhibition of mammalian DNA polymerase by the 5'- triphosphate of 1-β-D-arabinofuranosylcytosine and the 5'-triphosphate of 9-β-D-arabinofuranosyladenine. Cancer Res 28: 2061–2067
4. Huang P, Chubb S, Hertel L et al. (1990) Mechanism of action of 2',2'-difluorodeoxycytidine triphosphate on DNA synthesis. Proc Am Assoc Cancer Res 31: 426
5. Liliemark JO, Plunkett W (1986) Regulation of 1-β-D-arabinofuranosylcytosine 5'-triphosphate accumulation in human leukemia cells by deoxycytidine 5'-triphosphate. Cancer Res 46: 1079–1083
6. Gandhi V, Plunkett W (1988) Modulation of arabinosylnucleoside metabolism by arabinosylnucleotides in human leukemia cells. Cancer Res 48: 329–334
7. Gandhi V, Plunkett W (1989) Interaction of arabinosylnucleotides in K562 human leukemia cells. Biochem Pharmacol 38: 3551–3559
8. Tseng W-C, Derse D, Cheng Y-c et al. (1982) In vitro biological activity of 9-β-D-arabinofuranosyl-2-fluoroadenine and the biochemical actions of its triphosphate on DNA polymerase and ribonucleotide reductase from HeLa cells. Cancer Res 42: 2260–2264
9. Gandhi V, Plunkett W (1990) Cell cycle-dependent metabolism of arabinosylnucleosides in K562 human leukemia cells. Proc Am Assoc Cancer Res 31: 345
10. Gandhi V, Nowak B, Keating MJ et al. (1989) Modulation of arabinosylcytosine metabolism by arabinosyl-2-fluoroadenine in lymphocytes from patients with chronic lymphocytic leukemia: implication for combination therapy. Blood 74: 2070–2075
11. Clarkson B, Srife A, Freid J et al. (1970) Studies of cellular proliferation in human leukemia. Cancer 26: 1–19
12. Minden MD, Till JE, McCulloch EA (1978) Proliferative state of blast cell progenitors in acute myeloblastic leukemia (AML). Blood 52: 592–600
13. Griffin JD, Young D, Herrmann F et al. (1986) Effects of recombinant human GM-CSF on proliferation of clonogenic cells in acute myeloblastic leukemia. Blood 67: 1448–1453
14. Cannistra S, Groshek P, Griffin JD (1989) Granulocyte macrophage colony stimulating factor enhances the cytotoxic effects of cytosine arabinoside in acute myeloblastic leukemia and the myeloid blast crisis phase of chronic myelogenous leukemia. Leukemia 3: 328–334
15. Bhalla K, Birkhofer M, Arlin Z et al. (1988) Effect of recombinant GM-CSF on the metabolism of cytosine arabinoside in normal and

leukemic human bone marrow cells. Leukemia 2: 810–813

16. Estey E, Kantarjian H, Keating MJ et al. (1990) Use of GM-CSF prior to chemotherapy of AML: effects on circulating blast incorporation and ara-CTP formation. Blood 76 [Suppl 1]: 142 a

17. Plunkett W, Gandhi V, Grunewald R et al. (1990) Pharmacologically directed design of AML therapy. In: Gale RP (ed) Acute myelogenous leukemia: progress and controversies. Wiley/Liss, New York, pp 481–492

18. Plunkett W, Gandhi V, Chubb S et al. (1989) 2',2'-Difluorodeoxycytidine metabolism and mechanism of action in human leukemia cells. Nucleosides Nucleotides 8: 775–785.

19. Heinemann V, Xu Y-Z, Chubb S et al. (1990) Inhibition of ribonucleotide reduction in CCRF-CEM cells by 2',2'-difluorodeoxycytidine. Mol Pharmacol 38: 567–582

20. Grunewald R, Kantarjian H, Keating MJ et al. (1990) Pharmacologically directed design of the dose rate and schedule of 2',2'-difluorodeoxycytidine (Gemcitabine) administration in leukemia. Cancer Res 50: 6823–6826

21. Plunkett W, Liliemark JO, Adams TM et al. (1987) Saturation of 1-β-D-arabinofuranosylcytosine 5'-triphosphate accumulation in leukemia cells during high-dose 1-β-D-arabinofuranosylcytosine therapy. Cancer Res 47: 3005–3011

22. Wyllie AH, Kerr JFR, Currie AR (1986) Cell death: the significance of apoptosis. Int Rev Cytol 68: 755–785

23. Arends MJ, Morris RG, Wyllie AH (1990) Apoptosis. The role of the endonuclease. Am J Pathol 136: 593–608

24. Kaufmann SH (1989) Induction of endonucleolytic DNA cleavage in human acute myelogenous leukemia cells by etoposide, camptothecin, and other cytotoxic anticancer drugs: a cautionary note. Cancer Res 49: 5870–5878

25. Sorenson CM, Barry MA, Eastman A (1990) Analysis of events associated with cell cycle arrest at G_2 phase and cell death induced by cisplatin. J Natl Cancer Inst 82: 749

26. Gunji H, Kharbanda S, Kufe D (1991) Induction of internucleosomal DNA fragmentation in human myeloid cells by 1-β-D-arabinofuranosylcytosine. Cancer Res 51: 741–743

27. Keating MJ, Kantarjian H, Talpaz M et al. (1989) Fludarabine: a new agent with major activity against chronic lymphocytic leukemia. Blood 74: 19–25

28. Piro LD, Carrera CJ, Carson DA et al. (1990) Lasting remissions in hairy-cell leukemia induced by a single infusion of 2-chlorodeoxyadenosine. N Engl J Med 322: 1117–1121

29. Piro LD, Carrera CJ, Beutler E et al. (1988) 2-Chlorodeoxyadenosine: an effective new agent for the treatment of chronic lymphocytic leukemia. Blood 72: 1069–1073

30. Seto S, Carrera CJ, Kubota M et al. (1985) Mechanism of deoxyadenosine and 2-chlorodeoxyadenosine toxicity to nondividing human lymphocytes. J. Clin Invest 75: 377–382

Biochemical Basis for Combination Chemotherapy*

V. Gandhi, E. Estey, M. J. Keating, and W. Plunkett

Multiple drug treatment of malignant diseases has resulted in an increased frequency of response to chemotherapy and prolongation of disease-free survival. Combination drug therapy would ideally use the optimal schedule and doses of drugs for reinforcement of the therapeutic efficacy of one or more of the agents. Since combinations of chemotherapeutic drugs are necessary to potentially cure established cancers, it is rational to use drugs that interact via biochemical modulation to enhance the cell kill and thus to increase the cure rate [1]. We studied the combination of 9-β-D arabinofuranosylcytosine (ara-C) and 1-β-D-arabinofuranosyl-2-fluoroadenine (F-ara-A) to establish a biochemical basis for combination chemotherapy.

Ara-C is a deoxycytidine analogue effective in the treatment of adult acute leukemias. This is a prodrug and has to be phosphorylated to its triphosphate to exert cytotoxicity. The initial and rate-limiting step in the synthesis of the triphosphate (ara-CTP) is the phosphorylation of ara-C to its monophosphate. This step is catalyzed by deoxycytidine kinase, the activity of which is regulated by deoxynucleotides (dNTP), specifically dCTP. Because dCTP inhibits deoxycytidine kinase and consequently phosphorylation of ara-C, agents which can deplete or reduce deoxynucleotides might be expected to potentiate the metabolism of ara-C.

F-ara-A, an adenosine analogue that is also phosphorylated by deoxycytidine kinase, accumulates as its cytotoxic 5'-triphosphate, F-ara-ATP. Unlike ara-C, F-ara-A potentiates its own phosphorylation by lowering cellular deoxynucleotide pools. F-ara-ATP inhibits ribonucleotide reductase, and thereby blocks the de novo synthesis of deoxynucleotides. These actions support a biochemical rationale for combining F-ara-A and ara-C to modulate the metabolism of ara-C to achieve higher accumulation of ara-CTP.

Initial studies were conducted in K562 human leukemia cells. The cells were incubated with 100 μM F-ara-A for 3 h, washed, and incubated with 10 μM ara-C. The incubation with F-ara-A allowed these cells to accumulate F-ara-ATP and to decrease dNTP pools. Consistent with the hypothesis, the rate of ara-CTP accumulation (an indication of deoxycytidine kinase activity) increased threefold in K562 cells [2]. A similar level of potentiation was observed in another leukemia cell line, L1210 (Fig. 1). Further investigations in K562 cells demonstrated a relationship between F-ara-ATP and potentiation of ara-CTP accumulation. The magnitude of the stimulation of ara-C phosphorylation was dependent on the cellular concentrations of F-ara-ATP up to 75–100 μM, at which point no further increase in ara-CTP accumulation was seen (Fig. 2).

Department of Medical Oncology, University of Texas MD Anderson Cancer Center, 1515 Holcombe Boulevard, Houston, TX 77030, USA
* Research from the authors' laboratory was supported in part by Grants CA28596, CA32839, and CA53311 from the National Cancer Institute, DHHS, and Grant CH-130 from the American Cancer Society.

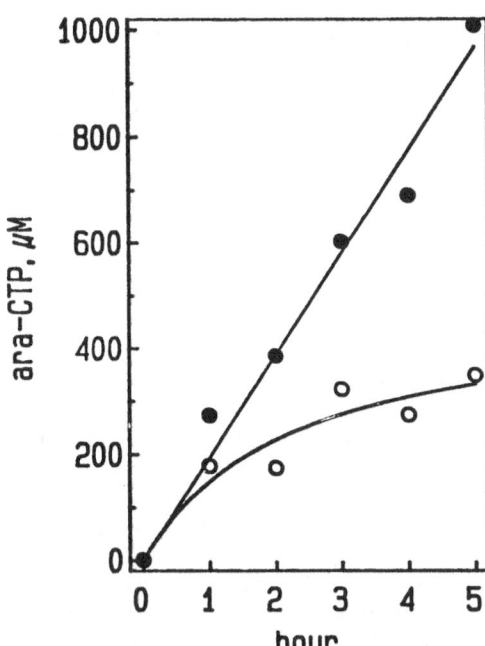

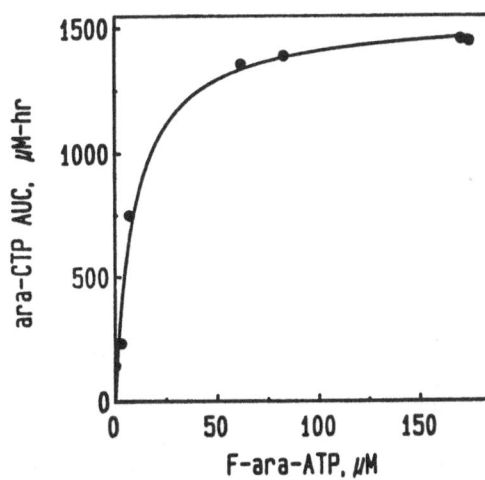

Fig. 2. Relationship between the cellular F-ara-ATP concentration and ara-CTP accumulation. K562 cells were incubated with 300 μM F-ara-A for 2.5 h to accumulate F-ara-ATP, and then washed into drug-free medium. At 0, 1, 2, 3, 12, and 18 h later, one portion of the culture was removed to determine the cellular concentration of F-ara-ATP, and ara-C (10 μM) was added to a second portion. The cellular concentration of ara-CTP was determined after 3 h. That value is plotted against the concentration of F-ara-ATP in the cells when ara-C was added

Fig. 1. Effect of F-ara-A incubations on ara-CTP accumulation in L1210 cells. The cells were incubated without *(open symbols)* or with 100 μM F-ara-A *(solid symbols)* for 3 h, washed in drug-free medium, and incubated with 10 μM ara-C. Aliquots are taken every hour up to 6 h, perchloric acid extracted, and levels of ara-CTP quantitated by HPLC assays

To understand the mechanistic basis for the potentiation of ara-CTP accumulation by F-ara-A, the rate of ara-C phosphorylation by K562 cell extracts was compared in different settings. The rate of ara-C phosphorylation in the reaction mixture that contained physiological concentrations of deoxynucleotides was less than the rate in those reactions that had lower deoxynucleotide levels observed in cells after F-ara-A treatment [2]. Interestingly, addition of 200 μM F-ara-ATP to the kinase reaction also stimulated ara-C phosphorylation. These results indicate that there may be a direct effect of F-ara-ATP on deoxycytidine kinase. F-ara-ATP-mediated inhibition of ribonucleotide reductase and lowering of deoxynucleotides suggest an indirect effect of F-ara-ATP on deoxycytidine kinase.

These observations were extended to fresh human lymphocytes isolated from patients with chronic lymphocytic leuke-

mia. Cells were incubated with ara-C either after in vitro F-ara-A treatment or after a therapeutic infusion of fludarabine phosphate [3]. A twofold incerase in the rate of ara-CTP accumulation was observed in the cells of 23 patients. Because of the indolent nature of this disease and the fact that leukemic lymphocytes have undetectable levels of deoxynucleotides, a direct effect of F-ara-ATP on the activity of deoxycytidine kinase measured as ara-CTP accumulation must be considered the leading hypothesis to explain this augmentation of ara-CTP metabolism. Furthermore, the modulatory effect of F-ara-ATP on ara-C metabolism is not limited to this analogue, but rather can be extended to other analogues phosphorylated by deoxycytidine kinase, such as 2-chlorodeoxyadenosine, 2'-deoxy-5-azacytidine, 2', 3'-dideoxycytidine, fazarabine, and 2', 2'-difluorodeoxycytidine [4].

Studies have indicated that the level and retention of ara-CTP in human leukemia

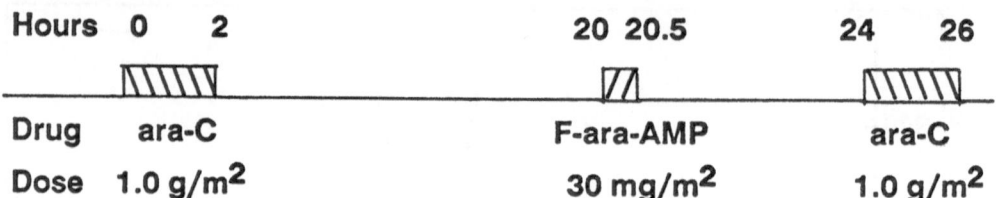

Fig. 3. First cycle of the treatment plan

cells in vitro [5] or during therapy [6, 7] are directly related to clinical response. This prompted us to design a protocol based on previous clinical, biochemical, and pharmacologic studies to test the modulation of ara-C metabolism by fludarabine phosphate in patients with AML in relapse. The first cycle of the treatment plan (Fig. 3) includes two doses of $1.0\,\mathrm{g/m^2}$ ara-C and one dose of 30 $\mathrm{mg/m^2}$ fludarabine phosphate (F-ara-AMP). The subsequent four cycles include one dose of fludarabine phosphate followed by one dose of ara-C. In the first cycle ara-C is given twice, before and after fludarabine phosphate, to permit comparison of the rate of accumulation of ara-CTP when ara-C is infused without prior treatment or after fludarabine phosphate. Thus, each patient served as his or her own "control" with respect to the effect of cellular F-ara-ATP on ara-CTP accumulation. The dose rate of ara-C, 0.5 $\mathrm{g/m^2}$ per hour (intermediate dose ara-C) [8–10], produced ara-CTP accumulation rates similar to those observed after high-dose ara-C therapy (3 # $\mathrm{g/m^2}$ over 2 h) in the same patients. These observations suggested that dCK was saturated at plasma ara-C levels ($>7\,\mu M$) [8] achieved with ara-C doses of 0.5 $\mathrm{g/m^2}$ per hour. Thus, the lower dose has the potential of producing equivalent responses, but with less toxicity. Ara-CTP concentrations 20 h after ara-C infusions are low [6, 7] and thus are unlikely to interfere with the metabolism of fludarabine phosphate infused at that time. This directed us to schedule the fludarabine phosphate infusion 20 h after the start of the ara-C infusion. Previous clinical studies using fludarabine phosphate at a dose rate of 25–30 $\mathrm{mg/m^2}$ per day for patients with CLL resulted in $>50\%$ response [11]. Since this dose is well tolerated by patients, we selected 30 $\mathrm{mg/m^2}$ per day of fludarabine phosphate for the present protocol. At this dose (25–30 $\mathrm{mg/m^2}$ per day), F-ara-ATP peaked within 4 h in CLL lymphocytes [12]. Our previous studies using human leukemia cells indicated that the augmentation of ara-CTP accumulation is directly related to the cellular concentration of F-ara-ATP. Therefore, ara-C infusions given 4 h after fludarabine phosphate infusions should optimize the conditions for ara-CTP modulation. Based on these studies, the protocol was designed to administer fludarabine phosphate 20 h after the first ara-C infusion; the second ara-C dose was given 4 h after fludarabine phosphate.

In vivo pharmacology of ara-C in plasma and ara-CTP in leukemic blasts from a patient with relapsed acute leukemia was analyzed to test the hypothesis that fludarabine infusion would enhance the metabolism of ara-CTP. The initial and linear rate of ara-CTP accumulation (0–2 h after start of ara-C infusion) was 189 $\mu M/h$ and 389 $\mu M/h$ during dose one and dose two of ara-C, respectively. The area under the concentration times time curve (AUC) was similarly increased by 1.8-fold during the second dose of ara-C. There was no significant difference in the rate of elimination of ara-CTP during these doses (1.9 h, first dose; 2.2 h, second dose), suggesting that the increase in ara-CTP AUC was due to potentiation of ara-C anabolism. Plasma pharmacology of ara-C and its deaminated metabolite, ara-U, remained similar during these doses. Consistent with our prediction, the concentration of ara-CTP 24 h after the first infusion was low (7 μM). As observed in the leukemic lymphocytes, the F-ara-ATP peaked 4 h after F-ara-A infusion to 28 μM.

These data clearly document that experimental strategies to potentiate ara-CTP accumulation have provided a basis for optimal combination sequence, schedule, and doses for the design of new protocols. Furthermore, protocols formulated on the basis of experimental, pharmacologic, and biochemical studies could be tested in a clinical setting.

References

1. Damon LE, Cadman EC (1988) The metabolic basis for combination chemotherapy. Pharmacol Ther 38: 73–127
2. Gandhi V, Plunkett W (1988) Modulation of arabionosylnucleoside metabolism by arabinosylnucleotides in human leukemia cells. Cancer Res 48: 329–334
3. Gandhi V, Nowak, B, Keating MJ, Plunkett W (1989) Modulation of arabinosylcytosine metabolism by arabinosyl-2-fluoroadenine in lymphocytes from patients with chronic lymphocytic leukemia: implications for combination therapy. Blood 74: 2070–2075
4. Gandhi V, Plunkett W (1990) Modulatory activity of 2', 2'-difluorodeoxycytidine on the phosphorylation and cytotoxicity of arabinosyl nucleosides. Cancer Res 50: 3675–3680
5. Preisler HD, Rustum Y, Priore R (1985) Relationship between leukemic cell metabolism of cytosine arabinoside and the outcome of chemotherapy for acute myelocytic leukemia. Eur J Cancer Clin Oncol 20: 1061–1066
6. Plunkett W, Iacoboni S, Estey E, Danhauser L, Liliemark JO, Keating MJ (1985) Pharmacologically directed ara-C therapy for refractory leukemia. Semin Oncol 12 [Suppl]: 20–30
7. Kantarjian HM, Estey EH, Plunkett W, Keating MJ, Walters RS, Iacoboni S, McCredie KB, Freireich EJ (1986) Phase I–II clinical and pharmacologic studies of high-dose cytosine arabinoside in refractory leukemia. Am J Med 81: 387–394
8. Plunkett W, Liliemark JO, Adams TM, Nowak B, Estey E, Kantarjian H, Keating MJ (1987) Saturation of 1-β-D-arabinosylcytosine 5'-triphosphate accumulation in leukemia cells during high-dose 1-β-D-arabinosylcytosine therapy. Cancer Res 47: 3005–3011
9. Estey E, Plunkett W, Keating MJ, McCredie KB, Freireich EJ (1988) Cytosine arabinoside (ara-C) in intermediate doses (IDAC) as therapy for patients (Pts) with acute myeloid leukemia (AML). Proc Am Assoc Cancer Res 29: 209
10. Plunkett W, Gandhi V, Grunewald H, Heinemann V, Estey E, Keating M (1990) Pharmacologically directed design of AML therapy. In: Gale RP (ed) Acute myelogenous leukemia: progress and controversies. Wiley/Liss, New York, pp 481–492
11. Keating MJ, Kantarjian H, O-Brien S, Koller C, Talpaz M, Schachner J, Childs CC, Freireich EJ, McCredie KB (1991) Fludarabine: a new agent with marked cytoreductive activity in untreated chronic lymphocytic leukemia. J Clin Oncol 9: 44–49
12. Danhauser L, Plunkett W, Keating MJ, Cabanillas F (1986) 9-β-D-arabinofuranosyl-2-fluoroadenine 5'-monophosphate pharmacokinetics in plasma and tumor cells of patients with relapsed leukemia and lymphoma. Cancer Chemother Pharmacol 18: 145–152

Interaction of Cytosine Arabinoside Accumulation and Cytosine Arabinoside Triphosphate Formation with Various Cytotoxic Drugs

G. Ehninger, B. Proksch, T. Wanner, H. Schmidt, E. Hallmen, E. Schleyer, K. Jaschonek, and W. Hiddemann

Introduction

Cytosine Arabinoside (ara-C) has proven to be one of the most active antileukemic agents although its optimal mode of administration and dosage are still controversial [1]. The antileukemic activity of ara-C requires its cellular uptake and the intracellular conversion to the active compound ara-C-triphosphate. At plasma concentrations below 5 µmol/l, transmembrane transport occurs by facilitated diffusion via a nucleoside carrier system. At higher plasma concentrations, which are reached during intermediate- to high-dose therapy, ara-C enters the cell by passive diffusion [2, 3]. The cytotoxicity of ara-CTP is mediated by the inhibtion of DNA polymerase and incorporation of ara-CTP into DNA. The cytotoxicity in tumor cells is well correlated with intracellular ara-CTP concentration and the amount incorporated into DNA [3–11]. The intracellular pool of active drug is decreased by an efflux of the parent compound and through deamination to the less toxic ara-U. Usually ara-C is used in combination chemotherapy. Less is known about the influence of various commonly used cytotoxic drugs on the accumulation and intracellular phosphorylation of ara-C. Our study was initiated to further explore this question.

Medizinische Universitätsklinik und Kinderklinik der Universität, Otfried-Müller-Str. 10, 7400 Tübingen, FRG

Methods

Blast cells from 16 patients with acute leukemia, predominantly at diagnosis, 2 with lymphoid, 13 with myeloid differentiation, 1 with a B-cell lymphoma in leukemic phase, were separated for our in vitro study. An assay for ara-C influx studies was developed. Tritium-labeled ara-C was used. [^{14}C] Sucrose was employed as a second radioactive compound as a marker for the extracellular space. After centrifugation, the uptake was calculated with channel counting, in the supernatant and cell pellet. Intracellular ara-CTP formation was measured by use of a high-performance liquid (HPLC) method developed by Schleyer [12]. Influx of ara-C into leukemic blast cells was determined without and with preincubation with various cytotoxic drugs. Results were compared by Student's two-tailed t test for paired observations. The drug concentrations used were taken from the literature and represent drug levels in the early distribution phase. Different concentrations were used when a compound was also administered in high-dose protocols.

Results

Figure 1 shows the ara-C influx at an extracellular concentration of 1 µmol ara-C. After incubation with ara-C alone, intracellular concentrations of 101 ± 64 pmol/million cells were measured. Doxorubicin, daunomycin, and mitoxantrone lowered the ara-C accumulation to 90 %. Asparagi-

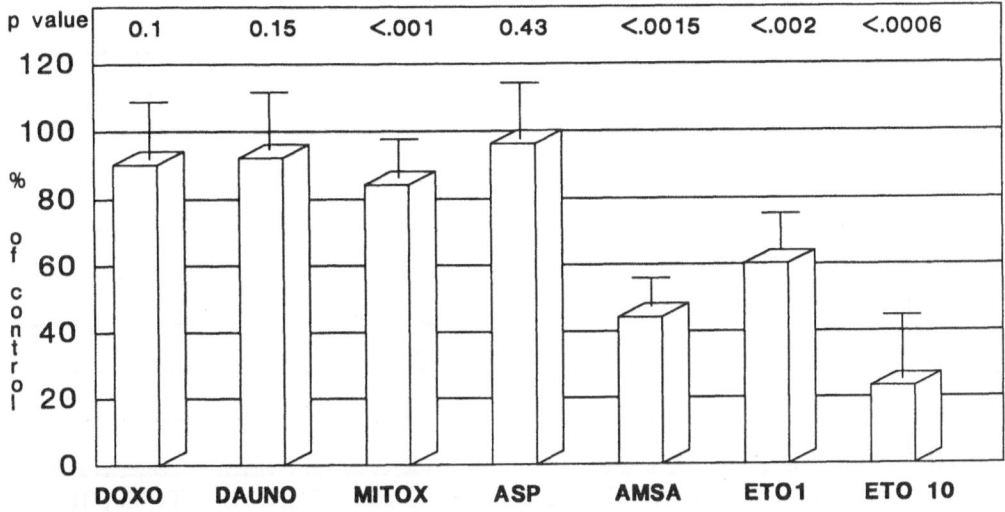

Fig. 1. Influence of various cytotoxic drugs on the accumulation of ara-C at an extracellular level of 1 μmol/l. Data are expressed a percentages of control. Uptake of control: 101 ± pmol ara-C/10^6 cells (n = 13). *ASP*, asparaginase; *DNR*, daunorubicin; *DOXO*, doxorubicin; *MXN*, mitoxantrone; *ETO 1*, etoposide 1 μg/ml; *ETO 10*, etoposide 10 μg/ml; *AMSA*, amsacrine

nase had no influence on uptake. In contrast, amsacrine and etoposide 1 μg/ml lowered uptake to about 50% that of controls. Higher etoposide concentrations of 10 μg/ml further inhibited ara-C uptake. These changes were highly significant.

Figure 2 shows the ara-C influx at an extracellular concentration of 10 μmol ara-C. After incubation with ara-C alone intracellular concentrations in controls were fivefold higher than at the lower ara-C concentration. Intracellular ara-C concen-

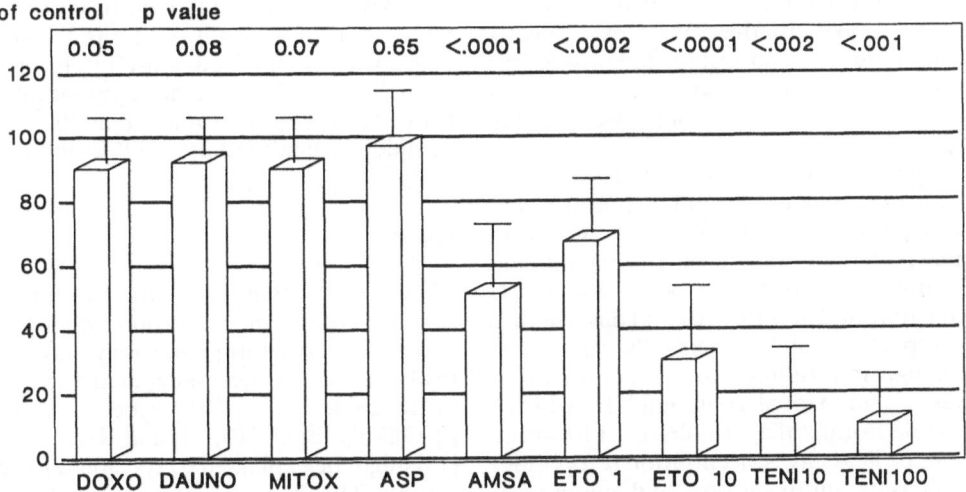

Fig. 2. Influence of various cytotoxic drugs on the accumulation of ara-C at an extracellular level of 10 μmo. Data are expressed as percentages of control. Uptake of control: 558 ± ?96 pmol ara-C/10^6 cells (n = 16) *ASP*, asparaginase; *DNR*, daunorubicin; *DOXO*, doxorubicin; *MXN*, mitoxantrone; *ETO 1*, etoposide 1 μg/ml; *ETO 10*, etoposide 10 μg/ml; *AMSA*, amsacrine

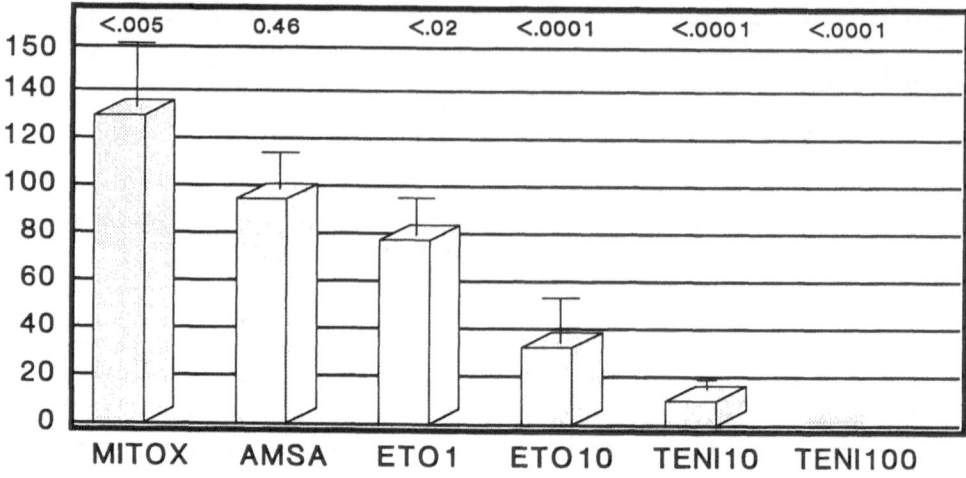

Fig. 3. Influence of various cytotoxic drugs on the formation of ara-CTP at an extracellular ara-C level of 10 µmol/l. Data are expressed as percentages of control. Uptake of control: 15 ± 8 ng ara-CTP/10^6 cells (n = 15). *MITOX*, mitoxantrone; *ETO 1*, etoposide 1µg/ml; *ETO 10*, etoposide 10 µg/ml; *AMSA*, amsacrine; *TENI 10*, teniposide 10 µg/ml; *TENI 100*, teniposide 100 µg/ml

trations of 550 ± 300 pmol/million cells were measured. Again, doxorubicin, daunomycin, and mitoxantrone lowered the ara-C concentration to 90 %. Asparaginase had no influence on uptake. Amsacrine and etoposide 1 µg/ml lowered uptake to about 50 % that of controls. Higher etoposide concentrations of 10 µg/ml further inhibited ara-C uptake. In this set of experiments teniposide was also tested. Teniposide was more potent than etoposide at decreasing ara-C uptake. These changes were highly significant.

Figure 3 shows the intracellular ara-CTP formation at an extracellular concentration of 10 µmol ara-C. At high ara-C concentrations, an impairment of transmembrane transport may not necessarily slow ara-C metabolism. Therefore, to find out whether transport was at least partially rate determining, intracellular ara-CTP formation was measured for all compounds for which a decrease of uptake was observed for more than 10 % at any concentration (etoposide, teniposide, mitoxantrone, and amsacrine). After incubation with ara-C alone, intracellular ara-CTP concentrations of 15 ± 8 ng/million cells were measured. Mitoxantrone increased the ara-CTP formation de-

spite slightly decreasing ara-C uptake. Amsacrine, which also lowered uptake, did not alter ara-CTP formation. This might be explained by the fact that mitoxantrone and amsacrine also inhibited catabolic pathways of ara-C and ara-CTP, for example of the deaminases. A quantity of 1 µg/ml etoposide lowered ara-CTP concentrations to 80 % that of controls whereas a higher concentration lowered ara-CTP levels to 30 %. Teniposide was a more potent inhibitor of ara-CTP formation and at 100 µg/ml completely inhibited ara-CTP formation.

Discussion

We are aware that, in addition to interactions on uptake and activation, other pharmacodynamic determinants may play a critical role. A sequence-dependent synergism of etoposide and ara-C described previously by Ohkubo et al. [13, 14] and Rivera et al. [15] might be explained by specific cell cycle activity. The sequence etoposide 6 h prior ara-C$_w$W was the most active combination. No activity was observed after simultaneous administration. This might be explained by our data and a decrease of

DNA synthesis by ara-C. This effects lasts for some hours, in which cells may remain in an etoposide-insensitive stage. An Australian group recently published a randomized investigation comparing etoposide added to daunorubicin and continuously administered ara-C [16]. A significantly improved remission duration but not survival was seen in a subgroup of patients. On the basis of our data and the animal studies described this result might have been less than optimal. Some leukemic cells might have been in an etoposide-insensitive stage and ara-C uptake and ara-CTP formation would have been decreased.

These data emphasize the need for thorough preclinical evaluations on possible interactions between cytotoxic agents. The present data may already justify the recommendation that the administration of etoposide and teniposide should not immediately precede or accompany ara-C administration in clinical trials.

References

1. Peters WG, Colly LP, Willemze R (1988) High-dose cytosine arabinoside: pharmacological and clinical aspects. Blut 56: 1–11
2. Wiley JS, Taupin J, Jamieson GP, Snook M, Sawyer WH, Finch LR (1985) Cytosine arabinoside transport and metabolism in acute leukemias and T cell lymphoblastic lymphoma. J Clin Invest 75: 632–422
3. Katarjian H, Estey EH, Plunkett W (1986) Phase I–II clinical and pharmacologic study of high-dose cytosine arabinoside in refractory leukemia. Am J Med 81: 387–394
4. Plunkett W, Iacoboni S, Estey E,, Danhauser L, Liliemark JO, Keating MJ (1985) Pharmacologically directed ara-C therapy for refractory leukemia. Semin Oncol 12: 20–30
5. Zittoun R, Marie JP, Delanian S, Suberville AM, Thevenin D (1987) Prognostic value of in vitro uptake and retention of cytosine arabinoside in acute myelogenous leukemia. Semin Oncol 14: 269–275
6. Preisler HD, Rustum YM, Azarnia N, Priore R (1987) Abrogation of the prognostic significance of low leukemic cell retention of cytosine arabinoside triphosphate by intensification of therapy and by alteration in the dose and schedule of administration of cytosine arabinoside. Cancer Chemother Pharmacol 19: 69–74
7. Chou T-C, Arlin Z, Clarkson BD, Philips FS (1977) Metabolism of 1-β-D-arabinofuranosylcytosine in human leukemic cells. Cancer Res 37: 3561–3570
8. Rustum Y (1978) Metabolism and intracellular retention of 1-β-D-arabinofuranosylcytarabine as predictors of response of animal tumors. Cancer Res 38: 543–548
9. Kufe DW, Spriggs D, Egan EM, Munroe D (1984) Relationships among ara-CTP pools, formation of (ara-C) DNA, and cytotoxicity of human leukemic cells. Blood 64: 54–58
10. Rustum Y, Preisler HD (1979) Correlation between leukemic cell retention of 1-β-D-arabinofuranosylcytarabine 5'-triphosphate and response to therapy. Cancer Res 39: 42–47
11. Iacoboni S, Plunkett W, Kantarjian H (1986) High dose cytosine arabinoside: treatment and cellular pharmacology of chronic myelogenous leukemia blast crisis. J Clin Oncol 4: 1079–1088
12. Schleyer E, Ehninger G, Zuhlsdorf M, Proksch B, Hiddemann W (1989) Detection and separation of intracellular 1-beta-D-arabinofuranosylcytosine-5-triphosphate by ion-pair high-performance liquid chromatography. J Chromatogr 497: 109–120
13. Ohkubo T, Hori H, Higashigawa M, Kawasaki H, Kamiya H, Sakurai M, Kagawa Y, Kakito E, Sumida K, Ooi K (1989) Synergistic interaction between etoposide and 1-beta-D-arabinofuranosylcytosine. Adv Exp Med Biol 253B: 355–362
14. Ohkubo T, Higashigawa M, Kawasaki H, Kamiya H, Sakurai M, Kagawa Y, Kakito E, Sumida K, Ooi K (1988) Sequence-dependent antitumor effect of VP-16 and 1-beta-D-arabinofuranosylcytosine in L1210 ascites tumor. Eur J Cancer Clin Oncol 24: 1823–1828
15. Rivera G, Avery T, Roberts D (1975) Response of L1210 to combination of cytosine arabinoside and VM-26 or VP16-213. Eur J Cancer 11: 639–639
16. Bishop JF, Lowentahl RM, Joshua D, Matthews JP, Todd D, Cobcroft R, Whiteside MG, Kronenberg H, Ma D, Dodds A, Herrmann R, Szer J, Wolf MM, Young G (1990) Etoposide in acute nonlymphocytic leukemia. Australian Leukemia Study Group. Blood 75: 27–32

Dose-Dependent Cellular and Systemic Pharmacokinetics of Cytosine Arabinoside

R. L. Capizzi and J. C. White

The proper selection of dose for any desired therapeutic effect must consider the drug's systemic and cellular pharmacokinetics. Pharmacokinetics, the measurement of drug concentration over time, is essential to the attainment of a desired pharmacodynamic effect. Correlation of cellular pharmacokinetics with systemic pharmacokinetics offers opportunities for optimal dosage and schedule selection so as to achieve the optimal therapeutic index.

Clinical research into the antileukemic efficacy of cytosine arabinoside (ara-C) over the past 25 years has spanned a wide dosage range from 10 mg/m^2 to >3000 mg/m^2. This has provided unique opportunities to relate dose to plasma concentrations which, in turn, have been related to cellular effects and, ultimately, the therapeutic index. A complete remission (CR) rate of 25 % is reported from the use of ara-C administered as a single agent at 100–200 mg/m^2 per day for 7 days (so-called standard dose ara-C or SDAC) in previously untreated patients with acute myeloid leukemia (AML) [1]. In contrast, recent trials with high-dose ara-C (HiDAC) in similar patients have resulted in a CR rate in the 70 %–80 % range [2], an effect equivalent to that achieved by the combined use of 100–200 mg/m^2 ara-C administered for 7 days in combination with three daily doses of an anthracycline antibiotic [3]. This paper will review the pharmacokinetic basis for this dose-related range in response rates.

The nucleoside ara-C enters leukemia cells via the nonconcentrative facilitated diffusion mechanism that is shared by naturally occurring nucleosides [4]. Once in the cell, ara-C is successively anabolized to the mono-, di-, and triphosphates. Ara-C triphosphate (ara-CTP) then polymerizes with normal nucleoside triphosphates and is incorporated into DNA, a process leading to cell death [4–7]. The two rate-limiting steps in this process are membrane transport [8] and the initial phosphorylation step to the nucleoside monophosphate, ara-CMP [4, 8]. Appropriate laboratory experiments can dissect the interrelationship and the relative importance of each of these steps.

The average number of nucleoside carrier molecules per cell can be quantified using the nucleoside analog, nitrobenzyl mercaptopurine riboside (NBMPR). NBMPR binds tightly to the nucleoside carrier ($K_d \cong 1$ nM [9, 10]) but is not translocated across the cell membrane. The cellular binding capacity for radiolabeled [³H]NBMPR is closely correlated with NBMPR-sensitive nucleoside transport rates. The number of NBMPR-binding sites and the rate of ara-C translocation across the cell membrane in a variety of cell lines and human leukemic blasts taken directly from patients (leukemic blasts) is shown in Table 1. Whereas various human and murine cell lines have an abundance of carrier molecules per cell (range of 59000–183000 sites/cell), leukemic blasts had at least an order of magnitude fewer sites/cell, average 4223 ± 4334, and markedly slower transport rates for ara-C

Comprehensive Cancer Center of Wake Forest University, Bowman Gray School of Medicine, 300 S. Hawthorne Road, Winston-Salem, NC 27103, USA

Table 1. Cytosine arabinoside transport rate and nucleoside carrier sites. (From White et al. [8])

	Rate[a]	NBMPR sites[b]
Patients		
Acute leukemia	14 ± 15	4223 ± 4334
	n = 45	n = 61
Human leukemia in cell culture		
ML-1	805	139000
HL-60	49	59000
CCRF-CEM	n.d.	183000
Mouse ascites tumors		
Ehrlich	272	94000
L5178Y	105	74000
P383	n.d.	137000

n.d., not determined
[a] pmol/min/10^6 cells at 50 μM [^{3}H] ara-C ± SD
[b] Maximal specific [^{3}H]NBMPR-binding sites per cell ± SD

14 ± 15 pmol/min per 10^6 cells for the leukemic blasts compared to 49–805 pmol/min per 10^6 cells for the cultured cell lines. Of note in this regard is the wide variability in NBMPR-binding sites and transport rates in leukemic blasts as reflected in the standard deviation for both parameters. Because of this wide interpatient variability, transport may assume variable importance as a determinant of ara-C's cellular pharmacology and on the optimal dosage for individual patients.

Cellular pharmacokinetic studies indicate that, at extracellular drug concentrations that are ≤ 1 M, membrane transport limits the net rate of cellular metabolism to phosphorylated metabolites. When transport capacity is low compared to phosphorylation capacity, intracellular ara-C will be metabolized as rapidly as it enters the cell. Table 2 lists the intracellular/extracellular concentration ratios for unchanged ara-C (i. e., as the nucleoside) when various cell types are exposed to 1 μM ara-C. Ehrlich ascites cells are typical of experimental cell lines in that they have very high nucleoside transport capacity (see Table 1). In these cells, ara-C very rapidly equilibrates across the cell membrane and the intracellular to extracellular ratio is close to 1. However, for leukemic blasts taken from five patients, the intracellular nucleoside concentration averages only 18 % of the extracellular concentration when the cells are exposed to 1 μM ara-C. This is because at 1 μM ara-C intracellular phosphorylation of ara-C takes place more rapidly than the capacity of the membrane carrier to translocate the drug across the cell membrane. This is significant because at this low concentration range the rate of phosphorylation is

Table 2. Dependence of intracellular ara-C (nucleoside) concentration on the extracellular ara-C level. (From White et al. [8])

Cells	Method[a]	[Intracellular ara-c] / [Extracellular ara-C]	
		1 μM	50 M
Patient 51	DEAE Sephadex	0.27	1.02
52	HPLC	0.14	0.53
52	DEAE Sephadex	0.12	0.41
53	DEAE Sephadex	0.37	0.76
54	DEAE Sephadex	0.10	0.38
55	HPLC	0.09	0.49
	Mean ± SD	0.18 ± 0.11	0.60 ± 0.25
Ehrlich	DEAE Sephadex	0.90	0.94

[a] Cells were incubated with [^{3}H]ara-C for 20 min, then extracted with tricarboxylic acid. Unchanged [^{3}H]ara-C (nucleoside) was separated from phosphorylated metabolites using minicolumns of DEAE-Sephadex A25 or anion-exchange HPLC.

approximately proportional to the intracellular concentration (effective intracellular K_m = approx. 1.5 µM [8, 11]. This limitation of the intracellular ara-C level is reflected in an increase in the apparent K_m for cellular uptake. An extracellular ara-C concentration of 4–5 µM is needed to achieve an intracellular concentration of 1.5 µM. As the extracellular concentration is increased to 50 µM, a concentration in the range of those achieved during a 3-h infusion of 3 g/m^2 (Table 3), the intracellular to extracellular ratio is increased to 0.6 with a range of 0.4–1.0. Intracellular/extracellular ratios approach unity, because leukemic blasts have a very high K_m for ara-C transport (>400 µM [8, 12]). Given this high K_m, the rate of ara-C transport into human blasts is essentially proportional to the plasma concentration in the standard to high dosage ranges, i.e., milligram to gram doses. However, the phosphorylation of intracellular ara-C is saturated at relatively low concentrations (K_m = 1.5 µM [8, 11]).

Table 3. Plasma levels of ara-C

	ara C level (µmol/l)	Reference
100 mg/m^2		
Bolus	20.0 (peak)	[18]
Continuous infusion	0.4	[18]
200 mg/m^2		
Continuous infusion	0.8	[31]
3000 mg/m^2	100.0	[21]

The impact of transport on cellular drug accumulation over a range of extracellular drug concentrations can be assessed by calculation of its "control strength" (C_t) [8]. C_t is a rather complex function of the K_ms and V_{max}s for transport and intracellular phosphorylation, and of the extracellular ara-C concentration [8]. This concept was developed to assess the impact of transport on cellular accumulation of nucleosides by Wohlhueter and Plagemann [13]. In this context, control strength defines the relative importance of membrane transport as a determinant of the net rate of cellular phosphorylation. A C_t of 1.0 would mean that the phosphorylation (or ara-CTP accumulation) rate was a direct function of the transport rate, while a C_t of zero would mean that the phosphorylation rate was independent of the transport rate. As illustrated in Fig. 1, transport control strength declines with increasing extracellular concentrations of ara-C. The solid line is based

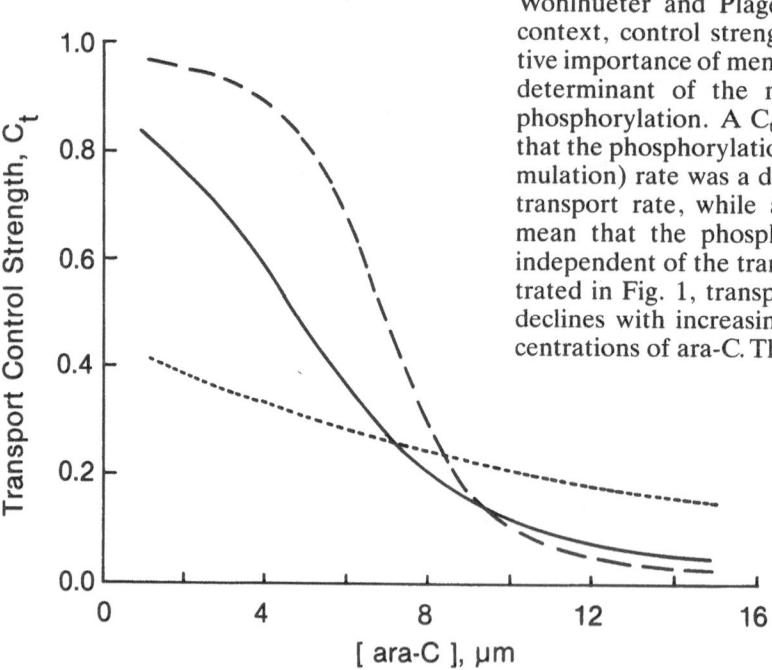

Fig. 1. Concentration dependence of transport control strength as a determinant of the rate of accumulation of ara-C in AML cells from patients. *Solid line* is based on median kinetic constants (see White et al. 1987). *Dashed and dotted lines* are derived from kinetic parameters of cells from two patients, which represent extremes of high and low sensitivity to transport capacity as a determinant of the rate of ara-C accumulation. *Solid line*, average AML; *dashed line*, patient 33; *dotted line*, patient 26. (From White et al. [8])

on the median kinetic constants for transport and phosphorylation from a group of 10–33 patients. The two broken lines are derived from kinetic parameters derived from cells taken from two patients which represent the extremes of high or low dependence on transport as a determinant of the phosphorylation rate. As indicated by the solid line, when median kinetic constants derived from the total patient population are used, transport is the rate-limiting step for cellular accumulation at ara-C concentrations achieved during the continuous infusion of SDAC (CI-SDAC) (see Table 3). This pharmacologic impediment can be eliminated by increasing the extracellular drug concentration to 1015 μM. This latter drug concentration is exceeded by current usage of 3 mg/m² (see Table 3).

The broken lines reflecting the two extremes in observations are of interest. For the patient depicted by the dotted line, transport is a relatively less important pharmacologic parameter. Even at low ara-C levels, an alteration in transport would have only a minor effect on the phosphorylation rate; transport capacity would not limit phosphorylation at either low or high doses. In contrast, the leukemic blasts in the patient depicted by the dashed line have a marked limitation in transport capacity at lower concentrations of ara-C typically achieved during CI-SDAC (Table 3). However, drug concentrations typical of HiDAC effectively eliminate this pharmacologic barrier. This pharmacologic characterization may typify the patient who failed to enter remission with an SDAC-containing protocol, but who could be induced into CR with HiDAC. These data would indicate that, from a purely cellular pharmacokinetic standpoint, an extracellular drug concentration of 10–15 μM would eliminate any transport limitation on the cellular accumulation of ara-C. This "optimal" concentration is much less than that achieved during the 3-h infusion of 3 g/m² wherein the mean plasma steady-state concentration (CPSS) is in the 50-μM range (Table 3). In an ongoing study of the population pharmacokinetics of ara-C, rather wide interpatient variability (four- to tenfold) in the CPSS has been observed at each dosage level [14].

This wide range of mean plasma concentrations associated with each dosage level may have substantial pharmacologic implications. These data would indicate that the ideal therapeutic practice would include plasma drug monitoring with appropriate dosage adjustments as needed to maintain the CPSS in the 10- to 15-μM range. However, even the most meticulous plasma drug monitoring and adjustment will not assure universal therapeutic success since ara-C is a pro-drug whose active form is an intracellular metabolite, ara-CTP; measurements of the latter are technically more cumbersome.

Cytosine arabinoside displays dose-dependent pharmacokinetic effects. The systemic pharmacokinetics of ara-C are primarily affected by systemic metabolism to ara-U (1-β-D-arabinofuranosyl uracil) by cytidine-deoxycytidine deaminase [15]. Ara-U is normally considered to be a metabolically inert, detoxification product. When administered as a bolus dose or following the termination of a continuous infusion as SDAC, the plasma elimination of ara-C has been described as a biexponential process [16–20] with a $t_{1/2\alpha}$ and β of 7–12 min and 111–157 min, [16, 20] respectively. In contrast, when administered as 3 g/m² the plasma elimination has been described as a triexponential process (Fig. 2) [21]. In this study, the observed steady-state plasma concentrations (CPSS) for ara-C varied from 60 to 166 μM, in ten courses in four patients; the average was 115 ± 32 μM [21]. In a larger, multicenter study the mean CPSS was 54 μM with a range of 20–80 μM in 16 patients. Clearly, the CPSS values associated with a 3-h infusion of 3 g/m² are larger than those required to optimize cellular transport and accumulation.

Metabolism to ara-U occurs within minutes of ara-C administration. Following the administration of 3 g/m² of ara-C, ara-U reaches peak plasma concentrations in the range of 310 ± 106 μM and is eliminated with an average apparent half-life of 3.75 ± 1.8 h (range 1.4–6.4 h) (Fig. 2). Nine hours after the termination of the HiDAC infusion, the time when a subsequent infusion of HiDAC would be started, the plasma concentration of ara-U averaged 83 ± 26

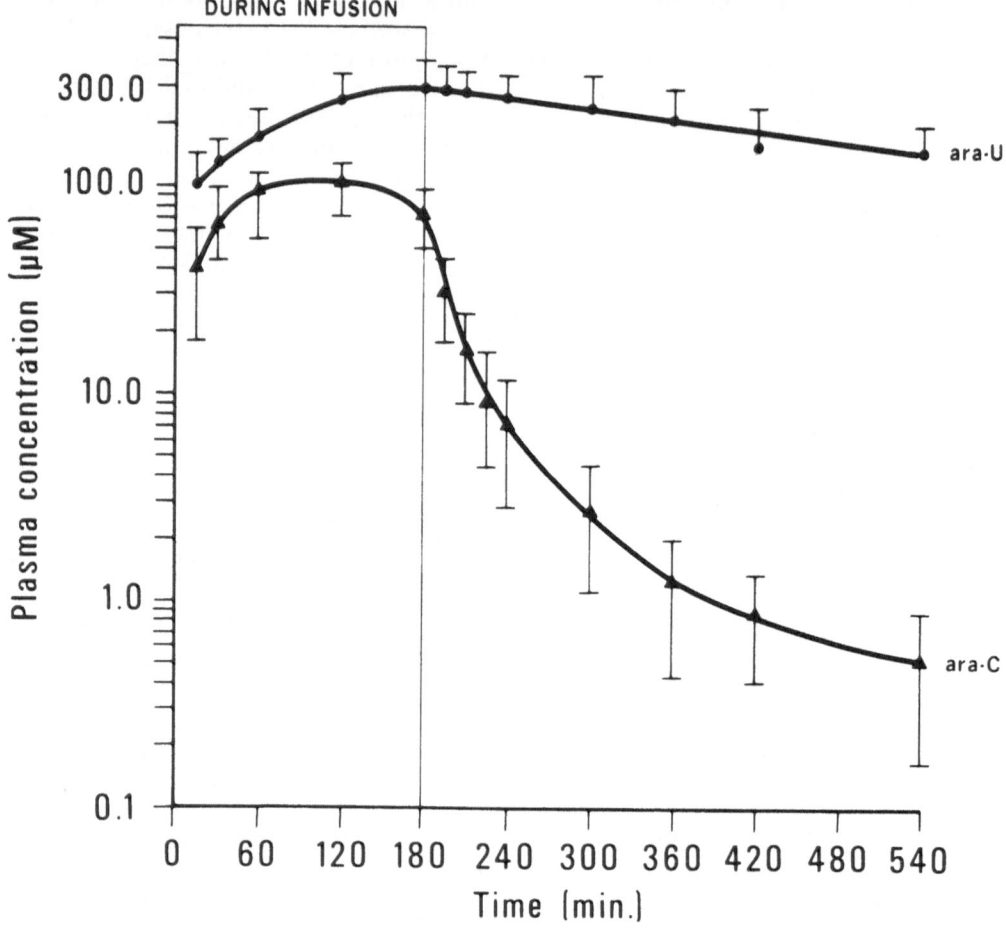

Fig. 2. Plasma-C and ara-U concentrations during and after a 3-h infusion of 3 g/m² ara-C administered every 12 h for four doses. *Points* represent the mean ± SD of ten studies in four patients. ?, ara-C; ?, ara-U. (From Capizzi et al. [21])

μM [21]. This rapid appearance of ara-U follwing the start of a HiDAC infusion and its long half-life raises several interesting questions relative to the effect of these high concentrations on the observed pharmacokinetics of HiDAC, especially as it departs from the observed pharmacokinetics of SDAC. It was conjectured that this dose-related effect was due to the inhibitory effect of ara-U on Cyd-dCyd deaminase. The inhibitory effect of ara-U on the activity of Cyd-dCyd deaminase derived from human leukemia cells is shown in Fig. 3. Increasing concentrations of ara-U interfere with deamination in a competitive fashion (product competitive inhibition)

with an apparent K_i of 5.6 μM. Limited data in the literature speak of dose-dependent pharmacokinetics for antimetabolites [22] and earlier investigations on ara-C metabolism noted a dose-related decrease in deamination [16].

This metabolite-drug (i. e., ara-U-ara-C) interaction was explored in vivo in leukemic mice. Mice bearing the L5178Y murine leukemia as an ascites tumor received a 48-h continuous infusion of ara-U. Table 4 details the plasma steady-state concentrations and the concentrations of ara-U in the liver and kidneys, the major catabolic sites for ara-C. Of interest is the substantial accumulation of ara-U in these organs in considerable

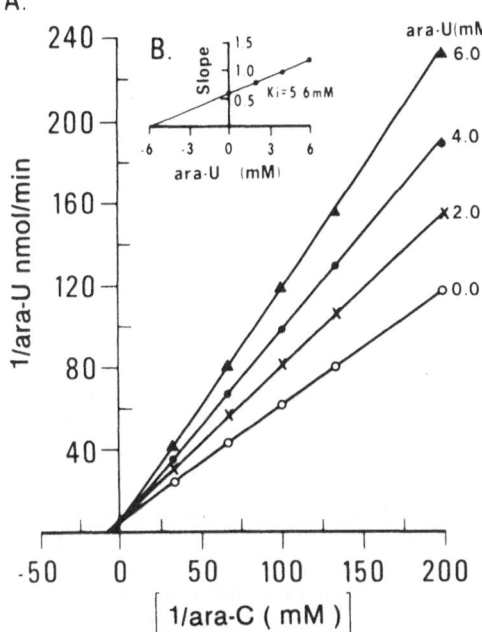

Fig. 3. Lineweaver-Burk plot indicating the inhibitory effect of ara-U on purified cytidine deaminase derived from human AML cells. The enzyme assays were performed using 0.7 units purified Cyd deaminase and the indicated concentrations of ara-U. The insert *(B)* shows a replot of the slope of the lines obtained from the double reciprocal plot *(A)* versus ara-U concentration. (From Capizzi et al. [21])

excess to that found in the plasma; these concentrations in the liver and kidneys exceed the K_i of ara-U for Cyd-dCyd deaminase. There may be some parallels in the tissue pharmacokinetics of ara-U and uridine. Dornowski and Handschumacher reported that, while a 250-mg/kg dose of uridine in mice increased the plasma con-

Table 4. Ara-U levels achieved during continuous infusion in mice. (From Chandrasekaran et al. [30])

Plasma SS	Liver	Kidney
723±31 μM (N=10)	10–29 MM	34–86 MM

K_i of ara-U for Cyd deaminase in liver and kidney was 11.2 and 18 MM, respectively

centration of uridine to over 1 mM for a brief period, the concentration of uridine increased 5-to 10-fold over the corresponding plasma concentration in most tissues, 20-fold in the spleen, and 70-fold in the kidney [23]. These findings suggest that, in normal tissues and explanted cells, pools of uridine are sustained by a concentrative transport mechanism and constitute a previously unrecognized reservoir. We observed a similar increase in ara-U concentration in these organs relative to the plasma concentration: up to 20-fold in the liver and 80-fold in the kidney. This organ accumulation relates to the concentration-dependent inhibitory effect of ara-U on Cyd-dCyd deaminase activity. This, in turn, retards ara-C catabolism, delaying its clearance from the plasma resulting in a larger area under the curve. At 240 min after ara-C administration, the plasma ara-C levels in the ara-U-treated group were approximately 11-fold (735 μM) higher than in the control group (65 μM). This, in turn, leads to higher concentrations of ara-C in the mouse leukemia cells. These studies have also shown that ara-U imparis the renal excretion of ara-C and results in a substantial accumulation of both ara-U and ara-C in plasma, ascites fluid, and L5178Y cells.

In addition to altering the systemic pharmacokinetic effects of ara-C, high concentrations of ara-U also have a significant effect on leukemia cytokinetics. Having noted the high plasma concentrations and long half-life of ara-U in patients treated with HiDAC, the repetitive infusion of HiDAC at 12-h intervals for 6–12 doses, as is commonly used in AML protocols, essentially provides a continuous infusion of ara-U. Twenty-four-hour exposure of murine leukemia L5178Y cells to high concentrations of ara-U in vitro causes an accumulation of cells in the S-phase of the cell cycle (Fig. 4) [24]. Similar effects are noted in the ara-U infusion studies in leukemic mice described above in the pharmacokinetic studies. These cytokinetic effects of ara-U have implications for ara-C pharmacology in that S-phase accumulation is associated with an increase in the specific activity of dCyd kinase, the rate-limiting enzyme in the cellular accumulation of ara-C [25–28].

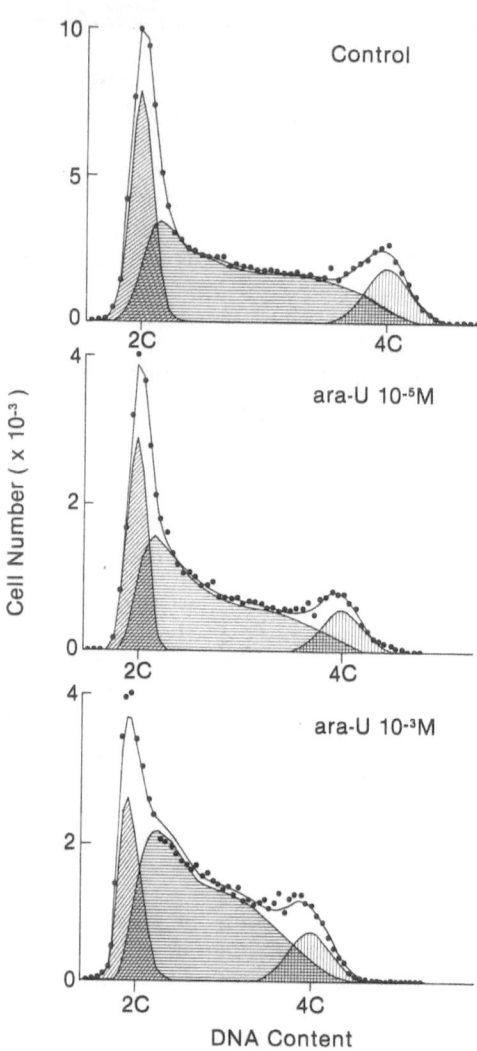

Fig. 4. DNA histogram analysis of L5178Y cells after 24-h treatment with ara-U. Cells were prepared and stained with propidium iodide and analyzed by flow cytometry as described in the references. (From Yang et al. [29])

ara-U and ara-C is associated with increased cytotoxicity to leukemia cells both in vitro [29] and in vivo [30]. Of interest is the apparent lack of increased toxicity to normal organs of the mouse [30]. Using isobologram analysis, Mueller and Zahn also noted pharmacologic synergy between ara-U and ara-C on L5178Y cells [24].

In summary, the cellular pharmacokinetics of ara-C are optimized at extracellular drug concentrations in the 10- to 15-μM range. At these concentrations transport rates are no longer rate limiting, and ara-C phosphorylation capacity is saturated. The prime determinants of the ara-C effect then shift to multiple intracellular events including anabolism to nucleotides, catabolism via deamination by Cyd-dCyd deaminase and dCMP deaminase, half-life of ara-CTP, the extent of incorporation into DNA, and the half-life of ara-CMP residues in DNA. When administered as repetitive doses of 3 g/m² over a 1- to 3-h period, systemic deamination of ara-C gives rise to high plasma concentrations of ara-U. This metabolite has a long plasma half-life and, at least in the mouse, is concentrated in the liver and kidneys. High concentrations in these organs retard the further catabolism of ara-C and thus increase the systemic AUC providing a longer exposure period to the drug. Additionally, by some as yet unknown mechanism, high concentrations of ara-U cause accumulation of cells in S-phase, the phase of the cell cycle wherein ara-C is maximally effective. These metabolite-drug interactions that occur when ara-C is given at high doses constitute a means for "self-potentiation" and may thus contribute to its overall therapeutic efficacy.

Since the subsequent nucleotide anabolic enzymes are present in excess, the cellular pool of ara-CTP is increased which, in turn, is associated with an associated increase in ara-C incorporation in DNA [29, 30]. Consistent with the well-described relationship between ara-C incorporation into DNA and cytotoxicity [4–7], this interaction between

References

1. Gale RP (1979) Advances in the treatment of acute myelogenous leukemia. N Engl J Med 300: 1189–1199
2. Capizzi RL, Powell BL (1987) Sequential high dose ara-C and asparaginase versus high dose ara-C alone in the treatment of patients with relapsed and refractory acute leukemias. Semin Oncol 14 [Suppl 1]: 40–50

3. Preisler HD, Davis RB, Kirshner J, Dupre E, Richards E 3d, Hoagland HC, Kopel S, Levy RN Carey R, Schulman P et al. (1987) Comparison of three remission induction regimens and two postinduction strategies for the treatment of acute nonlymphocytic leukemia: a Cancer and Leukemia Group B study. Blood 69: 1441–1449

4. Plagemann PGW, Marz R, Wohlhueter RM (1978) Transport and metabolism of deoxycytidine and 1-β-D-arabinofuranosylcytosine into cultured Novikoff rat hepatoma cells, relationship to phosphorylation, and regulation of triphosphate synthesis. Cancer Res 38: 978–989

5. Kufe D, Major P, Egan E, Beardsley P (1981) Incorporation of ara-C into L1210 DNA as a correlate of cytotoxicity. J Biol Chem 235: 3235–3239

6. Kufe D, Spriggs D, Egan EM, Munroe D (1984) Relationships among ara-CTP pools, formation of (ara-C)DNA, and cytotoxicity of human leukemic cells. Blood 64: 54–58

7. Major PP, Egan EM, Beardsley GP, Minden MD, Kufe D (1981) Lethality of human myeloblasts correlates with the incorporation of arabinofuranosylcytosine into DNA. Proc Natl Acad Sci USA 78: 3235–3239

8. White JC, Rathmell JP, Capizzi RL (1987) Membrane transport influences the rate of accumulation of cytosine arabinoside in human leukemia cells. J Clin Invest 79: 380–387

9. Cass CE, Gaudette LA, Paterson ARP (1974) Mediated transport of nucleosides in human erythrocytes. Specific binding of the inhibitor nitrobenzythioinosine to nucleoside transport sites in the erythrocyte membrane. Biochim Biophys Acta 345: 1–10

10. White JC, Hines LH, Rathmell JP (1985) Inhibition of 1-β-D-arabinofuranosylcytosine transport and net accumulation by teniposide and etoposide in Ehrlich ascites cells and human leukemic blasts. Cancer Res 45: 3070–3075

11. White JC, Capizzi RL (1991) A critical role for uridine nucleotides in the regulation of deoxycytidine kinase and the concentration dependence of 1-β-D-arabinofuranosylcytosine phosphorylation in human leukemia cells. Cancer Res (in press)

12. Wiley JS,, Jones SP, Sawyer WH, Paterson ARP (1982) Cytosine arabinoside influx and nucleoside transport sites in acute leukemia. J Clin Invest 69: 479–489

13. Wohlhueter RM, Plagemann PGW (1980) The roles of transport and phosphorylation in nutrient uptake in cultured animal cells. Int Rev Cytol 64: 171–240

14. Capizzi RL, Oliver L, Friedman H, Davis R, Mayer R, Schiffer C, Lunghofer B, Royer G (1988) Variations in ara-C plasma concentrations at steady-state (Cpss) during remission induction and intensification therapy of AML. A population pharmacokinetics study by CALGB. Proc Am Soc Clin Oncol 7: 57 (abstract)

15. Camiener GW (1968) Studies of the enzymatic deamination of ara-cytidine-V. Inhibition in vitro and in vivo by tetrahydrouridine and other reduced pyrimidine nucleosides. Biochem Pharmacol 17: 1981–1991

16. Ho DHW, Frei E (1971) Clinical pharmacology of 1-β-D-arabinofuranosylcytosine. Clin Pharmacol Ther 12: 944–954

17. Harris AL, Potter C, Bunch C (1979) Pharmacokinetics of cytosine arabinoside in patients with myeloid leukemia. Br J Clin Pharmacol 8: 219–227

18. Slevin ML, Piall EM, Aherne GW, Johnston A, Sweatman MC, Lister TA (1981) The pharmacokinetics of subcutaneous cytosine arabinoside in patients with acute myelogenous leukemia. Br J Clin Pharmacol 12: 507–510

19. Van Prooijen R, Van Der Kleijn E, Haanen C (1977) Pharmacokinetics of cytosine arabinoside in acute myeloid leukemia. Clin Pharmacol Ther 21: 744–752

20. Wan SH, Hoffman DH, Azarnoff DL (1974) Pharmacokinetics of 1-β-D-arabinofuranosylcytisone in humans. Cancer Res 34: 392–397

21. Capizzi RL, Yang J-L, Cheng E, Bjornson D, Sahasrabudhe D, Tan R-S, Cheng Y-C (1983) Alteration of the pharmacokinetics of high dose araC by its metabolite, high araU in patients with acute leukemia. J Clin Oncol 1: 763–771

22. Powis G (1983) Metabolism, therapeutic effect, on toxicity of anticancer drugs in man. Drug Metab Rev 14: 1145–1163

23. Darnowski JW, Handschumacher RE (1986) Tissue uridine pools: evidence in vivo of a concentrative mechanism for uridine uptake. Cancer Res 46: 3490–3494

24. Muller WEG, Zahn RK (1979) Metabolism of 1-β-D-arabinofuranosyluracil in mouse L5178Y cells. Cancer Res 39: 1102–1107

25. Liliemark JO, Plunkett W (1986) Regulation of 1-β-D-arabinofuranosylcytosine 5'-triphosphate accumulation in human leukemia cells by deoxycytidine 5'-triphosphate. Cancer Res 46: 1079–1083

26. Chiba P, Tihan T, Eher R, Koller U, Wallner C, Gobl R, Linkesch W (1989) Effect of cell growth and cell differentiation on 1-β-D-arabinofuranosylcytosine metabolism in myeloid cells. Br J Haematol 71: 451–455

273

27. Arner ES, Flygar M, Bohman C, Wallstrom B, Eriksson S (1988) Deoxycytidine kinase is constitutively expressed in human lymphocytes: consequences for compartmentation effects, unscheduled DNA synthesis, and viral replication in resting cells. Exp Cell Res 178: 335–342

28. Richel DJ, Colly LP, Arentsen-Honders MW, Starrenburg CWJ, Willemze R (1990) Deoxycytidine kinase, thymidine kinase and cytidine deaminase and the formation of Ara-CTP in leukemic cells in different phases of the cell cycle. Leuk Res 14: 363–369

29. Yang J-L, Cheng EH, Capizzi RL, Cheng Y-C, Kute T (1985) Effect of uracil arabinoside on metabolism and cytotoxycity of cytosine arabinoside in L5178Y murine leukemia. J Clin Invest 75: 141–146

30. Chandrasekaran B, Capizzi RL, Kute TE, Morgan T, Dimling J (1989) Modulation of the metabolism and pharmacokinetics of 1-β-D-arabinofuranosylcytosine by 1-β-D-arabinofuranosyluracil in leukemic mice. Cancer Res 49: 3259–3266

31. Weinstein HJ, Griffin TW, Feeney J, Cohen HJ, Propper RD, Sallan SE (1982) Pharmacokinetics of continuous intravenous and subcutaneous infusions of cytosine arabinoside. Blood 59: 1351–1353

Enhanced Accumulation of dFdC-Triphosphate in Tumor Cells with Short Retention of ARA-C Triphosphate

V. Heinemann[1] and W. Plunkett[2]

Introduction

The comparative analysis of cellular accumulation of 2', 2'-difluorodeoxycytidine 5'-triphosphate (dFdCTP) or 1-β-D-arabinofuranosylcytosine 5'-triphosphate (ara-CTP) has demonstrated a wide variation depending on which cell line was studied. Some cell lines show a nearly equal accumulation of dFdCTP and ara-CTP, while others accumulate dFdCTP to severalfold higher concentrations than ara-CTP. Both drugs, dFdC and ara-C, are activated by intracellular phosphorylation, a process in which deoxycytidine kinase (dCK) is rate limiting [1]. Intracellular accumulation and retention of ara-CTP and dFdCTP relate to cytotoxic drug activity. In contrast to ara-C, dFdC acts as an inhibitor of ribonucleotide reductase (RR) and deoxycytidylate deaminase (dCMPD) [2, 3]. Additionally, cellular elimination of dFdCTP is concentration dependent, while ara-CTP elimination occurs independently of cellular ara-CTP concentrations [1]. The present study set out to specify the mechanism responsible for differential accumulation of dFdCTP and ara-CTP. For this purpose the cell lines CCRF-CEM, K562, HL-60, and CHO were analyzed.

[1] Klinikum Grosshadern, Department of Internal Medicine and Hematology/Oncology, University of Munich, Marchioninistr. 15, 8000 Munich 70, FRG
[2] Department of Medical Oncology and Hematology, University of Texas MD Anderson Cancer Center, 1515 Holcombe Boulevard, Houston, Texas 77030, USA

Materials and Methods

dFdC, dFdU, dFdCMP, and [5-^{14}C]dFdC were synthesized at the Eli Lilly Research Laboratories (Indianapolis). Experiments were performed in human leukemia cell lines CCRF-CEM (T-lymphoblastic), HL-60 (promyelocytic), K562 (erythroblastic), and additionally in Chinese Hamster Ovary (CHO) cells. Analysis of acid-soluble cell extracts for nucleosides and nucleoside phosphates was performed by high-performance liquid chromatography (HPLC) as previously described [1]. Cellular dNTP concentrations were determined after degradation of NTP by periodate oxidation [3]. Activity of deoxycytidine kinase was assayed in broken cell extracts following the method of Saunders and Lai [4]. Deoxycytidylate deaminase activity was assayed in broken cell extracts according to the method reported by Fridland and Verhoef [5].

Results

Comparative Analysis of Cellular Accumulation of dFdCTP Versus ara-CTP

Four cell lines, CCRF-CEM, HL-60, K562, and CHO, were analyzed after separate incubation with 10 μM dFdC and ara-C respectively. Accumulation of nucleotide analogs was nearly parallel in CEM cells, where a dFdCTP/ara-CTP ratio of 1.2 was reached. By contrast, K562, HL-60, and CHO cells showed increasingly greater ratios of dFdCTP/ara-CTP (2.25, 6.6, and 17.3 respectively).

275

Comparative Analysis of dCK Activity in Cell Extracts

As an important factor of deoxycytine-analog phosphorylation, dCK activity was compared in extracts of CEM,, K562, HL-60, and CHO cells. dFdC was generally shown to have lower K_m values and higher V_{max} values than ara-C. $V_{maxdFdC}/V_{maxara-C}$ ratios of 2.3, 3.0, 2.6, and 2.0 were calculated for CEM, K562, HL-60, and CHO cells,, In fact, comparative analysis of these values did not yield a significant difference between cell lines. Additionally, no striking differences between cell lines were obtained when the efficacy of drug phosphorylation (V_{max}/K_m) was compared for dFdC and ara-C.

Effect of dFdC on Cellular dNTP Concentration

Perturbation of cellular dNTP pools was assayed in CEM, K562, and CHO cells after exposure to 10 µM dFdC. Control concentrations of dCTP in these cell lines were 30.1 µM, 3.5 µM, and 238 µM respectively. Exposure to dFdC resulted in a decrease of cellular dCTP pools to 6.6%, 23%, and 96% in CEM, K562, and CHO cells respectively.

Velocity of Drug Triphosphate Degradation

Elimination of dFdCTP in CEM, K562, and Hl-60 cells was linear at low dFdCTP concentrations (<50 µM), while biphasic elimination with a concentration-dependent increase of $t_{1/2}\beta$ was observed at greater dFdCTP concentrations. CHO cells showed only biphasic elimination kinetics. The time of inflection from $t_{1/2}\beta$ was essentially independent of dFdCTP concentration, and occurred at 4, 6, 2, and 2 h for CEM, K562, HL-60, and CHO cells, respectively. In CEM, K562, HL-60, and CHO cells, a $t_{1/2}\alpha$ of 3.3, 4.8, 2.0, and 3.9 h was observed.

Cytosine arabinoside triphosphate elimination, by contrast, was linear and independent of cellular ara-CTP concentrations. In CEM, K562, HL-60, and CHO cells ara-CTP half-lives ($t_{1/2}$) of 4.8, 2.3, 1.5, and 0.7 h were measured respectively. Apart from CEM cells, initital elimination of ara-CTP was faster than of dFdCTP.

Comparative Analysis of dFdCMP Deamination by dCMPD in Cell Extracts

Compared to ara-CMP, dFdCMP was a good substrate of dCMPD (data not shown). In CEM, K562, and HL-60 cells apparent K_m values of 0.063, 0.046, and 0.150 mM were calculated, with V_{max} values of 3.8, 1.7, and 0.8 nmol/min $\times$ 10^6 cells respectively. The effectivity of dFdCMP deamination was estimated to be 60.4, 37.4, and 5.5, respectively. No significant dCMPD activity was measured in CHO cells.

Effect of Hydroxyurea on Cellular ara-C Phosphorylation

To show the effect of inhibition of ribonucleotide reductase on dCK activity, cells were preincubated for 2 h with or without 5 mM hydroxyurea (HU). CEM and CHO cells were subsequently exposed to saturating concentrations of ara-C (10 and 100 µM respectively), and cellular ara-CTP accumulation was measured as a function of dCK activity. Pretreatment of CEM cells with HU induced only a minor increase of cellular ara-CTP accumulation from 364 to 374 µM (103%). By contrast, pretreatment of CHO cells resulted in a five fold increase of cellular ara-CTP accumulation.

Discussion

The superiority of dFdCTP over ara-CTP accumulation varied significantly between the cell lines CEM, K562, HL-60, and CHO. dFdCTP/ara-CTP ratios of 1.2, 2.25, 6.6, and 17.3 were achieved. These differences may originate in different characteristics of anabolism and/or catabolism of the respective drug triphosphates.

Deoxycytidine kinase plays an important role in the phosphorylation of dFdC and ara-C. The V_{max} of dFdC phosphorylation exceeded that of ara-C phosphorylation two- to threefold in cell extracts of all analyzed cell lines. In fact, there was no significant difference in the ratio of $V_{maxdFdC}/V_{maxara-C}$ between the cell lines. Neither dCK activity nor substrate properties of dFdC or ara-C were clearly responsible for the differences in analog triphosphate accumulation.

In contrast to ara-C, dFdC acts as an inhibitor of ribonucleotide reduction and depletes cellular dCTP pools [3]. A decrease in cellular dCTP concentrations was expected to reduce feedback inhibition of dCK, resulting in enhanced dCK activity [6]. However, dCTP depletion was least in CHO cells (96% of control) showing the greatest superiority of dFdCTP versus ara-CTP accumulation; dCTP depletion was greatest (6.6% of control) in CEM cells where dFdCTP and ara-CTP accumulation were nearly equal. The degree of cellular dCTP depletion consequently does not qualify as a predictor of superiority of dFdC over ara-C phosphorylation.

Also the velocity of drug triphosphate elimination contributes to the amount of dFdCTP or ara-CTP accumulation. Comparative analysis of the $T_{1/2}\beta$ of dFdCTP showed only minor differences between cell lines. By contrast, the $T_{1/2}$ of ara-CTP was longest in CEM cells (4.8 h) followed by K562 (2.3 h), HL-60 (1.5 h), and CHO (0.7 h). dCMPD activity was analyzed as an important determinant of dFdCTP and to a lesser extent of ara-CTP elimination. However, no correlation was found between dCMPD activity and the velocity of drug triphosphate elimination. We conclude that isolated analysis of phosphorylation or degradation of the respective drug triphosphates alone cannot explain the observed differences in nucleoside analog metabolism.

However, it appears that cell lines with the shortest $t_{1/2}$ of ara-CTP are the ones which will show the greatest advantage of dFdCTP accumulation. The following hypothesis may explain this observation. A short $t_{1/2}$ of ara-CTP may reflect a high turnover of dNTP for which dCMPD is presumably of less importance than deoxy-5'-nucleotidases. Cells with a high capacity of dCTP degradation need a comparatively high capacity to produce dCTP either through de novo synthesis (RR) or through the salvage pathway via dCK. If RR is inhibited, activation of the salvage pathway and consequently of dCK is correspondingly high [7]. By contrast, cells with a low dNTP turnover or a long $T_{1/2ara-CTP}$ respond to RR inhibition by a comparatively smaller degree of dCK activation. This hypothesis is supported by the observation that HU-mediated inhibition of RR enhanced dCK activity (as reflected by ara-CTP accumulation) by five fold in CHO cells ($T_{1/2}$ara-CTP) = 0.7 h), while ara-CTP accumulation was activated only to a minor extent (1.03-fold) in CEM cells ($T_{1/2}$ara-CTP = 4.8 h). In HL-60 cells a 2.4-fold increase of ara-CTP accumulation was observed after HU-mediated RR inhibition [7].

We conclude that enhancement of dFdC phosphorylation is expected to be greater in cells with short cellular ara-CTP retention compared to cells with long ara-CTP retention. In other words, cells with the unfavorable characteristic of short ara-CTP retention should be good candidates for dFdC treatment.

Summary

Several leukemia and animal tumor cell lines were analyzed for their respective ability to accumulate intracellular cytosine arabinoside triphosphate (ara-CTP) and 2', 2'-difluorodeoxycytidine 5'-triphosphate (dFdCTP). The superiority of cellular dFdCTP accumulation over ara-CTP accumulation after incubation with 10 µM drug is shown by the ratio of dFdCTP/ara-CTP, which was 1.2, 2.25, 6.6, and 17.3 in CEM, K562, H160, and CHO cells respectively. These differences in analog triphosphate accumulation could not be explained by different effects of dFdC-mediated inhibition of ribonucleotide reductase on dNTP pool size. Phosphorylation of dFdC or ara-C by deoxycytidine kinase in cell extracts was not significantly different between the cell lines. The ratios of $V_{maxdFdC}/V_{maxara-C}$ were nearly identical, at 2.3, 3.0, 2.6, and 2.0 for CEM, K562, HL60, and CHO respectively. Cellular elimination of dFdCTP alone did not account for the observed differences in dFdCTP accumulation ($T_{1/2\alpha\beta}$ = 3.3, 4.8, 2.0, 3.9). But an inverse relation was noted between ara-CTP retention and the ratio of dFdCTP/ara-CTP accumulation. The intracellular half-lives ($T_{1/2}$) of ara-CTP in CEM, K562, H160, and CHO were 4.8, 2.3, 1.5, and 0.7 h respectively. High dNTP turnover as reflected by a short $T_{1/2}$ of ara-CTP may necessitate a high activity of dNTP de novo synthesis. We hypothesize that dFdC-mediated inhibition of ribonucleotide reductase activates the salvage pathway and with it deoxycytidine kinase (dCK). Accordingly, activation of dCyd kinase-mediated dFdC phosphorylation may be greater in cells with high dNTP turnover.

References

1. Heinemann V, Hertel LW, Grindey GB, Plunkett W (1988) Comparison of the cellular pharmacokinetics and toxicity of 2', 2'-difluorodeoxycytidine and 1-β-D-arabinofuranosylcytosine, Cancer Res. 48: 4024–4031

2. Heinemann V, Hertel L, Grindey G, Plunkett W (1988) Cellular elimination of 2', 2'-difluorodeoxycytidine-5'-triphosphate (dFdCTP). Proc Am Assoc Cancer Res 29: 2004

3. Heinemann V, Xu Y-Z, Chubb S, Sen A, Hertel LW, Grindey GB, Plunkett W (1990) Inhibition of ribonucleotide reductase in CCRF-CEM cells by 2', 2'-difluorodeoxycytidine. Mol Pharmacol 38: 567–572

4. Saunders PP, Lai MM (1983) Nucleoside kinase activities of Chinese hamster ovary cells. Biochim Biophys Acta 761: 135–141

5. Fridland A, Verhoef V (1987) Mechanism for ara-CTP catabolism in human leukemic cells and effect of deaminase inhibitors on this process. Semin Oncol 14 [Suppl 1]: 262–268

6. Gandhi V,, Plunkett W (1990) Modulatory activity of 2', 2'-difluorodeoxycytidine on the phosphorylation and cytotoxicity of arabinosyl nucleosides. Cancer Res 50: 3675–3680

7. Kubota M, Takimoto T, Tanizawa A, Akiyama Y, Mikawa H (1988) Differential modulation of 1-β-D-arabinofuranosylcytosine metabolism by hydroxyurea in human leukemia cell lines. Biochem Pharmacol 37: 1745–1749

Intracellular Pharmacokinetics of Cytosine Arabinoside in Leukemic and Normal Blood Cells*

E. Schleyer, M. Zühlsdorf, C. Rolf, U. Kewer, C. Uhrmeister, B. Wörmann, T. Büchner, and W. Hiddemann

Introduction

The cytotoxic activity of ara-C has been shown to depend on its intracellular phosphorylation and the accumulation of its active metabolite ara-C 5' triphosphate (ara-CTP). Especially during high-dose regimens a long ara-CTP retention time was found to be related to the likelihood of achieving a complete remission and possibly even with remission duration [1–3]. These findings provided the means for a pharmacologically directed design of ara-C therapy attempting to optimize dose rates and treatment schedules according to the intracellular pharmacology of ara-CTP in leukemia blasts [4–7]. Preliminary data indicate that the investigation of intracellular ara-C pharmacokinetics may also enable the cytotoxic specificity of ara-C to be increased against leukemic cells since non-leukemic mononuclear cells were found to accumulate less ara-CTP and to eliminate it more rapidly than leukemic blasts. These findings may result from quantitative differences in the deoxyribonucleotide metabolism between the two cell populations as recently suggested by Bhalla and coworkers and Grant et al. [8–9]. The current study was initiated to expand on these investigations and to search for differences in intracellular ara-C pharmacokinetics between leukemic and nonleukemic mononuclear blood cells.

Patients, Material, and Methods

Patients

Pharmacokinetic investigations were performed in 32 patients with acute myeloid leukemia (AML) at initial diagnosis ($n = 6$) or first or second relapse ($n = 26$). In addition, two patients with acute lymphoblastic leukemia and high-grade non-Hodgkin's lymphoma were investigated during consolidation or salvage therapy.

Treatment Protocols

Patients with newly diagnosed AML received the TAD-9 induction regimen according to the first-line trial of the German AML Cooperative Group [10]. Treatment consisted of ara-C 100 mg/m² per day by continuous infusion over 24 h on days 1 and 2 followed by 30-min infusions of ara-C 100 mg/m² q 12 h on days 3–8 together with daunorubicin 60 mg/m² per day on days 3, 4, and 5, and 6-thioguanine 200 mg/m² per day orally on days 3–9. Patients with relapsed AML underwent the sequential HD ara-C-mitoxantrone (S-HAM) protocol [11, 12] comprising ara-C at either 1.0 or 3.0 g/m² q 12 h on days 1 and 2, and days 8 and 9 combined with mitoxantrone 10 mg/m² per

* This paper was supported by a grant from the Deutsche Krebshilfe, Dr. Mildred Scheel Stiftung für Krebsforschung, FRG, W 24/87/HI1.

279

day on days 3 and 4, and days 10 and 11. The identical regimen was also applied to the two patients with acute lymphoblastic leukemia and high-grade non-Hodgkin's lymphoma, respectively.

Measurements of Ara-C and Ara-U Plasma Pharmacokinetics

Plasma pharmacokinetics of ara-C and ara-U were determined in 30 patients. Blood samples were collected in Vacutainers containing 30 U heparin and 0.1 mM tetrahydrouridine (kindly provided by Pfizer Co., Karlsruhe). Ara-C and Ara-U plasma levels were measured by reverse-phase high-pressure liquid chromatography (HPLC) using a Spherisorb ODS C18 column (125 × 4.6 mm, Bischoff) with an isocratic eluent consisting of 50 mM phosphate buffer pH 6.9 with 2 % methanol [13]. The evaluation of measurements was performed using a computerized integration of peak areas (RAMONA, Nuclear Interphase, Münster).

Measurements of Intracellular Ara-CTP Concentrations

Measurements of intracellular ara-CTP levels were carried out on peripheral blood cells of 22 patients. In 13 cases leukemic blasts comprised more than 70 % of mononuclear blood cells while the remaining 9 patients revealed a normal composition of blood cells without evidence of circulating malignant cells. Heparinized blood samples were subjected to Ficoll-Hypaque gradient

separation (density, 1.078 g/ml) at 1000 g for 20 min at room temperature. Interphase cells were collected, washed, and resuspended in Hank's balanced salt solution (HBSS, Gibco). Ara-CTP measurements were performed by an ion-pair HPLC method using a reverse-phase C18 column as previously described in detail [14].

Pharmacokinetic Calculations

Analysis of pharmacokinetic results was based on the TOPFIT program providing an optimized adaption of coefficients of variation between the observed and calculated respective data [15].

Results

Plasma Ara-C and Ara-U Levels

Plasma ara-C concentration and area under curve (AUC) values are summarized in Table 1 and indicate a linear relation between the applied ara-C dose and the steady state concentration of plasma ara-C as well as of the respective (AUC) values. For the total tested dose range of 100–3000 mg/m² ara-C almost identical results were obtained for the plasma half-lives of ara-C following an open two-compartment model with $t_{1/2\alpha}$ of 6.0–6.6 min and $t_{1/2\beta}$ of 21–51 min while the respective values for ara-U were calculated according to a one-compartment model with $t_{1/2}$ values of 3.6–4.02 h. For both parameters little interpatient variation was observed.

Table 1. Plasma pharmacokinetic parameters of ara-C during conventional (100 mg/m² – TAD 9) or high-dose (1.0 or 3.0 g/m² – S-HAM) ara-C therapy

Regimen	n	Steady state (µg/ml)	AUC (µg × h/ml)	Clearance (ml/min)	$t_{1/2\alpha}$ (min)	$t_{1/2\beta}$ (min)
TAD-9 (0.1 g/m² ara-C)	5	–	1.43 ± 0.85	2735 ± 1368	6.0 ± 2.8	21 ± 10.1
S-HAM (1.0 g/m² ara-C)	17	4.7 + 1.5	14.8 ± 4.7	2352 ± 917	6.6 ± 3.8	51 ± 30.6
S-HAM (3.0 g/m² ara-C)	9	13.2 + 3.4	40.0 ± 10.4	2299 ± 505	6.1 ± 2.9	46 ± 22.1

Table 2. Intracellular ara-CTP pharmacokinetic parameters during conventional-dose (100 mg/m² – TAD 9) therapy in leukemic blasts

	$t_{1/2}$ (h)	AUC (ng h/10⁷ blasts)	Steady state ara-CTP concentration (ng/10⁷ blasts)
Mean	2.14	2329	51
Range	1.70–2.10	1179–4281	26–96

Intracellular Ara-CTP Concentrations in Leukemic Blasts

Measurements of the intracellular ara-CTP concentration were performed in peripheral leukemic blasts from 13 patients. Five patients were treated according to the TAD-9 protocol and received 100 mg/m² per day ara-C while the remaining eight patients were entered on the S-HAM regimen receiving two daily 3-h infusions of either 1.0 (*n* = 5) or 3.0 g/m² (*n* = 3) ara-C.

Intracellular Ara-CTP Concentrations in Leukemic Blasts During 48 h Continuous

Infusion of 100 mg/m² per Day Ara-C (TAD-9 Protocol). As indicated in Table 2 and Fig. 1, steady-state concentrations for ara-CTP were uniformly reached within 8–10 h after the start of ara-C therapy and differed by less than fourfold between individual patients as did the AUC values. Little variation was also observed for ara-CTP half-lives with $t_{1/2}$ values ranging from 1.70 to 2.50 h. In all cases ara-CTP levels declined rapidly after the end of the ara-C infusion (Fig. 2).

Intracellular Ara-CTP Concentrations in Leukemic Blasts During 3 h Infusions of 1.0

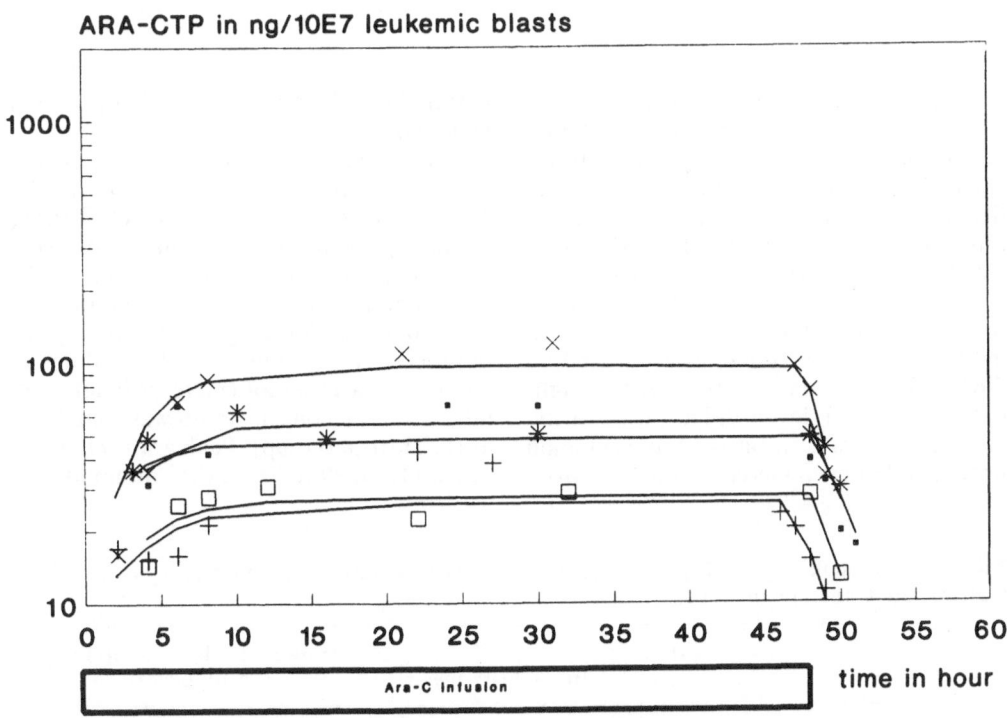

Fig. 1. Concentration of ara-CTP in leukemic blasts during 48-h continuous infusion of 100 mg/m² per day ara-C (TAD-9 protocol)

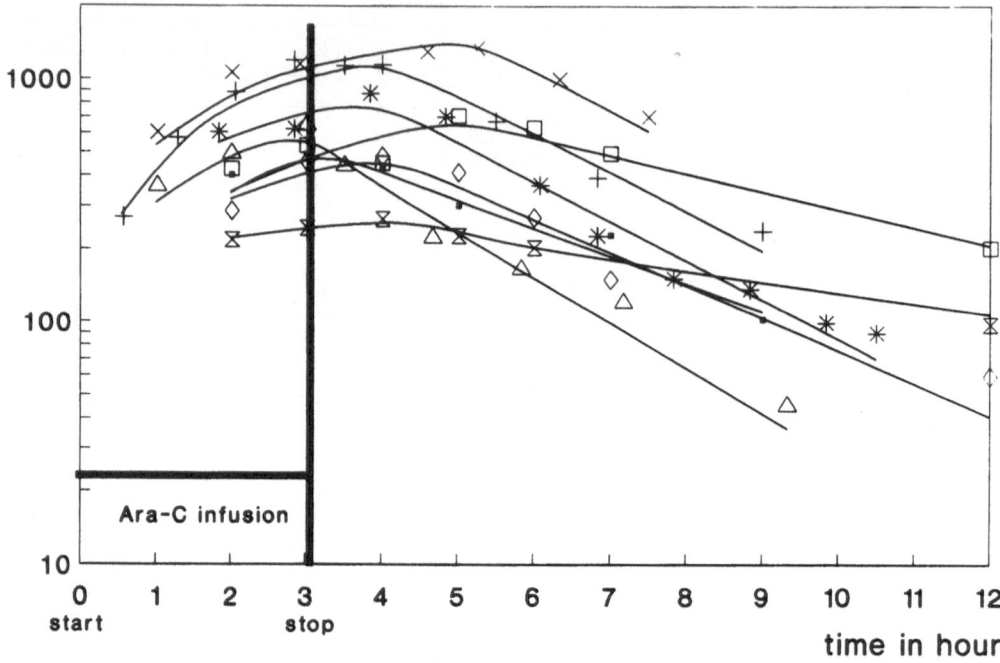

Fig. 2. Concentration of ara-CTP in leukemic blasts during 3-h infusion of 1.0 or 3.0 g/m² ara-C (S–HAM protocol)

or 3.0 g/m² Ara-C (S-HAM Protocol). Table 3 and Fig. 2 depict the respective detailed results and show a rapid increase in intracellular ara-CTP concentration within the first 15–30 min after the start of the ara-C infusion. Peak ara-CTP levels ranged from 200 to 1451 ng/10⁷ leukemic blasts with AUC values between 1116 and 8795 ng × h/10⁷ blasts differed substantially between individual patients ranging from 1.60 to 7.63 h. In addition, in seven of the eight patients ara-CTP levels did not drop at the end of the ara-C infusion but remained unchanged or even increased up to 1.5-fold within 1–2.5 h after the ara-C application (Fig. 2).

Intracellular Ara-CTP Concentrations in Normal Mononuclear Cells During 3-h Infusions of 1.0 or 3.0 g/m² Ara-C (S-HAM Protocol). Ara-CTP concentrations were measured in normal mononuclear cells from nine patients without circulating leukemic blasts undergoing S-HAM therapy as outlined before. Similar to the findings in leukemic blasts, a rapid increase in intracellular ara-CTP concentration was found after the start of therapy. Peak ara-CTP levels ranged from 89 to 747 ng/10⁷ mononuclear

Table 3. Intracellular ara-CTP pharmacokinetic parameters during high-dose (1.0 or 3.0 g/m² – S-HAM) ara-C therapy in leukemic blasts

	$t_{1/2}$ (h)	AUC (ng × h/10⁷ blasts)	Ara-CTP peak concentration (ng/10⁷ blasts)
Mean	2.97	4330	718
Range	1.61–7.63	1116–8795	200–1451

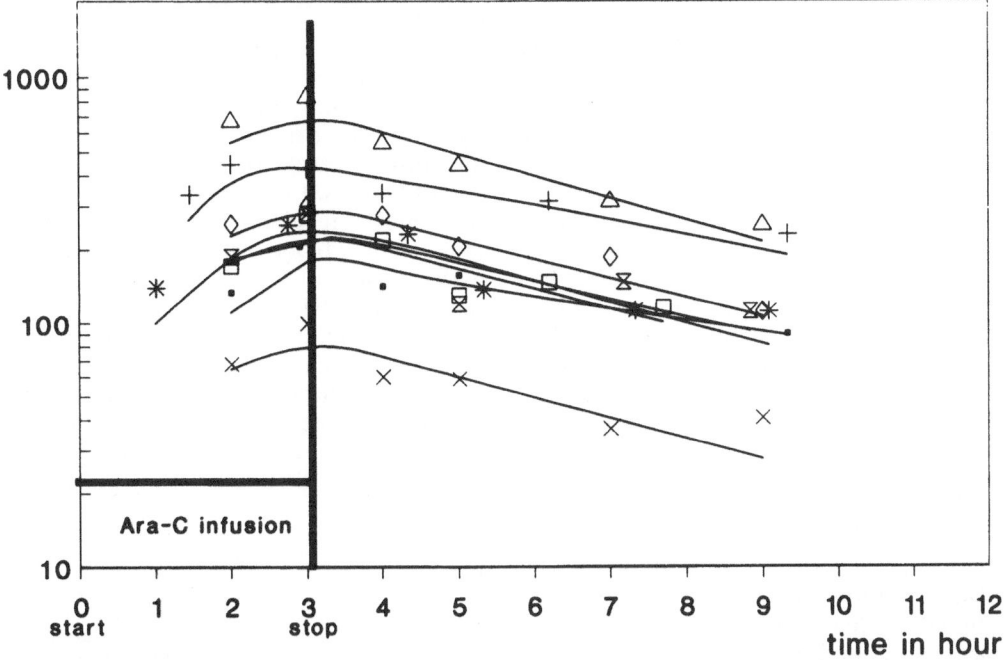

ARA-CTP in ng/10E7 normal cells

Fig. 3. Concentration of ara-CTP in normal mononuclear cells during 3-h infusion of 1.0 or 3.0 g/m^2 ara-C (S-HAM protocol)

cells with AUC values between 599 and 4843 ng × h/10^7 cells. In contrast to leukemic blasts, little interpatient variation was observed in ara-CTP retention times with $t_{1/2}$ ranging from 3.34 to 4.65 h. Most remarkably, however, intracellular ara-CTP levels dropped immediately after the end of the ara-C infusion in all analyzed cases (Fig. 3).

Discussion

The present study supports the approach of a pharmacokinetically directed ara-C therapy but, in addition, reveals differences in ara-C pharmacokinetics between leukemic blasts and normal blood cells. These findings may translate into an optimized scheduling of ara-C therapy with the aim of increasing its antileukemic activity without enhancing the cytotoxic effect on normal cells. The comparative analysis of ara-CTP pharmacokinetics in leukemic blasts and normal mononuclear cells during high-dose ara-C therapy indicates a substantial inter-

patient variation in ara-CTP retention times in leukemic blasts but not in normal mononuclear cells. More importantly, a uniform immediate decline in ara-CTP levels was observed in normal cells after the end of ara-C therapy while ara-CTP levels remained unchanged or even increased in the leukemic blasts of seven of eight patients during a post-treatment period of 1–2.5 h.

The latter finding has previously been reported by Plunkett and coworkers already and was thought to result from a sustained plasma ara-C concentration above 7–10 μmol/l, which is sufficient for a complete saturation of the ara-C-phosphorylating enzyme deoxycytidine kinase [16, 17]. This hypothesis, however, does not explain the differences in ara-CTP pharmacokinetics between normal and leukemic cells and is challenged by the rapid decline in ara-C plasma concentration as revealed by the respective concomitant measurements during the present investigation.

Hence, the observed findings most probably point to a prolonged availability of incompletely phosphorylated ara-C metabolites such as mono- or diphosphates which could result from differences in the activity of the deoxycytidine kinase complex between leukemic and normal cells and/or differences of deoxycytidine triphosphate concentrations. This assumption is supported by recent reports about the selective protection of normal hematopoietic cells from ara-C cytotoxicity by the coadministration of deoxycytidine [18] and the preferential outgrowth of normal hematopoietic precursor cells in suspension cultures after simultaneous exposure to ara-C and deoxycytidine [9]. Further studies are warranted to substantiate this hypothesis by the determination of ara-C mono- and diphosphate concentrations as well as of the activity of the pyrimidine nucleoside monophosphate and diphosphate kinases.

Independent of the underlying mechanism, the differences in ara-CTP between normal and leukemic cells may provide the basis for an optimized scheduling of ara-C therapy resulting in an increase of antileukemic activity without a concomitant enhancement of side effects and thus an improvement of the therapeutic index for ara-C. Further studies are underway to substantiate these findings and to elucidate its underlying mechanisms.

Summary

Pharmacokinetic analyses of intracellular cytosine arabinoside 5′ triphosphate (ara-CTP) levels and plasma ara-C and ara-U concentrations were performed in 32 patients with acute myeloid leukemia undergoing combination therapy including either standard (100 mg/m² per day) or high-dose (1.0 or 3.0 g/m²) ara-C. Plasma ara-C concentration showed a linear dependency from the applied ara-C dose but did not correlate with intracellular ara-CTP levels.

During conventional-dose ara-C therapy little interpatient variation was observed in ara-CTP retention times in leukemic blasts from five patients with $t_{1/2}$ values ranging from 1.70 to 2.50 h. In all cases ara-CTP levels declined rapidly after the end of treatment. Substantial differences in ara-CTP retention times were revealed, however, during 3-h infusions of either 1.0 or 3.0 g/m² ara-C in leukemic blasts from eight patients with $t_{1/2}$ values between 1.60 and 7.63 h. In addition, seven of the eight patients showed unchanged or even increasing ara-CTP levels for up to 2.5 h after the end of therapy. In contrast, ara-CTP retention times were relatively uniform in normal mononuclear blood cells from nine patients with $t_{1/2}$ values of 3.34–4.65 h. More importantly, ara-CTP levels dropped immediately after the high-dose ara-C infusion in all cases. These data strongly suggest differences in the intracellular pharmacokinetics of ara-C in leukemic and normal blood cells which may be used for the design of a more selective antileukemic ara-C application.

References

1. Plunkett W, Jacoboni S, Estey E, Danhauser L, Liliemark JO, Keating MJ (1985) Pharmacologically directed ara-C therapy for refractory leukemia. Semin Oncol 12 [Suppl 3]: 20–30
2. Rustum YM, Riva C, Preisler HD (1987) Pharmacokinetic parameters of 1-β-D-arabinofuranosylcytosine (ara-C) and their relationship to intracellular metabolism of ara-C, toxicity, and response of patients with conventional and high-dose ara-C. Semin Oncol 14 [Suppl 1]: 141–148
3. Estey E, Plunkett W, Dixon D, Keating M, McCredie K, Freireich EJ (1987) Variables predicting response to high-dose cytosine arabinoside therapy in patients with refractory acute leukemia. Leukemia 8: 580–583
4. Cappizzi RL, Yang JI, Rathmell JP, White JC, Cheng E, Cheng Y-C, Kute T (1985) Dose-related pharmacologic effects of high-dose ara-C and its self-potentiation. Semin Oncol 12 [Suppl 3]: 65–75
5. Riva CM, Rustum YM, Preisler HD (1985) Pharmacokinetics and cellular determinants of response to 1-β-arabinofuranosylcytosine (ara-C). Semin Oncol 12 [Suppl 3]: 1–8
6. Heinemann V, Estey E, Keating MJ, Plunkett W (1989) Patient-specific dose rate for continuous infusion high-dose cytarabine in relapsed acute myelogenous leukemia. J Clin Oncol 7: 622–628
7. Plunkett W, Heinemann V, Estey E, Keating M (1990) Pharmacologically directed design of leukemia therapy. In: Büchner T, Schellong G, Hiddemann W, Ritter J (eds) Acute

leukemias – prognostic factors and treatment strategies II. Springer, Berlin Heidelberg New York, pp 610–613

8. Bhalla K, Birkhofer M, Arlin Z, Grant S, Lutzky J, Graham G (1988) Effect of recombinant GM-CSF on the metabolism of cytosine arabinoside in normal and leukemic human bone marrow cells. Leukemia 2: 810–813

9. Grant S, Bhalla K, Arlin Z, Howe CWS (1990) The effect of a prolonged in vitro exposure to 1-β-D arabinofuranosylcytosine and deoxycytidine on the survival of normal (CFU-GM) and leukemic (L-CFU) human myeloid progenitor cells in suspension culture. Exp Hematol 18: 41–48

10. Büchner T, Urbanitz D, Hiddemann W, Rühl H, Ludwig WD, Fischer J, Aul HC, Vaupel HA, Kuse R, Zeile G, Nowrousian MR, König HJ, Walter M, Wendt FC, Sodomann H, Hossfeld DK, von Paleske A, Löffler H, Gassmann W, Hellriegel K-P, Fülle HH, Lunscken C, Emmerich B, Pralle H, Pees HW, Pfreundschuh M, Bartels H, Koeppen K-M, Schwerdtfeger R, Donhuijsen-Ant R, Mainzer K, Bonfert B, Köppler H, Zurborn K-H, Ranft K, Thiel E, Heinecke A (1985) Intensified induction and consolidation with or without maintenance chemotherapy for acute myeloid leukemia (AML): two multicenter studies of the German AML Cooperative Group. J Clin Oncol 3: 1583–1589

11. Hiddemann W, Maschmeyer G, Pfreundschuh M, Ludwig WD, Büchner T (1988) Treatment of refractory acute myeloid (AML) and lymphoblastic leukemia (ALL) with high-dose cytosine arabinoside (HD-ara-C) and mitoxantrone: indication of increased efficacy by sequential administration. Proc Am Soc Clin Oncol 5: 189

12. Hiddemann W, Schleyer E, Uhrmeister C, Aul C, Maschmeyer G, Heinecke A, Büchner T (1991) High-dose versus intermediate dose cytosine arabinoside in combination with mitoxantrone for the treatment of relapsed and refractory acute myeloid leukemia – preliminary clinical and pharmacological data of a randomized comparison. Cancer Treat Rev (in press)

13. Uhrmeister C, Schleyer E, Ehninger G, Büchner T, and Hiddemann W (1989) Pharmacokinetic measurements of Ara-C, Ara-U and intercellular Ara-CTP under sequential HAM therapy. Blut 59: 127

14. Schleyer E, Ehninger G, Zühlsdorf M, Proksch B, Hiddemann W (1989) Detection and separation of intracellular Ara-CTP by ion-pair high-performance liquid chromatography: a sensitive, isocratic, highly reproducible and rapid method. J Chromatogr 497: 109–120

15. Heinzel G, Hammer R, Wolf M, Koss FW, Bozler G (1977) Modellentwicklung in der Pharmakokinetik. Drug Res 27: 904–911

16. Liliemark JO, Plunkett W, Dixon DO (1985) Relationship of 1-β-D-arabinofuranosylcytosine in plasma to 1-β-D-arabinofuranosylcytosine 5′-triphosphate levels in leukemic cells during treatment with high-dose 1-β-D-arabinofuranosylcytosine. Cancer Res 45: 5952–5957

17. Plunkett W, Liliemark JO, Estey E, Keating MJ (1987) Saturation of ara-CTP accumulation during high-dose ara-C therapy: pharmacologic rationale for intermediate-dose ara-C. Semin Oncol 14 [Suppl 1]: 159–166

18. Bhalla K, MacLaughlin W, Cole J, Arlin Z, Baker M, Graham G, Grant S (1987) Deoxycytidine preferentially protects normal versus leukemic myeloid progenitor cells from cytosine arabinoside-mediated cytotoxicity. Blood 70: 568–571

Therapy of Relapsed Acute Myeloid Leukemia Using Targeted Plasma Concentrations of Cytosine Arabinoside and Etoposide*

J. Mirro, Jr., W. Crom, J. Belt, and M. Schell

Introduction

While the outcome for children with acute lymphocytic leukemia (ALL) has improved as a result of increased dose intensity, the same improvement has not occurred in acute myeloid leukemia (AML). Although approximately 85 % of children with AML achieve a complete remission (CR), the majority ultimately relapse and die of their disease [1–5]. Although bone marrow transplant (BMT) offers better disease control, patient selection and the timing of transplantation remains controversial [6–8]. Furthermore, because of the risk of early death and the development of graft-versus-host disease, clinical trials have not clearly demonstrated that BMT is the treatment of choice for AML in the first CR [9].

The major therapeutic problem in AML is effectively eliminating the residual leukemic cells after patients achieve a CR [5]. Explanations for treatment failure include: (1) the primary transforming event occurs in a hematopoietic stem cell; (2) the clonogeneic leukemic cells fail to enter the cell cycle, thus precluding the cytotoxic effects of S-phase-specific drugs; or (3) the devel-

opment of multidrug resistance, either classical or atypical in nature. Other possible hypotheses for treatment failure are insufficient exposure of leukemic cells to the active drug or inadequate conversion of the drug to its active metabolite within the cell [10, 11]. This study addresses the possibility that inadequate exposure of leukemic cells to the drug is responsible for treatment failure [12–14]. We reasoned that patients with rapid drug metabolism would have low plasma concentrations, a low systemic exposure, and therefore might fail therapy based on limited exposure of leukemic cells to the active agents [15, 16]. Alternatively, patients that are slow drug metabolizers may have high plasma concentrations and develop toxicity [13]. We therefore designed this protocol to increase the dose intensity of cytosine arabinoside (ara-C) and etoposide (VP-16) and reduce the interpatient variability.

In this protocol we targeted ara-C to a 1-μM steady-state plasma concentration (Cp$_{ss}$) and VP-16 to a 30 μM steady-state plasma concentration. The rationale for selecting an ara-C Cp$_{ss}$ of 1 μM was preliminary data suggesting that adequate levels of intracellular cytosine arabinoside triphosphate (ara-CTP) would be achieved at this extracellular concentration [10, 15]. We chose to administer the ara-C as a continuous infusion of 120 h since it is S-phase active. The administration of ara-C by continuous infusion also permitted better control of the plasma concentration.

We chose a 30μM plasma concentration for VP-16 based on therapeutic effects in an earlier front-line trial [5]. In that trial VP-16

Departments of Hematology-Oncology, Pharmacokinetics, Biochemical Pharmacology, and Biostatistics, St. Jude Children's Research Hospital, PO Box 318, Memphis, 38101-0318, USA
* Supported in part by USPHS grant CA-20180, NIH Cancer Center CORE Grant CA-21765, and by the American Lebanese Syrian Associated Charities (ALSAC).

concentrations of 12–15 μM were effective and nontoxic. A 96 h continuous infusion was selected because this drug is also S-phase active and a continuous infusion permitted easy control of the VP-16 plasma concentration [17].

Materials and Methods

The protocol consisted of two cycles of therapy (Fig. 1). In cycle 1, ara-C was administered as a continuous subcutaneous infusion for 120 h at a starting dose of 500 mg/m² per 24 h. Plasma concentrations were measured by HPLC at 1 and 6 h, and the dose was adjusted within 12 h to achieve a Cp_{ss} of 1 μM. The maximum dose of ara-C permitted on this protocol to limit toxicity was 750 mg/m² per 24 h. Twenty-four hours after the start of the ara-C in cycle 1, VP-16 was added. The VP-16 was administered as a continuous intravenous infusion for 96 h. To rapidly achieve the preselected plasma steady-state concentration of 30 μM, a loading dose of 70 mg/m² over 1 h was administered. The initial VP-16 infusion rate was 500 mg/m² per 24 h and within 12 h the VP-16 infusion was adjusted to achieve a 30μM plasma concentration (based on the levels at 1 and 6 h). Since this was a novel treatment approach, the maximum dose of VP-16 permitted was 750 mg/m² per 24 h.

All children had a bone marrow aspirate performed on day 10 to evaluate the response to cycle 1.

When toxicity resolved the patients were reevaluated; if they had progressive disease they were given cycle 2 immediately (20–35 days after cycle 1). If they had evidence of marrow recovery, cycle 2 was delayed and administered when they achieved a complete remission. Cycle 2 of this protocol consisted of a 120 h continuous infusion of ara-C at 1 μM plasma concentration with daunorubicin, 50 mg/m² per dose, given as a bolus on days 1 and 2 (Fig. 1).

All patients enrolled in this trial previously received intensive therapy with VP-16, ara-C, and daunorubicin but at lower doses. This trial was approved by the St. Jude Children's Research Hospital Clinical Trials Committee and all patients or parents gave informed consent as appropriate.

A diagnosis of AML was made by standard French-American-British (FAB) criteria based on morphology and cytochemical stains. Responses were evaluated by standard criteria. A complete response was defined as a cellular marrow aspirate with less than 5 % blasts and no identifiable leukemic cells, normal hematopoiesis, and normal performance status for >1 month. All toxicity was evaluated and graded by the National Cancer Institute Common Toxicity Criteria.

Fig. 1. Protocol therapy schema: Cycle 1 consisted of a continuous subcutaneous infusion of ara-C for 120 h with the infusion rate adjusted to achieve a 1μM plasma concentration. Exactly 24 h after starting therapy, VP-16 was administered for 96 h by continuous intravenous infusion to acheive a plasma concentration of 30 μM. The ara-C and VP-16 were administered simultaneously for 96 h and the infusions were stopped at the same time. Cycle 2 consisted of continuous infusion of ara-C at 1μM plasma concentration and two doses of daunorubicin. Cycle 2 was delayed until patients recovered from toxicity and achieved a CR or had progressive disease.

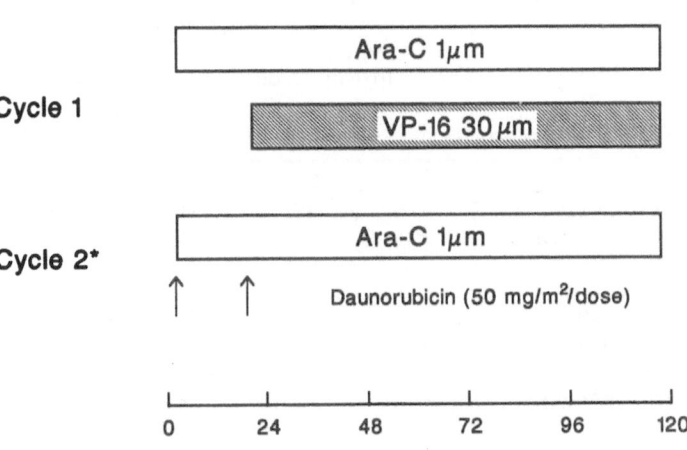

Results

There were 10 boys and 13 girls with a median age of 6.8 years (range, 1.0–16 years) enrolled on this trial. Twenty patients were in their first hematologic relapse, while three patients were in their second or subsequent hematologic relapse. Almost 80 % of the children (18 of 23) were receiving chemotherapy at the time they relapsed; one patient had undergone a bone marrow transplant and four were off treatment (Table 1). At the time of entry the median leukocyte count was $6.0 \times 10^9/l$ (range, $1–301 \times 10^9/l$). Most patients (57 %) had FAB M4 or M5 leukemia (Table 1).

Twenty-three patients received cycle 1 of therapy. The initial ara-C dose was 500 mg/m^2 per 24 h, but in most patients the dose was increased to a median of 550 mg/m^2 per 24 h (range, 412–750 mg/m^2 per 24 h) (Table 2). The VP-16 dose was also started at 500 mg/m^2 per 24 h and in most patients the infusion rate was increased to a median of 600 mg/m^2 per 24 h (range, 350–750 mg/m^2 per 24 h).

Table 1. Patient characteristics

Number of patients	23
Sex M:F	10:13
Median age (years)	6.8 (range, 0.1–16 years)
First hematologic relapse	20
Relapse while receiving therapy	18
Median leukocyte count (x10^9/l)	6.0 (range, 1.0–301)
CNS positive	3 (13 %)
Auer bodies	7 (30 %)
FAB class	
M1 + M2	9 (39 %)
M3	1 (4 %)
M4 + M5	13 (57 %)

Table 2. Dose of drug administered to achieve selected plasma concentrations

Drug	Cycle	daily dose (mg/m²) Median	Range
Ara-C	1	550	412–750
VP-16	1	600	350–750
Ara-C	2	600	350–759

The toxicity from cycle 1 was severe (Table 3). One patient died of sepsis and nine children developed documented infections. All 23 patients had leukocyte counts of $<1.0 \times 10^9/l$ and platelet counts of $<20 \times$

Table 3. Toxicity of targeted therapy

	Cycle 1 (n=23) Toxicity grade			Cycle 2 (n=16) Toxicity grade		
Toxicity/grade	0	1 or 2	3 or 4	0	1 or 2	3 or 4
Hematopoietic						
Leukocyte count	0	0	23	0	0	16
Platelet count	0	0	23	0	0	16
GI						
Mucositis	0	4	19	6	7	3
Diarrhea	13	9	1	14	2	0
Hepatotoxicity	7	9	7	7	5	4
Skin	6	13	4	12	2	2
Infections[a]	14	0	9	9	0	7

[a] One Patient died of *Escherichia coli* sepsis during cycle

10^9/l. Mucositis was also a major problem, with 19 of the 23 patients developing severe mucositis beginning on day 7 and resolving by approximately day 18. Hepatotoxicity was mild and manageable. Skin toxicity did occur on cycle 1 with the combination of ara-C and VP-16 and was generally diffuse erythema (Table 3).

Despite the severe toxicity, nine patients achieved a complete remission with cycle 1 alone. Two of these patients were then referred for bone marrow transplantation.

Sixteen patients then received cycle 2 of therapy. Six of these 16 had already achieved a complete remission while 10 had residual disease. The toxicity of cycle 2 (Table 3) was similar to cycle 1. Grade 4 hematopoietic toxicity developed in all the patients, and the incidence of infection was similar to cycle 1. Cycle 2 resulted in significantly less mucositis and skin erythema and possibly less hepatotoxicity. The median dose of ara-C administered during cycle 2 was 600 mg/m^2 per 24 h (range, 350–750 mg/m^2 per 24 h). Of the ten patients with residual disease that entered cycle 2, three additional patients achieved a complete remission. One of these patients was subsequently referred for transplantation.

The overall response rate was 52% (12 complete responders out of 23 patients). This CR rate is encouraging particulary since all these patients had received all three had agents previously, and most (18 children) had relapsed on therapy. The duration of complete response was also encouraging with a median CR of 4.9 months with a range of 1.8–8.2 months.

Discussion

This protocol was designed to determine if it was feasible to target plasma concentrations and standardize the total systemic exposure for ara-C and VP-16 in children. Additionally, the total doses of ara-C and VP-16 administered to these patients were significantly higher than generally administered during standard induction therapy. Although the doses were increased approximately two- to threefold, total systemic exposure was increased to a much greater extent (two- to tenfold). This approach yielded a higher and more uniform total drug exposure for all patients. This higher total exposure resulted in severe but predictable toxicity. Since all patients had received ara-C and VP-16 previously, the results in this relapse trial were encouraging. The results suggest that this combination is worthy of an upfront trial in previously untreated patients. The toxicity, however, suggests that the total systemic exposure should be decreased slightly.

This protocol was not designed to demonstrate a dose response relationship. The small number of patients does not permit meaningful statistical analysis between response to the initial AML induction therapy which included ara-C and VP-16 at lower doses and this therapy which was used at relapse.

Recent evidence suggests that the simultaneous administration of ara-C and VP-16 might decrease the therapeutic effects of each agent [18]. We did not study the cellular biochemical effects of these drugs on leukemic blasts in this protocol. Pharmacokinetic studies, however, did demonstrate that there was no change in Cp_{ss} of ara-C when VP-16 was administered.

This novel approach to individualizing antileukemic therapy is being used on our current front-line trial. On that trial with the Cp_{ss} of ara-C and VP-16 adjusted, the cellular pharmacology of ara-CTP and VP-16 is being studied to determine if they can predict initial response. This approach of targeting plasma steady-state concentrations and thereby the total systemic exposure is closer to defining an exact dose-intensity and should be considered for use in more clinical trials.

Summary

The plasma concentration of many antileukemic agents is highly variable when these drugs are administered at a dose per body surface area (mg/m^2). Since efficacy may be related to the total systemic exposure, we reduced interpatient variability in systemic exposure by adjusting the dose of cytosine arabinoside (ara-C) and etoposide (VP-16) administered to achieve a preselected steady-state plasma concentration (Cp_{ss}). Twenty-three children with acute myeloid leukemia (AML) in hematologic relapse were treated with ara-C at a Cp_{ss} of 1 μM for 120 h and VP-16 at a Cp_{ss} of 30 μM for 96 h (cycle 1). After patients recovered from toxicity (generally 20–35 days) they received a second cycle of therapy with ara-C at a 1μM Cp_{ss} × 120 h plus two doses of daunorubicin (50 mg/m^2 per dose).

Using a continuous infusion of these agents and a rapid high-performance liquid chromatography (HPLC) assay we were able to achieve the preselected levels within 12 h in most patients. The median dose of ara-C administered to achieve a 1μM plasma concentration was 550 mg/m^2 per 24 h (range, 412–750 mg/m^2 per 24 h) in cycle 1 and 600 mg/m^2 per 24 h (range, 350–750 mg/m^2 per 24 h) in cycle 2. The median dose of VP-16 administered to achieve the preselected Cp_{ss} of 30 μM was 600 mg/m^2 per 24 h (range, 350–750 mg/m^2 per 24 h). Some patients did not achieve the preselected Cp_{ss} because the protocol limited the maximum dose of ara-C and VP-16 to 750 mg/m^2 per 24 h. All children developed severe hematopoietic toxicity and 40 % developed documented infections. Mucositis was severe (grade 3 or 4) in 19 children (82 %) during cycle 1 but occurred in only 3 of 16 children during cycle 2. Despite the fact that all children received these agents previously, 12 children (52 %) achieved a complete remission (CR); with 9 of the 12 patients achieving a CR doing so after only cycle 1. These results indicate that administration of drugs at a preselected plasma concentration is possible and might be effective in previously untreated patients.

Acknowledgements. We wish to thank the medical and nursing staff of St. Jude Children's Research Hospital for patient care. We also wish to thank Ms. M. Rafferty for data analysis and Ms. P. Vandiveer for typing the manuscript.

References

1. Weinstein HJ, Mayer RJ, Rosenthal DS et al. (1983) Chemotherapy for acute myelogenous leukemia in children and adults: VAPA update. Blood 62: 315–319

2. Buckley JD, Lampkin BC, Nesbit ME et al. (1989) Remission induction in children with acute non-lymphocytic leukemia using cytosine arabinoside and doxorubicin or daunorubicin: a report from the Childrens Cancer Study Group. Med Pediatr Oncol 17: 382–390

3. Steuber CP, Civin C, Krischer J et al. (1991) A comparison of induction and maintenance therapy for acute nonlymphocytic leukemia in childhood: results of a Pediatric Oncology Group study. J Clin Oncol 9: 247–258

4. Creutzig U, Ritter J, Riehm H et al. (1985) Improved treatment results in childhood acute myelogenous leukemia: a report of the German Cooperative Study AML-BFM-78. Blood 65: 298–304

5. Kalwinsky D, Mirro J, Schell M et al. (1988) Early intensification of chemotherapy for childhood acute nonlymphoblastic leukemia: improved remission induction with a five-drug regimen including etoposide. J Clin Oncol 6: 1134–1143

6. Raimondi SC, Kalwinsky DK, Hayashi Y et al. (1989) The cytogenetics of childhood acute nonlymphocytic leukemia. Cancer Genet Cytogenet 40: 13–27

7. Kalwinsky DK, Raimondi S, Schell MJ et al. (1990) Prognostic importance of cytogenetic subgroups in de novo pediatric acute nonlymphocytic leukemia. J Clin Oncol 8: 75–83

8. Grier HE, Gelber RD, Camitta BM et al. (1987) Prognostic factors in childhood acute myelogenous leukemia. J Clin Oncol 5: 1026–1032

9. Dahl GV, Kalwinsky DK, Mirro J et al. (1990) Allogeneic bone marrow transplantation in a program of intensive sequential chemotherapy for children and young adults with acute nonlymphocytic leukemia in first remission. J Clin Oncol 8: 295–303

10. Liliemark JO, Plunkett W, Dixon DO (1985) Relationship of 1-β-*D*-arabinofuranosylcytosine in plasma to 1-β-*D*-arabinofuranosylcytosine 5′-triphosphate levels in leukemic cells during treatment with high-dose 1-β-*D*-arabinofuranosylcytosine. Cancer Res 45: 5952–5957

11. Rustum YM, Lawrence DD, Priore RL et al. (1986) Relationship between plasma pharmacokinetic parameters of arabinosylcytosine (ARAC) intracellular ARA-CTP, and toxicity of acute nonlymphocytic leukemia patients to treatment with high dose ARAC. Am Soc Clin Oncol 5: 164–171

12. Bertino JR (1987) Blood levels of chemotherapeutic agents and clinical outcome. J Clin Oncol 5: 996–997

13. Rodman JR, Abromowitch M, Sinkule JA et al. (1987) Clinical pharmacodynamics of continuous infusion teniposide: systemic exposure as a determinant of response in a Phase I trial. J Clin Oncol 5: 1007–1014
14. Preisler HD, Rustum YM, Azarnia N et al. (1987) Abrogation of the prognostic significance of low leukemic cell retention of cytosine arabinoside triphosphate by intensification of therapy and by alteration in the dose and schedule of administration of cytosine arabinoside. Cancer Chemother Pharmacol 19: 69–74
15. Plunkett W, Iacoboni S, Estey E et al. (1985) Pharmacologically directed ara-C therapy for refractory leukemia. Semin Oncol 3: 20–30
16. Karp JE, Donehower RC, Dole GB et al. (1987) Correlation of drug-perturbed marrow cell growth kinetics and intracellular 1-β-D-arabinofuranosylcytosine metabolism with clinical response in adult acute myelogenous leukemia. Blood 69: 1134–1140
17. Hande KR, Wedlund PJ, Noone RM et al. (1984) Pharmacokinetics of high-dose etoposide (VP-16-213) administered to cancer patients. Cancer Res 44: 379–382
18. Ehninger G, Proksch B, Wanner T et al. (1990) Cytosine arabinoside uptake and cytosine arabinoside triphosphate formation by leukemic blast cells is inhibited by etoposide and teniposide. Blood 76 (10) [Suppl 1]: 266a

Pharmacokinetics of High-Dose Etoposide Given in Diluted or Undiluted Form

G. Ehninger, P. Waidelich, B. Proksch, B. Eichel, H. Schmidt, C. Faul, U. Schuler, T. R. Spitzer, and J. Deeg

Introduction

The probability of relapse after allogeneic bone marrow transplantation is as high as 30 % in standard risk patients. Investigators have attempted to improve these results by combining total body irradiation (TBI) and etoposide [1–3]. However, the use of etoposide requires time-consuming dilution steps resulting in large fluid volumes that need to be administered. It was noted recently that the stability of etoposide in saline 0.9 % and dextrose 5 % is much greater than previously thought [4]. Lazarus et al. [5, 6] suggested administering etoposide without prior dilution. However, it is not clear whether administration in undiluted form alters bioavailability. Therefore, we conducted the present study to compare the pharmacokinetics of etoposide given as diluted or undiluted solution.

Patients and Methods

Fifteen patients with a high risk of relapse after allogeneic bone marrow transplantation were included in the clinicopharmacological study. Eight of them received etoposide at a dose of 30 mg/kg without prior dilution; in seven etoposide at various doses

Medizinische Universitätsklinik und Kinderklinik der Universität, Otfried-Müller-Str. 10, 7400 Tübingen, FRG

Fred Hutchinson Cancer Research Center, 1124 Columbia Street, Seattle, WA 98104, USA

Georgetown University, 3900 Reservoir Road NW, Washington DC 20007, USA

was diluted in sodium chloride 0.9 % for a final concentration of 1 mg/ml and infused at a rate of 500 ml/h as previously described [7]. The undiluted etoposide solution was administered by use of a perfusor (Secura FT; Braun, Melsungen, FRG) equipped with a 50-ml syringe made of polypropylene (Braun, Melsungen, No. 872881/0), an infusion line made of polyvinylchloride (Braun, Melsungen, No. 872296/0), and a dual- or triple-lumen central venous catheter (Quinton, Seattle, United States). The equipment was prefilled with etoposide solution; rinsing with other fluids was avoided.

Sample Treatment. Heparinized blood samples were collected from patients before treatment, at 4, 8, and 12 h during infusion, and 4, 8, 12, and 36 h following completion of the infusion. Plasma was removed after centrifugation for 10 min and immediately assayed or stored at −20 °C until use.

Determination of Etoposide by HPLC. Particularly for high-dose pharmacokinetic investigations a simple and rapid high-performance liquid chromatographic (HPLC) assay was developed, which allowed the determination of etoposide in plasma up to 48 h after the start of infusion.

Extraction and Analysis. In a 1.5-ml microcentrifuge tube, 300 μl plasma was mixed with an equal volume of acetonitrile, vortexed, and frozen at −20 °C to achieve a better deproteinization. After thawing the sample was centrifuged for 5 min in a microcentrifuge at 12 000 g. Twenty microliters of the supernatant was injected onto a HPLC system. Separation of etoposide was achieved isocratically using a Hypersil-Phenyl column (10 μm, 250 × 4 mm, Shandon), a mobile phase of water/methanol (50/50, v/v) containing 5 m*M* tetrabutylammonium phosphate, and a flow rate of 1 ml/min. Etoposide was detected at 254 nm (UV).

Quantitation, Calibration, Recovery, and Precision. Determination at 254 nm has shown sufficient sensitivity for the measurement of etoposide after high-dose administration. The external standard method was used for quantitation by plotting the peak area against known concentrations of standards. Pharmacokinetic data were calculated by use of the TOPFIT program [8]. Area under curve (AUC) values were calculated by use of the trapezoidal rule.

Results

The results are summarized in Tables 1 and 2. Plasma concentrations at the end of a 12-h infusion of eight patients receiving undiluted etoposide were between 32.4 and 108.1 μg/ml. AUC values of 764 ± 302 μg h/ml [= 41.8 ± 18.4 (μg min/ml)/(mg/m^2)] for etoposide were calculated. The results in patients receiving etoposide with prior dilution are given in Table 2. AUC values of 862 ± 354 μg h/ml [= 29.8 ± 8.2 (μg min/ml)/(mg/m^2)] for etoposide were calculated.

Table 1. Pharmacokinetic parameters of undiluted etoposide given as 12-h infusion

Patient	Dose (mg/kg)	Peak (μg/ml)	Half-life Terminal (h)	AUC (μg h/ml)	AUC/dose (μg h/ml)/ (mg/kg)	Clearance (ml/min)	VD (l)
1	30	48.4	2.9	525	17.5	63.8	16.0
2	30	41.4	2.8	644	21.5	59.3	13.2
3	30	108.1	4.0	1405	46.8	22.5	3.5
4	30	50.2	3.7	722	24.1	55.9	18.1
5	30	32.4		529	17.6	78.5	37.3
6	30	46.8	2.3	543	18.1	33.8	6.5
7	30	77.8	4.5	1116	37.2	28.9	11.2
8	30	42.7	13.6	626	20.9	53.6	17.6
Mean		56.0	4.8	764	25	49.5	15.4
Std		23.2	3.6	302	10	18.0	9.6

AUC, area under curve; VD, volume of distribution; Std, standard deviation

Table 2. Pharmacokinetic parameters of diluted etoposide

Patient	Dose (mg/kg)	Infusion time (h)	Peak (μg/ml)	Half-life terminal (h)	AUC (μg h/ml)	AUC/dose (μg h/ml)/ (mg/kg)	Clearance (ml/min)	VD (l)
1	23	7.25	53.7	2.6	414	18.2	117.6	26.8
2	30	4.16	174	15.4	566	18.9	20.1	5
3	65	10.85	112	4	1344	20.7	48.6	12.6
4	65	13	110	4.7	1064	16.4	54.8	22.3
5	65	8.38	110.8	3.7	1141	17.6	44.5	14.1
6	65	11.2	76.6	4.6	1080	16.6	71.5	21.5
7	30	4.75	63.2	3.4	428	14.3	66.9	13.1
Mean				5.5	862	17.5	60.6	16.5
SD				4.1	354	1.9	28.0	6.9

AUC, area under curve; VD, volume of distribution

Discussion

This study confirms that etoposide can be administered in undiluted form via a central venous catheter. Systemic availability of etoposide was as good as in patients who received diluted etoposide. The AUC values per dose were somewhat higher in patients receiving undiluted etoposide. Since the numbers of patients were small, it is possible that differences were due to interpatient variability. Comparing both drug formulations in a single patient on consecutive days might help to clarify this issue. In two other pharmacokinetic studies [9, 10] utilizing etoposide diluted in normal saline at doses of 30–70 mg/kg or 400–800 mg/m^2 for three consecutive days the AUC values were reported to be 36.9 (µg min/ml)/(mg/m^2) and 39.4 (µg min/ml)/ (mg/m^2), respectively. Our result of 41.8 $\pm$ 18.4 (µg min/ml)/(mg/m^2) in patients with undiluted etoposide is in good agreement with those. The administration of undiluted etoposide renders the therapy easier and less time consuming and avoids a high volume and saline load. Precipitations of etoposide were never detected if the infusion system was primed with etoposide solution and rinsing with other fluids was avoided. In addition to safety and practicability considerations, new schedules, which are attractive against the background of a schedule-dependent activity [11] of etoposide, will be more easily studied with this approach.

References

1. Schmitz N, Gassmann W, Rister M, Johannson W, Suttorp M, Brix F, Holthuis JJ, Heit W, Hertenstein B, Schaub J (1988) Fractionated total body irradiation and high-dose VP 16-213 followed by allogeneic bone marrow transplantation in advanced leukemias. Blood 72: 1567–1573
2. Blume KG, Forman SJ, O'Donnell MR, Doroshow JH, Krance RA, Nademanee AP, Snyder DS, Schmidt GM, Fahey JL, Metter GE, et al. (1987) Total body irradiation and high-dose etoposide: a new preparatory regimen for bone marrow transplantation in patients with advanced hematologic malignancies. Blood 69: 1015–1020
3. Zander AR, Culbert S, Jagannath S, Spitzer G, Keating M, Larry N, Cockerill K, Hester J, Horwitz L, Vellekoop L (1987) High dose cyclophosphamide, BCNU, and VP-16 (CBV) as a conditioning regimen for allogeneic bone marrow transplantation for patients with acute leukemia. Cancer 59: 1083–1086
4. Joel SP, Maclean MC, Slevin ML (1989) The stability of the intravenous preparation of etoposide in isotonic fluids. Proc Am Assoc Cancer Res 30: 244 (Abstract)
5. Lazarus HM, Creger RJ, Diaz D (1986) Simple method for the administration of high-dose etoposide during autologous bone marrow transplantation. Cancer Treat Rep 70: 819–820
6. Creger RJ, Fox RM, Lazarus HM (1990) Infusion of high doses of undiluted etoposide through central venous catheters during preparation for bone marrow transplantation. Cancer Invest 8: 13–16
7. Spitzer TR, Cottler-Fox M, Torrisi J, Cahill R, Greenspan A, Lynch M, Deeg HJ (1989) Escalating doses of etoposide with cyclophosphamide and fractionated total body irradiation or busulfan as conditioning for bone marrow transplantation. Bone Marrow Transplant 4: 559–565
8. Heinzel G, Hammer R, Wolf M (1977) Modellentwicklung in der Pharmakokinetik. Drug Res 27: 904–911
9. Newman EM, Doroshow JH, Forman SJ, Blume KG (1988) Pharmacokinetics of high-dose etoposide. Clin Pharmacol Ther 43: 561–564
10. Hande KR, Wedlund PJ, Noone RM, Wilkinson GR, Greco FA, Wolff SN (1984) Pharmacokinetics of high-dose etoposide (VP-16-213) administered to cancer patients. Cancer Res 44: 379–822
11. Slevin ML, Clark PI, Joel SP, Malik S, Osborne RJ, Gregory WM, Lowe DG, Reznek RH, Wrigley PF (1989) A randomized trial to evaluate the effect of schedule on the activity of etoposide in small-cell lung cancer. J Clin Oncol 7: 1333–1340

Clinical Implications of Idarubicin Pharmacology*

E. Berman, M. McBride, and B. Clarkson

Introduction

4-Demethoxydaunorubicin (idarubicin, IDR) is a new anthracycline that differs from its parent compound daunorubicin (DNR) by the deletion of a methoxy group at position 4 of the chromophore ring. This minor modification results in a compound that has a higher lipophilic coefficient and therefore more rapid cellular uptake [1]; in addition, IDR induces more single-strand breaks in tumor cells [2]. While both DNR and IDR are converted to alcohol metabolites, daunorubicin-ol (DNR-ol) and idarubicin-ol (IDR-ol), respectively, DNR-ol disappears from the plasma by hour 192 after three consecutive daily intravenous boluses while IDR-ol has a more prolonged plasma half-life with steady state levels measurable up to 216 h after the third bolus injection [3].

The cytotoxic activities of IDR and IDR-ol have been compared to that of DNR and another anthracycline epirubicin, and their respective metabolites in the leukemia cell lines K-562 and CCRF-CEM by Kuffel et al. [4]. IDR was three to five times more cytotoxic than the other parent anthracyclines and IDR-ol was 29- to 103-fold more cytotoxic than the other alcohol derivatives.

The Leukemia Service, Department of Medicine, Memorial Sloan Kettering Cancer Center, 1275 York Avenue, New York, NY 10021, USA
* This work was supported in part by American Cancer Society Research Career Development Award No. 89-124.

In order to determine whether these differences had significant clinical relevance, multiple centers in the United States and Europe designed prospective randomized trials comparing IDR and cytosine arabinoside (ara-C) with DNR and ara-C in adult patients with untreated acute myelogenous leukemia (AML) [5–7]. Results from three such trials in the United States are given in Table 1. It is important to note that the maximum age in the Memorial Sloan Kettering Cancer Center trial was 60 years while the other two trials had no age limit. In all three trials, however, patients on the IDR/ara-C arm had a higher incidence of remission.

Analysis of the Memorial data yielded two important features [5]. First, more than twice as many patients failed to achieve remission on the DNR/ara-C arm ($n = 25$) compared to the IDR/ara-C arm ($n = 12$). Twenty-one of the 25 (84 %) patients on the DNR/ara-C arm had persistent blasts after 2 induction courses compared to 8 of 12 patients on the IDR/ara-C arm (67 %) [5]. Second, patients on the IDR/ara-C arm had a probability of response approximating 80 % regardless of the initial white blood cell (WBC) count; while on the DNR/ara-C arm the incidence of response declined as the WBC increased [5].

These findings led us to compare the cellular uptake and retention characteristics of IDR and DNR in an anthracycline-resistant lymphoblastic leukemia cell line CEM-VBL. This particular cell line has been previously demonstrated to contain within its plasma membrane the ~170-kd glycoprotein pump (P-glycoprotein, Pgp)

295

Table 1. Clinical trials: IDR vs. DNR

Study	Age (years)	IDR/ara-C	DNR/ara-C	p value
MSKCC[a]	18–60	48/60(80%)	35/60(58%)	.005
Berman et al. [5]				
SEG[b]	>18	29/39(74%)	26/46(57%)	.09
Vogler et al. [6]	<60	16/20(80%)	14/22(64%)	NS
Multicenter[c]	>18	34/51(67%)	27/51(53%)	NS
Wiernik et al. [7]	≤60	31/38(815)	24/37(65%)	<.1

[a] IDR 12 mg/m²; ara-C 200 mg/m² CI × 5 days; DNR 50 mg/m²
[b] IDR 12 mg/m²; ara-C 100 mg/m² CI × 7 days; DNR 45 mg/m²
[c] IDR 13 mg/m²; ara-C 100 mg/m² CI × 7 days; DNR 45 mg/m²

that is responsible for the phenomenon of multidrug resistance (MDR) [8, 9]. The results of these preliminary studies suggest that IDR may not efflux from these cells in the same manner as DNR.

Materials and Methods

Cell Lines

The parent cell line CEM and its MDR-resistant subline were kept in the RPMI 1640 (Gibco) Laboratories, Grand Island, New York, supplemented with 10% (vol/vol) heat-inactivated fetal calf serum (FCS; Hyclone, Salt Lake City, Utah) and 1% L-glutamine (Gibco) and incubated at 37°C with 5% CO_2 and 95% humidified air.

Drugs

Verapamil has been shown to block Pgp by directly binding to Pgp [9]. Verapamil was obtained from Knoll Pharmaceuticals (Whippany, NJ), and was dissolved in sterile NaCl with 1.5% dimethylsulfoxide (DMSO) before each experiment (final concentration, 0.008%). The concentration of verapamil used in each of the experiments was 10 μM. Solutions containing verapamil were protected from light at all times by tinfoil wrapping. DNR and IDR wwere purchased from Adria Laboratories (Dublin, OH), dissolved in sterile water, and diluted with 10% fetal calf serum

(FCS) before each experiment. The final concentration of each anthracycline was 1 μg/ml.

Flow Cytometry

For determination of flow cytometric intracellular concentrations, a FACScan (Becton Dickinson, Mountain View, CA) equipped with an argon ion laser using a 488-nm line operating at 15 mW was used. Light was collected through a 585/42-nm filter in the DNR experiments and through a 545/20-nm filter in the IDR experiments.

Cell Uptake and Retention Studies

Cells were incubated at a concentration of 2 × 106 cells/ml and were exposed to DNR 1 μg/ml alone, IDR 1 μg/ml alone, or with combinations of the test drugs. At times 1, 5, 30, 45, and 60 min cells were washed twice in ice-cold phosphate-buffered saline (PBS) without CA^{2+} or Mg^{2+} (GIBCO) and resuspended in 0.5 ml ice-cold PBS with 5% FCS. IDR and DNR fluorescence was immediately measured using the FACScan.

Drug retention experiments were performed separately. Cells were incubated first with DNR 1 μg/ml, IDR 1 μg/ml, or the combination of anthracycline and test drug for 1 h. Samples were then washed twice in ice-cold medium and resuspended in 37°C in fresh medium containing the specific parameter. Either IDR or DNR fluorescence was measured at time 0, 5, 15, 30, 60, and 120 min using the same FACScan as in the uptake experiments.

Results

Rate of Anthracycline Uptake

Cells were incubated with either anthracycline alone at a concentration of 1 µg or anthracycline plus verapamil 10 µM. The fluorescent signals at the specific time points measured in the uptake experiments are given in Table 2. As can be seen, the rate of IDR intracellular uptake during the initial 10 min of incubation was nearly ten times more rapid than the rate of uptake for DNR (97/10 vs. 9/10).

Effect of Verapamil on DNR and IDR Uptake in CEM-VBL Cells

The difference in fluorescence at 60 min between cells incubated with DNR alone and cells incubated with DNR and verapamil is approximately fourfold (130:32), while the difference in signal between cells incubated with IDR alone and IDR plus verapamil was approximately 1.3-fold (293:233).

Effect of Verapamil on DNR and IDR Retention in CEM-VBL Cells

Cells were then incubated in either anthracycline alone at a concentration of 1 µg or anthracycline plus verapamil 10 µM. After a 1-h incubation, cells were washed and resuspended in either fresh medium or medium containing verapamil 10 µM. The fluorescent signals at the specified time points are outlined in Table 3. Approximately 73% of the IDR signal remained in the cell compared to 39% of the DNR signal (47/66 vs. 6/16). There was an approximate fivefold increase in DNR signal after cells were exposed to DNR plus verapamil and resuspended in fresh medium containing verapamil compared to a 2.6-fold increase in IDR signal after cells were exposed to IDR plus verapamil and resuspended in fresh medium containing verapamil (121/47 vs. 30/6).

Discussion

When prospectively compared to DNR in the clinical setting, IDR has been shown to induce remission in a greater percentage of adult patients with de novo AML [5–7]. In at least one study, the number of patients who had disease refractory to two courses of IDR/ara-C was significantly less than the number of patients refractory to two courses of DNR/ara-C [5]. While this may reflect the pharmacologic properties of both the parent drug and its biologically active metabolite IDR-ol, it is also possible that IDR exerts a different uptake pattern in drug-resistant cells.

Results of these preliminary experiments suggest that leukemia cells expressing the MDR phenotype accumulate IDR more rapidly than DNR. In addition, when verapamil is added to the medium, time-dependent accumulation of IDR is minimally increased from baseline values obtained when cells are incubated with IDR alone (Table 2). This is in marked contrast to cells simultaneously incubated with DNR plus

Table 2. Uptake of IDR and DNR in CEM-VBL cells incubated with or without verapamil

Parameter	Fluorescence measured at time (min)				
	5	15	30	45	60
0.1% M	6	7	6	6	7
DNR	11	20	30	31	32
DNR + V	14	22	56	90	130
IDR	52	149	193	212	233
IDR + V	39	182	256	287	293

Table 3. Retention of IDR and DNR in CEM-VBL cells incubated with or without verapamil

Parameter	Fluorescence measured at time (min)					
	0	5	15	30	60	120
0.1 %[a] →→ M	5	5	5	5	5	5
DNR + M →→ M	16	11	9	7	6	6
DNR + V →→ V	44	43	43	40	35	30
IDR + M →→ M	66	59	48	43	50	47
IDR + V →→ V	93	108	115	108	125	121

[a] Control medium is 0.1 % DMSO

verapamil. In this instance, the presence of verapamil increases the amount of intracellular DNR by approximately fourfold (Table 2).

Retention experiments also demonstrate that continued verapamil exposure doubles the intracellular IDR concentration (2.6 above baseline, Table 3). However, DNR intracellular concentration is increased by more than fivefold when verapamil is added to the medium.

In summary, IDR may not be transported out of MDR cells in the same manner as DNR. Insofar as the MDR phenomenon plays a role in clinical drug resistance, this finding may explain in part the superior clinical results of this anthracycline.

Summary

Clinical trials comparing idarubicin with daunorubicin in adult patients with acute mylelogenous leukemia suggest that idarubicin offers an improvement in remission incidence and overall survival. Additionally, in at least one study, more patients on the standard daunorubicin treatment arm proved resistant to two cycles of daunorubicin than patients on the idarubicin arm. In order to examine this phenomenon in vitro, we exposed multidrug resistant cell lines to both idarubicin and daunorubicin and measured anthracycline uptake and retention. Preliminary data suggest that idarubicin is taken up by the drug-resistant cells at a faster rate. Moreover, verapamil, an agent that reverses the multidrug resistant phenotype in vitro, did not significantly alter anthracycline uptake when co-incubated with idarubicin. This was in distinction to the markedly enhanced anthracycline uptake noted when both verapamil and daunorubicin were incubated together with the multidrug-resistant cells. Taken together, these results suggest that idarubicin is more effective in vitro in multidrug-resistant cells.

References

1. Supino A, Necca A, Dasdia T, Casazza AM, DiMarco A (1977) Relationship between effects on nucleic acid synthesis in cell cultures and cytotoxicity of 4-demethoxy derivatives of daunorubicin and adriamycin. Cancer Res 37: 4523
2. Schwartz HS, Kanter PM (1981) DNA damage by anthracycline drugs in human leukemia cells. Cancer Lett 13: 309
3. Speth PAJ, Van de loo FAJ, Linssen PCM, Wessels HMC, Haanen C (1986) Plasma and human leukemia cell pharmacokinetics of oral and intravenous 4-demethoxydaunorubicin. Clin Pharmacol Ther 40: 643
4. Kuffel MJ, Reid JM, Ames MM (1990) Characterization of cytotoxicity and DNA damage of idarubicin, idarubicin-ol and related anthracyclines and alcohol metabolites following incubation with leukemia cells. Am Assoc Cancer Res 31: 399
5. Berman E, Heller H, Santorsa J, McKenzie S, Gee TS, Kempin S, Andreeff M, Kolitz J, Gabrilove J, Reich L, Mayer K, Keefe D, Trainor K, Schluger A, Penenberg D, Raymond V, O'Reilly R, Jhanwar S, Young C, Clarkson B (1991) Results of a randomized trial comparing idarubicin and cytosine arabinoside with daunorubicin and cytosine arabinoside in adult patients with newly diagnosed acute myelogenous leukemia. Blood (in press)

6. Vogler WR, Velez-Garcia E, Omura G, Raney M (1989) A phase III trial comparing daunorubicin or idarubicin combined with cytosine arabinoside in acute myelogenous leukemia. Semin Oncol 16: 21

7. Wiernik PH, Case DC, Perimen PO, Arlin ZA, Weitberg AB (1989) A multicenter trial of cytarabine plus idarubicin or daunorubicin induction therapy for adult nonlymphocytic leukemia. Semin Oncol 16: 25

8. Kartner N, Riordan JR, Ling I (1983) Cell surface P-glycoprotein is associated with multidrug resistance in mammalian cell lines. Science 221: 1285

9. Willingham MC, Cornwell MM, Cardarelli CO, Gottesman MM, Pasten I (1986) Single cell analysis of daunomycin uptake and efflux in multidrug resistant and sensitive KB cells: effects of verapamil and other drugs. Cancer Res 46: 5942

10. Broggini M, Italia C, Colombo T, Marmonti L, Donelli M (1984) Activity and distribution of IV and oral 4-demethoxydaunorubicin in murine experimental tumors. Cancer Treat Rev 68: 739

Mitoxantrone: Pharmacokinetic and Pharmacodynamic Studies in Patients with Leukemia*

P. Muus, P. Linssen, R. Knops, H. Wessels, and T. De Witte

Introduction

Mitoxantrone is one of the newer drugs with cytotoxic activity against leukemic cells. The drug binds to DNA and it induces both single- and double-strand breaks and DNA-protein crosslinks within the cells. In addition the drug binds to the cellular cytoskeleton. It appears that binding of the drug in the various cellular compartments occurs at a different rate, with different affinity and most likely also with different cytotoxic significance. It is not known which of these or other events is responsible for the interference with the survival of the cell. Mitoxantrone is widely distributed through the body and also accumulates in nonhematologic tissue [1, 2].

Doses of mitoxantrone ranging from 5 to 14 mg/m^2 for 2–5 days are given in the treatment of leukemia. The drug is given in infusions of short duration or per continuous infusion. Decisions about dose schedules are hampered by lack of knowledge about the pharmacodynamics of the drug. We studied accumulation of mitoxantrone in vivo in plasma and blasts from patients who were treated for poor-risk leukemia. We also investigated the cellular level required to inhibit the clonogenic cell.

Department of Hematology, University Hospital Nijmegen, Nijmegen, The Netherlands
* Supported by Lederle Nederland B.V. and by the M & A de Kock Foundation.

Patients

Twenty-three patients with an unmaintained relapse ($n = 3$), a maintained relapse ($n = 3$), and primary refractory ($n = 3$) acute myeloid leukemia (AML) and myeloblastic transformation of chronic myeloid leukemia (CML) ($n = 14$) were treated with mitoxantrone 12 mg/m^2 per day per continuous infusion for 5 days and ara-C 200 mg/m^2/day in a continuous infusion for 7 days. Patients with myeloblastic transformation of CML received cryopreserved autologous peripheral stem cells following the treatment course ($n = 7$). Mitoxantrone was given on days 1, 3, 4, 5, and 6 [if no autologous stem cells, were available ($n = 7$) on days 1, 3, and 4 only] and ara-C on days 2–8. The median age of the AML patients was 55 (34–68) years; the CML patients had a median age of 46 (28–64) years.

Materials and Methods

In nine consecutive patients blood samples were drawn in heparinized tubes on ice at $t = 0$, and 0.5, 1.0, 6.0, 24, 48, 72, and 96 h after initiation of the mitoxantrone infusion. For in vitro experiments cryopreserved bone marrow blasts from leukemia patients and bone marrow and peripheral blood cells from healthy volunteers were used.

Ascorbic acid was added to the samples to a final concentration of 57 μM to prevent degradation of the mitoxantrone. Separation of the erythrocytes was performed by dextrane sedimentation according to Brons et al. [3]. The latter method has the advantage of minimizing the efflux of mitoxantrone from the cells. Peripheral nucleated cells and plasma were stored at $-20\,°C$ until analysis. Bone marrow cells were washed and subsequently separated in a density gradient (d: 1.085 g/ml) of Ficoll-Isopaque (Pharmacia, Uppsala, Sweden). The nucleated interphase cells were washed and resuspended in heat-inactivated fetal calf serum. Bone marrow cells were exposed to mitoxantrone for 2 h and 5 days. Medium consisted of Iscoves medium (Flow laboratories, Truine, Ayrshire, Scotland) supplemented with 5 % FCS, 50 IU/ml penicillin, and 50 µg/ml streptomycin (Flow Laboratories). Freshly prepared mitoxantrone solutions were added to final concentrations of 10^{-2} to 10^{+2} ng/ml. After extensive washing the survival of the clonogenic cells was assessed in the semisolid clonogenic CFU-GM or CFU-L assay as previously described [4]. Duplicate samples were frozen for later measurement of the cellular concentrations of mitoxantrone.

Mitoxantrone levels in plasma and cells were measured using a modification of the HPLC method of Reynolds et al. [5] and Choi et al. [6]. Amatrone was used as an internal standard. The detection limit was 0.5 ng/500 µl extraction volume. The amount of mitoxantrone in cells was measured per cell number. The cellular concentration was expressed per volume assuming that the volume of 560×10^6 cells is equal to one milliliter, for comparison of mitoxantrone levels in cells and plasma.

Treatment Results

In nine AML patients three complete and two partial responses were attained. One patient who had failed two remission induction courses consisting of conventional dose ara-C and daunorubicin entered a complete remission which has lasted 9 months. Also three out of 14 patients in myeloblastic transformation of CML entered a second chronic phase. These results indicate that certain poor-risk patients profit from mitoxantrone combined with conventional dose ara-C. The leukocytes were $<1.0 \times$ $10^9/l$ for a median of 23 days (11–45 days). The thrombocytes were $<20 \times 10^9/l$ for a median of 22 days (0–64 days). Four CML patients who did not receive autologous stem cells died in the seventh week of leukocytopenia. Two AML patients died in the second week of bone marrow hypoplasia. Nonhematological side effects were acceptable. No significant clinical cardiotoxicity occurred.

Plasma Levels of Mitoxantrone

Mitoxantrone levels in plasma rose quickly and in most patients a plateau was reached after 6 h. The plateau concentration in plasma ranged between 6 and 26 ng/ml in all patients ($n = 9$). When the mitoxantrone infusion was interrupted (day 2), plasma concentrations of mitoxantrone decreased by 73 %–95 % over 24 h ($n = 5$). Plasma levels, albeit very low, were measurable up to 1 week after the last dose of mitoxantrone in some patients, pointing to a long terminal half-life.

Mitoxantrone Concentrations in Blast Cells from Patients

Mitoxantrone was demonstrable in circulating blast cells in the peripheral blood of some patients as early as 30 min after initiation of the infusion. The cellular concentrations at this time point were in the range of plasma levels. In the course of the 1st day the cellular concentration increased to 103–476 ng/ml ($n = 6$). After interruption of the mitoxantrone infusion (day 2), the cellular level decreased by 22 %–78 % over the next 24 h in five patients and increased to 145 % in one. In contrast to plasma levels, blast cells continued to accumulate mitoxantrone during the subsequent days of treatment. No plateau concentrations were observed. Highest levels of 275–2458 ng/ml were measured on days 4 or 5. After completion of the mitoxantrone infusion considerable levels (118–506 ng/ml) of the drug remained present in the cells for at least 2 days in two patients who had enough leukocytes left in the peripheral blood to allow HPLC analysis.

Sensitivity of the Clonogenic Cells to Mitoxantrone for 2 h Vs. 5 days; the Extracellular Concentration

Sensitivity of leukemic clonogenic cells to mitoxantrone showed a wide interindividual variation. Prolongation of exposure to mitoxantrone from 2 h to 5 days resulted in a marked increase of cytotoxicity toward clonogenic cells. The concentration of mitoxantrone in the medium which inhibited 50 % of the clonogenic survival (ID^{50}) decreased from 100 to 7 ng/ml, from 32 to 1.6 ng/ml, and from 4.2 to 0.15 ng/ml in three different patients. Similar results were obtained for normal CFU-GM (data not shown).

Sensitivity of the Clonogenic cells to Mitoxantrone for 2 h Vs. 5 days; the Intracellular Concentration

Prolongation of the exposure time to mitoxantrone resulted in increased cellular accumulation. Cells had accumulated 325 ng/ml mitoxantrone when exposed to an extracellular concentration of 10 ng/ml for 2 h, 1355 ng/ml when exposed for 5 days, and 952 and 6082 ng/ml when exposed to 30 ng/ml for 2 h and 5 days respectively. No plateau was demonstrable for the cellular accumulation at either exposure time. In the CFU-GM assay, a cellular mitoxantrone concentration corresponded with a stronger inhibition of the clonogenic cells when that cellular level was attained in 5 days compared with 2 h. The intracellular mitoxantrone concentration at the start of the CFU-GM assay corresponding to 50 % inhibition of the clonogenic survival was 320 ng/ml when attained after 2 h of exposure and 120 ng/ml when attained after 5 days of exposure.

Discussion

Mitoxantrone in combination with ara-C per continuous infusion is effective in the treatment of certain poor-risk leukemia patients. Patients with myeloblastic transformation of CML appeared at risk of prolonged myelosuppression, particularly when no autologous stem cells were available for reinfusion. Nonhematologic toxicity of the schedule was acceptable.

Patients attained plasma (steady state) concentrations ranging between 6 and 26 ng/ml. These findings are in agreement with those reported by Kaminer at al. [7]. When the same dose of mitoxantrone is given to patients in a 30-min infusion, peak plasma levels of 400–960 ng/ml have been reported [5]. Avoiding high peak plasma levels may be important to restrict nonhematological toxicity.

With the present dose schedule, the maximum capacity for cells to accumulate mitoxantrone was not reached. Highest values in patients during the regimen ranged between 275 and 2458 ng/ml. In vitro after 5 days of exposure to 30 ng/ml mitoxantrone, cellular levels of 6082 ng/ml were found.

After completion of the infusion, cellular mitoxantrone decreased at a slower pace than plasma levels, and mitoxantrone remained detectable in the cells until hypoplasia occurred. A long terminal half-life has also been reported by Greidanus et al. [8], who demonstrated mitoxantrone in leukocytes up to 14 days after completion of a 21-day infusion of 1.1 mg/m^2 mitoxantrone per day.

This observation complicates the interpretation of in vitro dose-response curves comparing the percentage survival of clonogenic cells after incubation in drug-containing medium for various periods. Although the time of incubation in drug-containing medium is defined, the duration of intracellular exposure and as a consequence a possible continued cytotoxic effect can therefore not be accurately defined. Assuming that mitoxantrone remains present in the cells throughout the 10 days of the clonogenic assay at a constant concentration, the area under the concentration × time curve at the cellular concentration which inhibited the clonogenic survival by 50 % would be 77 440 ng.h/ml for a total exposure of $2+240$ h and 43 200 ng.h/ml for $120+240$ h. It was expected that the product of cellular mitoxantrone concentration and total exposure time would be comparable and that the curves are superimposable as is the case for doxorubicin (Adriamycin) [8].

Although these latter results need confirmation we like to make some preliminary speculations about their significance. One explanation could be that after 5 days the loosely bound mitoxantrone has disappeared from the cells. Apparently the more tightly bound mitoxantrone has more cytotoxic significance. An alternative explanation is that the clonogenic cells studied after 5 days of incubation represent earlier progenitor cells. It follows that the earlier progenitor cells would be more sensitive to mitoxantrone.

Summary

Twenty-three poor-risk leukemia patients received mitoxantrone (12 mg/m^2 per day) for 3–5 days and cytosine arabinoside (ara-C) (200 mg/m^2 per day) for 7 days both in a continuous infusion. Six complete and two partial responses were attained. The median duration of leukocytopenia (leukocytes $<1.0 \times 10^9$/l) was 23 days (range, 11–45 days). The median duration of thrombocytopenia ($<20 \times 10^9$/l) was 22 days (range, 0–64 days). Six patients died during early ($n = 2$) or persistent hypoplasia ($n = 4$). Particularly patients treated for myeloblastic transformation of CML were at risk for severe myelotoxicity. Steady state plasma concentrations of mitoxantrone ranged between 6 and 26 ng/ml. Blast cells continued to accumulate mitoxantrone. Highest cellular concentrations attained in vivo ranged between 275 and 2458 ng/ml. No cellular plateau could be demonstrated. Cellular levels decreased at a lower rate than plasma levels and mitoxantrone was detectable in the cells until hypoplasia occurred.

In vitro studies demonstrated a shift to the left of the dose response curves, relating the extracellular mitoxantrone concentration to the inhibition of the clonogenic survival when 2 h and 5 days of incubation in drug-containing medium were compared. Preliminary data suggest that after 5 days of incubation of cells in the presence of mitoxantrone the sensitivity of the clonogenic cells may have increased.

References

1. Ehninger G, Schuler U, Proksch B, Zeller K-P, Blanz J (1990) Pharmacokinetics and metabolism of mitoxantrone. Clin Pharmacokinet 18 (5): 365–380
2. Roberts RA, Cress AE, Dalton WS (1989) Persistent intra-cellular binding of mitoxantrone in a human colon carcinoma cell line. Biochem Pharmacol 38: 4283–4290
3. Brons PP, Wessels JM, Linssen PC, Haanen C (1987) Determination of amsacrine in human nucleated hematopoietic cells. J Chromatogr 422: 175–185
4. De Witte T, Plas A, Koekman E, Blankenborg G, Salden M, Wessels J, Haanen C (1983) Cell size monitored counter flow centrifugation of human bone marrow, resulting in clonogenic cell fractions substantially depleted of small lymphocytes. J Immunol Methods 65: 171–182
5. Reynolds DL, Sternson LA, Repta AJ (1981) Clinical analysis for the antineoplastic agent 1,4-dihydroxy-5,8-bis{[2-[2-hydroxy-ethyl]-amino]-ethyl]amino}-9,10-anthracenedione dihydrochloride in plasma. J Chromatogr 222: 225–240
6. Choi KE, Sinkele JA, Han DS, McGrath SC, Daly KM, Larson RA (1978) High-performance liquid chromatographic assay for mitoxantrone in plasma using electrochemical detection. J Chromatogr 420: 81–88
7. Kaminer LS, Choi KE Daley KM Larson RA (1989) Continuous infusion of mitoxantrone in relapsed acute nonlymphocytic leukemia. Cancer 65: 2619–2623
8. Greidanus J, Vries EG de, Mulder NH, Sleijfer DT, Uges DR, Oosterhuis B, Willemse PH (1989) A phase I pharmacokinetic study of 21-day continuous infusion mitoxantrone. J Clin Oncol 7: 790–797
9. Raijmakers R, Speth P, De Witte T, Linssen P, Wessels J, Haanen C (1987) Infusion-rate independent cellular concentration and cytotoxicity to human bone marrow clonogenic cells. Br J Cancer 56: 123–126

Pharmacological Sanctuaries in the Treatment of Acute Leukemia in the Rat*

K. Nooter, A. J. de Vries, A. C. M. Martens, and A. Hagenbeek

In most leukemia patients leukemic stem cells survive current chemotherapies. The high relapse rate in patients with acute myelocytic leukemia (AML) may, in part, be explained by the surviving leukemic cells being exposed to inappropriate drug concentrations. We used the Brown Norway acute myelocytic leukemia (BNML) model, which has been proven to resemble AML in humans in many characteristics. The BNML model has been studied extensively for more than a decade and for further reading the reader is referred to a recent review by Martens et al. [1].

In the study presented here we compared the pharmacokinetics and antitumor efficacy of daunorubicin in normal and leukemic rats [2]. Leukemic rats were treated with 7.5 mg/kg daunorubicin as an intravenous (i.v.) bolus dose, 13 days after transplantation of 10^7 leukemic cells. At various times after drug injection the rats were killed and the concentrations of daunorubicin and daunorubicinol were assayed by high-performance liquid chromatography (HPLC) in several organs [2].

We found that the femoral bone marrow accumulated less daunorubicin than did normal bone marrow, especially at the stage of a high leukemic cell burden (Fig. 1). However, the leukemia-infiltrated liver and spleen accumulated much larger amounts of drugs than normal liver and spleen (Figs. 2,

Institute of Applied Radiobiology and Immunology TNO, PO Box 5815, 2280 HV Rijswijk, The Netherlands
* This study was supported in part by the Netherlands Cancer Foundation.

3). Our explanation for the reduced anthracycline accumulation in the femoral bone marrow is the following: The inoculated anthracycline drug with its high affinity for cellular DNA is rapidly taken up by the large amount of easily accessible leukemic cells in liver and spleen and very little drug is left for the femoral bone marrow with its much slower uptake kinetics.

A strong suggestion for a role of the leukemic cell load in daunorubicin distribution is provided by the experiment in which we compared the pharmacokinetics of daunorubicin in leukemic rats, 13 days after transplantation, with those of leukemic rats 9 days after transplantation. It appeared that the amount of daunorubicin in the leukemic bone marrow is inversely proportional to the tumor load (data not shown).

These data suggest that lowering the tumor load prevents the formation of pharmacological sanctuaries. Subsequently, we performed experiments whereby the leukemic cell load was reduced by low-dose cyclophosphamide [3]. We investigated the effects of low-dose cyclophosphamide pretreatment on the daunorubicin concentrations in leukemic bone marrow. At day 12 after transplantation of the leukemia, rats were injected with cyclophosphamide (30 mg/kg i.p.). Two days later (d14) the leukemic rats received daunorubicin (7.5 mg/kg i.v.). The cyclophosphamide pretreatment led to a significant increase in daunorubicin concentration in the femoral bone marrow by a factor of about 7 (Fig. 1). The log leukemic stem cell kill (LCK) values, as estimated by a survival assay, were 1.8, 0.7, and 5.4 for the leukemic rats

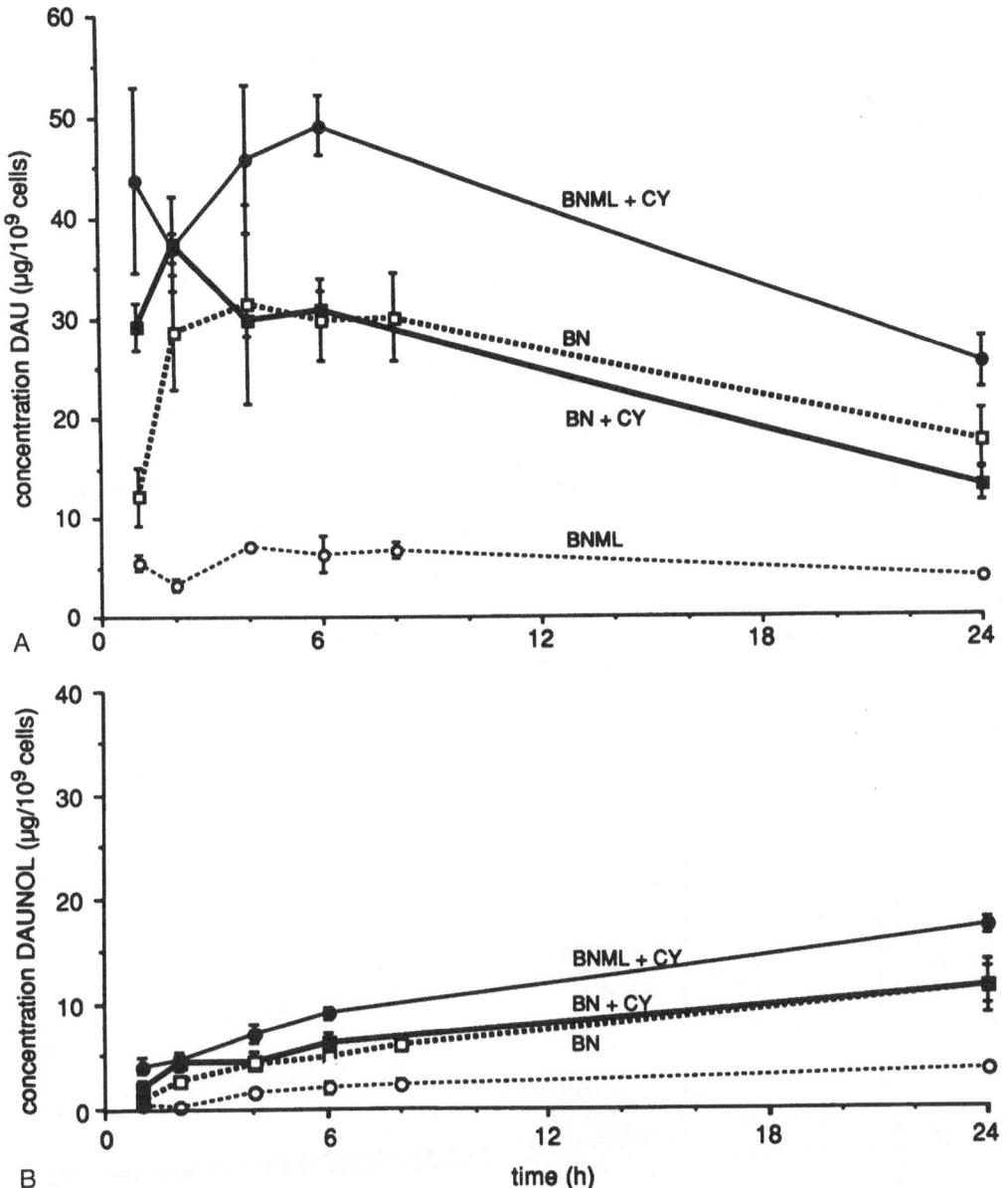

Fig. 1A, B. Bone marrow concentration/time course of daunorubicin (*DAU*)(*A*) and daunorubicinol (*DAUNOL*)(*B*) after daunorubicin 7.5 mg/kg in normal (*BN*)(□---□) and leukemic (*BNML*) rats (○---○) or after the same dose *DAU* combined with cyclophosphamide (*CY*) 30 mg/kg 2 days earlier in *BN* rats (■—■) and *BNML* rats (●—●). Mean and SD

injected with cyclophosphamide (d12), injected with daunorubicin (d14), or cyclophosphamide (d12) plus daunorubicin (d14), respectively (Fig. 4). The simultaneous administration of cyclophosphamide and daunorubicin at day 14 induced an LCK of 2.7, a value that is just the sum of the LCKs of cyclophosphamide and daunorubicin alone. These results indicate that low-dose cyclophosphamide pretreatment leads to an increased daunorubicin accumulation in femoral bone marrow of leukemic rats,

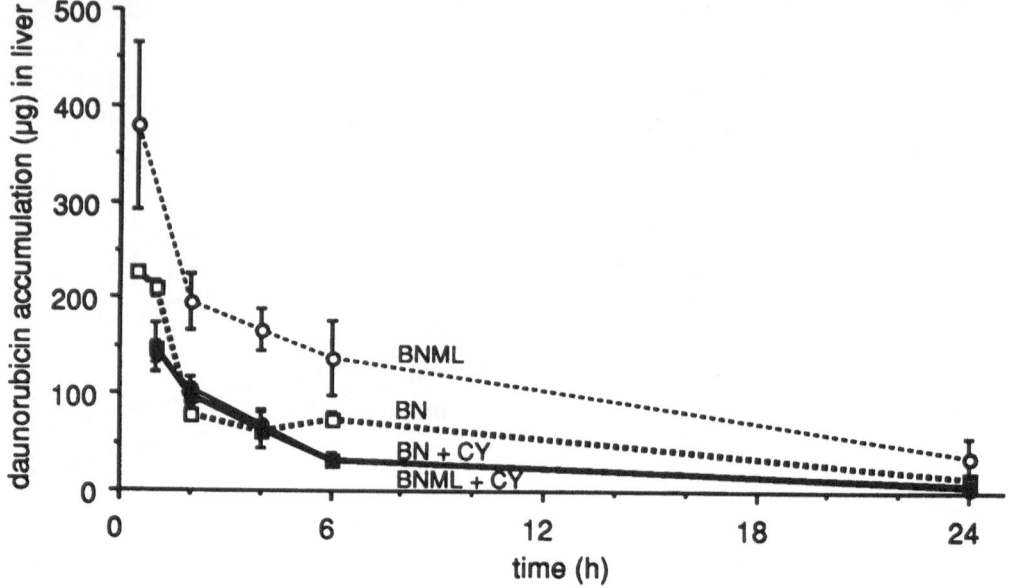

Fig. 2. Daunorubicin accumulation by liver in normal (*BN*) (□---□) and leukemic (*BNML*) rats (○---○) treated with daunorubicin or in *BN* rats (■—■) and *BNML* rats (●—●) treated with the same dose after cyclophosphamide 2 days earlier

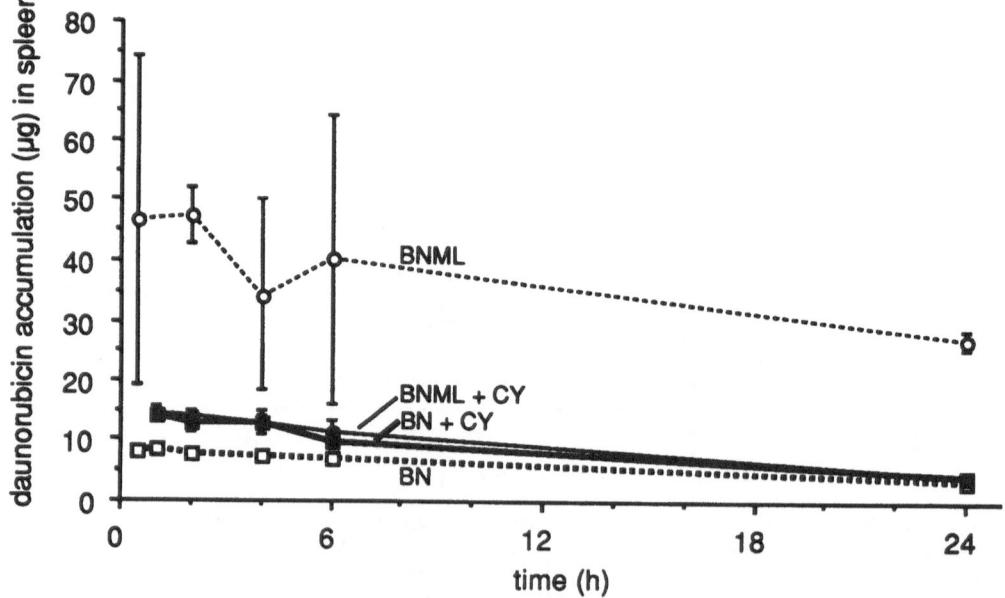

Fig. 3. Daunorubicin accumulation by spleen in normal (□---□) and leukemic rats (○---○). *Solid symbols* = after cyclophosphamide pretreatment

and has a clear synergistic effect on daunorubicin therapy.

The next question concerning the prevention of pharmacological sanctuaries with cytostatic agents was whether the effect of cyclophosphamide pretreatment resulted from a reduction in tumor load or is due to a specific effect of cyclophosphamide. To answer this question we used cytosine arabinoside (ara-C) instead of

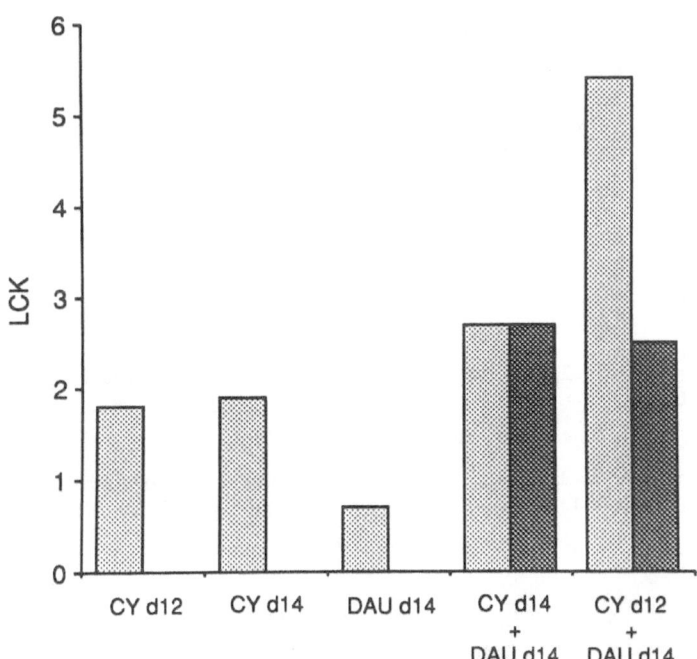

Fig. 4. Log leukemic stem cell kill (*LCK*) as estimated by survival for the different treatment groups. *Light bars* represent the LCK found experimentally, the *dark bars* represent the sum of the effects of the separate treatments

cyclophosphamide as a tumor load reducing agent. Leukemic rats were treated three times with ara-C (200 mg/kg, q12 h, i.v.), starting at day 12 after transplantation of the leukemia, followed by daunorubicin treatment on day 14. Normal rats were treated with the same treatment schedule. After tumor load reduction with ara-C the pharmacokinetic data in leukemic rats showed a complete restoration of the daunorubicin levels in the femoral bone marrow as compared to normal rats. From survival assays the LCK values estimated were 1.9, 0.3, and 4.4 for the leukemic rats treated with ara-C (start d12), treated with daunorubicin (d14), or treated with ara-C (start d12) plus daunorubicin (d14), respectively. In conclusion, these results indicate that tumor load reduction by either cyclophosphamide or ara-C leads to an increased daunorubicin accumulation in femoral bone marrow of leukemic rats, and has a clear synergistic effect on daunorubicin therapy.

In order to study whether the pharmacokinetics of other cytostatic drugs, related and unrelated to anthracyclines, are also influenced by the tumor load of the animal, we compared the pharmacokinetics of another DNA intercalator, mitoxantrone, with those of the antifolate methotrexate (MTX), in normal and leukemic rats. For that purpose we first developed a sensitive HPLC assay for the determination of mitoxantrone in bone marrow [4]. MTX was also determined by HPLC [5]. The bone marrow pharmacokinetics of mitoxantrone were studied by injection of mitoxantrone (2.5 mg/kg, i.v. bolus) in leukemic rats 13 days after transplantation. The rats were killed at various times after the injection, and the concentration of mitoxantrone in bone marrow was assayed. We found that the femoral bone marrow from leukemic rats contained about a factor 4.5 less mitoxantrone (per 10^9 nucleated cells) than did bone marrow from normal rats (Fig. 5a). The pharmacokinetics of MTX in bone marrow of both normal and leukemic (day 13) rats were studied after an intravenous bolus injection of MTX (25 mg/kg). The results showed that for MTX the phenomenon of decreased bone marrow drug accumulation was not observed (Fig. 5b). The most likely explanation is that DNA-intercalating drugs, which have a high affinity for cellular DNA, are rapidly taken up by the easily accessible leukemic cell load and

307

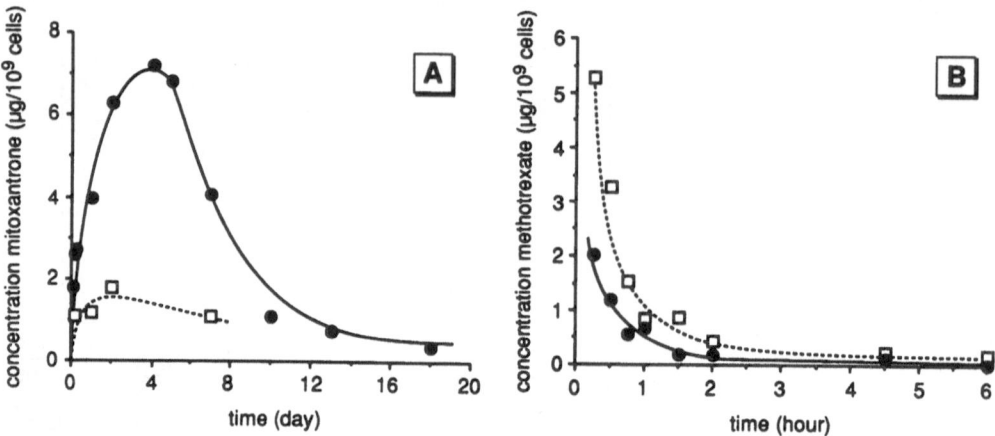

Fig. 5A, B. Bone marrow concentration/time curves of mitoxantrone (*MITOX*, 2.5 mg/kg)(*A*) and methotrexate (*MTX*, 25 mg/kg)(*B*) in normal (●—●) and leukemic (□---□) rats

that, as a consequence, the femoral bone marrow, which has much slower drug uptake kinetics, functions as a pharmacological sanctuary.

Removal of leukemic cell burden by chemotherapeutic pretreatment prevents the formation of pharmacological sanctuaries in the femoral bone marrow and dramatically potentiates the efficacy of anthracycline drugs. Extrapolation to man indicates that pretreatment of full-blown leukemia at diagnosis with low-dose effective chemotherapy may increase the efficacy of subsequent anthracycline-containing remission induction chemotherapy.

Summary

The total number of leukemic cells at the time of therapy may affect the tissue and target cell distribution and antitumor efficacy of cytotoxic drugs. We compared the pharmacokinetics and antitumor efficacy of the anthracycline drugs, daunorubicin and mitoxantrone in normal and leukemic rats and found that in the presence of a high leukemic cell load, the femoral bone marrow accumulated significantly less drug than normal bone marrow. Apparently, the femoral bone marrow can function as a pharmacological sanctuary.

Low dose cyclophosphamide pretreatment, which reduced the leukemic cell load

by about two log, led to a dramatic increase in anthracycline accumulation in the femoral bone marrow and to a strong potentiation of the anti-leukemic effect of the anthracycline drugs.

References

1. Martens ACM, Van Bekkum DW, Hagenbeek A (1990) The BN acute myelocytic leukemia (BNML) (a rat model for studying human acute myelocytic leukemia (AML). Leukemia 4: 241–257
2. Nooter K, Sonneveld P, Martens ACM (1985) Differences in the pharmacokinetics of daunomycin in normal and leukemic rats. Cancer Res 45: 4020–4025
3. Nooter K, De Vries AJ, Martens ACM, Hagenbeek A (1990) Effect of cyclophosphamide pretreatment on daunorubicin in rat acute leukaemia model. Eur J Cancer 26: 729–732
4. De Vries AJ, Nooter K (1990) Quantification of mitoxantrone in bone marrow by high performance liquid chromatography with electrochemical detection. J Chromatogr 563: 435–442
5. Storm AJ, Van der Kogel AJ, Nooter K (1985) Effects of X-irradiation on the pharmacokinetics of methotrexate in rats: alteration of the blood-brain barrier. Eur J Cancer Clin Oncol 21: 759–764

In Vitro Drug Resistance in Childhood Acute Lymphoblastic Leukemia in Relation to Age and Immunophenotype*

R. Pieters[1], G.J.L. Kaspers[1], E.R. van Wering[2], D.R. Huismans[1], A.H. Loonen[1], K. Hählen[2,3], and A.J.P. Veerman[1,2]

Introduction

The immunophenotype is one of the prognostic factors in children with acute lymphoblastic leukemia (ALL) [1–6]. B-ALL cases have the worst prognosis and patients with B-cell precursor ALL the most favorable prognosis. Among the patients with precursor B-ALL, those whose lymphoblasts have cytoplasmic μ heavy chain (cμ; preB ALL) and the small group of patients whose cells lack the common ALL (cALL) antigen characteristic of the earliest stage of B-cell differentiation (proB ALL) show poorer responses by comparison with the cALL+/cμ− cases (cALL). Also patients with T-ALL have an unfavorable prognosis. Part of these findings are still controversial because in some studies the immunophenotype is related to other clinical and biological features like white blood cell count (WBC) and organomegaly. Also, when effective treatments are used, the prognostic value of immunophenotype could be diminished [7–9].

Age is a well-established prognostic factor in childhood ALL [8]. Infants younger than 18 months have the worst prognosis [10–12]. Leukemia in these infants is char-

acterized by a high tumor load but also by a high incidence of the prognostically unfavorable proB phenotype [12]. Patients older than 10 years of age also have a relatively poor prognosis [8, 11, 13].

The cell biological basis for the associations between age and treatment outcome and between immunophenotype and treatment outcome is not understood. It has been shown that immunophenotype is correlated to karyotype but this itself does not elucidate the relationship with prognosis [14]. It is often suggested that differences in phenotype and karyotype reflect differences in drug resistance but no studies have been performed to support this hypothesis. Recently we adapted the MTT (3-[4,5-dimethylthiazol-2-yl]-2,5-diphenyl tetrazolium bromide) assay for in vitro drug sensitivity testing in ALL patient samples [15–17]. This assay shows good correlations between in vitro results and clinical response to chemotherapy [18–22]. We report here the relation of age and immunophenotype to in vitro drug resistance in children with ALL.

Materials and Methods

Cells

Bone marrow or peripheral blood cells from 84 children with untreated ALL were used. The data concerning the age of the children were derived from the central office of the Dutch Childhood Leukemia Study Group (DCLSG). In 46 cases cells had been cryopreserved in liquid nitrogen at −170 °C. Leukemic cells were isolated on a Ficoll

[1] Free University Hospital, Department of Pediatrics, De Boelelaan 1117, 1081 HV, Amsterdam, The Netherlands
[2] Dutch Childhood Leukemia Study Group, The Hague, The Netherlands
[3] Sophia's Children Hospital, Subdivision Haemato/Oncology, Erasmus University, Rotterdam, The Netherlands
* This study is supported by the Dutch Cancer Society (IKA 87–17 and 89–06).

309

Isopaque gradient (Lymphoprep 1.077 g/ml). The median percentage of malignant cells was 94% (range 66%–100%) and was not different between the immunological subtypes. Cryopreservation does not alter drug sensitivity [16] and bone marrow and peripheral blood cells did not differ as to drug sensitivity. Immunophenotyping was done in the research laboratory for Pediatric Hemato-Onco-Immunology of the Free University Hospital and in the laboratory of the DCLSG using an indirect peroxidase staining method. The samples of the B-lineage ALL, of which the B-cell origin was confirmed by the expression of CD19 and HLA-DR, were classified into four sequential differentiation stages: proB ALL cells were CD10$^-$, cytoplasmic μ chain$^-$ (cμ$^-$) and surface immunoglobulin (sIg$^-$); cALL cells CD10$^+$/cμ$^-$/sIg$^-$; preB ALL cells CD10^{+or-} / cμ$^+$/sIg$^-$; B-ALL cells CD10$^-$ / cμ$^-$/sIg$^+$.

Drug Sensitivity Assay

In vitro drug sensitivity was assessed with the MTT assay as described elsewhere [17]. Briefly, 96-well microculture plates contained 100 μl cell suspension with 6 duplicate concentrations of the following drugs: 6-thioguanine (6-TG), vincristine (VCR), prednisolone (Pred), daunorubicin (DNR), mafosfamide (Maf, an active derivative of cyclofosfamide), cytosine arabinoside (AraC), mustine HCl (Must) and L-asparaginase (L-Asp). Untreated control cells were set up in sixfold. After incubation in a humidified incubator in 5% CO_2 for 4 days at 37°C, 10 μl MTT solution was added for 6 h. MTT is reduced to a coloured formazan by living but not by dead cells. The formazan crystals were dissolved with 100 μl acid isopropanol. The optical density (OD) was measured with a microplate reader at 540 nm. The OD is linearly related to cell number. Leukemic cell survival (LCS) was calculated by the equation:

LCS = (OD treated well/mean OD control wells) × 100%.

The LC$_{50}$ is the drug concentration lethal to 50% of the cells.

Staining of the multidrug resistance p-glycoprotein with the monoclonal antibod-

ies C219 and JSB-1 and assessment of the effects of the resistance modifiers cyclosporin A (Sandimmune; CsA; 2 μg/ml) and verapamil (Vp; 5 μg/ml) upon leukemic cell kill by VCR and DNR with the MTT assay were done as described elsewhere [22].

Statistics

The Mann-Whitney U test (MWU) was used for two-tailed testing at a significance level of .05.

Results

Immunophenotype

Twenty patients had the T-ALL phenotype; 7 were proB-, 37 cALL, 17 preB- and 3 B-ALL. The relationship between immunophenotype and in vitro drug resistance is shown in Fig. 1 and Table 1. Several observations can be made from these data:

1. Large variations in sensitivity were detected with overlaps between the different immunological subtypes. In general, cALL and preB ALL cells had the lowest median LC$_{50}$ values, i.e., were the most chemosensitive cells. This was especially true for Pred and L-Asp.

2. T-ALL cells were significantly more resistant to Pred, DNR, AraC, Maf and L-Asp than cALL and preB ALL cells and more resistant to VCR than preB ALL cells. The largest absolute differences were for Pred and L-Asp: The median LC$_{50}$ values in T-ALL were respectively 180 and 12–25 times those in cALL and preB ALL. In 6/18 (33%) T-ALL cases the LC$_{50}$ for Pred was higher than the maximum concentration tested (250 μg/ml) compared to 2/43 (4%) cALL and preB ALL cases. In only 1/18 (6%) T-ALL cases was the LC$_{50}$ lower than the minimum concentration tested (0.1 μg/ml) compared to 16/43 (37%) cALL and preB ALL cases.

3. ProB ALL cells showed a significant resistance to 6-TG, Pred, DNR and a trend to resistance to L-Asp compared to cALL and preB ALL cells. ProB ALL

cells were more resistant to Maf than preB ALL cells. In 4/6 (67 %) proB ALL cases the LC$_{50}$ for Pred was higher than 250 µg/ml and in 0/6 proB cases lower than 0.1 µg/ml compared to respectively 2/43 (4 %) and 16/43 (37 %) cALL and preB ALL cases.

4. No differences were found between cALL and preB ALL cases with the exception of the alkylating drugs Maf

Table 1. Immunophenotype and drug resistance in childhood ALL

Drug	Pheno-type	LC$_{50}$ Median	Range	N	2-tailed p values T	ProB	cALL	PreB	B-ALL
6-TG	T-ALL	6.3	1.6–50.0	18			.074		
	ProB	10.1	2.5–17.9	7			.015	.057	
	cALL	4.9	1.6–15.3	30	.074	.015			
	PreB	5.0	2.1–14.9	15		.057			
	B		5.4–50.0	2					
VCR	T-ALL	5.7	.3–50.0	18				.047	.034
	ProB	2.1	.5–50.0	7				.050	
	cALL	2.9	.3–50.0	28				.011	
	PreB	2.0	.3–36.8	16	.047			.010	
	B	50.0	24.4–50.0	3	.034	.050	.011	.010	
Pred	T-ALL	53.4	.1–250.0	18			.005	.002	
	ProB	250.0	1.0–250.0	6			.006	.004	
	cALL	.3	.1–250.0	28	.005	.006			
	PreB	.3	.1–168.2	15	.002	.004			
	B	172.6	.1–250.0	3					
DNR	T-ALL	.193	.023–2.000	18			.025	.024	.027
	ProB	.275	.074–.863	7			.026	.014	.030
	cALL	.082	.002–.895	24	.025	.026		.009	
	PreB	.060	.002–.378	14	.024	.014		.008	
	B	1.385	.444–1.470	3	.027	.030	.009	.008	
AraC	T-ALL	.611	.018–2.500	14			.013	.004	
	ProB	.144	.029–.986	7					
	cALL	.169	.002–2.500	26	.013				
	PreB	.141	.002–.478	13	.004				
	B	.461	.082–2.266	3					
Must	T-ALL	12.4	1.7–60.0	6					
	ProB	38.5	4.7–48.5	5					
	cALL	38.0	1.1–115.4	18				.032	
	PreB	15.1	4.6–34.7	7		.032			
	B		.7–214.3	2					
Maf	T-ALL	18.0	3.3–100.0	14			.048	.0003	
	ProB	5.9	1.6–28.0	7				.035	
	cALL	5.4	.5–44.2	22	.048			.021	
	PreB	2.8	.2–15.6	12	.0003	.035	.021		
	B		.8–38.1	2					
L-Asp	T-ALL	1.20	.016–10.00	14			.024	.022	
	ProB	.93	.020–1.58	7			.073	.051	
	cALL	.05	.016–10.00	26	.024	.073			
	PreB	.10	.016–1.06	12	.022	.051			
	B		.80–10.00	2					

LC$_{50}$ values in micrograms per milliter (in units per milliliter for *L*-Asp). Two-tailed p values which were <.10 are shown

6-Thioguanine

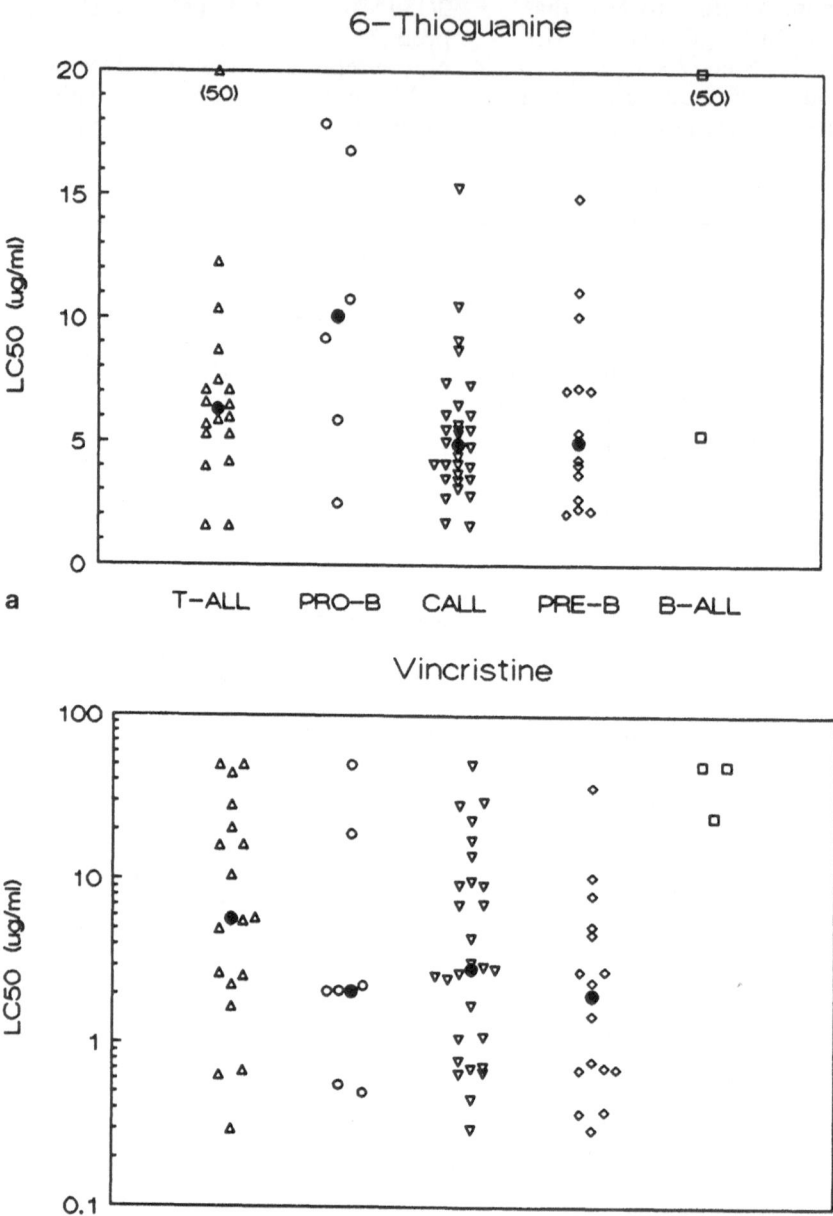

Fig. 1a–h. Relationship between immunophenotype and in vitro drug resistance in childhood ALL. LC_{50} values in μg/ml (for *L*-Asp in IU/ml). Symbols as in Fig. 2

and Must. PreB cells were more sensitive than cALL cells to these drugs with a two- to threefold difference in median LC_{50} values.

5. All three B-ALL cases were highly resistant to VCR and DNR compared to all other phenotypes. Staining for p-glycoprotein was negative. Verapamil and cyclosporin A did not increase the cytotoxic effect of VCR and DNR. Two out of three B-ALL cases were resistant to Pred. One B-ALL case was also highly

Prednisone

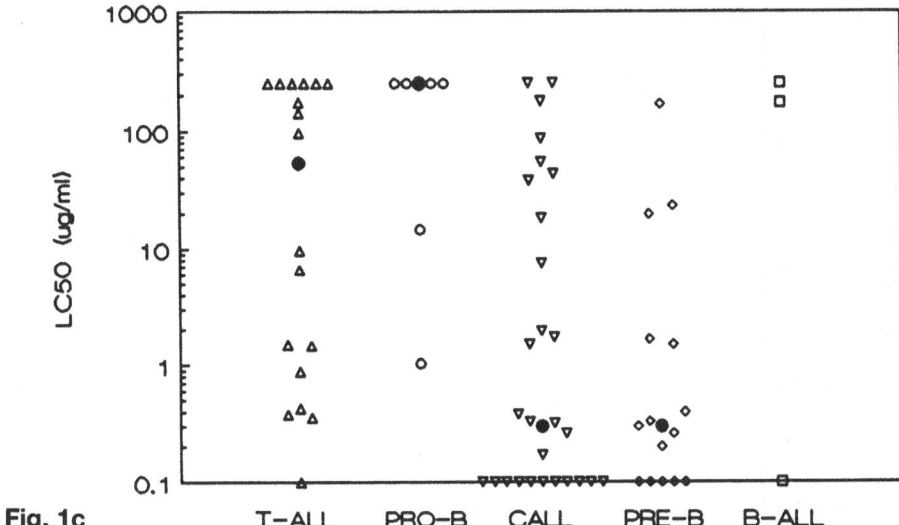

Fig. 1c

Daunorubicin

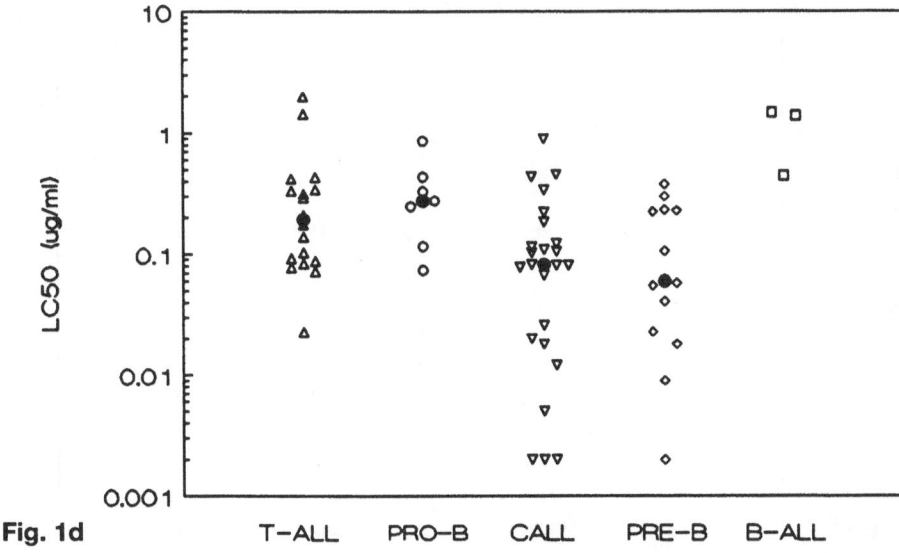

Fig. 1d

resistant to all other drugs tested while one other was relatively sensitive to these, especially to the alkylating drugs.

Age

The age was known in 82 patients. Eight patients were younger than 18 months at diagnosis. Of these children, four had proB-, two cALL and two preB ALL. Eighteen patients (six T-ALL, two proB-, eight cALL and two preB ALL) were older than 10 years at initial diagnosis. The drug resistance results of these cases are indicated in Table 2 and Fig. 2. The youngest group was significantly more resistant to Pred and DNR than the group of patients aged 18

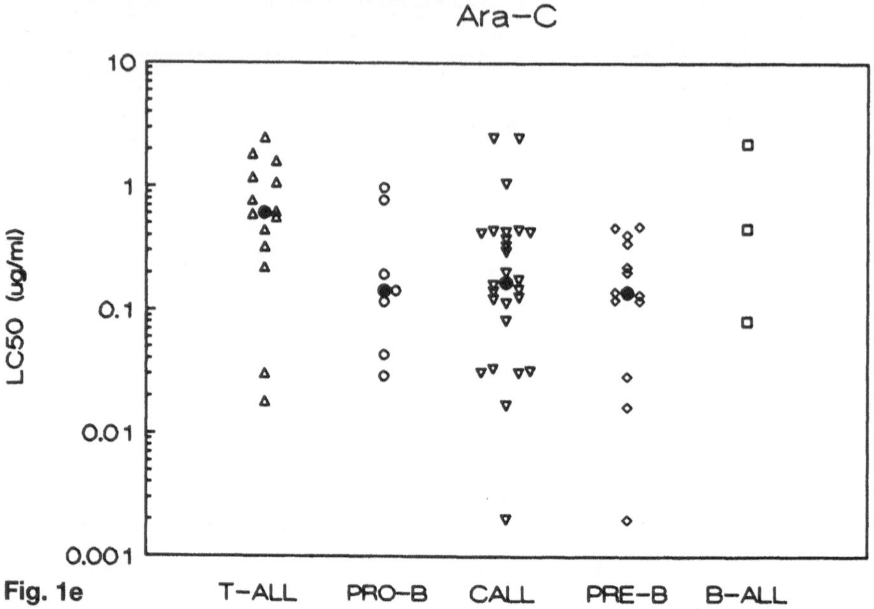

Ara–C

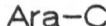

Fig. 1e

Mustine–HCl

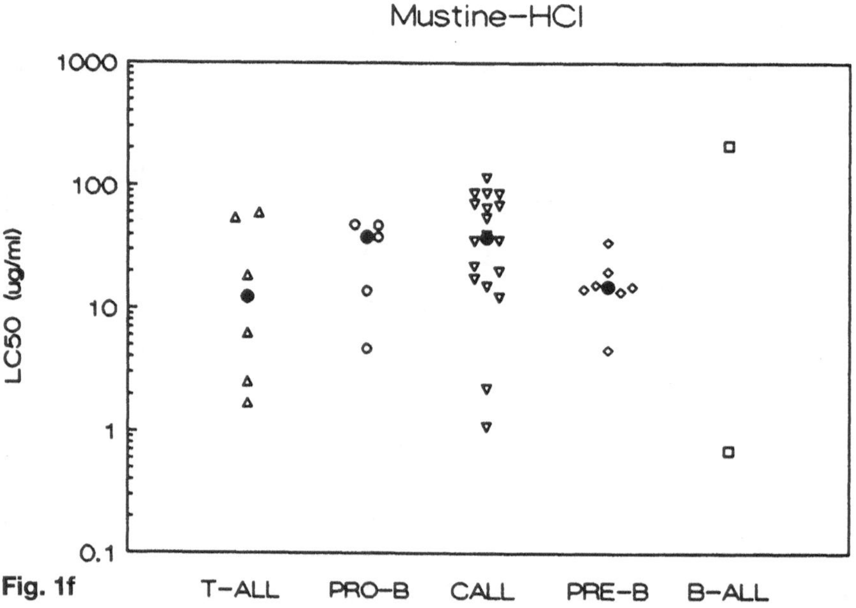

Fig. 1f

months to 10 years. The oldest group showed a significant resistance to Pred compared to the group aged 18 months to 10 years. The differences in L-Asp sensitivity were not statistically significant. If only patients with cALL and preB ALL were analyzed, still the same relationship was found between age and in vitro drug resistance to Pred and DNR but the groups

<18 months ($n = 3$) and >10 years ($n = 8$) were small. This is also reflected by the fact that the only two cALL/preB ALL cases with an LC_{50} >250 µg/ml for Pred fell in the youngest and oldest age group while the five cases in the intermediate age group with an LC_{50} >250 µg/ml for Pred were not of the cALL or preB phenotype. The largest absolute differences were observed again

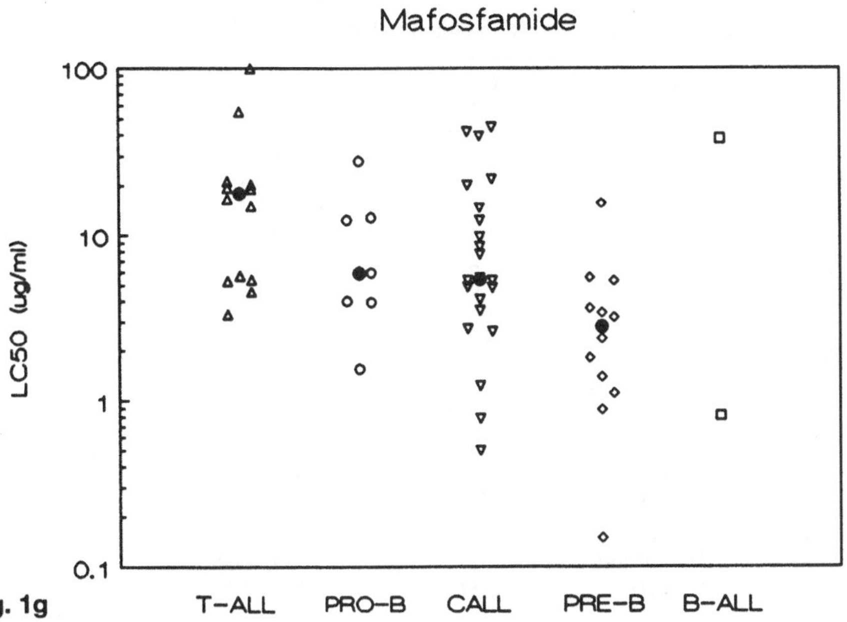

Mafosfamide

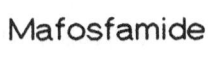

Fig. 1g

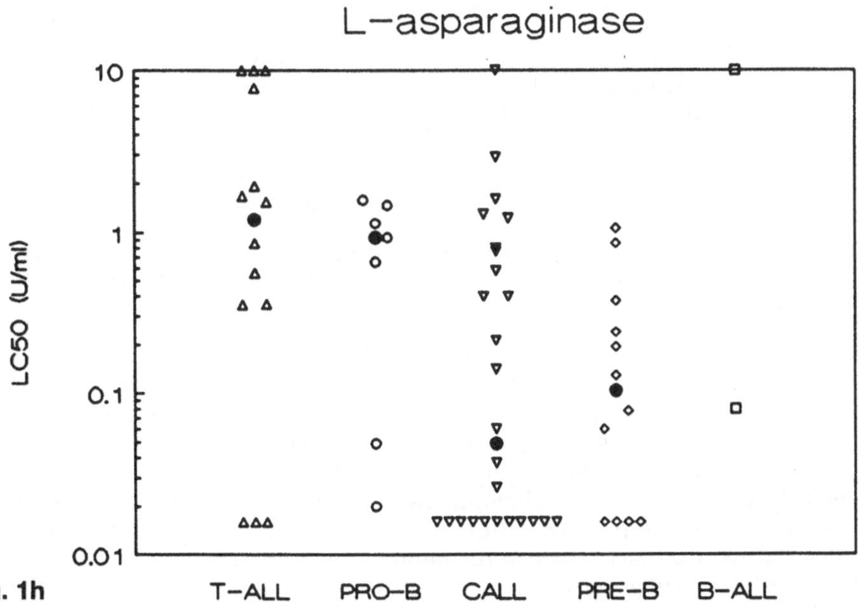

(scatter plot: LC50 (ug/ml), vertical axis from 0.1 to 100; groups: T-ALL, PRO-B, CALL, PRE-B, B-ALL)

L-asparaginase

Fig. 1h

(scatter plot: LC50 (U/ml), vertical axis from 0.01 to 10; groups: T-ALL, PRO-B, CALL, PRE-B, B-ALL)

for Pred and *L*-Asp: in the youngest and oldest group the median LC_{50} values for Pred were respectively >800 and 6 times and for <-Asp 9 and 3 times as high as those in the intermediate age group.

Discussion

Immunophenotype

With most treatment protocols for children with ALL, the immunophenotype has prognostic value. B-ALL cases have the worst and cALL the best prognosis. Compared to

315

Table 2. Age and drug resistance in childhood ALL

Drug	Age	LC$_{50}$		N	p
		Median	Range		
6-TG	<18 mths	5.7	2.3–16.8	7	
	18–120 mths	5.4	1.6–17.9	47	
	>10 yrs	5.8	1.6–50.0	16	
VCR	<18 mths	4.6	.5–19.0	6	
	18–120 mths	2.8	.3–50.0	48	
	>10 yrs	2.6	.6–50.0	16	
Pred	<18 mths	250.0	7.5–250.0	6	.004
	18–120 mths	.3	.1–250.0	46	
	>10 yrs	1.8	.1–250.0	16	.023
DNR	<18 mths	.289	.116– .436	6	.022
	18–120 mths	.084	.002–1.438	43	
	>10 yrs	.210	.005–2.000	15	
AraC	<18 mths	.144	.043–.986	5	
	18–120 mths	.312	.002–2.500	42	
	>10 yrs	.181	.016–2.500	14	
Must	<18 mths	26.8	4.7– 48.5	4	
	18–120 mths	35.2	1.1–115.4	24	
	>10 yrs	14.0	1.7– 86.5	8	
Maf	<18 mths	3.9	1.6–28.0	5	
	18–120 mths	5.3	.2–100.0	37	
	>10 yrs	9.8	2.6–100.0	13	
<-Asp	<18 mtsh	1.14	.020– 1.47	5	
	18–120 mths	.17	.016–10.00	40	
	>10 yrs	.47	.016–10.00	14	

LC$_{50}$ values in micrograms per milliliter (in units per milliliter for L-Asp). Two-tailed p values of the comparison of the youngest or oldest group with the intermediate age group which were <.10 are shown

cALL cases, T-, preB-, and proB ALL cases have a poorer outcome [1–9]. It is hypothesized that differences in cellular drug sensitivity may account for these differences in clinical responsiveness to chemotherapy. The present study reports on differences in in vitro drug resistance between the immunophenotypic subgroups of childhood ALL.

In general, cALL and preB ALL cells showed a higher chemosensitivity than cells of the other phenotypes. We did not find that preB ALL cells were more resistant to any of the drugs tested than cALL cells. PreB ALL cases were even more sensitive to the alkylating agents Maf and Must compared to cALL. This could suggest that sensitivity to alkylating drugs increases with B-cell maturation. We could not test

this hypothesis further because of the low number of B-ALL samples. One B-ALL sample was highly sensitive but the other highly resistant to Maf and Must. Single agent cyclofosfamide has been curative in some patients with advanced B-cell malignancies [23].

From the comparison of the T-, proB- and B-ALL cases with the cALL and preB ALL cases the following differences are evident:

– T-ALL cases showed a resistance to Pred, DNR, AraC, Maf and L-Asp. T-ALL cells were more VCR resistant than preB ALL cells.
– ProB ALL cases were resistant to 6-TG, Pred, DNR and L-Asp. ProB ALL cells were more Maf resistant than preB ALL cells.

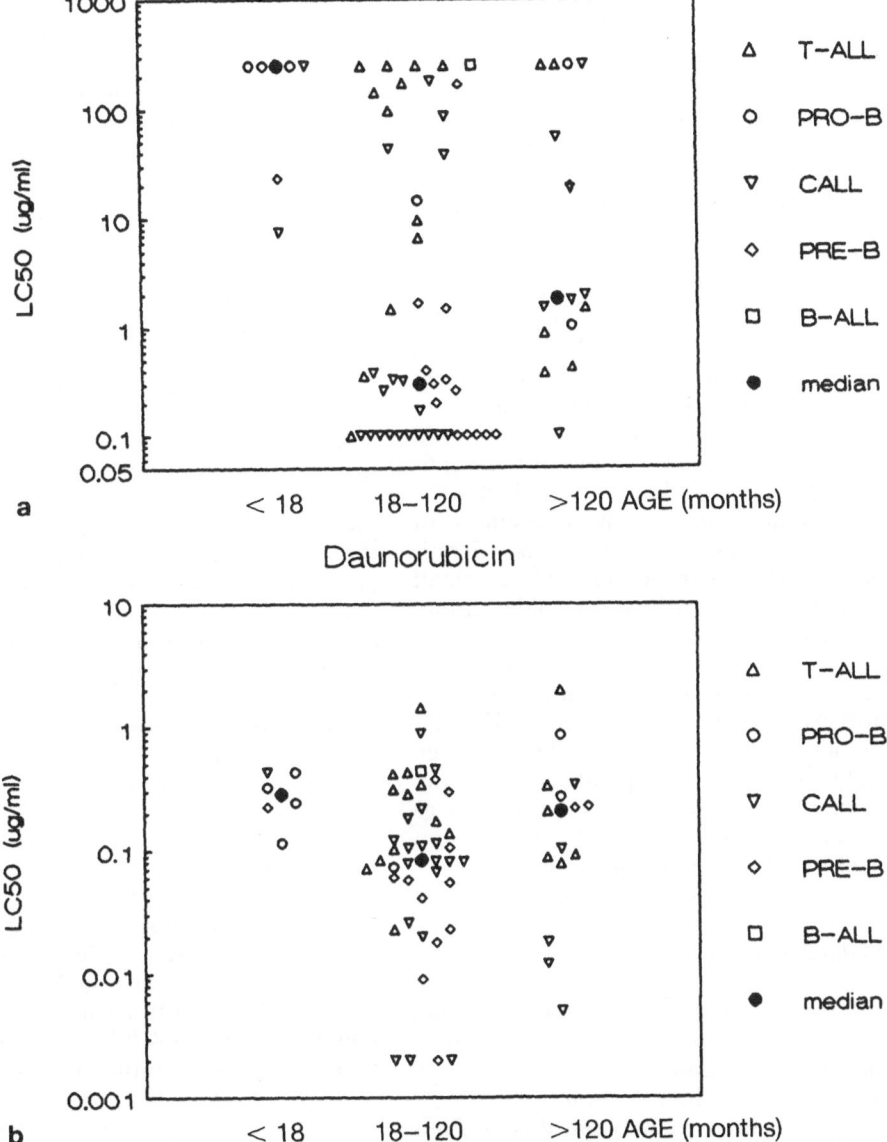

Fig. 2a, b. Relationship between age and in vitro drug resistance to Pred and DNR in childhood ALL. LC$_{50}$ values in μg/ml

- The number of B-ALL cases studied was too small to draw general conclusions. All three samples were resistant to VCR and DNR and two out of three also to Pred. For most other drugs only two samples could be evaluated, one showing a general resistance while cells from the other were relatively chemo-

sensitive especially to the alkylating agents. The VCR and DNR resistance in B-ALL was not due to the multidrug resistance (MDR) phenotype because:

a) VCR and DNR resistance was associated with resistance to drugs not involved in MDR;

b) p-glycoprotein could not be detected;

c) resistance modifiers did not increase the VCR- and DNR-induced cell kill.

Age

The youngest (<18 months) and oldest children (>10 years) have a poor prognosis compared to patients aged 18 months to 10 years [8, 10–13]. The youngest patients with ALL have an increased incidence of the earliest stage of precursor B-ALL, the cALL$^-$, cμ^- proB ALL [12]. This was also true in the present study in which 4/8 children aged <18 months had proB ALL while this phenotype was found in only 3/74 children aged >18 months. Cells from children <18 months were resistant to Pred and DNR. Although four out of five children <18 months had a relatively high LC$_{50}$ of >0.9 U/ml for L-Asp, the difference with the intermediate age group was not significant, which might be due to the small number of young patients. The oldest group of children (>10 years) also showed a resistance to Pred. Because the differences remained significant when only cALL and preB ALL cases were evaluated, the relationship between drug resistance and age might be partly independent from the immunophenotype. However, in the youngest group the member of patients was too small to draw a final conclusion.

Prednisone Resistance

The most important differences in drug resistance, both with respect to phenotype and age, were found for Pred. Three groups can be distinguished: a group of patients whose cells are extremely sensitive to Pred with the LC$_{50}$ value <0.1 µg/ml, the minimum concentration tested; on the other hand a group of patients whose cells are extremely resistant to Pred with the LC$_{50}$ value >250 µg/ml, the maximum concentration tested. The third category of patients shows an intermediate sensitivity to Pred with LC$_{50}$ values between these two cutoff points. Of the patients with T-ALL, proB ALL and B ALL, 41 % are categorized as extremely Pred resistant and only 7 % as extremely sensitive. Among cALL and

preB ALL cases these percentages were respectively 5 % and 37 %. Of patients <18 months, 67 % were extremely resistant and 0 % extremely sensitive. In patients >10 years, these percentages were respectively 25 % and 6 % and in the intermediate age group respectively 15 % and 47 %. Elsewhere we showed that ALL children with cells extremely sensitive to Pred have the best and children with cells extremely resistant to Pred have the worst prognosis. Also, six of ten relapsed ALL cases were extremely resistant and none of ten extremely sensitive to Pred, differing significantly from untreated ALL cases [22].

The finding that T- and B-ALL are relatively resistant to Pred correlates well with the fact that the number of glucocorticoid receptors differs among the phenotypes with a higher density in cALL and preB ALL than in T-ALL and B-ALL [24–26]. A low number of receptors usually implicates a Pred resistance but high numbers do not guarantee a response to this drug [27–31]. Therefore, studies to Pred resistance should incorporate a drug sensitivity assay, e.g., the MTT assay because this measures cell lysis which is the endpoint of all mechanisms of resistance instead of only the presence of receptors.

Conclusion

The prognostic value of age and immunophenotype might at least partly be explained by differences in drug sensitivity. This has to be confirmed in larger studies. It might then be possible to design more specific treatment protocols for the different risk groups.

Summary

Immunophenotype and age have prognostic value in childhood acute lymphoblastic leukemia (ALL) but it is not known why. In 84 children with ALL at initial diagnosis we studied the correlation between in vitro resistance to eight drugs, determined with the MTT assay, and immunophenotype and age. B-lineage ALL samples (CD19$^+$, HLA-DR$^+$) were classified into four differentiation stages: proB (CD10⁻, cytoplasmic μ⁻ [cμ⁻] and surface immunoglobulin [sIg⁻]; cALL (CD10⁺/cμ⁻/sIg⁻); preB (CD10⁺ᵒʳ⁻/cμ⁺/sIg⁻); B-ALL (CD10⁻/cμ⁻/sIg⁺). cALL cases are known to have the best prognosis; proB-, preB- and T-ALL cases show a worse and B-ALL the poorest prognosis. Patients aged <18 months and >10 years have a poor prognosis compared to patients in the intermediate age group. Our results showed that cALL and preB ALL cells were the most drug sensitive cells compared to the other phenotypes. No differences were found between cALL and preB ALL cases with the exception that preB cells were more sensitive to mustine and mafosfamide (Maf). Compared to cALL and preB ALL cases, T-ALL cases were significantly resistant to prednisolone (Pred), daunorubicin (DNR), *L*-asparaginase (*L*-Asp), cytosine arabinoside (AraC) and Maf; proB ALL cases to Pred, DNR, *L*-Asp and 6-thioguanine. The three B-ALL cases were resistant to VCR and DNR, which was not due to the multidrug resistance phenotype. Two out of three B-ALL cases were resistant to Pred. Compared to cells from patients aged 18 months to 10 years, cells from children <18 months were more resistant to Pred and DNR; cells from children >10 years were more resistant to Pred. We conclude that drug resistance patterns differed between different risk groups as defined by immunophenotype and age, which might at least partly explain the reported differences in responsiveness to chemotherapy.

Acknowledgements. We acknowledge the Dutch Childhood Leukemia Study Group (DCLSG) for their help in performing this study. Board members of the DCLSG are W.A. Kamps, K. Hählen, F.A.E. Nabben, J.A. Rammeloo, G.A.M. de Vaan, P.J. van Dijken, A.J.P. Veerman, R.S. Weening, E.Th. van 't Veer-Korthof, A. Postma, I. Risseeuw-Appel, J.P.M. Bökkerink, M.V.A. Bruin, F.C. de Waal, E.F. van Leeuwen, and M. van Weel-Sipman.

References

1. Crist WM, Grossi CE, Pullen J, Cooper M (1985) Immunologic markers in childhood acute lymphocytic leukemia. Semin Oncol 12: 105
2. Sallan SE, Ritz J, Pesando J, Gelber R, O'Brien C, Hithcock S, Coral F, Schlossman SF (1980) Cell surface antigens: prognostic implications in childhood acute lymphoblastic leukemia. Blood 55: 395
3. Greaves MF, Janossy G, Peto J, Kay H (1981) Immunologically defined subclasses of acute lymphoblastic leukemia in children: their relationship to presentation features and prognosis. Br J Haematol 48: 179
4. Pui CH, Williams DL, Raimondi SC, Melvin SL, Behm FG, Look AT, Dahl GV, Rivera GK, Kalwinsky DK, Mirro J, Dodge RK, Murphy SB (1986) Unfavorable presenting clinical and laboratory features are associated with calla-negative non-T, non-B lymphoblastic leukemia in children. Leuk Res 10: 1287
5. Crist W, Boyett J, Roper M, Pullen J, Metzgar R, van Eys J, Ragab A, Starling K, Vietti T, Cooper M (1984) Pre-B cell leukemia responds poorly to treatment: a Pediatric Oncology Group study. Blood 63: 407
6. Crist W, Boyett J, Jackson J, Vietti T, Borowitz M, Chauvenet A, Winick N, Ragab A, Mahoney D, Head D, Iyer R, Wagner H, Pullen J (1989) Prognostic importance of the pre-B-cell immunophenotype and other presenting features in B-lineage childhood acute lymphoblastic leukemia: a Pediatric Oncology Group study. Blood 74: 1252
7. Borowitz MJ (1990) Immunologic markers in childhood acute lymphoblastic leukemia. Hematol Oncol Clin North Am 4: 743
8. Poplack DG, Reaman G (1988) Acute lymphoblastic leukemia in childhood. Pediatr Clin North Am 35: 903
9. Miller DR (1988) Childhood acute lymphoblastic leukemia: 1. Biological features and their use in predicting outcome of treatment. Am J Pediatr Hematol Oncol 10: 163
10. Reaman G, Zeltzer P, Bleyer A, Amendola B, Level C, Sather H, Hammond D (1985) Acute lymphoblastic leukemia in infants less than one year of age: a cumulative experience of the Childrens Cancer Study Group. J Clin Oncol 3: 1513
11. Hammond D, Sather H, Nesbit M, Miller D, Coccoa P, Bleyer A, Lukens J, Siegel S (1986) Analysis of prognostic factors in acute lymphoblastic leukemia. Med Pediatr Oncol 14: 124

12. Crist W, Pullen J, Boyett J, Falletta J, van Eys J, Borowitz M, Jackson J, Dowell B, Frankel L, Quddus F, Ragab A, Vietti T (1986) Clinical and biologic features predict a poor prognosis in acute lymphoid leukemias in infants: a Pediatric Oncology Group study. Blood 67: 135

13. Crist W, Boyett J, Pullen J, van Eys J, Vietti T (1986) Clinical and biologic features predict poor prognosis in acute lymphoid leukemias in children and adolescents: a Pediatric Oncology Group review. Med Pediatr Oncol 14: 135

14. Pui C-H, Williams DL, Roberson PK, Raimondi SC, Behm FG, Lewis SH, Rivera GK, Kalwinsky DK, Abromowitch M, Crist WM, Murphy SB (1988) Correlation of karyotype and immunophenotype in childhood acute lymphoblastic leukemia. J Clin Oncol 6: 56

15. Pieters R, Huismans DR, Leyva A, Veerman AJP (1988) Adaptation of a rapid automated tetrazolium based (MTT-)assay for chemosensitivity testing in childhood leukemia. Cancer Lett 41: 323

16. Pieters R, Huismans DR, Leyva A, Veerman AJP (1989) Comparison of a rapid automated tetrazolium based (MTT-)assay with a dye exclusion assay for chemosensitivity testing in childhood leukemia. Br J Cancer 59: 217

17. Pieters R, Loonen AH, Huismans DR, Broekema GJ, Dirven MWJ, Heyenbrok MW, Hählen K, Veerman AJP (1990) In vitro drug sensitivity of cells from children with leukemia using the MTT assay with improved culture conditions. Blood 76: 2327

18. Santini V, Bernabei PA, Silvestro L, Dal Pozzo O, Bezzini R, Viano I, Gattei V, Saccardi R, Rossi Ferrini P (1989) In vitro chemosensitivity testing of leukemic cells: prediction of response to chemotherapy in patients with acute non-lymphocytic leukemia. Haematol Oncol 7: 287

19. Sargent JM, Taylor CG (1989) Appraisal of the MTT assay as a rapid test of chemosensitivity in acute myeloid leukaemia. Br J Cancer 60: 206

20. Hongo T, Fujii Y, Igarashi Y (1990) An in vitro chemosensitivity test for the screening of anti-cancer drugs in childhood leukemia. Cancer 65: 1263

21. Veerman AJP, Pieters R (1990) Drug sensitivity assays in leukemia and lymphoma. Br J Haematol 74: 381

22. Pieters R (1991) Drug resistance in childhood leukemia. Thesis, Free University, Amsterdam

23. Arseneau JC, Canellos GP, Banks PM, Berard CW, Gralnick HR, DeVita BT (1975) American Burkitt's lymphoma: a clinicopathologic study of 30 cases. I. Clinical factors relating to prolonged survival. Am J Med 58: 314

24. Costlow ME, Pui C-H, Dahl GV (1982) Glucocorticoid receptors in childhood acute lymphocytic leukemia. Cancer Res 42: 4801

25. Quddus FF, Leventhal BG, Boyett JM, Pullen DJ, Crist WM, Borowitz MJ (1985) Glucocorticoid receptors in immunological subtypes of childhood acute lymphocytic leukemia: a Pediatric Oncology Group study. Cancer Res 45: 6482

26. Vogler LB, Crist WM, Sarrif AM, Pullen J, Bartolucci AA, Falletta JM, Dowell B, Humphrey GB, Blackstock R, van Eys J, Metzgar RS, Cooper MD (1981) An analysis of clinical and laboratory features of acute lymphocytic leukemias with emphasis on 35 children with pre-B leukemia. Blood 58: 135

27. Pui C-H, Dahl GV, Rivera G, Murphy SB, Costlow ME (1984) The relationship of blast cell glucocorticoid receptor levels to response to single-agent steroid trial and remission response in children with acute lymphoblastic leukemia. Leuk Res 8: 579

28. Mastrangelo R, Malandrino R, Riccardi R, Longo O, Ranelletti FO, Iacobelli S (1980) Clinical implications of glucocorticoid receptor studies in childhood acute lymphoblastic leukemia. Blood 56: 1036

29. Pui C-H, Costlow ME (1986) Sequential studies of lymphoblast glucocorticoid receptor levels at diagnosis and relapse in childhood leukemia: an update. Leuk Res 10: 227

30. Thompson EB, Smith JR, Bourgeois S, Harmon JM (1985) Glucocorticoid receptors in human leukemias and related diseases. Klin Wochenschr 63: 689

31. Thompson EB, Harmon JM (1986) Glucocorticoid receptors and glucocorticoid resistance in human leukemia in vivo and in vitro. Adv Exp Med Biol 196: 111

Drug Resistance in Children with Relapsed Acute Lymphoblastic Leukemia*

R. Pieters[1], T. Hongo[2], A.H. Loonen[1], D.R. Huismans[1], H.J. Broxterman[3], K. Hählen[4], and A.J.P. Veerman[1]

Introduction

Nowadays the use of combination chemotherapy in children with acute lymphoblastic leukemia (ALL) results in a complete remission rate of more than 95 %. With the best currently available treatment, about two-thirds of these children will remain in continuous complete remission and can therefore be considered cured. Patients suffering from a relapse, however, have a cure rate which is much lower. One of the main causes of this poor prognosis is probably a resistance of the leukemic cells to a number of drugs used for treatment. At present the knowledge of drug resistance in childhood ALL is very limited. It is unknown for instance for which drugs resistance occurs and which mechanisms are of clinical importance. Currently, much attention is given to the multidrug resistance (MDR) phenomenon: a resistance to vincra alkaloids and anthracyclines, mediated by the drug efflux pump p-glycoprotein (-gp), which can at least be partially overcome by so-called resistance modifiers. Recently, we

and others adapted and improved assays to detect drug resistance of leukemic cells obtained from patients showing good correlations between in vitro results and clinical response to chemotherapy [1–8]. Because of the development of these short-term assays it has recently become possible to study drug resistance of patients with ALL. In the present study we assessed the resistance profiles of children with relapsed ALL and the clinical relevance of the MDR model in these patients.

Materials and Methods

Leukemic cells were obtained from bone marrow and peripheral blood samples taken for routine diagnostic procedures. Preparation of mononuclear cell suspensions and drug solutions have been described earlier [8]. In most cases, cells were used after cryopreservation. Patients with B-cell ALL characterized by the expression of surface immunoglobulins were excluded from the study. The percentage of malignant cells was 90.4 % ± 8.9 % (range, 65 %–100 %) and was not different between samples from untreated and relapsed ALL patients. Drug sensitivity was determined with the 4-day MTT assay as described earlier [8]. Briefly, 96-well microculture plates contained 100 µl cell suspension with 6 duplicate concentrations of the following drugs: 6-thioguanine (6-TG, 1.56–50 µg/ml); vincristine (VCR, 0.05–50 µg/ml); prednisolone (Pred, 0.08–250 µg/ml); daunorubicin (DNR, 0.002–2.0 µg/ml); mafosfamide (Maf,

[1] Department of Pediatrics, Free University Hospital, De Boelelaan 1117, 1081 HV Amsterdam, The Netherlands
[2] Department of Pediatrics, Hamamatsu University School of Medicine, Hamamatsu, Japan
[3] Department of Oncology, Free University Hospital, De Boelelaan 1117, 1081 HV Amsterdam, The Netherlands
[4] Sophia's Children Hospital, Subdivision Haemato/Oncology, Erasmus University, Rotterdam, The Netherlands
* This study is supported by the Dutch Cancer Society (IKA 87-17).

0.10–100 µg/ml), cytosine arabinoside (Ara-C, 0.0024–2.5 µg/ml), mustine HCl (Must, 0.16–500 µg/ml); L-asparaginase (L-Asp, 0.003–10 IU/ml). Untreated control cells were set up in sextuplicate. After incubation in a humidified incubator in 5 % CO_2 for 4 days at 37 °C, 10 µl MTT solution was added for 6 h. MTT is reduced to a colored formazan by living but not by dead cells. The formazan crystals were dissolved with 100 µl acid isopropanol. The optical density (OD) was measured with a microplate reader at 540 nm. The OD is linearly related to cell number. Leukemic cell survival (LCS) was calculated by the equation:

$$LCS = (OD \text{ treated well/mean OD control wells}) \times 100 \%.$$

The LC_{50} is the drug concentration lethal to 50 % of the cells.

The effects of the resistance modifiers cyclosporine A (CsA; 2 µg/ml), verapamil (Vp; 5 µg/ml) and lidocaine (40 µg/ml) upon leukemic cell kill by VCR and DNR were tested using the MTT assay. Accumulation studies were carried out with a radiochemical method as described elsewhere [9]. p-Glycoprotein staining of cytospun leukemic cells was done with the monoclonal antibodies C219 and JSB-1 using the Histostain-SP kit as described previously [10].

The Wilcoxon matched-paris signed-ranks test and the Mann-Whitney U test were used for two-tailed testing at a level of significance of 0.05.

Results and Discussion

Patient characteristics of the relapsed patients are shown in Table 1. Drug sensitivity profiles were evaluable in 41 untreated and 11 relapsed ALL patients. The LC_{50} values for DNR, VCR, Pred and L-Asp are shown in Fig. 1. Relapsed patients were significantly more resistant to 6-TG, Pred, DNR, Ara-C, Must, and Maf but not to VCR and L-Asp than untreated patients (Table 2). This suggests that L-Asp and VCR are not involved very often in drug resistance in children with relapsed ALL.

Since for some drugs the LC_{50} values of untreated patients show a nonparametric

Table 1. Characteristics of relapsed ALL patients

Patient No.	Comments
R1	Second BM relapse of T-ALL
R2	First BM relapse of T-ALL
R3a	Third BM testis and lymph node relapse of cALL
R3b	Fourth BM relapse 2 years after third relapse
R4	Third BM relapse of cALL
R5	First BM relapse of cALL
R6	Second BM relapse of cALL
R7	First BM relapse of T-ALL
R8	Third BM and CNS relapse of cALL
R9	First BM relapse of mixed lineage ALL/ANLL
R10	Second BM relapse of cALL
R11	First BM relapse of cALL
R12	Sixth BM relapse of cALL
R13	Fourth BM and CNS relapse of cALL
R14	First CNS relapse of T-ALL
R15	First BM and CNS relapse of cALL
R16	Third BM relapse of T-ALL
R17	Second BM relapse of T-ALL

BM, bone marrow; CNS, central nervous system; CR, complete remission

distribution (see, e.g., the Pred data in Fig. 1) the mean and standard deviations are less adequate parameters to describe these data. This problem can be circumvented by using percentiles. For example, a sample in the 90th percentile (P90) means that this sample is more resistant than 90 % of all samples tested. Using the P90 of untreated patients as the cutoff point of resistance, the resistance profiles of individual relapsed patients are presented in Table 3. Some patients (R3b, R7, R9) are resistant to almost all drugs tested while others (R1, R2, R8, R10, R12, R15, R16, R17) are resistant to only one to three drugs. This suggests that for some patients combinations of effective antileukemic drugs might be composed while this is not possible for those with a general resistance. On the other hand, the large overlaps in the ranges of LC_{50} values of untreated and relapsed patients might illustrate the fact that resistance of leukemic cells to anticancer drugs is only one of the factors contributing to the poor prognosis in relapsed leukemia. Inter-

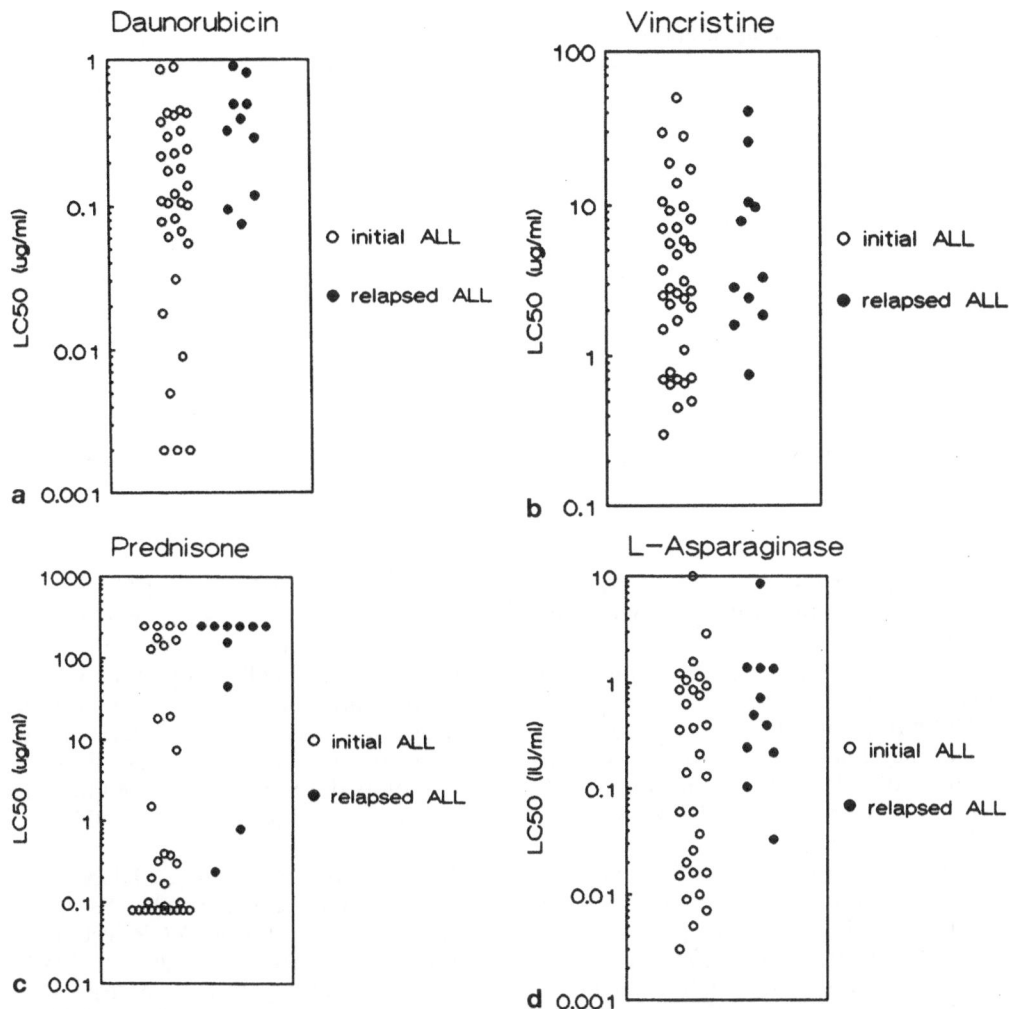

Fig. 1a–d. LC$_{50}$ values of cells from untreated and relapsed ALL patients, given in micrograms per milliliter for DNR, VCR, and Pred and in international units per milliliter for *L*-Asp

Table 2. LC$_{50}$ values of cells from newly diagnosed, initial patients ($n = 41$) and relapsed patients ($n = 11$) given in micrograms per milliliter with the exception of values for *L*-Asp, which is given in international units per milliliter. In some cases the LC$_{50}$ is higher than the highest concentration of a drug tested or lower than the lowest concentration tested

Drug	Median initial	Range relapse	Range initial	relapse	P
6-TG	4.4	11.9	1.6–14.9	4.7–16.1	.0004
AraC	.131	.460	.016–1.188	.114–2.500	.002
Asp	.177	.500	.003–10.000	.033–8.590	.091
DNR	.115	.363	.002–.895	.075–.910	.030
Maf	4.4	24.0	.5–50.0	13.1–54.4	.002
Must	22.2	90.3	1.1–87.0	16.2–198.4	.002
Pred	.3	250.0	.1–250.0	.2–250.0	.002
VCR	2.80	3.30	.30–50.0	.75–41.0	.358

Table 3. Resistance profile of individual ALL patients

Patient No.	6-TG	AraC	L-Asp	DNR	VCR	Pred	Maf	Must
R1	s	R	s	s	s	s	R	R
R2	R	R	s	s	s	R	s	s
R3b	R	R	s	R	R	R	R	R
R7	R	R	s	R	R	R	–	R
R8	R	s	s	s	s	s	R	R
R9	R	R	s	R	s	R	R	R
R10	–	s	s	s	s	R	–	s
R12	s	s	s	s	s	R	–	s
R15	R	s	s	s	s	(R)	–	s
R16	s	s	s	R	s	(R)	–	s
R17	s	R	R	s	s	–	–	R

R, LC_{50} value >P90 of untreated ALL patients; s, LC_{50} value <P90 of untreated ALL patients; –, not evaluable

patient pharmacokinetic variabilities are clearly related to the probability of oncolytic effects [11].

We studied several aspects of the MDR model:

1. Cross-resistance to vinca alkaloids and anthracyclines. As shown above the group of relapsed patients was significantly more resistant to DNR but not to VCR than the group of untreated ALL patients. Looking at individual cases (Table 3), a resistance to both VCR and DNR was found in two patients (R3b and R7) while in two others (R9, R16) cells were resistant to DNR but not to VCR. In all four cases, however, this was associated with resistance to other drugs which are not involved in the MDR model.

2. p-Glycoprotein expression. p-Glycoprotein staining was performed on cells from 28 untreated and 14 relapsed ALL samples (R1-3b, R7, R9-17). Cells from the positive control cell line 8226/Dox4, stained simultaneously, were clearly p-gp positive. All 42 cases, including the 4 patients who showed an in vitro resistance to DNR and VCR, were p-gp negative. This is in accordance with three recent studies that made clear that p-gp is infrequently found in childhood initial and relapsed ALL [12–14].

3. Resistance modifiers. Results of testing resistance modifiers were evaluable in 12 untreated and 8 relapsed samples. CsA alone decreased LCS to 88 % ± 38 % (mean ± SD), Vp to 96 % ± 12 % and lidocaine to 96 % ± 13 %. Figure 2 shows the ALL cell kill by combinations of resistance modifiers and cytostatic drugs corrected for the effect of the resistance modifiers alone. Addition of modifiers did not lead to a significantly increased cell kill by VCR and DNR.

Verapamil did not enhance DNR accumulation in ALL cells (mean 96.4 %, range 83 %–108 %; $n = 10$) while VCR accumulation was increased to a mean of 125 % (range 81 %–168 %). Cells from case R3b which were highly resistant to VCR ($LC_{50} = 41.0$ µg/ml) and DNR ($LC_{50} = 0.91$ µg/ml) did not accumulate less VCR or DNR than cells from nine other cases. Also, in this case, DNR and VCR accumulation and cytotoxicity were not influenced by resistance modifiers.

Altogether, these finding indicate that DNR and VCR resistance in children with relapsed ALL is not due to the mechanism of classic MDR but to other still unknown mechanisms. This is in accordance with the finding that decreased uptake and retention of vincra alkaloids and anthracyclines are not the only factors accounting for resistance to these classes of drugs [14, 15]. Diversion to some cellular compartment might play a role. Changes in topoisomerases or disturbed intracellular drug distributions are other possible explanations.

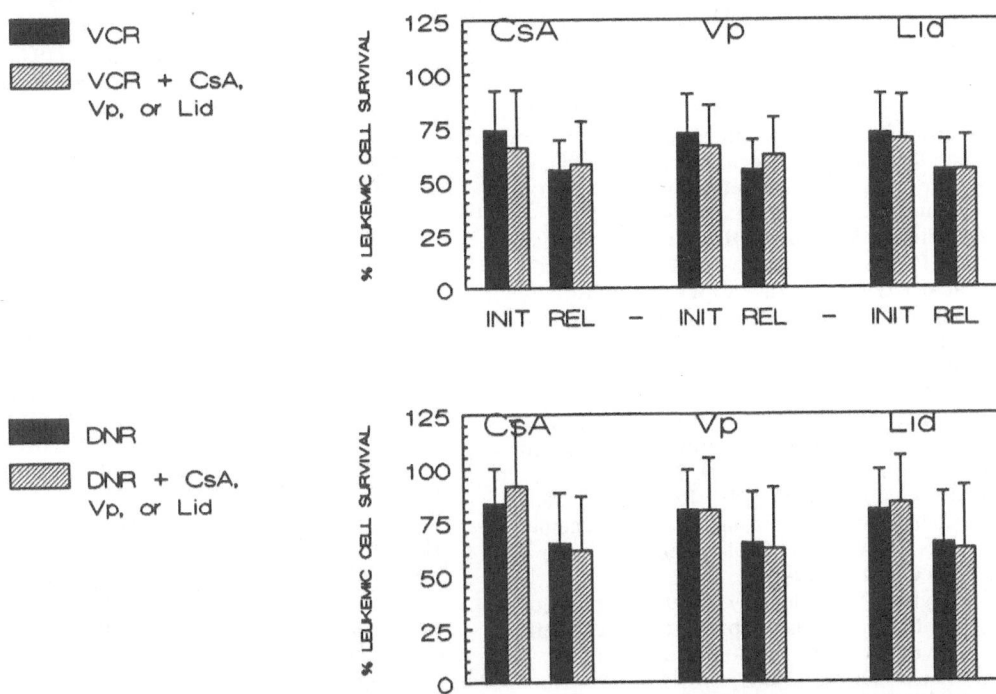

Fig. 2a, b. Leukemic cell survival values of cells from patients at initial diagnosis (*INIT*) and at relapse (*REL*) incubated with VCR or DNR with and without the addition of the resistance modfiers Vp, CsA and Lid. The LCS values are corrected for the effect of resistance modifier alone

Conclusions

We conclude that children with relapsed ALL show varying types of drug resistance. Notwithstanding the fact that large interindividual differences exist in degree of resistance and number of drugs to which a resistance is detected, significant differences between relapsed and untreated patients were found in sensitivity to DNR, 6-TG, Pred, Ara-C and alkylating drugs but not in sensitivity to VCR and *L*-Asp. DNR and VCR resistance in childhood relapsed ALL is not due to *p*-gp-mediated MDR which is not an important mechanism of drug resistance in these patients. Future studies on clinical drug resistance in ALL should not only focus on *p*-gp expression but should incorporate data of in vitro drug sensitivity testing because this measures the end result of all mechanisms of drug resistance.

Summary

Different aspects of drug resistance were studied in 17 children with relapsed acute lymphoblastic leukemia (ALL). The in vitro sensitivity profile was determined using the MTT assay. Cells from relapsed children were significantly more resistant to 6-thioguanine, prednisolone, cytosine arabinoside, daunorubicin (NR), mustine-HCl and mafosfamide but not to *L*-asparaginase and vincristine (VCR) than cells from 41 children with ALL at initial diagnosis. Some relapsed patients showed a general drug resistance while others were resistant to only one to three drugs. Resistance to anthracyclines and vinca alkaloids in childhood relapsed ALL appeared not to be due to p-glycoprotein-mediated multidrug resistance.

References

1. Hongo T, Fujii Y, Mizuno Y, Haraguchi S, Yoshida TO (1987) Anticancer drug sensitivity test using the short-term microplate culture and MTT dye reduction assay. Jpn J Cancer Chemother 14: 472–478
2. Pieters R, Huismans DR, Leyva A, Veerman AJP (1988) Adaptation of a rapid tetrazolium based (MTT-) assay for chemosensitivity testing in childhood leukemia. Cancer Lett 41: 323–332
3. Pieters R, Huismans DR, Leyva A, Veerman AJP (1989) Comparison of the rapid automated MTT-assay with a dye exclusion assay for chemosensitivity testing in childhood leukemia. Br J Cancer 59: 217–220
4. Twentyman PR, Fox NE, Rees JKH (1989) Chemosensitivity testing of fresh leukaemia cells using the MTT colorimetric assay. Br J Haematol 71: 19–24
5. Sargent JM, Taylor CG (1989) Appraisal of the MTT assay as a rapid test of chemosensitivity in acute myeloid leukaemia. Br J Cancer 60: 206–210
6. Santini V, Bernabei PA, Silvestro L, Dal Pozzo O, Bezzini R, Viano I, Gattei V, Saccardi R, Rossi Ferrini P (1989) In vitro chemosensitivity testing of leukemic cells: prediction of response to chemotherapy in patients with acute non-lymphocytic leukemia. Haematol Oncol 7: 287–293
7. Veerman AJP, Pieters R (1990) Drug sensitivity assays in leukaemia and lymphoma. Br J Haematol 74: 381–384
8. Pieters R, Loonen AH, Huismans DR, Broekema GJ, Dirven MWJ, Heyenbrok MW, Hählen K, Veerman AJP (1990) Detection of drug resistance in children with leukemia using the MTT assay with improved culture conditions. Blood 76: 2327–2336
9. Broxterman HJ, Kuiper CM, Schuurhuis GJ, Tsuruo T, Pinedo HM, Lankelma J (1988) Increase of daunorubicin and vincristine accumulation in multidrug resistant human ovarian carcinoma cells by a monoclonal antibody reacting with P-glycoprotein. Biochem Pharmacol 37: 2389–2393
10. Broxterman HJ, Pinedo HM, Kuiper CM, van der Hoeven JJM, de Lange P, Baak JJ, Scheper RJ, Keizer HG, Schuurhuis GJ, Lankelma J (1989) Immunohistochemical detection of P-glycoprotein in human tumor cells with a low degree of drug resistance. Int J Cancer 43: 340–343
11. Evans WE, Petros WP, Relling MV, Crom WR, Madden T, Rodman JH, Sunderland M (1989) Clinical pharmacology of cancer chemotherapy in children. Pediatr Clin North Am 36: 1199–1230
12. Tawa A, Ishihara S, Yumura K, Hara J, Inoue M, Muruyama F, Kawai S, Fujimoto T, Nobori U, Nishikawa A, Tsuruo T, Kawa-Ha K (1990) Expression of the multidrug-resistance gene in childhood leukemia. Jpn J Pediatr Hematol 4: 38–43
13. Rothenberg ML, Mickley LA, Cole DE, Balis FM, Tsuruo T, Poplack DG, Fojo AT (1989) Expression of the *mdr-1/p-170* gene in patients with acute lymphoblastic leukemia. Blood 74: 1388–1395
14. Ubezio P, Limonta M, d'Incalci M, Damia G, Masera G, Giudici G, Wolverto JS, Beck WT (1989) Failure to detect the *p*-glycoprotein multidrug resistant phenotype in cases of resistant childhood acute lymphocytic leukaemia. Eur J Cancer Clin Oncol 25: 1895
15. Rivera-Fillat MP, Pallares-Trujiloo J, Domenech C, Grau-Oliete MR (1988) Comparative uptake, retention and action of vincristine, vinblastine and vindesine on murine leukaemic lymphoblasts sensitive and resistant to vincristine. Br J Pharmacol 93: 902

Sensitivity of Childhood Acute Lymphoblastic Leukemia Cells to Prednisolone and Dexamethasone Assessed by the MTT Assay*

G.J.L. Kaspers[1], R. Pieters[1], C.H. Van Zantwijk[1], F.C. De Waal[1,2], E.R. Van Wering[2], and A.J.P. Veerman[1,2]

Introduction

Glucocorticoids like predniso(lo)ne and dexamethasone are well known for their antileukemic activity, especially in acute lymphoblastic leukemia (ALL). Several groups have investigated the sensitivity of malignant lymphoid cells to glucocorticoids (GCs) and possibilities to predict this sensitivity. Special attention was given to the correlation between GC receptor numbers and sensitivity to these drugs, with conflicting results [1–4]. The clinical response to an initial prednisone (PRD) monotherapy was shown to have prognostic value in childhood ALL, firstly in small patient-groups [3, 5], later in the large BFM-ALL 83 study [6]. Differences in GC sensitivity might be important to consider in the design of an optimal treatment for each individual. In vitro sensitivity testing is an attractive method to investigate these differences.

It is generally assumed that the treatment results are not influenced by the specific GC used, PRD or dexamethasone (DXM), provided PRD is given in about sevenfold higher dosages. This assumption is not based on studies which compared the antileukemic potency of these GCs, but rather their anti-inflammatory effects. Moreover, the factor seven was not found in several of these studies [7, 8]. To the best of our knowledge only two studies have compared the antileukemic effects of PRD and DXM [9, 10]. Even though "equivalent" dosages were used, treatment results were not identical with PRD and DXM.

We recently started a nationwide, prospective study in which the GC sensitivity in childhood ALL at initial diagnosis is investigated. In vitro sensitivity is determined with the short-term MIT assay. The results of this efficient and reliable assay have clinical relevance [11–15]. We report and discuss the results of the first 75 patients of this study regarding the in vitro sensitivity to PRD and DXM, with special attention given to the interindividual differences in GC sensitivity and the comparison of the antileukemic potency of these GCs.

Materials and Methods

Bone marrow (BM) or peripheral blood (PB) samples from 75 children with ALL at initial diagnosis were obtained from the laboratory of the Dutch Childhood Leukemia Study Group (DCLSG) for in vitro drug sensitivity testing. At the DCLSG laboratory immunophenotyping was done as described [16]. The MTT assay was successful in 60 out of the 75 (80%) patients, and in 57 cases PRD and/or DXM were successfully tested, cases and results which will be the subject of further discussion. There were 39 BM samples, with 92% ± 5% (mean ± SD) leukemic cells after isolation, and 19 PB samples with 90% ± 6% leukemic cells. The sample source, BM or PB, does not significantly influence test

[1] Department of Pediatrics, Free University Hospital, De Boelelaan 1117, 1081 HV Amsterdam, The Netherlands
[2] Dutch Childhood Leukemia Study Group, The Hague, The Netherlands
* Supported by the Dutch Cancer Society (IKA 87-17 and IKA 89-06).

results [17]. Sex was equally distributed (52% male), and most children were between 2 and 6 years old at diagnosis. The median white blood cell count was 24.9 (range, 2.5–729) $\times$ 10^9/l. Of 55 cases with known immunophenotypes there were 43 with precursor B-ALL, 1 with B-ALL, and 11 with T-ALL.

The MTT assay was done as described [13]. Briefly, 80 µl cell suspension (2×10^6 cells/ml) was added to wells of 96-well microculture plates, already containing 20 µl drug solution. Prednisolone disodium phosphate, dissolved in saline, and dexamethasone disodium phosphate, obtained in soluble form, were provided by our hospital pharmacy. Both GCs were tested in six concentrations in duplicate, PRD from 0.06 to 187.5 (later 0.05–1500) µg/ml, DXM from 0.0003 to 0.8 (later 0.0002–6) µg/ml. These concentrations refer to those of pure prednisolone and pure dexamethasone. The plates were incubated for 4 days at 37°C. Then MTT was added and the plates were incubated for another 6 h. The formed formazan crystals were dissolved with isopropanolol and the optical density (OD) of each well was determined using a spectrophotometer (Titertek Multiskan MCC 340). The OD is linearly related to the cell number [13]. The LC_{50}, the drug concentration lethal to 50% of the cells as compared to the control cell survival, was calculated from the dose-response curve and was used as a measure of in vitro drug sensitivity.

Wilcoxon's ranking test for unpaired data was used for two-tailed testing at a level of significance of $p < .05$. Correlation was expressed by the Spearman's rank correlation coefficient R_s.

Results

Dose-response curves were obtained in most cases. In the first samples tested a 50% cell kill was frequently not reached. Therefore, the highest concentrations of both PRD and DXM were increased as described. There were marked differences in sensitivity to both PRD and DXM (Table 1). The LC_{50} values for PRD ($n = 56$) ranged from <0.05 to >1500 µg/ml, those for DXM ($n = 48$) form <0.0002 to >6 µg/ml (Fig. 1). The median LC_{50} values were 1.38 µg/ml and 0.061 µg/ml for PRD and DXM respectively. In two precursor-B cases a growth stimulation was noted with both PRD and DXM. GC sensitivity was not correlated with sex or FAB classification (data not shown). The influence of age and immunophenotype on GC sensitivity is described elsewhere [14]. There was a significant ($p < .01$) correlation ($R_s = 0.89$) between sensitivity to PRD and DXM (Fig. 2). The antileukemic potency of PRD compared to that of DXM, expressed as the ratio of their respective LC_{50} values, also showed large differences (Fig. 3). In each case DXM was more potent than PRD and in 27/30 cases DXM was more than tenfold as active.

The ratios ranged in 30 cases from 4 to more than 5000, with a median of 38 (Table 1). In the remaining 17 cases in which both PRD and DXM were tested successfully, no ratio could be calculated because one or both LC_{50} values were outside the concentration range (if both, always at the same end of the range).

Table 1. In vitro sensitivity to prednisolone (PRD) and dexamethasone (DXM) in childhood ALL at initial diagnosis assessed by the MTT assay

| | LC_{50} values (µg/ml) and individual LC_{50} ratios | | |
	Range	Median	Number of samples
PRD	<0.05–>1500	1.38	56
DXM	<0.0002–>6	0.0608	48
PRD/DXM ratio	3.6–5208.8	37.7	30

* For the remaining samples the ration could not be calculated, because one on both LC_{50} values were outside the concentration ranges tested.

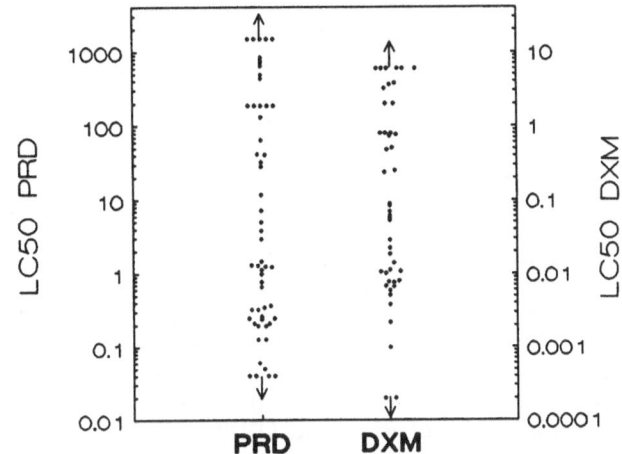

Fig. 1. LC$_{50}$ values of prednisolone (PRD, $n = 56$) and dexamethasone (DXM, $n = 48$) for 57 cases of childhood ALL at first diagnosis. *Arrows* indicate LC$_{50}$ values outside the concentration ranges tested

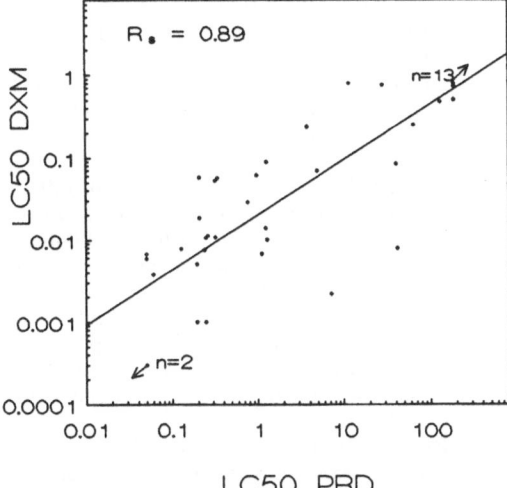

Fig. 2. Cross-sensitivity between PRD and DXM in 47 childhood ALL cases. *Arrows* indicate LC$_{50}$ values outside the concentration ranges tested

Discussion

In connexion with a nationwide, prospective study about clinical and in vitro GC sensitivity in childhood ALL at initial diagnosis, we assessed in vitro sensitivity to PRD and to DXM in 75 cases. The short-term, colorimetric MTT assay was used for this purpose. The results show large differences in sensitivity to both PRD and DXM (Fig. 1, Table 1), in agreement with the clinical experience [3, 5, 6]. We previously

showed that high-risk groups as defined by immunophenotype (ProB- and T-ALL) and age (children younger than 1.5 years or older than 10 years) are relatively resistant to PRD [14]. Furthermore, in vitro PRD resistance at diagnosis correlated with a relatively poor prognosis [15]. Good correlations have been reported between in vitro and in vivo GC sensitivity [1, 4, 18], although others could not confirm this [2].

Our results with respect to the in vitro antileukemic activity of DXM compared to that of PRD show marked interindividual differences (Fig. 3). However, DXM was always more potent than PRD, in 27/30 cases even more than tenfold more potent.

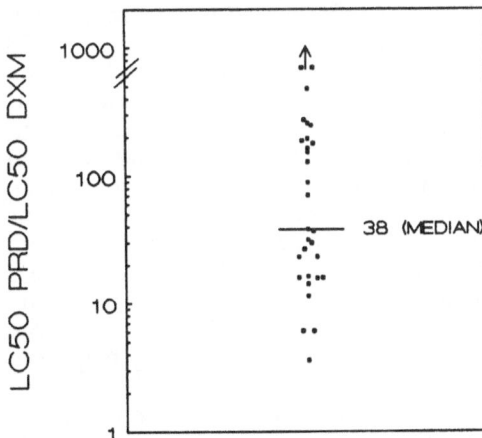

Fig. 3. The individual ratios of the LC$_{50}$ values for prednisolone and dexamethasone in 30 childhood ALL cases. The range is 3.6–5029

329

The median antileukemic potency of DXM was 38 times as high as that of PRD. It is generally assumed that PRD and DXM are GCs with identical antileukemic activities, if PRD is given at sevenfold higher dosages. This assumption is mainly based on studies investigating the anti-inflammatory effects of these GCs.

Although several times DXM was shown to be four to ten times as potent as PRD [19, 20], others found quite different ratios, e.g., with DXM being 39 [7] and even 67 [8] times as potent as PRD. Two clinical studies have specifically investigated the antileukemic activities of PRD and DXM in so-called equivalent doses, 40 mg/m^2 and 6 mg/m^2 every day respectively [9, 10]. Jones et al. [9] reported a significant reduction in CNS relapses, but not in BM relapses and deaths, when DXM was substituted for PRD in the treatment of childhood ALL. The Dutch ALL-VI study in which DXM was used was preceded by a pilot study in which PRD was used, the only difference between both protocols. The DXM-related toxicity was more pronounced than that of PRD. The treatment results with DXM seem to be better than with PRD, but longer follow-up is necessary for an appropriate comparison [10].

We conclude that it is possible to determine the in vitro sensitivity to PRD and DXM in childhood ALL, using the MTT assay. This sensitivity varies markedly, variance which has been reported to have clinical significance. The in vitro antileukemic activity of DXM is a median of 38 times as high as that of PRD, which contrasts to the generally assumed factor of 7. It would be interesting to compare the antileukemic potencies of PRD and DXM in childhood ALL, e.g., randomized as an initial monotherapy for 1 week. Our results suggest that in order to achieve optimal treatment with these drugs of each child with ALL, differences in GC sensitivity must be taken into account. In vitro drug sensitivity results could be very helpful in treatment modifications.

Acknowledgements. The laboratory of the Dutch Childhood Leukemia Study Group (DCLSG) provided the patient samples. Board members of the DCLSG are J.P.M. Bökkerink, M.V.A. Bruin, P.J. Van Dijken, K. Hählen, W.A. Kamps, E.F. Van Leeuwen, F.A.E. Nabben, A. Postma, J.A. Rammeloo, I. Risseeuw-Appel, G.A.M. De Vaan, E.Th. Van 'T Veer-Korthof, A.J.P. Veerman, F.C. De Waal, M. Van Weel-Sipman, and R.S. Weening.

References

1. Lippman ME, Konior G, Leventhal BG (1978) Clinical implications of glucocorticoid receptors in human leukemia. Cancer Res 38: 4251–4256
2. Homo F, Duval D, Harousseau JL et al. (1980) Heterogeneity of the in vitro responses to glucocorticoids in acute leukemia. Cancer Res 40: 2601–2608
3. Pui C-H, Dahl GV, Rivera G et al. (1984) The relationship of blast cell glucocorticoid receptor levels to response to single-agent steroid trial and remission response in children with acute lymphoblastic leukemia. Leuk Res 8: 579–585
4. Nanni P, Nicoletti G, Prodi G et al. (1982) Glucocorticoid receptor and in vitro sensitivity to steroid hormones in human lymphoproliferative diseases and myeloid leukemia. Cancer 49: 623–632
5. Mastrangelo R, Riccardi R, Corbo S et al. (1984) Prediction of clinical response to glucocorticoids in children with acute lymphoblastic leukemia. Eur Paediatr Haematol Oncol 1: 33–36
6. Riehm H, Reiter A, Schrappe M et al. (1986) Die Corticosteroidabhängige Dezimierung der Leukämiezellzahl im Blut als Prognosefaktor bei der akuten lymphoblastischen Leukämie im Kindesalter (Therapiestudie ALL-BFM 83). Klin Pädiatr 199: 151–160
7. Lerner LJ, Bianchi A, Turkheimer AR et al. (1964) Anti-inflammatory steroids: potency, duration and modification of activities. Ann N Y Acad Sci 116: 1071–1077
8. Nakai T (1961) Influences of small doses of various corticosteroids on the incidence of chemically induced subcutaneous sarcomas in mice. Cancer Res 21: 221–227
9. Jones B, Shuster JJ, Holland J (1984) Lower incidence of meningeal leukemia when dexamethasone is substituted for prednisone in the treatment of acute lymphoblastic leukemia – a late follow-up. Proc Am Soc Clin Oncol 3: 191 (abstract)
10. Veerman AJP, Hählen K, Kamps WA et al. (1990). Dutch Childhood Leukemia Study Group: early results of study ALL VI (1984–1988). In: Büchner T, Schellong G,

Hiddemann W, Ritter J (eds) Acute leukemias II. Springer, Berlin, Heidelberg New York, pp 473–477

11. Sargent JM, Taylor CG (1989) Appraisal of the MTT assay as a rapid test of chemosensitivity in acute myeloid leukemia. Br J Cancer 60: 206–210

12. Hongo T, Fujii Y, Igarashi Y (1990) An in vitro chemosensitivity test for the screening of anti-cancer drugs in childhood leukemia. Cancer 65: 1263–1272

13. Pieters R, Loonen AH, Huismans DR et al. (1990) In vitro drug sensitivity of cells from children with leukemia using the MTT assay with improved culture conditions. Blood 76: 2327–2336

14. Pieters R, Kaspers GJL, Van Wering ER et al. (1991) In vitro drug resistance in childhood acute lymphoblastic leukemia in relation to age and immunophenotype. This volume

15. Pieters R, Huismans DR, Loonen AH et al (1991). Relations of cellulas drug resistance to long-term clinical outcome in childhood acute lymphoblastic leukemia. Lancet 338: 399–403

16. Van Dongen JJM, Adriaansen HJ, Hooijkaas H (1987) Immunologic marker analysis of cells in the various hematopoietic differentiation stages and their malignant counterparts. In: Ruiter DJ et al. (eds) Application of monoclonal antibodies in tumor pathology. Nijhoff, Dordrecht, pp 87–116

17. Kaspers GJL, Pieters R, Van Zantwijk CH et al. (1991) In vitro drug sensitivity of normal peripheral blood lymphocytes and childhood leukaemic cells from bone marrow and peripheral blood. Bn J Canar 64: 469–474

18. Cline MJ, Rosenbaum E (1968) Prediction of in vivo cytotoxicity of chemotherapeutic agents by their in vitro effect on leukocytes from patients with acute leukemia. Cancer Res 28: 2516–2521

19. Cantrill HC, Waltman SR, Palmberg PF et al. (1975) In vitro determination of relative corticosteroid potency. J Clin Endocrinol Metab 40: 1073–1077

20. Berliner DL, Ruhmann AG (1967) Influence of steroids on fibroblasts. I. An in vitro fibroblast assay for corticosteroids. J Invest Dermatol 49: 117–122

Correlation of In Vitro Drug Resistance Assessed by the MTT Assay with Long-Term Clinical Outcome in Childhood Acute Lymphoblastic Leukemia*

R. Pieters[1], D.R. Huismans[1], A.H. Loonen[1], K. Hählen[2,3],
A. van der Does-van den Berg[3], E.R. van Wering[3], and A.J.P. Veerman[1,3]

Introduction

Clinical forms and mechanisms of drug resistance in childhood acute lymphoblastic leukemia (ALL) are poorly characterized. No studies have been reported on the relationship between initial chemosensitivity and final clinical outcome in ALL patients, most probably because of the lack of suitable in vitro assays. We recently reviewed the use of different assays in leukemic patients [1]: Clonogenic assays are not suitable for testing samples from patients with ALL. The short-term dye exclusion or differential staining cytotoxicity (DiSC) assay showed favorable clinical correlations and can be used in ALL patients but is too laborious for large-scale patient studies. We and others adapted the efficient MTT assay to study chemosensitivity in samples of leukemic patients and showed that the results of MTT and DiSC assays are comparable [1]. The MTT assay was found to predict initial response to chemotherapy in AML patients and to detect acquired drug resistance in ALL and AML patients. In this report we used the MTT assay to study the relation between drug sensitivity at initial diagnosis and the long-term clinical outcome in children with ALL.

Materials and Methods

Bone marrow or peripheral blood cells from 42 children with ALL at initial diagnosis who obtained complete remission were used. Standard risk patients were treated according to protocols of the Dutch Childhood Leukemia Study Group (DCLSG). High-risk patients, i.e., those with white blood cell counts (WBC) $>50 \times 10^9/l$, mediastinal enlargement and/or initial central nervous system leukemic involvement, were treated according to different institutional protocols. All patients were treated with prednisone, vincristine, L-asparaginas, 6-mercaptopurine, methotrexate, and in most cases with anthracyclines.

Isolation and immunophenotyping of leukemic cells were done as described before [2]. Mature B-ALL samples with immunoglobulins on their cell surface were excluded. Most samples were tested after cryopreservation in liquid nitrogen, which does not alter drug sensitivity [3]. The median percentage malignant cells was 95% (range 66%–100%). In vitro drug sensitivity was assessed with the MTT assay as described elsewhere [2]. Briefly, 96-well microculture plates contained 100 μl cell suspension with six duplicate concentrations of the following drugs: 6-thioguanine (6-TG, 1.6–50 μg/ml); vincristine (VCR, 0.05–50 μg/ml); prednisolone (Pred; 0.1–250 μg/ml); daunorubicin (DNR, 0.002–2 μg/ml); l-asparaginase (L-Asp;

[1] Free University Hospital, Department of Pediatrics, De Boelelaan 1117, 1081 HV Amsterdam, The Netherlands
[2] Sophia's Children Hospital, Subdivision Haemato/Oncology, Erasmus University, Rotterdam, The Netherlands
[3] Dutch Childhood Leukemia Study Group, The Hague, The Netherlands
* Supported by the Dutch Cancer Society (IKA 87-17).

0.016–10 IU/ml). Because of the instability of 6-mercaptopurine (6-MP) in vitro the results of 6-TG instead of 6-MP were analyzed [2]. Untreated control cells were set up in sixfold. After incubation in a humidified incubator in 5% CO_2 for 4 days at 37°C, 10 μl MTT solution was added for 6 h. MTT is reduced to a colored formazan by living but not by dead cells. The formazan crystals were dissolved with 100 μl acid isopropanol. The optical density (OD) was measured with a microplate reader at 540 nm. The OD is linearly related to cell number. Leukemic cell survival (LCS) was calculated by the equation:

LCS = (OD treated well/mean OD control wells) × 100%.

The LC_{50} is the drug concentration lethal to 50% of the cells.

The chi^2-test and the Mann-Whitney U test were performed at a two-sided significance level of 0.05. The Kaplan Meier method was used to estimate curves, which were compared with the logrank test at a one-sided significance level of 0.05: The null hypothesis is that the clinical outcome is equally good in the in vitro sensitive group and the in vitro resistant group; the alternative hypothesis is that the clinical outcome is poorer in the resistant group.

Results

The median and range of LC_{50} values are shown in Table 1. The results of the MTT assay were correlated with the clinical outcome. The median follow-up time was 49 months (range, 3–178 months).

Vincristine and L-asparaginase. Irrespective of the chosen cutoff point of sensitivity versus resistance, VCR-resistant and L-Asp-resistant cases did not have a lower probability of continuous complete remission (CCR) than respectively VCR-sensitive and L-Asp-sensitive cases (Fig. 1a, b).

6-Thioguanine. If 5 μg/ml was taken as the cutoff point between 6-TG sensitivity and resistance, patients with 6-TG resistance had a significantly lower probability of CCR (p <.01) than patients sensitive to 6-TG (Fig. 1c). Organomegaly, age, and immunophenotype did not differ between both groups but the proportion of boys and the white blood cell count (WBC) were higher in the 6-TG-resistant group. After stratification for sex and WBC, the prognostic value of 6-TG resistance was still significant ($p < .04$).

We studied whether leukemic cells from boys and girls differed in drug resistance. No significant differences were found if all phenotypes were analyzed but among patients with precursor B-ALL boys ($n = 21$) were significantly more resistant to 6-TG ($p = .037$) than girls ($n = 13$) but not to VCR, DNR, Pred, and L-Asp.

Prednisone. In some cases the LC_{50} values were higher than the maximum concentration tested (250 μg/ml) while in others the LC_{50} values were lower than the minimum concentration tested (0.1 μg/ml). The four patients with $LC_{50} > 250$ μg/ml had a lower probability of CCR ($p < .01$) than the 28 patients with LC_{50} values <250 μg/ml. Significant differences were also found if the cutoff point was lowered to 150 μg/ml ($p < .01$; fig. 1d). WBC, age, sex, immunophenotype and organomegaly were equally distributed between Pred sensitive and resistant groups. The tendency for a

Table 1. In vitro drug sensitivity data represented by LC_{50} values (micrograms per milliliter; for L-asparaginase in units per milliliter) of cells from children with ALL who obtained a complete remission

Drug	LC_{50} Median	LC_{50} Range	N
Vincristine	3.91	0.3–50.0	38
Prednisone	0.4	0.1–250.0	32
Daunorubicin	0.131	0.002–0.895	32
L-Asparaginase	0.213	0.016–10.000	29
6-Thioguanine	4.9	1.6–17.9	36

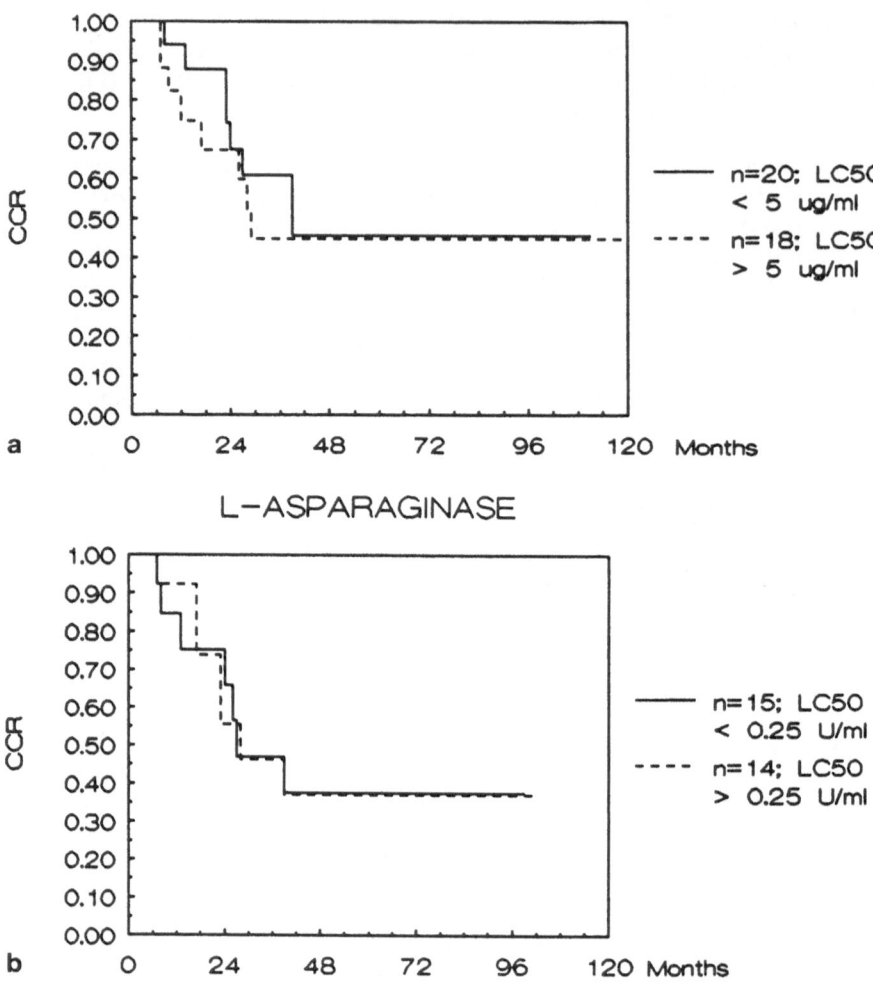

Fig. 1a–e. Relation between in vitro resistance to vincristine (**a**), *L*-asparaginase (**b**), 6-thioguanine (**c**), prednisone (**d**), and daunorubicin (**e**) and probability of continuous complete remission (CCR) in children with ALL. Patients are divived into drug-sensitive and drug-resistant groups based on the indicated LC_{50} values as cutoff points.

poorer prognosis going from the most sensitive group (LC_{50} <0.1 µg/ml) via the intermediate group (LC_{50} 0.1–150 or 0.1–250 µg/ml) to the most resistant group (LC_{50} >150 or 250 µg/ml) was significant (p <.05; Fig. 1d).

Daunorubicin. If patients treated with anthracyclnes were divided into a DNR-sensitive and -resistant group by the cutoff point of 0.150 µg/ml, the probability of CCR (Fig. 1e) was significantly lower in the DNR-resistant group (p <.02). Sex, orga-

nomegaly, immunophenotype, age, and WBC were comparable between both groups.

Discussion

Although clonogenic assays have long been considered to be the gold standard for in vitro chemosensitivity testing, short-term assays have been proven to be at least as valuable for the clinical situation of leu-

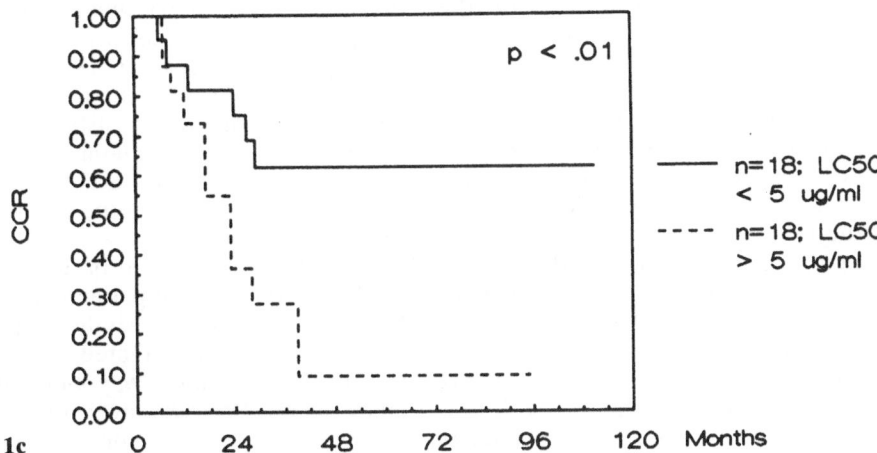

Fig. 1c

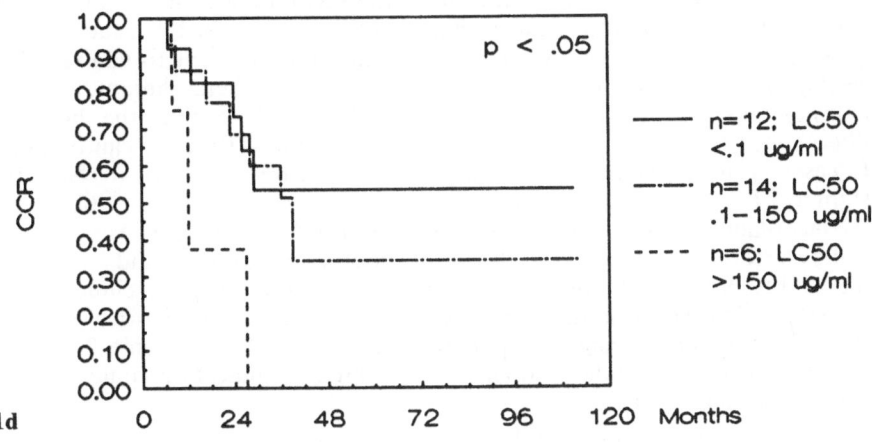

Fig. 1d

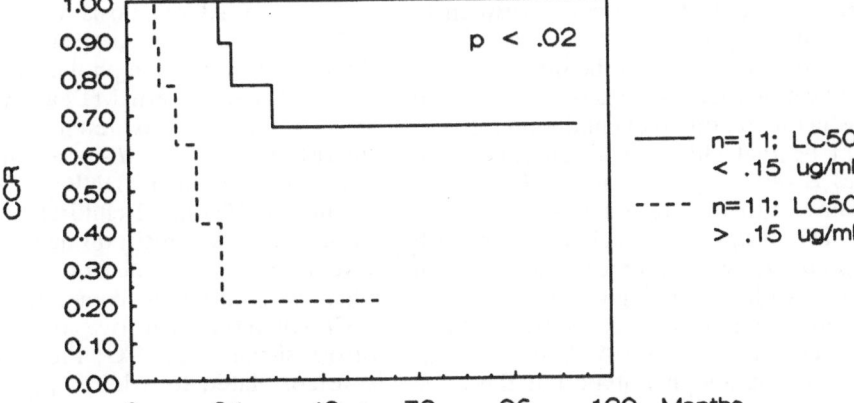

Fig. 1e

kemic patients [1, 3–5]. The present study uses the short-term MTT assay and is the first that correlates chemosensitivity with long-term clinical outcome in ALL patients. In vitro sensitivity to Pred appeared to be of prognostic value in childhood ALL. The prognosis worsened with a decreasing sensitivity of the cells to Pred. Patients whose cells were extremely resistant to Pred with the LC_{50} close to or higher than the maximum concentration tested had the poorest prognosis. This is in agreement with the findings of Riehm et al. [6], who showed that children with a poor response to 1 week monotherapy with prednisone have a poorer final clinical outcome than those with a good response to prednisone. Thus, cellular resistance to Pred seems to be a very important factor in the failure of response to chemotherapy in childhood ALL.

Patients whose cells were relatively resistant to 6-TG had a poorer prognosis than patients whose cells were 6-TG sensitive, suggesting that also cellular resistance to thiopurines has clinical implications in childhood ALL. Among the precursor B-ALL cases, cells from boys were more resistant to 6-TG than cells from girls, which is in concordance with the fact that cells from boys were found to form less 6-MP-derived cytotoxic nucleotides than cells from girls [7]. This suggests that a relative resistance to thiopurines might be part of the reason why in some studies boys have a poorer prognosis than girls.

Also DNR resistance appeared to be of prognostic value in childhood ALL. Although large interindividual variations in VCR- and L-Asp sensitivity were found, no correlation could be detected between in vitro sensitivity to these drugs and clinical outcome. This should not be interpreted as an indication that both drugs are of limited value in the treatment of childhood ALL. It might be that clinical resistance to these drugs is relatively uncommon. Elsewhere we showed that VCR and L-Asp were the only two drugs for which children with relapsed ALL were not more resistant than children with newly diagnosed ALL [3].

Many prognostic factors have been recognized in childhood ALL such as sex, age, and immunophenotype but the basis for this prognostic value is not understood.

Studying the prognostic value of in vitro drug sensitivity assays might lead to the recognition of a causal prognostic factor directly accounting for reported differences in prognosis. The present study gives evidence that cellular drug resistance is indeed a prognostic factor in childhood ALL. The patients in this study have been treated according to different protocols and have a relatively low overall 5 years CCR percentage ($\pm 50\%$), which can be explained by the high proportion of patients with a high WBC. A prospective study with larger numbers of patients treated according to one protocol is underway but will take many years. Also, we have to realize that oncolytic effects depend on two factors: In the first place the amount of effective drug that reaches the cells which is determined by pharmacokinetic parameters [8] and in the second place the cellular resistance to anticancer drugs. Both factors have to be taken into account to analyze the clinical response to chemotherapy.

We conclude that the highly efficient short-term MTT assay can be used to predict long-term response to chemotherapy in children with ALL: In vitro resistance to Pred, 6-TG and DNR was correlated to a poorer prognosis and may therefore account for the poor clinical outcome in part of the children with ALL. In vitro resistance to VCR and L-Asp was not related to clinical outcome.

Summary

The in vitro sensitivity to chemotherapeutic drugs at initial diagnosis was correlated with the long-term clinical outcome in children with acute lymphoblastic leukemia (ALL). The short-term MTT assay was used to assess sensitivity to prednisolone (Pred), vincristine (VCR), L-asparaginase (L-Asp), daunorubicin (DNR), and 6-thioguanine (6-TG) in 42 children with ALL. VCR- and L-Asp-resistant patients did not have a poorer outcome in terms of probability of continuous complete remission (CCR) than their sensitive counterparts. In vitro resistance to 6-TG, Pred, and DNR were correlated to a lower probability of CCR.

Acknowledgements. We acknowledge the Dutch Childhood Leukemia Study Group (DCLSG) for providing clinical data. Board members of the DCLSG are W.A. Kamps, K. Hählen, F.A.E. Nabben, J.A. Rammeloo, G.A.M. de Vaan, P.J. van Dijken, A.J.P. Veerman, R.S. Weening, E.Th. van 't Veer-Korthof, A. Postma, I. Risseeuw-Appel, J.P.M. Bökkerink, M.V.A. Bruin, F.C. de Waal, E.F. van Leeuwen, and M. van Weel-Sipman.

References

1. Veerman AJP, Pieters R (1990) Drug sensitivity assays in leukemia and lymphoma. Br J Haematol 74: 381–384
2. Pieters R, Loonen AH, Huismans DR, Broekema GJ, Dirven MWJ, Heyenbrok MW, Hählen K, Veerman AJP (1990) In vitro drug sensitivity of cells from children with leukemia using the MTT assay with improved culture conditions. Blood 76: 2327–2336
3. Pieters R (1991) Drug resistance in childhood leukemia. Thesis, Free University, Amsterdam.
4. McGuire WL, Kern DH, Von Hoff DD, Weisenthal LM (1988) In vitro assays to predict drug sensitivity and drug resistance. Breast Cancer Res Treat 12: 7–21
5. Weisenthal LM, Lippmann ME (1985) Clonogenic and nonclonogenic in vitro chemosensitivity assays. Cancer Treat Rep 69: 615–632
6. Riehm H, Feickert H-J, Schrappe M, Henze G, Schellong G (1987) Therapy results in five ALL-BFM studies since 1970: implications of risk factors for prognosis. In: Bücher T, Schellong G, Hiddemann W, Urbanitz D, Ritter J (eds) Acute leukemias. Prognostic factors and treatment strategies. Springer, Berlin Heidelberg New York, p 139
7. Lilleyman JS, Lennard L, Rees CA, Morgan G, Maddocks JL (1984) Childhood lymphoblastic leukaemia: sex difference in 6-mercaptopurine utilization. Br J Cancer 49: 703–707
8. Evans WE, Petros WP, Relling MV, Crom WR, Madden T, Rodman JH, Sunderland M (1989) Clinical pharmacology of cancer chemotherapy in children. Pediatr Clin North Am 36: 1199–1230

Prognostic Significance of Exposure to Intermediate-Dose Methotrexate in Children with Standard Risk ALL: The COALL 82/85 Experience

Jürgens H[1], G. Janka[2], M. Ibrahim[1], C. Tonert[2], K. Winkler[2], and U. Göbel[1]

Methotrexate is being widely used in doses ranging from 500 to 2 000 mg administered as prolonged infusion over 12–36 h followed by leucovorin rescue to consolidate remission of acute lymphoblastic leukemia

[1] Pediatric Hospital, Department of Hematology and Oncology, Heinrich Heine University, Düsseldorf, FRG, present address:
Pediatric Hospital, University of Münster,
Albert-Schweizer-Straße 33
W-4400 Münster, FRG
[2] Pediatric Hospital, University of Hamburg, Hamburg, FRG

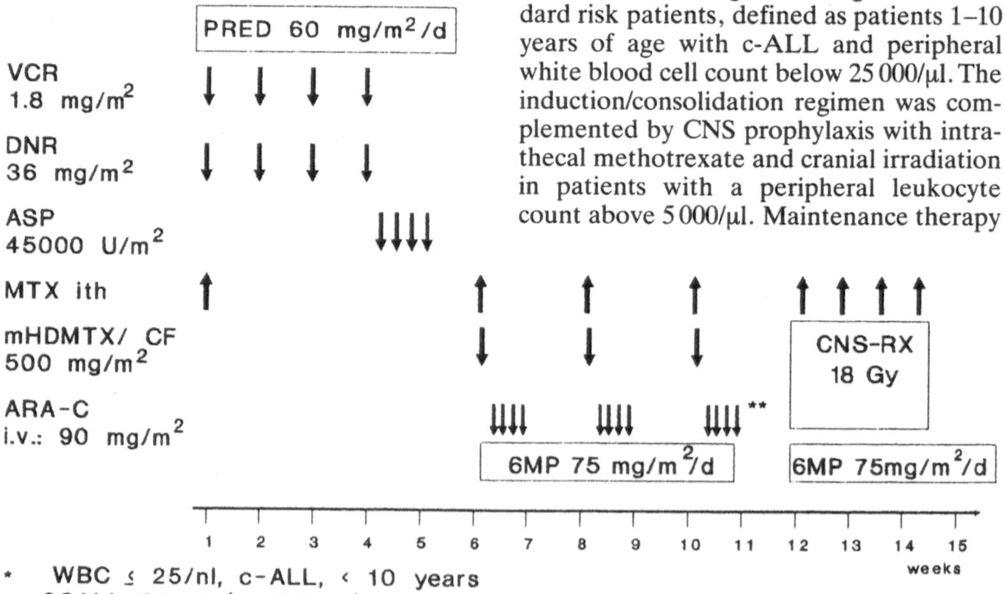

[1–4]. There is evidence that prolonged duration of exposure to methotrexate has a positive impact on the length of remission of ALL. Patients with a rapid systemic clearance of methotrexate have a higher risk of relapse [5–7].

In the COALL 82 and 85 studies induction with vincristine, prednisone, and daunorubicin was followed by consolidation with asparaginase, intermediate-dose methotrexate, and cytosine arabinoside (Fig. 1). Intermediate-dose methotrexate was administered as 24-h infusion of 500 mg/m², followed by three oral doses of 15 mg/m² leucovorin. This regimen was given to standard risk patients, defined as patients 1–10 years of age with c-ALL and peripheral white blood cell count below 25 000/µl. The induction/consolidation regimen was complemented by CNS prophylaxis with intrathecal methotrexate and cranial irradiation in patients with a peripheral leukocyte count above 5 000/µl. Maintenance therapy

Fig. 1. COALL 82 and COALL 85 treatment regimen for standard risk ALL patients: children between 1 and 10 years of age, c-ALL, UBC < 25000/µl

338

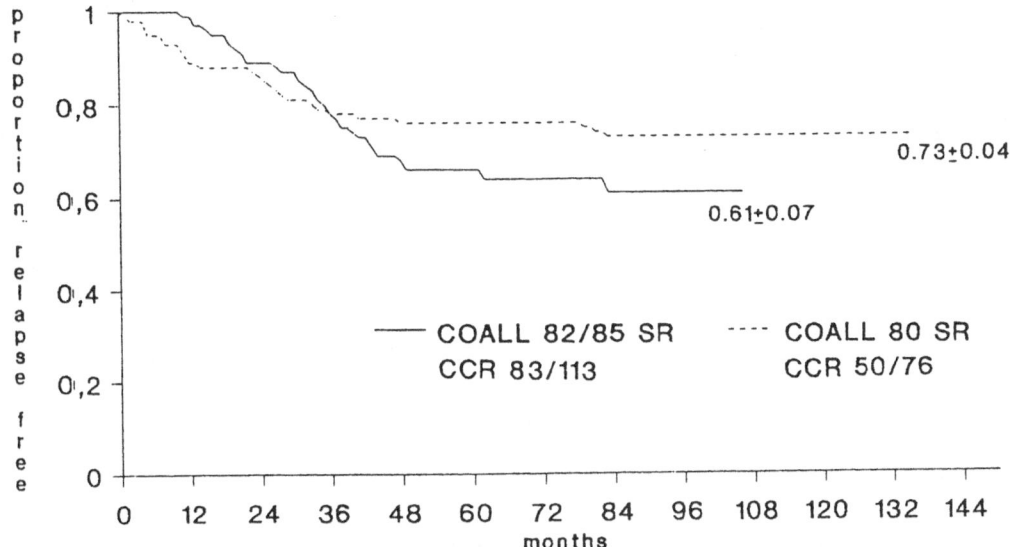

Fig. 2. Kaplan-Meier event-free survival of standard risk patients treated according to the COALL 80 protocol compared to patients treated according to the COALL 82 and 85 protocols. In COALL 80, cyclophosphamide 1200 mg/m^2 and reinduction

consisting of daily 6-mercaptopurine and weekly methotrexate was then administered for a total length of 24 months treatment from initial diagnosis [8].

Since disease-free survival of standard risk ALL patients treated according to the COALL 82/85 protocols had fallen behind results obtained for standard risk patients with the previous COALL 80 protocol (Fig. 2) [9], where cyclophosphamide was given instead of intermediate-dose methotrexate, an investigation was prompted to determine factors that might have influenced this outcome.

Patients and Methods

The records of 76 standard-risk ALL patients, ages ranging from 1 to 10 years, median 4,1 years, female to male ratio 1:1.1, diagnosed between January 1982 and December 1987 were available for review. To determine intraindividual differences in the handling of methotrexate and leucovorin administration, the following parameters were recorded:

- Serum methotrexate level at 24 h following the beginning of infusion, calculated as the mean of three courses

- Cumulative administered leucovorin dose per square meter body surface area (BSA), calculated as the mean of three courses
- Length of exposure to methotrexate defined as time from beginning of the methotrexate infusion to the first administered dose of leucovorin rescue (time to rescue), calculated as the mean of three courses

Results

As of 1 September 1990, 26/76 patients had relapsed. Fourteen patients presented with bone marrow relapse, six with CNS relapse, one with ovary relapse, two with combined bone marrow and CNS relapse, and three with combined bone marrow and testicular relapse.

According to the 24-h serum methotrexate level, 25 patients had levels below 5.0 µmol/l and 20 patients levels above 5.0 µmol/l. Kaplan-Meier life table analysis showed no significant difference between these two groups (Fig. 3).

With respect to the mean cumulative leucovorin dose per course, patients were

339

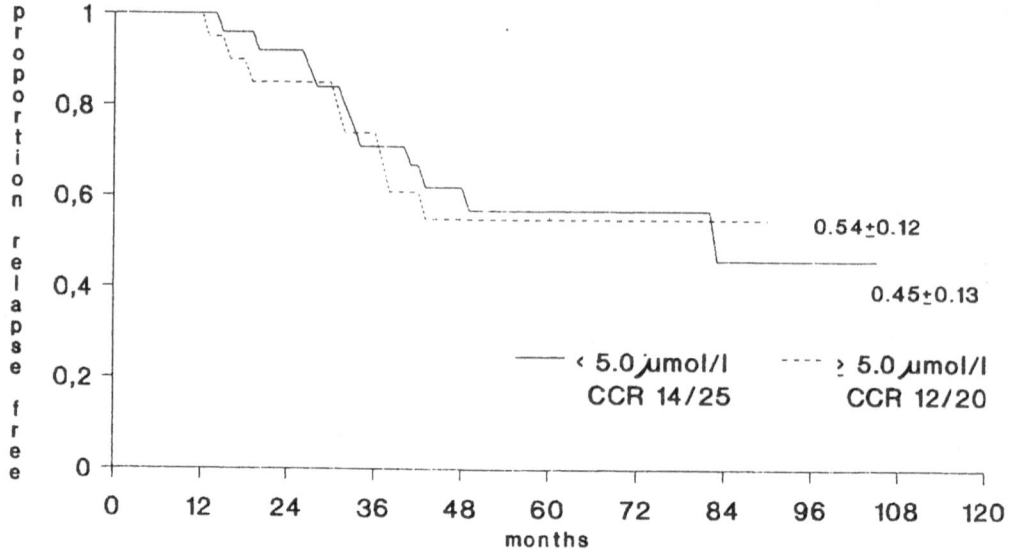

Fig. 3. Kaplan-Meier event-free survival according to the 24 h serum methotrexate level (mean of three courses) in COALL 82 and 85

grouped into three categories: below 50 mg/m², 22 patients, between 50 and 60 mg/m², 22 patients, and above 60 mg/m², 32 patients. According to Kaplan-Meier analysis there were no significant difference between these groups; however, there was a trend for patients with higher doses to have more relapses (Fig. 4).

According to time to rescue, 31 patients had received the first dose of leucovorin less than 43 h from the beginning of the methotrexate infusion, median 40 h. Forty-five patients had received their first dose of leucovorin later than 43 h since the beginning of the methotrexate infusion, median 48 h. Kaplan-Meier life table analyses

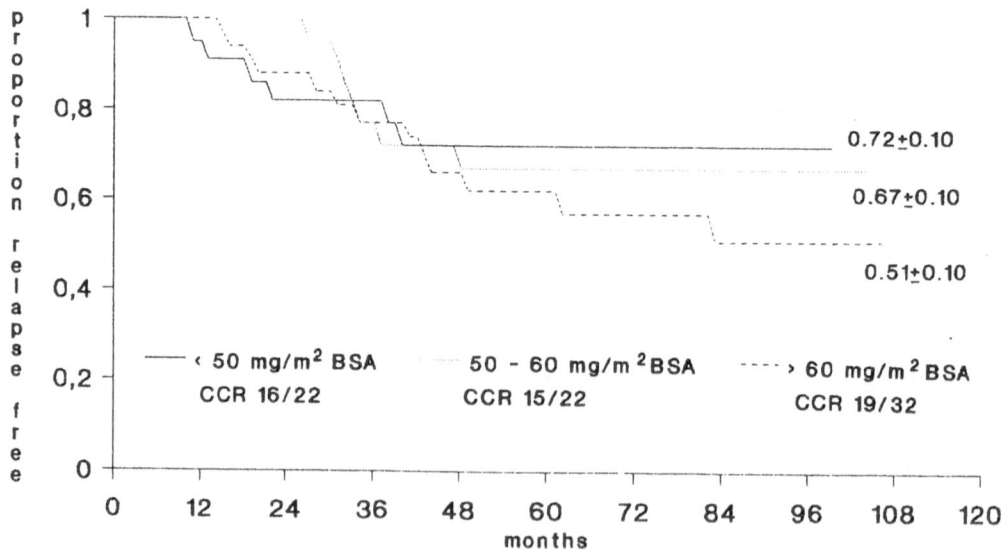

Fig. 4. Kaplan-Meier event-free survival according to the mean cumulative leucovorin dose/m² BSA (mean of three courses) in COALL 82 and 85

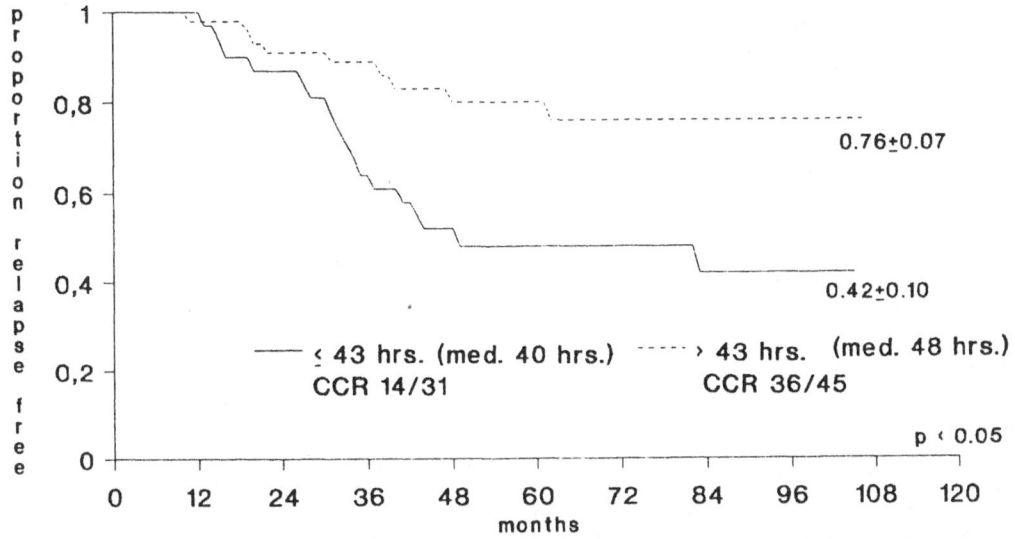

Fig. 5. Kaplan-Meier event-free survival according to time to rescue (interval between beginning of methotrexate infusion and first oral dose of leucovorin; mean of three courses) in COALL 82 and 85

showed a significant difference in favor of patients with prolonged exposure to methotrexate (76 % event-free survival) compared to patients with shorter duration of exposure (42 % surviving event-free (Fig. 5).

The increased number of relapses in patients with shorter exposure to methotrexate was mainly due to an increased rate of bone marrow relapses (10/17 versus 4/9).

Discussion

Although this investigation is not the result of a prospective randomized study, the results give evidence that the efficacy of intermediate-dose methotrexate correlates with the rescue regimen and that early rescue might jeopardize the effect of methotrexate on leukemic blasts and thus influence the quality of remission. These findings are in accordance with other published evidence [7, 10, 11]. Given a hidely accepted critical 48 h time threshold of folic acid deprivation to prevent severe toxicity [12], the optimal length of methotrexate infusion beyond 24 h has to be determined as well as the optimal rescue regimen

starting as late as possible and still avoiding severe toxicity.

According to these results, a methotrexate dose of 500 mg/m^2 should not be followed by leucovorin less than 48 h after the beginning of the methotrexate infusion. Further investigations to optimize the use of methotrexate with leucovorin factor rescue in ALL are strongly advocated.

Summary

Delayed plasma elimination of methotrexate (MTX) following intermediate-dose methotrexate (IDMTX) has been associated with improved disease-free survival (DFS) (Evans et al. 1986). IDMTX is widely used in combination chemotherapy for ALL to consolidate or maintain remission. Regimens differ in dose, length of infusion, hydration, and leucovorin rescue regimen. In view of the influence of delayed serum elimination, the effect of delayed rescue and hence prolonged exposure to MTX was retrospectively analyzed in patients treated according to the COALL 82 and 85 protocols, receiving three courses IDMTX 500 mg/m^2 as 24 h continuous infusion as consolidation following induction treatment. Standard risk patients only were reviewed since their treatment regimen was not complemented by reinduction. Of 76 standard risk ALL patients (c-ALL, WBC <25 000/μl, age range 1–10 years, median 3;10 years), 31 patients had received the first oral or i.v. dose of leucovorin between 38 and 42 h following the beginning of the MTX infusion and 45 patients between 46 and 48 h. Of 26 relapses, 17 occurred in the group of 31 patients with shorter MTX exposure and 9 in the group of 46 patients with prolonged exposure. According to Kaplan-Meier life table analysis, the difference between 81 % EFS and 45 % EFS is significant. Both groups are comparable according to age and sex distribution, there is, no difference in MTX serum levels at 24 and 48 h and hydration. It is concluded that in ALL delaying the leucovorin rescue following IDMTX is essential to ensure optimal efficacy of this regimen.

References

1. Freeman AI, Brecher ML, Wang JJ, Sinks LF (1979) Intermediate dose methotrexate (IDM) in childhood acute lymphocytic leukemia (ALL). Hämatol Bluttransfus 23: 115–123
2. Moe PJ, Seip M, Finne PH (1981) Intermediate dose methotrexate (IDM) in childhood acute lymphocytic leukemia in Norway. Preliminary results of a national treatment program. Acta Paediatr Scand 70: 73–79
3. Janka GE, Mack R, Helmig M, Haas R, Bidlingmaier F (1984) Prolonged methotrexate infusions in children with acute leukemia in relapse and in remission and with medulloblastoma. Pharmacokinetics, toxicity and clinical results. Oncology 41: 225–232
4. Jürgens H (1983) Hochdosierte Methotrexatbehandlung. Indikation, Risiken, Steuerung. Urban and Schwarzenberg, Munich
5. Evans WE, Stewart CF, Chen CH et al. (1984) Methotrexate systemic clearance influences probability of relapse in children with standard risk acute lymphoblastic leukemia. Lancet ß: 359–362
6. Borsi JD, Moe PJ (1987) Systemic clearance of methotrexate in the prognosis of acute lymphoblastic leukemia in children. Cancer 60: 3020–3024
7. Borsi JD, Moe PJ (1990) Pharmacokinetics of methotrexate and folinic acid in children: an update. In: Borsi JP, Riccardi R (eds.) Role of clinical pharmacology in pediatric oncology. Workshop Proceedings, Rome
8. Janka GE, Winkler K, Jürgens H, Göbel U. Gutjahr P, Spaar HJ (1986) Akute lymphoblastische Leukämie im Kindesalter: Die COALL-Studien. Klin Pädiatr 198: 171–177
9. Janka-Schaub GE, Winkler K, Jürgens H, Göbel U, Gutjahr P, Spaar HJ (1986) Intermediate-dose methotrexate in the treatment of childhood acute lymphocytic leukemia: lack of benefit during maintenance therapy following intensive induction therapy. Eur J Pediatr 145: 14–17
10. Bleyer WA (1989) New vistas for leucovorin in cancer chemotherapy. Cancer 63: 995–1007
11. Borsi JD, Sagen E, Romslo I, Moe PJ (1990) Rescue after intermediate and high-dose methotrexate: background, rationale, and current practice. Pediatr Hematol Oncol 7: 347–363
12. Bleyer WA (1978) The clinical pharmacology of methotrexate. New applications of an old drug. Cancer 41: 36–51

Protein Binding of Teniposide In Vitro and in Children with Acute Lymphoblastic Leukemia*

J. D. Borsi[1], W. P. Petros[2], J. H. Rodman[2], W. E. Evans[2], R. Koos[2], and D. Schuler[1]

Background and Objectives

Teniposide (VM-26)

Teniposide (VM-26) is an epipodophyllo-toxin anticancer drug, widely used as a single agent or in combination for the treatment of children with different malignancies (acute lymphoblastic leukemia, lymphomas, neuroblastoma). It is a phase-specific cytotoxic agent inducing premitotic block in the cell cycle by stabilizing the DNA-topoisomerase II complex. The dose-limiting toxicity of the drug is myelosuppression.

Pharmacokinetics and Clinical Effects

Several studies have demonstrated a relationship between the systemic pharmacokinetics and the clinical effects (response and toxicity) of VM-26. A significant correlation was found between the teniposide area under the curve (AUC) and decrease of circulating leukemic blasts (Sinkule 1984; Rodman JH, 1987), between state concentrations, systemic clearance, and oncolytic

response or toxicity (mucositis) (Rodman JH, 1987). This study also revealed a more than tenfold variability of systemic clearance, suggesting a similar variability of systemic exposure to the drug.

Plasma Protein Binding

A number of investigations have indicated that substantial interindividual variability in protein binding exists for many drugs. Pathologic conditions, including *cancer, kidney* or *liver disease,* or *concomitant drug therapy* have been shown to be major sources of this variability. The potential importance of these findings is derived from the fact that only free (unbound) drug can diffuse across biological membranes and interact with receptor sites. As only free drug is considered pharmacologically active, changes in protein binding may have direct clinical significance. For highly protein bound drugs (>90% bound), a small decrease of the protein-bound fraction results in a large increase in the active, free drug concentration.

Plasma Protein Binding of Epipodophyllotoxins

Etoposide (VP-16) is about 94%, teniposide (VM-26) is approximately 99%, bound to plasma proteins. Recent work by Stewart et al. (Stewart CF, 1989) has described altered protein binding of teniposide in adult cancer patients with abnormal liver function tests. In this study, patients with

[1] Second Department of Pediatrics, Semmelweis Medical School, Budapest, Hungary
[2] St. Jude Children's Research Hospital, Memphis, TN, USA
* Supported in part by the following grants from the U.S. Public Health Service, National Institutes of Health: R37 CA36401, Leukemia Program Project Grant CA20180, and Cancer Center CORE support grant CA21765 and by American Lebanese Syrian Associated Charities.

343

low serum total and/or high total bilirubin levels were found to have an increased etoposide free fraction. In addition, higher systemic clearance of the drug was observed in patients with low total protein concentrations. The plasma protein binding of teniposide has not been characterized in children or adults with cancer.

Primary Objectives of the Study

1. To characterize the protein binding of teniposide in vitro in human plasma
2. To examine the effect of other anticancer drugs on the protein binding of teniposide in vitro
3. To evaluate the protein binding of teniposide in vivo in children with acute lymphoblastic leukemia (ALL)
4. To analyze the effect of low serum total protein and/or high serum bilirubin levels on the protein binding of teniposide in selected samples from heavily pretreated children with relapsed ALL
5. To evaluate the effect of low serum total protein concentration on the clinical manifestation of bone marrow toxicity in patients receiving teniposide or etoposide therapy.

Patients, Materials, and Methods

Samples from 17 patients were analyzed. Nine patients were in first complete remission (CR) and eight children in second or third CR at the time of the study. All patients were treated with essentially similar induction therapy consisting of prednisone, vincristine, daunomycin, teniposide, cytosine arabinoside, and L-asparaginase. Teniposide (200 mg/m^2) was administered i.v. on days 22, 25, and 29 to newly diagnosed patients, and on days 30, 31, and 32 to relapsed patients. Relapsed patients also received 3×200 mg/m^2 teniposide in weekly intervals prior to the start of the reinduction therapy.

Maintenance therapy for patients in first remission consisted of daily 6-mercaptopurine and weekly methotrexate interrupted every 6 weeks for treatment with either high-dose methotrexate or teniposide (200

mg/m^2 i.v. days 1 and 3) with cytosine arabinoside (300 mg/m^2 i.v. days 1 and 3). Teniposide protein-binding studies were performed on samples taken during the first 2–6 months of maintenance therapy.

Maintenance therapy of relapsed patients (daily 6-mercaptopurine, weekly methotrexate, and biweekly PEG-asparaginase) was interrupted every 7 weeks for pulse therapy with 200 mg/m^2 i.v. teniposide with or without cytosine arabinoside. In these patients, teniposide protein-binding studies were performed in samples taken during the first 2–9 months of maintenance therapy.

Samples were taken pre-infusion, 1.5, 3.5, 8, and 24 h following the start of VM-26 infusion to determine total teniposide concentrations for calculation of systemic pharmacokinetic parameters of the drug.

Protein binding of teniposide was studied in selected serum samples from the above two groups of patients, with a comparable total teniposide level in the range of 16–53 µg/ml.

The effect of total protein concentrations on the development of bone marrow toxicity was studied in 32 children, following 111 treatments with VM-26 or VP-16.

In Vitro Studies

Sample Preparation

Pooled human plasma samples were spiked to achieve teniposide concentrations in the range of 10–350 µg/ml. Cytosine arabinoside (ara-C), mAMSA, or flavone acetic acid were added to the samples in concentrations shown in Figs. 3–4. After repeated centrifugation, the samples were left at room temperature for 2 h before analysis.

Binding Studies

Protein binding of teniposide was studied by *equilibrium dialysis* and/or *ultrafiltration*. The equilibrium dialysis apparatus consisted of 2×0.5 ml plexiglass cells (Mecca Inc., Aurora NY) separated by Spectra/Por 2, MWCO 12 000–14 000 (Spectrum Medical, Los Angeles, CA) membrane. Plasma samples were dialyzed against Sorenson's phosphate buffer (pH 7.4) at 37 °C for 6 h. Ultrafiltration was performed with the Amicon Centrifree TM micropartition system (Amicon Division of Grace Co. Danvers, MA). The dialysis and ultrafiltration equipment are illustrated in Fig. 1.

High-Performance Liquid Chromatography. Teniposide concentrations in plasma and buffer aliquots were determined with reverse-phase HPLC + electrochemical detection (applied potential, 0.75 V; range 5 nA (buffer) or 500 nA (plasma)). A Micro-Bondapack 25 cm phenyl column (Waters) and a mobile phase of water-ACN-acetic acid (70:30:2) were used in the system.

Calculations. Free fraction (f_u) is expressed as a percentage of total drug concentration. Measured free concentrations were corrected to colume shift, if they occurred during equilibrium dialysis, using the method of Huang (Huang J, 1988). Statistical calculations (Student's t test to compare group means, or nonparametric tests) were performed with standard methods.

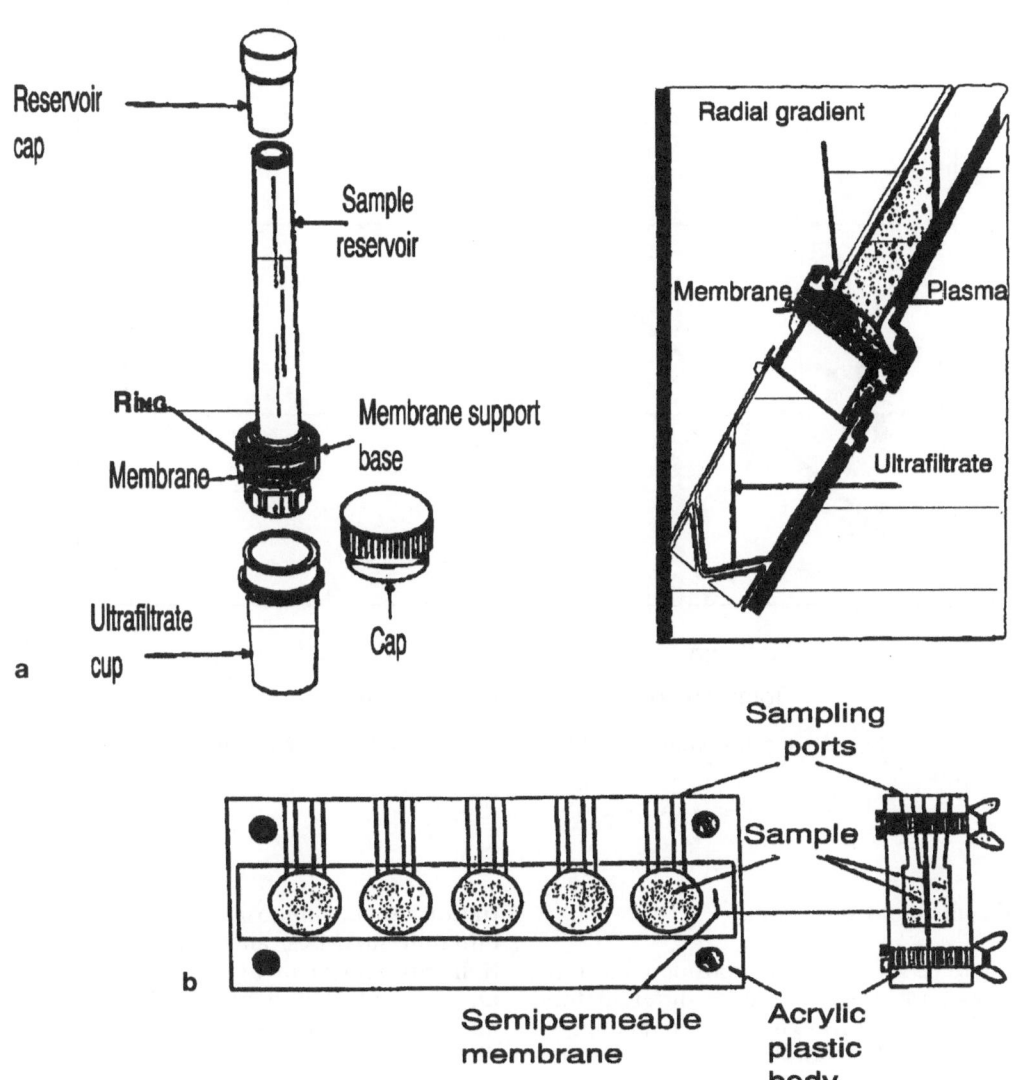

Fig. 1a,b. **a** Amicon Centrifree system. **b** Equilibrium dialysis chamber

345

Free Teniposide conc. (µg/ml)
Free fraction (%)

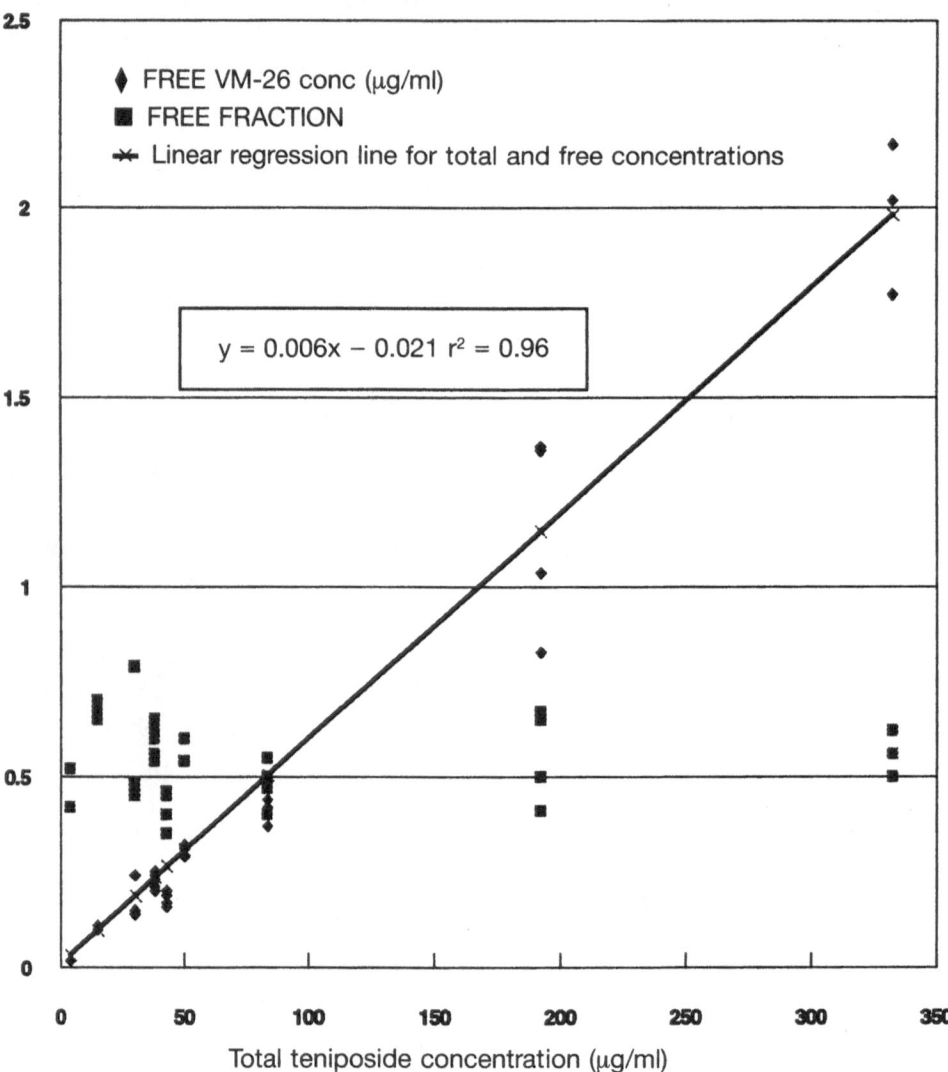

Fig. 2. Free teniposide concentrations and free fractions at different total teniposide levels

Results and Conclusions

Figure 2 shows free teniposide concentrations and free fractions at different total teniposide levels. The protein binding of teniposide does not depend on the concentration of the drug and does not become saturated in the clinically relevant concen-

tration range. Teniposide free fractions at different mAMSA and ara-C concentrations are shown in Fig. 3. mAMSA and ara-C do not displace teniposide from plasma proteins. Teniposide free fractions at different flavone acetic acid (FAA) levels are shown in Fig. 4. FAA seems to influence the protein binding of VM-26 in a concen-

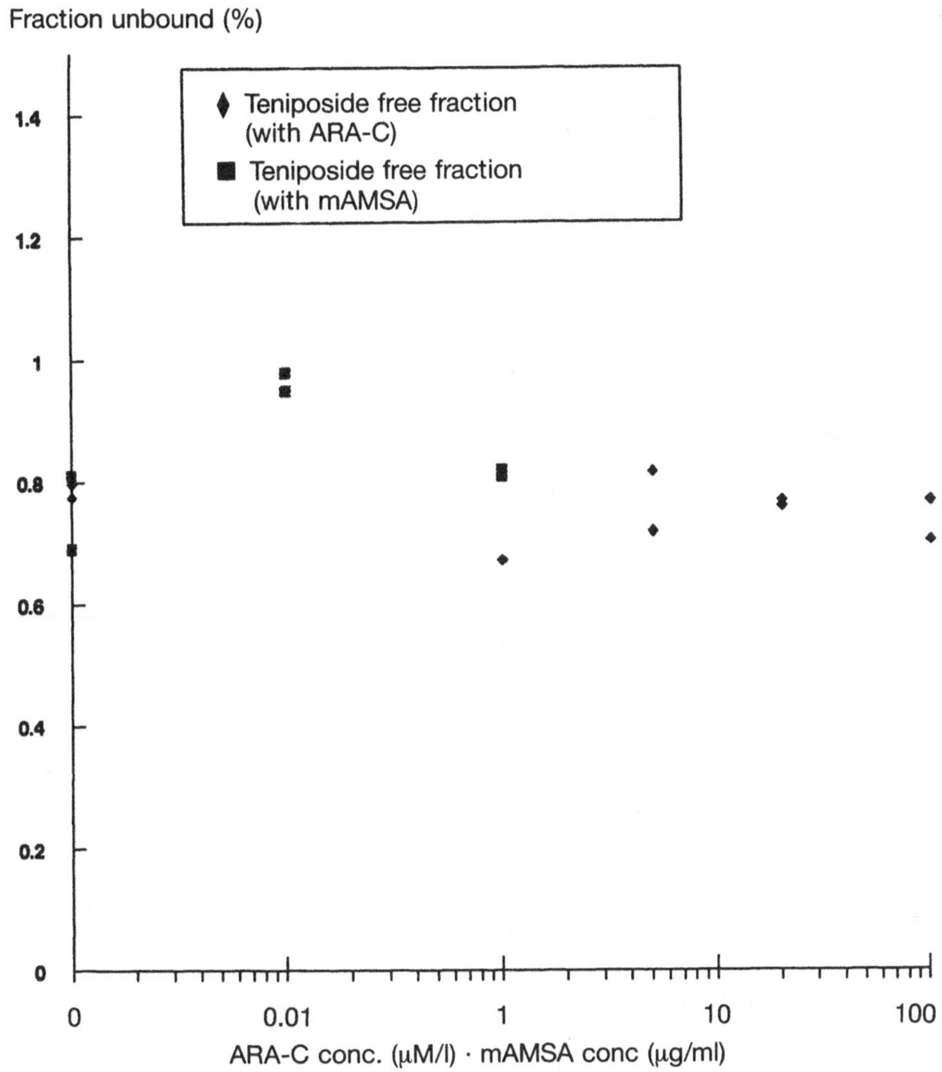

Fraction unbound (%)

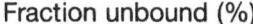

Fig. 3. Lack of displacement of teniposide from plasma proteins by mAMSA or ara-C

tration-dependent manner. Figure 5 shows Serum total protein and bilirubin levels of patients studied in first of subsequent remissions. Patients in the second group had lower serum total protein and higher bilirubin levels. The percentage unbound plasma teniposide levels in the two patient groups are shown in Fig. 6. The protein binding of VM-26 in patients seems to be characterized by four- to fivefold variability. Patients on relapse therapy with relatively lower serum total protein and higher serum bili-rubin levels have a significantly higher percentage of unbound teniposide. Figure 7 illustrates the relationship between white cell nadir and total protein concentration in serum following VM-26 and VP-16 treatments. All treatments given to patients with a total protein concentration <55 g/l were accompanied by bone marrow depression, whereas only 12 of 89 treatments caused a nadir below. 1.0 g/l in patients with a serum total protein concentration between 55 and 85 g/l.

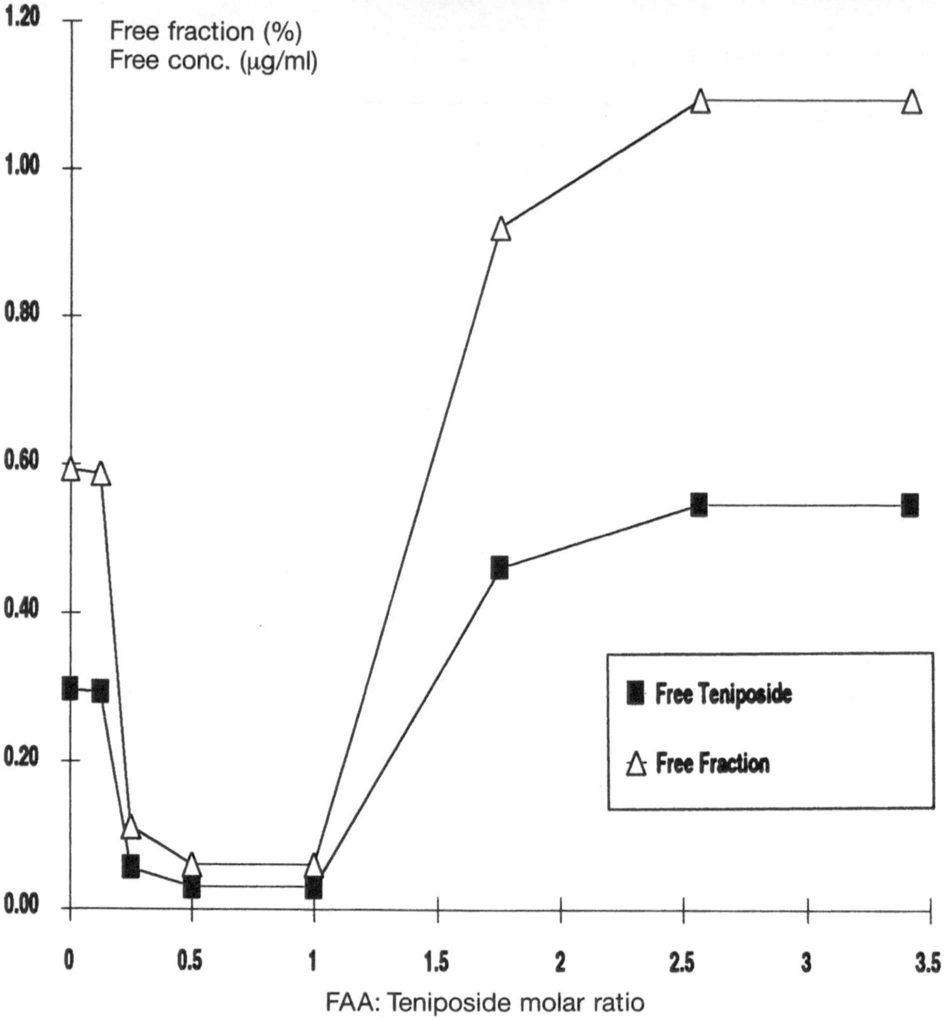

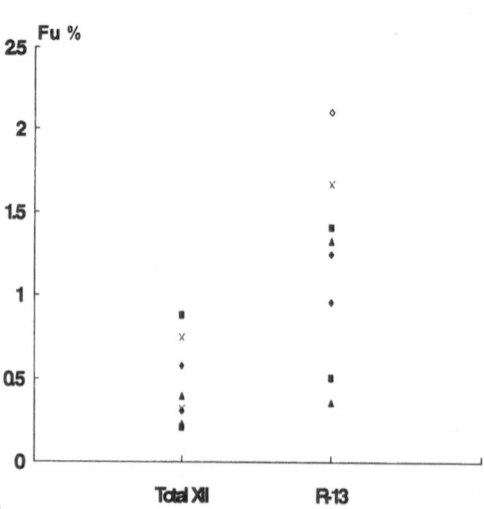

Fig. 4. Free teniposide levels and fractions unbound at different flavone acetic acid: teniposide molar ratios

Fig. 6. Percentage unbound plasma teniposide in patients with ALL in first (total XII) or subsequent remission (R-13)

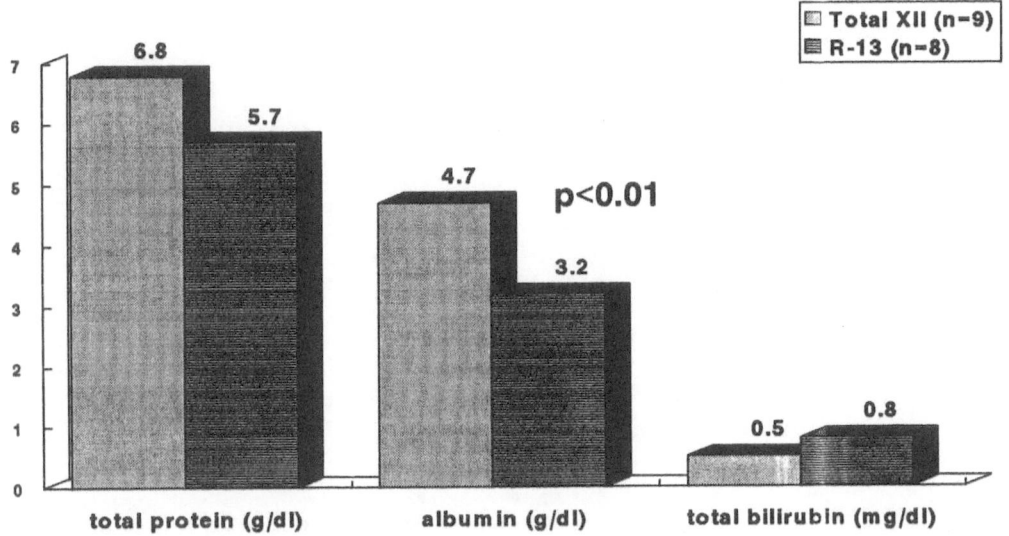

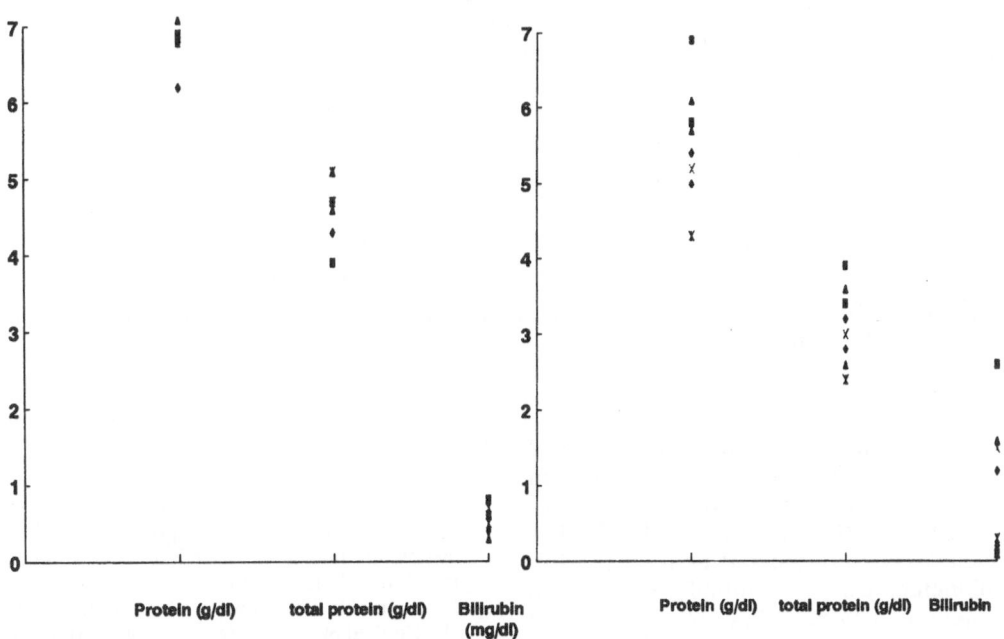

Fig. 5. Median serum total protein and bilirubin levels of patients in first or subsequent remissions

Summary

Teniposide is extensively (98%–99%) bound to plasma proteins, and its binding is not saturable in the clinically relevant concentration range. Coadministration of other drugs may influence the protein binding of teniposide. Reduction or increase of protein binding may have therapeutic consequences. There is a considerable interpa-

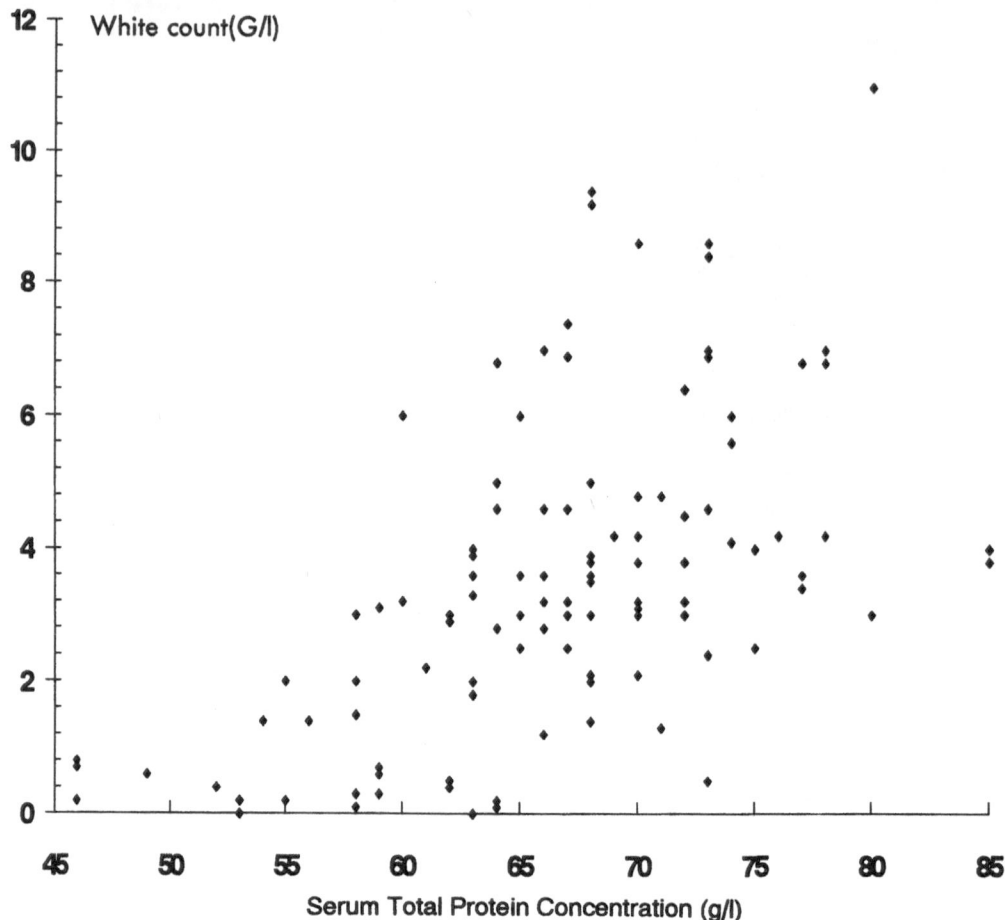

Fig. 7. Relationship between white cell nadir and total protein concentration in serum following vm-26 or VP-16 treatment

tient variability in the protein binding of VM-26. The influence of this variability on the pharmacokinetics and clinical effect (toxicity) on the drug has to be further studied. Hypoproteinemia and/or hyperbilirubinemia can substantially reduce the protein binding of VM-26. In a group of 32 patients, hypoproteinemia proved to be a significant predictor of myelotoxicity following the administration of epipodophyllotoxins.

References

1. Sinkule JA, Stewart CF, Crom WR; Melton ET, Dahl GV et al: Teniposide (VM-26) disposition in children with leukemia. Cancer Res 1984 44: 1235–1237
2. Rodman JH, Abromowith M, Sinkule JA, et al.: Clinical pharmacodynamics of continuous infusion teniposide: Systemic exposure as a determinant of response in a phase I trial. J Clin Oncol 1987. 5: 1007–14
3. Stewart CF, Pieper JA, Arbuck SG et al.: Altered protein binding of etoposide in patients with cancer. Clin Pharmacol Ther 1989. 45(1) 49–55
4. Huang J: Errors in estimating the unbound fraction of drugs due to the volume shift in equilibrium dialysis. J Pharm Sci 1983. 72: 1368–1369

Effect of Carboxymethylglucan-ara-C on Experimental Leukemia

L. Novotný, E. Balážová[1], V. Kéry[2], J. Sedlák[1], and V. Ujházy[1]

The substance 1-β-D-arabinofuranosylcytosine (ara-C) is one of the most effective drugs in the treatment of acute myeloblastic leukemia [1, 2]. However, its rapid deamination in vivo to almost inactive arabinosyluracil (i.e., 3) with its quick elimination from an organism [3, 4] is the main disadvantage for its practical use. This is the reason for the ongoing search for an ara-C derivative which cannot be deaminated and which possesses better pharmacokinetic parameters. Various pharmacokinetic and pharmacodynamic parameters of different compounds may be altered by various macromolecular carriers [5]. In our work we present the results of an ara-C and carboxymethylated glucan (CMG) conjugate preparation and an evaluation of its antileukemic activity.

The polysaccharide chosen for our work was β-D-glucan isolated from cell walls of the nonpathogenic yeast *Saccharomyces cerevisiae*, which is not degraded by any mammal enzyme and is less immunogenic than other types of microbial cell wall polysaccharide [6]. The yeast β-glucan possesses a pronounced chemical stability probably due to its compact crystalline structure, which is represented by (1-3)-β-D-glucan and (1-6)-β-D-glucan chains with a relative molecular weight of about 1 000 000 [7]. The carboxymethylation of the glucan molecule occurs predominantly

at C-6 of the glucose ring and makes the glucan soluble in water.

Coupling of ara-C to the carboxymethyl group of the CMG was performed using a general method for the formation of peptide bonds by isobutylchloroformiate condensation [8]. The presence of nitrogen in the synthesized CMG-ara-C conjugate which was indicated by the elementary analysis evidenced the binding of ara-C to the CMG. The same evidence of CMG-ara-C formation was obtained by UV and IR spectroscopy. It follows from the UV and IR spectroscopy results that ara-C was bonded to CMG carboxyl groups via its chromophoric part of the molecule (Fig. 1).

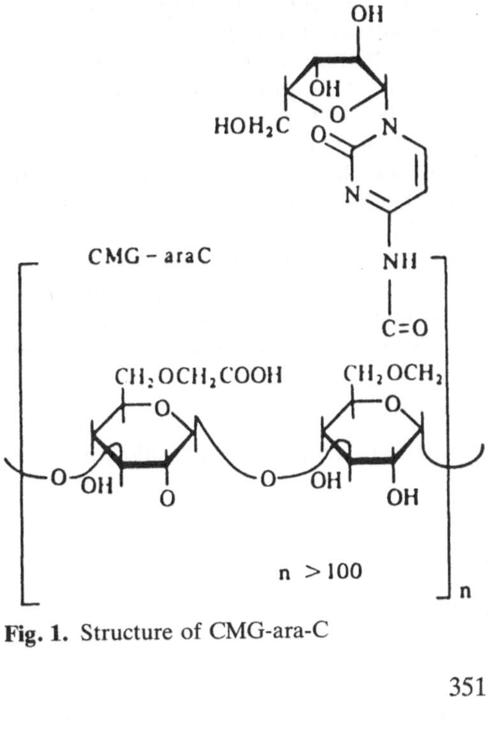

Fig. 1. Structure of CMG-ara-C

[1] Cancer Research Institute, Slovak Academy of Sciences, Spitalska 21, 812 32 Bratislava, Czechoslovakia
[2] Research Institute of Rheumatic Diseases, Piešťany, Czechoslovakia

351

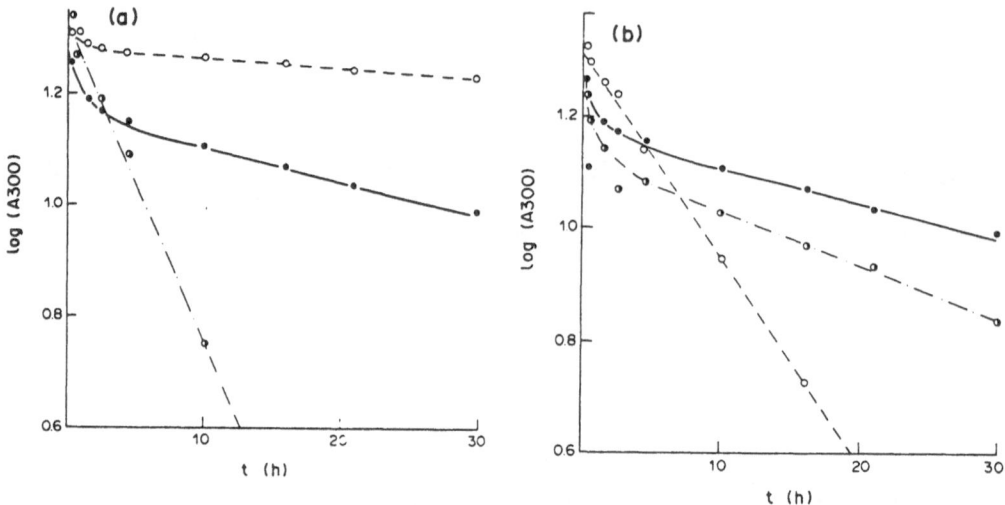

Fig. 2.a, b Hydrolysis of CMG-ara-C (1 mg/ml) in PBS, pH 7.4 (—), sodium acetate 0.1 mol/l, pH 4.0 (----), and sodium carbonate 0.1 mol/l, pH 9.0 (-.-.-) at 37 °C.
b Hydrolysis of CMG-ara-C (1 mg/ml) in PBS, pH 7.4 (—), and catalyzed by 0.1 mg/ml (----) and 0.01 mg/ml (-.-.-) trypsin at 37 °C

The bond between the amino group of ara-C and CMG should prevent deamination of ara-C in vivo.

The stability study showed that the hydrolysis of CMG-ara-C is not a simple process (Fig. 2a). The slow hydrolysis of the ara-C and CMG connecting bond is the reason for the prolonged release of ara-C into the blood stream in vivo. The consequence of these processes is an increase in therapeutic effectivity of this conjugate. The presence of trypsin under physiological conditions [in phosphate-buffered saline (PBS)] greatly enhanced the rate of hydrolysis (Fig. 2b). Chymotrypsin hydrolyzed CMG-ara-C only slowly. From these facts it follows that trypsin or trypsin-like proteases could participate in in vivo hydrolysis of CMG-ara-C. Carboxymethylated glu-can-ara-C was compared in all experiments with free ara-C and exerted higher activity in both suspension culture and in soft agar assay with L1210 cells (Table 1). CMG-ara-C had a better effect than free ara-C in vivo against P388 leukemia (Table 2) and especially against L1210 leukemia (Table 3). CMG-ara-C had absolutely no effect on the survival of leukemia L1210 resistant to ara-C-bearing mice (data not shown). From our data it seems clear, especially in the case of P388 leukemia experiments, that the repeated administration of CMG-ara-C increased the toxicity. This was probably due to the amount of polysaccharide administered and the percentage life span increase was then lowered. When the dose of CMG-ara-C was increased to 100 mg bound ara-C per kilogram body weight, the

Table 1. L1210 cell growth inhibition in suspension culture and in soft agar assay

Compound	Suspension culture (IC_{50}, μmol/l)	Soft agar assay (IC_{50}, μmol/l)
ara-C	0.08	0.23
CMG-ara-C	0.03	0.12

Table 2. The effectivity of ara-C and CMG-ara-C[a] (50 mg free ara-C or 50 mg ara-C bound to CMG per kilogram body w.) on the survival of leukemia P388 bearing mice[b].

Treatment	MST±SD (days)	% ILS	Significance[c]
None	22.5 ± 1.6	–	
CMG 500 mg/kg Days 1, 4, 7	22.8 ± 1.6	1	
Ara-C, day 1	29.3 ± 7.2	30	
CMG-ara-C, day 1	54.8 ± 8.0	144	0.001
Ara-C, days 1, 4	39.2 ± 12.8	16	
CMG-ara-C, days 1, 4	44.3 ± 17.4	97	n.s.
Ara-C, days 1, 4, 7	25.1 ± 2.5	12	
CMG-ara-C Days 1, 4, 7	36.3 ± 5.9	61	0.001

[a] Ten milligrams CMG bound to 1 mg ara-C
[b] Number of mice per group was five to seven
[c] Significance of the CMG-ara-C treatment results compared with the same treatment using free ara-C

Table 3. Effectivity of ara-C and CMG-ara-C[a] (50 mg free ara-C or 50 mg ara-C bound to CMG per kilogram body wt.) on the survival of leukemia L1210 bearing mice.

Treatment	MST ± SD (days)	% ILS	No of survivors	Significance[c]
None	8.8 ± 0.9	–	0/8	
CMG 500 mg/kg Days 1, 4, 7	8.0 ± 0.8	–9	0/8	
ara-C, day 1	9.5 ± 0.8	8	0/8	
CMG-ara-C, day 1	16.6 ± 3.4	89[b]	3/8	0.005
Ara-C, days 1, 4	11.0 ± 1.3	25	0/8	
CMG-ara-C Days 1, 4	38.0 ± 12.8	332[b]	4/7	0.05
Ara-C Days 1, 4, 7	12.3 ± 0.5	40	0/8	
CMG-ara-C Days 1, 4, 7	23.0 ± 9.3	161[b]	3/8	0.01

[a] 10 mg CMG bound to 1 mg ara-C
[b] Long-term survivors (more than 90 days) were not used in data evaluation
[c] Significance of the CMG-ara-C treatment results compared with the same treatment using free ara-C

toxic effect was evident (data not shown). Administration of the CMG alone produced no significant increase in life span (Tables 2, 3), and therefore it may be concluded that the increase in CMG-ara-C effectivity cannot be caused by the stimulation of the immune system in the experimental animals.

Inhibition of DNA synthesis was measured after the administration of both free and CMG-bound ara-C in the experiment with L1210-bearing mice (Fig. 3). The results clearly show that the duration of DNA synthesis inhibition following ara-C administration is approximately 5 h. Inhibition of DNA synthesis caused by CMG-ara-C had a duration of more than 24 h after administration. This fact explains the positive results of CMG-ara-C used in the in vivo treatment of the experimental leukemia.

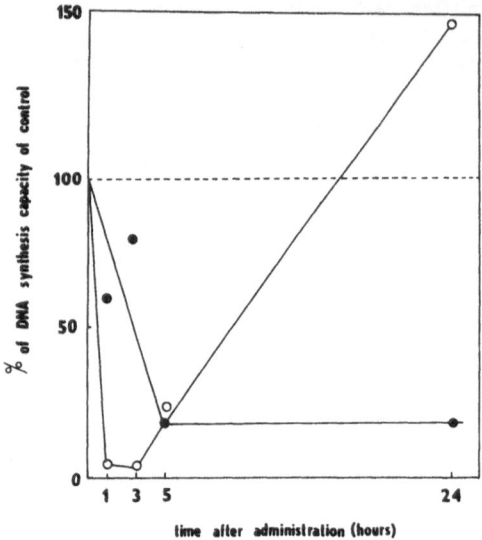

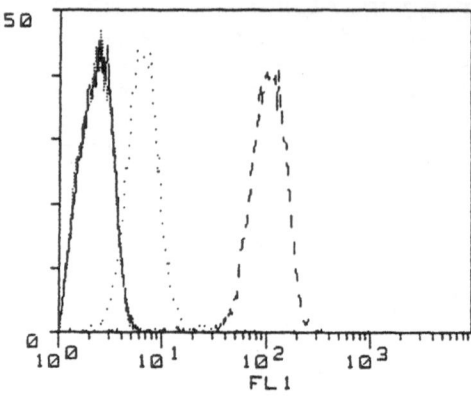

Fig. 3. Inhibition of DNA synthesis in leukemia L1210 cells in vivo by ara-C (o) and CMG-ara-C (●) after single-dose administration of 50 mg ara-C or equivalent per kilogram body wt

Fig. 4. FACS analysis of L1210 leukemia cells treated with CMG-phenylisothiocyanate demonstrates the fluorescence of the control cells (−) and the cells treated with CMG-phenylisothiocyanate at 0 °C (...) or at 37 °C (----)

The FACS analysis of the leukemia L1210 cell treated with phenylisothiocyanate-marked CMG was performed to better understand the possible mechanism of the CMG-ara-C antileukemic activity. It was shown that there is a 15 times higher concentration of CMG on the surface of the leukemia cell after the incubation at 37 °C compared with incubation at 4 °C in vitro (Fig. 4). It may be hypothesized on the basis of this experiment that the antileukemia effect of CMG-ara-C is based both on the slow hydrolysis of the bond between CMG and ara-C and on the concentration gradient of the administered polysaccharide on the cell surface.

References

1. Chabner BA (1982) Cytosine arabinoside. In: Chabner B (ed) Pharmacologic principles of cancer treatment. Saunders, Philadelphia, pp 387–401

2. Creasey VA (1975) Arabinosylcytosine. In: Sartorelli AC, Johns DG (eds) Antineoplastic and immunosuppressive agents, part 2. Springer, Berlin Heidelberg New York, pp 232–256 (Handbook of experimental pharmacology, vol 38)

3. Ho DHW, Freireich EJ (1975) Clinical pharmacology of arabinosylcytosine. In: Sartorelli AC, Johns DG (eds) Antineoplastic and immunosuppressive agents, part 2. Springer, Berlin Heidelberg New York, pp 257–284 (Handbook of experimental pharmacology, vol 38)

4. Novotný L, Farghali H, Janku I, Beránek J (1988) Comparative study of cyclocytidine and arabinosylcytosine disposition in rats. Neoplasma 35: 707–714

5. Poznansky MJ, Julianoi RL (1984) Biological approaches to the controlled delivering of drugs. Pharmacol Rev 36: 277–336

6. Yu RJ, Bishop CT, Cooper FP, Blank F, Hasenndever HF (1967) Glucans from *Candida albicans* (serotype B) and from *Candida parapsilosis*. Can J Chem 45: 2264–2267

7. Manners DJ, Masson AJ, Patterson JC (1973) The structure of a (1-3)-β-D-glucan from yeast cell walls. Biochem J 135: 19–30

8. Dean PDG, Rowe PH, Exley D (1972) Preparation of 6-oxoestriol-6-/O-(carboxymethyl)-oxime/- and 6-oxo-estrone-6-/O-(carboxymethyl)oxime/- bovine serum albumin conjugates. Steroids Lipids Res 3: 82–89

Plasma Pharmacology of Fludarabine and Cellular Bioavailability of Fludarabine Triphosphate*

A. Kemena, M. Keating, and W. Plunkett

Introduction

Fludarabine phosphate (F-ara-AMP) shows excellent response rates at low doses (18–30 mg/m^2 per day) in indolent lymphoid malignancies without major nonhematologic toxicity [1–5]. In high-dose regimens, however, it caused severe neurotoxic side effects [6–8]. This comparatively narrow therapeutic window requires precise pharmacokinetic studies for optimal dose scheduling. Further, as chronic lymphocytic leukemia (CLL) is the most frequent in this group of malignances, elderly patients are an important target population for treatment with fludarabine phosphate and might especially benefit from an oral formulation. Therefore studies of its bioavailability are needed. Finally, fludarabine phosphate is currently investigated as a biochemical modulator of cytosine arabinoside [9, 10]. As these nucleoside analogues exert close schedule dependent interaction, a careful pharmacokinetic analysis is essential. At low fludarabine phosphate doses comprehensive pharmacokinetic studies were limited by the sensitivity of assays based on UV detection [11–14]. We therefore developed a sensitive method based on the chemical condensation of F-ara-A with chloroacetaldehyde to a fluorescent derivative. Combined with a solid-phase extraction prior to derivatization, the quantitation limit was 2 pmol/ml plasma. In a clinical study designed to evaluate the oral bioavailability of fludarabine phosphate, we determined plasma F-ara-A levels over a period of 72 h in patients with relapsed CLL. Simultaneously the corresponding concentrations of the active metabolite fludarabine triphosphate (F-ara-ATP) were measured in circulating leukemic cells.

Materials and Methods

The chemical structure analysis of the fluorescent derivative of F-ara-A was carried out by Berlex Biosciences, Alameda, CA (United States).

Plasma samples were prepared from heparinized blood which contained 1 μM erythro-9-(2-hydroxy-3-nonyl)adenine to inhibit adenosine deaminase. Protein removal and sample concentration was accomplished by solid-phase extraction (SEP-PAK C$_{18}$ cartridge). The derivatization of F-ara-A was carried out in citrate buffer, pH 4.0 (final concentration 0.2 M), in the presence of 5.2 M chloroacetaldehyde. After incubation for 24 h at 50 °C the reaction products were separated by reverse-phase high-performance liquid chromatography (HPLC) (μBondapak C$_{18}$) under isocratic conditions. The mobile phase consisted of 2 % methanol and 5 % N,N-dimethylformamide in water. The fluorescent F-ara-A derivative (retention time about 10 min) was detected at an excitation wavelength of 296 nm and an

* This study is supported by a grant from the German Research Association (DFG) and by grant CA 32839 from the National Cancer Institute DHHS

emission wavelength of 410 nm. The methodology is described in detail elsewhere [15].

Intracellular nucleotide concentrations were determined by anion exchange HPLC in perchloric acid extracts of blood mononuclear cells [9].

Pharmacokinetic analyses were performed using the ESTRIP computer program [16].

Results

Optimization and Validation of the Test System

Published reaction conditions for the synthesis of etheno-adenine compounds [17–21] did not generate a fluorescent signal with the relatively inert fluorinated arabinosyladenine. Therefore modifications were required to yield 66.5 % ± 1.8 % fluorescing product in the optimized system using [8-³H]F-ara-A. Spectroscopic analysis of the fluorescent derivative confirmed its identity with arabinosyl-1,N^6-etheno-isoguanine. The reaction was shown to be specific for F-ara-A and its respective nucleotides, which could be derivatized with a comparable yield. Among the physiological nucleosides of adenine and cytosine which are known to form fluorescent etheno-derivatives [22], only adenosine and deoxyadenosine were detected at considerably lower relative sensitivities.

Table 1 shows the results of the validation of the fluorescence assay for F-ara-A quantitation in plasma. Processing (5 ml plasma per sample) consisted of solid-phase extraction, derivatization, and separation of the reaction products by HPLC.

Table 1. Validation of the fluorescence assay for F-ara-A quantitation in plasma

Limit of quantitation	2 pmol/ml plasma
Linearity	2 pmol – 2 nmol/ml plasma
Precision	3.0 % relative SD
Stability	0.5 % decay/h
Recovery	100 % (range 0.05–2 nmol/ml)
Protein binding	<0.03 %

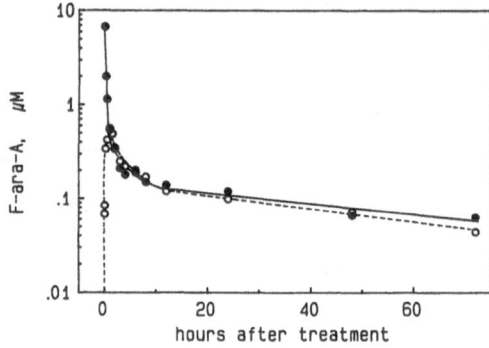

Fig. 1. Pharmacokinetics of F-ara-A in plasma after a 30-min i.v. infusion (*closed circles*, one patient) or oral application (*open circles*, one patient) of 60 mg fludarabine phosphate. Plasma (0.5–4 ml) was processed at each time point according to the procedure described in "Methods"

Quantitation of F-ara-A and Its Triphosphate in Patient Samples

Patients with refractory chronic lymphocytic leukemia received 60 mg fludarabine phosphate either as a 30-min i.v. infusion or as an aqueous solution orally. The pharmacokinetics of F-ara-A in plasma up to 72 h after treatment are shown in Fig. 1. F-ara-A was detected in plasma at 2 min following oral administration. After a 1.5- to 2-h accumulation phase, F-ara-A concentrations were comparable to those obtained by i.v. infusion. The triexponential elimination phases essentially paralleled after both routes of administration with similar terminal half-lives (31 and 32 h, $n = 5$ for each treatment group). F-ara-A plasma levels measured at 72 h were about 20–40 times above the quantitation limit of the fluorescence assay. Comparing the mean AUC values of five patients per treatment group, an oral bioavailability of about 80 % was determined.

Levels of F-ara-ATP in circulating leukemia cells (Fig. 2) showed similar accumulation and elimination kinetics after both routes of administration [$t_{1/2} = 36$ h (i.v.) and 32 h (oral)]. After oral ingestion of the drug, however, maximum F-ara-ATP con-

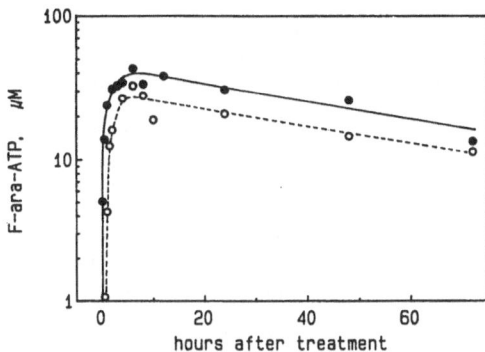

Fig. 2. Pharmacokinetics of F-ara-ATP in circulating leukemia cells after a 30-min i.v. infusion (closed circles, one patient) or oral application (open circle, one patient) of 60 mg fludarabine phosphate. Circulating mononuclear cells were processed at each time point according to the procedure described in "Methods"

centrations were generally lower, resulting in about 40% lower area under curve (AUC) values.

Discussion

Conventional UV-based methods for the quantitation of F-ara-A reach their limit of detection at 3–24 h after treatment with low-dose regimes of fludarabine phosphate [11–14]. We therefore developed an assay that employs fluorescence detection after HPLC. With a limit of quantitation of 2 pmol F-ara-A/ml plasma, it enables elimination kinetics to be monitored over a 72-h period after treatment with a fludarabine phosphate dose of 60 mg/m² per day given either by short-term i.v. infusion or orally. Measuring accumulation kinetics during absorption from the gastrointestinal tract, F-ara-A was detected 2 min following drug intake.

Our preliminary pharmacokinetic data from a study designed to evaluate the oral bioavailability of fludarabine phosphate suggest a triexponential elimination profile of F-ara-A with a terminal half-life of about 32 h. In previous reports, in which the less sensitive UV detection method was employed, biphasic or triphasic elimination kinetics with a terminal half-life of about 10

h were found after doses ranging from 18 to 80 mg/m² per day [11, 13, 14].

The oral bioavailability of the drug in plasma seems to be around 80%. The cellular "bioavailability" measured as nucleoside triphosphate was about 40% less after oral administration.

The derivatization reaction to a fluorescent compound may also be applied to the F-ara-A mono- and triphosphates and to arabinosyl-isoguanine, thereby providing several potential applications.

References

1. Grever MR, Kopecky KJ, Coltman CA et al. (1988) Fludarabine monophosphate: a potentially useful agent in chronic lymphocytic leukemia. Nouv Rev Fr Hematol 30: 457–459
2. Keating MJ, Kantarjian H, Talpaz M et al. (1989) Fludarabine: a new agent with major activity against chronic lymphocytic leukemia. Blood 74: 19–25
3. Leiby JM, Snider KM, Kraut EH, Metz EN, Malspeis L, Grever MR (1987) Phase II trial of 9-β-D-arabinofuranosyl-2-fluoroadenine 5'-monophosphate in non-Hodgkin's lymphoma: prospective comparison of response with deoxycytidine kinase activity. Cancer Res 47: 2719–2722
4. Von Hoff DD, Dahlberg S, Hartstock RJ, Eyre HJ (1990) Activity of fludarabine monophosphate in patients with advanced mycosis fungoides: a southwest Oncology Group study. J Natl Cancer Inst 82: 1353–1355
5. Kantarjian HM, Alexanian R, Koller CA, Kurzrock R, Keating MJ (1990) Fludarabine therapy in macroglobulinemic lymphoma. Blood 75: 1928–1931
6. Chun HG, Leyland-Jones BR, Caryk SM, Hoth DF (1986) Central nervous system toxicity of fludarabine phosphate. Cancer Treat Rep 70: 1225–1228
7. Spriggs DR, Stopa E, Mayer RJ, Schoene W, Kufe DW (1986) Fludarabine phosphate (NSC 312878) infusions for the treatment of acute leukemia: phase I and neuropathological study. Cancer Res 46: 5953–5958
8. Warrell RP Jr, Berman E (1986) Phase I and II study of fludarabine phosphate in leukemia: therapeutic efficacy with delayed central nervous system toxicity. J Clin Oncol 4: 74–79
9. Gandhi V, Plunkett W (1988) Modulation of arabinosylnucleoside metabolism by arabi-

nosylnucleotides in human leukemia cells. Cancer Res 48: 329–334

10. Gandhi V, Nowak B, Keating MJ, Plunkett W (1989) Modulation of arabinosylcytosine metabolism by arabinosyl-2-fluoroadenine in lymphocytes from patients with chronic lymphocytic leukemia: implications for combination therapy. Blood 74: 2070–2075

11. Malspeis L, Grever MR, Staubus AE, Young D (1990) Pharmacokinetics of 2-F-ara-A (9-β-D-arabinofuranosyl-2-fluoroadenine) in cancer patients during the phase I clinical investigation of fludarabine phosphate. Semin Oncol 17: 18–32

12. Noker PE, Duncan GF, El Dareer SM, Hill DL (1983) Disposition of 9-β-D-arabinofuranosyl-2-fluoroadenine 5'-phosphate in mice and dogs. Cancer Treat Rep 67: 445–456

13. Danhauser L, Plunkett W, Keating M, Cabanillas F (1986) 9-β-D-Arabinofuranosyl-2-fluoroadenine 5'-monophosphate pharmacokinetics in plasma and tumor cells of patients with relapsed leukemia and lymphoma. Cancer Chemother Pharmacol 18: 145–152

14. Hersh MR, Kuhn JG, Phillips JL, Clark G, Ludden TM, Von Hoff DD (1986) Pharmacokinetic study of fludarabine phosphate (NSC 312887). Cancer Chemother Pharmacol 17: 277–280

15. Kemena A, Fernandez M, Bauman J, Keating M, Plunkett W (1991) A sensitive fluorescence assay for quantitation of fludarabine and metabolites in biological fluids. Clin Chim Acta 200: 95–106

16. Brown RD, Manno JE (1978) ESTRIP, a BASIC computer program for obtaining initial polyexponential parameter estimates. J Pharm Sci 67: 1687–1691

17. Avigad G, Damle S (1972) Fluorimetric assay of adenine and its derivatives. Anal Biochem 50: 321–323

18. Perrett D (1987) Determination of adenosine ribo- and deoxyribonucleotides as their 1-N^6-etheno derivatives by reversed-phase ion-pair high-performance liquid chromatography. J Chromatogr 386: 289–296

19. Sonoki S, Tanaka Y, Hisamatsu S, Kobayashi (1989) High-performance liquid chromatographic analysis of fluorescent derivatives of adenine and adenosine and its nucleotides. Optimization of derivatization with chloroacetaldehyde and chromatographic procedures. J Chromatogr 475: 311–319

20. Mills GC, Schmalstieg FC, Trimmer KB, Goldman AS, Goldblum RM (1976) Purine metabolism in adenosine deaminase deficiency. Proc Natl Acad Sci USA 73: 2867–2871

21. Slegel P, Kitagawa H, Maguire MH (1988) Determination of adenosine in fetal perfusates of human placental cotyledons using fluorescence derivatization and reversed-phase high-performance liquid chromatography. Anal Biochem 171: 124–134

22. Barrio JR, Secrist JA III, Leonard NJ (1972) Fluorescent adenosine and cytidine derivatives. Biochem Biophys Res Commun 46: 597–604

Pharmacology of High-Dose 1,2,4-Triglycidylurazol in Preparative Regimens for Bone Marrow Transplantation: Preclinical Evaluation and First Clinical Results

[1]D. W. Beelen, [2]R. B. Schilcher, [1]R. Ehrlich, [1]K. Quabeck, [3]U. Schmidt, [4]D. Szy, [5]H. Grosse-Wilde, and [1]U. W. Schaefer

The racematic compound a/β-1,2,4-triglyci-dylurazol (TGU; NSC 332488) a triepoxide with alkylating properties, has a broad spectrum of anticancer activity in animal models including the L1210 and the P388 murine leukemias as well as the L5222 rat leukemia (reviewed in [1]). In a cyclophosphamide-resistant P388 leukemia subline, TGU exerted high antileukemic activity, which suggested that the compound might have non-cross-resistance with this group of alkylating agents. The pharmacokinetic profile of TGU is characterized by a rapid plasma clearance in animal models and humans. Clinical phase I/II trials in patients with solid tumors demonstrated that TGU has dose-dependent and dose-limiting myelotoxicity [2–7]. These pharmacologic properties of TGU imply that it might be useful in settings of high-dose therapy with bone marrow rescue. To elucidate its potential role in bone marrow transplantation (BMT), we performed dose escalation and pharmacokinetic studies using TGU in a beagle dog model. With regard to potential synergistic toxicities, combinations of TGU and total body irradiation (TBI) or high-dose busulfan (HD-BU) were used in animals receiving allogeneic bone marrow rescue. In an ongoing phase I/II trial TGU is currently being investigated in patients with refractory advanced hematologic malignancies prior to allogeneic marrow transplantation.

Materials and Methods

Preclinical Studies

Details of the studies in beagle dogs have been previously reported [8]. Generally, protective isolation and supportive therapy used in animal experiments resembled the situation of clinical marrow transplantation. Total body irradiation was performed in two daily fractions of 2 Gy over 3 days (total dose, 12 Gy) using a cobalt-60 source (dose rate, 6 cGy/min). Oral busulfan was given at a dose of 4 mg/kg body wt. per day in four divided doses over 4 days as a watery suspension of pulverized tablets. Adequate busulfan ingestion and absorption were controlled by measuring busulfan plasma levels twice daily during the treatment period. In animals receiving combinations of TGU with either TBI or HD-BU, the study drug was started 1 day after termination of the respective pretreatment (Table 1).

Human Studies

Patient characteristics and details of the preparative regimens prior to marrow transplantation are given in Table 2. Protective isolation and gnotobiotic care of patients as well as supportive therapy were performed as has been previously published [9].

[1] Departments of Bone Marrow Transplantation
[2] Internal Medicine (Tumor Research)
[3] Pathology, Radiotherapy, and Immunogenetics, University Hospital Essen, Hufelandstr. 55, 4300 Essen 1, FRG
Supported by Grant SFB 102 from Deutsche Forschungsgemeinschaft, TPC40

Table 1. Dose schedules of 1,2,4-triglycidyurazol (TGU) alone and combinations of TGU with total body irradiation (TBI) or high-dose busulfan (HD-BU) followed by allogeneic bone marrow rescue

Total TGU dose (mg/kg)	Dose/fraction (mg/kg)	Number of fractions	Number of animals
40	40	1	4
50	25	2	4
60	60	1	1
60	30	2	7
75	25	3	4
20+TBI	20	1	4
40+TBI	40	1	6
40+HD-BU	40	1	8

TBI, total body irradiation delivered by a cobalt-60 source in two daily fractions of 2 Gy (dose rate, 6 cGy/min) over 3 days; HD-BU, 1 mg/kg body wt. oral busulfan every 6 h over 4 days

Table 2. Patient characteristics, preparative regimens, and outcome of patients treated with TGU in combination with total body irradiation or high-dose busulfan prior to allogeneic marrow transplantation

UPN	Age/sex	Diagnosis	TGU dose mg/kg (mg/m²)	Additional therapy	Outcome (days after BMT)
318	32/M	ALL fourth relapse	30 (1200)	4 × 2.5 Gy TBI	Relapse (62), died (139)
341	26/F	NHL stage IV second relapse	30 (1200)	HD-BU	Cytomegalovirus pneumonia, died (18)
395	37/F	CML blastic phase	35 (1400)	4 × 2.5 GY TBI	Relapse (163), died (217)
403	33/M	AML second relapse	35 (1400)	4 × 2.5 Gy TBI	Relapse (38), died (164)
408	39/M	NHL stage IV second relapse	40 (1600)	HD-BU	Meningitis, pneumonia, died (132)

UPN, unique patient number; ALL, acute lymphoblastic leukemia; NHL, non-Hodgkin's lymphoma; CML, chronic myeloid leukemia; AML, acute myeloid leukemia; TBI, total body irradiation delivered by a cobalt-60 source in four daily fractions of 2.5 Gy (dose rate, 3 cGy/min); HD-BU, 1 mg/kg body wt. oral busulfan every 6 h over 4 days

Study Drug

Supplies of TGU were kindly made available by Asta Pharma AG, Frankfurt, Federal Republic of Germany, as a lyophilized powder with 20 mg D-mannitol/100 mg drug. It was reconstituted in 0.9 % saline to yield a final concentration of 10 mg/ml TGU solution. The required dose was given as a bolus injection over 1 min. In animal studies, the compound was injected into the right internal jugular vein. In patients a central venous catheter was used for injection of TGU.

Toxicologic Evaluation

For estimation of acute toxic effects on hematopoiesis, kidney, and liver functions, white blood cell (WBC) and platelet counts, and blood urea nitrogen (BUN), creatinine, transaminases (GOT, GPT) as well as alkaline phosphatase (AP) plasma levels were obtained on all week days during the observation period. Evaluation of gastrointestinal (GI) toxicity was based on the degree of oral mucositis and on frequencies of nausea and vomiting and/or diarrhea. Cardiovascular toxicity was monitored by ECG tracings and measurements of left-ventricular shortening fraction using cardias ultrasound in all patients. Adverse effects of the study drug were classified according to a graded toxicity scale [10]. In animals which died during experiments, complete autopsies with histologic examinations were performed.

Pharmacokinetic Analysis

Blood samples were collected in EDTA-containing tubes from a heparin lock placed in a peripheral vein at times 0, 1, 2, 5, 10, 15, 30, 45, and 60 min, 1.5, 2, 4, 6, 12, and 24 h. Specimens were chilled at $-1\,°C$ immediately after collection, centrifuged at 1270 g for 10 min, and the plasma stored at $-18\,°C$ until analysis. TGU was measured in plasma and organ extracts using high-pressure liquid chromatography (HPLC) as has been described previously [8, 11]. Predose samples did not contain interferences at the retention volume of TGU, and the lower limit of detection was 10 ng/ml probe volume.

Plasma concentration time data were analyzed using the AUTOAN computer program, supplied by Dr. J.G. Wagner (Upjohn Center for Clinical Pharmacology, Ann Arbor, MI, United States). The program used curve-stripping techniques to choose the most appropriate pharmacokinetic model.

Statistical Analysis

To detect differences in the pharmacokinetic profile of TGU in animals receiving the compound alone and those which were treated with combinations of TGU and either TBI or HD-BU, pharmacokinetic paramaters [area under curve (AUC), clearance, volume of distribution, and half-life time (t_{50}) values] in the different treatment groups were compared by Wilcoxon's rank sum test. These parameters were additionally compared in animals with and without lethal GI toxicity. Data base management, and descriptive and comparative statistics were performed on an IBM PS/2 Model 80 computer using SAS software (SAS Institute Inc, Cary, NC, United States).

Results

Preclinical Studies

The major adverse effects of TGU observed in beagle dogs were GI and hematologic toxicity. Gastrointestinal toxicity manifested as moderate to severe enteritis associated with serous or bloody diarrhea. The LD_{50} for this adverse effect was estimated to be in the range of 60 mg/kg TGU when given in two dose fractions of 30 mg/kg per day over 2 days. A single dose of 60 mg/kg led to a lethal generalized capillary leakage syndrome at 6 h after administration of TGU in one animal. The maximum tolerated single dose of TGU was 40 mg/kg and dose fractions of 25 mg/kg per day allowed dose escalations to a maximum cumulative dose of 50 mg/kg without lethal GI toxicity. Histopathological changes of the gut walls included areactive necrosis and denudation of the epithelium with concomitant thrombosis of submucosal veins and atrophy of lymphatic follicles. In addition, TGU led to dose-dependent toxic effects on liver function (Table 3). Other nonhematologic complications attributable to drug-related toxic effects were not observed.

Hematologic toxicity in animals surviving GI-toxic effects was severe and life-threatening. No clear-cut dose-response relationship existed between TGU dose and duration of leuko- or thrombocytopenia (Table 4). Although prolonged pancytopenia occurred in a dose range between 40 and 60 mg/kg TGU, all surviving dogs had complete hematopoietic recovery.

Table 3. Nonhematologic toxicity of TGU and combinations of TGU with total body irradiation (TBI) or high-dose busulfan (HD-BU)

TGU dose (mg/kg) Additional treatment	40	50	60	75	20 TBI	40 TBI	40 HD-BU
Number of animals	4	4	7	4	4	6	8
Gastrointestinal							
Diarrhea[a]	2–3	2–3	3–4	4	2–3	3–4	2–3
Lethal toxicity[b] (%)	0/4 (0)	0/4 (0)	4/7 (57)	4/4 (100)	0/4 (0)	4/6 (66)	0/8 (0)
Liver							
GOT (U/l)[c]	32 (24–75)	41 (29–75)	30 (22–140)	108 (49–187)	22 (16–103)	30 (15–291)	24 (16–34)
GPT (U/l)[c]	87 (32–180)	64 (41–132)	86 (39–256)	189 (77–269)	61 (39–216)	142 (31–1179)	52 (14–147)
AP (U/l)[c]	419 (231–5280)	290 (101–325)	1042 (109–3624)	1238 (887–2917)	203 (135–208)	846 (168–2224)	204 (102–678)
Kidney							
Creatinine (mg/dl)[c]	1.1 (0.9–3.2)	0.7 (0.6–1.0)	0.8 (0.7–3.9)	1.8 (1.3–2.9)	0.8 (0.7–0.9)	0.8 (0.7–0.9)	0.7 (0.7–1.2)
BUN (mg/dl)[c]	21 (18–69)	17 (14–25)	18 (15–55)	64 (22–79)	24 (10–26)	26 (18–66)	20 (15–24)

[a] Severity of organ involvement (graded toxicity scale), [b] Proportion of animals with lethal gastrointestinal toxicity as a consequence of necrotizing enteritis, [c] Median peak plasma concentrations (range)

The maximum tolerated single TGU dose in combination with TBI and allogeneic dog leukocyte antigen (DLA) identical marrow rescue was reduced by 50 % to 20 mg/kg. Again, a steep dose-response relationship was seen between TGU dose and GI toxicity with an estimated LD_{50} in the range of 30 mg/kg. Thus, the combination of TGU and TBI unequivocally showed cumulative toxic effects on the GI tract and liver function (Table 3).

In contrast, the combination of a single dose of 40 mg/kg TGU with high-dose busulfan and allogeneic marrow rescue was not associated with increased GI or liver toxicitiy (Table 3). Two of eight dogs died during marrow aplasia without significant laboratory or histopathological signs of toxicity. Two dogs receiving DLA-nonidentical unrelated marrow transplants rejected their grafts. In three of four dogs with DLA-identical related marrow donors, sustained engraftment could be demonstrated by sex chromosome analysis. Since DLA identical marrow engraftment cannot be attained by HD-BU alone in this model, it is justified to assume that the immunosuppressive properties of TGU allowed engraftment.

Plasma pharmacokinetic parameters are shown in Table 5. The best fit to the data was a one-compartment open-system model with an exponential decay (Fig. 1). Preceding TBI or HD-BU had no significant influence on these parameters in animals treated with 40 mg/kg TGU. Animals with lethal GI toxicity, however, showed markedly increased peak plasma levels and AUC values as well as reduced plasma clearance values in comparison to those which survived GI toxic effects (Table 6). This may reflect interindividual differences in drug metabolism contributing to the severity of this adverse effect. Significant TGU concentrations could be extracted from organs up to 7 days after administration of the drug, indicating extensive drug binding to tissues (data not shown; [8]).

Human Studies

The application of TGU was associated with moderate to severe nausea and vomit-

Table 4. Hematologic toxicity of TGU

TGU dose (mg/kg)	40	50	60	75
Number of animals	4	4	7	4
WBC nadir ($\times 10^9$/l)				
Median	0.1	0.15	0	0.1
Range	0–0.2	0.1–0.4	0–0.1	0.1–0.1
WBC nadir (day)				
Median	4	5	4	3
Range	4–7	4–5	3–6	3–6
WBC recovery (day)				
Median	25	28	28	n.e.
Range	16–35	22–30	25–33	n.e.
Platelet nadir ($\times 10^9$/l)				
Median	4	9	18	n.e.
Range	4–7	5–12	10–35	n.e.
Platelet nadir (day)				
Median	11	16	7	n.e.
Range	1–13	1–28	4–18	n.e.
Platelet recovery (day)				
Median	23	30	23	n.e.
Range	19–34	26–31	20–29	n.e.

n.e., not evaluable. All animals died from therapy-related toxicity prior to hematopoietic recovery

Table 5. Plasma pharmacokinetic parameters for animals treated with different dose levels of TGU

TGU dose (mg/kg)	No. of fractions	Peak plasma concentration (μg/ml)	AUC (μg10^{-2}/mlh)	Clearance (ml/min)	Volume of distribution (l)	t_{50} (min)
20	4	0.96(0.22)[a]	4.33(0.38)	109 432 (8 443)	137.7(88.7)	2.7(0)
25	12	3.15(0.99)	10.41(1.86)	88 846(12 939)	165.7(86.5)	2.9(0.1)
30	14	11.57(2.08)	38.37(7.04)	31 773(5 844)	154.4(40.9)	3.1(0.3)
40	18	8.00(1.31)	39.57(9.90)	51 078(7 795)	123.2(29.2)	3.1(0.1)
40	4	7.65(1.42)[b]	35.63(14.19)	58 106(22 707)	148.3(87.8)	2.9(0.1)
40+TBI	6	7.80(2.59)	44.20(22.76)	59 168(14 661)	161.8(58.9)	2.8(0.1)
40+HD-BU	8	8.37(1.54)	36.92(9.93)	39 475(7 405)	72.1(6.4)	3.5(0.3)

[a] Values of parameters represent the mean ($\pm$ standard error) of pharmacokinetics performed for each individual dose fraction. The number of fractions on which these calculations were based is indicated
[b] No significant differences were found between peak plasma concentrations, area under curve, clearance, volume of distribution, and half-life time values in animals receiving 40 mg/kg TGU alone or in combination with either TBI or HD-BU

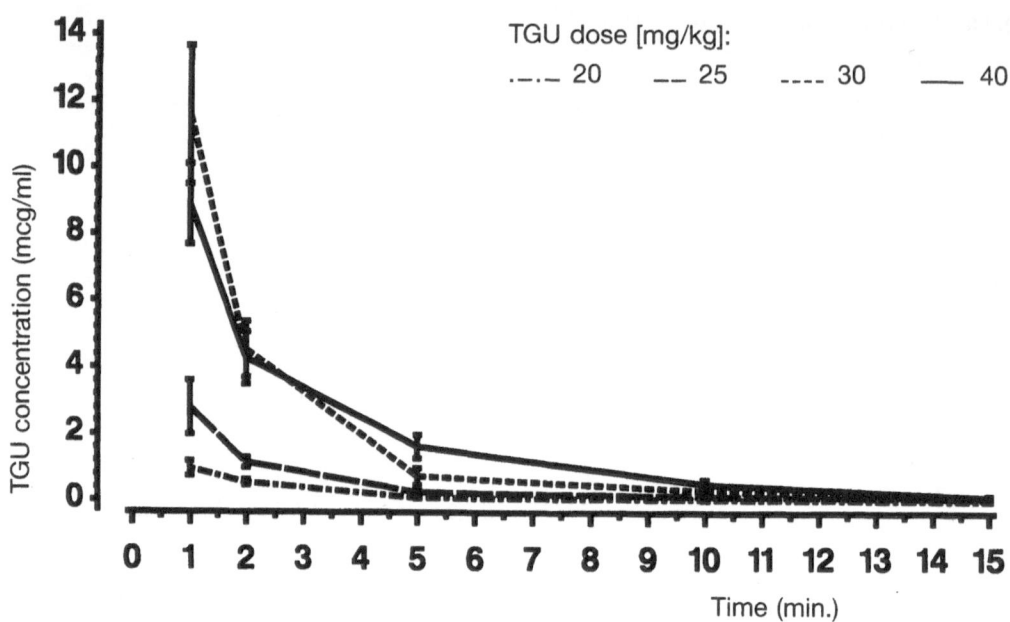

Fig. 1. Plasma levels of 1,2,4-triglycidylurazol (*TGU*) in beagle dogs

Table 6. Comparison of plasma pharmacokinetic parameters in animals with or without lethal toxic enteritis

TGU dose (mg/kg)	Outcome	Peak plasma concentration (μg/ml)	AUC (μg10⁻²/mlh)	Clearance (ml/min)	Volume of distribution (l)	t₁/₂ (min)
30(2)[a]	Alive (3)[b]	5.60[c] (1.02)	22.54(6.25)	46 343 (8 574)	248.8(77.9)	3.5(0.8)
30(2)	Dead (4)	16.06* (2.62)	50.25** (9.66)	20 846[+] (5 641)	84.4[+] (22.6)	2.8[++] (0)
40(1)+TBI	Alive (2)	3.95(0.95)	9.04(1.81)	99 854 (10 745)	399.4(42.9)	2.8 (0)
40(1)+TBI	Dead (4)	11.91(4.47)	80.20(39.41)	26 688 (13 021)	107.1 (52.4)	2.8(0.1)

$* \ p = 0.006; \ ** \ p = 0.06; \ + \ p = 0.02; \ ++ \ p = 0.04$

[a] Values represent the number of fractions of the indicated TGU dose applied to each animal
[b] Values represent the number of animals in which pharmacokinetics were studied
[c] Values represent means (± standard errors) of plasma pharmacokinetic parameters performed for each individual dose fraction in animals with or without lethal toxic enteritis. *P* values were derived from comparisons of these parameters by Wilcoxon's two-sample rank sum test

ing in all patients. Immediately after the second TGU dose, two patients developed supraventricular arrhythmias necessitating antiarrhythmic therapy. In one of these patients mycotic myocarditis was found at autopsy. The degree of oral mucositis and frequencies of diarrhea in the early post-transplant period appeared comparable to that of patients receiving our "standard"

preparative regimen of TBI (2.5 Gy/day over four consecutive days using a cobalt-60 source) in combination with cyclophosphamide (60 mg/kg per day over 2 days). Two patients developed two- and fivefold elevations of GOT plasma levels above baseline values (Table 7). Other adverse effects or toxic death attributable to the study drug were not observed.

Table 7. Nonhematologic toxicity (ECOG grades) in patients treated with combinations of TGU and total body irradiation or high-dose busulfan

Organ system / UPN	318	341	395	403	408
Gastrointestinal					
Nausea/vomiting	4	4	3	3	2
Stomatitis	4	4	4	1	4
Diarrhea	1	2	2	1	2
Liver					
SGOT/SGPT	0	0	0	3	1
Bilirubin	0	0	0	0	0
Cardiovascular					
Arrhythmia	4	4	0	0	0
LV function	0	0	0	0	0
Blood pressure	0	0	0	0	0

Three patients had massive leukemic marrow infiltrates prior to HLA-identical sibling marrow transplantation. Clearance of marrow involvement and allogeneic engraftment could be demonstrated by histologic and/or cytogenetic analysis in these patients. Unfortunately, leukemic relapse occurred at 38, 62, and 163 days after BMT. Two patients received an HLA-mismatched marrow transplant for treatment of intermediate or high-grade non-Hodgkin's lymphoma with marrow involvement. Both patients were treated in relapse after preceding unsuccessful autologous or allogeneic BMT. Marrow engraftment could be attained in these patients, who subsequently died due to infectious complications at 18 and 132 days after BMT.

Discussion

Our results obtained in a beagle dog model demonstrate that TGU has dose-dependent and dose-limiting gastrointestinal toxic effects with an estimated LD_{50} in the range of 60 mg/kg (corresponding to 2500 mg/m^2) given in two consecutive daily fractions of 30 mg/kg. This toxic effect was additionally characterized by a steep dose-response relationship. Animals with lethal toxicity had increased peak plasma levels and AUC

values in comparison to those without suggesting that interindividual differences in pharmacokinetics of the compound contributed to the severity of this adverse effect.

Myelosuppression as estimated by nadir values for WBC and platelets as well as time to reconstitution of peripheral blood counts was severe and life-threatening at all examined dose levels. Hematologic toxicity, however, was not clearly dose dependent, which is in contrast to one clinical trial, in which TGU showed dose-dependent myelosuppression in a dose range between 480 and 1250 mg/m^2 given in five fractions over 5 days [12]. Despite limitations in converting dosages between different species, TGU doses used in the animal studies were 2.5- to 3.5-fold higher than in the cited report, which may in part explain the lacking dose-toxicity relationship in this model.

Concerning combinations of TGU with the most frequently used modalities of myeloablation prior to BMT, i.e., TBI or HD-BU, cumulative gastrointestinal toxicity was restricted to the combination with TBI, and necessitated dose reductions of TGU by 50% to mitigate this adverse effect. The increase in gastrointestinal toxicity was not conditioned by changes in TGU pharmacokinetics as a consequence of preceding TBI.

The immunosuppressive properties of TGU in this model were impressive, since complete and sustained allogeneic DLA-identical marrow engraftment was attained in three of four recipient animals, which were pretreated by HD-BU, a compound with negligible immunosuppressive efficacy in settings of allogeneic BMT. Autopsy findings in animals which dies from gastrointestinal toxicity demonstrated complete atrophy of lymphatic follicles in lymph nodes, spleen, and gut walls, further supporting the substantial toxicity of TGU on the lymphatic system.

Our clinical results using TGU in a dose range between 30 mg/kg (1200 mg(m²) and 40 mg/kg (1600 mg/m²) in combination with TBI or HD-BU suggest that the compound can be administered with tolerable adverse effects in regimens preparatory for allogeneic BMT even in heavily pretreated patients. The severity of acute gastrointestinal toxicity appeared not to be increased in comparison to that of our "standard" TBI and cyclophosphamide regimen. Of concern is the observation that two patients developed cardiac arrhythmias in association with TGU application. Since both patients had been preexposed to cardiotoxic dosages of anthracyclines and oxazophosphorines, it remains uncertain whether this acute adverse effect can be related to arrhythmogenic or cardiotoxic properties of TGU. In addition, one of these patients showed acute infectious myocarditis at autopsy as a potentially contributing cause for arrhythmia. The clinical results in terms of eradicating the underlying disease are so far disappointing. It has to be emphasized, however, that marrow engraftment could even be attained in patients who had an increased risk of graft rejection. This further supports that TGU has potent immunosuppressive properties in regimens preparatory for BMT.

The pharmacokinetic profile of TGU in beagle dogs was characterized by a rapid plasma clearance with t_{50} values in the range of 2.7 and 3.5 min. Short plasma and systemic clearance rates of cytotoxic agents used in preparative regimes for BMT are of special importance to avoid cytotoxic effects on the transplanted marrow cells. In this regard, it appears of concern that

significant concentrations of TGU could be extracted from organs up to 7 days after administration of the compound, which indicates extensive drug binding to tissues. Kinetics of hematopoietic reconstitution, however, were apparently not delayed in the animal and human studies. Persistent binding of TGU to tissues thus appeared to have minor importance with regard to marrow graft function.

We conclude that the pharmacologic, myelotoxic, and immunosuppressive properties warrant further clinical studies to define the potential role or TGU in the framework of BMT.

References

1. Hilgard P, Peukert M, Pohl J (1984) a-/β-Triglycidyl-urazol (TGU, NSC 332488, I.N.N.: Anaxirone): a new chemotherapeutic agent. Cancer Treat Rev 11: 115
2. Bruntsch U, Dodion P, Ten Bokkel Huinink WW, Hansen HH, Pinedo HM, Hansen M, Renard J, Van Glabbeke M (1986) Primary resistance of renal adenocarcinoma to 1,2,4-triglycidylurazol (TGU, NSC 332488), a new triepoxide cytostatic agent–a phase II study of the EORTC early clinical trials group. Eur J Cancer Clin Oncol 22: 697
3. Cunningham D, Soukop M, Stuart JFB, Setanoians A, Gilchrist NL, Forrest GJ, Kaye SB (1986) A clinical and pharmacokinetic phase I study of 1,2,4-triglycidylurazol (TGU, NSC 332488). Eur J Cancer Clin Oncol 22: 1325
4. Cunningham D, Banham SW, Soukop M (1986) Small cell lung cancer: results of a phase II study of 1,2,4-triglycidylurazol. Cancer Chemother Pharmacol 17: 85
5. George M, Scotto V, Carnino F, Dodion P, Ten Bokkel Huinink WW, Rotmensz N, Vermorken JB (1987) Phase II trial of anxirone (1,2,4-triglycidylurazol, TGU) in patients with advanced ovarian carcinoma: an EORTC gynecological cancer cooperative group study. Eur J Cancer Clin Oncol 23: 867
6. Hansen SW, Bach F, Hansen HH, Kaplan S, Cavalli F (1985) Phase I trial of 1,2,4-triglycidylurazol (TGU, NSC 332488): a new triepoxide cytostatic agent. Eur J Cancer Clin Oncol 21: 301
7. Lund B, Hansen F, Hansen M, Hansen HH (1987) Phase II study of 1,2,4-triglycidylurazol (TGU) in previously untreated and

treated patients with small cell lung cancer. Eur J Cancer Clin Oncol 23: 1031

8. Beelen DW, Schilcher RB, Ehrlich R, Quabeck K, Schmidt U, Szy D, Grosse-Wilde H, Schaefer UW (1991) High dose 1,2,4-triglycidylurazol (TGU, NSC 332488) in regimens preparatory to bone marrow transplantation. Cancer Chemother Pharmacol 27: 361

9. Beelen DW, Quabeck K, Kaiser B, Wiefelspütz J, Scheulen ME, Graeven U. Grosse-Wilde H, Sayer HG, Schaefer UW (1990) Six weeks of continuous intravenous cyclosporin and short-course methotrexate as prophylaxis for acute graft-versus-host disease after allogeneic bone marrow transplantation. Transplantation 50: 421

10. Miller AB, Hoogstraten B, Staquet M, Winkler A (1981) Reporting results of cancer treatment. Cancer 47: 207

11. Schilcher RB, Young JD, Nowrousian MR, Hoffmann B, Schmidt CG (1986) Reversed-phase high-performance liquid chromatography determination of anaxirone in biological specimens. J Chromatogr 378: 248

12. Nicaise C, Rozencweig M, Crespeigne N, Dodion P, Gerard B, Lambert M, Decoster G, Kenis Y (1986) Phase I study of triglycidylurazol given on a 5-day iv schedule. Cancer Treat Rep 70: 599

2,2'-Difluorodeoxycytidine:
A New Antimetabolite with Inhibitory Activity Against Ribonucleotide Reduction and dCMP Deaminase

V. Heinemann[1], Y-Z Xu[2], A. Sen, and W. Plunkett[2]

Introduction

2',2'-Difluorodeoxycytidine (dFdC) is a new deoxycytidine analog (Fig. 1) in which both hydrogens of the 2'-carbon are replaced by fluorine atoms [1]. The prodrug dFdC is intracellularly phosphorylated by deoxycytidine kinase (dCK) and accumulates to the active 5'-triphosphate dFdCTP [2]. Cytotoxic activity of dFdC is related to intracellular accumulation and retention of dFdCTP [2, 3].

In several leukemia cell lines elimination of high dFdCTP concentrations was shown

2'−Difluorodeoxycytidine   2'−Deoxycytidine

(dFdC)   (dCyd)

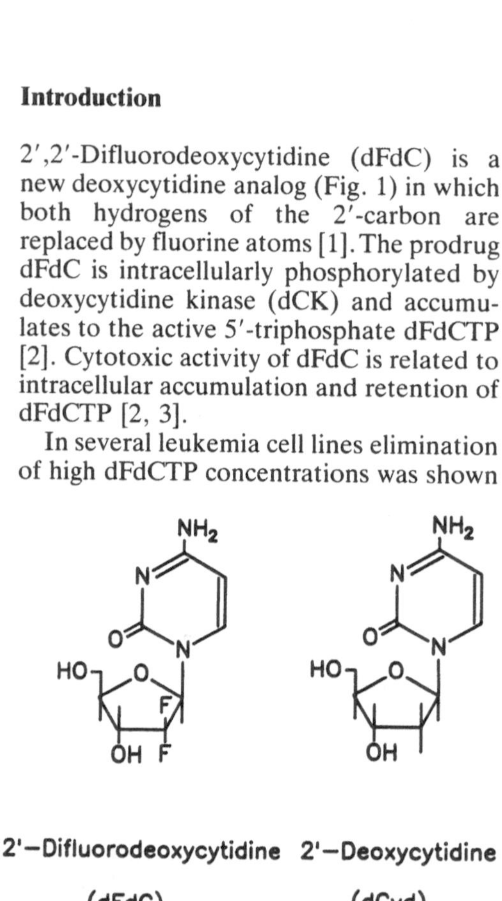

Fig. 1. Molecular structures of dFdC and dCyd

[1] Klinikum Grosshadern. Department of Hematology/Oncology, University of Munich, Marchioninistr. 15, 8000 Munich 70, FRG
[2] Department of Medical Oncology, University of Texas, MD Anderson Cancer Center, 1515 Holcombe Boulevard, Houston, TX, USA

to be biphasic with a short initial half-life followed by a second phase of considerably slower degradation [3–5]. Slow cellular elimination of dFdCTP is of interest since it relates to enhanced cytotoxicity of the drug. The present study investigates to what extent these elimination characteristics are defined by cellular dFdC metabolites or their interaction with cellular enzymes such as deoxycytidylate deaminase (dCMPD) and ribonucleotide reductase (RR). A mechanistic model is proposed which describes dFdC-mediated modulation of dCMPD and RR as determinants of dFdCTP elimination.

Materials and Methods

dFdU, dFdCMP, and [5−14V]dFdC were synthesized at the Eli Lilly Research Laboratories (Indianapolis, IN). 3,4,5,6-Tetrahydrouridine (THU) was provided by Dr. Ven Narayanan, Drug Synthesis and Chemistry Branch, National Cancer Institute. 3,4,5,6-Tetrahydrodeoxyuridine was obtained from Behring Diagnostics (La Jolla, CA). dFdCTP was synthesized from dFdCMP by Dr. Alina Sen.

All experiments were performed in triplicate using the human T-lymphoblast cell line CCRF-CEM. Analysis of acid-soluble cell extracts and culture medium for nucleosides and nucleoside phosphates was performed by high-performance liquid chromatography (HPLC) as previously describes [2]. Cellular dNTP concentrations were determined after degradation of NTP by periodate oxidation [6]. Deoxycytidylate deaminase activity was assayed in broken cell extracts according to the method reported by Fridland and Verhoef [7].

Incorporation of [5-³H]Cyd into DNA was measured as described by Jackson [8].

Results

Cellular dFdCTP Elimination. The effect of cellular dFdCTP concentration on the rate of dFdCTP elimination was analyzed after a 2-h exposure of CEM cells to 0.1 and 10 μM dFdC (cellular dFdCTP was 30 μM and 460 μM respectively). When drug washout was performed at a cellular dFdCTP concentration of 30 μM, dFdCTP elimination was linear with a $t_{1/2}\alpha$ of 3.3. h. However, at a dFdCTP concentration of 460 μM, dFdCTP elimination was biphasic with the inflection occurring at 4 h after washout. $T_{1/2}\alpha$ remained unaffected by the cellular dFdCTP concentration, while the terminal half-life ($t_{1/2}\beta$) was prolonged as cellular dFdCTP increased.

Modulation of dNTP Mediated by dFdC. After a 2-h incubation with 0.1 μM dFdC, cellular concentrations of dFdCDP and dFdCTP amounted to 1.34 ± 0.1 μM and 43.9 ± 5.4 μM respectively. At this time cellular pools of dCTP, dTTP, dATP, and dGTP were reduced to 21 %, 64 %, 54 %, and 52 %, respectively (Fig. 2). The ratio dTTP/dCTP in control cells was 2.4, while after a 2-h exposure to 0.1 μM and 10 μM dFdC this ratio increased to 6.7 and 8.1, respectively. Eight hours after washout of 0.1 μM dFdC, the dTTP/dCTP ratio had nearly normalized to a value of 3.2, while after washout of 10 μM dFdC this ratio remained elevated at 11.8.

Inhibition of dFdCDP Reduction Mediated by dFdC. The effect of dFdC and hydroxyurea (HU) on ribonucleotide reductase (RR) was analyzed by pulse treatment of cells with [³H]Cyd at the end of a 2-h drug exposure (Table 1). The incorporation of [³H]Cyd into dCTP and DNA was assayed as an estimate of RR activity. In fact, 0.1 μM dFdC reduced incorporation of [³H]Cyd into dCTP and DNA by 96.6 %

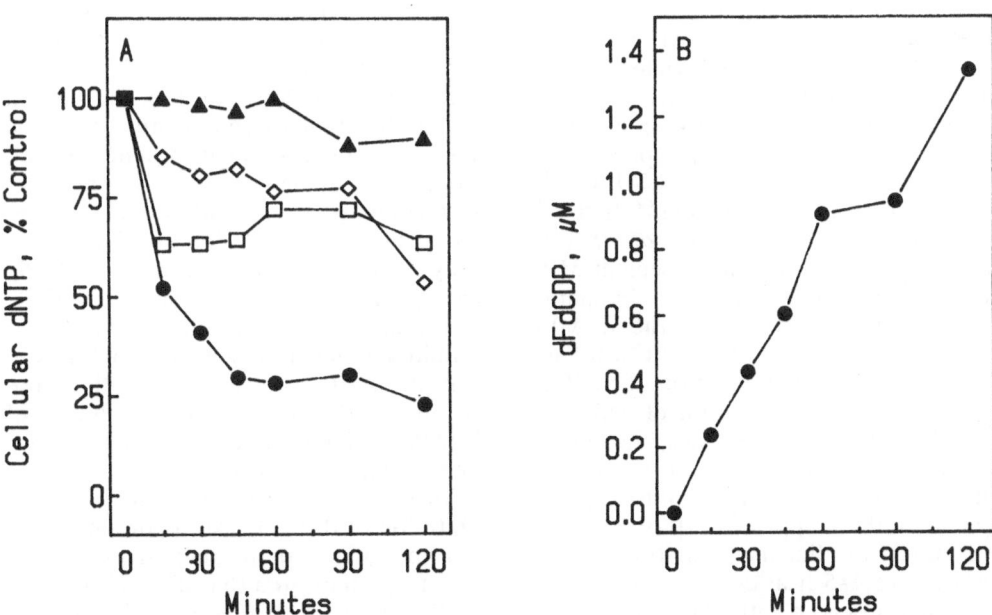

Fig. 2. Perturbation of dNTP pools in CEM cells induced by dFdC. CEM cells were exposed for 2 h to dFdC (0.01–10 μM), and dCTP (●), dTTP (▲), dATP (◇), and dGTP (□) were determined as a percentage of control. dNTP concentrations in control cells: dCTP 28 ± 2 μM, dTTP 64 ± 6.5 μM, dATP 76 ± 8 μM, and dGTP 51 ± 6.5 μM

Table 1. At the end of a 2-h exposure of CEM cells to indicated concentrations of dFdC or hydroxyurea, cells were pulsed with [³H]Cyd for 10 min. The radioactivity incorporated into the dCTP pool and into DNA was measured as an estimate of ribonucleotide reductase activity. Control incorporation was: dCTP, 11 240 dpm/5×10⁷ cells; DNA, 15 940 dpm/5×10⁷ cells

	[5-³H]Cyd incorporation	
	dCTP	DNA
Control	100 ± 5	100 ± 1
dFdC, 0.01 μM	42.3 ± 7.1	39.0 ± 2
dFdC, 0.1 μM	3.4 ± 3.6	3.2 ± 0.6
dFdC, 10 μM	0.7 ± 0.9	4.7 ± 1.2
Hydroxyurea, 5 mM	0	8.9 ± 0.1

and 96.8 % respectively. A further decrease of [³H]Cyd incorporation was noted after exposure to 10 μM dFdC. By comparison, after exposure to HU no radioactivity was determined in the dCTP pool and incorporation of [³H]Cyd into DNA was reduced by 91.1 %.

Modulation of dFdCMP Deamination by dCTP, dTTP, and dFdCTP. In broken cell extracts dCTP was found to be a necessary activator of dFdCMP deamination. dTTP inhibited dCMPD depending on the ratio of dTTP/dCTP. A 50 % inhibition of dFdCMP deamination was reached at a fourfold excess of dTTP over dCTP, while complete inhibition of dCMPD was achieved at a dTTP/dCTP ratio of 20. Also dFdCTP was inhibitory to dCMPD. In the presence of 5 μM dCTP, deamination of dCMP was inhibited with an IC_{50} of 0.46 mM dFdCTP.

dCMPD as a Determinant of dFdCTP Elimination. The relation between dCMPD activity and cellular dFdCTP elimination was investigated by use of the dCMPD inhibitor dTHU. After washout of 0.1 μM dFdC (2 h), linear elimination of dFdCTP was expected. Coincubation of cells with 100 μM dTHU induced a nearly complete inhibition of dCMPD [6] and transformed linear dFdCTP elimination into biphasic kinetics with an apparent $t_{1/2}\beta$ of 19 h. The inflection from linear elimination kinetics occurred at 4–5 h after drug washout, an effect not observed with THU, an inhibitor of Cyd/dCyd deaminase.

Discussion

Cellular dFdCTP elimination is unique in that it is characterized as a concentration-dependent process. Low dFdCTP concentrations (30 μM) at drug washout allowed linear elimination kinetics. However, biphasic dFdCTP elimination was observed at a dFdCTP concentration of 460 μM. While $t_{1/2}\alpha$ was not concentration dependent, $t_{1/2}\beta$ increased as a function of cellular dFdCTP concentration. Comparable kinetics of drug triphosphate elimination have not been observed with ara-CTP, ara-ATP, or F-ara-ATP [2, 9].

To better understand the mechanism behind the biphasic elimination kinetics, the extracellular products of dFdCTP catabolism were studied. Since activity of cytidine deaminase is insignificant in CEM cells, extracellular accumulation of dFdU essentially occurred as a function of dCMPD activity. In fact, it was observed that dFdU excretion into the extracellular medium was inhibited at high intracellular dFdCTP concentrations (data not shown). We therefore hypothesized that a relative inhibition of dCMPD activity may occur at high cellular concentrations of dFdCTP.

Several mechanisms of dFdC-mediated inhibition of dCMPD can be proposed:
1. Experiments performed in crude cell extracts indicated that dFdCTP inhibits dCMPD with an IC_{50} of 0.46 mM;
2. dFdCMP deamination by dCMPD is subject to allosteric regulation by dCTP as an activator, and dTTP as an inhibitor.

dCMPD inhibition was dependent on the ratio of dTTP/dCTP, and complete inhibition was achieved at a 20-fold excess of dTTP over dCTP.

The importance of these considerations became evident in view of dFdC-mediated perturbations of cellular dNTP (Fig. 2). In fact, dFdC inhibits ribonucleotide reduction (RR) comparable to the effect of hydroxyurea [10]. dFdC-mediated RR inhibition resulted in a greater depletion of dCTP than of dTTP and accordingly increased the ratio of dTTP/dCTP. The degree of dTTP/dCTP elevation as well as the velocity of recovery from an elevated dTTP/dCTP ratio were dependent on the cellular concentration of dFdCTP or its metabolites (data not shown).

Consequently, dFdCTP may inhibit its own catabolism by a concentration-dependent modulation of dCMPD activity. In accordance with this hypothesis, dTHU-mediated inhibition of dCMPD changed linear elimination of dFdCTP into biphasic kinetics similar to those seen at high dFdCTP concentrations. We conclude that inhibition of dCMPD and RR is part of the self-potentiative activity of dFdC which is responsible for delayed cellular elimination and increased cytotoxicity of dFdCTP.

Summary

Cellular pharmacodynamics of 2,2'-difluorodeoxycytidine (dFdC) are characterized by the ability of dFdC metabolites to inhibit dCMP deaminase (dCMPD) and ribonucleotide reductase. Elimination of dFdCTP from CCRF-CEM cells is regulated by the activity of dCMPD, an enzyme which effectively deaminates dFdCMP to the nontoxic product dFdUMP. As cellular dFdCTP concentrations increased ≥ 100 μM (after 2 h exposure to dFdC ≥ 0.3 μM), dFdCTP elimination was transformed from monophasic to biphasic kinetics and thus to a slower catabolism. In fact, high concentrations of dFdCTP ($IC_{50} = 0.46$ mM) were inhibitory to dCMPD in cell extracts. Inhibition of dCMPD was also induced by a depletion of the allosteric activator dCTP or an excess of the allosteric inhibitor dTTP, resulting in an elevated ratio of dTTP/dCTP. Perturbation of dNTP pools, specifically an elevation of the dTTP/dCTP ratio, was induced by dFdCDP-mediated inhibition of RR. Exposure of CEM cells to dFdC predominantly depleted the dCTP pool, while the pool sizes of dTTP, dATP, and dGTP were less affected. A 2-h exposure to 0.1 μM or 10 μM dFdC increased the dTTP/dCTP ratio by 6.7- and 8.1-fold respectively. In CEM cell extracts dCMPD activity was reduced by 50 % at a fourfold excess of dTTP over dCTP. Additionally, inhibition of ribonucleotide reductase activates the dNTP salvage pathway and with it phosphorylation of dFdC to dFdCTP. We conclude that dFdC-mediated modulation of dCMPD and RR contribute to an increased accumulation and prolonged elimination of cellular dFdCTP.

References

1. Hertel LW, Boder GB, Kroin JS, Rinzel SM, Poore GA, Todd GC, Grindey GB (1990) Evaluation of the antitumor activity of gemcitabine (2',2'-difluorodeoxycytidine). Cancer Res 50: 4417–4422
2. Heinemann V, Hertel LW, Grindey GB, Plunkett W (1988) Comparison of the cellular pharmacokinetics and toxicity of 2',2'-difluorodeoxycytidine and 1-β-D-arabinofuranosylcytosine. Cancer Res 48: 4024–4031
3. Heinemann V, Hertel L, Grindey G, Plunkett W (1988) Cellular elimination of 2',2'-difluorodeoxycytidine-5'-triphosphate (dFdCTP). Proc Am Assoc Cancer Res 29: 2004
4. Chubb S, Heinemann V, Novotny L, Hertel LW, Nowak B, Mineishi S, Grindey GB, Plunkett W (1987) Metabolism and action of 2',2'-difluorodeoxycytidine in human leukemic cells. Proc Am Assoc Cancer Res 28: 324
5. Plunkett W, Gandhi V, Chubb S, Nowak B, Heinemann V, Mineishi S, Sen A, Hertel LW, Grindey GB (1989) 2',2'-Difluorodeoxycytidine metabolism and mechanism of action in human leukemia cells. Nucleosides Nucleotides 8: 775–785
6. Heinemann V, Plunkett W (1989) Modulation of deoxynucleotide metabolism by the deoxycytidylate deaminase inhibitor 3,4,5,6-tetrahydrodeoxyuridine. Biochem Pharmacol 38: 4115–4121
7. Fridland A, Verhoef V (1987) Mechanism for ara-CTP catabolism in human leukemic cells and effect of deaminase inhibitors on this

process. Semin Oncol 14 [Suppl 1]: 262–268

8. Jackson RC (1978) The regulation of thymidylate biosynthesis in Novikoff hepatoma cells and the effects of amethopterin, 5-fluorodeoxyuridine, and 3-deazauridine. J Biol Chem 253: 7440–7446

9. Plunkett W, Chubb S, Alexander L, Montgomery JA (1980) Comparison of the toxicity and metabolism of 9-β-*D*-arabinofuranosyl-2-fluoroadenine and 9-β-*D*-arabinofuranosyladenine in human lymphoblastoid cells. Cancer Res 40: 2349–2355

10. Heinemann V, Xu Y-Z, Chubb S, Sen A, Hertel LW, Grindey GB, Plunkett W (1990) Inhibition of ribonucleotide reductase in CCRF-CEM cells by 2′,2′-difluorodeoxycytidine. Mol Pharmacol 38: 567–572

Screening of 19 Monoclonal Antibodies for their Potential as Ricin A-Chain Immunotoxins Against Myeloid Leukemia Cell Lines*

A. Engert[1,2], A. Brown[1], V. Diehl[2], and P. Thorpe[1]

Introduction

Second-generation ricin A-chain immuno-toxins have better stability, higher purity, and home to the liver much less rapidly than their predecessors [1, 2]. They have been demonstrated in vitro and in vivo to have potent antitumor activity against B-cell lymphomas, T-cell lymphomas, and Hodg-kin's disease tumors [3–5] and are currently undergoing clinical evaluation in man [6]. Few attempts have been made hitherto to evaluate immunotoxins for the treatment of AML [7]. In the present study we screened 19 monoclonal antibodies (MoAbs) for their potential as ricin A-chain immunotox-ins against four myeloid cell lines.

Material, Methods, and Results

The characteristics of the 19 MoAbs are listed in Table 1. Most of the antibodies tested bind to myeloid antigens (CD 13, CDw17, CD33, CD34) whereas the remain-der recognize activation antigens (CD25, CD30, CD71) which are present on both myeloid and nonmyeloid cell types. The four myeloid cell lines used as targets were K562, U937, HL60, and KG1.

FACS analysis performed by standard techniques indicated that CD13, CD15, CD33, and CD71 antibodies strongly stained U937, HL60, and KG1 cells where-as the CD36 antibody and the E1, E2, and E3 antibodies against unclustered determi-nants stained these cells weakly (Table 2). The K562 cell line showed variable and generally weaker staining with all the anti-bodies except the CD71 (anti-transferrin receptor) antibodies.

The potential of the MoAbs to form ricin A-chain immunotoxins was screened by an indirect cytotoxicity assay in which the target cells are incubated first with the test antibody and then with an affinity-purified goat Fab'prime immunotoxin directed against mouse immunoglobulin. The doub-le-layer immunotoxin enters the target cell as would the direct-linked immunotoxin and the assay therefore reliably predicts the potency of any given MoAb as ricin A-chain immunotoxin [8]. As shown in Table 3, only the CD71 MoAbs, MEM75 and 120-2A3, formed effective immunotoxins against the myeloid target cell lines. Indirect immuno-toxins prepared from all the other antibod-ies in the panel were completely ineffective against U937, HL60, and KG1 cells. Addi-tionally, they were mostly ineffective against K562 cells with only 1G10 (CD15), T5A7 (CD17), and 5F1 (CD36) showing weak toxicity.

Discussion

The major finding to emerge from the present study was that human myeloid leukemia cell lines are poorly susceptible to killing by ricin A-chain immunotoxins. Only CD71 MoAbs which recognize the

[1] Drug Targeting Laboratory, ICRF, Lincoln's Inn Fields, London, WC2A 3PX, UK
[2] First Medical Clinic, University of Cologne, J. Stelzmannstr. 9, 5000 Cologne 41, FRG
* Supported in part by DFG grant En 179 1/1.

Table 1. Monoclonal antibodies evaluated in the present study

	Antibody	Reactivity	Isotype	Source
Myeloid antigens	My7	CD13	IgG2b	Coulter Imm.
	WM15	CD13	IgG1	Sera Lab.
	1G10	CD15	IgM	Bernstein
	T5A7	CDw17	IgM	Bernstein
	My9	CD33	IgG2b	Coulter Imm.
	WM53	CD33	IgG1	Sera Lab
	p67-7	CD33	IgG1	Bernstein
	12.8	CD34	IgM	Bernstein
	E1	Unclustered	n.k.	Bernstein
	E2	Unclustered	n.k.	Bernstein
	E3	Unclustered	n.k.	Bernstein
Activation antigens	B-B10	CD25	IgG1	Wijdenes
	HRS-3	CD30	IgG1	Pfreundschuh
	MEM-75	CD71	IgG1	Horejsi
	120-2A3	CD71	IgG1	Villela
Various	RFB4	CD22	IgG1	Chen
	5F1	CD36	IgM	Bernstein
	1B3	Unclustered	IgG2a	Bernstein
	TDR31.1	MHC classII	IgG1	Bodmer

n.k., not known

Table 2. FACS analyses on myeloid cell lines

Antibody	Specificity	Intensity of staining			
		K562	U937	HL60	KG1
My7	CD13	−	++	++	++
WM15	CD13	−	++	+++	++
1G10	CD15	+	++	++	++
T5A7	CD17	+	−	++	++
RFB4	CD22	−	−	+	−
B-B10	CD25	−	++	−	−
HRS-3	CD30	++	+	+	−
My9	CD33	+	++	++	++
WM53	CD33	+	++	+++	+++
p67-7	CD33	+	+++	+++	+++
12.8	CD34	−	+	−	++
5F1	CD36	+	+	+	+
1B3	Unclustered	−	+	+	+
E1	Unclustered	−	+	+++	+++
E2	Unclustered	−	++	+	++
E3	Unclustered	−	+	+	+
TDR31.1	MHC class II	+	+	−	++
MEM75	CD71	+++	+++	+++	+
120-2A3	CD71	+++	+++	+++	++

−, MFI <20 U; +, MFI 21–70 U; ++, MFI 71–120 U; +++, MFI >120 U

374

Table 3. Potency of ricin A-chain immunotoxins as predicted by an indirect cytotoxicity assay on myeloid cell lines

Antibody	Specificity	Predicted cytotoxic potency			
		K562	U937	HL60	KG1
My7	CD13	−	−	−	−
WM15	CD13	−	−	−	−
1G10	CD15	+	−	−	−
T5A7	CD17	+	−	−	−
RFB4	CD22	−	−	−	−
B-B10	CD25	−	−	−	−
HRS-3	CD30	−	−	−	−
My9	CD33	−	−	−	−
WM53	CD33	−	−	−	−
p 67-7	CD33	−	−	−	−
12.8	CD34	−	−	−	−
5F1	CD36	+	−	−	−
1B3	Unclustered	−	−	−	−
E1	Unclustered	−	−	−	−
E2	Unclustered	−	−	−	−
E3	Unclustered	−	−	−	−
TDR31.1	MHC class II	−	−	−	−
MEM-75	CD71	+ +	+	+	+
120-2A3	CD71	+ +	+	+	+ +

−, $IC_{50} > 10^{-8}M$; +, IC_{50} $10^{-8}-10^{-9}M$; + +, IC_{50} $10^{-9}-10^{-10}M$

transferrin receptor (TfR) showed significant toxicity to four myeloid leukemia cell lines. CD71 immunotoxins, however, are probably unsuitable for clinical use in the systemic treatment of AML since TfR is expressed on vital tissues such as liver, pancreas, and brain endothelium [9]. Importantly, ricin A-chain immunotoxins against CD22, CD25, and CD30, which have been demonstrated previously to be extremely effective at killing B cells, T cells, and Hodgkin's cells [3–5] failed to kill myeloid target cells, suggesting that myeloid cells tend to have a lower susceptibility to killing by immunotoxins than nonmyeloid cells.

Immunotoxins containing ricin A-chain are known to differ in their potency depending on the affinity of the immunotoxin to the target antigen [3], the density of the target antigen on the target cell [10], the location of the epitope recognized by the immunotoxin on the target antigen [11], and the rate and route of endocytosis of the antigen-immunotoxin complex [12]. Kinetic studies performed on HL60 cells with an effective CD71 immunotoxin, 120-

2A3.dgA, and an ineffective CD33 immunotoxin, p67-7.dgA, demonstrated that p67-7.dgA was more rapidly endocytosed and, in comparison, about twice as rapidly degraded to TCA-soluble material [13]. These data suggest that myeloid cells might degrade ricin A-chain immunotoxins rather than transport the A-chain to the cytosol where it acts by catalytically inactivating ribosomes.

We are currently investigating improved immunotoxins for AML including the use of substances that block the rapid lysosomal degradation or potentiate the entry of A-chain into the lysosomes.

References

1. Thorpe PE, Wallace PM et al. (1988) Improved antitumor effects of immunotoxins prepared with deglycosylated ricin A-chain and hindered disulfide linkages. Cancer Res 48: 6396
2. Blakey DC, Watson GJ et al. (1987) Effect of chemical deglycosylation of ricin A-chain on the in vivo fate and cytotoxic activity of an immunotoxin composed of ricin A-chain and

an anti-Thy 1.1 antibody. Cancer Res 47: 947

3. Shen GL, Li JL et al. (1988) Evaluation of four CD22 antibodies as ricin A-chain containing immunotoxins for the in vivo therapy of human B-cell leukemias and lymphomas. Int J Cancer 42: 792

4. Hertler AA, Schlossman DM et al. (1989) An immunotoxin for the treatment of T-acute lymphoblastic leukemic meningitis: studies in rhesus monkeys. Cancer Immunol Immunother 28: 59

5. Engert A, Martin G et al. (1990) Antitumor effects of ricin A-chain immunotoxins from intact antibodies and Fab'fragments on solid human Hodgkin's disease tumors in mice. Cancer Res 50: 2929

6. Vitetta E, Stone M et al. (1991) A phase I immunotoxin trial in patients with B-cell lymphoma. Cancer Res 51: 4052

7. Myers DE, Uckun FM et al. (1988) Immunotoxins for ex vivo purging in autologous bone marrow transplantation for acute non-lymphocytic leukemia. Transplantation 46: 240

8. Till M, May RD et al. (1988) An assay that predicts the ability of monoclonal antibodies to form potent ricin A-chain containing immunotoxins. Cancer Res 48: 1119

9. Schwarting R, Stein H (1989) Cluster report CD71. In: Knapp W et al. (eds) Leucocyte typing IV. Oxford University Press, New York, pp 455–560

10. Preijers FWMB, Tax WJM et al. (1988) Different susceptibilities of normal T cells and T cell lines to immunotoxins. Scand J Immunol 27: 533

11. Press OW, Martin PJ et al. (1988) Ricin A-chain immunotoxins directed against different epitopes on the CD2 molecule differ in their ability to kill normal and malignant T cells. J Immunol 141: 4410

12. Preijers FWMB, Taw WJM et al. (1988) Relationship between internalization and cytotoxicity of ricin A-chain immunotoxins. Br J Haematol 70: 289

13. Engert A, Brown A, Thorpe PE (1991) Resistance of myeloid leukemia cell lines to ricin A-chain immunotoxins. Leuk Res (in press)

Clinical Trials in Relapsed
and Refractory Acute Myeloid Leukemia

Patterns of Failure in Salvage Therapy for Acute Myelogenous Leukemia

M.J. Keating, H. Kantarjian, S. O'Brien, E. Estey, C. Koller, M. Beran,
K.B. McCredie, and E.J. Freireich

Introduction

The advent of cytosine arabinoside and daunorubicin into clinical practice in the late 1960s converted acute myelogenous leukemia (AML) from an incurable to a potentially curable disease [1]. In the last 20 years, the complete remission rates for combinations of therapy as initial induction regimens have been of the range of 50%–80% [2–4]. Despite a variety of postremission strategies, the majority of patients who enter remission relapse with a median of 12–15 months [2–5]. Between 20% and 30% of patients appear to be cured of their disease if they achieve a remission as they remain free of disease for periods in excess of 5 years. Treatment of patients who either fail to achieve a complete remission (primary refractory) or who relapse following a remission (relapsed patients) is unsatisfactory. The majority of studies which are reported are conducted on selected patients with a variety of combinations. For similar regimens such as high-dose cytosine arabinoside, the response rates vary from 25% to 60% [6–8]. While this may be a result of the chemotherapy offered to these patients, an alternate explanation is that the characteristics of the patients entered on studies is different. Very few comparative trials of various regimens have been conducted in salvage therapy for AML so that the best approach to reinduction therapy has not been es-

University of Texas, MD Anderson Cancer Center, 1515 Holcombe Blvd., Box 38, Houston, Texas 77030, USA

tablished. With the advent of new agents such as amsacrine, mitoxantrone, etoposide, and idarubicin and various schedules of high-dose cytosine arabinoside, a variety of treatment programs are now being recommended for management of refractory or relapsed AML patients [9–11].

The purpose of this study was to evaluate the response to treatment of refractory and relapsed patients with AML. Factors predictive for either probability of achieving a complete remission or dying during remission induction have been sought. The outcome of treatment over different time periods in the last 15 years has also been compared. The purpose of this study was to get a sense as to whether any treatment regimen is more or less likely to obtain complete remission or whether the outcome of patients after failing their initial attempt at cure is determined predominantly by treatment or by the biology of their leukemia.

Patient Population

All patients who have received their initial remission induction therapy at the MD Anderson Cancer Center and were classified either as primary refractory (failing to achieve complete remission on initial remission induction therapy) or relapsed (recurrent leukemia after having achieved a complete remission) were evaluated. A total of 1211 patients underwent remission induction therapy between 1975 and 1990. Of this group, 151 were considered primary refractory to treatment and 476 achieved a complete remission and subsequently relapsed. Of the primary refractory patients, 105 (70%) went on to receive salvage therapy at our institution and of those patients that relapsed 405 (85%) went on to receive salvage therapy. Thus a total of 510 patients underwent salvage therapy at the MD Anderson Cancer Center between 1975 and 1990. Twenty-one percent of these patients were primary refractory, 46% had an initial remission duration of less than 12 months, and 33% had an initial CR duration of greater than 12 months. The patient characteristics are illustrated in Table 1. A substantial number of patients had prior malignancies or prior myelodysplastic syndrome. A small proportion of the patients had organ dysfunction and poor performance status which would have interdicted their being treated on most salvage protocols.

Table 1. Characteristics of salvage AML population: 1974–1991

Total	510
Male/female	55% : 45%
Age <50 years	56%
Primary refractory	21%
	>67%
CR duration <12 months	46%
Prior malignancy	9%
Prior MDS	20%
Creatinine >2 mg%	3%
Bilirubin >2 mg%	4%
Performance status 3–4	6%

A variety of treatment options were used during the time period under discussion. Conventional dose ara-C (50–200 mg/m^2 per day for 5–10 days), used either alone or combined with other agents such as anthracyclines, amsacrine, or mitoxantrone, was administered to one-sixth of the patients. A variety of high-dose and intermediate-dose ara-C regimens have been used either alone or combined with the above-mentioned agents. Intermediate dose ara-C is defined as being in the range of 500 to 1 000 mg/m^2 given every 12 h. High-dose cytosine arabinoside is 3 g/m^2 given over 2 h every 12 h. In addition, a number of patients received

continuous infusion therapy with high-dose ara-C (doses of 1.5–3 g/m^2 per day for 4–5 days). These regimens respectively are classified as intermediate- and high-dose ara-C ± other drugs. Approximately one-fourth of the patients received such regimens. A number of patients received an anthracycline or amsacrine as a single agent and a small number received mitoxantrone either as a single agent or combined with etoposide (VP-16) as their initial salvage therapy. Six percent of patients underwent transplant. Approximately one-fourth of the patients received a variety of phase I/II studies as their first salvage therapy and are classified as miscellaneous (Table 2).

Table 2. Regimens used in first salvage AML treatment, 1974–1991

Regimens	No.	Percent
Conventional dose ara-C/others	84	16.5
High- and intermediate-dose ara-C/others	137	26.9
Anthracyclines	67	13.1
Amsacrine	45	8.8
Mitoxantrone ± VP-16	23	4.5
Transplant	31	6.1
Miscellaneous	121	23.7

Before combining such diverse patient populations together, the outcome of therapy during various time periods was evaluated. The patients were split into the time periods of 1974–1980, 1981–1985, and 1986–1991 and compared for outcomes. As seen in Table 3, the complete remission rate, the proportion of patients dying on study, and the proportion of patients who were resistant were very similar during the observed time periods. In addition, as illustrated in Fig. 1, the survival of patients during the same three time periods was almost identical.

Results

Of the 510 patients treated, 155 (30%) obtained a complete remission; 129 (25%)

Table 3. Response to initial salvage treatment of AML by time period

Time period	No. pts.	% CR	% Died	% Resistant
1974–1980	181	29	25	46
1981–1985	153	31	26	43
1986–1991	176	31	25	44

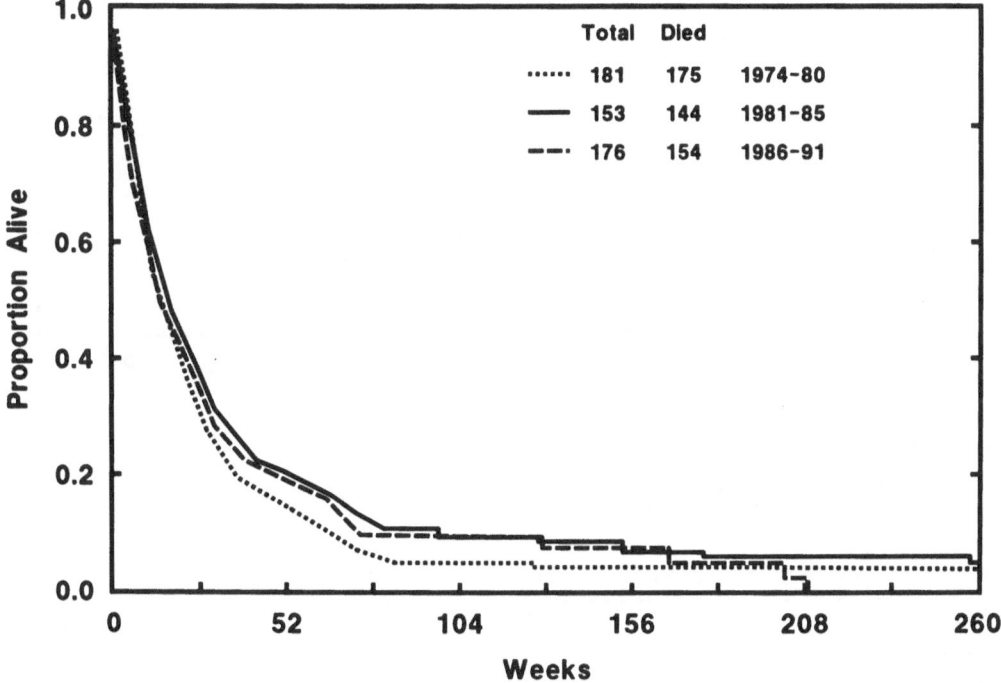

Fig. 1. Survival AML first salvage by time period

died during their salvage treatment attempt and 226 (44%) were resistant but survived their remission induction therapy. The times to either achieving complete remission or dying are illustrated in Fig. 2. Eighty-five percent of the patients who were classified as complete remission or died had reached that status by 8 weeks.

The response rate according to the different treatment regimens used is illustrated in Table 4. There was a variation in treatment outcome with complete remission rates of 24%–52%, death rates of 19%–35%, and resistance of 19%–48%. The exception to this was in the miscellaneous group of studies where patients received a variety of phase I–II regimens. In

this group the complete remission rate was only 7%. The proportion of patients who were resistant to these therapies is also higher than for regimens of proven activity.

A number of characteristics associated with probability of achieving a complete remission or probability of dying following salvage therapy for AML were evaluated. The results are illustrated in Table 5. Overall, there was a fairly good correlation with the probability of different patient characteristics predicting for the outcomes of complete remission or inversely death. For example, patients with a long initial complete remission had a high probability of achieving a complete remission and a low

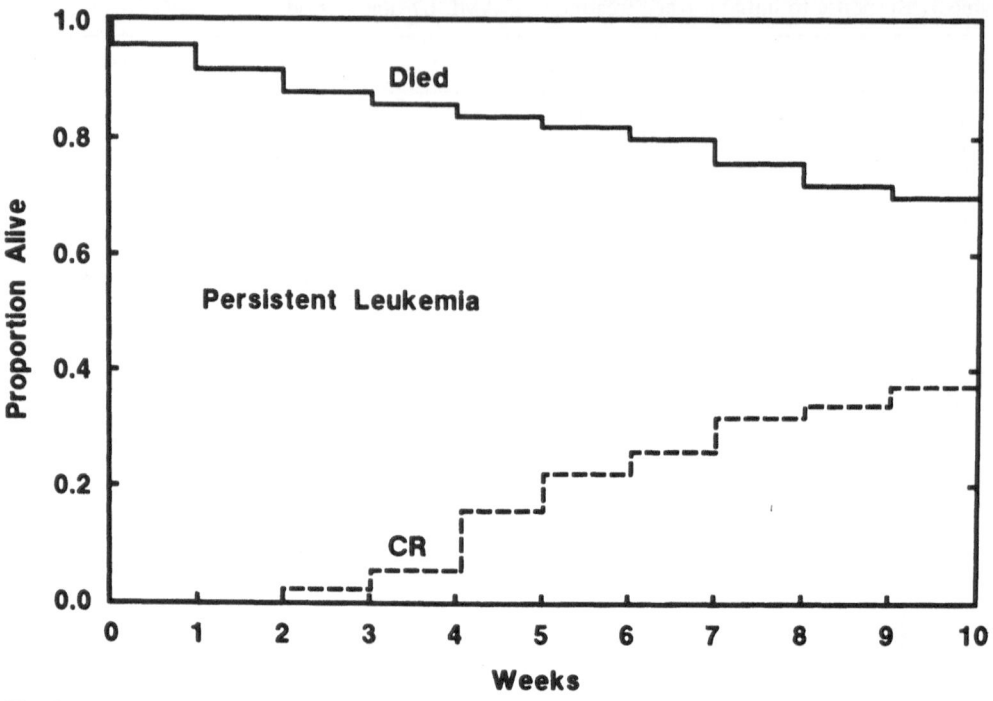

Fig. 2. Time to response: first salvage AML

Table 4. Outcome of salvage therapy according to regimen used

Regimen	Patient	% CR	% Died	% Resistant
Conventional ara-C	84	39	19	42
High-dose ara-C	140	42	25	33
Anthracycline	67	24	28	48
Amsacrine	45	29	27	44
Mitoxantrone ± VP-16	23	39	35	26
Transplant	31	52	29	19
Miscellaneous	121	7	25	69

probability of dying during remission induction therapy. A similar pattern was noted for various cytogenetic groups. Patients who were older had a lower likelihood of obtaining a complete remission and a higher probability of dying during salvage therapy. Other parameters such as the LDH level, liver, and renal function, infection status at the time of initiating treatment, performance status, height of the white blood cell count, history of prior myelodys-plastic syndrome, hemoglobin level, and platelet count were all predictive for outcome.

The strongest predictor for probability of achieving remission was the duration of the initial remission duration or whether the patients were primary refractory to remission induction therapy (Table 6). Probability of CR, resistance, and death for patients who are primarily refractory or had remission duration of 1–6 months or 7–12 months

Table 5. Characteristics associated with probability of CR with salvage therapy of AML

	CR	Death
1. Duration of initial CR	+++	+++
2. Karyotype	+++	+++
3. Age	+++	+++
4. LDH level	++	++
5. Organ function	+++	+++
6. Infection status	+	+++
7. Albumin level	++	+++
8. Performance status	+++	+++
9. WBC count	++	+++
10. Prior MDS	+++	+++
11. Hemoglobin level	--	+
12. Platelet count	+	+++

+, $p<.05$; ++, $p<.01$; +++, $p<.001$

was very similar. There was a fairly high proportion of patients who were primary refractory who died during their initial salvage attempt. There has been a steep increase in probability in achieving complete remission on salvage therapy for those who had been in remission for more than 12 months and in particular those who had been in remission for more than 18 months.

We have previously published a logistic regression model which is able to calculate an expectation for the probability of achieving complete remission on first salvage therapy [12]. The factors included in this model are the initial CR duration, the age of the patient, and the serum LDH value. This model was applied to the whole patient population (Table 6) and to the different treatment regimens. After adjusting for these characteristics, the observed vs. expected number of complete remissions was highest for the high-dose ara-C regimens and the mitoxantrone ± VP-16 regimens (Table 7). No predictive model has been developed for risk of dying during salvage therapy. The conventional dose ara-C regimens failed to match their expectation as did the anthracycline regimens. If the CR rates are compared for patients

Table 6. Prognostic factors for response to first salvage therapy

Characteristic	Value	Patients	% CR	% Died	% Resistant
Age (years)	<40	196	38	17	44
	40–49	89	33	18	49
	50–59	85	22	31	47
	≥60	141	20	38	41
Karyotype	inv16	28	64	4	32
	t(15;17)	23	70	17	13
	t(8;21)	35	37	20	43
	Diploid	227	32	20	48
	+8	35	14	51	34
	−5/−7	47	4	47	49
	Misc.	76	24	21	55
	Insufficient metasphases	35	20	40	40
Duration of initial CR (weeks)	0 (Refractory)	105	19	35	46
	4–25	109	17	25	59
	26–51	124	22	25	53
	52–77	86	43	20	37
	≥78	86	59	20	21
Probability of CR first salvage	<0.1	82	7	41	51
	0.1–0.19	97	16	36	49
	0.2–0.29	151	24	22	53
	0.3–0.39	36	39	17	44
	≥0.4	147	55	14	31

Table 7. Observed vs. expected CR rates for categories of treatment

Regimen	O/E ratio	
	CR	Death
Conventional ara-C	0.90	?
High-dose ara-C	1.23	?
Anthracyclines	0.82	?
Amsacrine	1.02	?
Mitoxantrone ± VP-16	1.38	?
Transplant	1.04	?
Miscellaneous	0.32	?

whose initial remission duration was short or long, it can be seen that all of the treatment regimens had their greatest activity in patients whose initial remission duration was prolonged (Table 8). A similar observation can be made for those with favorable cytogenetic categories such as t(8;21), t(15;17), and inv16. The diploid and miscellaneous groups of patients were intermediate; patients with trisomy of chromosome number 8 or loss of all or part of chromosomes 5 or 7 had a disappointing response whatever treatment regimen was offered to them.

The survival of patients who underwent first salvage therapy is strongly influenced by their response to the initial salvage therapy. Patients who were resistant to salvage attempts had a significantly worse outcome than those who achieved a complete remission on initial salvage treatment. Of those patients who did achieve a complete remission, 16% are alive at 5 years (Fig. 3). The duration of first complete remission is strongly associated with survival following the first salvage therapy. The only patients who were identified to have a reasonable probability of being alive at 5 years with a potential for cure on salvage therapy were those whose initial CR duration was greater than or equal to 18 months.

Discussion

This study reviews their outcome following first salvage therapy for AML at a major singular institution over a period of 15 years. The consistency of treatment outcomes for first salvage therapy and the consistency of the survival curves for three discrete time periods over that 15 years suggest that there has been no major advance in management of relapsed or refractory patients with AML over this time period. An uncontrolled variable in this analysis is the intensity of the treatment that the patients have received prior to being exposed to salvage therapy. On the other hand, no dramatic improvement in response rate or survival following salvage therapy occurred after the introduction of high-dose ara-C regimens or the use of agents such as amsacrine and mitoxantrone.

Table 8. Response to various treatment approaches: first salvage therapy for AML according to initial CR duration

Treatment	Refractory	Duration of initial CR (weeks)		
		4–51	52–77	≥78
Conventional ara-C ± others	0/4 (−)	3/30 (10)	9/19 (47)	19/30 (63)
High + Intermediate ara-C ± others	8/28 (29)[a]	14/54 (26)	16/27 (59)	20/32 (63)
Anthracyclines	2/7 (29)	9/42 (21)	2/14 (14)	3/4 (75)
Amsacrine	1/15 (7)	7/20 (35)	3/6 (50)	2/4 (50)
Mitoxantrone ± VP-16	2/5 (40)	6/14 (43)	0/3 (−)	1/1 (100)
Transplant	4/7 (57)	4/8 (50)	5/9 (56)	3/6 (50)
Miscellaneous	2/41 (5)	3/67 (4)	1/7 (14)	2/6 (33)
Total	20/107 (19)	46/235 (20)	36/85 (42)	50/83 (60)

[a] CR/total (%)

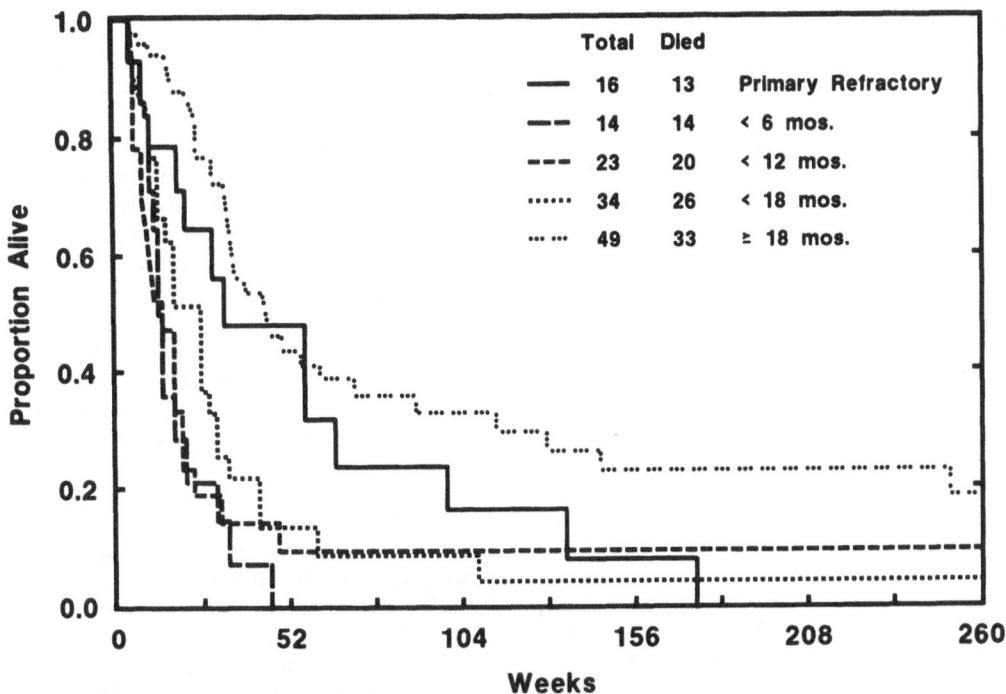

	Total	Died	
——	16	13	Primary Refractory
— —	14	14	< 6 mos.
– – –	23	20	< 12 mos.
·······	34	26	< 18 mos.
···· ···	49	33	≥ 18 mos.

Fig. 3. Complete remission duration AML first salvage by duration first CR

The major determinant of outcome on initial salvage therapy is the prior history of responsiveness of the patient to initial therapy [12, 13]. Patients who were refractory to their initial treatment regimen have a low probability of responding to any salvage program. Likewise, patients who had an initial response to treatment but relapsed in less than 12 months presumably have a substantial proportion of their leukemia cell population at time of initial diagnosis that has a resistant phenotype. Whether this is based on multi-drug resistance or some other phenotypic expression of resistance is uncertain. However, it is obvious that patients with more sensitive disease, namely those whose initial remissions lasted for more than 12 months, have the highest salvage response rate. This finding is similar to that of Hiddemann et al., where patients with long initial remissions had a high response rate and this superior survival compared with patients with refractory disease or short initial remissions [13]. They, however, found that patients whose initial remissions were between 6 and 12 months had a superior response rate than those with

shorter remissions. This discordance may be due to differences in prior treatment experience of the patient groups or favorable subsets of patients being included on different studies.

The major outcomes following initial remission induction therapy are complete remission and death during induction. The proportion of patients that are refractory to initial remission induction is approximately 10%. However, in salvage therapy, resistance emerges as a major feature. In even the most intensive regimens which include high-dose cytosine arabinoside alone or together with other treatments, one-third of the patients are refractory and many patients who die during salvage therapy have a substantial amount of residual leukemia at the time of death. This area appears to be a fertile ground for investigation of strategies for overcoming the resistant phenotype in AML.

While the duration of initial remission is strongly correlated with response and survival, the biologic determinant of karyotype cannot be overlooked. It is now well established that patients with inv16 or t(15;17) have long initial remission durations following initial therapy while patients who are t(; 21) or diploid have intermediate CR durations and those with other karyotypes have inferior CR durations [14]. Thus the karyotype is closely correlated with initial remission duration and is probably the major determinant of responsiveness to various chemotherapy regimens. The dismal response rate and survival of patients with abnormalities in chromosomes number 5 and 7 or trisomy of chromosome number 8 following salvage therapy reflects the low response rate and short initial remission duration following their first treatment regimen of these subsets [14]. It is obvious that new treatment approaches need to be undertaken for such patients.

Studies have been undertaken predicting the probability of early mortality in initial remission induction [15]. These factors include the age of the patient, organ function, performance status, infection status, neutrophil count, platelet count, hemoglobin level, etc. Similar features appear to apply to patients undergoing salvage therapy. The large number of factors that are associated with probability of complete remission and probability of dying during salvage therapy suggests that predictive models could be developed which can be prospectively applied and used as monitoring methods for sequential analysis of clinical trials. The prognostic factor model, which we developed and published [12], is useful prospectively in identifying probability of achieving complete remission.

The majority of treatment regimens which have been published as being very effective are single arm studies [6–11, 16, 17]. A major deficiency in these studies is that the pool of patients from which they have been derived is uncertain. For example, what proportion of patients refractory to initial treatment regimens actually go on to receive the reported salvage regimen? Likewise, are patients who have had short remissions less likely to return for aggressive chemotherapeutic approaches or are they more likely to be treated with palliative regimens. While it is important to develop regimens which are active and well tolerated, there is a deficiency in the salvage literature of comparative studies or efforts to provide meaningful information regarding the pretreatment characteristics of the patient population such as the number of patients who were refractory to initial remission induction therapy or had short remissions. One solution to this predicament could be the development of predictive models for complete remission and dying during therapy. However, an alternate method may be comparative studies. It is unlikely that the biology of leukemia is changing substantially but there are certainly consistent changes in referral practice to different institutions. Additionally entry criteria of patients onto protocols are more tightly defined now than previously. Unless particular attention is paid to detail, single arm studies, or comparisons with literature or historical controls are fraught with difficulty.

The fact that all of the treatment regimens are more effective in patients with long initial remission durations suggests that the actual treatment regimens that are offered are less important than the biologic determinants of the disease. Part of this may be due to the fact that there has been more intensive use of agents such as cytosine arabinoside and anthracyclines, mitoxantrone, etc. in recent years during the initial remission induction and intensification phases of patient's treatment histories. This factor may have a negative impact on the response to salvage therapy and survival after salvage therapy.

One challenging area is the concept of conducting phase I/II trials in first salvage patients. As is obvious from our analysis, the miscellaneous group of treatment regimens which include a number of phase I/II studies is associated with a low response rate and a high proportion of patients failing because of resistant disease. It appears reasonable to offer phase I/II studies to patients who were initially refractory to remission induction therapy or had remission durations of less than 12 months as the possibility of such patients achieving a complete remission on best conventional therapy is less than one in three and the chance of being cured with chemotherapy is almost nil. Thus, new approaches to treatment would seem best offered to this subset of patients. However, patients whose initial remission duration was greater than 18 months are very similar to patients who present with de novo disease with a high response rate to salvage therapy and a similar probability of long-term survival following relapse as de novo presentations of acute leukemia. This subset of patients might best be treated for cure on the treatment regimens being studied for front-line patients. Salvage therapy research is essential for us to develop new agents or combinations. In addition, it appears to be the most opportune area to investigate mechanism of overcoming resistance to established agents in AML.

References

1. Keating MJ, McCredie KB, Bodey GP, Smith TL, Gehan E, Freireich E (1982) Improved prospects for long-term survival in adults with acute myelogenous leukemia. JAMA 248: 2481–2486
2. Weinstein HJ, Mayer RJ, Rosenthal DS, Coral FS, Camitta BM, Gelber RD (1983) Chemotherapy for acute myelogenous leukemia in children and adults: VAPA update. Blood 62: 315–319
3. Keating MJ, Gehan EA, Smith TL, Estey EH, Walters RS, Kantarjian HM, McCredie KB, Freireich EJ (1987) A strategy for evaluation of new treatments in untreated patients: application to a clinical trial of AMSA for acute leukemia. J Clin Oncol 5: 710–721
4. Phillips GL, Reece DE, Shepherd JD, Barnett MK, Brown RA, Frei-Lahr DA, Klingemann H-G, Bolwell BJ, Spinelli JJ, Herzig RH, Herzig GP (1991) High-dose cytarabine and daunorubicin induction and postremission chemotherapy for the treatment of acute myelogenous leukemia in adults. Blood 77: 1429–1435
5. Buechner T and Hiddemann W (1990) Treatment strategies in acute myeloid leukemia (AML). Blut 60: 61–67
6. Keating MJ, Estey E, Plunkett W, Iacoboni S, Walters R, Kantarjian H, Andersson B, Beran M, McCredie KB, Freireich EJ (1985) Evolution of clinical studies with high-dose cytosine arabinoside at the M.D. Anderson Hospital. Semin Oncol 12: 98–104
7. Herzig RH, Wolff SN, Lazarus HM, Phillips GL, Karanes C, Herzig GP (1983) High-dose cytosine arabinoside therapy for refractory leukemia. Blood 62: 361–369
8. Preisler HD, Epstein J, Barcos M, Priore R, Raza A, Browman GP, Vogler R, Winton E, Grunwald H, Rai K, Brennan J, Bennett J, Goldberg J, Gottlieb A, Chervenick P, Joyce R, Miller K, Larson R, D'Arrigo P, Doeblin T, Stein M, Bloom M, Steele R, Lee H (1984) Prediction of response of acute non-lymphocytic leukaemia to therapy with "high dose" cytosine arabinoside. Br J Haematol 58: 19–32
9. Hiddemann W, Kreutzmann H, Straif K, Ludwig WD, Mertelsmann R, Donhuijsen-Ant R, Lengfelder E, Arlin Z, Buchner T (1987) High-dose cytosine arabinoside and mitoxantrone: a highly effective regimen in refractory acute myeloid leukemia. Blood 69: 744–749
10. Ho AD, Lipp T, Ehninger G, Illiger H-J, Meyer P, Freund M, Hunstein W (1988) Combination of mitoxantrone and etoposide in refractory acute myelogenous leukemia – an active and well-tolerated regimen. J Clin Oncol 6: 213–217
11. Hines JD, Oken MM, Mazza JJ (1984) High-dose cytosine arabinoside and m-AMSA in effective therapy in relapsed acute nonlymphocytic leukemia. J Clin Oncol 2: 545–549
12. Keating MJ, Kantarjian H, Smith TL, Estey E, Walters R, Andersson B, Beran M, McCredie KB, Freireich EJ (1989) Response to salvage therapy and survival after relapse in acute myelogenous leukemia. J Clin Oncol 7: 1071–1080
13. Hiddemann W, Büchner T (1990) Treatment strategies in acute myeloid leukemia (AML). Blut 60: 163–171
14. Keating MJ, Smith TL, Kantarjian H, Cork A, Walters R, Trujillo JM, McCredie KB, Gehan EA, Freireich EJ (1988) Cytogenetic pattern in acute myelogenous leukemia: a major reproducible determinant of outcome. Leukemia 2: 403–412
15. Estey E, Smith TL, Keating MJ, McCredie KB, Gehan EA, Freireich EJ (1989) Prediction of survival during induction therapy in patients with newly diagnosed acute myeloblastic leukemia. Leukemia 3: 257–264
16. Bjorkholm M, Bjornsdottir J, Stenke L, Grimfors (1990) Mitoxantrone, etoposide and cytarabine in the treatment of acute nonlymphocytic leukemia. Oncology 47: 112–114
17. Harrousseau JL, Reiffers J, Hurteloup P, Milpied N, Guy H, Riga-Huguet F, Facon T, Dufour P, Ifrah N for the French Study Group of Idarubicin in Leukemia (1989) Treatment of relapsed acute myeloid leukemia with idarubicin and intermediate-dose cytarabine. J Clin Oncol 7: 45–49

Cancer and Leukemia Group B Studies in Relapsed AML

E. J. Lee, P. C. Amrein, P. A. Paciucci, and C. A. Schiffer

In the past 20 years, substantial progress has been made in the treatment of acute myeloid leukemia (AML), previously a uniformly fatal diseae. Initial treatment usually consists of a combination of cytosine arabinoside (Ara-C) and daunorubicin, and complete remission (CR) is achieved in approximately 65 % of patients with somewhat higher response rates in younger patients. Once CR is achieved, further chemotherapy is necessary to produce long term disease free survival. However, the majority of patients will relapse; despite the use of these two active drugs as postremission therapy in schedules that have included a 30-fold increase in the dose of Ara-C, there has been, at best, only a modest improvement in survival. Thus, despite 15 year of use of the combination of daunorubicin and Ara-C, the fraction of patients cured with chemotherapy remains in the range 20 %–25 % [1–5]. Substantial improvement in long-term disease-free survival has been elusive.

Once relapse occurs, further use of the anthracycline/Ara-C combination rarely results in prolonged relapse-free survival. For this reason, many patients in first relapse of AML have been treated with chemotherapeutic agents not previously tested in AML. The possibility exists that new drugs may have different mechanisms of action and may not be cross-resistant with standard drugs. This lack of cross-resistance may be suggested by the ability to obtain CR in patients who have not achieved CR following Ara-C and daunorubicin (patients with refractory AML), by the demonstration of cure in patients who achieved CR but were not cured with standard initial treatment, and by the occurrence of longer remission durations following treatment with newer agents when compared to the duration of CR following initial treatment.

Cancer and Leukemia Group B (CALGB) and the University of Maryland Cancer Center (UMCC) have conducted a series of phase I and II studies in patients with relapsed and refractory AML, and have identified new drugs and combinations of new drugs that may not be cross resistant with anthracycline-Ara-C. The goal of such studies was to improve outcome for patients with AML in relapse, and to identify new active regimens for subsequent use in newly diagnosed patients with AML.

Diaziquone (AZQ) is a lipophilic aziridinylquinone synthesized with the goal of producing an agent with alkylating activity that could penetrate the central nervous system [6]. Initially, no activity was seen in patients with relapsed AML using a once daily schedule [7]. Based on pharmacokinetic data that showed a short plasma half-life in vivo, and in vitro studies suggesting that prolonged exposure was necessary for optimal cytotoxic effect [8], a continuous infusion trial was performed at the University of Maryland Cancer Center which documented a CR rate of 23 % [9]. There was little nonhematologic toxicity, with minimal mucositis. In the initial continuous infusion study at the UMCC, AZQ was given at a dose of 28 mg/m^2 per day for 7 days. Two patients treated on this initial

University of Maryland Cancer Center, 22 S. Greene St., Baltimore, Maryland 21201, USA

phase I study continue in unmaintained CR at 6.5 and 8 years after having relapsed following initial treatment with standard "3 + 7" induction and intensive, ara-C based, postremission chemotherapy. Half of the six patients who achieved CR had unmaintained CRs that were longer than those that followed primary treatment for AML.

Nonetheless, bone marrow aplasia was quite prolonged in this group of patients receiving a 7-day infusion, with a median of 48 days to granulocyte recovery (>500 PMN/μl). A second study was then done within CALGB with the duration of infusion reduced to 5 days. The CR rate for the 55 patients with AML treated in first relapse was 22 % with a median time to granulocyte recovery of 37 days [10]. Because there was again minimal nonhematologic toxicity, this drug seemed suitable for combination chemotherapy with other newly identified active agents.

Initially, AZQ was combined with m-AMSA [11] with acceptable toxicity but the combination did not seem to offer any advantage over the use of either drug alone. Subsequently, studies with etoposide and mitoxantrone have been done with the goal of identifying regimens for use as consolidation treatment for patients with AML in first remission.

A phase I trial of the combination of AZQ and etoposide at the University of Maryland Cancer Center [12], and two CALGB phase I trials of etoposide and mitoxantrone [13] and mitoxantrone and AZQ [14] were conducted simultaneously. These trials tested variable doses of AZQ and etoposide in combination with mitoxantrone at 12 mg/m^2 per day for 3 days. The two major dose-limiting toxicities encountered were prolonged bone marrow aplasia and mucositis, the latter particularly at dose of etoposide in excess of 150 mg/m^2 per day for 5 days by continuous infusion. The maximum tolerated doses of these drugs when used in combination were: AZQ 28 mg/m^2 per day for 5 days as a continuous infusion; etoposide 150 mg/m^2 per day for 5 days as a continuous infusion; mitoxantrone 12 mg/m^2 per day for 3 days as a bolus infusion.

In the study of AZQ/etoposide at the UMCC, more than half of the patients with AML in first relapse achieved unmaintained CR durations with the new combination that exceeded their initial CR duration following intensive postremission Ara-C based treatment, and one patient remains disease free at 3.5 years without any postremission therapy.

Subsequently, a randomized phase II study was initiated by CALGB to define the activity and toxicity of all three different couplets. Patients with relapsed or refractory AML were randomized to receive two of three drugs at the following doses: AZQ 28 mg/m^2 per day for 5 days by continuous infusion; etoposide 150 mg/m^2 per day for 5 days by continuous infusion; mitoxantrone 12 mg/m^2 per day for 3 days by bolus infusion. The preliminary results suggest that the major toxicity was performed myelosuppression, and that the combination of AZQ/mitoxantrone may be superior in patients in first relapse. The CR rats was 44 % for AZQ/mitoxantrone compared to 21 % and 22 % for the other combinations. Nonhematologic toxicity was relatively minimal with a small fraction of patients with significant mucosal toxicity [15].

A recent report by Brown et al. suggested that the combination of cyclophosphamide and etoposide in doses usually used with bone marrow transplantation has significant activity in patients with AML resistant to induction chemotherapy with high-dose Ara-C and daunorubicin, and that this regimen can be administered without bone marrow transplantation [15]. A CR rate of 42 % was reported for all patients with relapsed or refractory AML treated with this regimen, and a CR rate of 30 % was noted in patients who had failed to achieve CR following initial induction with high-dose Ara-C and daunorubicin. This level of activity is unusual in this highly resistant group of patients, and this regimen was thought to be a reasonable choice to combine with AZQ/mitoxantrone in the treatment of newly diagnosed, previously untreated patients. The combination of AZQ/mitoxantrone was chosen so as to provide maximum exposure to different chemotherapeutic drugs.

With the hope of improving the prognosis for newly diagnosed patients with AML, CALGB has planed and carried out a sequence of trials in untreated patients less than 60 years of age. The initial trial utilized what were felt to be "full" doses of potentially non-cross-resistant postremission therapy: AZQ 28 mg/m^2 per day for 5 days by continuous infusion and mitoxantrone 12 mg/m^2 per day daily for 3 days; cyclophosphamide (Cytoxan) 50 mg/kg daily for 4 days and etoposide 2.4 g/m^2 given at a dose rate of 70 mg/m^2 per hour. Many patients could not receive both of the planned courses of treatment, and myelosuppression was excessive with prolonged granulocytopenia. Of the 46 patients entered, there were five deaths from complications of postremission therapy.

A subsequent pilot study was then begun using attenuated doses of these agents: Cytoxan 50 mg/kg per day for 2 days and etoposide 1.8 g/m^2 by continuous infusion, followed by AZQ 28 mg/m^2 per day for 3 days by continuous infusion and mitoxantrone 12 mg/m^2 per day for 3 days, as well as a course of high-dose Ara-C (3 g/m^2 over 3 h twice daily on days 1, 3, and 5). There are, as yet, no data available about the toxicity of this sequence.

With the completion of this pilot study, the next trial is planned to be a phase III comparison in which newly diagnosed patients less than 60 years of age are treated with a standard daunorubicin/Ara-C induction followed by randomization between: the three cycle treatment currently being piloted using high-dose Ara-C followed by the two potentially non-cross-resistant regimens; the "best" arm of the current phase III study [4] which compares three different dose levels of Ara-C as postremission therapy (100 or 400 mg/m^2 given as continuous infusions for 5 days or high-dose Ara-C 3 g/m^2 given twice daily on days 1, 3, and 5).

References

1. Cassileth PA, Begg CB, Silber R, Spiers A, Burkart PT, Scharfman W, Knospe WH, Bennett JM, Mazza JJ, Oken MM, Keller AM, O'Connell MJ (1987) Prolonged unmaintained remission after intensive consolidation therapy in adult acute nonlymphocytic leukemia. Cancer Treat Rep 71: 137–140

2. Dutcher JP, Wiernik PH, Markus S, Weinberg V, Schiffer CA, Harwood KV (1989) Intensive maintenance therapy improves survival in adult acute nonlymphocytic leukemia: an eight-year follow-up. Leukemia 2: 413–419

3. Rees JKH, Gray RG, Swirsky D, Hayhoe FGJ (1986) Principal results of the Medical Research Council's 8th acute myeloid leukemia trial. Lancet II: 1236–1241

4. Schiffer CA, Mayer RJ for the CALGB (1990) Cancer and Leukemia Group B (CALGB) Studies in acute myeloid leukemia. In: Gale RP (ed) Acute myelogenous leukemia: progress and controversies. Wiley/Liss, New York, pp 313

5. Wolff SN, Marion J, Stein RS et al. (1985) High-dose cytosine arabinoside and daunorubicin as consolidation therapy for acute nonlymphocytic leukemia in first remission: a pilot study. Blood 65: 1407–1411

6. Bachur NR, Collins JM, Kelley JA, Van Echo DA, Kaplan RS, Whitacre M (1982) Diaziquone, 2,5-diaziridinyl-3,6-biscarboethoxy-amino-1,4-benzoquinone, plasma and cerebrospinal fluid kinetics. Clin Pharmacol Ther 31: 650–655

7. Van Echo DA, Schulman P, Budman DR, Ferrari A, Wiernik PH (1982) A phase I trial of aziridinylbenzoquinone (NSC 182986) in patients with previously treated acute leukemia. Am J Clin Oncol 5: 405–410

8. Egorin MJ, Fox BM, Spiegel JF, Gutierrez PL, Friedman RD, Bachur NR (1985) Cellular pharmacology in murine and human leukemic cell lines of diaziquone (NSC 182986). Cancer Res 45: 992–999

9. Lee EJ, Van Echo DA, Egorin MJ, Nayar B, Shulman P, Schiffer C (1986) Diaziquone given as a continuous infusion is an active agent for relapsed adult acute nonlymphocytic leukemia. Blood 67: 182–187

10. Schulman P, Davis R, Lee E, Ellerton J, Staszweski H for the Cancer and Leukemia Group B (1987) Phase II study of continuous-infusion diaziquone in relapsed/refractory acute nonlymphocytic leukemia. Cancer Treat Rep 71: 755–757

11. Schiffer CA, Davis RB, Mayer RJ, Peterson BA, Lee EJ (1987) Combination chemotherapy with diaziquone and amsacrine in relapsed and refractory acute nonlymphocytic leukemia: a Cancer and Leukemia Group B study. Cancer Treat Rep 71: 879–880

12. Lee EJ, Reck K, Schiffer C (1990) Continuous infusion diaziquone and etoposide: a phase I study in adult patients with acute leukemia. Leukemia 4: 189–192

13. Paciucci PA, Davis RB, Holland JF et al. (1990) Mitoxantrone and constant infusion etoposide for relapsed and refractory acute

myelocytic leukemia. Am J Clin Oncol 13: 516–519

14. Amrein PC, Davis RB, Mayer RJ, Schiffer CA (1990) Treatment of relapsed and refractory acute myeloid leukemia with diaziquone and mitoxantrone: a CALGB phase I study. Am J Hematol 35: 80–83

15. Lee EJ, Paciucci A, Amrein P, Schulman P, Davis R, Schiffer CA (1990) A randomized phase II trial of three regimens in the treatment of relapsed or refractory acute myeloid leukemia (AML) in adults: a CALGB study. Blood 76 [Suppl]: 294a

16. Brown RA, Herzig RH, Wolff SN, Frei-Lahr D, Pineiro L, Bolwell BJ, Lowder JN, Harden EA, Hande KR, Herzig GP (1990) High-dose etoposide and cyclophosphamide without bone marrow transplantation for resistant hematologic malignancy. Blood 76: 473–479

Clinical Trials in Adults with Relapsed and Refractory Acute Myelogenous Leukemia: The ECOG and the University of Rochester Experience*

J. M. Rowe[1], M. M. Oken[2], P. A. Cassileth[3], W. Andersen[4], J. M. Bennett[1], and P. H. Wiernik[5]

Introduction

The treatment of relapsed or refractory acute myelogenous leukemia remains mostly unsatisfactory. Although many patients can achieve a complete remission, the response duration is usually short and very few, if any, of these patients can be cured using chemotherapy alone. Bone marrow transplantation, allogeneic or autologous, offers the only hope for long-term survival. Results of such transplantation for refractory patients depend, to a significant degree, on the status of the patients at the time of transplantation; those in complete remission have a far better prognosis. While certain experimental agents are being studied, it is important to attempt to define a group of patients that are truly refractory and are less likely to respond to a standard salvage regimen. This report summarizes clinical trials conducted by the Eastern Cooperative Oncology Group (ECOG) and at the University of Rochester Medical Center for relapsed and refractory acute myelogenous leukemia (AML) patients and also discusses future directions of clinical trials in this group of patients.

Materials and Methods

EST 5483

This was a major ECOG study for relapsed and refractory AML patients with, additionally, randomization to determine if postremission maintenance therapy could affect the CR duration (Table 1).

Table 1. EST 5483: relapsed or refractory AML

		Maintenance
ARA-C 3 g/m² q12 h Days 1–6		ARA-C 10 mg/m² s.c.b.i.d. × 21 days
+	if CR	Repeat every 8 weeks to relapse
m-AMSA 100 mg/m² qd Days 7–9		*No Maintenance*

URCC 2482M

This was a study conducted at the University of Rochester and designed as a non-cross-resistant regimen for highly refractory patients (Table 2). No patients were treated

[1] University of Rochester, Hematology Unit (JMR) and Cancer Center (JMB), Rochester, NY (CA 11083), USA
[2] VA Medical Center, Minnepolis, MN, USA
[3] University of Pennsylvania Cancer Center, Philadelphia, PA, USA
[4] Dana Farber Cancer Institute, Boston, MA, USA
[5] Albert Einstein Cancer Center, Bronx, NY, USA
* This work was conducted by the Eastern Cooperative Oncology Group and supported in part by Public Health Service Grants (CA-21115) from the NCI, NIH, Department of Health and Human Services.

Table 2. URCC 2482M: AML

Relapsed (2nd, 3rd, or 4th)	Aclacinomycin A 60 mg/m^2 daily × 5 days
or	
Refractory	VP-16-213 100 mg/m^2 daily × 5 days

in first relapse unless they had failed reinduction at that stage. Additionally the study was unusual in that it did not exclude patients with hepatic or renal dysfunction or those with poor performances status and more than half of the patients had active infections at the start of therapy.

EST 1487

This is another ECOG study for relapsed or refractory AML patients (Table 3). It was initially designed as a non-cross-resistant regimen for relapsed patients who had previously received high-dose cytosine arabinoside as consolidation (EST 3483) or as treatment for relapse (EST 5483). The concept behind this combination is based on the demonstrated activity and apparent synergism using aclacinomycin A and VP-16-213 in URCC 2482M.

Table 3. ECOG 1487: AML

Relapsed (1st or 2nd)	Mitoxantrone 12 mg/m^2 daily × 5 days
or	
Refractory	VP-16-213 100 mg/m^2 daily × 5 days

For both URCC 2482M and for EST 1487 no maintenance therapy was included, although a considerable number of patients received some form of postremission therapy (including bone marrow transplantation).

Results

EST 5483

Very preliminary results indicate a very good response rate to this regimen of high-dose cytosine arabinoside followed by amsacrine for relapsed patients (Table 4). The response rate appeared comparable for first or second relapse patients who had not previously received this drug combination. Additionally there was a very significant response in truly refractory patients. Very preliminary analysis of the postremission randomization appears to show a significant benefit in terms of remision duration for those patients randomized to receive low-dose Ara-C 10 mg/m^2 sub-q bid for 21 days (repeated every 8 weeks) [1]. The patients who received this maintenance therapy had a median CR duration of approximately 8 months compared with 3 months for those patients who did not receive any maintenance therapy.

Table 4. EST 5483: relapsed or refractory AML, preliminary results

	N	CR rate
Relapsed (1st or 2nd)	163	57 %
Primary refractory	70	30 %

URCC 2482M

Results of this study have been published [2]. Of the 35 patients treated, there was an overall response rate of 40 %. This was considered a very satisfactory treatment result considering the extraordinarily high risk group of patients entered into this study, many of whom were accepted for "end-of-the-line" therapy.

EST 1487

This study is still ongoing and accruing patients in second relapse. Preliminary ana-

393

Table 5. EST 1487: AML, preliminary results

	N	Response rate	Median CR duration (days)
First relapse	35	57 %	121
Refractory (primary or secondary)	34	21 %	67

lysis, shown in Table 5, indicates a good response for patients who entered the study in first relapse. A less satisfactory response was obtained for refractory patients, although some of the observed responders had been completely refractory also to high-dose cytosine arabinoside. Further very preliminary analysis of the patients in first relapse indicates a significant difference in outcome based on a duration of the first remission (Table 6).

Table 6. EST 1487: AML, preliminary results

	Initial CR duration		
	<6 months	>6 months	
CR rate	3/13 (23 %)	15/22 (68 %)	$p = 0.009$

Discussion

Preliminary results from EST 5483 clearly demonstrate the efficacy of cytosine arabinoside and amsacrine in relapsed and refractory patients, although it is not clear what benefit, if any, was obtained by the addition of amsacrine and whether the latter served to increase the toxicity of this regimen. The preliminary data on the effect of maintenance therapy on the median CR duration is important as it may be the first time in a large prospective randomized trial that any form of maintenance therapy has been shown to affect the CR duration for relapsed or refractory patients. Additionally, if these data are confirmed, it will probably no longer by ethical to include a "no maintenance" arm in future clinical trials for relapsed or refractory AML patients. The synergistic effects of VP-16-213 with aclacinomycin A were demonstrated in URCC 2482M and the somewhat similar regimen that was used in 1487 – employing mitoxantrone with VP-16-213. The preliminary analysis of this latter regiment indicates that, while this combination proved highly effective for patients in first relapse, the response rate for refractory patients was clearly lacking although there was definite activity in some patients who were completely refractory to high-dose cytosine arabinoside.

Preliminary analysis of the response rate for patients treated in first relapse seem to indicate that there was a significant difference in outcome depending on the duration of the initial first CR. Specifically, those patients who entered the study after a short CR (<6 months) had a CR rate of only 23 % – similar to the response for refractory patients – while those who entered the study after a longer CR (>6 months) had a CR rate of 68 % – roughly comparable to the induction results in de novo AML. These preliminary results are important in that they suggest that patients who relapse after a short CR are more appropriately considered as truly refractory and should be so included in the future study designs as has been suggested by others [3]. Additionally, the results for patients who relapsed after a longer CR are not likely to be improved using new experimental agents, and the investigational use of these in AML should be reserved for patients who appear to be truly refractory. Other agents are being studied in an attempt to improve the results in remission induction for refractory AML patients. In a recently completeled study carboplatin was evaluated; it appears to have definite activity in refractory AML patients although the precise data are not yet available.

Future ECOG studies include evaluation of new agents such as menogaril and taxol, as well as an evaluation of the combination of cytosine arabinoside, mitoxantrone, and VP-16-213 for truly refractory patients. The use of hemopoietic growth factors, such as GM-CSF and IL-3, to stimulate the leukemic clone is also likely to be included in some future AML studies [4]. Future ECOG studies of postremission therapy for refractory patients are likely to include low-dose Ara-C as maintenance therapy while evaluating the use of other agents including interleukins (IL2) and, possibly, interferons. The overwhelming majority of relapsed or refractory patients will die, using chemotherapy alone. At the present time bone marrow transplantation offers the only therapy with curative potential and major efforts are clearly directed at improving the results of this mode of therapy for relapsed and refractory patients, as well as making it a therpeutically feasible option for a greater number of patients.

References

1. Oken MM, Kim K, Mazza JJ, Hines JD, Bennett JM, Cassileth PA, O'Connell MJ (1991) Maintenance low dose Ara-C (LDAC) improves complete remission (CR) duration from salvage induction therapy for relapsed and refractory acute myelogenous leukemia (AML) (abstract). ASCO (submitted)
2. Rowe JM, Chang AYC, Bennett JM (1988) Aclacinomycin A and etoposide (VP-16.213): an effective regimen on previously treated patients with refractory acute myelogenous leukemia. Blood 71: 992
3. Hiddemann W, Büchner T (1990) Treatment strategies for relapsed acute myelogenous leukemia – a proposal based on the definition of refractoriness against conventional chemotherapy. In: Gale RP (ed) Acute myelogenous leukemia: progress an controversies. Wiley/Liss, New York, pp 363
4. Estey E, Kurzrock R, Talpaz M, McCreadie K, Keating M, Kantarjian H, Freireich E, Gutterman J, Deisseroth A (1990) Use of C-CSFs in AML. In: Gale RP (ed) Acute myelogenous leukemia: progress and controversies. Wiley/Liss, New York, p 441

Intermediate-Dose Cytarabine in the Treatment of Relapsed or Refractory Leukemias

J. L. Harousseau and N. Milpied

High-dose cytarabine (HD ARA-C) has been extensively used in relapsed acute myeloid leukemia (AML), either alone [1] or in combination with asparaginase [2], daunorubicin (DNR) [3], amsacrine (AMSA) [4], or mitoxantrone [5]. With this high-dose regimen (3 g/m² twice daily for 4–6 days), high remission reinduction rates have been achieved, but at the expense of significant toxicity, in particular cerebellar toxicity [6]. This complication, which may be irreversible and/or fatal, is dose related and precludes total doses over 48 g/m² per cycle. It is mainly encountered for total doses of 36 g/m² (3 g/m² for 12 doses) or more. The incidence of severe cerebellar toxicity is also related to age, patients >50 years of age having a greater incidence than younger patients [6]. In order to reduce the major toxicities of HD ARA-C, some investigators have used combinations of AMSA or mitoxantrone (MTZ) at optimal dosage with ARA-C at lower cumulative doses [7, 8]. Van Prooijen et al. treated 15 relapsed AML patients with cytarabine (500 mg/m² every 12 h for 6 days) in combination with doxorubicin and vincristine and obtained 80 % CR [9]. Moreover, infusions of ARA-C at doses lower than the standard dose of 3 g/m² maintain plasma ARA-C levels sufficient to saturate the cellular ARA-CTP accumulation [10]. Thus, cytarabine could be used at intermediate-dose (ID ARA-C) with the same efficacy but less toxicity than in HD ARA-C containing regimens.

For several years, we have used ID ARA-C in the treatment of relapsed and refractory acute leukemias. We present here the results of three consecutive multicenter trials with ID ARA-C.

Patients and Methods

In these three studies, ID ARA-C was used at the dose at 1 g/m² q12 h (2 h infusion). In study 1, 35 patients with AML in first hematologic relapse received the IDA-RUB-ID ARA-C protocol [11], consisting of idarubicin (IDR) 8 mg/m² per day, days 1–5 and ID ARA-C 1 g/m² for 6 doses (days 1–3). In study 2, 30 patients with high-risk AML (refractory: 8 patients; in first relapse: 20 patients; chemoinduced: 2 patients) received a combination of mitoxantrone (MTZ) and ID ARA-C [12]. MTZ was given at the dose of 12 mg/m² per day for 5 consecutive days and ID ARA-C was given for 6 doses (7 patients) or 10 doses (23 patients). In study 3, 43 patients with relapsed (39 patients) or refractory (4 patients) ALL received the PAME protocol: prednisone 0.5 mg/k/day, days 1–5, ID ARA-C for 10 doses, MTZ 12 mg/m² per day, days 1–5, etoposide 200 mg/m² per day, days 6–8 [13]. The clinical characteristics of the 108 patients included in these three studies are listed in Table 1.

Results

The results are shown in Table 2. The overall CR rates were respectively 60 %, 57 %, and

Table 1. Clinical characteristics of the 108 patients

	Study 1 IDARUB – IDARA-C	Study 2 MTZ – IDARA-C	Study 3 PAME	
Total No. of patients (M/F)	53 (21/14)	30 (10/20)	43 (24/19)	
Median age (range)	56 (23–78)	51 (2–65)	28 (15–58)	
FAB classification	M1-2-3-6:27 M4-5 :8	M1-2-3-6:12 M4-5 :12	Immuno- phenotype	Common ALL 26 T ALL 8 ND 9

Initial WBC count (10 × l)
  Median
  Range
	
	15
	0.8–314
		
		6.8
		1.4–83
			
			8
			1–100	

Initial platelet count (10 × l)
  Median
  Range
	
	48
	12–440
		
		60
		6–212
			
			107
			11–490	

Disease status
  First relapse
  Refractory
  Chemoinduced
	
	35
	–
	–
		
		20
		8
		2
			
			39
			4
			–	

Duration of CR1[a] (months)
  Median
  Range
	
	16
	1–86
		
		10
		7–78
			
			5
			1–102	

Prior cumulative dose of
DNR (mg/m^2)
  Median
  Range
	
	280
	150–650
		
		270
		0–600
			
			270
			0–570	

Prior treatment with HD ARA-C	5/35	14/30	–	

[a] For patients in first relapse

Table 2. Results

	No. of patients	No. of CRs (%)	No. of PRs	Death during treatment or in aplasia	No. of failures
Study 1 (IDARUB – IDARA-C)	35	21 (60)	4	4	6
Study 2 (MTZ – IDARA-C)	30	17 (57)	–	5	8
Study 3 (PAME)	43	30 (70)	–	5	8

70% in the three studies. For patients in first hematologic relapse the CR rates were respectively 60% (21/35), 60% (12/20), and 72% (28/39). We have studied the influence on the therapeutic outcome of the following parameters: age, sex, FAB classification in study 1 and 2 (4–5 versus other subgroups) or immunophenotype in study 3, white blood cell count, platelet count, duration of first CR, cumulative dose of

DNR, and when appropriate (study 2) previous treatment with HD ARA-C.

In study 1, the only prognostic factor was the duration of the first CR. In the case of early relapse (before the median duration of 16 months) the CR rate was 35 % whereas it was 83 % in late relapse ($p = 0.003$).

In study 2, when relapses occurred after the median duration of the first CR (10 months) the CR rate was 78 % versus 50 % in early relapses. This difference was not significant ($p = 0.1$). The only predictive factor in this study was the previous use of HD ARA-C (as part of postremission consolidation therapy). Out of the 14 patients previously treated with HD ARA-C, only 21 % achieved CR, versus 87 % for the 16 patients who had not received this treatment ($p < 0.001$).

In study 3, none of the studied factors had a significant influence on the therapeutic outcome. The CR rate was not affected by the duration of the first CR (<5 months: 72 %, >5 months 71 %).

Toxicity

Hematologic Toxicity

In patients achieving CR, the duration of neutropenia ($<0.5 \times 10^9$/l) was 15–38 days (median 23 days) in study 1, 17–49 days (median 24) in study 2, and 10–52 days (median 24) in study 3. The median durations of thrombocytopenia ($<30 \times 10^9$/l) were respectively 19, 24, and 20 days. There were four infectious deaths in study 1, four in study 2 and five in study 3.

Extrahematologic Toxicity

A summary of extrahematologic side effects is given in Table 3. In study 1, diarrhea, skin toxicity, and hepatic disturbances which are complications of HD ARA-C therapy were rare and mild. No ocular or cerebellar toxicity was recorded. The overall extrahematologic tolerance was good with only 17 % severe mucositis. In study 2, apart from nausea and vomiting, the main side effect was mucositis scored as grade 3–4 of the WHO classification in 31 % of the cases. Grade 3–4 diarrhea and hepatic toxicity were more frequent than in study 1 (17 % and 20.5 %). Skin reactions were noted in 34.5 % of the cases but were always mild transient. Reversible cerebellar toxicity was noted in three patients. In study 3, mucositis was the most pronounced side effect with 46 % of the patients experiencing WHO grade 3 or 4. No significant ocular or skin toxicity was recorded and only one patient had reversible cerebellar toxicity. Overall, 13 cardiac events (12 %) were reported, including 3 congestive heart failures (2 in study 2, 1 in study 3). None of them was fatal.

Discussion

In these three consecutive studies, ID ARA-C was used at the same dosage (1

Table 3. Extrahematologic toxicity (WHO grade)

Toxicity	Study 1 IDARUB–IDARA-C	Study 2 MTZ–IDARA-C	Study 3 PAME
Nausea/vomiting	71.5 (28.5)	89.5 (41)	91 (21)
Diarrhea	20 (0)	62 (17)	NA
Mucositis	28.5 (17)	86 (31)	88 (46)
Hepatic	29 (3)	55 (20.5)	46 (5)
Cardiac	11.5 (0)	7 (7)	16 (2)
Cutaneous	3 (0)	34.5 (0)	0 (0)
Cerebellar[a]	0 (0)	10 (3)	2.5 (2.5)

Numbers refer to percentages of recorded side effects and number in parentheses to percentages of WHO grade 3–4
[a] Herzig grading [1]

g/m^2 q12 h) for 3 or 5 days (six or ten doses) in combination with IDR (study 1), MTZ (study 2) or MTZ, etoposide and prednisone (study 3). The incidence of side effects described with HD ARA-C containing regimens was low. There was no conjunctivitis and no severe or fatal cerebellar toxicity even in patients over the age of 50 years. Diarrhea, skin toxicity, and hepatic disturbances were rare and mild except in study 2. The cardiac tolerance of IDR and MTZ in patients pretreated with anthracyclines were good with only 13 cardiac events and three congestive heart failures. In fact the major side effect was mucositis, noted in all three studies and severe in almost half of the patients in study 3. This side effect was attributed mainly to IDR, MTZ and/or VP16.

Thus, these ID ARA-C containing protocols appeared to be well tolerated, even in patients >50 years of age, and as a result of this good tolerance the CR rate was not affected by age. All three regimens were very effective in relapsed leukemias with CR rates of 60%, 60%, and 72%. The number of refractory leukemias treated was too small to draw any conclusion in this indication but 5 out of 12 refractory patients achieved CR. It is difficult to compare the results obtained in published trials because of differences in the age of the patients, the status of the disease (refractory or not), the length of first CR, and the nature of prior treatments. However, the results of these three studies appear comparable to those achieved with HD ARA-C containing regimens in AML [1–6, 8, 14] or ALL [15]. These protocols are now used in frontline therapy of acute leukemias as induction or consolidation treatments.

Two prognostic factors appeared: the duration of first CR in study 1 and prior treatment with HD ARA-C in study 2. The current protocols, at least in AML, frequently include intensive consolidation therapy with HD ARA-C. In these protocols, the relapses occur early, mainly within 1 year of CR. In the future, this will probably raise again the issue of relapse management. More aggressive combination protocols will certainly increase the toxicity. Thus new directions must be explored, such as potentialization of drug-induced cyto-toxicity by hemopoietic growth factors or drug-resistance gene expression reversal.

References

1. Herzig RH, Wolff SN, Lazarus HM et al. (1983) High dose cytosine arabinoside therapy for refractory leukemia. Blood 62: 361–369
2. Capizzi RL, Poole M, Cooper MR et al. (1984) Treatment of poor risk acute leukemia with sequential high dose ARA-C and asparaginase. Blood 63: 654–700
3. Herzig RH, Lazarus HM, Wolff SN et al. (1985) High dose cytosine arabinoside with and without anthracycline antibioties for remission induction of acute non lymphoblastic leukemia. J Clin Oncol 3: 992–997
4. Hines JD, Oken MM, Mazza J et al. (1984) High dose cytosine arabinoside and M-AMSA is effective therapy in relapsed acute nonlymphocytic leukemia. J Clin Oncol 2: 545–549
5. Hiddemann W, Kreutzmann H, Strait K et al. (1987) High dose cytosine arabinoside and mitoxantrone: a highly effective regimen for refractory adult acute myeloid leukemia. Blood 69: 744–749
6. Herzig RH, Hines JD, Herzig GP et al. (1987) Cerebellar toxicity with high dose cytosine arabinoside. J Clin Oncol 5: 927–932
7. Marcus RE, Catovsky D, Goldman J et al. (1985) Mitoxantrone and high dose cytarabine in adult acute myeloid leukemia. Lancet i: 1384
8. Arlin ZA, Ahmed T, Mittelman A et al. (1987) A new regimen of amsacrine with high-dose cytarabine is safe and effective therapy for acute leukemia. J Clin Oncol 5: 371–375
9. Van Prooijen HC, Dekker AW, Punt K (1984) The use of intermediate dose cytosine arabinoside (ID ARA-C) in the treatment of acute non lymphocytic leukaemia in relapse. Br J Haematol 57: 291–299
10. Plunkett W, Lillemark JO, Adams T et al. (1987) Saturation of 1-βD arabinoside/cytosine 5'-triphosphate accumulation in leukemia cells during high dose 1-βD arabinofuranoside/cytosine therapy. Cancer Res 47: 3005–3011
11. Harousseau JL, Reiffers J, Hurteloup P, Milpied N, Guy H, Rigal-Huguet F, Facon T, Dufour P, Ifrah N for the French Study Group of Idarubicin in Leukemia (1989) Treatment of relapsed acute myeloid leukemia with idarubicin and intermediate-dose cytarabine. J Clin Oncol 7: 45–49

12. Harousseau JL, Milpied N, Brière J, Desablens B, Ghandour C (1990) Mitoxantrone and intermediate-dose cytarabine in relapsed or refractory acute myeloblastic leukemia. Nouv Rev Fr Hematol 32: 227–230
13. Milpied N, Gisselbrecht C, Harousseau JL, Sebban C, Witz F, Troussard X, Gratecos N, Michallet M, Le Blond V, Auzanneau G, Fiere D (1990) Successful treatment of adult acute lymphoblastic leukemia after relapse with prednisone, intermediate-dose cytara-bine, mitoxantrone and etoposide (PAME) chemotherapy. Cancer 15: 627–631
14. Zittoun R, Bury J, Stryckmans P et al. (1985) Amsacrine with high dose cytarabine in acute leukemia. Cancer Treat Rep 69: 1447–1448
15. Arlin ZA, Feldman E, Kempin S et al. (1988) Amsacrine with high-dose cytarabine is highly effective therapy for refractory and relapsed acute lymphoblastic leukemia in adults. Blood 72: 433–435

Mitoxantrone, Etoposide, and Intermediate-Dose Cytosine Arabinoside (MEC): An Effective Regimen for Refractory Acute Myeloid Leukemia

S. Amadori, A. M. Testi, M. Vignetti, A. Spadea, P. Fazi, A. P. Iori, G. Isacchi, and F. Mandelli

Treatment of acute myeloid leukemia (AML) frequently induces complete remission (CR) with initial induction chemotherapy. However, long-term disease-free survival is achieved in only a minority of patients, since the majority ultimately relapse [1]. The prognosis of patients who fail to achieve an initial CR or who experience recurrence of their leukemia remains dismal. Results of salvage therapy have been generally disappointing with low response rates and occasional long-term survivors in most studies [2]. Recently, we reported that a combination of intermediate-dose cytosine arabinoside (Ara-C) and mitoxantrone could induce CR in 24/36 (67%) patients with advanced AML, without undue toxicity [3]. Responses were observed in 85% of patients whose initial remission lasted for more than 6 months, but in only 28% and 33% of those with primary refractory disease and shorter remission duration, respectively.

In an attempt to improve on the results of salvage therapy for patients with poor-risk advanced AML, a modified regimen (MEC) was developed at our institution with the addition of VP-16 to the basic intermediate-dose Ara-C and mitoxantrone combination, and applied to 32 patients with refractory AML.

Materials and Methods

Between February 1988 and March 1990, 32 consecutive eligible patients with refractory AML were entered into the study after informed consent was obtained. Clinical characteristics of the patients are detailed in Table 1. All patients were recruited from the current Italian multicenter trials (EORTC-GIMEMA AML-8 for adults; AIEOP LAM-87 for children) and had received a standardized induction treatment with daunorubicin and conventional-dose Ara-C. For the purpose of this study, definition of refractory AML was made according to the following criteria: (1) failure to enter CR after two induction courses, or earlier evidence of absolute drug resistance as defined by the reappearance of circulating blasts and/or persistence of a hypercellular leukemic marrow 14–21 days from start of therapy; (2) relapse occurring within 6 months from initial CR; (3) relapse after bone marrow transplantation (autologous or allogeneic). The MEC

Table 1. Patient characteristics

No. of patients	32
Male/female	19/13
Median age in years (range)	24 (5–56)
Morphology (FAB)	
M1–M3	10
M4–M5	22
Disease status	
Primary resistance	18
Early relapse	8
Relapse after BMT	6

Section of Hematology, Department of Human Biopathology, University La Sapienza, Via Benevento 6, 00161 Rome, Italy

regimen consisted of a single 6-day course of mitoxantrone 6 mg/m², etoposide 80 mg/m² and intermediate-dose Ara-C 1 g/m² daily on days 1–6. The three drugs were administered intravenously according to the following sequence: the 6-h infusion of Ara-C was preceded by a short (1 h) infusion of VP-16 and followed, 3 h later, by a bolus of mitoxantrone. Patients who achieved CR were given a second 4-day course of MEC as consolidation and then submitted to an individualized program of postremission therapy.

Results

Of the 32 patients entered on study, 21 (66 %) achieved CR; 2 patients (6 %) died during marrow hypoplasia of infection, and 9 (28 %) had resistant disease. The median time from initiation of treatment to documentation of CR was 33 days (range 25–55 days). Of the various pretreatment variables examined, only age was significantly correlated with attaining CR (Table 2). Patients younger than 50 years of age had a CR rate of 76 % compared to 29 % for older patients ($P = 0.03$). Though not statistically significant, a difference was seen in response rate when patients were grouped by status of disease. Primary resistant patients

Table 2. Response by patient characteristics

Character-istics	No. of CR/Total	% CR	P value
Age (years)			
<50	19/25	76	0.03
>50	2/7	29	
Sex			
Male	12/19	63	NS
Female	9/13	69	
FAB			
M1–M3	8/10	80	NS
M4–M5	13/22	59	
Disease status			
Primary resistance	10/18	56	
Early relapse	7/8	87	NS
Relapse after BMT	4/6	67	

had a CR rate of 56 % compared to 87 % for patients who presented in early relapse and to 67 % for those relapsing after a bone marrow transplant. The median remission duration was 16 weeks (range 6–119+) and three patients are presently alive in continuous complete remission after 47–119+ weeks. Overall, relapse has occurred in 17 patients 6–117 weeks from CR (median 15 weeks); one additional patient died in CR at 32 weeks of massive intracranial bleeding while persistently thrombocytopenic following a bone marrow autograft. The overall median survival for the 32 patients on study was 36 weeks (range 2–124+ weeks).

Severe myelosuppression was documented in all patients, resulting in fever or documented infections in 91 % of patients. Nonhematologic toxicity was minimal, consisting mainly of tolerable nausea and vomiting, and mild to moderate mucositis.

Discussion

The results of this study indicate that the MEC regimen is a very effective and tolerable salvage chemotherapy program for patients with refractory AML. Overall, 66 % of patients entered CR after a single induction course. Toxicity was acceptable with an induction mortality rate of only 6 %.

These results compare favorably with those of recent salvage trials for AML in which inclusion criteria similar to ours were adopted [4, 5], as well as with our past experience involving the use of intermediate-dose Ara-C and mitoxantrone for patients with poor-risk advanced AML [3]. Addition of a third active drug such as VP-16 apparently resulted in a potentiation of the antileukemic activity of the basic intermediate-dose Ara-C and mitoxantrone combination, without adding too much toxicity. CR rates of 56 % and 87 %, respectively, for patients with primary resistant and early relapsed AML are among the best ever reported in the literature. Furthermore, the 67 % CR rate obtained in patients relapsing after bone marrow transplantation confirms the high antileukemic activity of the MEC regimen, which may be superior to the previous salvage program.

These encouraging results warrant its investigation in front-line AML therapy.

References

1. Champlin RE, Gale RP (1987) Acute myelogenous leukemia: recent advances in therapy. Blood 69: 1551–1562
2. Hiddemann W, Büchner T (1990) Treatment strategies in acute myeloid leukemia (AML). B. Second line treatment. Blut 60: 163–171
3. Amadori S, Meloni G, Petti MC, Papa G, Miniero R, Mandelli F (1989) Phase II trial of intermediate dose Ara-C (IDAC) with sequential Mitoxantrone (MITOX) in acute myelogenous leukemia. Leukemia 3: 112–114
4. Hiddemann W, Kreutzmann H, Straif K, Ludwig WD, Mertelsmann R, Donhuijsen-Ant R, Lengfelder E, Arlin Z, Büchner T (1987) High-dose cytosine arabinoside and mitoxantrone: a highly effective regimen in refractory acute myeloid leukemia. Blood 69: 744–749
5. Ho AD, Lipp T, Ehninger G, Illiger H-J, Meyer P, Freund M, Hunstein W (1988) Combination of Mitoxantrone and Etoposide in refractory acute myelogenous leukemia. An active and well-tolerated regimen. J Clin Oncol 6: 213–217

Intermediate-Dose Arabinoside and Amsacrine: An Effective Regimen in Relapsed and Refractory Acute Leukemia

V. Heinemann and U. Jehn

Introduction

Adequate treatment of poor prognosis acute myeloid (AML) and lymphocytic leukemia (ALL) such as refractory and relapsed acute leukemia still remains a major challenge of research. High-dose cytosine arabinoside (ara-C) (HD ara-C) containing regimens were introduced because of their non-cross-resistance to conventional-dose ara-C. Monotherapy with HD ara-C in relapsed patients was effective to a similar degree as combination regimens containing anthracyclines or mAMSA [1]. However, combination regimens appeared preferable specifically in the treatment of refractory leukemia [1–4]. Pharmacological considerations led to the use of intermediate-dose ara-C (ID ara-C), which promised a decrease in treatment-associated toxicity while therapeutic efficacy was maintained [5]. We present an updated [6] evaluation of our experience using ID ara-C and mAMSA as reinduction treatment for relapsed and refractory AML and ALL.

Patient Characteristics and Methods

Patients of all age groups and French-American-British (FAB) subtypes with relapsed, primary or secondary refractory AML ($n=45$) and ALL ($n=3$) were included in this phase II study. *Pretreatment*

Department of Internal Medicine and Hematology/Oncology Klinikum Grosshadern, University of Munich, Marchionistr. 15, D-800-Munich 70, FRG

in relapsed patients consisted of either intensive or conventional or no maintenance. The majority of patients in first relapse experienced their relapse during or after completion of intensive maintenance treatment according to the EORTC-AML 6 programm [7, 8]: they had been randomized to either six courses of the induction type (DNR 45 mg/m^2 i. v. day 1 plus ara-C 100 mg/m^2 s. c. days 1–5) or to six courses of a non-cross-resistant drug combination alternating mAMSA (150 mg/m^2 i. v. day 1) plus ara-C (3 g/m^2 i. v. q 12 h days 1 and 2) with AMSA plus 5-azacytidine (150 mg/m^2 i. v. days 1–3). Conventional maintenance included for AML patients the EORTC-AML 5 program [9] or for ALL patients the German Cooperative Adult ALL study [10]. Patients relapsing without prior maintenance had either a 3/7-type regimen or TAD 9 [11] for induction. Patients in second relapse were pretreated either with a 3/7-type regimen or a combination of ID ara-C/AMSA [12] or of HD ara-C/AMSA/5-AZA [13] during first relapse. *Refractory patients* were defined as being resistant to one (6×AML, 1×ALL) or two courses (6×AML) of an anthracycline-containing induction regimen totaling a minimum of three and a maximum of six doses of DNR (45 mg/m^2) combined – for AML – with 7 or 14 doses of ara-C (200 mg/m^2). Patients with a history of myelodysplastic syndrome (MDS) or a second malignancy were included.

The *reinduction regimen* consisted of ID ara-C 1 g/m^2 i. v. every 12 h by a 2-h infusion for 6 days and mAMSA 120 mg/m^2 as a 1-h infusion on days 5, 6, and 7. One or two cycles for induction were given. When CR was reached, one course of intensive consolidation was administered consisting of HD ara-C 3 g/m^2 every 12 h by a 2-h infusion for 4 days and mAMSA 120 mg/m^2 i.v. day 5. The treatment-free interval between two induction cycles was 3–4 weeks. The interval between the kind of induction and the beginnung of consolidation was 4-5 weeks. No further therapy was given thereafter.

Disease-free survival (DFS) was measured from complete remission (CR) to relapse or death in CR. Duration of survival was calculated either from diagnosis or from CR to death. Transplanted patients or patients lost-to-follow-up were either censored as having relapsed or died at the time of bone marrow transplantation (BMT) or lost-to-follow-up or not censored at time of BMT. Survival curves were calculated according to the Kaplan-Meier method. Tests of statistical significance for difference in survival curves were performed using the two-tailed logrank test.

Results

A total of 48 consecutive patients (45 AML, 3 ALL) with either refractory ($n=13$) or relapsed ($n=35$) acute leukemia entered the study. The median age of refractory patients was 54 years, of relapsed patients 46 years. The median age of all patients was 49 years with a range of 18–67 years.

Four of the relapsed and one of the refractory patients who reached remission with this program received the identical regimen a second time at subsequent relapse yielding a total of 40 relapses, 31 first and 9 second relapses. One relapsed and two refractory patients had a previous history of MDS, another patient suffered in addition to refractory AML from cervical cancer stage II–III, one relapsed patient of stage I breast cancer. Median duration of the preceding first remission in relapsed patients was 9 months, of the preceding second remission 6 months. Median time from last chemotherapy to relapse was 4 months in all relapsed patients. The patient's characteristics are shown in Tables 1 and 2.

Table 1. Patient characteristics

Total (n)	48
Median age (years, range)	49 (18–67)
FAB	
M1 (1× mixed)	3
M2 (1× 2E)	15
M3	4
M4 (1× hybrid)	16
M5	5
M6	2
ALL (1× hybrid)	3
Refractory pts. (n)	13
Primary resistant	12
(11× AML, 1× ALL)	
Resistant second relapse	1
(1× AML)	
Median age (years)	54
Relapsed pts.	35
Median age (years)	46
Relapses	40
First	31
Second	9

Table 2. Pretreatment characteristics of relapsed patients

Duration of preceding remission (all) (median, months)	8.5
First	9
Second	6
Time from last chemotherapy to relapse (median, months)	4
Type of preceding chemotherapy (first relapse)	
Intensive maintenance (EORTC AML 6)	
Induction type (DNR/ara-C)	13
Alternating type (HD ara-C, AMSA/5-AZA)	7
Conventional maintenance	
AML (EORTC AML 5)	1
ALL (German Coop)	2
No maintenance	
3/7 type	7
ID ara-C/AMSA	1
Type of preceding chemotherapy (second relapse)	
ID ara-C/AMSA	4
3/7 type	4
HD ara-C/AMSA/5-AZA	1

Six out of 13 *refractory* patients (46%) reached CR, 5 after one cycle of ID ara-C/AMSA and 1 patient after 2 cycles. Five of 6 patients who achieved CR were older than 50 years. Four patients remained refractory and three died in hypoplasia. One patient died 10 days after reaching CR of a lung hemorrhage due to aspergillosis (Table 3). DFS of the six responders was 2.5 months, survival from time of CR 4.1 months. The overall survival of the six responders and the remaining seven nonresponding patients ($n=13$) from time of diagnosis was 5.3 months (Table 5). None of the responding refractory patients received a BMT.

Twenty-four out of 31 patients in first *relapse* (77.4%) and 7/9 in second relapse

(77.8%) reached CR, 29 after 1 cycle of ID ara-C/AMSA and 2 patients after 2 cycles regardless of the type of prior treatment. Response to reinduction treatment was independent of age in that 11/31 responding patients were aged ≥50 years as compared to 3/8 nonresponders.

One out of 40 patients reached a stable partial remission, 5/40 patients remained refractory, 3 were in first and 2 in second relapse. Three out of 40 patients died during hypoplasia without evidence of leukemic regrowth, all in first relapse. One patient died at the time of treatment evaluation in CR of a sudden lung hemorrhage due to aspergillosis. Four patients – three after first and one after second relapse – died in CR during hypoplasia following intensive consolidation with HD ara-C/AMSA. Four patients were transplanted within 1–3 months after reaching a second remission; two of them received an allograft and are in continued CR 37+ and 39.5+ months after BMT. Two patients received an autograft, one of which died shortly thereafter, and one is in continued CR at 22+ months (Table 3).

Table 3. Response to treatment

Total (n)	48	
Refractory	13	
Complete remission (primary resistant)		
One cycle	4	(46%)
Two cycles	1	
Complete remission (resistant relapse)		
One cycle	1	(46%)
Failure (refractory)	4	
Hypoplastic death	3	
Death in CR	1	
Relapses	40	
Complete remission (first relapse)	24/31	(77%)
One cycle	22	
Two cycles	2	
Complete remission (second relapse)	7/9	(78%)
One cycle	7	
Partial remission	1	
Failure (refractory)		
First	3	
Second	2	
Hypoplastic death, first	3	
Death in CR (after induction)	1	
Hypoplastic death in CR (after consolidation)	4	

Table 4. Remission incidence according to pretreatment characteristics

Relapses total	40
Complete remission	31
Duration of preceding first remission (median, months)	10.5
second remission (median, months)	9.5
Time from last chemotherapy to first relapse (median, months)	5
second relapse (median, months)	5.5
Failure	9
Duration of preceding first remission (median, months)	4.5
second remission (median, months)	3.5
Time from last chemotherapy to first relapse	2
second relapse	2.7

Table 5. Response to treatment

	BMT censored[a]		not censored	
DFS (median, months)				
Relapses (n=31)	3		3.5	
Refractory (n=6)	2.5		–	
Relapses + refractory (n=37)	3		2.9	
With consolidation (n=28)	3.3	p=.049	4.6	p=.032
Without consolidation (n=9)	1.9		2.2	
Survival CR[b]				
Relapses (n=31)	4.9		9.3	
Refractory (n=6)	4.1		–	
Relapses + refractory (n=37)	5		8.8	
Survival, all[c]				
Relapses (n=40)	5.8		7.2	
Refractory (n=13)	5.3		–	
Relapses + refractory (n=53)	5.7		6.4	
Responder (n=37)	6.1	p=.011	9.5	p=.004
Nonresponder (n=16)	2.4		4.4	

[a] Four patients receiving BMT within 3 months after achieving CR and one patient lost-to-follow-up at 3 months CR were censored
[b] Time from remission until death
[c] Time from diagnosis until death

Table 4 shows that responding patients after first and second relapse had a longer duration of preceding first and second remission than nonresponders (10.5 vs. 4.5 and 9.5 vs. 3.5 months). Similarly, the time from last chemotherapy to first or second relapse was longer in responding as compared to nonresponding patients (5 vs. 2 and 5.5 vs. 2.7 months). The type of preceding chemotherapy had no impact on whether another remission was or achieved or not.

Median DFS of 312 responding relapsed patients was 3 months when BMT patients were censored at the time of BMT, and 3.5 months without censoring. Correspondingly, survival from time of CR was 4.9 months (9.3 months without censoring at BMT). The median overall survival of responding plus nonresponding relapsed patients (n=40) was 5.8 months (7.2 months without censoring at BMT) (Table 5). A total of 37 *refractory and relapsed* patients reached CR after one or two cycles of induction. Their median DFS was 3 months. Nine out of these 37 patients did not receive intensive

consolidation after achieving CR because of patient refusal or toxicity during induction. Their median DFS was 1.9 months as compared to 3.3 months (p=0.049) of the 20 consolidated patients (Table 5). This difference was significant whether patients were censored at BMT or not. The overall survival of responding (n=37) and nonresponding (n=16) relapsed and refractory patients (n=53) was 5.7 months (6.4 months without censoring at time of BMT). The survival advantage of responding relapsed and refractory patients as compared to nonresponders became evident when both groups were compared (Table 5): responding patients (n=37) survived 6.1 months (9..5 months without censoring at BMT) while nonresponders had a median overall survival of 2.4 months (4.4 months without censoring at BMT). This difference was significant (p=0.011) for both censored or not censored cohorts. The major *toxicity* seen in this study was a noncardiogenic pulmonary edema due to ara-C as substantiated in detail elsewhere [14]. Eleven out of 48 patients (23 %) experienced this type

Table 6. Lung toxicity

Total	11/48 (23 %)
Recovery	7
Death	4
Type of preceding maintenance	
Intensive (EORTC AML 6)	3/11
DNR, ara-C, (induction type)	3/11
HD ara-C/AMSA/5-AZA (alternating)	3/11
Conventional (EORTC AML 5)	1/11
No Maintenance	4/11

of lung toxicity: seven patients recovered and four died. From our data, the incidence of pulmonary edema was not related to the type of preceding treatment and therefore independent of the cumulative dose of ara-C (Table 6). Lethal fungal infections were observed in three instances: twice asperigillosis of the lung and once a candida septicemia.

Discussion

Treatment with intermediate-dose ara-C/mAMSA was evaluated as induction therapy for refractory and relapsed acute leukemia. Complete remission was achieved in 46 % (6/13) of refractory patients. Comparable results were reported by others using high-dose ara-C for remission induction [15–17]. The patient's age did not serve as a prognostic factor for remission induction. Median DFS in this patient group was 2.5 months including one patient who died of a lung hemorrhage 10 days after reaching CR. While ID ara-C/AMSA proved to be effective in inducing remissions, remission duration was short indicating that follow-up treatment is needed in this cohort of patients. Such an attempt seems worth undertaking since the overall survival of responders and nonresponders was 5.3 months.

In relapsed patients, an overall CR rate of 77.5 % (31/40) was reached which compares favorably to other studies using high – or intermediate-dose ara-C [18–20]. In comparison, remission reinduction with a conventional-dose ara-C containing regimen yielded a CR rate of 59 % [21]. Remission was achieved independent of prior treatment or patient's age. In fact, remission rates were identical when patients were treated at first or second relapse (77 % vs. 78 %). The majority of patients (22/24) reached remission after one cycle of treatment, an observation which demonstrates high sensitivity of relapsed leukemia to intermediate-dose ara-C/AMSA. In accordance with previous reports, the probability of remission induction at relapse was positively correlated to initial remission duration (Table 4).

Median DFS of relapsed patients was short (3 months) and not significantly different from the refractory group. DFS was essentially independent of whether BMT patients were censored or not (3.0 vs. 3.5 months). It should be noted, however, that 5/31 patients died in CR, 4 of whom following intensive consolidation with HD ara-C, while one patient was lost-to-follow-up 2 months after reaching CR (20 %). These circumstances may have contributed to the short DFS.

Interestingly, while CR rates were significantly higher for relapsed than for refractory patients (77.5 % vs. 46 %), DFS (3 vs. 2.5 months) and survival of responders (4.9 vs. 4.1 months) were comparable for both groups. This finding may suggest that responding patients in relapsed and refractory leukemia share similar disease characteristics, particularly with regard to regrowth kinetics of leukemic cells. In good agreement with this hypothesis is the fact that the overall survival of responders plus nonresponders in relapsed and refractory patients is similar (5.8 vs. 5.3 months) (Table 5).

When refractory and relapsed patients were analyzed together, a DFS of 3 months was calculated. Patients who received consolidation treatment after remission induction showed a significantly ($p=0.049$) longer DFS (3.3 months) than patients who were not consolidated (1.9 months) (Fig. 1). Note again that a DFS of 3.3 months of the consolidated group includes 4/28 (15 %) patients who died in CR following consolidation with HD ara-C. Still, this observation appears to support the importance of consolidation treatment. However, it should be pointed out that the median DFS advantage of consolidated patients (1.4 months) was nearly identical to the time needed for the consolidation treatment itself. It may be concluded that ID ara-C/AMSA does induce apparent remissions, but leukemic regrowth after the end of treatment cannot effectively be prevented. Therefore, alternative approaches for post-remission therapy are warranted. Despite short DFS, treatment of refractory and relapsed leukemia provides a realistic benefit for the patient. In fact, ID ara-C/AMSA therapy clearly ($p=0.011$) yielded a survival advantage for responding patients (6.1 months) compared to nonresponding patients (2.4 months) (Fig. 2).

Four patients were transplanted in the relapsed group and none in the refractory cohort. Survivals of responding refractory and relapsed patients were nearly identical (4.1 vs. 4.9 months) when patients were censored at BMT. In contrast, when censoring was omitted, a survival advantage became apparent for the relapsed group where BMT was a treatment option once

patients had reached remission (4.1 vs. 9.3) (Table 5). However, this difference was not significant ($p=0.668$).

Because of the small number of responding refractory patients ($n=6$), relapsed patients were compared when censoring was performed at BMT versus no censoring (Fig. 3). Again, no significant difference was observed ($p=0.178$). Despite the lack of significance for median survival, the curves suggest that BMT seems beneficial as one option of postremission treatment, particularly when the individual patient is considered.

Toxicity of treatment was acceptable. Treatment-associated mortality amounted to an overall 25% (12/48) including six patients with hypoplastic death after induction and four patients with hypoplastic death in CR after intensive consolidation with HD ara-C. Pulmonary toxicity was observed as noncardiogenic pulmonary edema in 23% (11/48) of patients resulting in a fatal outcome in four patients. The modality of prior treatment had no impact on the incidence of pulmonary toxicity. In agreement with others [22], a relation between the cumulative dose of ara-C and the development of pulmonary toxicity could not be demonstrated (Table 6).

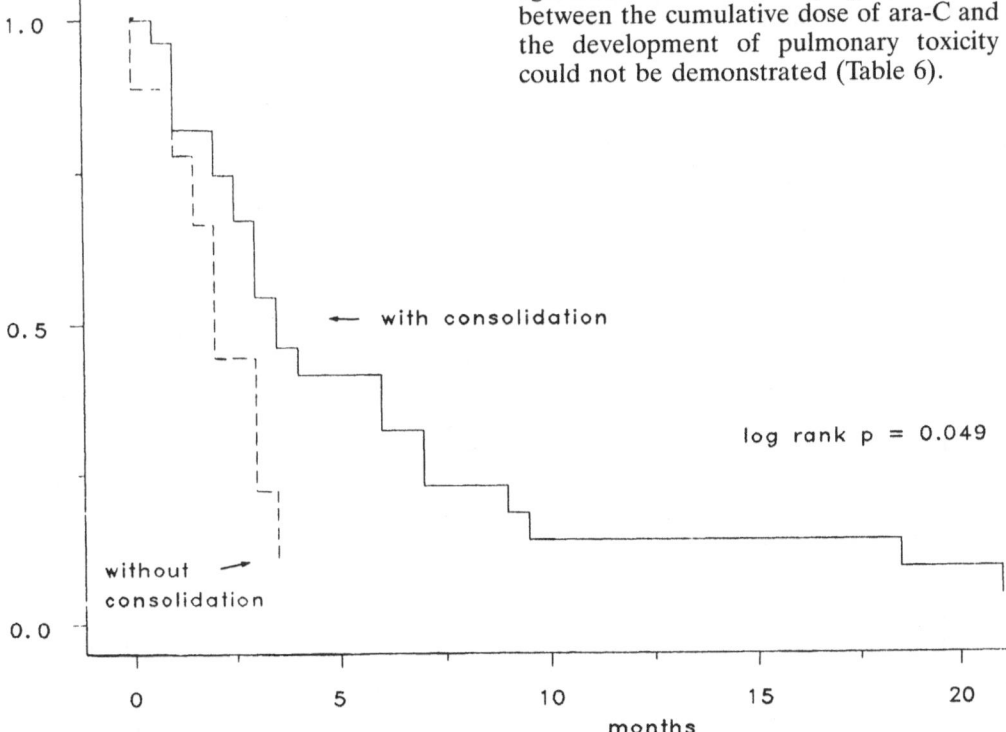

Fig. 1. DFS of relapsed and refractory pts receiving consolidation or not

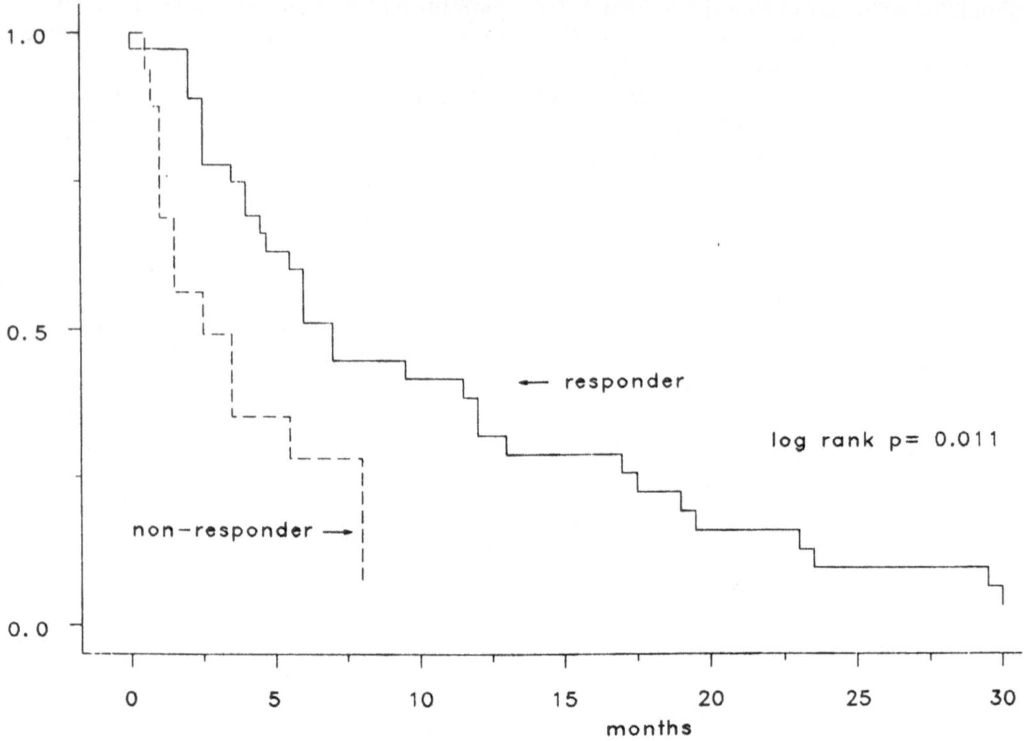

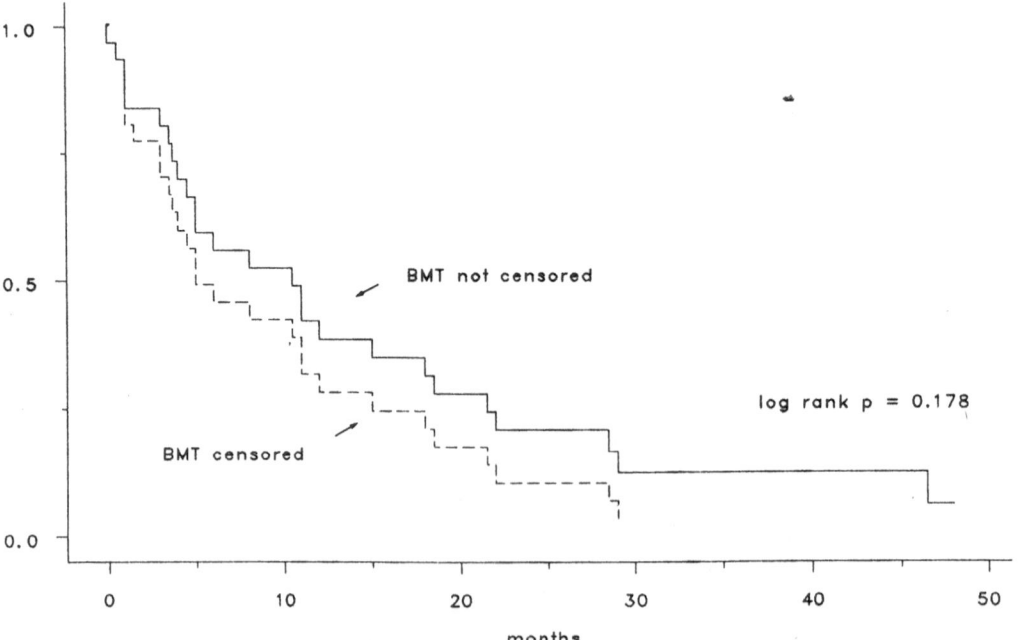

Fig. 2. Survival of responding and non-responding (relapsed and refractory) pts.-BMT was censored.

Fig. 3. Survival of responding relapsed pts. comparing when BMT was censored vs not censored.

References

1. Herzig RH, Lazarus HM, Wolff SN et al. (1985) High-dose cytosine arabinoside therapy with and without anthracycline antibiotics for remission induction of acute non-lymphoblastic leukemia. J Clin Oncol 3: 992–997
2. Kantarjian H, Estey E, Plunkett W et al. (1986) Phase I–II clinical and pharmacologic studies of high-dose cytosine arabinoside in refractory leukemia. Am J Med 81: 387–394
3. Decker RW, Ho WG, Champlin RE (1987) Phase II study of amsacrine and high-dose cytarabine for resistant acute myelogenous leukemia. Cancer Treat Rep 71: 881–882
4. Willemze R, Zwaan FE, Colpin G, Keuning JJ (1982) High-dose cytosine arabinoside in the management of acute leukemia. Scand J Haematol 29: 141–146
5. Heinemann V, Jehn U (1990) Rationales for a pharmacologically optimized treatment of acute non-lymphocytic leukemia with cytosine arabinoside. Leukemia 4: 790–796
6. Jehn U, Heinemann V, Wilmanns W (1989) Intermediate-dose ara-C/mAMSA for remission induction and high-dose ara-C/AMSA for intensive consolidation in relapsed and refractory adult acute myelogenous leukemia (AML). Anticancer Res 9: 119–124
7. Jehn U, Zittoun R, for the EORTC Leukemia Lymphoma Study Group (1985) AML-6 Studie zum Wert einer zyklisch alternierenden Chemotherapie während der Remission bei akuter myeloischer Leukämie. Onkologie 8: 94
8. Zittoun R, Jehn U, Fiere D et al. (1989) Alternating vs. repeated postremission treatment in adult acute leukemia: a randomized study of the EORTC Leukemia Cooperative Group. Blood 73: 896
9. Hayat M, Jehn U, Willemze R et al. (1986) A randomized comparison of maintenance treatment with androgens, immunotherapy, and chemotherapy in adult acute myelogenous leukemia. A Leukemia-Lymphoma Group Trial of the EORTC. Cancer 58: 617–623
10. Hoelzer D, Thiel E, Löffler H et al. (1984) Intensified therapy in acute lymphoblastic and acute undifferentiated leukemia in adults. Blood 64: 38–47
11. Büchner T, Urbanitz D, Hiddemann W et al. (1985) Intensified induction and consolidation with or without maintenance chemotherapy for acute myeloid leukemia (AML): two multicenter studies of the German AML Cooperative Group. J Clin Oncol 3: 1583–1589
12. Willemze R, Jäger U, Jehn U et al. (1989) Intermediate and high-dose ara-C and mAMSA for remission and consolidation treatment of patients with acute myeloid leukemia: an EORTC Leukemia Cooperative Group Phase II study. Eur J Cancer Clin Oncol 24: 1721–1725
13. Zittoun R, Bury J, Stryckmans P et al. (1985) Amsacrine with high-dose cytarabine in acute leukemia. Cancer Treat Rep 69: 1447–1448
14. Jehn U, Göldel N, Rienmüller R, Wilmanns W (1988) Non-cardiogenic pulmonary edema complicating intermediate and high-dose Ara-C treatment for relapsed acute leukemia. Med Oncol Tumor Pharmacother 5: 41–47
15. Herzig RH, Wolff SN,, Lazarus HM et al. (1983) High-dose cytosine arabinoside therapy for refractory leukemia. Blood 62: 361–369
16. Willemze R, Fibbe WE, Zwaan FE (1983) Experience with intermediate and high dose cytosine arabinoside in refractory leukemia. Onkologie 6: 201–204
17. Hiddemann W, Kreutzmann H, Straif K et al. (1987) High-dose cytosine arabinoside and mitoxantrone: a highly effective regimen in refractory acute leukemia. Blood 69: 744–749
18. Hines JD, Oken MM, Mazza JJ et al. (1984) High-dose cytosine arabinoside and m-AMSA is effective therapy in relapsed acute leukemia. J Clin Oncol 2: 545–549
19. Van Prooijen HC, Dekker AW, Punkt K (1984) The use of intermediate dose cytosine arabinoside (ID-ara C) in the treatment of acute non-lymphocytic leukemia at relapse. Br J Haematol 57: 291–299
20. Willemze R, Peters WG, van Hennik MB et al. (1985) Intermediate and high-dose ara-C and mAMSA (or daunorubicin) as remission and consolidation treatment for patients with relapsed acute leukemia and lymphoblastic non-Hodgkin lymphoma. Scand J Haematol 34: 83–87
21. Hiddemann W, Martin WR, Sauerland CM et al. (1990) Definition of refractoriness against conventional chemotherapy in acute myeloid leukemia: a proposal based on the results of retreatment by thioguanine, cytosine arabinoside, and daunorubicin (TAD 9) in 150 patients with relapse after standardized first-line therapy. Leukemia 4: 184–188
22. Andersson BS, Luna MA, Yee C et al. (1990) Fatal pulmonary failure complicating high-dose cytosine arabinoside therapy in acute leukemia. Cancer 65: 1079–1084

411

High-Dose Versus Intermediate-Dose Cytosine Arabinoside Combined with Mitoxantrone for the Treatment of Relapsed and Refractory Acute Myeloid Leukemia: Results of an Age-Adjusted Randomized Comparison*

W. Hiddemann[1], C. Aul[2], G. Maschmeyer[3], R. Schönrock-Nabulsi[4], W. D. Ludwig[5], A. Bartholomäus[6], P. Bettelheim[7], K. Becker[8], L. Balleisen[9], B. Lathan[10], H. Köppler[11], T. Grüneisen[12], R. Donhuijsen-Ant[13], A. Reichle[14], A. Heinecke[15], C. Sauerland[15], and T. Büchner[1]

Introduction

In the treatment of relapsed and refractory acute myeloid leukemia (AML), cytosine arabinoside (AraC) is unanimously considered a highly active single agent when given in repeated doses of more than 500 mg/m² up to 3000 mg/m². Major dispute continues about the optimal dosage of AraC required for a most effective killing of leukemic blasts without undue toxicity to normal tissues. Based on pharmacokinetic investigations, AraC doses between 500 and 1000 mg/m² seem to be most appropriate since the intracellular enzyme deoxycytidine kinase which transforms AraC into the active phosphorylated form AraCTP is already saturated [1, 2]. The further increase in AraC dosage may therefore not translate into an enhanced antileukemic activity but rather into more pronounced toxicity to other organs.

Cellular mechanisms of drug resistance against AraC, however, such as an increase in the AraCTP-inactivating enzyme cytidine deaminase, an inhibition of AraC uptake into the cell by a hampered capacity of the respective transmembrane transport system, a decrease in AraCTP incorporation into the DNA molecule, or a more rapid and effective repair of DNA damage, may interfere with AraCTP formation and its intracellular metabolism and may require higher doses of AraC for a most effective antileukemic activity [3–11]. To date, no definite conclusion can be drawn about the clinical relevance of these and other mechanisms resulting in resistance against conventional doses of AraC or about the appropriate dosage which might be necessary to overcome these conditions. In an attempt to approach this question the German AML Cooperative Group initiated a prospective randomized clinical trial in patients with relapsed or refractory AML comparing high-dose with intermediate dose Ara-C with an adjustment for age on the basis of the previously established sequential high-dose Ara-C/mitoxantrone regimen (S-HAM) [12].

Patients, Protocol, and Methods

Eligibility criteria included the diagnosis of AML according to the FAB classification in relapse or with refractoriness against standardized first-line regimens applied in the

Departments of Hematology and Oncology, University of Münster[1], Düsseldorf[2], Berlin[5], Vienna[7], Hamburg[8], Cologne[10], Marburg[11], Munich[14]; Evangelisches Krankenhaus, Essen-Werden[3]; Krankenhaus St. Georg, Hamburg[4]; St. Bernward Krankenhaus, Hildesheim[6]; Evangelisches Krankenhaus, Hamm[9]; Städtisches Krankenhaus, Neukölln-Berlin[12]; St. Johannis-Hospital, Duisburg-Hamborn[13]; Department of Biostatistics, University of Münster[15], FRG
* Supported in part by a grant from the Deutsche Krebshilfe, Dr. Mildred Scheel Stiftung W 24/87/Hi 1.

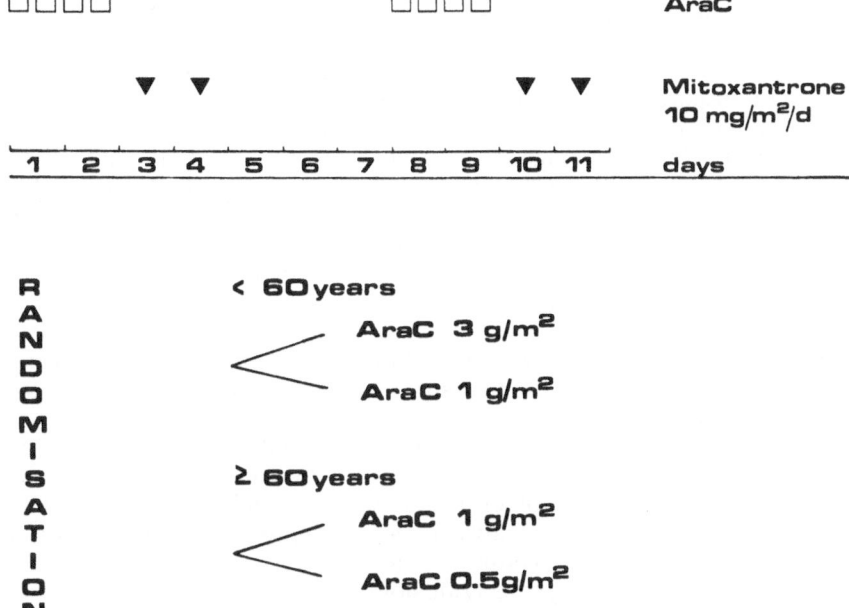

□□□□   □□□□   AraC

▼ ▼   ▼ ▼   Mitoxantrone
10 mg/m²/d

1 2 3 4 5 6 7 8 9 10 11   days

R
A
N
D
O
M
I
S
A
T
I
O
N

< 60 years
     AraC 3 g/m²
     AraC 1 g/m²

≥ 60 years
     AraC 1 g/m²
     AraC 0.5g/m²

Fig. 1. Sequential HD AraC and mitoxantrone (S-HAM)

multicenter trials of the German AML Cooperative Group [13, 14]. Therapy according to the S-HAM protocol consisted of AraC on days 1, 2, 8, and 9 and mitoxantrone on days 3, 4, 10, and 11, respectively (Fig. 1). While patients of all ages received mitoxantrone at a uniform dose of 10 mg/m² per day the randomized comparison of different doses for AraC was adjusted to age as follows:

Patients younger than 60 years of age were randomly assigned to receive either 3.0 mg/m² or 1.0 g/m² AraC per application while older patients were randomized to either 1.0 g/m² or 0.5 g/m² AraC per single dose (Fig. 1). In order to avoid selection of patients with different prognoses, the randomization was balanced for the following stratification criteria:

1. Type of first-line treatment
2. Primary resistance against induction therapy
3. Duration of the preceding remission
4. Number of relapses

All patients received glucocorticoid eye drops during the AraC administration for the prophylaxis of photophobia and con-junctivitis. Antiemetic therapy and prophy-lactic antibiotic regimens were applied at the discretion of the participating centers. Antileukemic response was judged accord-ing to CALGB criteria and side effects were evaluated following WHO definitions. The interval between the onset of therapy and the posttreatment achievement of more than 20 000 thrombocytes/mm³ and more than 500 granulocytes/mm³ was defined as time to recovery (TR). Patients achieving a complete remission were scheduled to receive two (≤ 60 years) or one (> 60 years) 4-week cycles of prolonged consolidation therapy consisting of conventional dose AraC, m-AMSA, vincristine, prednisone, 6-thioguanine, and cyclophosphamide as previously described in detail [15, 16].

Results

At present, 170 patients have been entered into the study from 14 participating centers in Germany and Austria. From the 137 patients who have completed the S-HAM cycle and in whom complete documenta-tion is available, 12 cases had to be excluded because of a preceding myelodysplastic syndrome, protocol violation, death before therapy or relapse after autologous bone marrow transplantation. Of the remaining 125 evaluable patients, 88 were younger than 60 years while 37 belonged to the older age group. Overall, 58 (47%) of the 125 patients achieved a complete remission, 28 patients (22%) were nonresponders, and 39 patients (31%) died within the first 6 weeks after the start of treatment (early deaths = ED).

No significant differences were found in CR rates between the different treatment groups being 49% versus 45% for the 3.0 versus 1.0 g/m² AraC regimens in patients <60 years and 47% versus 44% after 1.0 versus 0.5 g/m² AraC in older patients (Tables 1, 2). No differences between the respective regimens emerged either for the time to CR (median 46 days) or remission duration (median 4.5 months). The evaluation of initial cytoreduction in the bone marrow 7 days after completion of chemotherapy, however, revealed the tendency towards a higher proportion of cases with an adequate blast clearance to less than 5% residual leukemic cells after the high-dose as compared to the intermediate-dose AraC protocols in patients <60 years of age. In this group, less than 5% blasts were found in 80% versus 65% after 3.0 g/m² versus 1.0 g/m² AraC. In the older age group blast cell clearance was similar with 71% after 1.0 g/m² AraC and 78% after 0.5 g/m² AraC. Analysis of treatment failures demonstrated a significantly higher rate of nonresponders after the lower dose regimens in both age groups of 37% and 28% versus 11% and 11% in patients receiving AraC at higher dose ($p < 0.01$). Correspondingly, more early deaths were observed in the latter groups of 40% and 42% as compared to 18% and 28%, respectively, ($p < 0.05$) (Tables 1, 2).

Nonhematologic toxicity consisted mainly of nausea and vomiting, diarrhea, mucositis, and liver enzyme elevations. CNS symptoms were observed in 16 of 91 treatment courses in the younger age group (17%) and in 8 of 36 courses (22%) in older patients. While in the latter age group toxicities were not different in severity and frequency between the different AraC dose groups, a significantly higher frequency of CNS toxicity was observed in younger patients receiving 3.0 g/m² AraC (28% versus 7%, $p < 0.01$). Except for this difference toxicities were otherwise comparable.

Table 1. Treatment results in evaluable patients <60 years ($n = 88$)

AraC dose (g)	CR	ED	NR + PR	n
3.0	22 (49%)	18 (40%)	5 (11%)	45
1.0	19 (45%)	8 (18%)	16 (37%)	43
	41 (47%)	26 (29%)	21 (24%)	88
		$p < 0.05$	$p < 0.01$	

Table 2. Treatment results in evaluable patients >60 years ($n = 37$)

AraC dose (g)	CR	ED	NR	n
1.0	9 (47%)	8 (42%)	2 (11%)	19
0.5	8 (44%)	5 (28%)	5 (28%)	18
	17 (46%)	13 (35%)	7 (19%)	37

From the 28 patients achieving a complete remission 8 patients subsequently underwent autologous or allogeneic bone marrow transplantation. Seventeen patients were treated by a prolonged consolidation chemotherapy as derived from a pediatric AML trial previously reported in detail [15, 16]. Since three patients died from severe infections during consolidation because of prolonged aplasia, consolidation was stopped, prematurely. Of the 50 patients not undergoing bone marrow transplantation 32 have relapsed after 1–18 months, and 15 are in ongoing remission for 1+ to 11+ months. Overall, the median remission duration is 4.5 months and overall median survival is calculated for 5 months.

Discussion

The present study addresses for the first time the question of intermediate-versus high-dose cytosine arabinoside in the treatment of relapsed and refractory acute myeloid leukemia in way of a prospective randomized comparison. Pharmacokinetic investigations suggest that this issue is settled already in favor of intermediate doses of AraC in the range of 500–1000 mg/m^2 per single application. These doses were shown to saturate the intracellular enzyme deoxycytidine kinase transforming AraC into its active from AraCTP [1, 2], suggesting that higher doses will not result in increased antileukemic activity but more pronounced side effects, only. Various mechanisms of cellular resistance against AraC, however, such as an increase in the AraCTP-inactivating enzyme cytidine deaminase, a reduction of AraCTP incorporation into the DNA molecule or more effective repair of AraC-induced DNA damage may require application of higher doses of AraC for optimal antileukemic activity [3–11]. This thesis is supported by two consecutive studies by Willemze et al. in refractory acute myeloid leukemias. In the first trial, 10 of 20 patients achieved a complete remission after treatment with 12 doses of 3.0 g/m^2 AraC whereas in a subsequent study none of 8 patients responded to 12 doses of 1.0 g/m^2 AraC [17]. A similar difference was

not observed, on the other hand, by Herzig and coworkers when comparing 2.0 vs. 3.0 g/^{2} AraC both given twice daily for 6 days [18].

Since side effects of AraC treatment were convincingly shown to correlate with AraC dosage [18–20] and the possible therapeutic advantage of shorter retention of AraCTP in normal hematopoietic cells as compared to leukemic blasts seems to be abolished at higher AraC doses [1], it is essential for the optimal treatment of patients with relapsed or refractory acute leukemia to define the dosis of AraC which can be applied safely without losing antileukemic activity.

In the current prospectively randomized multicenter trial of the German AML Cooperative Group no major differences in overall response rates were observed which seems to support the use of intermediate doses of AraC as derived from pharmacokinetic investigations. A more detailed investigation of the present results, however, reveals some remarkable differences in outcome. Hence, a significantly higher rate of patients with persistent leukemia was observed in the patient group receiving the lower AraC dose while early death rates were significantly enhanced in the high-dose AraC treatment arms. The impression that higher doses of AraC might have a higher antileukemic effect which does not translate into a higher response rate because of an increased treatment-associated toxicity is emphasized by the analysis of blast cell clearance from the bone marrow one week after the completion of therapy. This parameter indicates in fact a higher clearance rate after the application of 3.0 g/m^2 versus 1.0 g/m^2 AraC in younger patients (80 % versus 65 %). In the older age group, receiving 1.0 g/m^2 or 0.5 g/m^2 AraC, a similar difference was not found.

In general, these data emphasize that the question of the most appropriate and effective dose of AraC in relapsed and refractory acute myeloid leukemia still remains open at the present time. The data of the current study strongly suggest that an increase in AraC dose may be associated with an enhancement of AraC antileukemic activity, which, however, does not translate into an improved remission rate due to a higher rate of early deaths predominantly from uncontrollable infections. Hence, at the present time intermediate-dose AraC represents the recommended dose in the sequential S-HAM regimen for the treatment of advanced AML. Improved control of infectious complications by the use of hematopoietic growth factors, however, may allow dose escalation for more effective antileukemic therapy in the near future [21].

Summary

One hundred and seventy patients with relapsed or refractory acute myeloid leukemia (AML) were entered into a prospective randomized comparison of high-dose versus intermediate-dose cytosine arabinoside (AraC) both combined with mitoxantrone (mitox) according to the previously established sequential HD-AraC/mitox regimen (S-HAM). AraC was administered by 3 h inf. q12 h on days 1, 2 and 8, 9 at randomly assigned doses of either 3.0 versus 1.0 g/m^2 in patients <60 years of age or 1.0 versus 0.5 g/m^2 in older patients. Mitox was given to all cases at a dose of 10 mg/m^2 per day on days 2, 4 and 10, 11. Randomization was stratified for primary refractoriness against induction therapy and the length of first remission in relapsed cases (<6 months, 6–18 months, >18 months). From 125 presently evaluable cases, 58 patients (47%) achieved a complete remission (CR), 28 patients (22%) were nonresponders (NR) and 39 patients (31%) died within the first 6 weeks after the start of treatment (early death = ED). No significant differences were found in CR rates, being 49% and 45% for the 3.0 versus 1.0 g/m^2 AraC regimens in patients <60 years and 47% and 44% after 1.0 versus 0.5 g/m^2 AraC in older patients. No differences between the respective regimens emerged either for the time to CR (median 46 days) or remission duration (median 4.5 months). In patients <60 year, evaluation of initial cytoreduction in the bone marrow 7 days after completion of chemotherapy, however, revealed a tendency towards a higher proportion of cases with adequate blast clearance (<5%) after 3.0 g/m^2 AraC of 80% as compared to 65% after the lower

AraC dose. In this context, analysis of treatment failures demonstrated a significantly higher rate of NR after the lower dose regimens in both age groups of 37% and 28% versus 11% and 11% in patients receiving AraC at higher doses ($p < 0.01$). Correspondingly, more EDs were observed in the latter groups. These data suggest a dose response relation of AraC antileukemic activity which does not translate into an improved remission rate due to a higher rate of ED predominantly from uncontrollable infections.

References

1. Riva CM, Rustum YM, Preisler HD (1985) Pharmacokinetics and cellular determinants of response to 1-β-arabinofuranosyl-cytosine (AraC). Semin Oncol 12 [Suppl 3]: 1–8
2. Plunkett W, Liliemark JO, Adams TM, Nowak B, Estey E, Kantarjian H, Keating MJ (1987) Saturation of 1-β-arabinofuranosylcytosine 5′-triphosphate accumulation in leukemic cells during high-dose 1-β-D-arabinofuranosylcytosine therapy. Cancer Res 47: 3005–3011
3. Chu MY, Fischer GA (1965) Comparative studies of leukemic cells sensitive and resistant to cytosine arabinoside. Biochem Pharmacol 4: 333–341
4. Kessel D, Hall TC, Wodinsky I (1967) Transport and phosphorylation as factors in the antitumor action of cytosine arabinoside. Science 156: 1240–1241
5. Chu MY, Fischer GA (1968) The incorporation of ^{3}H-cytosine arabinoside and its effects on murine leukemia cells. Biochem Pharmacol 17: 753–767
6. Momparler RL, Chu MY, Fischer GA (1968) Studies on a new mechanism of resistance of L 5178 Y murine leukemia cells to cytosine arabinoside. Biochim Biophys Acta 161: 481–487
7. Stewart CD, Burke PJ (1971) Cytidine deaminase and development of resistance to arabinosyl cytosine. Nature 223: 109–110
8. DeSaint-Vincent RB, Buttin G (1973) Studies of 1-β-arabinofuranosylcytosine-resistant mutants of Chinese-hamster fibroblasts. Eur J Biochem 37: 481–487
9. Tattersall MHN, Ganeshaguru K, Hoffbrand AV (1974) Mechanisms of resistance of human acute leukemia cells to cytosine arabinoside. Br J Haematol 27: 39–46
10. Wiley JS, Jones SP, Sawyer WH (1983) Cytosine arabinoside transport by human

leukemic cells. Eur J Cancer Clin Oncol 19: 1067–1074

11. Abé I, Sato S, Honi K, Suzuki M, Sato H (1982) Role of dephosphorylation in accumulation of 1-β-arabinofuranosylcytosine 5'-triphosphate in human lymphoblastic cell lines with reference to their drug sensitivity. Cancer Res 42: 2846–2851

12. Hiddemann W, Büchner T, Essink M, Koch O, Stenzinger W, van de Loo J (1988) High-dose cytosine arabinoside and mitoxantrone: preliminary results of a pilot study with sequential application (S-HAM) indicating high antileukemic activity in refractory acute leukemias. Onkologie 11: 10–12

13. Büchner T, Urbanitz D, Hiddemann W, Rühl H, Ludwig WD, Fischer J, Aul HC, Vaupel HA, Kuse R, Zeile G, Nowrousian MR, König HJ, Walter M, Wendt FC, Sodomann H, Hossfeld DK, von Paleske A, Löffler H, Gassmann W, Hellriegel KP, Fülle HH, Lunscken C, Emmerich B, Pralle H, Pees HW, Pfreundschuh M, Bartels H, Koeppen KM, Schwerdtfeger R, Donhuijsen-Ant R, Mainzer K, Bonfert B, Köppler H, Zurborn KH, Ranft K, Thiel E, Heinerle A (1985) Intensified induction and consolidation with or without maintenance chemotherapy for acute myeloid leukemia (AML): two multicenter studies of the German AML Cooperative Group. J Clin Oncol 3: 1583–1589

14. Büchner T, Hiddemann W, Blasius S et al. (1990) Adult AML: the role of chemotherapy intensity and duration. Two studies of the AML Cooperative Group. In: Büchner T, Schellong G, Hiddemann W, Ritter J (eds) Acute leukemias II. Prognostic factors and treatment strategies. Springer, Berlin Heidelberg New York, pp 261–266

15. Creutzig U, Ritter J, Riehm H, Langermann HJ, Henze G, Kabisch H, Niethammer D, Jürgens H, Stollmann B, Lasson U, Kaufmann U, Löffler H, Schellong G (1985) Improved treatment results in childhood acute myelogenous leukemia: a report of the German Cooperative Study AML-BFM-78. Blood 65: 298–304

16. Ritter J, Creutzig U, Schellong G (1990) Improved treatment results in the myelocytic subtypes FAB M1–M4 but not in FAB M5 after intensification of induction therapy: results of the German Childhood AML Studies BFM-78 and BFM-83. In: Büchner T, Schellong G, Hiddemann W, Ritter J (eds) Acute leukemias II. Prognostic factors and treatment strategies. Springer, Berlin Heidelberg New York, pp 185–192

17. Willemze R, Fibbe WE, Zwaan FE (1983) Experience with intermediate and high-dose cytosine arabinoside in refractory acute leukemia. Onkologie 6: 200–204

18. Herzig RH, Hines JD, Herzig GP, Wolff SN, Cassileth PA, Lazarus HM, Adelstein DJ, Brown RA, Coccia PF, Strandjord S, Mazza JJ, Fay J, Phillips GL (1987) Cerebellar toxicity with high-dose cytosine arabinoside. J Clin Oncol 5: 927–932

19. Herzig RH, Wolff SN, Lazarus HM, Phillips GL, Karanes C, Herzig GP (1983) High-dose cytosine arabinoside therapy for refractory leukemia. Blood 62: 361–369

20. Lazarus HM, Herzig RH, Herzig GP, Phillips GL, Roessmann D, Fishman J (1981) Central nervous system toxicity of high-dose systemic cytosine arabinoside. Cancer 48: 2577–2582

21. Büchner T, Hiddemann W, Koenigsmann M, Zühlsdorf M, Wörmann B, Böckmann A, Aguion Freire E, Innig G, Maschmeyer G, Ludwig WD, Sauerland MC, Heinecke A, Schulz G (1991) Recombinant human granulocyte-macrophage colony-stimulating factor following chemotherapy in patients with acute myeloid leukemia at higher age or after relapse. Blood (in press)

Treatment of Refractory and Relapsed Childhood Acute Myelogenous Leukemia with High-Dose Cytosine Arabinoside and Mitoxantrone (HAM): Results of the AML Relapse Study BFM-85

J. Ritter, U. Creutzig, and G. Schellong for the AML-BFM Group

Introduction

In spite of intensive induction polychemotherapy and subsequent intensive postremission chemotherapy nearly one-half of the children with acute myelogenous leukemia (AML) still relapse with their disease and ultimately die of drug-resistant leukemia. High secondary remission rates have recently been reported by the application of high-dose cytosine arabinoside (HD ARA-C) alone or in combination with anthracyclines, asparaginase or m-AMSA [1, 3–5, 7, 8, 11]. Especially patients with AML refractory against conventional-dose ARA-C were shown to benefit from the use of HD ARA-C [6]. In 1985 Hiddemann and coworkers reported on the high antileukemic activity in refractory and relapsed AML in adults using the combination of HD ARA-C plus mitoxantrone [5]. In the same year the German multicenter AML-BFM study group decided to use this drug combination in *children* with refractory and relapsed AML. This report gives an update of the pediatric HD ARA-C/mitoxantrone study.

Patients, Treatment Protocol and Methods

Twenty-five children with refractory and relapsed AML were treated with the combination of HD ARA-C and mitoxantrone.

University Children's Hospital Münster, Albert-Schweitzer-Str. 33, W-4400 Münster, FRG

All children were initially treated according to protocol AML-BFM-83 [10]. Table 1 shows some patient characteristics of the 25 children. The male : female ratio was slightly higher than in first line patients in study BFM-83. The distribution according to the FAB subtypes was similar to the first line patients [2]. Eight children were refractory to induction and consolidation treatment according to study AML-BFM-83 [10]. Eleven children relapsed within the 1 year after diagnosis, whereas the remaining six children relapsed in the 2 year after diagnosis. Therapy consisted of HD ARA-C 3 g/m² every 12 h by a 3-h continuous infusion on days 1–4. Mitoxantrone was given at a dose of 12 mg/m² per day on days 3, 4, and 5. Suportive care included glucocorticoid eye-

Table 1. Patient characteristics and entry criteria

N	25
Sex (male : female)	17 : 8
Age	9 mos – 16⁵/₁₂ years (median: 8⁴/₁₂ years)
FAB M1	6
M2	4
M3	1
M4	8
M5	3
M6	2
M7	1
Entry criteria:	
Primary nonresponse (protocol BFM-83)	8
Early relapse (<12 mos)	11
Late relapse (>12 mos)	6

Table 2. Treatment results of HD ARA-C/Mitox in children

	N	ED	NR	CR	In CR
Refractory AML	8	1	4	3	1 (30+)
Early relapse (<12 mos)	11	2	4	5	1 (52+ after BMT)
Late relapse (>12 mos)	6	1	–	5	2 (42+; 18+)
	25	4	8	13	4

drops and oral vitamin B6. The evaluation of the antileukemic efficacy was based on CALGB criteria [12].

Results

Treatment results of the 25 children are given in Table 2. Three out of eight children who did not respond to induction/consolidation treatment of study BFM-83, 5/11 children with early relapse, and 5/6 children with late relapse achieved a complete remission, the CR rate being 52 %. Four out of 25 children (16 %) died early within the first 6 weeks in bone marrow aplasia and 8/25 (32 %) did not respond to the HAM protocol. The main toxicity of the HAM protocol was hematotoxicity, as shown in Table 3. All children needed platelet support, and all children developed fever in bone marrow aplasia. Two of 15 children with documented infections and 2 of 10 children with fever of unknown origin died during bone marrow aplasia despite every type of supportive care including artificial ventilation. The median time to recovery of peripheral blood counts (WBC <500/μl; platelets <20 000/μl) of the responding

Table 3. Hematologic toxicity of the HAM protocol

Platelet support	25/25
Life-threatening bleeding	1/25
Fever	25/25
Documented infections	15/25
Bacterial	10
Fungal	5
Fever of unknown origin	10/25

children was 28 days with a range of 24–36 days. Five of the 13 responding children underwent bone marrow transplantation in second remission. One of these children is in long-lasting second remission (52+ months), whereas two children died early after transplantation. Two children relapsed after bone marrow transplantation. The remaining eight responding children received different forms of maintenance treatment. Three of them are in long-lasting second CR (18+; 30+; 42+ months). The eight children who did not respond to the HAM protocol died after 1–6 months due to refractory leukemia.

Discussion

The treatment results of the present childhood study using the combination HD ARA-C and mitoxantrone revealed a CR rate of 52 %. These results are in the same range as treatment results in adults using the same combination. Markus et al. [9] described 10/18 complete remissions (56 %), whereas Hiddemann et al. [7] described 21/40 complete remissions (53 %) using the HAM protocol. All children in the present childhood HAM study were recruited from the multicenter trial AML-BFM-83 [2], and had therefore received a standardized first-line treatment with ADE induction and seven-drug/8-week consolidiation [2]. The hematologic effects of HD ARA-C and mitoxantrone were comparable to the ADE induction treatment of the AML-BFM-83 protocol [2]. The time to recovery of WBC <500/μl and platelets <20 000/μl was 28 days and thus in the same range as in a comparable study in adult patients [7]. Furthermore, the time to recovery was in the same range as after ADE induction according to study BFM-83 [2]. Based on the standardized intensive first-line treatment, the present study demonstrtes a high antileukemic efficacy of the combination HD ARA-C and mitoxantrone in refractory and relapsed childhood AML.

References

1. Capizzi RL, Poole M, Cooper MR. Richards FII, Stuart JJ, Jackson DVJr, White DR, Spurr CL, Hopkins JO, Muss HB. Rudnick SA, Wells R, Gabriel D, Ross D (1984) Treatment of poor risk acute leukemia with sequential high-dose Ara-C and asparaginase. Blood 63: 694–700
2. Creutzig U, Ritter J, Schellong G for the AML-BFM Study Group (1990) Identification of two risk groups in childhood acute myelogenous leukemia after therapy intensification in study AML-BFM-83 as compared with study AML-BFM-78. Blood 75: 1932–1940
3. Herzig RH, Wolff SN; Lazarus HM, Phillips GL, Karanes C, Herzig GP (1983) High-dose cytosine arabinoside therapy for refractory leukemia. Blood 62: 361–369
4. Herzig RH, Lazarus HM, Wolff SN, Phillips GL, Herzig GP (1985) High-dose cytosine arabinoside therapy with and without anthracycline antibiotics for remission reinduction of acute nonlymphoblastic leukemia. J Clin Oncol 3: 992–997
5. Hiddemann W, Kreutzmann H, Ludwig WD, Aul HC, Donhuisen-Ant R, Lengelder E, Büchner T (1985) Mitozantrone and high-dose cytarabine in refractory adult acute myeloid leukaemia. Lancet ii: 508–509
6. Hiddemann W, Kreutzmann H, Straif K, Ludwig WD, Mertelsmann R, Donhuijsen-Ant R, Lengfelder E, Arlin Z, Büchner T (1987) High-dose cytosine arabinoside and mitoxantrone: highly effective regimen in refractory acute myeloid leukemia. Blood 69: 744–749
7. Hiddemann W, Büchner T (1990) Treatment strategies in acute myeloid leukemia (AML). Blut 60: 163–171
8. Hines JD, Oken MM, Mazza JJ, Keller AM, Streeter RR, Glick JH (1984) High-dose cytosine arabinoside and m-AMSA is effective therapy in relapsed acute nonlymphocytic leukemia. J Clin Oncol 2: 545–549
9. Marcus DE, Catovsky D, Goldman JM, Galton DAG, Newland AC, Slocombe G, Hegde U (1985) Mitoxantrone and high-dose cytarabine in adult acute myeloid leukaemia. Lancet; 1384–1385
10. Ritter J, Creutzig U, Schellong G (1990) Improved treatment results in the myelocytic subtypes FAB M1-M4 but not in FAB M5 after intensification of induction therapy: Results of the German AML Studies BFM-78 and BFM-83. In: Büchner T, Schellong G, Hiddemann W, Ritter J (eds) Acute Leukemias II. Springer, Berlin Heidelberg New York, pp 185–192
11. Willemze R, Zwaan FE, Colpin G, Keuning JJ (1982) High-dose cytosine arabinoside in the management of refractory acute leukaemia. Scand J Haematol 29: 141–146
12. Yates J, Glidewell O, Wiernik P et al. (1982) Cytosine arabinoside with daunorubicin or adriamycin for therapy of acute myelocytic leukemia: a CALGB study. Blood 60: 454–462

Sequential Standard-Dose Cytosine Arabinoside/Mitoxantrone Therapy (SAM) in Adults with Acute Myeloid Leukemia*

H. Radtke[1], J. Schwamborn[1], H. Daus[1], D. Hufnagl[2], R. Herboth[3], J. Preiß[4], and H. W. Pees[1]

Introduction

During the last 2 decades different treatment strategies have been tested as remission induction therapy in acute myeloid leukemia (AML) in adults in several large trials. The present standard regimen includes cytosine arabinoside (200 mg/m^2 per day) for 7 days and an anthracycline derivate like daunorubicin (60 mg/m^2 per day) for 3 days [1]. The double-induction strategy with repetition of two identical chemotherapy courses prolongs disease-free survival [2]. Recently the new anthraquinone derivate mitoxantrone has been introduced in the therapy of refractory and relapsed AML. In combination with high-dose cytosine arabinoside or etoposide, a high efficacy of the drug could be demonstrated [3, 4]. However, experience using mitoxantrone in primary therapy of AML is still limited. In randomized trials Phillips et al. [5] and Arlin et al. [6] demonstrated a marginal, not significant superiority of mitoxantrone compared to daunorubicin. In 1980 Burke et al. [7] reported the results of a sequential chemotherapy modality timed to coincide with enhanced tumor

proliferation after initial aplasia induction. On this basis, Capizzi et al. [8] and Hiddemann et al. [9] applied high-dose cytosine arabinoside in a sequential mode and showed an enhanced efficacy compared to conventional chemotherapy. In a prospective multicenter trial we are currently evaluating the efficacy and toxicity of a double-induction therapy with standard-dose cytosine arabinoside and mitoxantrone in a sequential mode (SAM protocol) in adults with untreated AML.

Patients and Therapy

Four hospitals in southwest Germany are participating in this ongoing trial. All adults with newly diagnosed AML have been included since July 1988. Patients with secondary leukemia (preceeding myelodysplasia or chemotherapy) or aged over 65 years are excluded. Up to now 24 patients have been treated in this trial, 22 patients have been evaluable (10 men, 12 women), and two patients have not yet finished induction therapy. Age ranged from 16 to 65 with a median of 52 years. Six patients presented with monoblastic differentiation (FAB M5), four of these having widespread monoblastic cutaneous infiltration.

In the SAM protocol cytosine arabinoside (100 mg/m^2) is given twice daily as 1-h infusion on days 1–5 and days 8–10, mitoxantrone (12 mg/m^2) is applied daily as a short infusion on days 3–5 and day 9 (Fig. 1). After restoration of peripheral blood counts, therapy is repeated with the same dosage. Bone marrow is examined on

[1] Medizinische Universitätsklinik, Innere Medizin I, 6650 Homburg/Saar, FRG
[2] Caritas-Krankenhaus Lebach, 6610 Lebach, FRG
[3] Kliniken der Stadt Saarbrücken-Winterberg, 6600 Saarbrücken, FRG
[4] Caritasklinik St. Theresia-Rastpfuhl, 6600 Saarbrücken, FRG
* Supported by Lederle Arzneimittel GmbH & Co, Wolfratshausen, FRG.

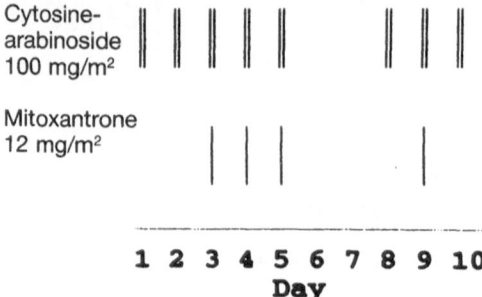

Cytosine-arabinoside 100 mg/m²

Mitoxantrone 12 mg/m²

1 2 3 4 5 6 7 8 9 10
Day

Fig. 1. Schema of the SAM protocol (sequential standard-dose cytosine arabinoside/mitoxantrone)

day 17 of the first therapy cycle, and remission state is obtained after both therapy cycles when the leukocyte count reaches a value above 3000/mm³.

Results

Twenty-two of 24 patients completed two cycles of induction therapy. Fourteen out of 22 patients (64%) achieved a complete remission, 10 of these 14 already after 1 cycle of chemotherapy. One patient (5%) achieved a partial remission, two patients (9%) were nonresponders. Five patients (23%) died after onset of therapy: three of cerebral bleeding (one on day 2 of first

Table 1. Overall responses in 22 patients with newly diagnosed AML treated with sequential standard-dose cytosine arabinoside and mitoxantrone

Complete remission (CR)	14/22	64%
Partial remission (PR)	1/22	5%
Nonresponder (NR)	2/22	9%
Early death (ED)	5/22	23%

Table 2. Adverse effects of sequential standard-dose cytosine arabinoside and mitoxantrone (WHO grade)

	First × SAM ($n = 22$)				Second × SAM ($n = 17$)			
WHO grade	1	2	3	4	1	2	3	4
Nausea/vomiting	9	3	2	0	4	1	3	0
Diarrhea	0	1	0	1	0	0	0	0
Obstipation	0	0	0	0	0	0	0	0
State of consciousness	1	0	0	0	0	0	0	0
Cutaneous toxicity	1	1	0	0	1	0	0	0
Mucositis	1	5	2	1	1	3	1	0
Drug fever	0	0	0	0	0	0	0	0
Infection	2	13	3	2	3	2	5	1
Hepatotoxicity	2	2	0	1	2	2	0	0
Nephrotoxicity	2	0	0	0	0	0	0	0
Pulmonary toxicity	2	0	0	0	0	0	0	0
Cardiotoxicity	1	1	0	0	0	0	0	0
Neurotoxicity	1	0	0	0	0	0	0	0

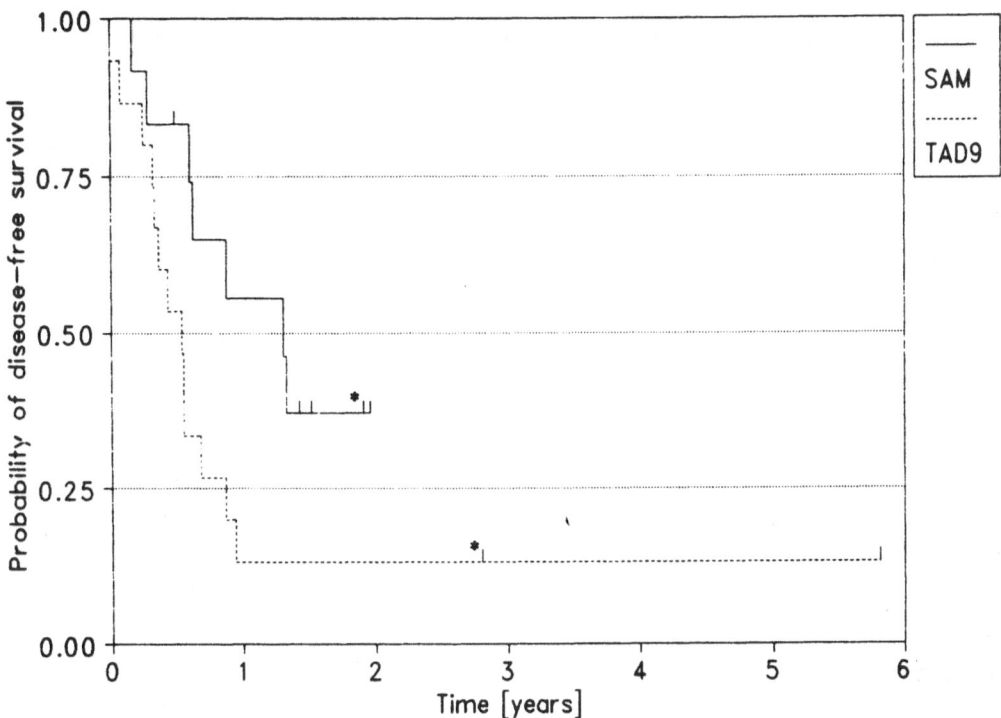

Fig. 2. Kaplan-Meier plot of disease-free survival for 14 patients treated with SAM protocol compared to 15 patients treated with the TAD9 regimen as a historical control (* = bone marrow transplantation)

therapy!), one of infection, and one succumbed to pneumonia, liver dysfunction and untractable diarrhea (Table 1). Duration of aplasia (leukocyte count $<1000/mm^3$) ranged from 8 to 32 days in first therapy with a median of 20 days and from 3 to 38 days in second therapy with a median of 17 days. Toxicity is summarized in Table 2. The main problem was infection due to bone marrow aplasia; other adverse effects were tolerable.

Figure 2 shows a Kaplan-Meier plot of disease-free survival compared to the results of our hospital with the TAD9 protocol [2] as a historical control. Median duration of disease-free survival for the 14 patients achieving complete remission after therapy with SAM protocol was 414 days. Seven patients are still at risk. Median disease-free survival for the 15 patients achieving complete remission after treatment with TAD9 protocol was 177 days. The difference is not yet significant ($p =$

0.0502). Therapy after achieving complete remission was different and is presented in Table 3.

Discussion

The preliminary results of this multicenter trial demonstrate an encouragingly high efficacy of the SAM protocol with low toxicity. Compared to our own experience with the TAD9 regimen, the remission rate is significantly higher ($p < 0.01$ in chi^2 test) and the disease-free survival is longer ($p = 0.0502$ in logrank test). Duration of aplasia seems to be slightly longer compared with conventionally timed chemotherapy probably due to the sequential application mode. A longer follow-up in this trial will contribute additional information to the question of whether mitoxantrone is superior to daunorubicin in the treatment of AML.

Table 3. Further therapy of the 14 patients achieving complete remission after induction therapy with SAM protocol (from Caplizzi et al. [8])

	n	Comment
No further therapy	6	Four patients in continuous remission on day 179+, 519+, 553+, 716+
Allogenic BMT	1	Patient died in remission due to GvHD
Autologous BMT	1	Patient in continuous remission on day 697+
Consolidation therapy	2	Both patients relapsed
Maintenance therapy	1	Patient relapsed and died due to aplasia during maintenance therapy
Other	3	One patient relapsed before BMT, 2 patients still under therapy

References

1. Gale RP, Foon KA (1986) Acute myeloid leukemia: recent advances in therapy. Clin Haematol 15: 781–810
2. Büchner T, Urbanitz D, Hiddemann W et al. (1985) Intensified induction and consolidation with or without maintenance chemotherapy for acute myeloid leukemia (AML): two multicenter studies of the German AML Cooperative Group. J Clin Oncol 3: 1583–1589
3. Hiddemann W, Kreutzmann H, Striaf K et al. (1987) High-dose cytosine arabinoside and mitoxantrone: a highly effective regimen in refractory acute myeloid leukemia. Blood 69: 744–749
4. Ho AD, Lipp T, Ehninger G et al. (1986) Mitoxantrone and VP-16 in refractory acute myelogenous leukemia. Onkologie 9: 148–150
5. Phillips MJ, Johnson SA, Prentice AG (1988) Randomised study of mitoxantrone/cytosine arabinoside (2 + 5) and daunorubicin/cytosine arabinoside (2 + 5) in the treatment of acute myelogenous leukemia. In: Proceedings 3rd United Kingdom Novantrone Symposium. Wiley, Chichester, pp 9–14
6. Arlin Z, Case DC Jr, Moore J et al. (1988) Randomized multicenter trial of cytosine arabinoside with mitoxantrone or daunorubicin in previously untreated adult patients with acute nonlymphocytic leukemia (ANLL). Leukemia 4: 177–183
7. Burke PJ, Vaughan WP, Karp JE (1980) A rationale for sequential high-dose chemotherapy of leukemia timed to coincide with induced tumor proliferation. Blood 55: 960–968
8. Capizzi RL, Poole M, Cooper MR et al. (1984) Treatment of poor risk acute leukemia with sequential high-dose ARA-C and asparaginase. Blood 63: 694–700
9. Hiddemann W, Büchner T, Essink M et al. (1988) High-dose cytosine arabinoside and mitoxantrone: preliminary results of a pilot study with sequential application (S-HAM) indicating a high antileukemic activity in refractory acute leukemias. Onkologie 11: 10–12

Acute Myeloid Leukemia: An Update of Treatment Results with High-Dose Ara-C Consolidation Therapy*

G. Heil[1], M. Freund[2], H. Link[2], P. Mitrou[3], D. Hoelzer[3], H. Wandt[4], G. Ehninger[5], E. Fackler-Schwalbe[6], G. Schlimok[6], A. Lösch[7], W. Queißer[7], B. Löffler[8], and E. Kurrle[1]

Introduction

Substantial progress in chemotherapy and supportive care made it possible in 60%–80% of adult patients suffering from de novo acute myeloid leukemia (AML) to achieve a complete remission (CR) of the disease [1]. Despite this progress not more than about 20% of the complete responders remain in long-term remission and are probably cured. The vast majority, however, relapse with their disease mostly within the first 2 years after achievement of CR [2]. The outcome of AML patients might be improved not only by alternate treatment strategy in remission induction therapy but also in postremission therapy [3]. The latter view is supported by the superior outcome of patients who underwent allogeneic bone marrow transplantation [4, 5]. Unfortu-

nately bone marrow transplantation as a postremission therapy is restricted to only a minority of patients younger than 50 years with an HLA identical sibling. To improve outcome of the remaining patients two alternate treatment modalities are of basic interest. The patients received either long-term postremission therapy including cycles of myelosuppressive drug combinations [3]. On the other hand promising results were obtained by treatment of patients with one or two cycles of an aggressive postremission therapy with 8–12 doses of high-dose cytosine arabinoside (HD Ara-C) either alone or in combination with an anthracycline, amsacrine or etoposide without further maintenance therapy [6, 7]. Despite the fact that the antileukemic effect of various high-dose cytosine arabinoside combinations had also been shown to be effective in relapsed and refractory AML patients, the definite role in postremission therapy remained to be further elucidated since some selection in studies so far presented could not be excluded [8, 9]. It was the aim of a multicenter trial of the Süddeutsche Hämoblastosegruppe initiated in 1985 to analyze the influence of high-dose cytosine arabinoside/daunorubicin (HD Ara-C/NDR) consolidation therapy on unmaintained continuous complete remission of patients with de novo AML. Furthermore, the toxicity of an HD Ara-C/NDR therapy was to be analyzed in patients 50 years old or younger. This treatment modality was restricted to this age group since an increase in toxicity especially CNS toxicity was reported in patients over 50 years old [10].

[1] Department of Internal Medicine III, University of Ulm, Ulm, FRG
[2] Department of Hematology and Oncology, University of Hannover, Hannover, FRG
[3] Department of Hematology and Oncology, University of Frankfurt, Frankfurt, FRG
[4] Department of Internal Medicine, Klinikum Nürnberg, Nürnberg, FRG
[5] Department of Internal Medicine/Hematology, University of Tübingen, Tübingen, FRG
[6] Department of Internal Medicine, Zentralklinikum Augsburg, Augsburg, FRG
[7] Oncology Center, University of Mannheim, Mannheim, FRG
[8] Department of Internal Medicine, Robert-Bosch-Krankenhaus Stuttgart, Stuttgart, FRG
* A study of the Süddeutsche Hämoblastosegruppe. The study was supported by the Deutsche Krebshilfe (contract M37/85 He2).

Patients and Methods

Patient Selection

Between May 1985 and April 1990 149 patients suffering from de novo AML (FAB M1–M6) were included in the multicenter trial [11, 12]. The median age of all patients under study was 37 years (range 15–50 years). Exclusion criteria were as follows: age over 50 years; secondary leukemia or history of myelodysplastic syndrome, aplastic anemia or smoldering leukemia; severe disease of heart, lung, liver, kidneys or CNS; severe complications of the leukemia if not treatable successfully.

Treatment

Induction therapy comprised two cycles of a three-drug combination (DAV I/II) including cytarabine, daunorubicin and VP 16-213. Patients in complete remission received one additional course of the DAV combination theory (DAV III) as early consolidation after recovery of the neutrophil count to over 1000/l and thrombocytes to over 100 000/l (Fig. 1). Patients in complete remission who were not candidates for allogeneic bone marrow transplantation received one or two courses of HD Ara-C/DNR as late consolidation therapy (Fig. 1) 4 weeks after recovery from early consolidation therapy. Patients with severe complications during the first course of HD Ara-C/DNR such as severe infections or prolonged aplasia did not receive the second course. None of the patients received maintenance therapy.

Supportive Care

The patients were treated under conventional ward conditions in single or two-bed rooms. Prophylactic platelet transfusion and antibiotic therapy were given as previously described [11].

Evaluation

Toxicity was quantitated according to the World Health Organization (WHO) grad-ing system [13]. The evaluation of the antileukemic efficacy was based on CALGB criteria [14]. Duration of CR was analyzed from the achievement of CR until relapse. Survival was determined from the beginning of treatment until death. Patients who underwent bone marrow transplantation were censored at time of transplantation. Life tables were calculated according to the method of Kaplan and Meier. The closing date for statistical evaluation was 01.04.90.

Results

Induction Therapy

One hundred and four out of the 149 patients (70%) included in the trial achieved a complete remission, 7 patients achieved a partial remission (4.7%), 24 patients (16%) were treatment failures, and 14 patients (9.3%) died during induction therapy.

Late Consolidation Therapy

Fifty-nine out of 104 patients (57%) in CR received one or two courses of HD Ara-C/DNR as late consolidation therapy. Of the remaining cases seven patients relapsed prior to onset of HD Ara-C/DNR therapy and 17 patients were transplanted. Hematologic and nonhematologic toxicity of late consolidation therapy was profound in all cases under study with a median duration of critical neutropenia of 24 days. Nonhematologic toxicity was mainly due to infectious complications. Of the treatment courses 49% were associated with WHO III/IV infectious complications and two patients died due to fatal septicemia. CNS toxicity was mild to moderate with only one patient displaying grade IV (WHO) symptoms, which were reversible after cessation of therapy. The probability of survival of all 149 patients under study after 57 months is 37% with a median survival time of 23 months. Median remission duration of all 104 complete responders is 25 months and of those with late consolidation therapy 37 months.

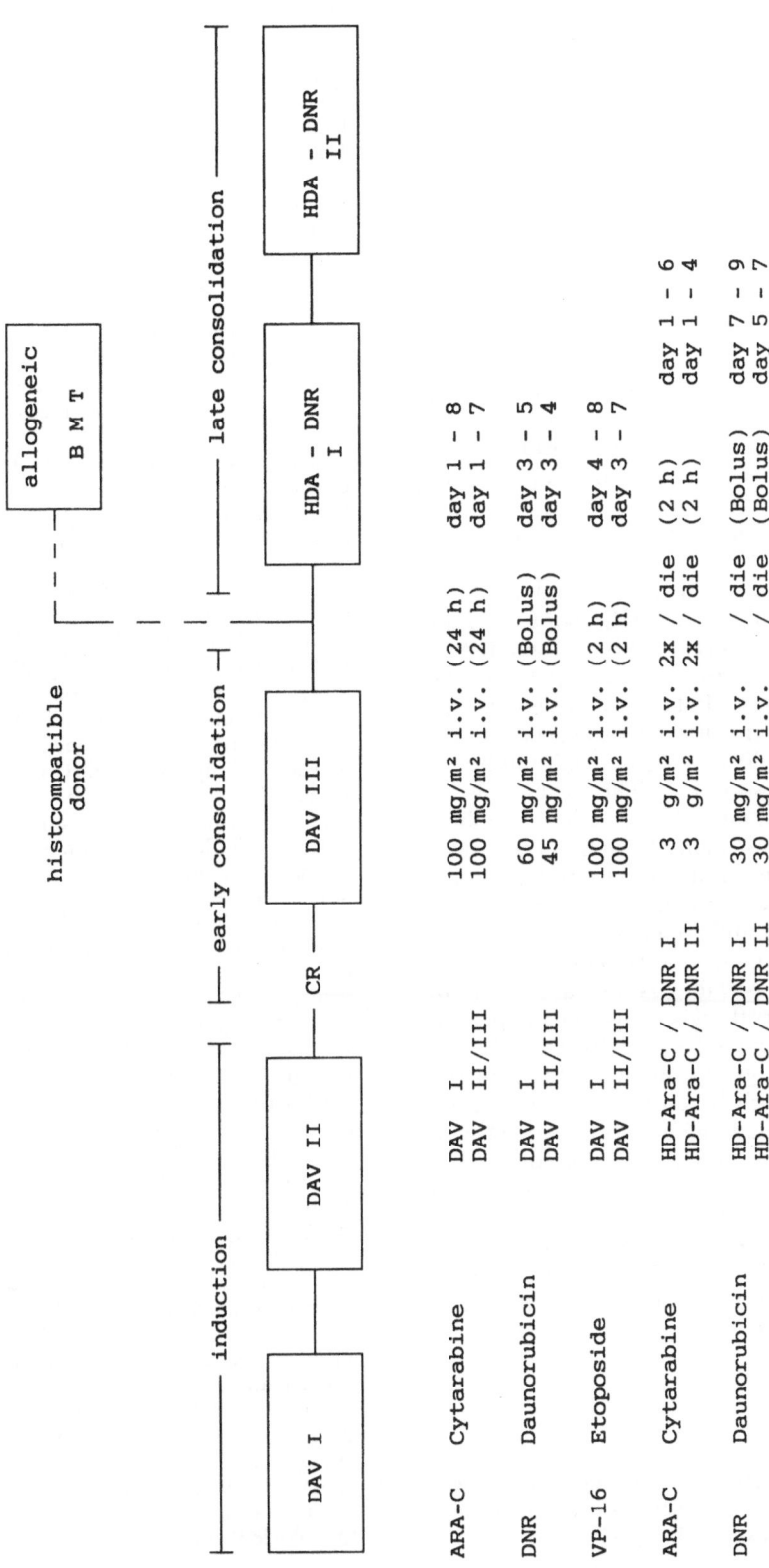

Fig. 1. Protocol therapy for acute myelogenous leukemia (FAB M1–M6). Age ≤50 years

Discussion

The role of HD Ara-C/DNR treatment in postremission therapy was analyzed in a multicenter trial from May 1985 to April 1990 in patients aged 50 years or younger after an identical induction and early consolidation therapy. The outcome of 59 HD Ara-C/DNR consolidation patients was found to be substantially improved compared with that of a historical control group [15].

These data provide additional evidence that long-term postremission chemotherapy including repeated myelosuppressive cycles might be successfully replaced by aggressive short-term postremission chemotherapy [16]. One has to take into consideration, however, that only about one-half of the complete responders of this study were eligible for HD Ara-C therapy so that a selection cannot be excluded. As a consequence a larger series of patients and a longer period of observation seem necessary to confirm these data and to analyze the optimal dose of Ara-C and number of courses necessary [17]. The toxicity of this high-dose therapy with a lethal complication rate of less than 5 % makes this strategy feasible in this age group, though infectious complications in particular need careful attention and sophisticated supportive care. It remains questionable, however, whether this strategy is also applicable to patients over 50 years of age, who appear to suffer from an increased toxicity [2, 18]. This patient group might profit from the same approach by either using a reduced dosage or by adding hematopoietic growth factors to shorten the period of critical neutropenia and the incidence of infectious complications [19].

Acknowledgement. The authors wish to thank Mrs. D. Oesterle for her excellent assistance in documentation and her secretarial support.

References

1. Gale PR, Büchner T (1989) Acute leukemias: prognostic factors and treatment strategies. Leukemia 3: 758–761
2. Welborn JL, Lewis JP, Meyers F (1989) Impact of reinduction regimens on the clinical course of adult acute nonlymphocytic leukemia. Leukemia 11: 711–716
3. Büchner T, Hiddemann W (1990) Treatment strategies in acute myeloid leukemia (AML) A. First line chemotherapy. Blut 60:61–67
4. Appelbaum FR, Dahlberg S, Thomas ED, Buckner CD, Cheever MA, Clift RA, Crowley J, Deeg HJ, Fefer A, Greenberg PD, Kadin M, Smith W, Stewart P, Sullivan K, Storb R, Weiden P (1984) Bone marrow transplantation or chemotherapy after remission induction for adults with acute nonlymphoblastic leukemia. Ann Intern Med 101: 581–588
5. Champlin R, Ho W, Winston D, Decker R, Greenberg P, Burnison M, Holly FE, Gale RP (1987) Treatment of adults with acute myelogenous leukemia: prospective evaluation of high-dose cytarabine in consolidation chemotherapy and with bone marrow transplantation. Semin Oncol 14 [Suppl 1]: 1–6
6. Wolff SN, Herzig RH, Phillips GL, Lazarus HM, Greer JP, Stein RS, Ray WA, Herzig GP (1987) High-dose cytosine arabinoside and daunorubicin as consolidation therapy for acute nonlymphocytic leukemia in first remission: an update. Semin Oncol 14 [Suppl 1]: 12–17
7. Takaku F, Urabe A, Mizoguchi H, Hoshino S, Toyama K, Tanaka K, Nomura T, Dan K, Fujioka S, Saito T, Ogawa T, Mutch Y, Yamaguchi H (1987) High-dose cytosine arabinoside in the consolidation therapy of acute nonlymphocytic leukemia in remission. Semin Oncol 14 [Suppl 1]: 55–57
8. Willemze R, Peters WG, Hennik MB van, Fibbe WE, Kootte AMM, Berkel M van, Lie R, Rodenburg CJ, Veltkamp JJ (1985) Intermediate and high-dose ARA-C and m-AMSA (or daunorubicin) as remission and consolidation treatment for patients with relapsed acute leukaemia and lymphoblastic non-Hodgkin lymphoma. Scand J Haematol 34: 83–87
9. Willemze R, Zwaan FE, Colpin G, Keuning JJ (1982) High dose cytosine arabinoside in the management of refractory acute leukaemia. Scand J Haematol 29: 141–146
10. Herzig RH, Lazarus HM, Herzig PF, Coccia PF, Wolff SN (1985) Central nervous toxicity with high-dose cytosine arabinoside. Semin Oncol 12 [Suppl 3]: 233–236
11. Kurrle E, Ehninger G, Freund M, Heil G, Hoelzer D, Link H, Mitrou PS (1986) Age adapted induction and intensified consolidation therapy in acute myelogenous leukemia. Onkologie 9: 141–143

12. Kurrle E, Ehninger G, Fackler-Schwalbe E, Freund M, Heil G, Hoelzer D, Link H, Löffler B, Lösch A, Mitrou PS, Oehl S, Queisser W, Schlimok G, Wandt H (1990) Consolidation therapy with high-dose cytosine arabinoside. Experiences of a prospective study in acute myeloid leukaemia. Haematol Blood Transfus 33: 254–260

13. World Health Organization (1979) WHO handbook for reporting results of cancer treatment. WHO, Geneva (WHO publ no 38)

14. Yates J, Glidewell O, Wiernik P, Cooper MR, Steinberg D, Dosik H, Levy R, Hoagland C, Henry P, Gottlieb A, Cornell C, Berenberg J, Hutchinson JL, Raich P, Nissen N, Ellison RR, Frelick R, James GW, Falkson G, Silver RT, Haurani F, Green M, Henderson E, Leone L, Holland JF (1982) Cytosine arabinoside with daunorubicin or adriamycin for therapy of acute myelocytic leukemia: a CALGB study. Blood 60: 454–462

15. Link H, Kurrle E, Frauer HM, Heil G, Heimpel H, Waller HD, Ostendorf P, Wilms K, Hoelzer D (1986) TAD-induction therapy for 175 adults with acute myeloid leukemia followed by consolidation and maintenance therapy. Onkologie 9: 135–138

16. Wolff SN, Herzig RH, Fay JW, Philips GL, Lazarus HM, Flexner JM, Stein RS, Greer JP, Cooper B, Herzig GP (1989) High-dose cytarabine and daunorubicin as consolidation therapy for acute myeloid leukemia in first remission: long term follow-up and results. J Clin Oncol 7: 1260–1267

17. Rustum YM, Riva C, Preisler HD (1987) Pharmacokinetic parameters of 1-β-D-arabinofuranosylcytosine (ara-C) and their relationship to intracellular metabolism of ara-C, toxicity, and response of patients with acute nonlymphocytic leukemia treated with conventional and high-dose ara-C. Semin Oncol 14: 141–148

18. Champlin RE, Gajewski JL, Golde DW (1990) Treatment of acute myelogenous leukemia in the elderly. Semin Oncology 16: 51–56

19. Brandt SJ, Peters WP, Atwater SK, Kurtzberg J, Borowitz MJ, Jones RB, Shpall EJ, Bast RC, Gilbert CJ, Oette DH (1988) Effect of recombinant human granulocyte-macrophage colony stimulating factor on hematopietic reconstitution after high-dose chemotherapy and autologous bone marrow transplantation. N Engl J Med 318: 869–876 (abstract)

Continuous Infusion of Mitoxantrone Combined with High-Dose Cytarabine (c-HAM) in Acute Myeloblastic Leukemia

W. Linkesch and I. Grassl

The cellular mitoxantrone concentration with continuous infusion is about twice as high as with a bolus infusion of an equal myelotoxic dose. Mitoxantrone could be detected in plasma for at least 5 days after the end of a 21-day infusion period and in leukocytes for at least 14 days [1]. In our previous study using continuous infusion of mitoxantrone combined with high-dose cytarabine (c-HAM) the mean plasma concentration of mitoxantrone remained constant and ranged around 200 ng/ml 15 days after onset of therapy [2]. Cell kinetic studies revealed a conditioning effect of cytosine arabinoside (Ara-C) for the subsequent administration of daunorubicin or mitoxantrone [3–5]. Experimental results indicate a time-dependent synergistic effect of high-dose cytosine arabinoside (HD Ara-C) and mitoxantrone [6].

A significant antileukemic activity of a combination chemotherapy consisting of HD Ara-C and mitoxantrone (HAM) could be demonstrated in patients with refractory acute myeloblastic leukemia (AML) by achieving complete remissions (CR) in 30%–53% of the patients [7, 8]. That original HAM protocol revealed a remarkably low rate of resistant leukemias (12%), but an unacceptably high early death rate of 33% [7]. In an attempt to reduce early death rates and nonhematological toxicity we developed a modified protocol (c-HAM) including continuous infusion of mitoxantrone combined with HD Ara-C. Administering a c-HAM regimen to patients with refractory/relapsed AML we observed a CR rate of 64% with no cases of early death and a remarkably low nonhematological toxicity [1, 9]. That high therapeutic index of our c-HAM protocol encouraged us to apply that regimen as induction and/or consolidation therapy in patients with AML.

The study comprised 23 patients (median age 57; range 17–80 years, 18 female, 5 male) from our clinic. Nineteen patients suffered from de novo AML, three having an antecedent myelodysplastic syndrome which turned into an over AML, and one patient had a secondary AML. The c-HAM treatment regimen consisted of HD Ara-C 2 g/m² (patients <60 years) or 1 g/m² (patients >60 years) every 12 h by a 3-h infusion on day 1–3 combined with mitoxantrone 10 mg/m² given by 18-h infusion on day 1–3. Seventeen patients received one induction course with DAT (daunorubicin 50 mg/m² × 3, cytarabine 200 mg/m² × 5 continuous infusion, thioguanine 100 mg/m² × 12 h × 10 p.o.) followed by two to three cycles of c-HAM. Two patients received two cycles of idarubicin 12 mg/m² × 3 and cytarabine 200 mg/m² × 5 continuous infusion followed by one to two cycles of c-HAM. Four patients with contraindication to anthracyclines (arrhythmia) received only c-HAM (three to four cycles). Toxicity was assessed according to the WHO criteria [10], while the antileukemic efficacy was judged according to the cooperative acute leukemia group 3 (CALGB) criteria [11].

Second Department of Internal Medicine, University of Vienna, Garnisongasse 13, 1090 Vienna, Austria

Results

All 23 consecutive patients enrolled into the study are evaluable, as we observed no case of early death. Nineteen of 23 patients (83%) achieved a complete remission, two patients a partial remission, and two patients were nonresponders. Survival rates and therapeutic results are shown in Table 1. Six patients underwent successful bone marrow transplantation (four allogeneic, one syngeneic, one autologous) with survivals of 43+ 22+, 23+, 29+, 21+,

Table 1. Myelosuppression during therapy with c-HAM (*n* = 21)

Time to:		Days	(Median, range)
Leukocytes (10⁹/l)	< 500	7	(2–15)
Nadir of leukocytes		9	(2–15)
Granulocytes	> 500	22	(16–50)
Leukocytes	> 1 000	20	(7–42)
Leukocytes	> 2 000	25	(15–50)
Thrombocytes	>20 000	17	(10–57)

and 17+ months. Three patients with an antedecent myelodysplastic syndrome achieved complete remission. Severe side effects with toxicity grades 3 and 4 according to the WHO criteria were seen in three patients suffering mainly from diarrhea, nausea, vomiting, and mucositis. We observed no significant toxicity (grades 3 + 4) concerning kidney, liver, CNS, or heart. The results of hematological toxicity after 21 cycles of a c-HAM regimen are illustrated in Table 2. A decrease in leukocytes <500 μl was achieved after 7 (2–15) days and nadir of leukocytes occurred after 9 (2–15) days. The median time for recovery of granulocytes to values above 500/μl was 22 (16–50) days for a platelet count above 20 000/μl 17 (10–57) days from the onset of therapy.

Discussion

Similar to our previous study [2] the preliminary results demonstrate again a high antileukemic effect of the c-HAM regimen. The

Table 2. Induction/postremission therapy with c-HAM in ANLL

Initials	Age/sex	Diagnosis	Survival (months)	Outcome
O. B.	58/f	AML M4	25	CR
T. M.	34/f	AML M1	7	NR
R. M.	76/m	AML M4	11	PR
L. V.	27/f	AML M1	5	NR
R. S.	23/f	RAEB-t	43+	CR-all. BMT
F. W.	60/m	AML M2	26+	CR
Ö. H.	39/m	AML M2	22+	CR-all. BMT
W. L.	20/f	AML M1	28	CR-all. BMT
S. T.	77/f	AML M1	12	CR
W. R.	46/m	AML M5	29+	CR-au. BMT
B. K.	55/m	AML M5	9	CR
T. J.	32/f	AML M2	21+	CR-syn. BMT
S. H.	57/f	AML M2	16+	CR
R. R.	80/f	AML M2	6	CR
S. T.	77/f	AML (MDS)	5	CR
S. H.	78/f	AML M1	8	PR
G. M.	80/f	AML M4	16+	CR
B. R.	45/f	AML (sec.)	6	CR
W. M.	44/f	AML M2	17+	CR-all. BMT
G. J.	74/f	AML (MDS)	8	CR
W. L.	17/f	AML M4	12+	CR
K. P.	72/f	AML M2	9+	CR
H. M.	70/f	AML M4	4+	CR

(sec), Secondary AML

response rate of 83 % CR compares favorably with other HD Ara-C combinations especially regarding patients of that age. For bolus administration of mitoxantrone it has been demonstrated that a plasma level of mitoxantrone 60 min after infusion decreased to below mean lethal concentration repeated for human cells exposed for 1 h in vitro [12]. Patients who achieved a CR had higher plasma levels of mitoxantrone at their daily nadir than those patients who manifested resistant disease [13]. Using a very sensitive HPLC method we demonstrated a constant plasma concentration of mitoxantrone with a mean range of about 200 ng/ml 15 days after onset of c-HAM therapy [9, 14].

Therefore we succeeded not only in a significant increase of the daily nadir but also in achieving a constant level of the drug above a concentration necessary to kill human cells in vitro [12].

As in a previous study we did not observe a case of early death. Nonhematological toxicity compared favorably with similar treatment protocols [7, 15]. Response rates of this study compared favorably to results we achieved with induction/consolidation therapy using DAT (daunorubicin, cytarabine, thioguanine) or AAT (daunorubicin, cytarabine, thioguanine) regimens [16, 17].

Patients with contraindications to a therapy with anthracyclines (arrhythmia) tolerated the c-HAM regimen very well and achieved CR.

In conclusion, in our opinion the c-HAM protocol offers advantages compared to the original HAM or to the sequential HAM protocol: a constant long-lasting plasma level of mitoxantrone, a low nonhematological toxicity, and a high therapeutic index.

References

1. Greidanus J, de Vries E, Mulder N, Steijfer D, Uges D, Oosterhuis B, Willemse P (1989) A phase I pharmacokinetic study of 21 day continuous infusion mitoxantrone. J Chir Oncol 7 (6): 790–797
2. Linkesch W, Thaler J, Gattringer C, Konwalinka G (1990) Continuous infusion of mitoxantrone combined with high-dose cytarabine in refractory/relapsed acute myeloblastic leukemia and blast crisis of chronic myelogenous leukemia. Haematol Blood Transfus 33: 330–332
3. Büchner T, Barlogie B, Asseburg U, Hiddemann W, Kamanbroo D, Göhde W (1974) Accumulation of S-phase cells in the bone marrow of patients with acute leukemia by cytosine arabinoside. Blut 28: 299
4. Edelstein M, Vietti T, Valeriote F (1974) Schedule dependent synergism for the combination of 1-β-D-arabinofuranosylcytosine and daunorubicin. Cancer Res 34: 293
5. Colly LP, van Bekkum DW, Hagenbeek A (1984) Enhanced tumor load reduction after chemotherapy induced recruitment and synchronization in a slowly growing rat leukemia model (BNML) for human acute myelocytic leukemia. Leuk Res 8: 953
6. Fountzilas G, Ohnuma T, Okano T, Greenspan EM, Holland JF (1983) Schedule-dependent synergism of cytosine arabinoside (Ara-C) with mitoxantrone in human acute myelogenous leukemia cell line HL 60. Proc Am Assoc Cancer Res Am Soc Clin Oncol 2: 179 (abstr)
7. Hiddemann W, Kreutzmann H, Straif K, Ludwig WD, Mertelsmann R, Donhuijsen-Ant R, Lengfelder E, Arlin Z, Büchner T (1987) High-dose cytosine arabinoside and mitoxantrone: a highly effective regimen in refractory acute myeloid leukemia. Blood 69 (3): 744–749
8. Brito-Babapulle F, Catovsky D, Slocombe G et al. (1987) Phase II study of mitoxantrone and cytarabine in acute myeloid leukemia. Cancer Treat Rep 71: 161–163
9. Linkesch W, Czejka M, Georgopoulos A (1988) Kontinuierliche Mitoxantrontherapie kombiniert mit hochdosiertem Cytosin-Arabinosid (C-HAM): Pharmakokinetische und klinische Ergebnisse. In: Lutz D, Heinz R, Nowotny H, Stacher A (eds) Leukämien und Lymphome – Fortschritte und Hoffnungen. Urban and Schwarzenberg, Munich, pp 76–77
10. World Health Organization (1979) WHO handbook for reporting results of cancer treatment. WHO, Geneva
11. Ohnuma T, Rosner F, Levy RN et al. (1971) Treatment of adult leukemia with L-asparaginase. Cancer Chemother Rep 55: 269
12. Dewinko B, Yang LY, Barlogie B et al. (1983) Comparative cytotoxity of bisamtrene, mitoxantrone, ametrantone, dihydroxy-anthracenedione, dihydroxyanthracenedione-diacetate and doxorubicin on human cells in vitro. Cancer Res 43: 2648–2653

13. Larson RA, Daly KM, Kyung E et al. (1987) A clinical and pharmacokinetic study of mitoxantrone in acute nonlymphocytic leukemia. J Clin Oncol 5: 391–397
14. Czejka M, Georgopoulos A (1988) Mitoxantrone determination using high-performance liquid chromatography: improved sensitivity by loop-column injection for dual dose pharmacokinetic studies. J Chromatogr 425: 429–434
15. Hiddemann W, Büchner T, Essink M, Koch O, Stenzinger W, van de Loo J (1988) High-dose cytosine arabinoside and mitoxantrone: preliminary results of a pilot study with sequential application (S-HAM) indicating a high antileukemic activity in refractory acute leukemias. Onkologie 11: 10–12
16. Linkesch W, Michlmayr G, Gerhartz H, Illinger H, König H, Düllmann J, Keilhauer R, Moldrzyk D (1989) Amsacrine, cytarabine and thioguanine (AAT) vs. daunorubicin, cytarabine, thioguanine (DAT) in adults with untreated acute non-lymphoblastic leukemia (ANLL): Austrian-German results. Onkologie I 12: 8–10
17. Linkesch, Domingo-Albos A, Hoffmann R, Schulof R, Makavy A, Amare M, Rickles F (1989) A randomised comparative trial of amsacrine, cytarabine and thioguanine (AAT) vs. daunorubicin, cytarabine and thioguanine (DAT) as front-line therapy for ANLL. Proc Am Soc Clin Oncol 8: 204

Treatment of Refractory and Relapsed Acute Leukemias with Cytosine Arabinoside and Mitoxantrone

T. Rozmysłowicz[1], G. Pałynyczko[1], J. Mazur[1], R. Konecki[1], D. Apel[1], B. Mariańska[1], S. Maj[1], J. Holowiecki[2], E. Rudzka[2], T. Ławniczek[2], Ł. Kachel[2], J. Wojnar[2], S. Krzemień[2], L. Konopka[1], and S. Pawelski[1]

Introduction

In the last few years several new agents for the treatment of acute leukemia have been studied. These have included amsacrine, idarubicin, mitoxantrone, homoharringtonine and most recently diaziquone [1]. Mitoxantrone is a relatively new synthetic anthracenedione derivative with strong antineoplastic activity in vitro and in vivo against solid tumors and leukemias [2].

Clinical studies have shown that acute leukemias resistant to doxorubicin and other anthracyclines are only partially resistant to mitoxantrone [3]. The incomplete cross-resistance with other anticancer agents has also been reported [4]. The elimination half-life of mitoxantrone is very long, based on the body content of drug 35 days after dosing. The most important route of mitoxantrone elimination appears to be fecal [5]. Mitoxantrone binds to DNA but cardiotoxicity is less pronounced than after other anthracycline antibiotics [6]. Previously reported clinical symptoms of toxicity (excluding myelosuppression) like nausea, vomiting, stomatitis and alopecia are usually of limited clinical significance [7].

The possible synergistic antileukemic effect of mitoxantrone and cytosine arabinoside has led to combination chemotherapy particularly in refractory and relapsed acute leukemias [1].

Patients, Materials, and Methods

At the Institute of Hematology in Warsaw and at the Department of Hematology, Medical Academy, Katowice, 49 patients (mean age 33 years) with refractory and relapsed acute leukemias (35 patients with acute nonlymphoblastic leukemia, ANLL, and 14 patients with acute lymphoblastic leukemia, ALL) were treated with cytosine arabinoside (ARA-C) (Alexan; Mack, FRG) in combination with mitoxantrone, which was obtained partly from Lederle Lab., United States (Novantrone) and from Polfa Co., Poland (Mitoksantrone).

According to cytochemical examination based on FAB classification and using monoclonal antibodies (in all cases immunophenotyping of leukemic cells was performed using monoclonal antibodies obtained from Becton-Dickinson, United States) the following types of ANLL were diagnosed: M_0, 1; M_1, 2; M_2, 25; M_3, 3; M_4, 2; M_6, 2 and ALL: L_1 (common), 3; L_2 (null), 11 (Table 1). Therapy consisted of three different doses of ARA-C: I, 3 g/m^2 every 12 h during 3-h infusion on days 1–4; II, 1 g/m^2 every 12 h during 3-h infusion on days 1–4; III, 100 mg/m^2 in continuous infusion on days 1–7. Mitoxantrone in combination with high doses of ARA-C (3 g/m^2 and 1 g/m^2) was used in doses of 10 mg/m^2 on das 3–5 and in low doses of ARA-C (100 mg/m^2) on days 1–3. The induction phase consisted of one or two cycles of therapy during 2–3 months.

[1] Institute of Hematology, Chocimska str. 5, 00-957 Warsaw, Poland
[2] Department of Hematology, Medical Academy, Reymonta str. 40-029 Katowice, Poland

Table 1. Patient characteristics

Number of patients	49
Female : male	26 : 23
Age (years)	16–65 (mean 33)
ANLL (No.)	35
FAB classification	
M_0	1
M_1	2
M_2	25
M_3	3
M_4	2
M_6	2
ALL (No.)	14
L_1 (common)	3
L_2 (null)	11

Results

Treatment results are shown in Table 2. Out of the 49 patients, 24 (49%) responded to the treatment. Seventeen (35%) patients achieved complete remission (CR) and 7 (14%) partial remission (PR). Of the 35 cases with ANLL, CR was obtained in 13 (37%) and PR in 4 (11%) patients. In the ALL group CR was achieed in four (29%) patients and PR in three (21%) patients respectively. The median duration of complete remission was 7 months (range 2–12 months) and the median survival time for all treated patients was 24 months (Kaplan-Meier analysis). Twenty-five (51%) patients

Table 2. Results of combination chemotherapy: cytosine arabinoside plus mitoxantrone in refractory and relapsed acute leukemias

Diagnosis	Patients	
	No.	%
ANLL		
CR	13	37
PR	4	11
ALL		
CR	4	29
PR	3	21
Total CR	17	35
PR	7	14

did not respond to the treatment and nine (18%) died soon after one course of induction therapy with severe thrombocytopenic purpura and neutropenia with subsequent sepsis. Four (8%) patients died during the subsequent 7 months with recurrent or progressive disease.

All patients were evaluated for toxicity. The most important side effects were myelosuppression and pancytopenia (Table 3) observed in all the patients with subsequent bacterial infections (49%). Severe neutropenia (<0.5/nl) lasted at least 10 days (range 0–33 days) and thrombocytopenia (<20/nl) 13 days respectively (range 0–37 days). All patients required intravenous antibiotics and antimycotic treatment. Other substantial side effects were moderate (nausea, vomiting, 47%; alopecia, 39%). No cardiac toxicity was observed.

Table 3. Toxicity of cytosine arabinoside plus mitoxantrone therapy in acute leukemias

Toxicity	Number of patients and mean value (score) grading according to WHO
Nausea and vomiting	17 (2°), 6 (3°)
Cardiac toxicity	2 (1°)
Documented bacterial infections	14 (2°), 3 (3°), 7 (4°)
Diarrhea	3 (2°), 2 (3°)
Hemorrhage and thrombocytopenia	49 (4°)
Leukopenia	49 (4°)
Neurotoxicity	2 (1°)
Alopecia	13 (1°), 6 (2°)

Discussion

As a single agent at 12 mg/m^2 daily $\times$ 5 mitoxantrone was demonstrated in patients with ANLL in relapse and defined as an active antileukemic agent. A CR rate was 35% (25 of 71 patients) [8]. Subsequent addition of cytosine arabinoside increased the CR rate significantly to 70% (range 33%–74%) in relapsed and refractory acute leukemias. In the group of ALL patients a lower CR rate was obtained [9–13]. Comparing the results of all the trials it is difficult to find any difference in efficacy of the combinations whatever the dose of cytosine arabinoside used (100 mg/m^2, 0.5 g/m^2, 1 g/m^2 and 3 g/m^2) [1, 3].

The results of this study indicate that combination therapy consisting of cytosine arabinoside and mitoxantrone seems to have a significant activity in refractory or relapsed acute leukemias. However, in comparison to other data our CR rates were lower mainly in ALL patients (29 %) but the total response rate was 49 % (CR + PR). Because of the small group of patients, a much larger study would be needed.

The substantial side effects can limit wider application of the presented drug combination. The major toxicity is myelosuppression and subsequent cytopenia. The addition of colony-stimulating growth factors may further improve prognosis in such patients [14].

References

1. Arlin ZA (1990) Current status of mitoxantrone combination chemotherapy programs: a personal view. Leukemia Lymphoma 1: 301–305
2. Durr FE, Wallace RE, Citarella RV (1983) Molecular and biochemical pharmacology of mitoxantrone. Cancer Treat Rev 10 [Suppl B]: 3–11
3. Rozmysłowicz T, Pałynyczko G, Mazur J, Konopka L (1991) Mitoxantrone in the treatment of malignant haematological disorders (in Polish). Terapia i Leki 10: 255–262
4. Dalton WS, Cress AE, Alberts DS (1988) Cytogenetic and phenotypic analysis of a human colon carcinoma cell line resistant to mitoxantrone. Cancer Res 48: 1882–1888
5. Alberts DS, Peng Y-P, Leigh S et al. (1983) Disposition of mitoxantrone in patients. Cancer Treat Rev 10 [Suppl B]: 23–27
6. Benjamin RS, Chawla SP, Ewer MS et al. (1985) Evaluation of mitoxantrone cardiotoxicity by nuclear angiography and endomyocardial biopsy: an update. Invest New Drugs 3: 117–121
7. Arlin ZA, Silver R, Cassileth P et al. (1985) Phase I–II trial of mitoxantrone in acute leukaemia. Cancer Treat Rep 69: 61–64
8. Arlin ZA, Dukart G, Schoch I et al. (1985) Phase I–II trial of mitoxantrone in acute leukemia: interim report. Invest New drugs 3: 213–217
9. Paciucci P, Dutcher J, Cuttner J et al. (1987) Mitoxantrone and Ara-C in previously treated patients with acute myelogenous leukemia. Leukemia 1 (7): 565–567
10. Hiddemann W, Kreutzmann H, Straif K et al. (1987) High-dose cytosine arabinoside and mitoxantrone: a highly effective regimen in refractory acute leukemia. Blood 69: 744–749
11. Rozmysłowicz T, Pałynyczko G, Mazur J et al. (1990) Mitoxantrone in treatment of refractory acute leukemias. Blood 76 (10) [Suppl 1]: 315a
12. Arlin ZA, Case D, Moore J et al. (1988) Randomized trial of mitoxantrone and daunorubicin-based therapy in untreated acute myelogenous leukemia. Am Soc Clin Oncol 7: 186
13. Hiddemann W, Büchner T, Heil G et al. (1990) Treatment of refractory acute lymphoblastic leukemia in adults with high dose cytosine arabinoside and mitoxantrone (HAM). Leukemia 4 (9): 637–640
14. Kantarijan HM, Walters RL, Keating MJ et al. (1990) Mitoxantrone and high-dose arabinoside for the treatment of refractory acute lymphocytic leukemia. Cancer 65: 5–8

Mitoxantrone and VP-16,213 (MVP16) in AML Patients Refractory to Cytosine Arabinoside with Daunorubicin and High-Dose Cytosine Arabinoside with Amsidine: Preliminary Results

S. Daenen, B. Löwenberg, P. Sonneveld, G. Verhoeff, P. Huygen, and L. Verdonck, for the Dutch Hematologie-Oncologie Vereniging Volwassenen Nederland (HOVON)

Introduction

Patients with acute myeloid leukemia (AML) refractory to standard remission induction therapy consisting of cytosine arabinoside (AraC) and daunorubicin have a dismal outcome. Both high-dose AraC with amsacrine (HDAraC-AMSA, [1]) and VP-16,213 with mitoxantrone [2] are among the few chemotherapy courses which have been shown to produce remissions in refractory and relapsing AML. It is conceivable that both regimens could be effective in the same subpopulation of patients and that any of them would be ineffective whenever the other fails to induce a complete remission (CR). Evaluation of the response of patients treated with one of these regimens after failure of the other can give some insight into the behavior of refractory AML.

In an ongoing Dutch multicenter trial, newly diagnosed adults with AML were treated consecutively with three chemotherapy courses:
a) AraC with daunorubicin,
b) HDAraC – AMSA, and
c) VP-16,213 with mitoxantrone (MVP16).

After the third course, patients in CR since the second course were randomized between autologous bone marrow trans-

Department of Haematology, University of Groningen, Oostersingel 59, 9713 EZ Groningen, The Netherlands

plantation (ABMT) and no further therapy. As part of this study patients who were not in CR after the second course still received the third course, not as consolidation but as salvage therapy. The aim was to examine the efficacy and the toxicity of MVP16 in this homogeneous population of highly pretreated AML patients.

Study Design

This was an open study for AML patients refractory to AraC-dauno and to HDAraC-AMSA who are considered candidates for further intensive chemotherapy. Patients are given one or two courses of:
– VP-16,213 100 mg/m^2 per day for 5 days
– Mitoxantrone 10 mg/m^2 per day for 5 days

After one or two courses patients in CR were free to continue with any additional therapy at the discretion of the physician. Supportive care included antibiotic prophylaxis and blood products as required.

Preliminary Results

Twenty-four patients are evaluable at the time of this writing. Nine patients attained CR after one course of MVP16 and one patient after two courses. One nonresponder to previous chemotherapy attained a partial remission (PR), giving a response rate of 45.8%. Four patients, including the two who had a PR after one course, received two courses of MVP16 and one patient underwent a successful ABMT.

In four of the CR patients duration of the remission was only 4 months but the seven others are still in CR 7$^+$ to 28$^+$ months after MVP16. The median survival of the responders was 12$^+$ months (range 8–34$^+$ months), compared to 6 months in the nonresponders (range 3–13$^+$ months).

Responders were mainly among the patients who showed at least some reaction to the previous therapy: 10 of the 11 responders had a PR after the HDAraC-AMSA therapy. Nevertheless, five of these did not improve from the first to the second course and three even deteriorated in that they could not consolidate a CR which was reached after the first course. In contrast, 9 of 13 nonresponders had shown no response at all to the previous therapy.

Toxicity was mainly hematological with a median duration of leukocytopenia of 45 days (range 29–160 days) and thrombocytopenia of >60 days (range 41 days to indefinite) for responders. The blood counts of nonresponders mostly did not recover completely. Surprisingly, three nonresponders had a remarkably short period of thrombocytopenia from 18 to 20 days. Infections and febrile episodes occurred in nine patients; five of them had two infectious episodes. Five patients had pulmonary infection, often fungal in origin, and five had gram-positive bacteremia. Other side effects were negligible with only occasionally severe nausea and vomiting.

Discussion

The AML patients in this small study belong to a homogeneous group with an extremely bad prognosis because they did not attain a CR after a standardized treatment with two different courses of intensive remission induction therapy. Nevertheless, almost half of them reached a CR which was durable in a considerable number and which allowed one patient to proceed to a successful ABMT. These results suggest that refractoriness of AML to cytostatic therapy can be overcome by other cytostatic drugs and is not always due to absolute drug resistance or unfavorable cytokinetic characteristics. Even so, the probability of attaining CR was highest in those patients who had shown some response to the previous chemotherapy. Most of the patients who did not respond at all to the earlier courses did not respond to the MVP16 either.

There were remarkably few nonhematological side effects. The infections were rarely severe. However, three nonresponders showed a very short duration of thrombocytopenia. This suggests that in some nonresponder patients an alteration of, e.g., the pharmacokinetics of the cytostatics could be more important than cellular refractoriness for the lack of susceptibility of the leukemic process.

In comparison to Ho et al. [2], who examined the value of the same cytostatic regimen in a larger group of 61 patients, the response rate in the present study is somewhat lower (41.6 % CR plus 4.1 % PR versus 42.6 % CR plus 11.7 % PR) but the remission duration is much better (9$^+$ versus 4.7 months). Reasons for these differences are not obvious but are probably due to differences in patient populations. The patient population in the study of Ho et al. [2] was less homogeneous with respect to earlier chemotherapy and stage of disease.

References

1. Zittoun R, Bury J, Stryckmans P et al. (1985) Amsacrine (AMSA) with high dose cytarabine in acute leukemia. Cancer Treat Rep 69: 1447–1448
2. Ho AD et al. (1988) Mitoxantrone and VP-16 in refractory acute myelogenous leukemia. J Clin Oncol 6: 213–217

Induction Therapy for Acute Myelogenous Leukemia with Idarubicin/Cytosine Arabinoside and Mitoxantrone/Etoposide in "Response-Adapted" Sequence

R. Haas[1], A. Schneeweiß[1], B. Brado[1], B. Witt[1], W. Hunstein[1], F. Del Valle[2], M. Goebel[3], and A. D. Ho[4]

Introduction

With conventional induction chemotherapy 47%–72% of adult patients with acute myelogenous leukemia (AML) achieve complete remission (CR). However, the probability of continuous CR ranges from 8% to 45% at 3 years [1]. Most of the chemotherapeutic protocols for induction treatment consist of cytosine arabinoside (Ara-C) combined with an anthracycline such as daunorubicin. One possibility to improve the induction remission rate is the administration of new agents with higher antileukemic activity. Furthermore, for patients not responding to the first-line chemotherapy, an alternate regimen with non-cross-resistant cytostatic drugs should be considered in the early phase of induction treatment.

Idarubicin (4-demethoxydaunorubicin; IDA) is a new chemotherapeutic agent that lacks the methoxyl group in position 4 of the aglycon of daunorubicin. In preclinical studies, Casazza et al. demonstrated that idarubicin was four- to fivefold more effective than daunorubicin or doxorubicin when evaluated against a variety of experimental leukemias [2]. Vogler et al. [3] report an 86% complete remission rate with idarubicin/Ara-C versus an 80% complete CR rate with daunorubicin/Ara-C in patients

with de novo AML. Berman et al. [4] demonstrated that idarubicin/Ara-C is at least as effective as standard therapy with Ara-C daunorubicin in adult patients with newly diagnosed AML.

It was the aim of this study to evaluate the remission induction rate and toxicity of a "response-adapted" sequential therapy with idarubicin/Ara-C (IDAC) followed by mitoxantrone/etoposide (NOVE) in adult patients with de novo AML. The rationale for this clinical trial was to design a treatment protocol with non-cross-resistant chemotherapeutic agents to obtain a higher complete remission rate for patients not responding to one cycle of IDAC.

Patients and Methods

From January 1989 to September 1990, a total of 31 patients (age between 15 and 58 years) with previously untreated AML were included in this trial. The cutoff date for this report was 31 January 1991. The study was approved by the local Ethical Review Committee. A written informed consent was obtained from all patients. Exclusion criteria included bilirubin >2 mg/dl, creatinine >2 mg/dl, a cardiac ejection fraction less than 50% and pregnancy. The study design is shown in Fig. 1. The chemotherapy consisted of Ara-C (100 mg/m^2 per day) as a continuous 7-day infusion and idarubicin (12 mg/m^2 per day) as a 1-hour i.v. infusion on each of the first 3 days of treatment. Patients achieving a complete or partial remission received a second cycle of IDAC, whereas those failing to respond to IDAC

[1] Department of Internal Medicine, University of Heidelberg, Hospitalstr. 3, 6900, FRG
[2] Städtische Klinik Oldenburg, FRG
[3] Farmitalia Freiburg, FRG
[4] Northeastern Ontario Oncology Program, Sudbury, Ontario, Canada

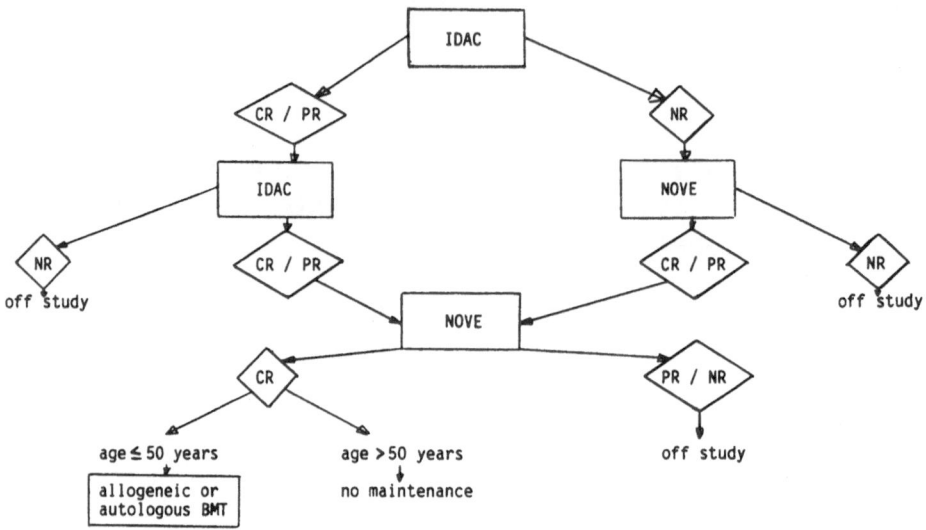

Fig. 1. Study design

received mitoxantrone (10 mg/m^2 per day) as i.v. infusion and etoposide (100 mg/m^2 per day) as i.v. infusion, both from day 1 to day 5. Patients not responding to NOVE were taken off study and treated with high-dose Ara-C and Crasnitin (asparaginase). All patients achieving CR or PR after either two cycles of IDAC or one cycle of IDAC and NOVE received a subsequent cycle of NOVE as early consolidation therapy. Thereafter, patients were either followed without any maintenance therapy or included in a bone marrow transplant program. Patients with an HLA-compatible sibling received an allogeneic BMT whereas patients without a suitable donor underwent autologous BMT with mafosfamide-purged bone marrow. The characteristics of the 31 patients entered on this treatment protocol are shown in table 1.

Results

Response Rate

Of the 31 patients who entered this clinical trial, 1 patient died on the 4th day of chemotherapy due to an acute respiratory distress syndrome. Therefore, treatment response was evaluable in 30 patients. After

2 cycles of IDAC, 25 of 30 patients had attained a CR (83%), wihile the majority (22 of 30 patients) had obtained CR already after the first course of IDAC (73%). Of the five initial nonresponders to IDAC, three achieved CR after the first cycle of NOVE. Thus, 28 of 30 patients (93%) achieved CR after a sequential induction therapy with either two cycles of IDAC or one cycle with IDAC followed by NOVE. The median time required to achieve CR in these 28 patients was 31 days (range, 17–78 days). The two patients not responding to IDAC/NOVE were subsequently treated with high-dose Ara-C and Crasnitin and achieved a CR. However, both patients relapsed shortly after they underwent bone marrow transplantation.

Toxicity

Severe myelosuppression was observed in all patients under both chemotherapy regimens (Table 2). The median time of neutropenia following the first cycle of IDAC with neutrophils <0.5/nl was 25 days (range, 6–46 days) and the phase of thrombopenia with platelets <50.0/nl was 21 days (median, range, 11–47 days). In comparison, the phase of severe myelosuppression

Table 1. Patient characteristics

Number of Patients	
Total	31
Evaluable for toxicity	31
Evaluable for efficacy	30
Age (median, range) (years)	41 (15–58)
Female/male	19/12
Classification according to FAB	
M1	4
M2	6
M3	4
M4	12
M5	4
M6	1

Hematological parameters at entry

	Median	Range
WBC (/nl)	13.0	0.4–432.0
Hemoglobin (g/dl)	9.3	6.0–12.9
Platelets (/nl)	47.0	5.0–183.0

FAB, French-American-British; WBC, white blood count

Table 2. Duration of severe cytopenia

| | IDAC | | NOVE |
	First cycle	Second cycle	.All cycles
Number of patients	30	23	29
Days of neutrophils <0.5/nl			
Median	25	17	24
Range	6–46	11–30	12–61
Days of platelets <50.0/nl			
Median	21	14	22
Range	11–47	6–40	5–44

was shorter after the second cycle of IDAC with 17 days (median, range, 11–30 days) for neutrophils <0.5/nl and 14 days (median, range, 6–40 days) for platelets <50.0/nl. The patients treated with NOVE had a median time of 24 days (range, 12–61 days) with a neutrophil count <0.5/nl and a median period of 22 days (range, 5–44 days) with a platelet count <50.0/nl.

One treatment-related death occurred during consolidation therapy with NOVE due to an overwhelming gram-negative septicemia. Besides that, no significant complications – especially no major cardiac toxicity – occurred during this sequential induction chemotherapy.

Response Duration and Survival

With respect to disease-free survival (DFS), 28 patients were evaluable. Eight

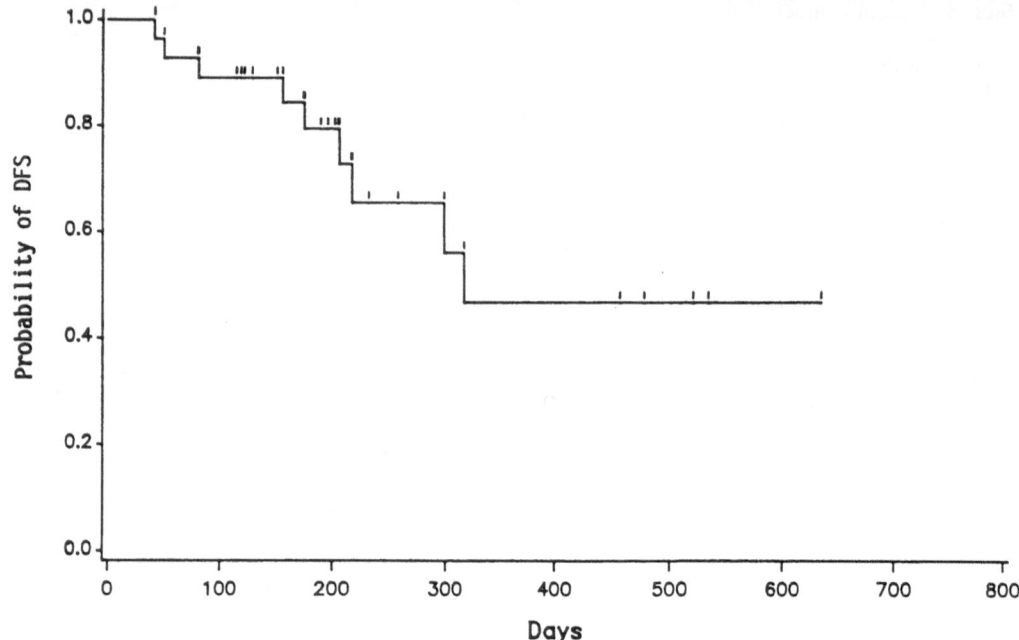

Fig. 2. Disease-free survival in patients achieving CR after sequential therapy with IDAC and NOVE (*n* = 28). Eight BMT patients were censored at time of transplantation

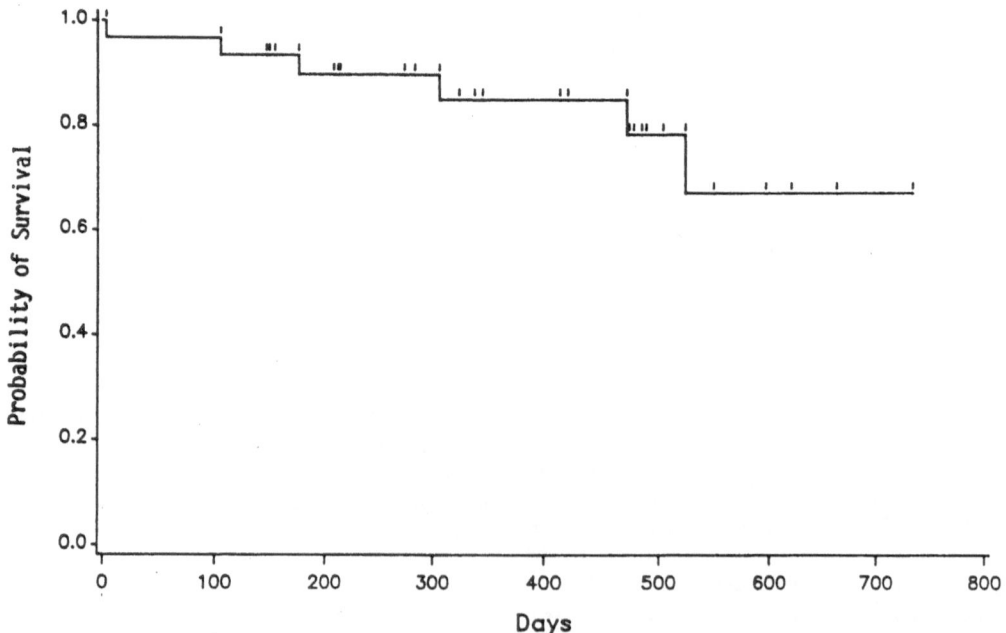

Fig. 3. Time of survival of all patients (*n* = 31) treated with IDAC and NOVE. For this analysis the BMT patients were not censored

patients were censored because of bone marrow transplantation. Of the remaining 20 patients, 8 relapsed after a median time of 191 days (range, 50–317 days). One patient died due to septicemia during the neutropenic phase after the early consolidation therapy with NOVE. The remaining 11 patients are in CR with a median disease-free survival of 258 days (range, 115–636 days) (Fig. 2). It is worth noting that in two of the relapsed patients a second complete remission could be achieved by chemotherapy. The Kaplan-Meier analysis for the overall survival of the 31 patients is shown in Fig. 3. With a longest follow-up of 734 days, there is a 67% probability of survival.

Bone Marrow Transplantation

Eight patients in first CR were included in a bone marrow transplantation protocol. All of them were female. The median age was 38 years with a range from 15 to 49 years. Two patients had an HLA-identical sibling donor and could undergo allogeneic BMT. In the remaining six patients an autologous BMT with mafosfamide-purged bone marrow was performed. The duration of the remission before BMT was 165 days (median, range, 20–210 days). The median follow-up after BMT is 290 days (range, 77–584 days).

Five patients (four after autologous BMT/one after allogenic BMT) are in unmaintained complete remission for a median time of 288 days (range, 77–584 days). One patient with allogenic BMT died of GvH-related complications, whereas two patients relapsed after autologous BMT.

Discussion

In this clinical trial idarubicin combined with Ara-C was studied as induction therapy for patients with previously untreated AML. Furthermore, its therapeutic benefit within a sequential "response adapted" therapy protocol was evaluated. Therefore, patients not responding to IDAC were treated consecutively with a combination of mitoxantrone and etoposide. With this new therapeutic concept we achieved a complete response rate of 93%, which is very high compared to a usual CR rate of up to 72% in the conventional standard protocols [1]. It is worth noting that 25 patients attained a CR after two cycles of IDAC therapy alone (83%), demonstrating the therapeutic efficacy of the new anthracycline analogue idarubicin. These data are comparable with a report by Wiernik et al. [5] showing that idarubicin/Ara-C may be more effective than daunorubicin/Ara-C as induction therapy for previously untreated adults with AML. A similar observation has been made by Berman et al. [4] with a better survival rate in patients treated with idarubicin/Ara-C compared to patients with daunorubicin/Ara-C. With respect to toxicity, both regimens, IDAC and NOVE, were well tolerated with expected toxicities like nausea, vomiting, stomatitis and alopecia. One patient died due to a respiratory distress syndrome on the 44th day of treatment and another patient died in the phase of severe pancytopenia during consolidation therapy with NOVE due to an overwhelming septicemia. In conclusion, the induction therapy with IDAC and NOVE in a response-adapted sequential application is highly effective in AML. Furthermore, a high rate of complete remissions has an important impact on the number of patients eligible for bone marrow transplantation.

Summary

It was the aim of this study to evaluate the remission induction rate and toxicity of a sequential therapy with idarubicin/cytosine arabinoside (IDAC) followed by mitoxantrone/etoposide (NOVE) in patients with de novo acute myelogenous leukemia (AML). Idarubicin 12 mg/m^2 per day was given as i.v. short infusion (day 1–3) and Ara-C 100 mg/m^2 per day as continuous infusion (day 1–7). NOVE consisted of mitoxantrone 10 mg/m^2 per day and etoposide 100 mg/m^2 per day (both day 1–5). From January 1989 until September 1990, 31 patients (p) were included in the study. Their distribution according to the FAB classification was as follows: M1: 4 p, M2: 6 p, M3: 4 p, M4: 12 p, M5: 4 p, M6: 1 p.

Nineteen patients were female and 12 patients male. The median age was 41 years (range, 15–58 years). Because of 1 early death, only 30 patients were evaluable for response. Patients achieving complete remission (CR) or partial remission (PR) received another cycle of IDAC followed by one cycle of NOVE as early consolidation therapy. The nonresponders after the initial IDAC cycle received NOVE. Twenty-five patients attained a CR after two cycles of IDAC (83 %). Three of the five nonresponders to IDAC achieved a CR after one cycle of NOVE. Thus, 28 of 30 patients (93 %) achieved a CR. With respect to disease-free survival (DFS), 8 patients were censored because of bone marrow transplantation (BMT). Of the remaining 20 patients, 11 are in CR, whereas 8 patients relapsed and one patient died of a septicemia during the neutropenic phase after the consolidation therapy with NOVE. The median DFS for the 11 patients in CR is 258 days (range, 115–636 days). In conclusion, induction treatment with IDAC and NOVE in "response adapted" sequential application is highly effective in patients with de novo AML. Whether this chemotherapy results in a longer DFS than after standard therapy remains to be seen.

References

1. Büchner T et al. (1987) Postinduction and preremission chemotherapy alternatives for adult AML: three multicenter studies of the AML cooperative group. In: Büchner T et al. (eds) Acute leukemias. Springer, Berlin Heidelberg New York, pp 57–63 (Haematology and blood transfusion, vol 30)
2. Casazza AM, Pratesi G et al. (1980) Antileukemic activity of 4-demethoxydaunorubicin in mice. Tumori 66: 549–564
3. Vogler WR, Velez-Garcia E et al. (1989) A phase-three trial comparing daunorubicin or idarubicin combined with cytosine arabinoside in acute myelogenous leukemia. Semin Oncol 16 [Suppl 2]: 21–24
3. Berman E, Raymond V et al. (1989) Idarubicin in acute leukemia: results of studies at Memorial Sloan-Kettering Cancer Center. Semin Oncol 16 [Suppl 2]: 30–34
5. Wiernik PH, Case DC Jr et al. (1989) A multicenter trial of cytarabine plus idarubicin or daunorubicin as induction therapy for adult nonlymphocytic leukemia. Semin Oncol 16 [Suppl 2]: 25–29

Use of AMSA Combination Chemotherapy in Patients with Acute Myelogenous Leukemia Unsuitable for Anthracycline or Mitoxantrone Treatment

G. Maschmeyer, K. Willborn, and W. Heit

Introduction

Cardiotoxic drugs such as anthracyclines or mitoxantrone are essential components of most established chemotherapy regimens for the treatment of acute myelogenous leukemia (AML). In large multicenter trials, up to 20 % of patients <60 years and more than 50 % of patients >60 years of age must be primarily excluded from treatment mostly due to their history or clinical signs of congestive heart failure or significant arrhythmias. In addition, many patients with relapsed or refractory disease have been heavily pretreated with anthracyclines and thus are not suitable for further administration of these substances. Studies on this poor-risk subgroup of AML patients are rare and focus on the use of low-dose cytosine arabinoside or other less aggressive drug regimens. Amsacrine has been reported as an effective antileukemic drug from numerous clinical trials since 1980. When administered in a total dose of about 600 mg/m² in combination with conventional or high-dose cytosine arabinoside, response rates of up to 70 % have been observed [1–10]. We therefore conducted a clinical study on the use of amsacrine in combination with cytosine arabinoside for first-line or reinduction chemotherapy in AML patients unsuitable for anthracycline or mitoxantrone treatment.

Evangelic Hospital, Essen-Werden, Department of Hematology and Oncology, Pattbergstr. 1–3, 4300 Essen 16, FRG

Materials and Methods

From May 1985 to November 1990, a total of 48 patients (32 male, 16 female) with acute myelogenous leukemia were treated with AMSA combination chemotherapy. Their median age was 60 years with a range from 19–74 years. Demographic data are shown in Table 1. Diagnosis was made by morphological and cytochemical analysis of blood and bone marrow smears using the FAB classification of acute leukemias [11] and was confirmed by immunophenotyping of blast cells with monoclonal antibodies using immunofluorescence microscopy and flow cytometry. Contraindications to the use of cardiotoxic substances were confirmed by two-dimensional echocardiography and by radionuclide ventriculography. Patients with hepatic dysfunction defined by the elevation of liver enzymes or bilirubin above double the normal range were excluded from AMSA treatment. AMSA was combined with conventional-dose cytosine arabinoside and 6-thioguanine (TA-AMSA), with high-dose cytosine arabinoside (HA-AMSA) or sequentially with high-dose cytosine arabinoside (sequential HA-AMSA). The three applied regimens and the administered dosage of AMSA are listed in Table 2. Complete remission was defined by a marrow blast count below 5 %, absence of blasts in peripheral blood smears, resolution of eventual extramedullar leukemic infiltrates, peripheral granulocyte counts above 1500/mm³, and thrombocyte counts above 100 000/mm³. Partial remission was defined by a marrow blast count of 5 %–25 %, peripheral granulocyte

Table 1. Demographic data

	n	%
Patients	48	
Median age in years (range)	60 (19–74)	
Sex		
Male	32	66.7
Female	16	33.3
FAB type		
M1	11	22.9
M2	10	20.8
M3	–	
M4	15	31.2
M5	9	18.8
M6	1	2.1
Hybrid	2	4.2
Stage of disease		
First remission induction	22	45.8
First relapse	17	35.4
Second relapse	4	9.1
Third relapse	2	4.2
Primary nonresponse	3	6.2
Pretreatment[a]		
TAD-9	20	41.7
HAM	13	27.1
COAP	3	6.2
TA-AMSA	3	6.2
HA-AMSA	2	4.2
No pretreatment	22	45.8
Indication for AMSA		
Congestive heart failure	35	72.9
Cumulative cardiotoxicity of anthracyclines	5	10.4
Primary nonresponse / early relapse	8	16.7

[a] Superadditive

counts above 500/mm^3 and thrombocyte counts above 25 000/mm^3. Aplasia was defined by severe hypocellular bone marrow without morphological evidence of residual blast cells.

Side effects were graded according to the criteria of the World Health Organization (WHO). All patients were treated in one- to three-bed rooms on a separate hematological ward and received a cooked hospital diet. For infection prevention, all patients were given oral antimicrobial prophylaxis (ciprofloxacin or cotrimoxazole plus colis-tin, both in combination with a polyene antifungal). Empirical antimicrobial therapy and blood cell support was administered according to standard guidelines.

Results

In 29 out of 48 patients (60.4 %), a response to treatment with AMSA combination chemotherapy could be observed. Complete remission was achieved in 19 (39.6 %), partial remission in 4 (8.3 %), and another 6 patients (12.5 %) died in aplasia. Nineteen patients (39.6 %) did not respond (Table 3). Twenty-eight patients (58.3 %) received TA-AMSA, 16 (33.3 %) HA-AMSA, and 4 (8.3 %) sequential HA-AMSA. Twenty-two patients were treated for first remission induction, all due to congestive heart failure. They had a response rate of 63.6 %; however, 5 out of 14 responders (22.7 % of total) died in aplasia (Table 4). In patients with complete remission, the median time to granulocyte recovery above 1000/mm^3 was 32 days with a range from 22–60 days.

Table 3. Overall treatment results

	n	%
Patients	48	
Response	29	60.4
Complete remission	19	39.6
Partial remission	4	8.3
Death in aplasia	6	12.5
Nonresponse	19	39.6

Table 4. Results of first-line treatment

	n	%
Patients	22	
Responders	14	63.6
Complete remision	8	36.7
Partial remission	1	4.5
Death in aplasia	5	22.7
Nonresponders	8	36.4

Table 2. Applied AMSA regimens

TA-AMSA		
AMSA	210 mg/m² i.v. (2 h)	Days 3–5
6-TG	200 mg/m² p.o.	Days 3–9
Ara-C	100 mg/m² i.v. (24 h)	Days 1 and 2
	100 mg/m² q 12 h i.v. (30 min)	Days 3–8
HA-AMSA		
AMSA	210 mg/m² i.v. (2 h)	Days 2–4
Ara-C	3 g/m² q 12 h i.v. (3 h)	Days 1–4
Sequential HA-AMSA		
AMSA	150 mg/m² i.v. (2 h)	Days 3 and 4
		Days 10 and 11
Ara-C	3 g/m² q 12 h i.v. (3 h)	Day 1 and 2
		Days 8 and 9

AMSA, m-amsacrine; 6-TG, 6-thioguanine; Ara-C, cytosine arabinoside

Table 5. Characteristics of complete responders

No. of patients with complete remission	19
(% of total)	(39.6)
AMSA regimen	
TA-AMSA	13
HA-AMSA	4
Sequential HA-AMSA	2
Median time to granulocyte recovery	
>1.0/nl (days)	32
(range)	(22–60)
Median duration of relapse-free	
survival (days)	199
(range)	(44–1092+)
Number of patients receiving	
Consolidation therapy	4
Maintenance therapy	9

Median time of relapse-free survival was 199 days with a range of 44–1092+ days. Four patients received consolidation and nine patients maintenance therapy (Table 5). Nonresponse was seen in 8 out of 22 patients in first remission induction therapy, 6 out 17 patients treated for first relapse, 2 out of 4 for second relapse, both two patients for third relapse, and 1 out of 3 primary nonresponders. Adverse treatment effects are listed in Table 6. Nausea and vomiting were seen in 73%, diarrhea in 44%, and hepatotoxicity in 29% of patients, while cardiotoxic effects were observed in 6 patients, one of whom had WHO grade III. All drug-related side effects were reversible; a lethal complication due to AMSA was not recorded.

Table 6. Side effects

Side effect[a]	Total		WHO I/II		WHO III/IV	
	(n)	(%)	(n)	(%)	(n)	(%)
Nausea/vomiting	35	72.9	19	39.6	16	33.3
Diarrhea	21	43.7	10	20.8	11	22.9
Hepatotoxicity	14	29.2	12	25.0	2	4.2
Cardiotoxicity	6	12.5	5	10.4	1	2.1
Rash	3	6.2	3	6.2	–	
Drug fever	1	2.1	1	2.1	–	
Neuropathy	1	2.1	1	2.1	–	

[a] Superadditive

Discussion

The results of this monocenter study on patients with acute myelogenous leukemia and contraindications for established remission induction of reinduction treatment protocols demonstrate the efficacy of amsacrine combination chemotherapy in this high-risk subgroup. In patients with first relapse, the results are comparable to those achieved with high-dose cytosine arabinoside in combination with mitoxantrone [12], whereas in patients treated for first remission induction the CR rate of 37 % and the rate of patients with lethal complications during aplasia (23 %) is markedly worse than reported for standard regimens. However, data focussing on this subgroup of patients who are generally excluded from treatment with these standard regimens are not available. Thus, our study results obtained in patients under first-line treatment should be considered with respect to the results of mild chemotherapy, e.g., with low-dose cytosine arabinoside [13, 14], or data on patients without effective antileukemic treatment whose median survival is in the range of 8 weeks [15]. Cardiac arrhythmia was observed in 6 out of 48 patients (12.5 %) and appeared to be related to serum potassium levels, as has been described in reviews on amsacrine, also for rare cases of amsacrine-related seizures [16–18]. A history of congestive heart failure or myocardial infarction thus does not represent an obstacle to this aggressive remission induction chemotherapy; however, the median time to granulocyte recovery of more than 4 weeks observed in our patients with complete remission might be deleterious for these patients. Optimal support with blood cell preparations and prompt empirical antimicrobial treatment of fever and infection should be available, and serum electrolyte levels monitored carefully during amsacrine administration. It appears promising to conduct a prospective trial on amsacrine in combination with conventional-dose cytosine arabinoside and 6-thioguanine (TAA) or with high-dose cytosine arabinoside (HAA) in patients with AML who are considered for aggressive chemotherapy

but are not suitable for treatment with potentially cardiotoxic substances.

Conclusions

1. In high-risk AML patients with contraindications for standard remission induction therapy, anthracyclines or mitoxantrone might be replaced by AMSA.
2. AMSA in combination with conventional or high-dose Ara-C appears to be effective for the treatment of first or second relapses following first-line therapy with standard regimen or AMSA combination therapy. In addition, it might be effective also in patients with primary nonresponse to standard treatment regimens.
3. The toxicity of AMSA combination therapy focusses on (reversible) gastrointestinal and hepatic side effects, whereas severe cardiotoxicity is to be expected only rarely.
4. These data suggest that a prospective trial should be conducted in order to study AMSA in combination with conventional or high-dose Ara-C as standard regimen for the treatment of AML in patients unsuitable for anthracycline or mitoxantrone therapy.

References

11. Arlin ZA, Flomenberg N, Gee TS, Kempin SJ, Dellaquila C, Mertelsmann R, Straus DJ, Young CW, Clarkson BD (1981) Treatment of acute leukemia in relapse with 4'-(9-acridinyl-amino)methanesulfon-m-anisidide (AMSA) in combination with cytosine arabinoside and thioguanine. Cancer Clin Trials 4: 317–321
2. Arlin ZA, Ahmed T, Mittelman A, Feldman E, Mehta R, Weinstein P, Rieber E, Sullivan P, Baskind P (1987) A new regimen of amsacrine with high-dose cytarabine is safe and effective therapy for acute leukemia. J Clin Oncol 5: 371–375
3. Boccia R, Zighelboim J, Champlin RE, Kim CC, Gale RP (1984) AMSA: a phase II trial in resistant and recurrent acute myelogenous leukemia. Med Pediatr Oncol 12: 178–179
4. Dhaliwal HS, Shannon MS, Barnett MJ, Prentice HG, Bragman K, Malpas JS, Lister TA (1986) Treatment of acute leukaemia with

m-AMSA in combination with cytosine arabinoside. Cancer Chemother Pharmacol 18: 59–62

5. Estey EH, Keating MJ, Smith TL, McCredie KB, Legha SS, Walters RS, Bodey GP, Freireich EJ (1984) Prediction of complete remission in patients with refractory acute leukemia treated with AMSA. J Clin Oncol 2: 102–106

6. Hines JD, Oken MM, Mazza JJ, Keller AM, Streeter RR, Glick JH (1984) High-dose cytosine arabinoside and m-AMSA is effective therapy in relapsed acute nonlymphocytic leukemia. J Clin Oncol 2: 545–549

7. Hines JD, Mazza JJ, Oken MM, Adelstein DJ, Keller A, Bennett JM, O'Connell MJ (1987) Prolonged survival after high-dose cytosine arabinoside and amsacrine induction in patients with previously untreated de novo acute nonlymphocytic leukemia. Semin Oncol 14 [Suppl 1]: 37–39

8. Kahn SB, Spiers A, Knospe WH, Soojian M, Glick JH (1987) Amsacrine (4'-(9-acridinylamino)-methanesulfon-m-anisidide) (m-AMSA) and 5-azacytidine (AZA) for remission induction in patients with relapsed adult acute nonlymphocytic leukemia. Am J Clin Oncol 10: 78–81

9. Legha SS, Keating MJ, McCredie KB, Bodey GP, Freireich Ej (1982) Evaluation of AMSA in previously treated patients with acute leukemia: results of therapy in 109 adults. Blood 60: 484–490

10. Zittoun R, Bury J, Stryckmans P, Löwenberg B, Rozendaal KY, Haanen C, Kerkhofs M, Jehn U, Willemze R (1985) Amsacrine with high-dose cytarabine in acute leukemia. Cancer Treat Rep 69: 1447–1448

11. Bennett JM, Catovsky D, Daniel MT, Flandrin G, Galton DAG, Gralnick HR, Sultan C (1976) Proposals for the classification of the acute leukaemias: French-American-British (FAB) Co-operative Group. Br J Haematol 33: 451–458

12. Hiddemann W, Kreutzmann H, Straif K, Ludwig WD, Mertelsmann R, Donhuijsen-Ant R, Lengfelder E, Arlin Z, Büchner T (1987) High-dose cytosine arabinoside and mitoxantrone: a highly effective regimen in refractory acute myeloid leukemia. Blood 69: 744–749

13. Mufti GJ, Oscier DG, Hamblin TJ, Bell AJ (1983) Low doses of cytarabine in the treatment of myelodysplastic syndrome and acute myeloid leukemia. N Engl J Med 309: 1653–1654

14. Winter JN, Variakojis D, Gaynor ER, Larson RA, Miller KB (1985) Low-dose cytosine arabinoside (ara-C) therapy in the myelodysplastic syndromes and acute leukemia. Cancer 56: 443–449

15. Wiernik PH, Serpick AA (1970) Factors affecting remission and survival in adult acute nonlymphocytic leukemia (ANLL). Medicine 49: 505–513

16. Louie AC, Issell BF (1985) Amsacrine (AMSA) – a clinical review. J Clin Oncol 3: 562–593

17. Weiss RB, Grillo-López AJ, Marsoni S, Posada JG Jr, Hess F, Ross BJ (1986) Amsacrine-associated cardiotoxicity: an analysis of 82 cases. J Clin Oncol 4: 918–928

18. Mittelman A, Arlin ZA (1983) AMSA-induced seizures in patients with hypokalemia. Cancer Treat Rep 67: 102–103

Treatment of High-Risk Relapsing or Refractory AML with M-AMSA and ID-ARAC

M. Freund[1], S. Giller[1], F. Hinrichs[2], A. Baars[2], J. Meran[1], A. Körfer[1], H. Link[1], and H. Poliwoda[1]

Introduction

The prognosis of patients with refractory or relapsing acute myeloid leukemia (AML) is poor. Easy to handle treatment regimens with high effectivity and tolerable toxicity are warranted. High-dose cytosine arabinoside (HD ara-C) is effective in relapsing or resistant AML [1–9]. However, doses of 3000 mg/m² ara-C are associated with significant mucositis, cutaneous, liver, and CNS toxicity. Pharmacological data indicate that intermediate doses of ara-C may be as effective as high doses [10]. The therapeutic effect of HD ara-C can be enhanced substantially by combination with anthracyclines [6, 11–17] but this may involve the risk of cumulative cardiotoxicity in heavily pretreated and elderly patients. The antineoplastic, DNA-topoisomerase II-reactive DNA intercalating acridine derivative 4′(9-acridinylamino) methanesulfon-m-anisidine (m-AMSA) is active in AML [18–25]. M-AMSA may be combined with ara-C without a significant negative effect on ara-CTP accumulation, elimination, or total intracellular exposure with ara-CTP [26]. As a single agent m-AMSA is as effective as HD ara-C [3]. In combination with conventional ara-C it is at least as effective as daunorubicin [27, 28]. Against this background we have studied a condensed 5-day combination of m-AMSA and intermediate-dose ara-C (ID ara-C) in a population of patients with high-risk AML.

Patients and Methods

Between January 1987 and January 1990, 22 patients [15 male, 17 femle; median age, 48.3 years (range 26–70 years)] with relapsing or refractory AML were enrolled. The study was approved by the ethics committee of the Hannover Medical School and informed consent was obtained from patients prior to admission to the study. The morphology of AML according to FAB [29, 30] was as follows: 2 M1, 8 M2, 9 M4, 2 M4 Eo, 1 M5a. The pretreatment status of the patients was classified in six subgroups:
1. patients resistant to two courses of aggressive chemotherapy,
2. patients with no second complete remission after one course of chemotherapy,
3. patients with first relapse and less than 6 months of preceding remission,
4. patients with high-risk first relapses less than 6 months after HD ara-C consolidation or after autologous BMT,
5. other patients with first relapse, and
6. patients with second or following relapse

The 5-day treatment consisted of ara-C 1000 mg/m² administered over 3 h twice daily in 250 ml glucose 5%, and in m-AMSA 100 mg/m² given over 1 h in 500 ml glucose 5%. A first course of consolidation with an identical course of ID ara-C and m-AMSA was given to six patients and

[1] Department of Hematology and Oncology, Hannover Medical School, Konstanty-Gutschow-Str. 8, 3000 Hannover 61, FRG
[2] Evangelisches Krankenhaus, Oldenburg, FRG

a second one to three patients. There was no maintenance therapy. One patient had an allogeneic and another an autologous BMT in complete remission (CR). Both were censored by the time of the transplantation. The toxicity was quantified according to the WHO criteria [31]. Responses were evaluated according to the criteria of the CALGB [32]. Durations of survival, granulopenia, and thrombopenia were calculated according to Kaplan and Meier [33].

Results

Response to Therapy

Twenty-four courses of ID ara-C and m-AMSA were administered for induction (one patient received three induction cycles). The overall treatment results are summarized in Table 1. The overall complete remission rate was 54 % with all CRs being entered after the first treatment course. In seven patients with resistant AML (subgroups 1 and 2), three complete remissions were obtained (43 %). Nine out of 15 patients with relapsing AML achieved a complete remission (60 %). The median remission duration was 9.0 months and the median survival 8.1 months with six patients being censored after a median time of 7.3 months (Fig. 1, 2).

Toxicity

Toxic side effects are summarized in Tables 2 and 3. The main toxicity was hematologic. The median duration of granulopenia below 500/µl was 20 days and the duration of thrombopenia below 20 000/µl 28 days (Fig. 3, 4). In patients entering a complete remission the durations were 15 and 25 days respectively. Only few patients experienced severe infections or bleeding.

Table 1. Treatment results

Status of refractoriness		N	Result
(1)	Resistant to two courses of aggressive chemotherapy (1 pt. with secondary AML)	6	3 CR (1, 1+[a], 32+ mo), 1 PR, 2 NR
(2)	No second CR after one course of aggressive chemotherapy	1	1 PR
All resistant patients		7	3 CR (43 % [CI: 35 %–85 %]) 2 PR (28 %) 2 NR (28 %)
(3)	Early first relapse (<6 mo) (1 pt. with secondary AML)	6	2 CR (6, 12 mo), 1 PR, 3 NR
(4)	High-risk first relapse <6 mo after HD AraC consolidation or after autologous BMT	3	3 CR (4+[b], 5, 7 mo)
(5)	Other first relapses	2	1 CR (12 mo), 1 NR
(6)	Second or following relapse	4	3 CR (2, 7+, 9 mo), 1 ED
All relapsing patients		15	9 CR (60 %; [CI: 10 %–76 %]) 1 PR (7 %) 5 NR (33 %)
All patients		22	12 CR (54 % [CI: 33 %–76 %]) 3 PR (14 %) 7 NR (32 %)

CI, 95 % confidence interval
[a] Censored, allogeneic BMT in CR
[b] Cebsored, autologous BMT in CR

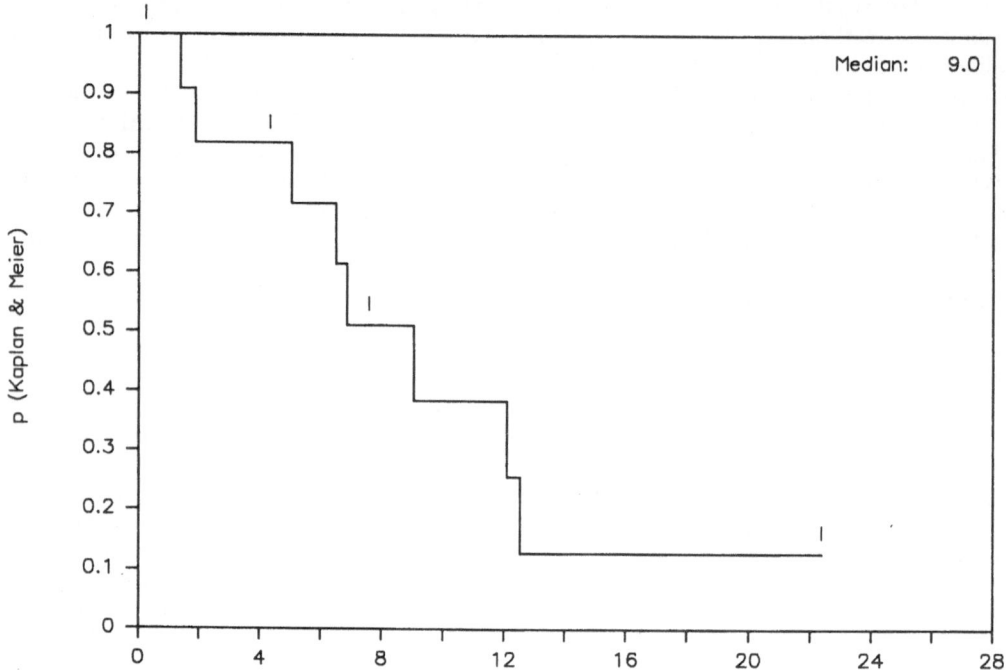

Fig. 1. Remission duration (two patients are censored at 1+ and 4+ months because of allogeneic or autologous BMT)

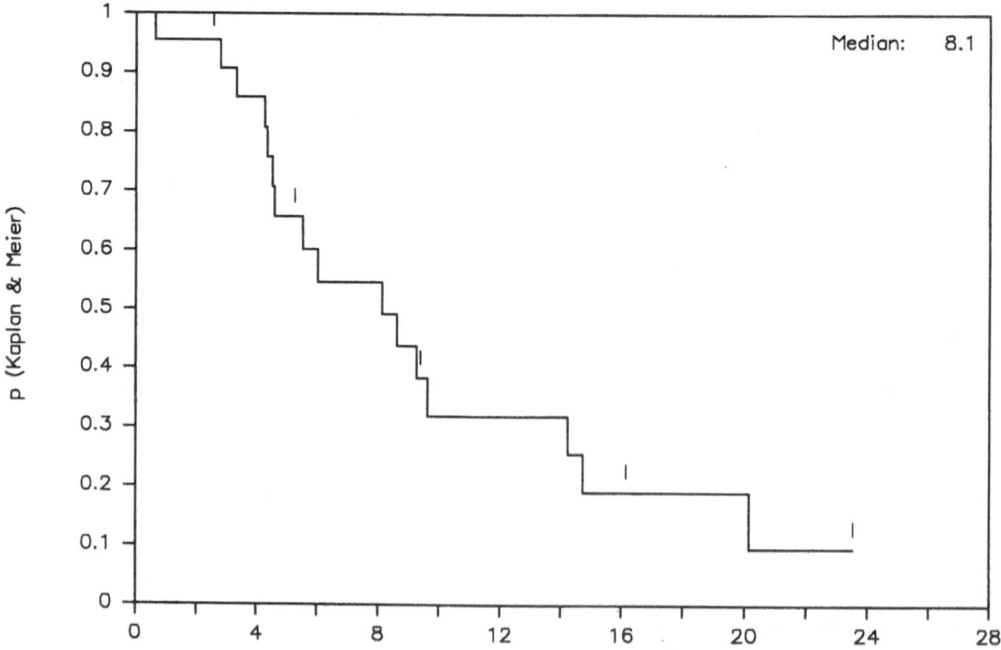

Fig. 2. Total survival

452

Table 2. Toxicity in 24 induction cycles

Toxicity (WHO)	0 (%)	1 (%)	2 (%)	3 (%)	4 (%)
Granulopenia	–	–	–	–	100
Thrombopenia	–	–	–	–	100
Bleeding	54	4	25	17	–
Bilirubin	73	18	–	9	–
Alkaline phosphatase	75	17	4	4	–
GOT/GPT	46	21	25	8	–
Nausea, vomiting	–	–	50	50	–
Mucositis	67	8	8	4	13
Diarrhea	25	25	25	25	–
Creatinin	92	8	–	–	–
Pulmonal	92	–	4	4	–
Cutaneous	42	17	33	4	4
Alopecia	–	–	–	100	–
Local infection	33	17	50	–	–
Sepsis	67	4	21	4	4
FUO	33	8	46	13	–
Cardiac rhythm	96	4	–	–	–
Cardiac function	96	–	–	–	4
Eye	92	4	4	–	–
Cerebellar	100	–	–	–	–

Table 3. Toxicity in nine consolidation cycles

Toxicity (WHO)	0 (%)	1 (%)	2 (%)	3 (%)	4 (%)
Granulopenia	–	–	–	–	100
Thrombopenia	–	–	–	–	100
Bleeding	63	–	13	25	–
Bilirubin	88	13	–	–	–
Alkaline phosphatase	88	13	–	–	–
GOT/GPT	50	13	25	–	13
Nausea, vomiting	–	–	44	44	11
Mucositis	88	–	13	–	–
Diarrhea	–	63	25	13	–
Creatinine	75	25	–	–	–
Pulmonal	88	13	–	–	–
Cutaneous	38	38	25	–	–
Alopecia	–	–	–	100	–
Local infection	78	11	11	–	–
Sepsis	100	–	–	–	–
FUO	22	33	44	–	–
Cardiac rhythm	88	13	–	–	–
Cardiac function	75	–	–	25	–
Eye	89	–	11	–	–
Cerebellar	100	–	–	–	–

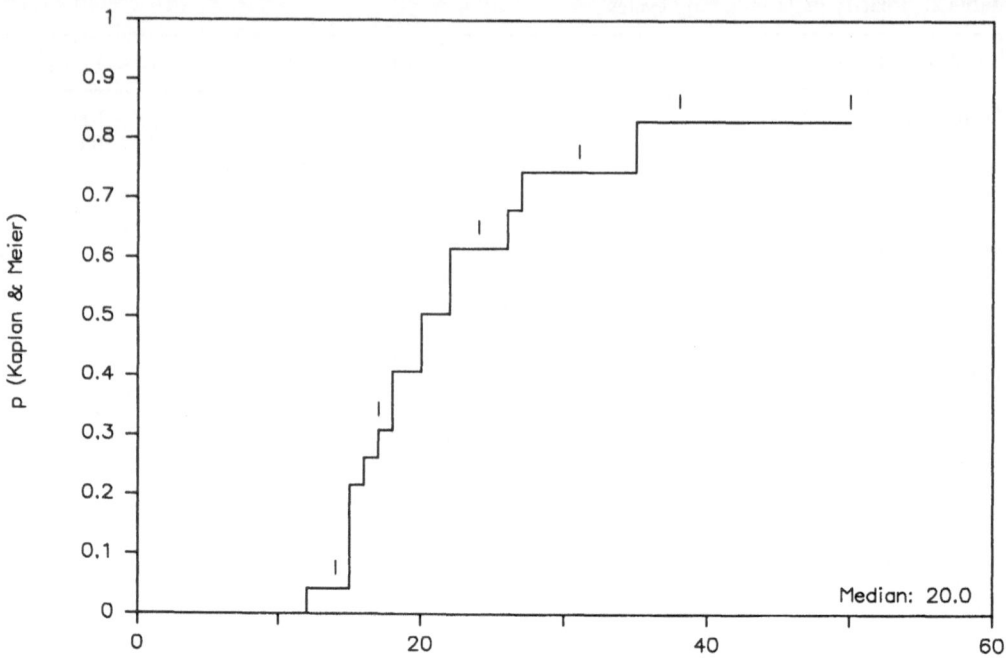

Fig. 3. Duration of granulopenia in induction (patients are considered without respect to the result of the induction)

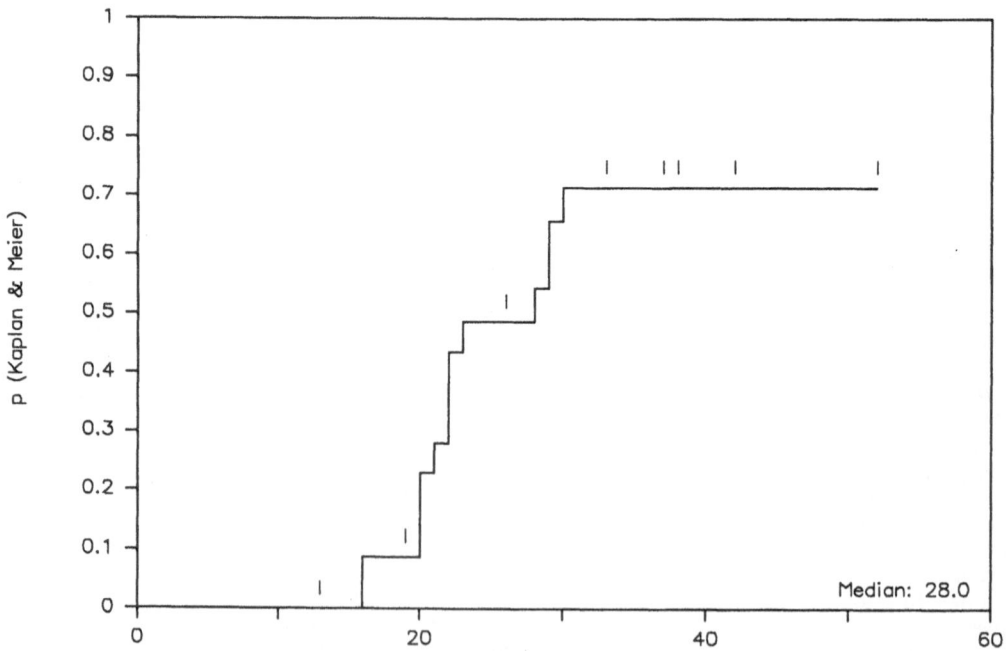

Fig. 4. Duration of thrombopenia in induction

There was one treatment-related hypoplastic death. Gastrointestinal side effects were seen in some patients with nausea, diarrhea, and mucositis. Conjunctivitis was infrequent and usually mild. No cerebellar toxicity was experienced. There were similar side effects in nine consolidation cycles with a median duration of granulopenia and thrombopenia of 22 and 23 days.

Discussion

Eight studies have been reported with high-dose or intermediate-dose ara-C and m-AMSA. A total of 310 patients have been treated for relapsing or refractory AML with a complete remission rate of 51.9 %. In five studies high-dose ara-C was given up to 6 days [34–38]. Three other studies were designed with ID ara-C for 6 days [39–41] with a total duration of treatment up to 7 days. Comparing HD ara-C schedules with ID ara-C-containing regimens a favorable trend for the intermediate-dose treatment is obvious (CR rate 48.0 % vs. 59.1 %; $p = 0.052$).

In patients with high-risk relapsing or refractory AML 5-day m-AMSA and ID ara-C is very effective and has mild organ toxicity. The overall results are fully comparable to previous results with high-dose ara-C and m-AMSA which showed that 51.9 % complete remissions were induced in resistant and relapsing AML [34–38]. The 5-day schedule has the same activity as longer-lasting schedules with intermediate-dose ara-C, which resulted in 40.0 % (CI, 15 %–65 %) CR in resistant AML [39, 41] and in 65.8 % (CI, 57 %–75 %) CR in relapsing AML [39–41]. The effect of 5-day m-AMSA and ID ara-C compares favorably with combinations of HD ara-C and anthracyclines [6, 11–17] or VP16 [42–44], which were reported to induce 50 % and 53.5 % complete remissions in 204 and 83 patients. We conclude that 5-day m-AMSA and intermediate-dose ara-C is a powerful induction therapy in relapsing or refractory AML. The toxic side effects are tolerable and the treatment is easy to handle. The schedule should be further evaluated in elderly and heavily pretreated patients.

Summary

Twenty-two patients with a median age of 48.3 years (range, 26–70 years; 10 m, 12 f) were treated with m-AMSA 100 mg/m^2 and ara-C 2×1000 mg/m^2 i.v. day 1–5. There were 2 AML M1, 8 M2, 9 M4, 2 M4 Eo, and 1 M5a. Twenty-four cycles of therapy were given for induction. Twelve patients achieved a complete remission, three a partial remission and six did not respond. The median remission duration was 9.0 months and the median overall survival 8.1 months. Side effects of induction consisted mainly of hematologic toxicity and infections with a median duration of WHO grade 4 granulopenia and thrombopenia of 20 and 28 days respectively. Organ toxicity was mild with mucositis, cutaneous and liver toxicity being experienced by only a few patients. There was one treatment-related death. Five-day m-AMSA and intermediate-dose ara-C is an easy to handle condensed treatment schedule with tolerable toxicity. Its effectivity in relapsed and refractory AML is comparable to combinations of high-dose ara-C with anthracyclines or etoposide.

Acknowledgements. We are indebted to our colleagues Drs. A. Engert, G. Exeriede, J. Pieper, M. Sosada, J. Tischler, to the Hannover Medical School nursing staff caring for the patients, and to Mr. H. G. Layda for his support in preparing the manuscript.

References

1. Herzig RH, Wolff N, Lazarus HM, Phillips GL, Karanes C, Herzig GP (1983) High-dose cytosine arabinoside therapy for refractory leukemia. Blood 62: 361–369
2. Breithaupt H, Pralle H, Eckhardt T, von Hattingberg M, Schick J, Loeffler H (1982) Clinical results and pharmacokinetics of high dose cytosine arabinoside (HD ARA-C). Cancer 50: 1248–1257
3. Vogler WR, Preisler HD, Winton EF, Gottlieb AJ, Goldberg J, Brennan J, Grunwald H, Rai K, Bowman G, Miller KB, Chervenick P, Azarnia N (1986) Randomized trial of high-dose cytosine arabinoside versus amsacrine in acute myelogenous leukemia in relapse: a Leukemia Intergroup study. Cancer Treat Rep 70: 455–459

4. Rudnick SA, Cadman EC, Capizzi RL, Skeel RT, Bertino JR, McIntosh S (1979) High dose cytosine arabinoside in refractory acute leukemia. Cancer 44: 1189–1193
5. Kantarjian HM, Estey EH, Plunkett W, Keating M, Walters RS, Iacoboni S, McCredie KB, Freireich EJ (1986) Phase I–II clinical and pharmacologic studies of high-dose cytosine arabinoside in refractory leukemia. Am J Med 81: 387–391
6. Willemze R, Fibbe WE, Zwaan FE (1983) Experience with intermediate and high dose cytosine arabinoside in refractory acute leukemia. Onkologie 4: 200–204
7. Rohatiner A, Slevin ML, Dhaliwal HS, Malpas JS, Lister TA (1984) High-dose cytosine arabinoside: response to therapy in acute leukemia and non-Hodgkin's lymphoma. Cancer Chemother Pharmacol 12: 90–93
8. Early AP, Preisler HD, Slocum H, Rustum YM (1982) A pilot study of high-dose 1-β-D-arabinosylcytosine for acute leukemia and refractory lymphoma: clinical response and pharmacology. Cancer Res 42: 1587–1594
9. Takaku F, Urabe A, Mizoguchi H, Yamada O, Wakabayashi Y, Miura Y, Sakamoto S, Yoshida M, Miwa S, Asano S, Morisaka T, Nomura T, Toyama K, Aoki I, Murase T, Maekawa T, Miyawaki S, Murakami H, Yamada H, Ohno R, Kawashima K, Yokomaku S, Kinogasa K, Adachi Y, Mori M, Ise T, Mutoh Y, Yamaguchi H (1985) High-dose cytosine arabinoside in refractory acute leukemia. Semin Oncol 12 [Suppl 3]: 144–150
10. Plunkett W, Liliemark JO, Adams TM, Nowak B, Estey E, Kantarjian H, Keating MJ (1987) Saturation of 1-beta-d-arabinofuranosylcytosine 5′-triphosphate accumulation in leukemia cells during high-dose 1-beta-d-arabinofuranosylcytosine therapy. Cancer Res 47: 3005–3011
11. Walters RS, Kantarjian HM, Keating MJ, Plunkett WK, Estey EH, Andersson B, Beran M, McCredie KB, Freireich EJ (1988) Mitoxantrone and high-dose cytosine arabinoside in refractory acute myelogenous leukemia. Cancer 62: 677–682
12. Hiddemann W, Kreutzmann H, Straif K, Ludwig WD, Mertelsmann R, Donhuijsen-Ant R, Lengfelder E, Arlin Z, Büchner T (1987) High-dose cytosine arabinoside and mitoxantrone: a highly effective regimen in refractory acute myeloid leukemia. Blood 69: 744–749
13. Hiddemann W, Maschmeier G, Pfreundschuh M, Ludwig WD, Büchner T (1988) Treatment of refractory acute myeloid (AML) and lymphoblastic leukemia (ALL) with high-dose cytosine arabinoside (Hd Ara-C) and mitoxantrone: indication of increased efficacy by sequential administration. Proc Am Soc Clin Oncol 7: A731 (abstr)
14. Amadori S, Papa G, Miniero R, Meloni G, Petti MC, Mandelli F (1988) Intermediate-dose ara-C (IdAC) with sequential mitoxantrone (Mitox) in acute myeloid leukemia (AML). Proc Am Soc Clin Oncol 7: A670 (abstr)
15. Van Prooyen HC, Dekker AW, Punt K (1984) The use of intermediate dose cytosine arabinoside in the treatment of acute non-lymphocytic leukemia in relapse. Br J Haematol 57: 291–299
16. Brito-Babapulle F, Catovsky D, Newland AC, Goldman JM, Galton DAG (1987) Treatment of acute myeloid leukemia with intermediate-dose cytosine arabinoside and mitoxantrone. Semin Oncol 14 [Suppl 1]: 51–52
17. Sanz MA, Martinez J, Borrego D, Martin-Aragonés G, Lorenzo I, Sanz G, Sayas MJ, Jarque I, Pastor E, Rafecas J (1987) High-dose cytosine arabinoside and mitoxantrone in high-risk acute nonlymphoblastic leukemia. Semin Oncol 14 [Suppl 1]: 18–20
18. Dupont J, Garay G, Scaglione C, Wooley P, Pavlovski S (1981) A phase II trial of m-AMSA in acute leukemia. Proc Am Assoc Cancer Res Am Soc Clin Oncol 22: 477 (abstr)
19. Van Echo DA, Markus SD, Schimpff SC, Wiernik PH (1981) A phase II trial of 4′(9-acridinylamino-methanesulfon-M-anisidine in adult relapsed acute leukemia. Proc Am Assoc Cancer Res Am Soc Clin Oncol 22: 230 (abstr)
20. Issell BF (1980) Amsacrine. Cancer Treat Rev 7: 73–83
21. Lawrence HJ, Ries CA, Reynolds RD, Levis JP, Kroetz MM, Torti FM (1982) AMSA – a promising new agent in refractory acute leukemia. Cancer Treat Rep 66: 1475–1478
22. Legha SS, Keating MJ, Zander AR, McCredie KB, Bodey GP, Freireich FJ (1980) 4′(9-acridinylamino) methanesulfon-m-anisidine: a new drug effective in the treatment of adult acute leukemia. Ann Intern Med 9: 17–21
23. Slevin ML, Shannon MS, Prentice HG, Goldman AJ, Lister TA (1981) A phase I and II study of m-AMSA in acute leukemia. Cancer Chemother Pharmacol 6: 137–140
24. Tan CTC, Hancock C, Steinherz PG, Sorell M, Chan KW, Mondora A, Miller DR (1982) Phase II study of 4′(9-acridinylamino) methanesulfon-m-anisidine (NSC-249992) in children with acute leukemia and lymphoma. Cancer Res 42: 1579–1581

25. Winton EF, Volger WR, Rose KL (1980) Phase II study of acrinidyl anisidine (NSC-249992) in refractory adult acute leukemia. Proc Am Assoc Cancer Res Am Soc Clin Oncol 21: 437 (abstr)
26. Plunkett W, Nowak B, Keating MJ (1987) Effect of amsacrine on ara-CTP cellular pharmacology in human leukemia cells during high-dose cytarabine therapy. Cancer Treat Rep 71: 479–483
27. Berman E, Arlin ZA, Gaynor J, Miller W, Gee T, Kempin SJ, Mertelsmann R, Andreeff M, Reich L, Nahmias N et al. (1989) Comparative trial of cytarabine and thioguanine in combination with amsacrine or daunorubicin in patients with untreated acute nonlymphocytic leukemia: results of the L-16M protocol. Leukemia 3: 115–121
28. Keating MJ, Gehan EA, Smith TL, Estey EH, Walters RS, Kantarjian HM, McCredie KB, Freireich EJ (1987) A strategy for evaluation of new treatments in untreated patients: application to a clinical trial of AMSA for acute leukemia. J Clin Oncol 5: 710–721
29. French-American-British (FAB) Co-Operative Group, Bennett JM, Catovsky D, Daniel MT, Flandrin G, Galton DAG, Gralnick HR, Sultan C (1976) Proposals for the classification of the acute leukaemias. Br J Haematol 33: 489–496
30. Bennett JM, Catovsky D, Daniel MT, Flandrin G, Galton DAG, Gralnik HR, Sultan C (1985) Proposed revised criteria for the classification of acute myeloid leukemia. A report of the French-American-British cooperative group. Ann Intern Med 103: 626–629
31. Miller AB, Hoogstraten B, Staquet M, Winkler A (1981) Reporting results of cancer treatment. Cancer 47: 207–214
32. Ohnuma T, Rosner S, Levy RN, Cuttner J et al, Moon JH, Silver RT, Blom J, Falkson G, Burningham R, Glidewell O, Holland JF (1971) Treatment of adult leukemia with l-asparaginase. Cancer Chemother Rep 55: 269–275
33. Kaplan EL, Meier P (1958) Nonparametric estimation from incomplete observations. J Am Stat Assoc 53: 457–481
34. Hines JD, Oken MM, Mazza JJ, Keller AM, Streeter RR, Glick JH (1984) High-dose cytosine arabinoside and m-AMSA is effective therapy in relapsed acute non lymphocytic leukemia. J Clin Oncol 2: 545
35. Zittoun R, Bury J, Strykmans P, Löwenberg B, Peetermens M, Rozendaal KY, Haanen C, Kerkhofs M, Jehn U, Willemze R (1985) Amsacrine with high-dose cytarabine in acute leukemia. Cancer Treat Rep 69: 1447–1448
36. Decker RW, Ho WG, Champlin RE (1987) Phase II study of amsacrine and high-dose cytarabine for resistant acute myelogenous leukemia. Cancer Treat Rep 71: 881–882
37. Witz F, Olive D, Lederlin P, Bordigoni P, Troussard X, Grosbois B, Schaison G, Cornu G (1987) Intérêt des hautes doses de cytosine-arabinoside dans letraitement des leukcémies aiguës résistantes. Presse Med 16: 159–162
38. Arlin ZA, Ahmed T, Mittelman A, Feldman E, Mehta R, Weinstein P, Rieber E, Sullivan P, Baskind P (1987) A new regimen of amsacrine with high-dose cytarabine is safe and effective therapy for acute leukemia. J Clin Oncol 5: 371–375
39. Peters WG, Willemze R, Colly LP (1988) Results of induction and consolidation treatment with intermediate and high-dose cytosine arabinoside and m-AMSA of patients with poor-risk acute myelogenous leukaemia. Eur J Haematol 40: 198–204
40. Willemze R, Jager U, Jehn U, Stryckmans P, Bury J, Suciu S, Solbu G, Zittoun R, Burghouts J, Loewenberg B, Abels J, Cauchie C (1988) Intermediate and high dose ara-C and m-AMSA for remission induction and consolidation treatment of patients with acute myeloid leukemia: an EORTC Leukemia Cooperative Group phase II study. Eur J Cancer Clin Oncol 24: 1721–1725
41. Jehn U, Heinemann V (1990) Intermediate-dose Ara-C/m-AMSA for remission induction and high-dose Ara-C/m-AMSA for intensive consolidation in relapsed and refractory adult acute myelogenous leukemia. Hamatol Bluttransfus 33: 333–338
42. Gore M, Powles R, Lakhani A, Milan S, Maitland J, Goss G, Nandi A, Perren T, Forgeson G, Treleaven J, Zuiable A, Porta F (1989) Treatment of relapsed and refractory acute leukaemia with high-dose cytosine arabinoside and etoposide. Cancer Chemother Pharmacol 23: 373–376
43. Cheng PN, Leung TW, Shiu WC (1987) Etoposide, high dose ara-C and asparaginase in poor risk acute leukaemias in Hong Kong. EORTC Symposium on Recent Advances in Cancer Management 14–15 (abstr)
44. Gryn J, Conroy J, Crilley P, Topolsky D, Kahn SB, Brodsky I (1989) High-dose cytarabine (ADAC) and VP-16 for refractory or relapsed ANLL. Proc Am Soc Clin Oncol 8: 202 (abstr)

Aclacinomycin A/Etoposide Combination Therapy for Advanced Relapsed Acute Myeloid Leukemia: A Phase II Study of the Arbeitsgemeinschaft Internistische Onkologie

W. Hiddemann[1], K. Becker[2], A. Grote-Metke[3], R. Kuse[4], A. Bartholomäus[5],
A. Reichle[6], I. Meuthen[7], R. Schlag[8], R. Fuchs[9], H. G. Fuhr[10], D. Leimer[11],
D. K. Hossfeld[2], and T. Büchner[1]

Introduction

In spite of the substantial advances in the chemotherapy of acute myeloid leukemia (AML) within recent years, the majority of patients still relapse with their disease and only 20%–30% of patients experience long-term disease-free survival [1, 2]. Primary or secondary resistance of the leukemic blasts against the applied therapeutic agents is considered the main reason for the ultimate failure of antileukemic treatment. In order to overcome this resistance and in the search for more effective antileukemic agents, the German AML Cooperative Group has carried out several phase I/II studies in refractory AML during the last 10 years. Besides the combination of AMSA and VP-16, a monotherapy trial with high-dose cytosine arabinoside (HD-AraC) and studies of HD-AraC combined with mitoxantrone were evaluated [3–5]. The appropriate basis for these investigations is provided by standardized regimens for first line and second line therapy which allow for a clear definition of refractoriness against conventional treatment modalities [6–9].

_____

Departments of Internal Medicine, Universities of Münster[1], Hamburg[2], München rechts der Isar[6], München-Innenstadt[8]; Evangelisches Krankenhaus, Hamm[3]; Krankenhaus St. Georg, Hamburg[4]; St. Bernward Krakenhaus, Hildesheim[5]; Städt. Krankenhaus Holweide, Köln[7]; St. Antonius-Hospital, Eschweiler[9]; Städt. Krankenanstalten, Wiesbaden[10]; Städt. Krankenanstalten, Kaiserslautern[11], FRG

Among the aforementioned studies for the treatment of refractory AML, HD-AraC and mitoxantrone (HAM) proved to have the highest efficacy with a remission rate of 53% [3]. Hence, this combination was subsequently incorporated into first line treatment as part of the double induction strategy [7]. A timed sequential modification of HAM, S-HAM, is furthermore evaluated in a randomized multicenter trial in relapsed AML, addressing the question of high-dose versus intermediate-dose AraC in terms of efficacy and toxicity [10]. This regimen is currently the standard salvage protocol for relapsed cases. Patients not responding to S-HAM treatment or relapsing again after successful second line therapy could not be offered an additional alternative approach. Recently, however, Rowe and coworkers reported promising results with aclacinomycin A and etoposide in a similarly pretreated group of patients [11, 12]. Of 35 patients with advanced AML, 12 achieved a complete remission and two additional patients obtained a partial response. The median remission duration was 99 days. Besides well-known side effects of intensive antileukemic therapy, a higher frequency of severe mucositis was observed. Considering the intensive prior therapy and the advanced disease status, these results suggest a high antileukemic activity of Acla/VP-16. They are further supported by preceding single-agent studies indicating the efficacy of both agents in less heavily pretreated cases [13–17]. These data prompted us to evaluate the Acla/VP-16 combination in the German AML Cooperative Group in patients with advanced relapsed AML.

Patients, Material and Methods

The present study comprised 31 patients with heavily pretreated advanced AML at ages 20–71 years with a median age of 43 years. Their pretreatment characteristics are outlined in Tables 1 and 2. All patients were recruited from the respective trials of the German AML Cooperative Group and had received a standardized first line treatment comprising double-induction therapy as initial therapy [6, 7] and sequential high-dose AraC and mitoxantrone (S-HAM) as the treatment of first relapse [10]. One additional patient was included with a relapse after autologous bone marrow transplantation.

Prior to therapy all patients gave their informed consent after having been advised about the purpose and investigational na-

ture of the study as well as of potential risks.

Therapy consisted of Acla 60 mg/m^2 per day by a 30-min infusion on days 1–5. VP-16 was given immediately thereafter at a dose of 100 mg/m^2 per day as a 30-min infusion also on days 1–5.

Toxicity was quantitated according to the World Health Organization (WHO) grading system. Evaluation of antileukemic efficacy was based on CALGB criteria. Complete remission was definded by the disappearance of leukemic blasts from the bone marrow and blood as well as from possible extramedullary sites and required the normalization of peripheral blood counts to thrombocytes >100 000/mm^3 and granulocytes >1500/mm^3. The duration of critical cytopenia was evaluated by the time for granulocyte recovery to >500/mm^3 and thrombocytes >20 000/mm^3 from the onset of treatment.

Results

Twenty-seven of the 31 patients were treated with one course of Acla/VP-16, four patients receied a second cycle of the same regimen.

Nonhematologic Toxicity

A summary of the nonhematologic side effects is given in Table 3. Nausea and vomiting, mucositis and liver enzyme elevations were the most frequent side effects. In

Table 1. Patient characteristics

n	31
Age	20–71 years (median 43)
⩾60 years	6
Sex	
– Female	16
– Male	15
FAB subtypes	
M1	7
M2	5
M3	–
M4	12
M5	5
M6	–
Undifferentiated	2

Table 2. Patient characteristics

resistant	
first relapse	10
second relapse	18
>second relapse	2
relapse after ABMT	1

Table 3. Side effects

	WHO I/II	WHO III/IV
Nausea/vomiting	19 (54%)	9 (26%)
Mucositis	12 (34%)	18 (51%)
Hepatic	22 (63%)	4 (11%)
Diarrhea	17 (49%)	6 (17%)
Cardiac	7 (20%)	–
Skin	6 (17%)	3 (9%)
CNS	1 (3%)	
Renal	4 (11%)	1 (3%)
Infection	12 (34%)	18 (51%)

35 cources = 100%

459

addition, severe infections were observed during 51 % of treatment cycles.

Hematologic Effects and Antileukemic Efficacy

Ten patients (32 %) achieved a complete remission, and another three patients achieved a partial remission with a normalization of peripheral blood counts but a residual leukemic subpopulation in the bone marrow of 15 %–18 % blasts, respectively. In ten patients (32 %) the leukemic blasts persisted or recovered after bone marrow aplasia; they were therefore considered nonresponders. Eight patients (26 %) died during the treatment-induced phase of aplasia (early deaths).

In patients achieving a CR or PR the median time to the recovery of granulocyte counts >500/mm^3 and thrombocyte counts >20000/mm^3 was 23 days (15–35 days), the median time to remission being 32 days (21–44 days). Of the 13 patients in CR or PR, 3 were subsequently transplanted, one of them relapsing immediately thereafter. Five additional patients relapsed after 1–10 months, respectively, and five patients are in ongoing remission at 1$^+$–6$^+$ months.

Discussion

In refractory and relapsed acute leukemias clinical phase I/II studies are performed not only as salvage therapy for patients with advanced disease but also in the search for new agents or drug combinations with significant antileukemic activity that might subsequently be incorporated into first line treatment for more effective initial therapy. In order to facilitate the comparability of clinical phase I/II studies in AML and to judge the efficacy of various combinations on the basis of comparable prerequisites, criteria for the definition of refractoriness against concentional chemotherapy were identified by the German AML Cooperative Group [8,, 9] and provided the basis for several subsequent clinical phase I and II trials [3–5]. The current protocol of Accla/VP-16 was restricted to a heavily pretreated group of patients with AML at advanced relapse. All patients had relapsed after standardized first line treatment and had failed on or relapsed after a uniform salvage regimen at first relapse comprising HD-AraC and mitoxantrone [10]. The observed response rate of ten complete remissions and three partial remissions in this highly unfavorable group of patients indicates a significant antileukemic activity of Acla/VP-16 and suggests a lack of cross-resistance to the previously applied agents. In our opinion, the observed high rate of early deaths is not a reflection of a high toxicity of the two-drug combination but rather of the advanced disease status at which patients were entered on this protocol. The distribution and frequency of overall side effects were not different from other intensive regimens except for a higher frequency of severe mucositis and reversible bluish changes in skin color which were more irritating than truly disturbing.

The current data are comparable to previous reports about the two-drug combination in less intensively pretreated patients [11, 12] and also confirm the previously observed spectrum of side effects.

In summary, the preliminary data of the present study indicate a significant antileukemic activity of Acla/VP-16 in heavily pretreated patients with advanced relapsed AML and encourage the continuing application of this combination to substantiate the observed findings.

Summary

In a clinical phase II study aclacinomycin A (Acla) and etoposide (VP-16) were given in combination to 31 patients with acute myeloid leukemia (AML) in advanced relapse. All patients had received a standardized first line and second line treatment and were in refractory first relapse ($n=10$), second, third or fourth relapse ($n=20$) or in relapse after bone marrow transplantation ($n=1$). Therapy consisted of Acla 60 mg/m^2 per day and VP-16 100 mg/m^2 per day both given from days 1 to 5. Complete remission (CR) was achieved in ten patients (32 %), and three patients achieved partial remission (PR) (10 %). Ten patients did not respond (32 %) and eight patients died within 6 weeks after the onset of treatment (26%) and were considered as early deaths. Toxicity consisted mainly of nausea and vomiting, mucositis, severe infections, and liver enzyme elevations. Recovery of blood counts occurred at a median of 23 days; the median time to CR or PR was 32 days. These data indicate a significant antileukemic activity of Acla/VP-16 in heavily pretreated patients with advanced relapsed AML and encourage the continuing application of the two-drug combination to substantiate these preliminary findings.

References

1. Büchner T (1984) Gegenwärtiger Stand der Behandlung der akuten Leukämie. Intern Welt 7: 366–405
2. Gale RP (1979) Advances in the treatment of acute myelogenous leukemia. N Engl J Med 300: 1189–1199
3. Hiddemann W, Kreutzmann H, Straif K, Ludwig WD, Mertelsmann R, Donhuijsen-Ant R, Lengfelder E, Arlin Z, Büchner T (1987) High-dose cytosine arabinoside and mitoxantrone: highly effective regimen in refractory acute myeloid leukemia. Blood 69: 744–749
4. Hiddemann W, Büchner T, van de Loo J (1989) Grundlagen der Rezidivtherapie bei akuter myeloischer Leukämie. Dtsch Med Wochenschr 114: 599–605
5. Hiddemann W, Urbanitz D, Preusser P, Achterrath W, Büchner T (1989) Treatment of refractory acute myeloid leukemia with mAMSA and VP-16-213 in combination: results of a clinical phase I/II study. Hematol Oncol 7: 267–273
6. Büchner T, Urbanitz D, Hiddemann W, Ludwig WD, Fischer J, Aul HC et al. (1985) Intensified induction and consolidation with or without maintenance chemotherapy for acute myeloid leukemia (AML): two multicenter studies of the German AML Cooperative Group. J Clin Oncol 3: 1583–1589
7. Büchner T, Hiddemann W, Blasius S, Koch P, Maschmeyer G, Tirier C et al. (1990) Adult AML: the role of chemotherapy intensity and duration. Two studies of the AMLCG. In: Büchner T, Schellong G, Hiddemann W, Ritter J (eds) Acute leukemias II. Springer, Berlin Heidelberg New York, pp 26 (Haematology and blood transfusion, vol 33)
8. Hiddemann W, Martin WR, Büchner T (1987) Definition of refractoriness to conventional therapy in advanced myeloid leukemia: an essential prerequisite for clinical phase I/II studies. Proc Am Soc Clin Oncol 6: 156
9. Hiddemann W, Martin W-R, Sauerland C-M, Heinecke A, Büchner T (1990) Definition of refractoriness against conventional chemotherapy in acute myeloid leukemia – a proposal based on the results of retreatment by thioguanine, cytosine arabinoside and daunorubicin (TAD 9) in 150 patients with relapse after standardized first line therapy. Leukemia 4: 184–188
10. Hiddemann W, Aul C, Maschmeyer G, Lathan B, Koeppler H, Hoffmann R et al. (1989) High dose versus intermediate dose cytosine arabinoside with mitoxantrone in the treatment of relapsed and refractory acute myeloid leukemia. Blut 59: 316
11. Rowe JM, Chang AYC, Bennett JM (1986) Aclacinomycin A (ACA) and Etoposide (VP-16-213) in heavily pretreated patients with acute non-lymphocytic leukemia (ANLL): a phase II study. Proc Am Soc Clin Oncol 5: 635
12. Rowe JM, Chang AYC, Bennett JM (1988) Aclacinomycin A and etoposide (VP-16-213): an effective regimen in previously treated patients with refractory acute myelogenous leukemia. Blood 71: 992–996
13. Bennett JM, Lymann GM, Cassileth PA, Glick JH, Oken MM (1984) A phase II trial of VP-16 in adults with refractory acute myeloid leukemia. An ECOG study. Am J Clin Oncol 7: 471–473
14. Van Echo DA, Wiernik P, Aisner J (1980) High dose VP-16-213 for the treatment of patients with previously treated acute leukemia. Can Clin Trials 3: 325–328
15. Mitrou PS, Kuse R, Anger H, Hermann R, Bonfert B, Pralle H, Thiel E, Westerhausen M, Mainzer K, Bartels H (1985) Aclarubicin (aclacinomycin A) in the treatment of relapsing acute leukemias. Eur J Cancer Clin Oncol 21: 919–923
16. Pedersen-Bjergaard J, Brincker H, Ellegaard J, Drivsholm A, Freund L, Jensen KB, Jensen MK, Nissen NI (1984) Aclarubicin in the treatment of acute nonlymphocytic leukemia refractory to treatment with daunorubicin and cytarabine: a phase II trial. Cancer Treat Rep 68: 1233–1238
17. Yamada K, Nakamura T, Tsuruo T, Kitanara T, Maekawa T, Ozaka Y et al. (1980) A phase II study of aclacinomycin A in acute leukemia in adults. Cancer Treat Rev 7: 177–182

Therapeutic Choices Influencing Duration of Complete Remission in Acute Myelogenous Leukemia

G. Lambertenghi-Deliliers, C. Annaloro, A. Oriani, R. Mozzana, and E. E. Polli

Introduction

Complete remission (CR) can be achieved in up to 80% of all adults with acute myelogenous leukemia (AML) [1, 2]. However, the majority of available studies agree that the relapse rate in patients stopping therapy soon after achieving CR is nearly 100%, and that maximum disease-free survival (DFS) does not exceed 1 year [3, 4].

In the effort to reduce residual leukemic population several postremission strategies have been designed at different times. Conventional consolidation includes the delivery of one or more cycles of about the same doses of the same drugs used during induction, which may or may not be followed by long-term maintenance [4]. This approach has led to a significant prolongation of DFS and an increase in the rate of long-term survivors to 20% [5].

An alternative option is the development of intensive postremission schedules along two main lines: the use of either non-cross-resistant myelosuppressive drugs or high-dose (HD) chemotherapy. The real usefulness of the first strategy is still controversial and largely depends on the investigated drugs used; the most promising results have come from the introduction of VP-16 [6].

In several comparative, though generally nonrandomized, studies, HD cytosine arabinoside (Ara-C) significantly increased the percentage of patients in long-term continuous CR [7, 8].

The precise role of HD chemotherapy followed by either allogeneic or autologous bone marrow transplantation (BMT) is not easy to understand because of the difficulty in satisfactorily designing prospective randomized trials [9]. More consistent long-term data favor allogeneic BMT [10], but this procedure can be used in only a minority of patients. Controversy still exists concerning the real effectiveness of autologous BMT (ABMT) in prolonging DFS and this debate is made more complicated by the number of variables involved in performing an optimal ABMT [11, 12].

The present report deals with the long-term results of an adult AML protocol including idarubicin (IDA) in the induction and consolidation phases and intensive postremission chemotherapy followed by ABMT in nonrandomized, selected patients.

Materials and Methods

From April 1986 to January 1990, 49 consecutive hospitalized patients with previously untreated AML entered this study. Their essential characteristics are listed in Table 1.

All patients received a course of IDA 12 mg/m^2 i.v. daily for three consecutive days, followed by a 1-h i.v. infusion of Ara-C 120 mg/m^2 every 12 h on days 4–10. No further induction therapy was given when the myelogram showed CR, although patients showing more than 5% of residual blasts

Institute of Medical Science, University of Milan, Via Francesco Sforza 35, 20122 Milan, Italy

Table 1. Patient characteristics

No. of patients		49		
Age (years)	median:	44	range:	16–64
M/F		31/18		
WBC	median:	8 800	range:	800–138 000
Hb	median:	9.7	range:	5–14.9
Plts	median:	51 000	range:	10–417 000
WBC >50 000		6		
FAB:	M0	3		
	M1	13		
	M2	14		
	M3	6		
	M4	4		
	M5	7		
	M6	1		
	M7	1		

received a second induction course of IDA and Ara-C. Patients were considered resistant if, after two courses, there was an inadequate clearance of bone marrow leukemic cells, a regrowth of marrow blasts after recovery from aplasia, or if CR lasted less than 1 month.

For patients achieving CR, a consolidation program was used which consisted of two courses of IDA (8 mg/m^2 per day i.v. for two consecutive days) and Ara-C (150 mg/m^2 subcutaneously every 12 h for 5 days) alternately administered with two courses of VP-16 (150 mg/m^2 per day i.v. for three consecutive days) and Ara-C (as above).

Late intensification treatment with HD Ara-C or BMT (allogeneic or ABMT) was given depending on the patient's age (under or over 50 years) and availability of an HLA-compatible donor. DFS curves were calculated according to the life table method and compared by means of Wilcoxon's test.

Results

The outcome of induction therapy is shown in Table 2: 41 of the 49 patients (83.6%) attained CR, 7 of them requiring two courses of therapy. Three patients died of sepsis in the aplastic period without any bone marrow evidence of leukemia. The remaining five patients were classified as

Table 2. Outcome of induction therapy

Induction		Pts.	%
	Evaluable	49	100
	CR	41	83.7
	After one course	34	82.9
	After two courses	7	17.1
	Resistant	5	10.2
	Early death	3	6.1
Post-remission	(Max. follow-up = 54 months)		
	Pts in CCR	19	46.3
	Deaths in CR	4	9.8
	Relapse (median = 8 months)	18	43.9

resistant because of blastic regrowth after recovery from aplasia.

As of November 1990, 19 (46.3%) of the 41 patients who achieved CR were still in CR after a follow up of 10–54 months, 18 (43.9%) had relapsed after a median of 8 months (range 3–27 months) and 4 (9.8%) had died of causes unrelated to leukemia (3 during consolidation and 1 during the late intensification phase).

As shown in Fig. 1, the median DFS of all 41 patients who achieved CR is now 26 months (curve A). The median duration of CR is longer in the 34 patients in CR after

463

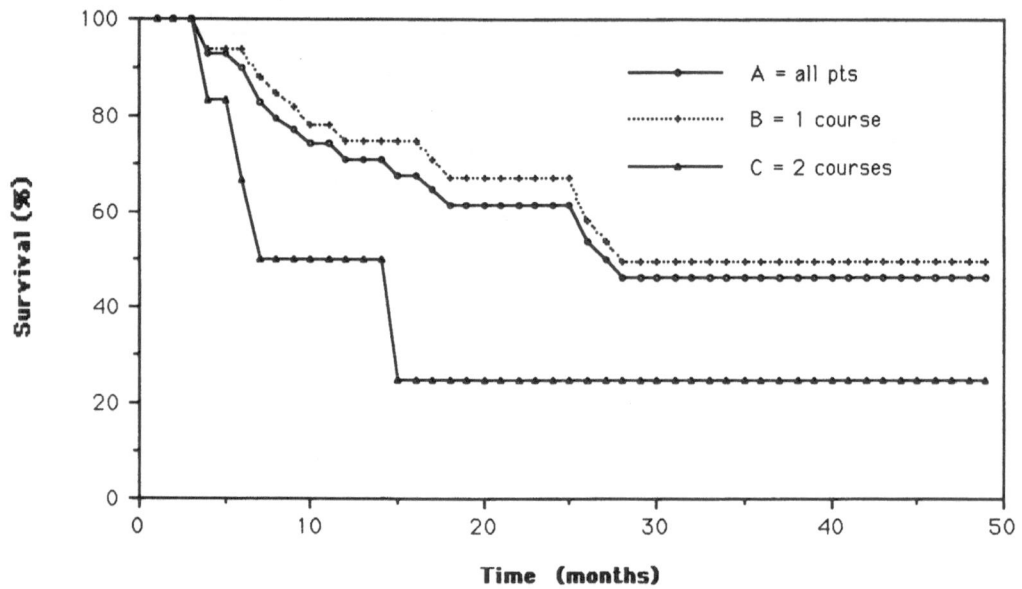

Fig. 1. Disease-free survival curve of 41 adult AML patients: *curve A*, all patients; *curve B*, 34 patients achieving CR after 1 course; *curve C*, 7 patients achieving CR after 2 courses

one induction course: 27 (curve B) versus 14 (curve C) months, while 4-year DFS chances are 49.3% and 25% respectively.

Eight patients received ABMT as late intensification after 7–14 months of CR (median 11 months). One of them relapsed after a DFS of 17 months; seven are still in first CR after a follow-up of 14–49 months.

When the patients are considered in terms of the late intensification regimen, there is a favorable trend for ABMT, with median DFS not reached after 48 months and a 4-year DFS chance of 87.5%. The median DFS of the patients not submitted to autografting is 25 months. If only the patients of this last group, with at least 11 months in CR, are considered, the 4-year DFS chance is 51.9% although the median has not yet been reached after 48 months.

Discussion

The results of this single-institution study are encouraging in terms of both CR rate and DFS [1, 2]. Our data confirm the primary role of the induction phase in determining the CR rate and the duration of DFS [13]. IDA improved the quality of response by increasing the speed of cytoreduction, as testified by the high rate of CR achieved after only one course [14]. The analysis of DFS highlights the fact that induction with IDA delayed the occurrence of relapse, since the duration of CR was much longer in patients who achieved it after only one induction cycle.

In the consolidation phase, we selected the approach of adding VP-16, as the most promising non-cross-resistant, nonintercalating drug [6, 15]. The rate of therapy-related deaths could thus be minimized, although perhaps at the expense of some early relapse.

High-dose chemotherapy was employed in the late intensification phase and the cases subsequently receiving ABMT deserved their better survival. However, no clear-cut conclusions can be drawn since there was no randomization, the patients amenable to ABMT were younger and some eligible patients were discarded because of early relapse. Difficulties in properly designing the control group are shared by most of the clinical trials but, nevertheless, the best results are generally reported when ABMT is performed late after CR [10, 12]. As a trend favoring ABMT persists after the exclusion of cases relapsing within 1 year, it could be cautiously inferred, also from our data, that ABMT exerts an effective influence in prolonging DFS and that late intensification is perhaps

References

1. Champlin RE, Gale RP (1987) Acute myelogenous leukemia. Blood 69: 1551–1562
2. Mayer RJ (1987) Current chemotherapeutic treatment approaches to the management of previously untreated adults with de novo acute myelogenous leukemia. Semin Oncol 14: 384–396
3. Büchner T, Urbanitz D, Hiddemann D et al. (1985) Intensified induction and consolidation with or without maintenance chemotherapy for acute myeloid leukemia (AML): two multicenter studies of the German AML Cooperative Group. J Clin Oncol 3: 1583–1589
4. Cassileth P, Harrington D, Hines J et al. (1986) Maintenance therapy in adult acute nonlymphoblastic leukemia (ANLL) prolongs initial complete remission duration. Blood 8 [Suppl 1]: 220a (abstr 758)
5. Rees JKH, Gray RG, Swinsky D et al. (1986) Principal results of the Medical Research Council's 8th acute myeloid leukaemia trial. Lancet II: 1236–1241
6. Bishop JF, Lowenthal RM, Joshua D et al. (1990) Etoposide in acute nonlymphocytic leukemia. Blood 75: 27–32
7. Wolff SN, Herzig RH, Fay JW et al. (1989) High dose cytarabine and daunorubicin as consolidation therapy for acute myeloid leukemia in first remission: long term follow-up and results. J Clin Oncol 7: 1260–1267
8. Champlin R, Gajewski J, Nimer S et al. (1990) Postremission chemotherapy for adults with acute myelogenous leukemia: improved survival with high-dose cytarabine and daunorubicin consolidation treatment. J Clin Oncol 8: 1199–1206
9. Begg CB, Pilote L, Mc Glave PB (1989) Bone marrow transplantation versus chemotherapy in acute nonlymphocytic leukemia: a meta-analytic review. Eur J Cancer Clin Oncol 25: 1519–1523
10. Hermans J, Suciu S, Stijnen T et al. (1989) Treatment of acute myelogenous leukemia. An EBMT-EORTC retrospective analysis of chemotherapy versus allogeneic or autologous bone marrow transplantation. Eur J Cancer Clin Oncol 25: 545–550
11. Mc Millan AK, Goldstone AH, Linch DC et al. (1990) High dose chemotherapy and autologous bone marrow transplantation in acute myeloid leukemia. Blood 76: 480–488
12. Mandelli F, Rees JKH, Gorin NC et al. (1990) Postremission treatment in acute myeloid leukemia: chemotherapy or autologous or allogeneic bone marrow transplantation. Haematological (Pavia) 75: 203–211
13. Büchner T, Hiddemann W, Maschmeyer G et al. (1990) How to improve therapy for adult acute myeloid leukemia: studies of the AML Cooperative Group in the Federal Republic of Germany. 21st Symposium of the Gesellschaft zur Bekämpfung der Krebskrankheiten Nordrhein-Westphalen (GKP), Düsseldorf, June 1989. Cancer Res Clin Oncol 116: 97–99
14. Gottlieb AJ, Weinberg V, Ellison RR, Henderson ES et al. (1984) Efficacy of daunorubicin in the therapy of adult acute nonlymphocytic leukemia: a prospective randomized trial by cancer and leukemia Group B. Blood 64: 267–274
15. Stadtmauer EA, Cassileth PA, Gale RP (1989) Etoposide in leukemia, lymphoma and bone marrow transplantation. Leuk Res 13 (8): 639–650

Intensive Antileukemic Treatment for Advanced Primary Myelodysplastic Syndromes: Analysis of 30 Patients

V. Runde, C. Aul, A. Heyll, and W. Schneider

Introduction

Myelodysplastic syndromes (MDS) are clonal malignant bone marrow disorders, characterized by both quantitative and qualitative defects of all hematopoietic cell lines. In the majority of cases, they have a fatal course within months to years owing to infections, hemorrhages or transition to acute myeloid leukemia (AML). Prognosis is particularly poor in patients with refractory anemia with excess of blasts (RAEB), RAEB in transformation (RAEB/T) and chronic myelomonocytic leukemia (CMML) who, according to recent studies, have a median survival of only 4.5 – 18 months [1–3].

With the possible exception of bone marrow transplantation in younger patients [4], no treatment modality is known that can clearly alter the natural course of MDS. Despite favorable results in some patients, treatment with immunosuppressive drugs, androgens, inducers of myeloid differentiation, interferons or low-dose chemotherapy is generally not effective in these disorders [5–8]. The role of hematopoietic growth factors (e.g., GM-CSF, G-CSF, Multi-CSF) which may lead to an improvement of peripheral blood cytopenias has not been fully examined [9]. Aggressive chemotherapy has yielded conflicting results in MDS. Based on earlier reports [10], this approach has been regarded as ineffective or even dangerous because of the risk of severe and prolonged bone marrow aplasia. Furthermore, the low remission rates obtained in MDS have been explained by a reduced responsiveness of the preleukemic cell clone to chemotherapy, and/or by the suppression or absence of normal progenitor cells required for regeneration of hematopoiesis. Armitage et al. [11], however, presented data according to which younger patients might respond more favorably to intensive chemotherapeutic protocols. Encouraging results have also been found in other studies usually involving small groups of patients [12, 13]. To evaluate the chances of aggressive induction chemotherapy in preleukemia, we treated a total of 30 patients in advanced stages of MDS (RAEB, RAEB/T and MDS/AML) with standard AML protocols. We also describe the clinical course of four patients who underwent bone marrow transplantation after achievement of complete remission.

Patients and Methods

Patients

From April 1981 to November 1990, 30 patients (18 male, 12 female) with an initial diagnosis of MDS were treated with aggressive combination chemotherapy. Their median age was 54 years (range, 17–64 years). In none of the cases was there a past history of myelotoxic chemotherapy and/or radiation. MDS was classified according to French-American-British (FAB) criteria. The median time from diagnosis to initiation of aggressive chemotherapy was 1

Department of Internal Medicine, Hematology and Oncology Division, Heinrich Heine University, Moorenstraße 5, W-4000 Düsseldorf 1, FRG

Table 1. Clinical and hematological features of 30 patients with advanced MDS treated with aggressive chemotherapy

	MDS	n	MDS/AML	n
Morphological	RAEB	1	M 1	4
diagnosis	RAEB/T	14	M 2	6
			M 4	3
			M 5	1
			M 6	1
Age (years)	53 (17–64)[a]		54 (32–64)[a]	
WBC ($\times 10^9$/l)	3.3 (0.8–21.6)[a]		6.6 (0.6–310)[a]	
Platelets ($\times 10^9$/l)	80 (9–196)[a]		40 (7–143)[a]	
Presence of Auer rods		6 (40%)		4 (27%)
Normal karyotype		4/7		6/6
Single abnormalities		1/7		
Multiple abnormalities		2/7		–
Previous treatment with low-dose Ara-C		–		5

[a] Median (range)

month (Range, 0–21 months). FAB categories at the start of treatment were RAEB in 1 and RAEB/T in 14 cases. Fifteen patients had already transformed to overt AML (MDS/AML). The clinical and hematological features of the patients are shown in Table 1. Bone marrow cytogenetic analysis was performed in 13 patients of whom 10 had a normal karyotype, 1 a single chromosomal aberration and 2 multiple chromosomal abnormalities. The Karnofsky score ranged from 60% to 90% (median, 80%). Six patients had previously been treated with low-dose cytosine arabinoside (Ara-C). Three patients achieved a short-lived remission (range, 6–11 months), whereas the others were refractory to low-dose Ara-C.

Treatment Regimens

Chemotherapeutic protocols used for remission induction are shown in Table 2. Twenty-eight patients were treated with a single induction course (TAD-9). In addition, one patient received a double induction regimen in which the initial TAD-9 cycle was followed on day 21 by a second TAD-9 course (TAD-9/TAD-9). In another patient treated with double induction the second part of the protocol consisted of a combination of high-dose Ara-C and mitoxantrone (TAD-9/HAM). Complete remission (CR) and partial remission (PR) were defined according to the CALGB criteria. In general, postremission chemotherapy included consolidation (TAD-9) and regu-

Table 2. Chemotherapeutic protocols used for remission induction

TAD-9	Ara-C 100 mg/m^2	c.i.v.	day 1+2
	Ara-C 100 mg/m^2	i.v. 2x/d	day 3–8
	Thioguanine 100 mg/m^2	p.o. 2x/d	day 3–9
	Daunorubicin 60 mg/m^2	i.v. 1x/d	day 3–5
HAM	Ara-C 3000 mg/m^2	i.v. 2x/d	day 1–3
	Mitoxantrone 10 mg/m^2	i.v. 1x/d	day 3–5

c.i.v., continuous intravenous infusion; Ara-C, cytosine arabinoside

Table 3. Results of intensive chemotherapy in 30 patients with advanced MDS

	MDS ($n = 15$)	MDS/AML ($n = 15$)
TAD-9	14	14
TAD-9/HAM	0	1
TAD-9/TAD-9	1	0
Aplasia period after		
TAD-9 in patients entering CR (days)	17 (6–39)[a]	19 (14–21)[a]
Responses		
CR after first course	13/15	6/15
CR after second course	0/2	1/4
PR	0/15	2/15
NR	2/15	4/15
ED	0/15	2/15
BMT		
Autologous in first CR	1	
Allogeneic in first CR	2	
Allogeneic in second CR (MUD)	1	

CR, complete remission; PR, partial remission; NR, no response; ED, early death; BMT, bone marrow transplantation; MUD, matched unrelated donor
[a] Median (range)

lar maintenance chemotherapy, as recommended by the German AML Study Group [14]. Two patients in first CR received an allogeneic bone marrow graft from a histocompatible sibling, one patient in first CR received an autologous bone marrow graft, and one patient was transplanted in second CR with a bone marrow graft from a matched unrelated donor.

Results

Induction Chemotherapy

The results of induction chemotherapy are shown in Table 3. Seventeen (61%) out of 28 patients treated with TAD-9 entered CR. Early death from infection occurred in two cases. One patient with a partial response entered CR after a second cycle of TAD-9. Five out of six patients refractory to the initial TAD-9 treatment received a second course of induction chemotherapy, either with TAD-9 (three patients) or HAM (two patients). None of these cases entered remission. One patient not responding to two cycles of TAD-9 received a modified HAM protocol (sequential HAM) without achieving CR. Both patients receiving a

double induction protocol (TAD-9/TAD-9 or TAD-9/HAM) as primary treatment of MDS entered CR.

The following pretreatment characteristics appeared to be related to the outcome of chemotherapy: (1) the percentage of marrow blast cells, as suggested by a higher CR rate in patients with RAEB or RAEB/T (87%) than in patients with overt AML (47%), (2) the presence of Auer rods which could be demonstrated in 40% of the complete responders as compared to 20% of nonresponding patients, and (3) the age of patients (Table 4).

No unusual toxicities of induction chemotherapy were noted. Twenty-seven of 30 induction cycles were complicated by episodes of fever ($> 38.5 °C$) necessitating systemic antibiotic therpy. Microorganisms found in blood cultures or bronchoalveolar lavage material included gram-positive coc-

Table 4. Complete remission rates according to age and morphological diagnosis

	<45 years	≥45 years
MDS	5/5 (100%)	8/10 (80%)
MDS/AML	2/3 (67%)	5/12 (42%)

ci in four, gram-negative bacilli in three, *Mycobacterium tuberculosis* in one, and *Candida* or *Aspergillus* species in two patients. One patient developed life-threatening pseudomembranous enterocolitis while being treated with broad-spectrum antibiotics because of fever of unknown origin. The median duration of bone marrow aplasia (leukocytes $< 1.0 \times 10^9/l$ and/or platelets $< 20 \times 10^9/l$) for patients achieving CR after one cycle of TAD-9 was 18 days (range, 6–39 days). Not surprisingly, patients treated with a double induction protocol experienced much longer periods of bone marrow aplasia (27 and 51 days, respectively).

Postremission Treatment

After induction of CR, 11 of 20 patients received consolidation (TAD-9) and regular maintenance chemotherapy according to the recommendations of the German AML Study Group (14). Meanwhile, ten patients have relapsed (median follow-up, 24 months). The median duration of complete remissions in this subgroup of patients was 13 months (range, 5+ –41 months). Patients not receiving postremission treatment had a poor prognosis with a median remission duration of only 2 months. It should be noted that three out of nine patients retreated with aggressive chemotherapy at the time of relapse entered a second remission which lasted between 2 and 4 months. For the entire group of patients, the median survival after the onset of chemotherapy was 16 months, and at the time of writing five patients are still alive.

Four patients in first and second remission, respectively, were treated with various forms of bone marrow grafts. Of these, three are in continuous CR 6, 8 and 23 months after BMT with a Karnofsky score of 100 %, while one patient succumbed to infectious complications (cerebral toxoplasmosis) in the posttransplant period (10 months after BMT). The age of these patients varied from 21 to 43 years. Up to now, the longest remission (23 months) is observed in a patient who received an unpurged autologous marrow graft 4 months after achievement of CR.

Discussion

As shown by a number of studies, prognosis of MDS primarily depends on the bone marrow blast cell count at the time of diagnosis. Median survival for these disorders progressively shortens from over 30 months in RA to 11 months in RAEB and 5 months in RAEB/T. At present, no treatment modality is known that can clearly alter the natural course of MDS.

Aggressive chemotherapy as used in de novo AML is usually not recommended for patients with MDS. Such reluctance stems from earlier studies according to which these patients have a low probability of entering remission, but often succumb to complications of chemotherapy-induced bone marrow aplasia [10, 15]. In selected patients, however, intensive chemotherapeutic protocols have been shown to produce CR rates of up to 50 % [12]. The clinical relevance of this approach becomes even more important because MDS is not just a disease of the elderly, but is increasingly diagnosed in younger patients who can be expected to tolerate the side effects of more intense treatment [16].

In this study, 30 patients with advanced primary MDS (RAEB, RAEB/T, and MDS/AML) were treated with standard AML protocols. In contrast to other series [11], all but two patients received an identical induction protocol, including cytosine arabinoside and daunorubicin. In the overall population, the complete remission rate was 67 %. Response to chemotherapy was particularly good (87 %) in patients with RAEB and RAEB/T, whereas patients already transformed to overt leukemia had a much lower CR rate (47 %). It may, therefore, be assumed that with progression of MDS to acute leukemia the chances for successful remission induction decrease. Other pretreatment characteristics that appeared to influence the remission probability in our study were the presence of Auer rods as well as the age of patients. In addition, other authors have emphasized the prognostic importance of cytogenetic findings. In the study by Fenaux et al. [17], for example, patients with a normal karyotype had both higher CR rates and longer remissions than patients with chromosomal abnormalities. Bloomfield, who recently performed a metaanalysis on 73 intensively treated patients with secondary MDS or AML, also observed a close relationship between cytogenetic findings and outcome of chemotherapy. Remission rates were particularly poor in patients with abnormalities of chromosome 5 (13 %), whereas 43 % of patients with a normal karyotype achieved CR [18]. In our study, the number of patients analyzed was too small to draw any firm conclusions on the prognostic role of cytogenetics.

Primary drug resistance of the preleukemic cell clone, as suspected by many authors [19], was not a major problem in our series. Only 6 (20 %) of the 30 patients had refractory disease, and except for 1 patient with MDS/AML all complete remissions were obtained after a single induction course. It should also be emphasized that in most patients induction chemotherapy was well tolerated. Much in contrast to other studies in which treatment-related mortality was as high as 35 % [17], we observed only two cases of early death (7 %). We surmise that differences in patient numbers, inclusion criteria, timing and design of chemotherapy as well as supportive measures account for the variant clinical results of aggressive chemotherapy in MDS.

Our study further demonstrates that the duration of hematological remissions in MDS is generally short. Only two patients in our series survived more than 2 years without relapse of their disease. Administration of consolidation and maintenance chemotherapy appeared to have a beneficial effect on the remission lenght. However, even in this subgroup of patients overall results were much worse than those reported for patients with de novo AML [14]. With rare exceptions [13, 20] other authors have reported similar discouraging results, suggesting that cure of MDS by conventional chemotherapy is hardly achievable.

In selected patients, bone marrow transplantation may be a more promising approach to treatment of MDS. In our series four younger patients were transplanted in first and second remission, respectively. At present, three patients are alive without recurrence of MDS 6–23 months after transplantation. Appelbaum et al. [21] have recently analyzed their results of allogeneic BMT in a consecutive series of 59 patients with MDS or closely related bone marrow disorders (aplastic anemia with clonal cytogenetic abnormalities). They found a disease-free survival of 45 % 3 years from transplant. Although younger patients with a low medullary blast cell count at the time of BMT were shown to have the best disease-free survival, long-term remissions were also observed in two of four patients over the age of 50 years. From their data, Appelbaum et al. [21] concluded that patients up to an age of 55 years should be considered candidates for allogeneic BMT, supposing their performance status is adequate and a histocompatible donor is available.

References

1. Tricot G, Vlietinck R, Boogaerts MA, Hendrickx B, De Wolf-Peeters C, Van den Berghe H, Verwilghen RL (1985) Prognostic factors in the myelodysplastic syndromes. Importance of initial data on peripheral blood counts, bone marrow cytology, trephine biopsy and chromosomal analysis. Br J Haematol 60: 19–32
2. Aul C, Schneider W (1988) Myelodysplastic syndromes. A prognostic factor analysis of 221 untreated patients. Blut 57: 234 (abstr)
3. Sanz GF, Sanz MA, Vallespi T, Canizo MC, Torrabadella M, Garcia S, Irrigiuble D, San Miguel JF (1989) Two regression models and a scoring system for predicting survival and planning treatment in myelodysplastic syndromes. A multivariate analysis of prognostic factors in 370 patients. Blood 74: 395–408
4. De Witte T, Zwaan F, Gratwohl A, Vernant J, Kolb HJ, Vossen et al. (1989) Timing of marrow transplantation in secondary leukemias and myelodysplastic syndromes. Transplant Proc 21: 2958–2959
5. Aul C, Heyll A (1990) Therapie der myelodysplastischen Syndrome. Dtsch Med Wochenschr 115: 1842–1850
6. Aul C, Gattermann N, Schneider W (1991) Treatment of advanced myelodysplastic syndromes with recombinant interferon-alfa2b. Eur J Haematol 46: 11–16
7. Koeffler HP, Heitjan D, Mertelsmann R, Kolitz JE, Schulman P, Itri L, Gunter P, Besa E (1988) Randomized study of 13-*cis* retinoic

acid v placebo in the myelodysplastic syndromes. Blood 71: 703–708

8. Aul C, Schneider W (1989) The role of low-dose cytosine arabinoside and aggressive chemotherapy in advanced myelodysplastic syndromes. Cancer 64: 1812–1818

9. Negrin RS, Haeuber DH, Nagler A, Olds LC, Donlon T, Souza LM, Greenberg PL (1989) Treatment of myelodysplastic syndromes with recombinant human granulocyte colony-stimulating factor. A phase I–II trial. Ann Intern Med 110: 976–984

10. Cohen J, Creger W, Greenberg PL, Schrier SL (1979) Subacute myeloid leukemia. A clinical review. Am J Med 66: 959–966

11. Armitage JO, Dick FR, Needleman SW, Burns CP (1981) Effect of chemotherapy for the dysmyelopoietic syndrome. Cancer Treat Rep 65: 601–605

12. Tricot G, Boogaerts MA (1986) The role of aggressive chemotherapy in the treatment of the myelodysplastic syndromes. Br J Haematol 63: 477–483

13. Murray C, Cooper B, Kitchens LW (1983) Remission of acute myelogenous leukemia in elderly patients with prior refractory dysmyelopoietic anemia. Cancer 52: 967–970

14. Büchner T, Hiddemann W, Koch P, Pielken H, Urbanitz D, Kreutzmann H et al. (1989) The role of maintenance chemotherapy, immunotherapy, induction dose reduction in elderly patients and double induction in the treatment of adult acute myeloid leukemia. Four randomized studies of the AML Cooperative Group. Beitr Onkol 36: 1–10

15. Dreyfus B (1976) Preleukemic states: I. Definition and classification. II. Refractory anaemia with an excess of myeloblasts in the bone marrow (smoldering acute leukemia). Blood Cells 2: 33–35

16. Aul C, Schneider W (1988) Epidemiological and aetiological aspects of primary myelodysplastic syndromes. Blut 57: 233 (abstr)

17. Fenaux P, Lai JL, Jouet JP, Pollet JP, Bauters F (1988) Aggressive chemotherapy in adult primary myelodysplastic syndromes. Blut 57: 297–302

18. Levine EG, Bloomfield CD (1986) Secondary myelodysplastic syndromes and leukaemias. Clin Haematol 15: 1037–1080

19. Cheson BD (1990) The myelodysplastic syndromes: current approaches to therapy. Ann Intern Med 112: 932–941

20. Hoyle FC, De Bastos M, Wheatley K, Sherrington PD, Fischer PJ, Rees JKH, Gray R, Hayhoe FGJ (1989) AML associated with previous cytotoxic therapy, MDS or myeloproliferative disorders: results from the MFC's 9th AML trial. Br J Haematol 72: 45–53

21. Appelbaum FR, Barrall J, Storb R, Fisher LD, Schoch G, Ramberg RE et al. (1990) Bone marrow transplantation for patients with myelodysplasia. Pretreatment variables and outcome. Ann Intern Med 112: 590–597

Treatment of Relapsed or Refractory Adult Acute Lymphocytic Leukemia

M. Freund[1], H. Diedrich[1], A. Ganser[2], G. Heil[3], A. Heyll[4], M. Henke[5],
W. Hiddemann[6], R. Haas[7], R. Kuse[8], P. Koch[6], H. Link[1], G. Maschmeyer[9],
M. Planker[10], W. Queißer[11], C. Schadeck-Gressel[12], N. Schmitz[13], U. von Verschuer[9],
S. Wilhelm[14], and D. Hoelzer[2]

Introduction

The primary treatment of acute lympho-cytic leukemia (ALL) has been considerably improved. In the first German multicenter study, 01/81 complete remissions have been induced in 272 of 368 patients (73.9 %), and in the second study 02/84 in

[1] Abteilung Hämatologie und Onkologie, Medizinische Hochschule Hannover, Hannover, FRG
[2] Abteilung Hämatologie, Zentrum Innere Medizin, Universität Frankfurt, Frankfurt, FRG
[3] Abteilung Innere Medizin III, Zentrum Innere Medizin, Universität Ulm, Ulm, FRG
[4] Abteilung Hämatologie/Onkologie, Medizinische Klinik und Poliklinik, Universität Düsseldorf, Düsseldorf, FRG
[5] Medizinische Universitätsklinik Freiburg, Freiburg, FRG
[6] Abteilung Hämatologie/Onkologie, Medizinische Universitätsklinik Münster, Münster, FRG
[7] Medizinische Universitäts-Poliklinik Heidelberg, Heidelberg, FRG
[8] Hämatologische Abteilung, Allgemeines Krankenhaus St. Georg, Hamburg, Hamburg, FRG
[9] Medizinische Abteilung, Evangelisches Krankenhaus Essen-Werden, Essen-Werden, FRG
[10] Medizinische Klinik II, Städtische Krankenanstalten Krefeld, Krefeld, FRG
[11] Onkologisches Zentrum der Fakultät für Klinische Medizin, Mannheim, Mannheim, FRG
[12] Medizinische Klinik II, St. Johannes-Hospital Duisburg, Duisburg, FRG
[13] II. Medizinische Universitäts- und Poliklinik Kiel, Kiel, FRG
[14] Schwerpunkt Hämatologie/Onkologie, II. Medizinische Klinik, Klinikum Karlsruhe, Karlsruhe, FRG

350 of 442 (79.2 %) [1]. Though 35 % of the patients remain disease free after 7.5 years in the first study and 48 % after 3 years in the second, relapsing and refractory disease is still the most prevalent problem in ALL. The development of effective salvage therapies is warranted. Against this background the German Multicenter ALL Study Group has evaluated an intensive protocol for patients with relapsed or refractory ALL.

Patients and Methods

Between May 1986 and June 1990 66 patients with relapsing or refractory ALL (49 male, 17 female) with a mean age of 30.2 years (range 16–62 years) were enrolled in 16 centers[1]. All patients were pretreated with the BMFT regimen. The study was conducted in accordance with the Helsinki declaration and was reviewed and approved by the ethical committee of the Hannover Medical School. Informed consent was obtained prior to admission. Patients with severe concomitant diseases, without response to platelet transfusions and with severe unmanageable complications of leukemia, were not admitted. Forty patients had cALL, 21 t-ALL, 3 O-ALL, and in 2 information on immunotyping was missing.

Induction phase I consisted of prednisone (60 mg/m^2 p.o. day 1–21), vindesine (3 mg/m^2 i.v. day 1, 8, 15), daunorubicin (45 mg/m^2 i.v. days 1, 8, 15), *erwinia* asparaginase (10 000 U/m^2 i.v. day 7, 8, 14, 15), and MTX i.t. (15 mg day 1, 8). In patients with no detectable remaining blastic infiltration hemopoietic recovery was allowed before the start of the second induction phase. Patients with remaining blastic infiltration were started with phase II of induction after recovery from organ toxicity and after stabilization of the clinical status. Phase II of induction consisted of high-dose cytarabine (3000 mg/m^2 3 h infusion twice daily day 1–4), and etoposide (100 mg/m^2 i.v. day 1–5). In patients over 50 years of age intermediate-dose cytarabine was given (1000 mg/m^2 twice daily day 1–5).

After complete remission patients were assigned to two different consolidation regimens. Consolidation A consisted of dexamethasone 3×5 mg/m^2 p.o. day 1–5, MTX 1500 mg/m^2 infusion 1 h day 1, teniposide 80 mg/m^2 i.v. day 1–3, cytarabine 300 mg/m^2 i.v. day 1–3, and folinic acid 15 mg/m^2 p.o. 6 h day 2–4. In consolidation B ifosfamide 5000 mg/m^2 infusion 24 h day 1 with mesna and vindesine (3 mg/m^2 i.v. day 2) was given. 15 milligrams MTX was injected i.t. on day 1 of consolidation A and B.

Evaluations with physical examination, standard laboratory tests, and bone marrow aspirations were done early after induction phase I, prior to phase II, after phase II and prior to every consolidation chemotherapy. Toxicities were evaluated according to WHO criteria [2] and responses according to the criteria of the CALGB [3]. Survival analyses were done according to Kaplan and Meier [4] and statistical significance was calculated by the chi-square test and the Mantel Cox log rank test. Patients with bone marrow transplantation were censored for calculated disease-free survival and overall survival. Multivariate analysis was performed by the Cox model (BMDP statistical package).

Results

Sixty-six patients have been treated. Of these 54 had their first relapse. Four patients had no complete remission after primary BMFT induction phases I and II, four had a second relapse, two had a relapse after autologous BMT, and one each after allogeneic and syngeneic BMT.

Treatment and Side Effects

Sixty-six courses of induction phase I, and 47 courses of induction phase II were given. In complete remission 4 courses of consolidation A, and 8 courses of consolidation B were given to 11 patients (for a detailed information on the treatment status see table 1). The number of treatment courses evaluable for toxicity was 57/66 and 37/47 for induction phases I and II and 1/4, resp. 3/8 in consolidation A and B. Side effects of induction phase I consisted of hematotoxicity with subsequent infections and gastrointestinal toxicity. Details are given in table 2. The median duration of granulopenia grade 4 WHO was 16 days. Thrombopenia grade 4 WHO was encountered by 50% of the patients. In induction phase II some patients experienced additional cutaneous, ocular, and hepatic toxicity (table 3). Granulopenia grade 4 WHO lasted for a median of 15 days and thrombopenia for a median of 11 days. The toxicity of the consolidation regimen was generally mild.

Table 1. Status of treatment

	Ongoing	Discontinued	Reasons for discontinuation					
			BMT	Side effects	Death	Refractory	Relapse	Others
Induction 1	2	17	3	4	5	–	1	4
Induction 2	2	36	10	2	1	14	7	2
Consolidation 1	2	4	1	–	–	–	3	–
Consolidation 2	3	–	–	–	–	–	–	–
Totals	9	57	14	6	6	14	11	4

Table 2. Toxicity in 57 cycles of induction phase I

WHO	Grade 0		Grade 1		Grade 2		Grade 3		Grade 4	
	n	%	n	%	n	%	n	%	n	%
Granulopenia	2	4	1	2	–	–	4	7	48	87
Thrombopenia	6	11	3	5	7	13	12	21	28	50
Bleeding	38	68	8	14	7	13	1	2	2	4
Bilirubin	34	60	20	35	3	5	–	–	–	–
Alkaline phos-phatase	46	81	7	12	4	7	–	–	–	–
GOT/GPT	21	37	14	25	13	23	5	9	4	7
Nausea, vomiting	27	47	16	28	7	12	6	11	1	2
Mucositis	36	64	7	13	5	9	8	14	–	–
Diarrhea	47	84	5	9	4	7	–	–	–	–
Creatinine	54	95	2	4	1	2	–	–	–	–
Pulmonal	52	91	3	5	1	2	–	–	1	2
Drug fever	54	95	1	2	2	4	–	–	–	–
Cutaneous	55	96	1	2	–	–	–	–	1	2
Alopecia	12	22	6	11	20	37	16	30	–	–
Local infection	43	75	4	7	5	9	4	7	1	2
Sepsis	49	86	1	2	2	4	4	7	1	2
FUO	53	93	–	–	4	7	–	–	–	–
Cardiac rhythm	48	87	4	7	3	5	–	–	–	–
Cardiac function	55	96	–	–	2	4	–	–	–	–
Peripheral neuropenia	48	84	7	12	2	4	–	–	–	–
Constipation	51	89	4	7	–	–	2	4	–	–

Thirty-four (63%) of 54 patients in first relapse achieved a CR (25 after phase 1, and 9 after phase 2 of induction). Two patients had a partial remission, and 13 patients did not respond. Five died during therapy or in aplasia: two with sepsis, one with candida pneumonia, and two with bleeding. The median duration of disease-free survival (DFS) was 2.9 months (Fig. 1) and the median overall survival (OAS) 6.6 months (Fig. 2). The CR rate was superior in patients with c-All compared to those with t-ALL (70% vs. 47%, statistically not significant), and in patients with a preceding CR of more than 18 months versus those with a shorter preceding remission (81% vs. 46%, $p < 0.01$) (see table 4). The duration of survival and disease-free survival was not significantly different for patients with c-All and t-All though there was more early mortality in patients with t-All. Patients with a preceding remission of less than 18 months had an inferior overall survival (Fig. 3) compared to those with longer preceding remissions. A multivar-iate analysis for survival was done in the patients with first relapse including sex, risk factor at initial diagnos age, duration of preceding CR, WBC at relapse, and immunotyping as predictive factors. The duration of preceding remission was the strongest predictor ($p = 0.001$). WBC at relapse was a second significant predictor ($p = 0.012$), but it was not statisically independent from the duration of first remission. A negative correlation was found in patients with c-ALL between the log of WBC at relapse and duration of preceding remission ($r = 0.38$).

Of 12 patients with second relapse, relapse after BMT or refractory disease, 7 (58%) achieved a complete remission. Four patients entered a complete remission after induction phase I and three after induction phase II. One patient suffered early death from sepsis, three patients had nonresponding disease and another patient was not evaluable for response. The duration of disease-free survival was 2, 2+, 3, 3, 3+, 5+, and 8+ months.

Table 3. Toxicity in 37 cycles of induction phase II. Only cycles with high-dose ara-C (3 000 mg/m^2 twice daily day 1–4) are considered

WHO	Grade 0		Grade 1		Grade 2		Grade 3		Grade 4	
	n	%	n	%	n	%	n	%	n	%
Granulopenia	–	–	–	–	–	–	–	–	37	100
Thrombopenia	–	–	–	–	–	–	1	3	36	97
Bleeding	22	59	6	16	7	19	2	5	–	–
Bilirubin	31	84	4	11	2	5	–	–		
Alkaline phosphatase	28	76	7	19	1	3	1	3	–	–
GOT/GPT	14	38	7	19	9	24	7	19	–	–
Nausea, vomiting	1	3	6	17	14	39	15	42	–	–
Mucositis	13	36	8	22	2	6	10	28	3	8
Diarrhea	13	36	7	19	8	22	8	22	–	–
Creatinine	37	100	–	–	–	–	–	–	–	–
Pulmonal	34	92	1	3	–	–	2	5	–	–
Drug fever	32	86	1	3	4	11	–	–	–	–
Cutaneous	22	59	9	24	5	14	1	3	–	–
Alopecia	4	11	–	–	5	14	28	76	–	–
Local infection	20	57	3	9	6	17	4	11	2	6
Sepsis	25	71	–	–	1	3	5	14	4	11
FUO	26	74	–	–	8	23	1	3	–	–
Cardiac rhythm	29	78	8	22	–	–	–	–	–	–
Cardiac function	37	100	–	–	–	–	–	–	–	–
Peripheral neuropenia	35	95	–	–	2	5	–	–	–	–
Eye	29	78	4	11	4	11	–	–	–	–
Cerebellar	34	92	2	5	–	–	1	3	–	–

Table 4. Selected risk factors and treatment results in patients with first relapse

	NR	PR	CR all	CR Ph1	CR Ph2	NE	ED
ALL	26 %	2 %	60 %	40 %	19 %	–	12 %
AUL	25 %	–	75 %	75 %	–	–	–
No information	13 %	13 %	75 %	63 %	13 %	–	–
C-ALL	24 %	3 %	70 %	52 %	18 %	–	3 %
T-ALL	24 %	6 %	47 %	35 %	12 %	–	24 %
O-ALL	33 %	–	67 %	67 %	–	–	–
No information	–	–	100 %	–	100 %	–	–
Low risk[a]	23 %	–	77 %	55 %	23 %	–	–
High risk[a]	25 %	6 %	53 %	41 %	13 %	–	16 %
First CR <18 mo.	32 %	7 %	46 %	36 %	11 %	–	14 %
First CR >18 mo.	15 %	–	81 %	58 %	23 %	–	4 %

[a] At first diagnosis

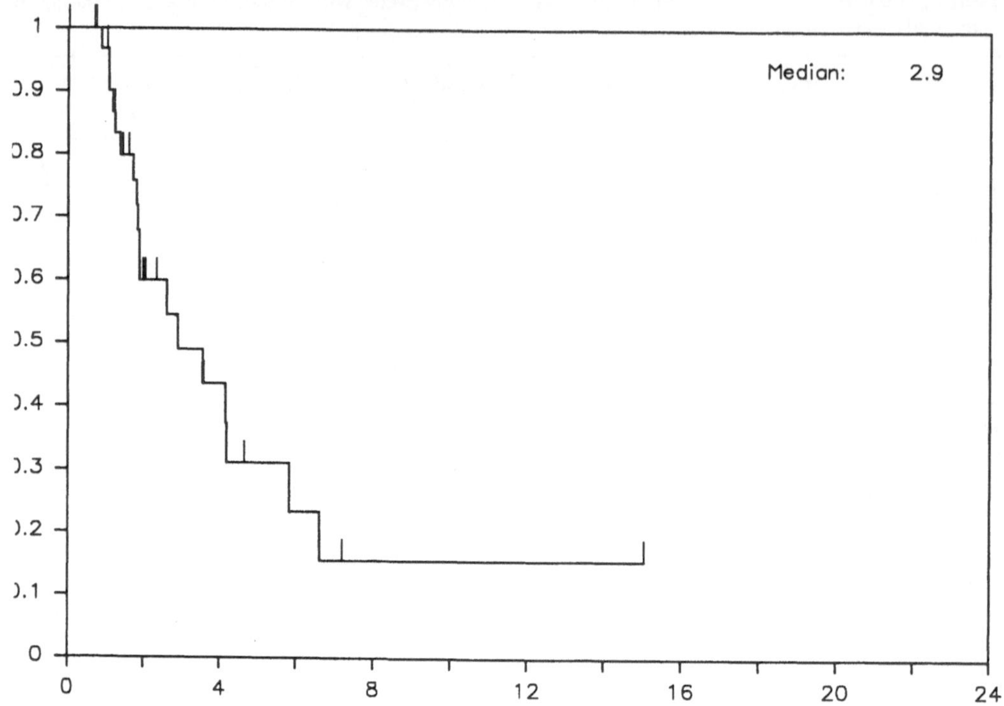

Abb. 1. Disease-free survival (months) after treatment for first relapse. (Patients with autologous or allogeneic BMT in CR were censored)

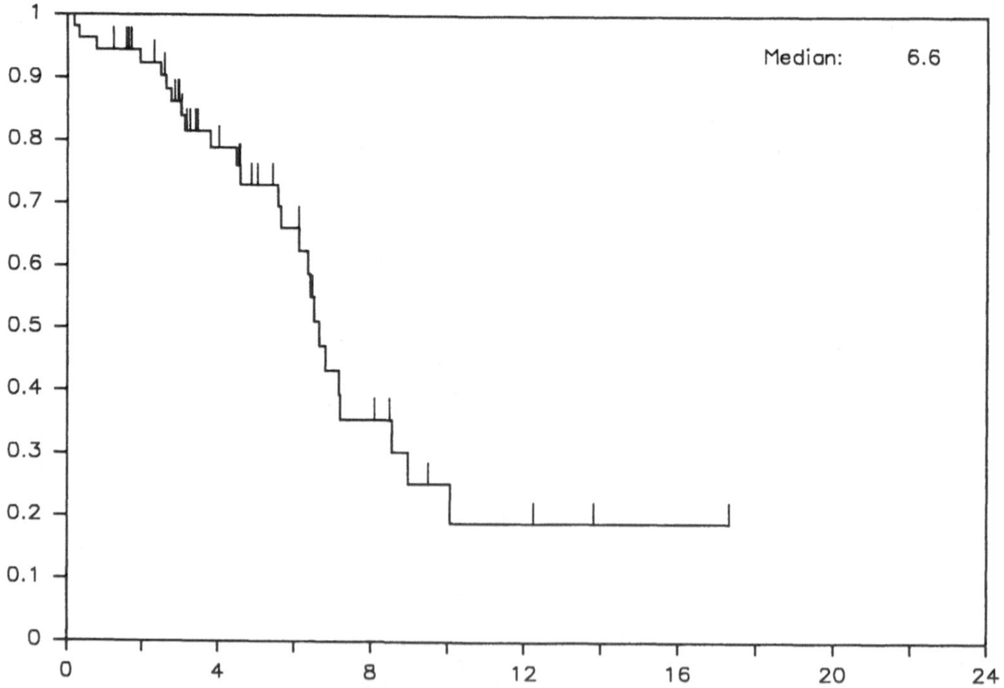

Fig. 2. Overall survival (months) after treatment for first relapse. (Patients with autologous or allogeneic BMT in CR are censored)

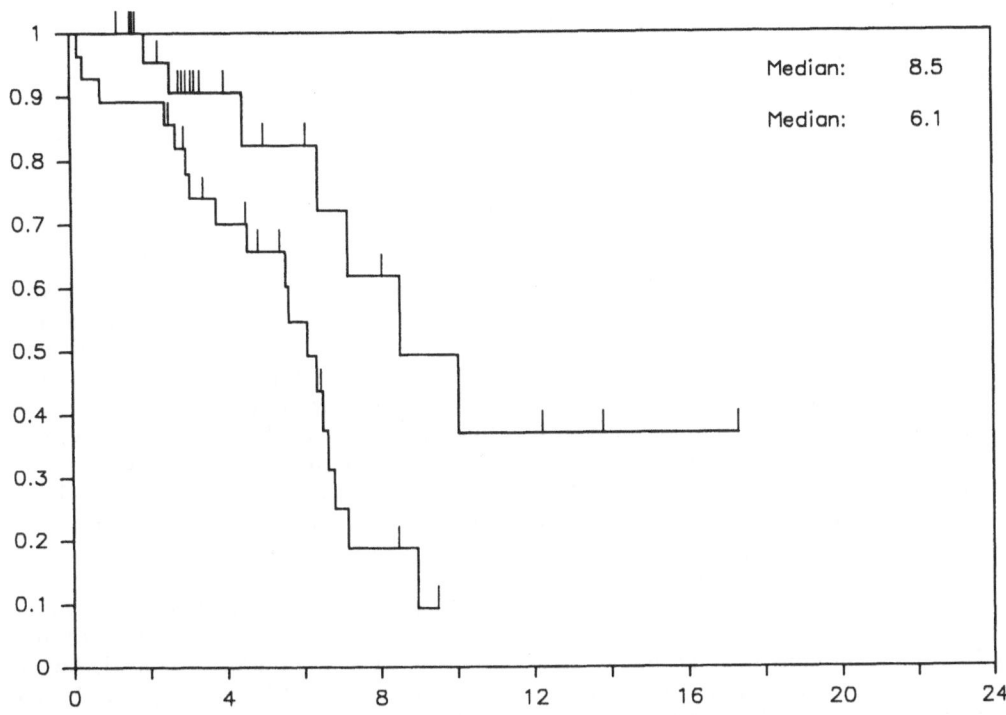

Fig. 3. Overall survival after treatment for first relapse according to the duration of the preceding remission. The upper curve shows patients with a preceding remission of more than 18 months

Table 5. Duration of disease-free survival in 22 patients with BMT

	n	Disease-free survival
Allogeneic BMT in CR	8	(2, 2+, 3, 4, 6, 7, 13+, 18+)
Autologous BMT in CR	7	(1, 4, 4, 5, 7, 8, 12)
Allogeneic BMT later	5	(1+, 1, 1, 8, 15+)
Autologous BMT later	2	(2, 3)

Twenty-two patients had a bone marrow transplantation (BMT): 8 had an allogeneic, 7 an autologous BMT in CR, 5 had an allogeneic, and 2 an autologous BMT after another relapse or with refractory disease. Five patients with allogeneic BMT are alive and well (see table 5).

Discussion

The prognosis of relapsing adult acute lymphocytic leukemia is poor. Therefore it is controversial whether a palliative or a curative concept should be favored in patients without HLA-matched bone marrow donor. Combinations of vinca alcaloids, prednisone, anthracycline ± asparaginase have induced remissions in 74% of patients with relapsing All [5–9]. High-dose cytosine arabinoside is an effective monotherpy [10–16] or has been given successfully in combination with AMSA [17–20], anthracyclines [21], anthrachinones [22–24], asparaginase [25–27], or podophyllotoxins [28–31]. The rationale of our study was to improve treatment results in patients with relapsing ALL by combining both principles in a treatment strategy first reducing tumor burden by a modified ViDAP regimen and intensification by a combination with high-dose cytosine arabinoside.

Eight studies including more than 20 patients with relapsing or refractory adult ALL have been published with complete remission rates of 26% and 75% [18, 22, 23, 32–36]. Some of these studies cannot be fully compared because of poor information on pretreatment and state of refractoriness. Our study includes the so far largest group of patients. All patients were pretreated with the BMFT regimen. In first relapse 64% of patients entered a complete remission. There is only one study so far published with a higher remission rate [18], but Ph^1-positive patients have been excluded.

The major problem in relapsing ALL is short duration of disease-free survival (DFS), which was 2.9 months in our patients. Median times for DFS were reported previously between 2.2 and 7 months [18, 22, 23, 32–36]. Some of the studies with long remission duration had poor results in induction chemotherapy [34, 36]. This may result in a positive selection of patients with a better remission duration. However, patients in studies with intensive maintenance and consolidation [33, 34, 36] had longer remission durations than patients who were treated by intensive induction only [18, 22, 23, 32]. On our study only 11 of the 34 patients with complete remission received consolidation treatment. This deficit may contribute to the short duration of DFS. An intensification of this treatment element should be part of future studies.

Summary

Sixty-six [49 m, 17 f, mean age 30.2 years (16–62 years)] were treated for relapsing or refractory ALL. Induction phase I consisted of vindesine 3 mg/m² i.v. day 1, 8, 15; DNR 45 mg/m² i.v. day 1, 8, 15; *Erwinia* asparaginase 10 000 U/m² i.v. day 7, 8, 14, 15; and prednisone 60 mg/m² p.o. day 1–21. For induction phase II cytarabine 2 × 3 000 mg/m² i.v. day 1–4 (in patients >50 years 1 000 mg/m²) and VP16 100 mg/m² i.v. day 1–5 were given. Eleven patients received consolidation therapy. Thirty-four (64%) of 54 patients with first relapse achieved a CR (25 after phase I, and 9 after phase II of induction). The median disease-free survival was 2.9 months and the median overall survival 6.6 months. In patients with first relapse the CR rate was superior in patients with c-ALL compared to those with t-ALL (70% vs. 47%, statistically not significant), and in patients with a preceding CR of more than 18 months (81% vs. 46%, $p < 0.01$). Survival and remission duration was similar in patients with c-ALL compared to those with t-ALL. Patients with a preceding remission of less than 18 months had a statistically significant inferior survival compared to those with a longer preceding remission. The duration of the preceding remission was the major prognostic factor for survival in a multivariate analysis. Seven of 12 patients with primary refractory disease, second relapse, or relapse after BMT achieved a complete remission. Side effects of induction phase I consisted predominantly of hematologic toxicity with subsequent infections and of gastrointestinal toxicity. In phase II some patients additionally experienced cutaneous, ocular, and hepatic toxicity. Six patients died during induction. We conclude that the treatment efficiently induces remissions in relapsing adult ALL with tolerable toxicity but the remission duration has to be improved by intensifying consolidation and maintenance.

References

1. Hoelzer D, Thiel E, Loeffler H, Büchner T, Ganser A, Heil G et al. (1988) Intensivierte Konsolidierungstherapie für ALL-Hochrisikopatienten. Onkologie 11: 18–24
2. Miller AB, Hoogstraten B, Staquet M, Winkler A (1981) Reporting results of cancer treatment. Cancer 47: 207–214
3. Ohnuma T, Rosner S, Levy RN, Cuttner J, Moon JH, Silver RT, Blom J, Falkson G, Burningham R, Glidewell O, Holland JF (1971) Treatment of adult leukemia with L-asparaginase. Cancer Chemother Rep 55: 269–275

4. Kaplan EL, Meier P (1958) Nonparametric estimation from incomplete observations. J Am Stat Assoc 53: 457–481
5. Woodruff RK, Lister TA, Paxton AM, Whitehouse JMA, Malpas JS (1978) Combination chemotherapy for haematological relapse in adult acute lymphoblastic leukaemia. Am J Hematol 4: 173–177
6. Mandelli F, Testi AM, Aloe Spiriti MA, Giona F, Meloni G,Moleti ML, Amadori S, Pacciarini MA (1986) Evaluation of a polychemotherapeutic regimen including Idarubicin (4-demethoxydaunorubicin) in relapsed acute lymphocytic leukemia. Haematologica (Pavia) 71: 34–38
7. Elias L, Shaw MT, Raab SO (1979) Reinduction therapy for adult acute leukemia with adriamycin, vincistine, and prednisone: a Southwest Oncology Group Study. Cancer Treat Rep 63: 1413–1415
8. Reaman GH, Ladisch S, Eichelberger C, Poplack DG (1980) Improved treatment results in the management of single and multiple relapses of acute lymphoblastic leukemia. Cancer 45: 3090–3094
9. Paciucci PA, Cuttner J, Holland JF (1984) Mitoxantrone as a single agent and in combination chemotherapy in patients with refractory acute leukemia. Semin Oncol 11: 36–40
10. Herzig RH,Wolff SN, Lazarus HM, Phillips GL, Karanes C, Herzig GP (1983) High-dose cytosine arabinoside therapy for refractory leukemia. Blood 62: 361–369
11. Rudnick SA, Cadman EC, Capizzi RL, Skeel RT, Bertino JR, McIntosh S (1979) High dose cytosine arabinoside in refractory acute leukemia. Cancer 44: 1189–1193
12. Kantarjian HM, Estey EH, Plunkett W, Keating M,Walters RS, Iacoboni S, McCredie KB, Freireich EJ (1986) Phase I–II clinical and pharmacologic studies of high-dose cytosine arabinoside in refractory leukemia. Am J Med 81: 387–391
13. Rohatiner A, Slevin ML, Dhaliwal HS, Malpas JS, Lister TA (1984) High-dose cytosine arabinoside: response to therapy in acute leukemia and non-Hodgkin's lymphoma. Cancer Chemother Pharmacol 12: 90–93
14. Marsh W, Wozniak A, McCarley D (1987) Therapy of relapsed acute lymphocytic leukemia. Proc Am Soc Clin Oncol 6: 147 (abstr)
15. Early AP, Preisler HD, Slocum H, Rustum YM (1982) A pilot study of high-dose 1-β-d-arabinofuranosylcytosine for acute leukemia and refractory lymphoma: clinical response and pharmacology. Cancer Res 42: 1587–1594
16. Takaku F, Urabe A, Mizoguchi H,Yamada O, Wakabayashi Y, Miura Y et al. (1985) High-dose cytosine arabinoside in refractory acute leukemia. Semin Oncol 12 [Suppl 3]: 144–150
17. Peters WG, Willemze R, Colly LP (1986) Results of induction and consolidation treatment with intermediate and high-dose ara-C and m-AMSA containing regimens in patients with primarily failed or relapsed acute leukemia and non-Hodgkin's lymphoma. Scand J Haematol [Suppl] 44: 7–16
18. Arlin ZA, Feldman E, Kempin S, Ahmed T, Mittelman A, Savona S, Ascensao J, Baskind P, Sullivan P, Fuhr HG, Mertelsmann R (1988) Amsacrine with high-dose cytarabine is highly effective therapy for refractory and relapsed acute lymphoblastic leukemia in adults. Blood 72: 433–435
19. Zittoun R, Bury J, Strykmans P, Löwenberg B, Peetermens M, Rozendaal KY, Haanen C, Kerkhofs M, Jehn U, Willemze R (1985) Amsacrine with high-dose cytarabine in acute leukemia. Cancer Treat Rep 69: 1447–1448
20. Peters WG, Willemze R, Colly LP (1987) Intermediate and high-dose cytosine arabinoside-containing regimens for induction and consolidation therapy for patients with acute lymphoblastic leukemia and lymphoblastic non-Hodgkin's lymphoma: The Leyden experience and review of the literature. Semin Oncol 14 [Suppl 1]: 86–91
21. Ishii E, Hara T, Ohkubo K, Matsuzaki A, Takeuchi T, Ueda K (1986) Treatment of childhood acute lymphoblastic leukemia with intermediate-dose cytosine arabinoside and adriamycin. Med Pediatr Oncol 14: 73–77
22. Hiddemann W, Buchner T, Heil G, Schumacher K, Diedrich H, Maschmeyer G, Ho AD, Planker M, Gerith Stolzenburg S, Donhuijsen Ant R et al. (1990) Treatment of refractory acute lymphoblastic leukemia in adults with high dose cytosine arabinoside and mitoxantrone (HAM). Leukemia 4: 637–640
23. Kantarjian HM, Walters RL, Keating MJ, Estey EH, O'Brien S, Schachner J, McCredie KB, Freireich EJ (1990) Mitoxantrone and high-dose cytosine arabinoside for the treatment of refractory acute lymphocytic leukemia. Cancer 65: 5–8
24. Leclerc J, Rivard G, Blanchet M, Benoit P, David M, Demers J, Hume H, Langevin AM (1988) The association of once a day high-dose ara-C followed by mitoxantrone for three days induces a high rate of complete remission in children with poor prognosis acute leukemia. Blood 72 [Suppl]: 210a (abstr)

25. Capizzi RL, Poole M, Cooper MR (1984) Treatment of poor risk leukemia with sequential high-dose ara-C and asparaginase. Blood 63: 694

26. Amadori S, Papa G, Avvisati G, Fenu S, Monarca B, Petti MC, Pulsoni A, Mandelli F (1984) Sequential combination of high-dose ara-C and asparaginase for the treatment of advanced acute leukemia and lymphoma. Leuk Res 8: 729–735

27. Wells RJ, Feusner J, Devney R, Woods WG, Provisor AJ, Cairo MS, Odom LF, Nachman J, Jones GR, Ettinger LJ, Capizzi RL (1985) Sequential high dose cytosine arabinoside-asparaginase treatment in advanced childhood leukemia. J Clin Oncol 3: 998–1004

28. Gore M, Powles R, Lakhani A, Milan S, Maitland J, Goss G, Nandi A, Perren T, Forgeson G, Treleaven J, Zuiable A, Porta F (1989) Treatment of relapsed and refractory acute leukaemia with high-dose cytosine arabinoside and etoposide. Cancer Chemother Pharmacol 23: 373–376

29. Larson RA, Gaynor ER, Shepard KV, Daly KM (1985) High-dose ara-C plus VM-26 in adult acute lymphoblastic leukemia. Eur J Cancer Clin Oncol 21: 1261–1263

30. Hohl RJ, Daly KM, LeBeau MM, Larson RA (1989) High dose ara-C (HDAC) with VM-26 as salvage therapy for adults with acute lymphoblastic leukemia (ALL). Proc Am Soc Clin Oncol 8: 206 (abstr)

31. Freund M, Link H, Diedrich H, LeBlanc S, Wilke H, Poliwoda H (1991) High-dose ara-C and etoposide in refractory or relapsing acute leukemia. Cancer Chemother Pharmacol (in press)

32. Garay G, Milone J, Dibar E, Pavlovsky S, Kvicala R, Sackmann Muriel F, Montres Varela D, Eppinger-Helft M (1983) Vindesine, prednisone, and daunomycin in acute lymphoblastic leukemia in relapse. Cancer Chemother Pharmacol 10: 224–226

33. Yap BS, McCredie KB, Keating MJ, Bodey GP, Freireich EJ (1981) Asparaginase and methotrexate combination chemotherapy in relapsed acute lymphoblastic leukemia in adults. Cancer Treat Rep [Suppl 1] 65: 83–87

34. Terebolo HR, Anderson K, Wiernik PH, Cuttner J, Cooper RM, Faso L, Berenberg JL (1986) Therapy of refractory adult acute lymphoblastic leukemia with vincristine and prednisolone plus tandem methotrexate and L-asparaginase. Results of a Cancer and Leukemia Group B Study. Am J Clin Oncol 9: 411–415

35. Yap BS, McCredie KB (1978) Refractory acute leukemia in adults treated with sequential colaspace and high dose methotrexate. Br Med J 2: 791–793

36. Kantarjian HM, Walters RS, Keating MJ, Barlogie B, McCredie KB, Freireich EJ (1989) Experience with vincristine, doxorubicin, and dexamethasone (VAD) chemotherapy in adults with refractory acute lymphocytic leukemia. Cancer 64: 16–22

Mitoxantrone and Continuous Infusion of Cytosine Arabinoside in the Treatment of Relapsed and Refractory Acute Leukemia

V. Liso, G. Specchia, V. Pavone, S. Capalbo, A. Iacobazzi, and N. Pansini

Introduction

Despite an improved remission rate in patients with acute leukemia (AL) following the introduction of intensive chemotherapy programs, the incidence of relapsed and refractory patients still remains an important clinical problem. High-dose cytosine arabinoside (ARA-C) has been employed in patients with refractory or relapsed acute leukemia, alone or in combination with asparaginase [1], amsacrine [2] or idarubicin [3]. Recently, several clinical studies, investigating the combined use of mitoxantrone (MITOX) and ARA-C, have shown encouraging results in the treatment of relapsed or refractory acute leukemia [4–7]. In this work, we have investigated the efficacy and toxicity of MITOX in combination with continuous infusion of ARA-C in patients with refractory and relapsed acute leukemia.

Materials and Methods

Forty-six patients with relapsed or refractory AL were entered in the study. Twenty had acute lymphoblastic leukemia (ALL) and 26 had acute nonlymphoid leukemia (ANLL). Bone marrow and peripheral blast cells were categorized on the basis of FAB classification [9], cytochemical investigations [10], and cytoplasmic Ig and surface

Hematology Service, University of Bari, Bari, Italy
Supported in part by MURST and Prog. Fin. Regione Puglia Mz. B. Calabrese is fully acknowledged

marker analysis. Patients were considered eligible for the study if they had a performance status of 0–2 (WHO criteria), normal liver and renal functions and no evidence of severe cardiac dysfunction. Clinical characteristics of patients are shown in Table 1.

Patients with ALL

Fourteen patients had been treated with GIMEMA Protocol 0183 (10) and 6 with GIMEMA Protocol 0288 including daunorubicin followed on day 32 by MITOX 10 mg/m² for 3 days in the induction phase. Of the 20 patients, 6 were refractory to first line treatment, 9 had relapsed within 12 months of complete remission (CR) and 5 had relapsed more than 12 months after achieving the first CR.

Patients with ANLL

Twenty-one patients (age <60 years) had been previously treated for remission induction with daunorubicin 45 mg/m² per day for 3 days and ARA-C 200 mg/m² per day continuous infusion for 7 days (GIMEMA Protocol) [11]. Five patients (age >60 years) had been treated with daunorubicin 45 mg/m² per day for 1–2 days and cytosine arabinoside 200 mg/m² for 1–5 days. Of the 26 patients, 11 showed primary resistance to two courses of intensive first line treatment with daunorubicin and ARA-C, 3 had relapsed within the first 6 months of CR (early relapse) and 12 had relapsed off

Table 1. Characteristics of patients with acute leukemia

Patients	No.	46
Sex	Male	25
	Female	21
Age (years)	Range	15–76
	Median	38
ALL		20
Disease status	Refractory	6
	Relapsed	14
First line treatment	GIMEMA protocol 0183	14
	GIMEMA protocol 0288	6
FAB classifikation	L1	5
	L2	13
	L3	2
AnLL		
Disease status	Refractory	11
	Relapsed	15
First line treatment	GIMEMA protocol 8201	21
	DAUNO (2) +ARA-C (5)	5
FAB classification	M1	2
	M2	12
	M4	2
	M5	7
	M6	1
	M7	2

therapy more than 6 months after achieving the first CR (late relapse); median CR duration was 8.5 months (range 7–17 months). Prior cumulative dose of daunorubicin was between 180 and 500 mg/m^2 (median 270 mg/m^2).

Treatment

All patients received a two-course induction therapy consisting of MITOX, 12 mg/m^2 per day, by intravenous infusion on day 1, 2 and 3 and ARA-C 200 mg/m^2 per day by continuous infusion on day 1–7. The second reinduction course was administered 7–10 days after the first. Therapy response was evaluated after the second reinduction course. Response to therapy and toxicity were assessed using the conventional criteria of the Cancer and Leukemia Group [12] and WHO [13] respectively. After achieving CR, the patients received one course of the same protocol as consolidation therapy.

Results

Overall results of treatment with MITOX plus continuous infusion of ARA-C in refractory and relapsed AL are summarized in Table 2. Complete remission was observed in 10 of 20 patients (50%) with ALL. Of the ten patients who obtained CR, three were refractory to the first line of treatment and seven were in first relapse. The median remission duration for the entire group (ten patients) was 5 months (range 2–9 months). In responsive ALL patients, the median duration of leukocytopenia ($<0.5 \times 10^9$l) was 14 days (range 12–23 days) and that of thrombocytopenia ($<20 \times 10^9$ l) was 12 days (range 10–20 days) after the two reinduction courses. Partial remission was observed in two relapsed patients. Five patients had persistent leukemia and three had hypoplasia or aplastic bone marrow after reinduction treatment but with rapid increase in leukemic cells. One patient died of cerebral hemorrhage in aplasia. Four documented

Table 2. Results in 46 patients with acute leukemia treated with MITOX and continuous infusion of ARA-C

	No.	CR	PR	F	Induction deaths	CR duration median	(months) Range
All patients	46	27 (58.6%)	2	15	2	5	2–16
All							
Refractory	6	3 (50%)	–	3	–	5	3–6
Relapsed	14	7 (50%)	2	4	1	5	2–9
AnLL							
Refractory	11	6 (54.5%)	–	4	1	5	2–13
Relapsed	15	11 (73.3%)	–	4	–	4.5	2–16

infections (two clinical and two bacteriological) were observed in four patients. Out of 26 patients with ANLL, 17 (65.3%) achieved CR. The cytotypes of 17 responder patients were 2M1, 7M2, 6M5 and 2M7. Particularly two patients with M7, failing first line treatment, obtained CR by one course with MITOX plus ARA-C; they are still in CR after 8 and 7 months respectively. Of the 17 AnLL patients who obtained CR, 11 were in first relapse, and 6 were refractory to the first line of treatment including daunorubicin and ARA-C. The median remission duration for the entire group (17 patients) was 5 months (range 2–16 months). In responsive AnLL patients, the median duration of granulocytopenia (<05 $\times 10^9$l) and thrombocytopenia (<20 $\times 10^9$l) was 14 days (range 10–25 days). One patient died of cerebral hemorrhage, in aplasia, while infections were documented in five patients (Table 3). Extrahematologic toxicity was acceptable, side effects tolerable, nausea and vomiting mild, and moderate stomatitis and reversible hepatic function abnormalities were observed. No cardiac toxicity was observed (Table 3).

Discussion

In recent years many protocols including MITOX alone [14, 15] or in combination with ARA-C high dose, intermediate dose or conventional dose [5–8, 16] showed encouraging results in the treatment of relapsed or refractory patients with AL. The two agents have different biochemical mechanisms of action [17] without overlapping reported toxicities. The efficacy of MITOX and ARA-C compared with other salvage regimens (high-dose ARA-C alone or in combination with other agents such etoposide, amsacrine, asparaginase or idarubicin) is difficult to determine due to the heterogeneity of the reported studies [1–5, 16–19].

Paciucci [16] also supports a comparative trial of MITOX with either high-dose or conventional-dose ARA-C. Analysis of

Table 3. Extrahematologic toxicity in 46 patients with acute leukemias treated with MITOX and ARA-C

	WHO				
	0	1	2	3	4
Nausea and vomiting	31	9	4	2	0
Alopecia	23	13	7	3	0
Diarrhea	35	7	4	0	0
Mucositis	33	10	3	0	0
Liver toxicity	42	2	2	0	0
Cardiac toxicity	46	0	0	0	0
Infections	37	7	2	0	0

available data seems to indicate that while the use of megadose ARA-C combined with daily doses of MITOX does not necessarily translate into a greater antileukemic effect, it will, however, definitely increase the frequency and severity of toxic complications.

The results of our study indicate that the sequential combination of MITOX and conventional-dose ARA-C in continuous infusion is an effective and tolerable regimen for refractory and relapsed AL cases. Of the 26 patients with pretreated ANLL, 17 (65.3 %) (6 refractory and 11 relapsed) achieved CR with a median CR duration of 5 months. Concerning ALL, 10 of 20 (50 %) adult ALL patients (3 refractory and 7 in first relapse) obtained CR with a median CR duration of 5 months.

These results are comparable with the majority of data reported in the literature [4–6, 16, 18] and demonstrate the antileukemic activity of this combination with no documented evidence of clinical cross-resistance with induction regimens based on standard-dose ARA-C and anthracyclines. In our experience, using MITOX and ARA-C in continuous infusion at conventional doses, nonhematologic toxicity was minimal, consisting mainly of tolerable nausea and mild vomiting, moderate stomatitis and reversible liver dysfunction. The regimen toxicity was acceptable without any observed new or synergistic toxicity with the combination treatment. In responders, the duration of pancytopenia was not larger than usually seen after conventional chemotherapy as indicated by the median recovery times of granulocytes and platelets. Because of acceptable toxicity, MITOX plus continuous infusion of standard dose of ARA-C could be considered for reinduction of relapsed or refractory AL, particularly in AL patients eligible for intensive programs post second CR.

Summary

Forty-six patients with relapsed or refractory AL (20 with ALL and 26 with AnLL) received a regimen employing two courses of mitoxantrone 12 mg/m^2 by rapid intravenous infusion on days 1, 2 and 3 and cytosine arabinoside 200 mg/m^2 per day by continuous infusion on days 1–7. Of 20 patients with ALL, 10 (50 %) (3 refractory and 7 relapsed) achieved complete remission (CR). Median duration of CR was 5 months (range 2–9 months). CR was achieved in 17 of 26 (65.3 %) patients with ANLL (8 refractory and 9 relapsed). Median duration of CR was 5 months (range 2–16 months). The treatment was associated with minimal extrahematologic toxicity with noncardiac toxicity.

References

1. Capizzi R, Davis R, Powell B, Cuttner J, Ellison RR, Cooper MR, Dillman R, Major WB, Dupre E, Mc Intyre OR (1988) Synergy between high-dose cytarabine and asparaginase in the treatment of adults with refractory and relapsed acute myelogenous leukemia. A Cancer and Leukemia Group B study. J Clin Oncol 6 (3) 499–508
2. Arlin ZA, Feldman E, Kempin S, Ahmed T, Mittelman A, Savona S, Ascensao J, Baskind P, Sullivan P, Fuhr HG, Mertelsmann R (1988) Amsacrine with high dose cytarabine is highly effective therapy for refractory or relapsed lymphoblastic leukemia in adults. Blood 72: 433–435
3. Giona F, Testi AM, Amadori S, Meloni G, Carotenuto M, Resegotti L, Colella R, Leoni P, Carella AM, Grotto P, Miniero R, Mandelli F (1990) Idarubicin and high-dose cytarabine in the treatment of refractory and relapsed acute lymphoblastic leukemia. Ann Oncol 1: 51–55
4. Hiddemann W, Kreutzmann H, Straif K, Ludwig WD, Mertelsmann R, Planker M, Donhuijsen-Ant R, Lengfelder E, Arlin Z, Buchner T (1987): High-dose cytosine arabinoside in combination with mitoxantrone for the treatment of refractory acute myeloid and lymphoblastic leukemia. Semin Oncol 14 [Suppl 1]. 73–77
5. Amadori S, Meloni G, Petti MC, Papa G, Miniero R, Mandelli F (1989): Phase II trial of intermediate dose ARA-C (IDAC) with sequential mitoxantrone (MITOX) in acute myelogenous leukemia. Leukemia 3(2) 112–114
6. Lejeune C, Tubiana N, Gastaut JA, Maraninchi D, Richard B, Launay MC, Sainty D, Sebahoun G, Carcassonne Y (1990): High-dose cytosine arabinoside and mitoxantrone in previously treated acute leukemia patients. Eur J Haematol 44: 240–243

7. Arlin ZA (1990): Current status of mitoxantrone combination chemotherapy programs: a personal view. Leukemia Lymphoma 1: 301–305

8. Bennett JM, Catovsky D, Daniel MT, Flandrin G, Galton DAG, Gralnick HR, Sultan C (1976): Proposal for the classification of the acute leukemias. Br J Haematol 33: 451

9. Liso V, Troccoli G, Specchia G, Magno M (1977) Cytochemical normal and abnormal eosinophils in acute leukemias. Am J Hematol 2: 123–131

10. Gimema Cooperative Group: Gimema ALL 0183 (1989): A multicentric study on adult acute lymphoblastic leukaemia in Italy. Br J Haemat 71: 377–383

11. Mandelli F, Petti MC, Avvisati G, Amadori S, Broccia G, Carella AM, Carotenuto M, Di Raimondo F, Floritoni G, Lazzarino M, Leone G, Martelli M, Mirto S, Pete A, Petti M, Resegotti L, Specchia G, Vegna ML for the Cooperative Group Gimema (1990): Experience in the treatment of adult acute myelogenous leukemia. In: Acute myelogenous leukemia. Progress and controversies Wiley Liss, New York, pp 273–291

12. Cancer and Leukemia group B (1974) Criteria for evaluating acute leukemia.

13. Herzig RH, Wolff SN, Lazarus HM, Phillips GL, Karanes C, Herzig GP (1984): High dose cytosine arabinoside therapy for refractory leukemia. Blood 62: 361–369

14. Paciucci PA, Cuttner J, Holland JF (1984): Mitoxantrone as a single agent and in combination chemotherapy in patients with refractory acute leukemia. Semin Oncol 11 [Suppl 1]: 36–40

15. Bezwoda WB, Bernasconi C, Hutchinson RM, Winfield DA, De Bock R, Mandelli F (1990): Mitoxantrone for refractory and relapsed acute leukemia. Cancer 66: 418–422

16. Paciucci PA, Dutcher JP, Cuttner J, Strauman II, Wiernik PH, Holland IF (1987): Mitoxantrone and ARA-C in previously treated patients with acute myelogenous leukemia. Leukemia 1 (7): 565–567.

17. Heinemann V, Murray D, Walters R, Meyn RE, Plunkett W (1988): Mitoxantrone induced DNA damage in leukemia cells is enhanced by treatment with high-dose arabinosyl cytosine. Cancer Chemother Pharmacol 22: 205–210.

18. Lazzarino M, Morra E, Alessandrino EP, Orlandi E, Pagnucco G, Morante S, Bernasconi P, Inverardi D, Bonfichi M, Bernasconi C (1989): Mitoxantrone and etoposide: an effective regimen for refractory or relapsed acute myelogenous leukemia. Eur J Haematol 43: 411–416

19. Milpied N, Gisselbrecht C, Harousseau JL, Sebban C, Witz F, Troussard X, Gratecos N, Michallet M, Leblond V, Auzanneau G, Fiere D (1990): Successful treatment of adult acute lymphoblastic leukemia after relapse with prednisone, intermediate-dose cytarabine, mitoxantrone, and etoposide (PAME) chemotherapy. Cancer 66: 627–631

Oral Idarubicin in Pretreated Pediatric Acute Leukemia*

S. Bielack[1], U. Bode[2], M. Goebel[3], P. Gutjahr[4], R. Haas[5], N. Kuhn[6], H. Siewert[7], and R. Erttmann[1]

Introduction

Anthracyclines are among the most useful drugs in the treatment of both lymphoblastic (ALL) and nonlymphoblastic (ANLL) acute leukemias of childhood. However, the benefit of the most commonly used anthracyclines daunorubicin and doxorubicin is limited by their cardiotoxicity [1] and by resistance against these compounds. The daunorubicin analog idarubicin (4-demethoxydaunorubicin) might be less cardiotoxic and has shown greater antileukemic efficacy in some preclinical and clinical trials [2]. In addition, the chemical structure of idarubicin leads to appreciable resorption of active drug after oral application [3, 4], allowing therapy in an outpatient setting. We therefore conducted an open, multicenter trial assessing the toxicity and efficacy of oral idarubicin in refractory acute leukemia in children.

[1] Abteilung für pädiatrische Hämatologie und Onkologie, Universitätskinderklinik, Hamburg, FRG
[2] Universitätskinderklinik, Bonn, FRG
[3] Farmitalia Carlo Erba GmbH, Freiburg, FRG
[4] Universitätskinderklinik, Mainz, FRG
[5] Universitätskinderklinik, München, FRG
[6] Kinderklinik Wuppertal, Klinikum Barmen, Wuppertal, FRG
[7] Universitätskinderklinik RWTH, Aachen, FRG

* Supported by Farmitalia Carlo Erba GmbH, Freiburg

Patients and Treatment Protocol

The study was open to pediatric patients with hematologic manifestation of recurrent or primarily refractory ALL or ANLL treated at German pediatric oncology centers. Informed consent was obtained from all patients or their legal guardians. Bilirubin >2 mg/dl, creatinine >2 mg/dl, a fractional shortening rate (FS) of <28% on m-mode echocardiography or previous cardiac disorders were exclusion criteria, as were predictable intolerable side effects, presence of concomitant severe diseases, or a Karnofsky status <40%, while pretreatment with other anthracyclines was permitted.

Idarubicin was given p.o. at a single dose of 13.3–30 mg/m^2 per day before meals on each of three consecutive days (total dose = 40–90 mg/m^2). No concomitant chemotherapy was allowed with the first course of idarubicin. Patients responding to therapy were eligible to receive additional courses at 21- to 28-day intervals, depending on blood counts.

Partial remission was assumed when the peripheral blood was free of blasts and showed normal counts, and blasts in the bone marrow were reduced to less than 10%. Complete response was defined as the peripheral blood being free of blasts and showing normal counts, the bone marrow had to be of normal cellularity with <5% blasts.

Toxicity was graded as mild (I), moderate (II), severe (III), or life-threatening (IV) according to a modified WHO toxicity score: Hematologic toxicity, leukocytes/nl: $\geq 4.0 = 0, 2.0–3.9 = I, 1.0–1.9 = II, 0.5–0.9 = III, <0.5 = IV$; platelets/nl: $\geq 100 = 0, 60–99 = I, 30–59 = II, 10–29 = III, <10 = IV$. Nonhematologic toxicity, hepatic: bilirubin (mg/dl) $<1.25 = 0, 1.26–2.5 = I, 2.6–5.0 = II, 5.1–10.0 = III, >10 = IV$; all other toxicity graded according to standard WHO criteria.

Fisher's exact test was used for statistical analysis of the influence of idarubicin dose on response and leukopenia.

Results

Patients

Idarubicin p.o. was given to 20 pediatric patients aged 2–18 years (median 13 years) with relapsed ($n = 19$; $5 \times$ 1st, $9 \times$ 2nd, $4 \times$ 3rd, $1 \times$ 4th relapse) or primarily refractory ($n = 1$) ALL ($n = 18$) or ANLL ($n = 2$) (patient characteristics see Table 1). Prior

anthracycline therapy reached cumulative doses of 38–880 mg/m^2 (Table 2). Thirteen patients received one course, seven more than one (two to eight) courses of idarubicin.

Toxicity

Bone marrow suppression was the most frequent and most severe side effect (Table 3). The leukocyte nadir was reached between days 5 and 21 (median = day 11), counts of less than 1 (0.5)/nl were documented in 13 (6) of 17 patients evaluable for hematological toxicity. One patient (No. 2) died of sepsis during prolonged cytopenia. The frequency of severe leukopenia was clearly dose related, with six of nine after more than 60 mg/m^2, but only one of eight evaluable patients after lower doses reaching leukocyte nadirs of <0.5/nl ($p = 0.036$, Fisher's exact test). Thrombocytopenia <30 (10)/nl was documented in 12 (5) patients.

Table 1. Patient characteristics. Clinical data of 20 patients treated with oral idarubicin. All patients showed hematological evidence of acute leukemia

Patient	Age (years)	Sex	Diagnosis	Relapse
1	6	Female	C-ALL	Second
2	16	Male	T-ALL	Third[a]
3	17	Male	C-ALL	Second
4	13	Female	C-ALL	Second
5	10	Female	C-ALL	Fourth
6	4	Male	C-ALL	First[b]
7	16	Male	ALL	Third
8	14	Male	ALL	Second
9	15	Male	C-ALL	First
10	2	Female	ANLL-M5	Second
11	18	Male	C-ALL	Second
12	7	Female	C-ALL	Second
13	2	Male	ANLL-M5	Ini.[c]
14	13	Female	C-ALL	Third
15	3	Female	C-ALL	Second
16	15	Female	C-ALL	First
17	13	Male	C-ALL	Third
18	9	Male	T-ALL	First
19	15	Female	C-ALL	Second
20	10	Male	T-ALL	First

[a] Plus CNS, skin and testicular involvement
[b] Additional testicular involvement
[c] Refractory to initial therapy
Age, age in years at start of idarubicin treatment; diagnosis: ALL, acute lymphoblastic leukemia; ANLL, acute nonlymphoblastic leukemia

Table 2. Anthracycline pretreatment

Patient	Daunorubicin	Doxorubicin	Mitoxantrone	Total
1	144	–	–	144
2	240	–	–	240
3	281	108	–	389
4	207	145	–	352
5	800	80	–	880
6	91	–	–	91
7	227	100	–	327
8	221	88	–	309
9	60	60	30	150
10	87	145	22	254
11	160	–	–	160
12	316	–	–	316
13	184	90	–	274
14	231	28	–	259
15	38	–	–	38
16	217	97	–	314
17	92	181	–	273
18	110	113	–	213
19	283	–	–	283
20	65	69	–	134

Cumulative doses (mg/m^2) of daunorubicin, doxorubicin, and mitoxantrone given to participating patients prior to idarubicin treatment

Table 3. Summary of side effects observed after the first idarubicin treatment cycle given to 20 pediatric patients with acute leukemia. See text for grading of toxicity

Grade	Nausea Vomit	Stomatitis	Diarrhea	Hepatic	Cardiac	Infection	Leukopenia	Platelets
0	11	13	16	14	17	14	0	3
I	1	1	2	2	0	0	0	0
II	7	3	1	1	0	3	4	3
III	1	2	0	1	1	0	6	7
IV	0	0	0	0	0	1[a]	7	4
NE[b]	0	1	1	2	2	2	3	3

[a] One death due to sepsis during prolonged pancytopenia
[b] Not evaluable due to early death ($n=1$) or missing data ($n=2$)

Otherwise, idarubicin was generally well tolerated. However, one girl (No. 14), pretreated with 259 mg/m^2 anthracyclines, developed congestive heart failure responsive to appropriate medical intervention after 76 mg/m^2 idarubicin. In addition, one case of reversible hyperbilirubinemia (3.7 mg/dl, No. 4), one case of severe nausea and two cases of severe mucositis were observed (Table 3).

Antileukemic Activity

Remission was achieved in 7/20 patients (4 CR, 3 PR) (Table 4). Those patients who reached CR did so after the first (No. 14, 19), second (No. 4) or third (No. 6) cycle. Five of nine patients receiving more than 60 mg/m^2 responded, compared to only 2 of 11 treated with lesser doses ($p = 0.102$, Fisher's exact test).

Table 4. Therapeutic efficacy. Response to oral idarubicin in 20 pediatric patients with relapsed or refractory acute leukemia. See text for definition of complete (CR) and partial remission (PR)

Patient	Dose (mg/m^2)*	Remission
1	40	None
2	62	None
3	44	None
4	90	Complete[b]
5	90	None
6	86	Complete[c]
7	50	None
8	58	None
9	44	None
10	55	None
11	65	None
12	60	None
13	59	Partial
14	76	Complete[a]
15	50	Partial
16	53	None
17	41	None
18	71	Partial
19	74	Complete[a]
20	73	None
Total		4 CR; 3 PR

* Dose of initial cycle. (Patients were eligible for administration of more than one treatment cycle, if at least a partial remission was achieved after the first dose). Patients who did so reached complete remission after the first (a), second (b), or sixth (c) idarubicin course

Discussion

The daunorubicin analog idarubicin (4-demethoxydaunorubicin) has been advocated for the treatment of acute leukemia in children and adults [2, 5], In vitro data have suggested an increased antileukemic efficacy of idarubicin compared to daunorubicin in some assays [6], as well as increased penetration into leukemic cells [7].

Clinical activity of single agent intravenous idarubicin has been demonstrated in relapsed and refractory acute leukemia in adults [8–10] and children [11, 12]. A recent review of six randomized studies has shown idarubicin to be at least as effective or even better than doxorubicin or daunorubicin during remission induction in primary ANLL (all combined with cytosine arabinoside) [2]; the same result was found in a pediatric trial of reinduction after first relapse of ALL [13]. Myelotoxicity has emerged as the dose-limiting side effect of phase I studies, while cardiotoxic effects of idarubicin might even be lower than those of equieffective doses of either doxo- or daunorubicin [2]. As a major advantage over the other anthracyclines, oral administration of idarubicin is feasible, with a bioavailability of some 25%–30% [3, 4], allowing oral drug administration in the outpatient setting. Phase I studies of oral idarubicin in leukemic children reported a maximum tolerated dose (MTD) in the range of 3 × 40 mg/m^2 [14, 15].

We therefore conducted a trial of oral idarubicin at a dose of 13.3–30 mg/m^2 on each of three consecutive days in heavily (anthracycline) pretreated pediatric patients with relapsed or refractory acute leukemia, mainly ALL. In this setting, 7 of 20 patients achieved at least a partial remission, including 4 complete responses. Extramedullary toxicity was generally well tolerable. The only case of clinically obvious cardiotoxicity was reversible after appropriate therapy. However, idarubicin induced severe, sometimes protracted myelosuppression, particularly after treatment with more than 60 mg/m^2 per course. One patient died of sepsis during prolonged cytopenia. Therefore, the application of the high idarubicin doses suggested by Tan et al. [14] and Pui et al. [15] was not feasible in our study. Trials of oral idarubicin in adult patients also point towards a lower MTD [16, 17]. A reduction of the idarubicin dose, however, might also compromise antileukemic efficacy, as responses in our study were primarily seen after treatment with doses above 60 mg/m^2.

Conclusions

Oral idarubicin can induce remissions in some children with relapsed or refractory acute leukemia. Due to severe myelotoxicity at higher doses, no more than 60 mg/m^2 per course should be given to this patient group; however, this might reduce therapeutic efficacy.

Summary

Idarubicin was given p.o. to 20 pediatric patients suffering from relapsed or primarily refractory anthracycline pretreated acute lymphoblastic ($n = 18$) or nonlymphoblastic leukemia ($n = 2$). The dose per cycle was 40–90 mg/m^2, given as 13.3–30 mg/m^2 on three consecutive days. Severe toxicity was mainly hematologic, with seven patients reaching leukocyte nadirs of $<0.5 \times 10^9/l$, including one case of fatal sepsis during cytopenia. Nausea and vomiting (1), mucositis (2), hepatic (1) and cardiac (1) dysfunction contributed to grade III toxicity. Complete remission (CR) was documented in four patients (20%); in addition, three patients (15%) achieved partial remission (PR).

References

1. Von Hoff DD, Rosencweig M, Piccart M (1980) The cardiotoxicity of anticancer agents. Semin Oncol 9: 23
2. Carella AM, Berman E, Maraone M, Ganzina F (1990) Idarubicin in the treatment of acute leukemias. An overview of preclinical and clinical studies. Haematologica (Pavia) 75: 1–11
3. Smith DB, Margison JM, Lucas SB, Wilkinson PM, Howell A (1987) Clinical pharmacology of oral and intravenous 4-demethoxydaunorubicin. Cancer Chemother Pharmacol 19: 138–142
4. Gillies HC, Herriot D, Liang R, Ohashi K, Rogers HJ, Harper PG (1987) Pharmacokinetics of idarubicin (4-demethoxydaunorubicin; IMI-30; NSC 256439) following intravenous and oral administration in patients with advanced cancer. Br J Clin Pharmacol 23: 303–310
5. Wiernik P (ed) (1989) Idarubicin: a new presence in leukemias. Semin Oncol 16 [Suppl 2]: 1–36
6. Casazza AM, Pratesi G, Giuliani F, DiMarco A (1980) Antileukemic activity of 4-demethoxydaunorubicin in mice. Tumori 66: 549–552
7. Erttmann R, Bode U, Erb N, Forcadell de Dios P, Gutjahr P, Haas R, Kuhn N, Siewert H, Landbeck G (1988) Antineoplastische Wirksamkeit und Toxizität von Idarubicin (4-Demethoxydaunorubicin) bei rezidivierten akuten Leukämien des Kindesalters. Klin Pädiatr 200: 200–204
8. Daghestani AN, Arlin ZA, Leyland-Jones B, Gee TS, Kempin SJ, Mertelsmann R, Budman D, Schulman P, Baratz R, Williams L, Clarkson BD, Young CW (1985) Phase I and II clinical and pharmacological study of 4-demethoxydaunorubicin (idarubicin) in adult patients with acute leukemia. Cancer Res 45: 1408–1412
9. Carella AM, Santini G, Martinengo M, et al. (1985) 4-Demethoxydaunorubicin in refractory or relapsed acute leukemias. A pilot study. Cancer 55 1452–1454
10. Harrousseau JL, Hurteloup P, Reiffers J, et al. (1987) Idarubicin in the treatment of relapsed or refractory acute myeloid leukemia. Cancer Treat Rep 71: 991–995
11. Tan CTC, Hancock C, Steinherz P, Bacha DM, Steinherz L, Luks E, Winick N, Meyers P, Mondora A, Dantis E, Niedzwiecki D, Stevens YW (1987) Phase I and clinical pharmacological study of 4-demethoxydaunorubicin (idarubicin) in children with advanced cancer. Cancer Res 47: 2990–2995
12. Madon E, Grazia G, De Bernardi B, Comelli A, Carli M, Sainati L, Paolucci G, Canino R, Colella R, Bagnulo S, Di Pietro N (1987) Phase II study of idarubicin administered iv to pediatric patients with acute lymphoblastic leukemia. Cancer Treat Rep 71: 855–856
13. Harris R, Feig S, Baum E, Holcenberg J, Pendergrass T, Bleyer A, Holt C, Krailo M, Hammond D (1988) Idarubicin (IDR) vs daunomycin for reinduction of relapsed childhood ALL – a CCSG study. Proc Am Soc Clin Oncol 7: 189
14. Tan C, Bacha D, Hancock C (1984) New anthracyclines in childhood cancer. 14th International Congress of Chemotherapy. (abstr No 104)
15. Pui CH, de Graaf SS, Dow LW, Rodman JH, Evans WE, Alpert BS, Murphy SB (1988) Phase I clinical trial of orally administered 4-demethoxydaunorubicin (idarubicin) with pharmacokinetic and in vitro drug sensitivity testing in children with refractory leukemia. Cancer Res 48: 5348–5352
16. Lowenthal RM (1987) A possible special role for oral idarubicin in the treatment of leukemia following myelodysplastic syndrome. In: Mandelli F, Polli E, Clarkson B (eds) Proceedings of the session in idarubicin in the treatment of acute leukemia. 4th International Symposium on Therapy of Acute Leukemia. Excerpta Medica, Amsterdam, pp 50–55
17. Hochster H, Green M, Liebes L, Speyer JL, Wernz J, Blum R, Muggia F (1990) Good tolerance of weekly oral idarubicin: a phase I study with pharmacology. Cancer Chemother Pharmacol 26: 297–300

Involvement of the CNS in Childhood AML: Experiences of the AML-BFM Studies -78, -83, and -87*

U. Creutzig, J. Ritter, and G. Schellong for the AML-BFM Study Group

As children with acute myelogenous leukemia (AML) used to have an overall lower incidence of central nervous system (CNS) involvement than those with acute lymphoblastic leukemia (ALL), prophylactic treatment has not been routine. However, the improvement in the rate of long-term survival in childhood AML has been accompanied by an increase in CNS relapses if children receive no CNS prophylaxis [1]. In the following we present our analysis of CNS leukemia (initial and relapse) based on the three German BFM (Berlin-Frankfurt-Münster) studies AML-78, -83, and -87.

* Supported by the Bundesministerium für Forschung und Technologie, and Deutsche Krebshilfe, FRG.

Univ.-Kinderklinik, Albert-Schweitzer-Str. 33, D-4400 Münster, FRG

Treatment

The first two BFM studies AML-78 and -83 employed cranial irradiation combined with intrathecal methotrexate (MTX) or cytosine arabinoside (ARA-C, four times) for all patients during consolidation treatment. Dosages were determined according to age and initial cerebrospinal fluid (CSF) blast count (Table 1). Patients of study AML-BFM-87 without initial CNS involvement and white blood count (WBC) < 70 000/mm³ were randomized for CNS irradiation during the first 2.5 years of the trial. Thereafter, randomization was abandoned. Prophylactic CNS treatment consisted of ARA-C i.th. and high-dose ARA-C ($3 \text{ g/m}^2 \times 6$) which was applied during two intensification courses.

Patient and Methods

From December 1978 to December 1990, 510 AML patients under 17 years of age

Table 1. Dosages for cranial irradiation and intrathecal drug administration in CNS treatment (studies AML-BFM-78 and -83)

Age (years)	Cranial irradiation "Prophylactic" (GY)	"Therapeutic" (GY)	MTX i.th. (study -78) (mg/m²)	ARA-C i.th. (study -83) (mg)
< 1	12	20		20
≥1–2	15	24		26
≥2–3	18	30	12.5	34
≥3	18	30		40

ᵃ Children with initial CNS involvement (> 10 blast cells in the CSF) additionally received spinal cord irradiation with 15 Gy (< 1 year), 20 Gy (1–2 years), and 24 Gy (≥2 years)

491

entered the three studies BFM-78, -83, and -87, the latter being still open for patient entry. The initial diagnosis of AML and its subtypes was established according to the FAB classification [2, 3]. Criteria for CNS involvement were: more than ten blast cells/mm³ in the CSF or evidence of cerebral leukemic infiltration at biopsy or operation.

Results

AML-BFM-78 and -83 Studies

Twenty-three out of 316 children with CSF examinations presented with CNS involvement initially. As shown in Table 2, extramedullary organ involvement at other sites was frequent in children with initial CNS involvement ($p = 0.13$). Meningeal leukemia occurred more often in children with hyperleukocytosis (WBC $\geq$ 100 000/mm³) compared to children with a lower WBC ($p < 0.04$). Especially children with FAB M4 showed an elevated initial blast count in the CSF (FAB M4 vs. other FAB types $p < 0.0001$).

Treatment results in children of studies -78 and -83 with or without initial CNS leukemia are presented in Table 3. The patients of both groups were equally likely to achieve remission (CR), but the relapse rate was higher in initially CNS-positive patients. Life-table estimates for a 7-year duration of the event-free interval (EFI, Fig. 1) were 35 % (SD 12 %) in initially CNS-positive and 54 % (SD 3 %) for CNS-negative patients ($p < 0.05$).

Sixteen of 101 relapses occurred either isolated in the CNS ($n = 5$) or in combination with other relapse sites ($n = 11$) (Table 4). Children with initial CNS leukemia had a higher frequency of CNS relapses than CNS-negative patients ($p < 0.03$).

There were no isolated or combined CNS relapses in patients with FAB M2, whereas the incidence in FAB M5 was high ($n = 7$; Table 5). When relapses with CNS involvement were censored, the difference in prognosis between initially CNS-positive and -negative patients disappeared (Fig. 2).

Outcome After CNS Relapse

Table 6 gives an overview on treatment and outcome after CNS relapse. Survival after CNS relapse was short, at a median of

Table 2. Initial data of patients with or without initial CNS involvement: studies AML-BFM-78 and -83

	Without CNS involvement (%)	CNS involvement (%)	p-value X² test
Boys	52	61	
Extramedullary organ involvement	24	41	
Liver > 5 cm bcm	16	26	
Spleen >5 cm bcm	14	9	
WBC ≥100 000/mm³	19	39	0.04
FAB M1	22	26	
FAB M2	23	4	
FAB M3	3	0	
FAB M4	23	61	0.0001
FAB M5	25	9	
FAB M6	3	0	
No. of patients	294	23	

In 16 children initial CNS involvement was doubtful or no data were submitted
bcm, below costal margin

492

Table 3. Treatment results in children with or without CNS involvement (Studies AML-BFM-78 and -83)

	No CNS involvement	CNS involvement
No. of patients treated	294	23
Early deaths prior to therapy	7	1
Patients treated	287	22
Deaths during induction therapy	24	2
Nonresponders	28	3
CR achieved	235 (82%)	17 (77%)
Death in CCR	8	1
Relapses	91	10
In CCR	123	6

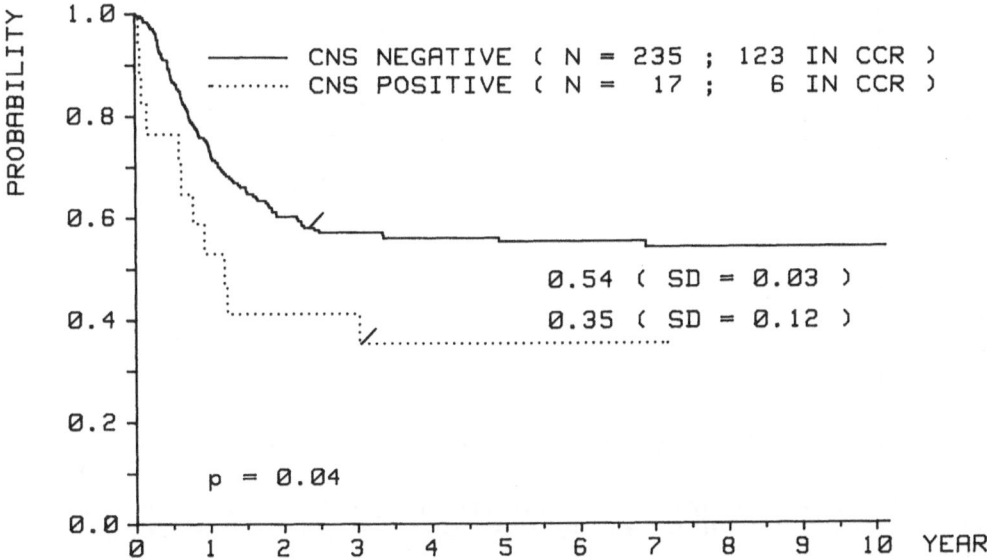

Fig. 1. Probability of event-free interval (EFI) duration in patients with or without initial CNS involvement. Studies AML-BFM-78 and -83. /, last patient entering the group

Table 4. Isolated and combined CNS relapses in children with initial CNS involvement (Studies AML-BFM-78 and -83)

Initial	n	Relapse without CNS involvement	Relapse in CNS		Percentage of CNS relapses
			Isolated	Combined	
CNS positive	23	6	2	2	40% (10)
					p ≤0.03
CNS negative	287	81	3	7	11% (91)

Out of 16 patients with unknown initial CNS status two relapsed with CNS leukemia

Table 5. Isolated and combined CNS relapses according to FAB types in studies AML-BFM-78 and -83

	Isolated CNS relapse	Combined CNS relapse	CNS relapse Total
FAB M1	1	4	5
FAB M2	–	–	–
FAB M4	1	3	4
FAB M5	3	4	7
Other	–	–	–
No. of patients	5	11	16

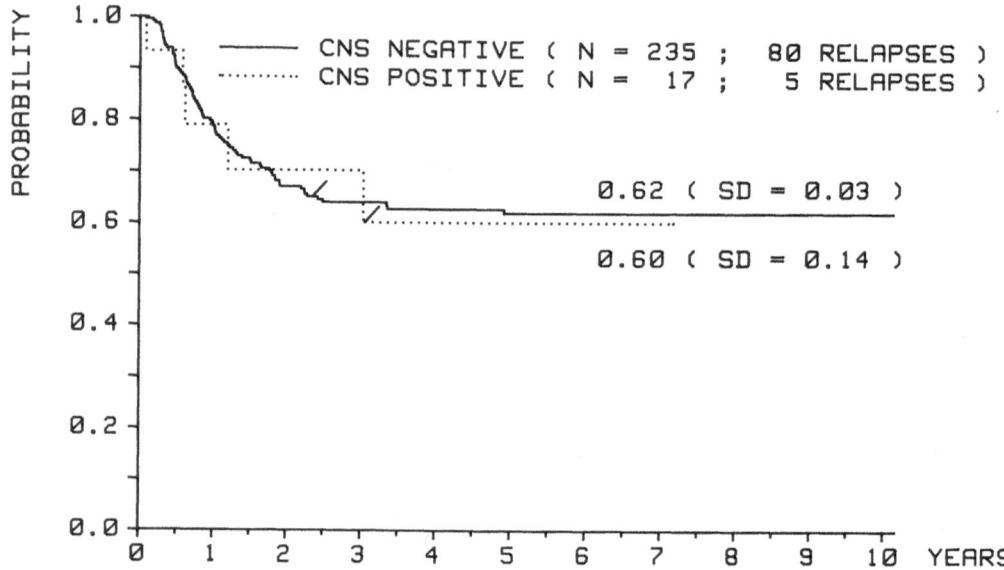

Fig. 2. Probability of relapse-free interval (RFI) duration in patients with or without initial CNS involvement. Studies AML-BFM-78 and -83. CNS relapses censored. /, last patient entering the group

6.1 months; only one child, who was treated with implantation of radiogold after isolated CNS relapse, has remained in second remission for 7 years.

AML-BFM-87 Study

Due to the low number of CNS relapses in initially CNS-negative patients of study BFM-87, CNS irradiation which had been randomized during the first 2.5 years was abandoned. CNS prophylaxis consisted of ARA-C i.th. and highdose ARA-C, which is known to undergo slower elimination in the CSF than in the periphery. Currently, after a follow-up of 4–48 months, four combined CNS relapses have occurred. Two of these children were among the group of 40 initially CNS-negative patients who received CNS irradiation, and two belonged to the nonirradiated group ($n = 73$). So far, none of the children with initial CNS involvement and irradiation after CR ($n = 13$) have relapsed in the CNS. Three of the four CNS relapses occurred in children with FAB type M5.

Table 6. Outcome after CNS relapse

	Pat. No.	Therapy	Outcome
Isolated CNS relapse	1	OP	Early death, cerebral bleeding
tumorous	2	OP + RT 45 Gy	CNS relapse, 5 months
In the CSF	3	MTX i.th.	PR, progress 5 months
	4	RT spinal 29 Gy	Hematologic relapse, 6 months
	5	Implantation of radiogold	In CCR, 7 years
Combined CNS relapse	6	Palliative	Early death, infection
	7	Palliative	Early death, infection
	8	Palliative	PR, progress, 1.5 months
	9	Palliative	PR, progress, 2.5 months
	10	Palliative with RT	Relapse, 12 months
	11	BFM-78 protocol	PR, progress 14 months
	12	BFM-83 protocol	Relapse, 5 months
	13	RT 24 Gy + BFM-83	Relapse, 2 years
	14	Autologous BMT in PR	Relapse, 1 year
	15	Autologous BMT	Relapse, 3 months
	16	Allogenic BMT	Death in CCR after 2 years

BMT, bone marrow transplantation; OP, operation; RT, radiotherapy

Discussion

The incidence of CNS leukemia at the time of diagnosis is higher in AML than in ALL. Five pediatric studies [4] cite an incidence of 5%–14%; we found 7%–12% in our trials. On the other hand, CNS leukemia in relapse was less often seen. This may be a reflection of the shorter disease-free survival time of children with AML, since the occurrence of CNS leukemia was higher in studies with better long-term results [1]. On the other hand the value of CNS "prophylaxis" in AML is not clear. Dahl et al. [5] reported that 24 Gy craniospinal irradiation significantly reduced the incidence of late CNS leukemia, but there was no advantage in duration of remission. In the CCG-251 protocol [6] with prophylactic treatment of radiotherapy and MTX i.th. the CNS relapse rate was low; only 6 of 399 patients (2%) achieving remission had subsequent isolated CNS relapses. Four of them occurred in patients prior to bone marrow transplantation, who did not receive cranial irradiation. Thus, it seems that some form of prophylaxis is necessary.

Our rate of CNS relapses (6% isolated and combined) in studies BFM-78 and -83 was also low. In these studies, CNS "pro-phylaxis" consisted of intrathecal doses of MTX (BFM-78) and ARA-C (BFM-83) as well as radiotherapy. In order to avoid long-term sequelae of CNS irradiation one question of the ongoing trial BFM-87 is, whether a different form of CNS treatment with i.th. and high-dose ARA-C might be sufficient in preventing CNS relapses. Longer follow-up and larger patient numbers will be needed to prove the assumption.

The finding of an increased risk of CNS relapse, especially in children with FAB M5, was noted in other pediatric studies [1, 7, 8] as well as in our own. Therefore, a more aggressive CNS treatment with cranial irradiation may be of benefit not only for the group of initially CNS-positive patients but also for those with a monocytic component.

Participating Members of the AML-BFM Study Group: A. Gnekow (Augsburg); G. F. Wündisch (Bayreuth), G. Henze (Berlin); U. Bode (Bonn); H.-J. Spaar, P. Lieber (Bremen); W. Andler, I. Meyer (Datteln); U. Göbel, H. Jürgens (Düsseldorf); W. Havers, B. Stollmann-Gibbels (Essen); J.-D. Beck (Erlangen); B. Kornhuber, V. Gerein (Frankfurt); M. Brandis, A. Sutor (Freiburg); F. Lampert (Gießen); G. Prindull, M. Lakomek (Göttingen); H. Kabisch (Hamburg); H. Riehm, P. Weinel, A. Reiter (Hannover); H. Ludwig (Heidelberg); N. Graf, M. Müller (Homburg/Saar); G. Nessler (Karlsruhe); H. Wehinger (Kassel); R. Schneppenheim (Kiel); F. Berthold (University of Cologne); W. Sternschulte (Cologne); J. Otte, P. Buscsky (Lübeck); P. Gutjahr (Mainz); O. Sauer (Mannheim); C. Eschenbach (Marburg); Ch. Bender-Götze (Munich Poliklinik); K.-D. Tympner, P. Klose (Munich Harlaching); R. Haas, P. Schmidt (Munich von Haunersches Children's Hospital); St. Müller-Weihrich (Munich-Schwabing); W. Schuster (Nurenberg, Cnopf'sche); U. Schwarzer (University of Nurenberg); J. Treuner (Stuttgart); D. Niethammer (Tübingen); G. Gaedicke (Ulm); T. Luthardt (Worms); J. Kühl (Würzburg).

References

1. Grier HE, Gelber RD, Camitta BM. Delorey MJ, Link MP, Price KN, Leavitt PR, Weinstein HJ (1987) Prognostic factors in childhood acute myelogenous leukemia. J Clin Oncol 5: 1026–1032
2. Bennett JM, Catovsky D, Daniel M-T, Flandrin G, Dalton DAG, Gralnick HR, Sultan C (1976) Proposals for the classification of the acute leukaemias. Br J Haematol 33: 451–458
3. Bennett JM, Catovsky D, Daniel M-T, Flandrin G, Dalton DAG, Gralnick HR, Sultan C (1985) Proposed revised criteria for the classification of acute myeloid leukemia: a report of the French-American-British Cooperative Group. Ann Intern Med 103: 626–629
4. Lampkin BC, Woods W, Strauss R, Feig St, Higgins G. Bernstein I, D'Angio G, Chard R, Bleyer A, Hammond D (1983) Current status of the biology and treatment of acute non-lymphocytic leukemia in children (Report from the ANLL Strategy Group of the Children's Cancer Study Group). Blood 61: 215–228
5. Dahl GV, Simone JV, Hustu HO, Mason C (1978) Preventive central nervous system irradiation in children with acute nonlymphocytic leukemia. Cancer 42: 2187–2198
6. Buckley, JD, Chard RL, Baehner RL, Nesbit ME. Lampkin BC, Woods WG, Hammond GD (1989) Improvement in outcome for children with acute nonlymphocytic leukemia. A report from the children's cancer study group. Cancer 63: 1457–1465
7. Pui CH, Dahl GV, Kalwinsky DK, Look AT, Mirro J, Dodge RK, Simone JV (1985) Central nervous system leukemia in children with acute nonlymphoblastic leukemia. Blood 66: 1062–1067
8. Chessels JM, O'Callaghan U, Hardisty RM (1986) Acute myeloid leukaemia in childhood: clinical features and prognosis. Br J Haematol 63: 555–564

Modified REZ BFM 87 Protocol in Relapsed Childhood ALL: A Preliminary Report

T. Urasinski, J. Peregud-Pogorzelski, and A. Brodkiewicz

Introduction

As reported elsewhere, treatment results in childhood acute lymphoblastic leukemia (ALL) achieved in our institution are still unsatisfactory (T. Urasinski and J. Pogorazelski, unpublished data). After the median follow-up time of 33 months the probability of event-free survival (p-EFS) is 0.429 and relapses are the main reason for treatment failures. Thus the problem of relapsed ALL is of vital importance for us.

The outcome for children with relapsed ALL has remained very poor [1, 2]. Bone marrow transplantation can be a curative procedure for selected patients only and in some cases is connected with long-term effects [3]. It has been proven during the last decade that intensive chemotherapy, containing non-cross-reacting agents, can offer the chance of prolonged second remission and it seems that the best results have been achieved by the BFM Group [4, 5].

This report summarizes our preliminary experiences with the use of the modified REZ BFM 87 protocol. The original protocol was kindly provided by Prof. G. Henze [6].

Patients and Method

The study comprised 12 children with ALL, who relapsed between December 1987 and

First Pediatric Department, Pomeranian Medical Academy, ul. Unii Lubelskiej 1, 71-344 Szczecin, Poland

October 1989. These were eight boys and four girls aged 50–113 months (median 75 months). All children had been previously treated using the BFM 79 protocol, modified by the Polish Leukemia Study Group. All patients suffered from late relapses (as defined by the BFM Study), after remission lasting from 9 to 38 months (median, 29 months). Nine of the children were still on treatment, while three relapsed after treatment cessation. There were ten isolated (five bone marrow, four CNS and one testicular) and two combined (bone marrow plus testicular) relapses.

All patients were treated using the modified REZ BFM 87 protocol. The protocol's modification comprised a twofold dose reduction of MTX. Details of the treatment are given in Fig. 1). Treatment results were evaluated using the Kaplan-Meyer method. The minimum follow-up time was 12 months.

Results

Two patients did not achieve remission and died 1 and 2 months from diagnosis. One patient died in remission from massive gastrointestinal bleeding. Five patients relapsed after remission lasting 2–21 months. Only four patients remain in second remission 11, 11, 24, and 25 months respectively. Among those who relapsed there were four isolated recurrences in bone marrow and one combined bone marrow and testicular relapse. The probability of event-free survival (p-EFS) was 0.250 and the probability of survival (p-S) was 0.333.

497

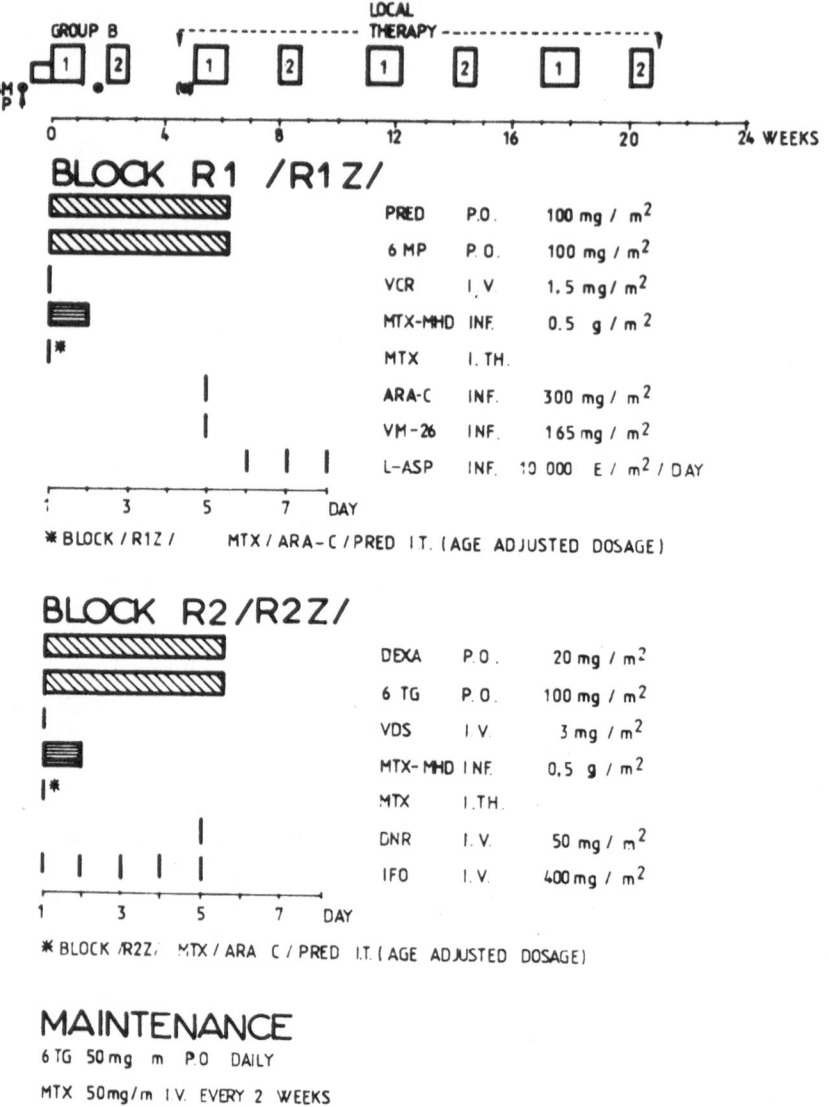

Fig. 1. BFM REZ 87 modified protocol

Treatment results are given in Figs. 2 and 3.

Discussion

Different mechanisms responsible for relapses of acute lymphoblastic leukemia and implications for their treatment were discussed by Henze et al. [5]. These include the necessity of local plus systemic therapy, high-dose rapid altering therapy with new drugs incorporated and prolonged intensive therapy. Protocols designed in this fashion are more successful but are also more myelotoxic and severe infections due to granulocytopenia are the major cause of death in leukemic patients [5, 7]. Having no experience in such aggressive chemotherapy and taking into consideration the fact

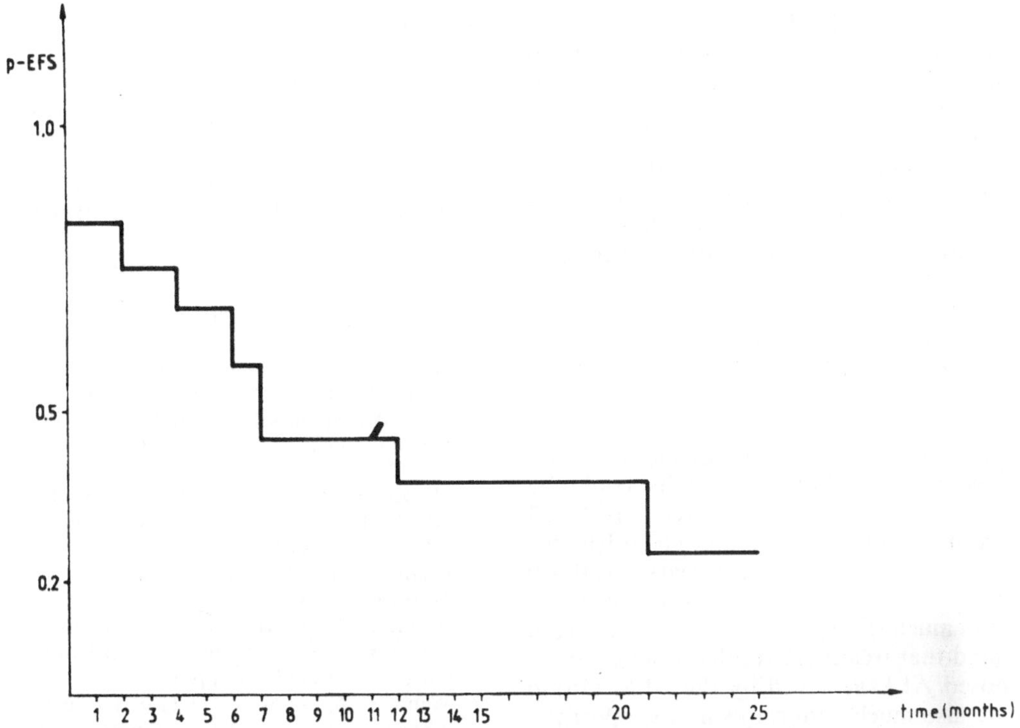

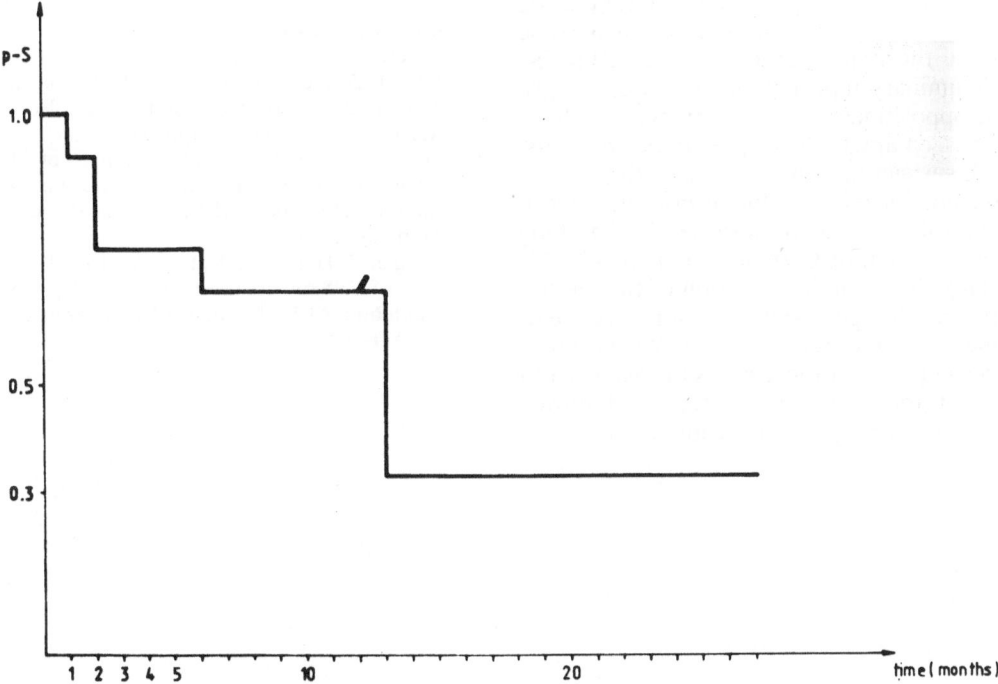

Fig. 2. *p*-EFS for patients treated with the modified BFM REZ 87 protocol (*n*=12)

Fig. 3. *p*-S for patients treated with the modified BFM 87 protocol (*n*=12)

that infections in children with acute lymphoblastic leukemia are still difficult to manage in our institution, we decided to modify the REZ BFM 87 protocol by reducing the dose of intravenous methotrexate, but maintaining the schedule and dosage of other agents. The group studied comprised patients with late relapses only, occurring later than 6 months after the end of initial treatment. Our awareness of side effects of methotrexate was supported by data from the literature; methotrexate at higher dosage is known to cause bone marrow depression and its associated consequences [8].

Because of the dosage of methotrexate used in this study our results could be compared to those of the REZ BFM 83 protocol for late relapses [5]. The p-EFS for patients followed-up for 3 years was 0.640 compared to 0.250 achieved in our group with much shorter observation. Keeping in mind that treatment results of newly diagnosed ALL achieved by the BFM Group are also much better, this may support the opinion of Rivera et al. that among children who do not have access to large treatment centers and who are treated in suboptimal conditions the proportion of failures may be higher [9]. Our results are also much worse than those presented in REZ BFM 85 preliminary reports [10, 11]. Interestingly, in opposition to this observation we have not seen any CNS relapses in our patients. We suspect that the dose of methotrexate, 0.5 g/m^2 in 24 h infusion, is not sufficient to control bone marrow disease, thus masking the problem of CNS involvement. We also think that twofold reduction of the methotrexate dosage resulted in our poor treatment results of relapsed ALL. We have thus decided that in these cases the REZ BFM 87 protocol should be properly followed with strict prophylaxis of infections.

References

1. Chessells JM, Breatnach F (1981) Late marrow recurrences in childhood acute lymphoblastic leukaemia. Br Med J 238: 749–751
2. Chessells JM, Cornbleet M (1979) Combination chemotherapy for bone marrow relapse in childhood lymphoblastic leukaemia (ALL). Med Pediatr Oncol 6: 359–365
3. Niethammer D, Dopfer R, Klingebiel T et al. (1989) Actual role and perspectives of BMT in children. Bone Marrow Tranplantat 4: 7–11
4. Rivera GK, Buchanan G, Bovett JM et al. (1986) Intensive retreatment of childhood acute lymphoblastic leukemia in first bone marrow relapse. N Engl J Med 315: 273–278
5. Henze G, Buchmann S, Fengler R et al. (1987) The BFM relapse studies in childhood ALL: concepts of two multicenter trials and results after 2 1/2 years. Haematol Blood Transfus 30: 147–155
6. Henze G (1986) Studie zur Behandlung von Kindern mit Rezidiv einer akuten lymphoblastischen Leukämie. pp 5–15
7. Wendt F, Maschmeyer G (1987) Infection prevention and immediate antibiotic therapy in the neutropenic patient. Haematol Blood Transfus 30: 175–181
8. Bleyer WA (1978) The clinical pharmacology of methotrexate. New applications of an old drug. Cancer 41: 36–51
9. Rivera GK, Santana V, Mahmoud H et al. (1989) Acute lymphoblastic leukemia in childhood: the problem of relapses. Bone Marrow Transplant 4 [Suppl 1]: 80–85
10. Henze G, Fengler R, Hartmann R et al. (1990) BFM Group treatment results in relapsed childhood ALL. Haematol Blood Transfus 33: 619–626
11. Fengler R, Hartmann R, Bode U et al. (1990) Risk of CNS relapse after systemic relapse of childhood ALL. Haematol Blood Transfus 33: 511–515

Platelet Transfusion in Patients with Bone Marrow Aplasia

V. Weisbach, J. Zingsem, T. Zeiler, H. G. Heuft, H. Baurmann and R. Eckstein

Introduction

Thrombocytopenia and the necessity of platelet transfusions for prevention of hemorrhagic complications present major problems in the management of patients with bone marrow aplasia (e.g., during multiple chemotherapy or bone marrow transplantation). The avoidance of HLA immunization with possibly resulting platelet transfusion refractoriness is of particular importance. We report the results of our transfusion strategy in patients with bone marrow aplasia with special respect to this problem.

Materials and Methods

Our transfusion strategy for preventing HLA immunization consists of the exclusive transfusion of filtered/leukocyte-poor packed red cell concentrates, prophylactic transfusion of HLA-A,B-matched single donor platelet concentrates (PC) at a thrombocyte count of less than 20 000/µl and therapeutic platelet transfusions in disseminated intravascular coagulation or acute bleeding.

Single donor platelet concentrates (PC) were prepared by different cell separators (Haemonetics V50, Cobe Spectra, Fresenius AS 104 OR Fenwal CS 3000). We report

Blutbank, Abteilung Innere Medizin und Poliklinik m. S. Hämatologie und Onkologie, Universitätsklinikum Rudolf Virchow, Standort Charlottenburg, Freie Universität Berlin, Spandauer Damm 130, 1000 Berlin 19, FRG

data concerning 1016 platelet transfusions in 144 hematologic patients, receiving 1–37 HLA-A,B-Matched single donor PC. Posttransfusion response was analyzed calculating the corrected count increment (CCI) 1 and 16–24 h posttransfusion according to the following formula: CCI

$$= \frac{\text{Absolute increment} \times \text{body surface area}}{\text{Number of transfused platelets} \times 10^{11}}.$$

Crossmatching was done by the lymphocytotoxicity test (LCT).

Results

A positive LCT predicted a significantly ($p < 0.01$) lower platelet increment 1 h after transfusion (Table 1). Thirty-three out of 144 patients, i.e., 23% of the patients

Table 1. Predictive value of a positive crossmatch in LCT for success of platelet transfusions (CCI 1 and 16–24 h after transfusion)

	CCI after 1 h		CCI after 16–24 h	
	x̄	SD	x̄	SD
LCT Positive (n=51)	8100	9400	6100	9400
	p <0.01		n.s.	
Negative (n=487)	13300	14900	8200	10300

501

studied, developed HLA antibodies, only 14 of them becoming refractory to platelet transfusions (a patient is designated refractory when three consecutive transfusions resulted in a 1-h CCI <4500 in the absence of clinical factors impairing the increment (i.e., septicemia, DIC, surgery) [1, 2].

Discussion

The significantly reduced CCI 1 h after platelet transfusion associated with a positive crossmatch corroborates the well-known major role of lymphocytotoxic antibodies and of LCT in platelet transfusion practice. In our opinion the number of refractory patients according to the given definition is of as doubtful value as the definition itself. Only a small group of patients are without any clinical factor impairing platelet increment and very few patients will not develop clinical problems after several platelet transfusions followed by small increments. The incidence of HLA antibodies in our patients (23 %), exclusively supported with HLA-A,B-matched PC, seems to be low compared to HLA antibody incidences of 40 %–50 % in patients with acute leukemia receiving random pooled/random single donor PC, as reported in the literature [3–5]. We therefore feel encouraged to continue the development of our transfusion concept.

References

1. Gmur J, Felten A von, Osterwalder B, Honegger H, Hormann A, Sauter C, Deubelbeiss K, Berchtold W, Metaxas M, Scali G, Frick PG (1983) Delayed alloimmunization using random single donor platelet transfusions: a prospective study in thrombocytopenic patients with acute leukemia. Blood 62: 473–479
2. Tosato G, Applebaum FR, Deisseroth AB (1978) HLA-matched platelet transfusion therapy of severe aplastic anemia. Blood 52: 846–854
3. Messerschmidt GL, Makuch R, Appelbaum F, Ungerleider RS, Abrams R, O'Donnell J, Holohan TV, Fontana J, Wright D, Anagnon NP (1988) A prospective randomized trial of HLA-matched versus mismatched single-donor platelet transfusions in cancer patients. Cancer 62: 795–801
4. Pamphilon DH, Farrell DH, Donaldson C, Raymond PA, Brady CA, Bradley BA, (1989) Development of lymphocytotoxic and platelet reactive antibodies: prospective study in patients with acute leukemia. Vox Sang 57: 177–181
5. Howard JE, Perkins HA (1978) The natural history of alloimmunization to platelets. Transfusion 18: 496–503

Renal Failure in Acute Leukemia: Incidence, Cause and Clinical Outcome

R. Munker[1,2], U. Mann[1], U. Jehn[1], R. Baumgart[1], and H. J. Kolb[1,2]

Introduction

Renal failure is one possible complication of acute leukemia [1, 4], especially in children with acute lymphoblastic leukemia [9]. In adults, no exact data with regard to its incidence, pathogenesis and clinical implications exist; therefore we studied these parameters in an unselected group of patients who were treated by chemotherapy or bone marrow transplantation.

Material and Methods

We reviewed the records of 220 consecutive patients who were treated at our center between January 1985 and August 1989 with either chemotherapy (166 patients) or bone marrow transplantation (54 patients). Cast follow-up was July 1990. Diagnosis of acute leukemia was established with standard methods. Refractory leukemia was diagnosed when 2 months of standard chemotherapy failed to induce remission. Three categories of renal impairment in acute leukemia were distinguished:
1. Acute renal failure requiring hemodialysis (ARF)
2. Moderate renal impairment (serum creatinine ≥ 2 mg/dl)
3. Minor renal impairment (serum creatinine $\geq 1.4 < 2$ mg/dl)

[1] Medizinische Klinik III, Universitätsklinikum Großhadern, 8000 Munich 70, FRG
[2] GSF Institut für Klinische Hämatologie, Marchioninistr. 15, 8000 Munich 70, FRG

Renal failure occurring as part of multi-organ failure within 7 days before death was excluded from analysis. For statistical comparison the groups were analyzed by the t test, and survival was calculated by Kaplan-Meier analysis.

Results

Patients Treated with Chemotherapy

At diagnosis, 2/166 patients presented with ARF, 6/166 patients with a moderate and 29/166 patients with a minor impairment of renal function. During the later course of disease ARF occurred in seven patients and moderate and minor complications in seven patients and moderate and minor complications in 10 and 16/166 patients. In summary, 22.3 % of the patients had an impaired renal function at diagnosis and 19.9 % during the later course of disease. Combining these data, at least 67 complications occurred in 57 patiens (34.3 %). Statistically, only few correlations were found with the type of leukemia (see Table 1). Several risk factors for renal complications were identified: Patients with a history of kidney disease (chronic pyelonephritis, nephrolithiasis, hydronephrosis, etc.) more often had renal complications at diagnosis (50 % vs. 18 %, $p < 1$ %) and during the later course (45 % vs. 16 %, $p < 1$ %). Patients with refractory leukemia more often had renal complications at diagnosis compared to patients who reached complete remission (37 % vs. 16 %, $p < 1$ %). Further risk factors for complications at diagnosis were (see Table

Table 1. Incidence of renal complications in acute leukemia

Type/Subtype	At diagnosis		During treatment/ beyond
AML	$n=126$	21.4%	19.8%
Smoldering	$n=14$	0 %[a]	21.4%
FAB-M1	$n=8$	12.5%	0 %
FAB-M2	$n=20$	25 %	25 %
FAB-M3	$n=18$	38.9%	27.8%
FAB-M4	$n=38$	18.4%	18.4%
FAB-M5	$n=24$	29.2%	20.8%
FABM6/7	$n=4$	0 %	0 %
ALL/AUL	$n=40$	25 %	20.0%
c-ALL	$n=20$	15.0%	20.0%
T-ALL	$n=11$	18.2%	27.3%
B-ALL	$n=5$	40 %	20 %
AUL	$n=4$	75 %[a]	0 %

No significant difference between types of leukemia
[a] Borderline decreased/increased incidence ($p < 5\%$)

Table 2. Risk factors for renal complications in acute leukemia

Impaired renal function	At diagnosis		Later	
	Yes	No	Yes	No
Mean WBC (g/l)	119	35***	49	58[a]
Mean age (years)	59.7	50.2*	56.0	51.5[a]
Male sex (%)	81	43**	64	49[a]

Significant differences: $+++\ p < 0.01\%$, $++\ p < 0.1\%$, $*\ p < 1\%$
[a] No significant differences

2): initial WBC, age, male sex. Complications at diagnosis predisposed the patients for later complications (data not shown). Among the causes of renal impairment at diagnosis paraneoplastic mechanisms ranged first (leukostasis or renal infiltration, tubular damage by myoglobin, urates or lysozyme). During the later course septicemias or antibiotic/antimycotic treatment were major causes. No tumor lysis syndrome or direct renal toxicity of cytostatic drugs was observed. During the terminal phase renal failure was part of multiorgan failure in 44/135 patients (33%). At autopsy renal infiltration was recognized in

5/14 patients (36%). When patients with renal complications (any degree) are compared at diagnosis with patients without renal failure, no significant difference of survival was found (see Fig. 1). It should be noted, however, that both patients with ARF at diagnosis died within 1 month. During the later course of disease with more severe and fewer minor complications the presence of renal impairment predicted shortened survival (see Fig. 2). Among the 166 patients reviewed, 3 had a coincident urothelic cancer and one an advanced prostatic cancer.

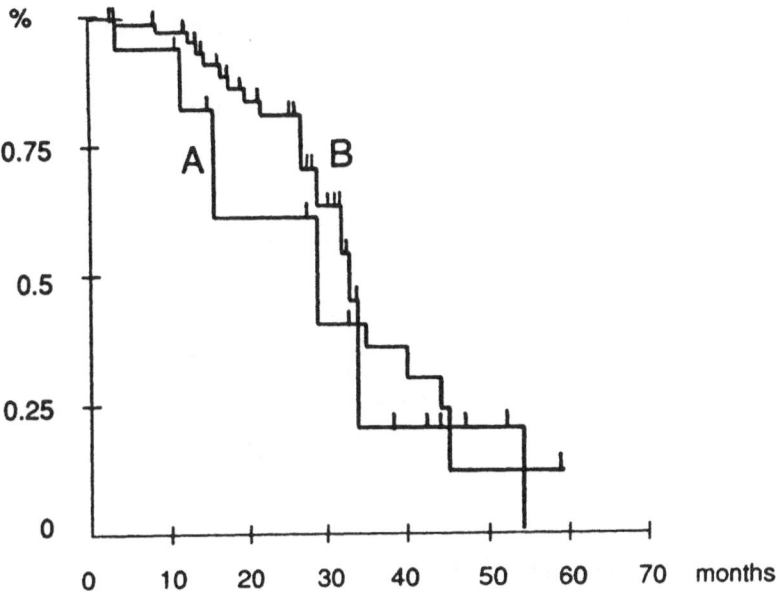

Fig. 1. Survival of patients with renal complications (any degree) at diagnosis (*A*) compared to patients with no complications (*B*)

complications (B)

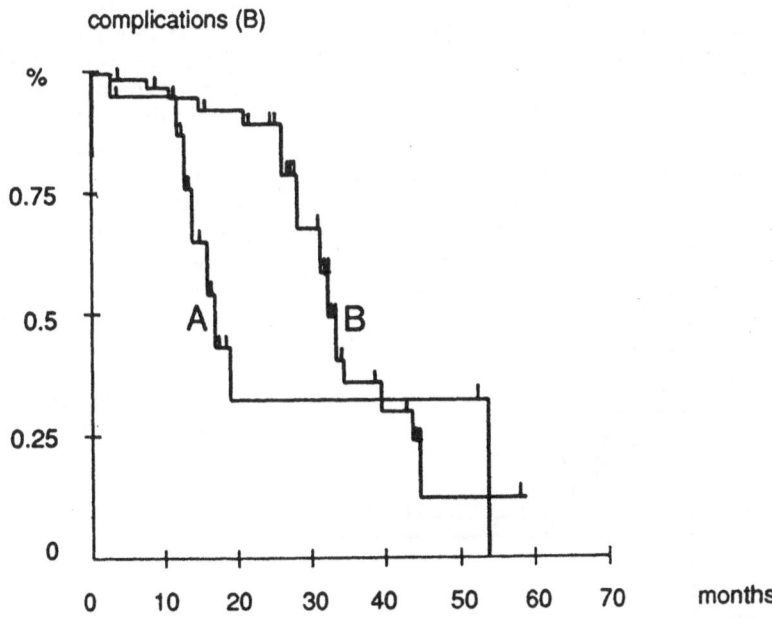

Fig. 2. Survival of patients with renal complications (any degree) during later course of disease (*A*) compared to patients with no complications (*B*)

Patients Treated with Bone Marrow Transplantation

Among the 54 patients studied, 1 had a moderate and 5 a minor impairment of renal function before transplantation. During conditioning until day 100 after transplantation, four patients had ARF, 6 a major and 13 a minor complication (total incidence, 42.6%). The only risk factor

Table 3. Risk factors for renal complications during initial period after bone marrow transplantation

Parameter		Incidence of complications	
Allogenic	$n=44$	50%	
Autologous	$n=10$	10%	p <5%
Stable remission	$n=38$	50%	
Refractory	$n=16$	25%	n.s.
ALL/AUL	$n=14$	50%	
AML	$n=40$	40%	n.s.
Renal history	$n=\ 9$	22%	
No history	$n=45$	47%	n.s.

predicting renal complications was an allogenic compared to an autologous transplant, whereas no correlations existed for age, sex, ALL/AUL vs. AML, refractory leukemia vs. stable remission, and renal history vs. no history (see Table 3). Of the causes of renal complications until day 100, infections and treatment with antimycotics or antibiotics and cyclosporininduced toxicities figure first with about 30% each. Two patients had a severe hemolytic uremic syndrome. The survival of patients suffering from renal complications until day 100 after bone marrow transplantation was not different from patients without renal complications (see Kaplan-Meier plot in Fig. 3). Again the prognosis of patients who developed ARF was poor: the four patients observed died within 0 and 2 months. Beyond day 100 after bone marrow transplantation, 8 out of 45 patients had renal complications (17.8%). If early and late complications are combined, 30 out of 56 patients had 46 episodes of impaired renal function.

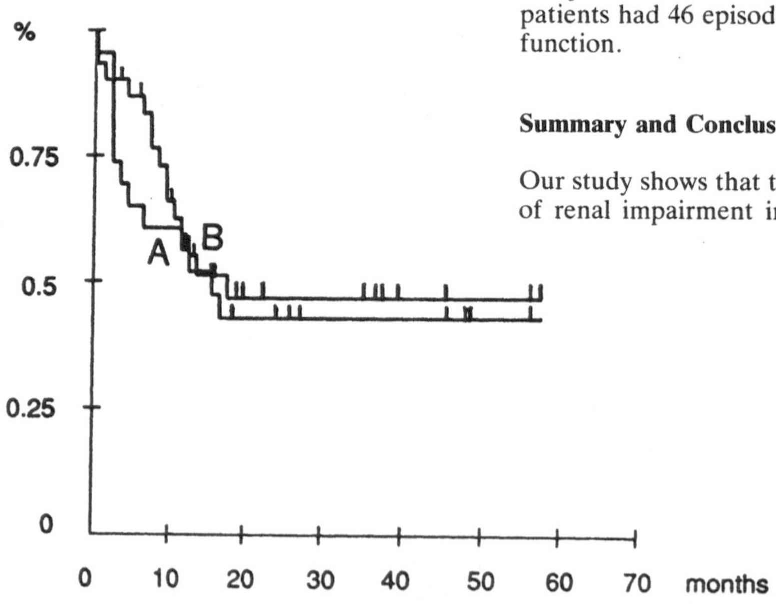

Summary and Conclusions

Our study shows that the overall incidence of renal impairment in acute leukemia is

Fig. 3. Survival of patients with renal complications (any degree) during initial phase after BMT (*A*) compared to patients with no complications (*B*)

more common than previously recognized: about 20%–30% of patients have some degree of renal impairment. Late but not early complications predict survival. Risk factors for early complications are leukocyte counts, a history of kidney disease, refractory leukemia, age and male sex. Some [3, 8] but not all [5, 6] earlier studies characterized renal impairment as an adverse prognostic factor. The majority of early complications are related to a preexisting impairment of renal function or are paraneoplastic. Since the prognosis of untreated leukemia is very poor, the cytostatic treatment should not be delayed in the context of decreased renal function. Among all groups of patients, acute renal failure has a short survival; therefore the prevention of renal complications is most important. After bone marrow transplantation, renal impairment occurs in more than 40% of the patients investigated, particularly in allogeneic transplants. Earlier studies mentioned the importance of cyclosporin toxicity and microangiopathy after bone marrow transplantation [2, 7]. However, when cases of acute renal failure are excepted and if toxicities are carefully monitored, a decrease of renal function has no impact on survival.

Acknowledgement. The statistical support of S. Maag is acknowledged.

References

1. Ardaillou R, Slama R (1961) Les complications rénales des hémopathies malignes. pathol Biol 9: 1049–1060
2. Holler E, Kolb JH et al. (1989) Microangiopathy in patients on cyclosporin prophylaxis who developed acute graft-versus-host disease after HLA-identical bone marrow transplantation. Blood 73: 2018–2024
3. Keating MJ, Smith TL et al. (1982) A prognostic factor analysis for use in development of predictive models for response in adult acute leukemias. Cancer 50: 457–465
4. Merrill D, Jackson H (1943) The renal complications of leukemia. N Engl J Med 228: 271–276
5. Passe S, Miké V et al. (1982) Acute nonlymphoblastic leukemia prognostic factors in adults with long-term follow-up. Cancer 50: 1462–1471
6. Schwartz RS, Mackintosh FR et al. (1984) Multivariate analysis of factors associated with outcome of treatment for adults with acute myelogenous leukemia. Cancer 54: 1672–1681
7. Shulman H, Striker G et al. (1981) Nephrotoxicity of cyclosporin A after allogeneic bone marrow transplantation. N Engl M Med 305: 1392–1395
8. Smith TL, Gehan EA et al. (1982) Prediction of remission in adult acute leukemia development and testing of predictive models. Cancer 50: 466–472
9. Stapleton FB, Strother DR et al. (1988) Acute renal failure at onset of therapy for advanced stage Burkitt lymphoma and B cell acute lymphoblastic leukemia. Pediatrics 82: 863–869

Post Remission Therapy

Marrow Transplantation in Patients with Acute Myeloid Leukemia in First Remission, First Relapse or Second Remission*

R. A. Clift, C. D. Buckner, F. R. Appelbaum, and F. B. Petersen for the Seattle Marrow Transplant Team

Allogeneic marrow transplantation from HLA-identical siblings for patients with acute myeloid leukemia (AML) in first remission results in approximately 50% survival. Data reported by the Seattle team and the International Bone Marrow Transplant Registry indicate that most transplant regimens are associated with a 30% probability of transplant-related deaths, a 20% probability of relapse and 50% long-term survival [1, 2]. Most patients with AML in first remission have received unmodified allogeneic marrow after preparation with a regimen of cyclophosphamide (CY) plus total body irradiation (TBI). Many approaches have been investigated in an attempt to improve these results.

One approach has been to substitute BU for TBI. The Johns Hopkins marrow transplant team originally reported results with a regimen of BU 16 mg/kg followed by CY 200 mg/kg and recently reported a survival of 64% in 22 patients transplanted for AML in first remission [3]. Tutschka et al. [4] suggest that the BU/CY regimen is less toxic and just as effective if the CY dose is reduced to 120 mg/kg following BU 16 mg/kg. Other agents such as melphalan have been substituted for CY followed by

TBI without apparent benefit [5]. TBI followed by high-dose etoposide appears to be an effective combination in patients transplanted for AML [6].

Another approach has been to decrease transplant-related morbidity by reducing the incidence and severity of graft-versus-host disease (GVHD). T-cell depletion of donor marrow decreases the incidence and severity of acute GVHD, but has been associated with an increased rate of graft failure and relapse, resulting in no improvement in survival [7, 8]. Similarly, when cyclosporine (CSP) and methotrexate (MTX) were used in combination for prophylaxis of GVHD the incidence and severity of acute GVHD were markedly reduced but the probability of relapse doubled, negating any benefit on survival [1, 9]. The observation that elimination of GVHD led to an increased incidence of relapse has centered attention on the need for more effective preparative regimens. For patients with AML in first remission receiving MTX plus CSP, the increase in relapse rate associated with improved GVHD control was prevented by increasing the dose of TBI from 12.0 Gy to 15.75 Gy [9]. However, a consequence of the higher TBI dose was an increase in transplant-related deaths.

Many patients with AML have been transplanted in first relapse. Previous analyses have indicated that for patients not transplanted while in first remission this is the optimal time for transplant [1, 10]. It is important that studies of transplantation for patients in first relapse exclude patients who have received therapy aimed at achieving another remission because such therapy

* This work was supported by PHS grant numbers CA 15704, CA 18029, CA 18221, and CA 09515 awarded by the National Cancer Institute, DHHS.

The Fred Hutchinson Cancer Research Center, Veterans Administration Medical Center and the University of Washington School of Medicine, Seattle, USA

will remove from consideration those patients who achieve second remission and thereby increase the proportion of patients with resistant disease.

This report will consider recent Seattle experience in transplanting patients with AML in first remission, untreated first relapse or second remission.

Transplants in First Remission

Between April 1985 and September 1988, 71 consecutive patients with AML in first remission were registered in a protocol for allogeneic marrow transplantation from HLA-identical siblings. All patients received CY 60 mg/kg intravenously on each of two successive days followed by TBI from opposing ^{60}Co sources at a dose rate of 6–7 Cgy/min. Thirty-four patients were randomized to receive 12.0 Gy TBI in 2.0-Gy daily fractions for 6 days, and 37 patients were randomized to receive 15.75 Gy TBI administered as 2.25-Gy fractions daily for 7 days. All patients received GVHD prophylaxis with a combination of MTX and CSP.

The probabilities of relapse, nonrelapse mortality, and relapse – free survival for both groups of patients are presented in Figs. 1–3. The probability of developing moderate to severe acute GVHD was 0.21 for the 12.0 Gy group and 0.48 for the 15.75 Gy group ($p=0.02$). Patients in the 15.75

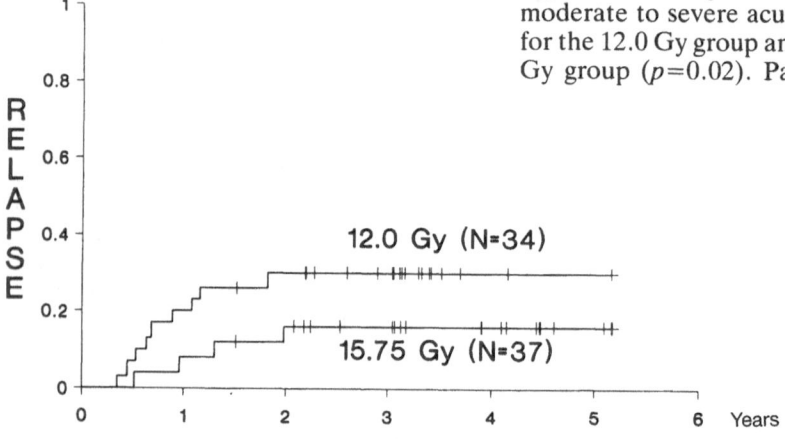

Fig. 1. The probability of relapse for patients randomized to receive 12.0 Gy fractionated TBI versus 15.75 Gy fractionated TBI ($p=.06$). Patients with AML transplanted in first remission

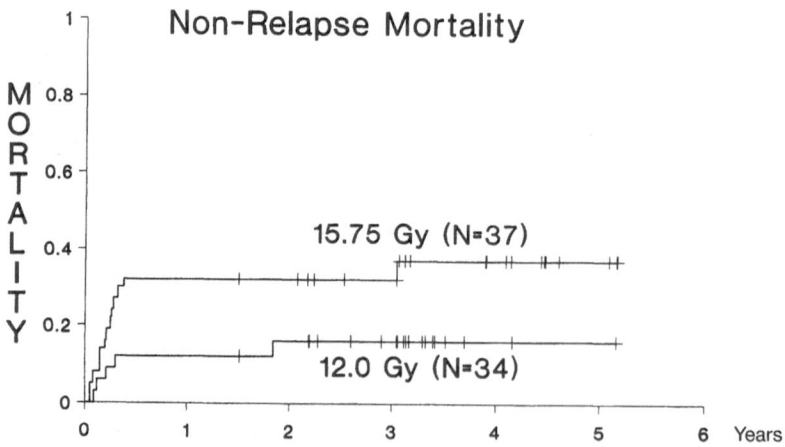

Fig. 2. Patients with AML transplanted in first remission. The probability of posttransplant death from causes other than relapse in patients randomized to receive 12.0 Gy fractionated TBI versus 15.75 Gy fractionated TBI ($p=.04$)

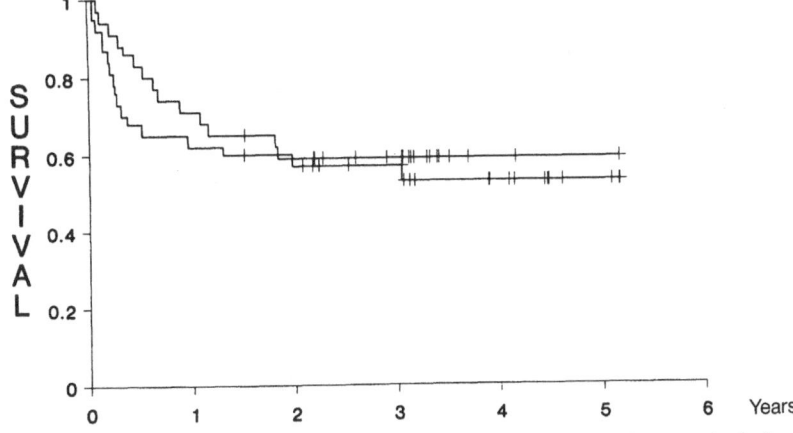

Fig. 3. Patients with AML transplanted in first remission. The probability of relapse-free survival after transplantation for patients randomized to receive 12.0 Gy fractionated TBI versus 15.75 Gy fractionated TBI

Gy group received less of the prescribed MTX and CSP than patients in the 12.0 Gy group, presumably as a consequence of toxicity from the irradiation schedule. It is possible that the increase in risk of developing serious acute GVHD in the 15.75 Gy group resulted from this reduced prophylaxis. Alternatively, increased tissue damage from the higher dose of TBI may have predisposed to GVHD or enhanced the clinical manifestations of acute GVHD.

Seventeen patients in the 12.0 Gy group and 12 in the 15.75 Gy group received 100 % of the prescribed MTX and more than 80 % of the prescribed CSP during the first 28 days posttransplant. Only one of these patients developed significant acute GVHD (grade 2) but clinical extensive chronic GVHD occurred in eight (six in the 12.0 Gy group and two in the 15.75 Gy group). Among these 29 patients there were 6 relapses and 5 deaths (all in relapsed patients) in the 17 patients of the 12.0 Gy group, and no relapses or deaths in the 12 patients who received 15.75 Gy. This pattern suggests that the additional 3.75 Gy of TBI had a significant antileukemic effect independent of the development of GVHD. However, the decrease in relapse rate following 15.75 Gy TBI was offset by an increase in transplant-related deaths, which were almost all associated with acute

GVHD. There was neither transplant-related mortality nor acute GVHD in the patients who received GVHD prophylaxis as prescribed. Thus the increased mortality associated with increased exposure to TBI was in part a consequence of increased acute GVHD in patients whose GVHD prophylaxis was inhibited by TBI-induced tissue damage.

Transplants in Untreated First Relapse

From 1975 through 1988, 98 patients received marrow transplants from HLA identical siblings while in untreated first relapse using a variety of regimens. Three regimens involved enough patients to permit useful comparison of outcome. In all three regimens CY 60 mg/kg was given on each of two successive days before TBI. Nineteen patients received 12.0 Gy TBI given as six daily fractions, followed by a combination of MTX and CSP. Twenty-two patients received 15.75 Gy TBI given in 2.25-Gy daily fractions followed by MTX and CSP. Twenty-nine patients received 15.75 Gy TBI but the GVHD prophylaxis was with MTX only. The probabilities of relapse, transplant-related mortality and survival are shown in Figs. 4–6. Patients who received 15.75 Gy TBI followed by

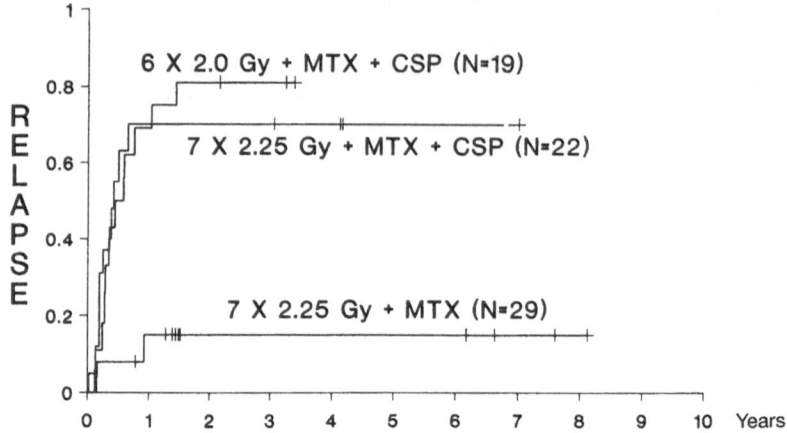

Fig. 4. The probability of posttransplant relapse in patients with AML transplanted in untreated first relapse

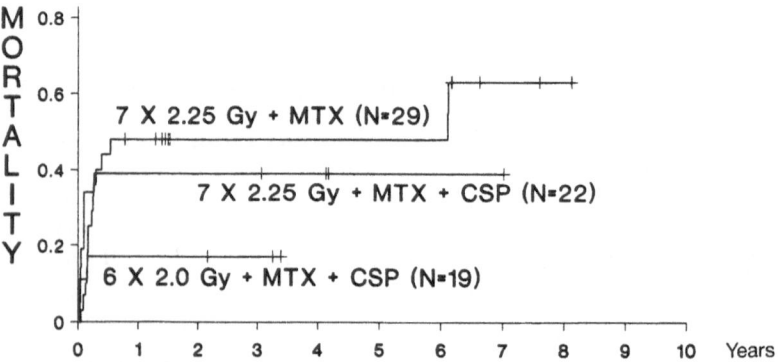

Fig. 5. The probability of posttransplant death from causes other than relapse in patients with AML transplanted in untreated first relapse

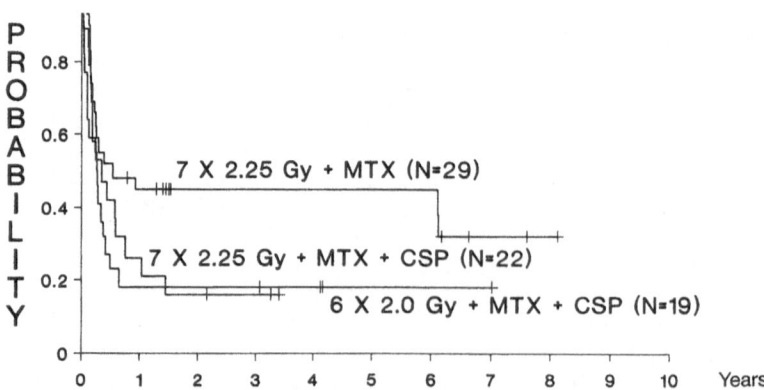

Fig. 6. The probability of relapse-free survival after transplantation for AML in untreated first relapse

514

MTX without CSP had a transplant-related mortality of 40 % during the first 100 days posttransplant, but this regimen was associated with the best disease-free survival due to a relatively low probability of relapse.

Transplants in Second Remission

Between April 1985 and July 1990, 13 patients with AML in second remission have been transplanted using a variety of regimens and unmodified marrow. Figure 7 depicts the probabilities of survival and relapse for these patients.

Influence of Phase

Figure 8 presents the relapse-free survival of patients transplanted in the three phases considered here. It is clear that there is no advantage to transplantation in second remission rather than first relapse. Only a minority of relapsed patients will achieve second remissions sufficiently durable to enter the transplantation procedure in good clinical condition and very few will achieve prolonged disease-free survival without transplantation. The posttransplant survival probability for second remission patients is disappointingly small and the relapse probability is high. However, Fig. 4 shows that patients transplanted in untreated first relapse using certain regimens do no better and the effect of regimen on the results of transplantation in second remission has been inadequately explored.

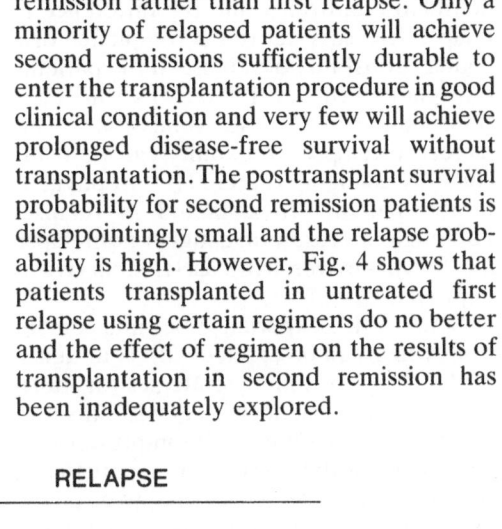

Fig. 7. The probabilities of posttransplant relapse and relapse-free survival for patients with AML transplanted in second remission transplanted between April 1985 and July 1990

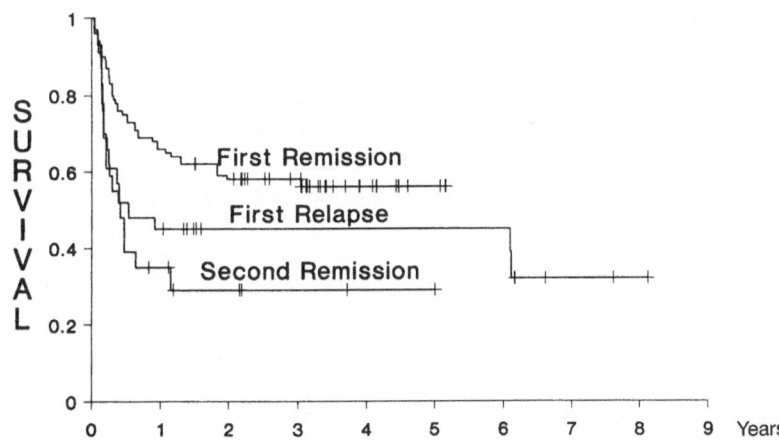

Fig. 8. The probability of relapse-free survival for patients with AML transplanted in first or second remission between April 1985 and July 1990 or in untreated first relapse using a regimen of CY + 15.75 Gy fractionated TBI + MTX

515

The disease-free survival after transplantation in first relapse is clearly worse than after transplantation in first remission. When the patients treated with the same regimen (15.75 Gy TBI + MTX + CSP) are compared, there is no difference in the nonrelapse mortality and the difference in relapse-free survival is a consequence of a higher probability of relapse in the patients transplanted in first relapse than in those transplanted in first remission. This increased relapse probability can be overcome by changing the GVHD prophylaxis in the patients transplanted in relapse. Although this results in a higher nonrelapse mortality, the overall disease-free survival is improved.

None of this experience permits conclusions which can be applied with confidence to the design of timing strategies for transplantation in patients with AML. This topic, of course, assumes more importance as cure by chemotherapy becomes more than a theoretical possibility. A strategy of delaying transplantation until patients relapse avoids the need to assess the prospects of primary cure. Figure 9 compares the results of transplantation in first remission with the projected results of delaying transplantation until first relapse. It uses the first remission duration statistics generated by the AML Coop Group Study (BMFT)[11] and the disease-free posttransplant survival

statistics for patients transplanted in first relapse in Seattle. The model demonstrates that there is very little difference in disease-free survival between the two options. However, the strategy of delay has never been tested in a clinical study, and there are many reasons why the practical outcome of a strategy of delay might be disappointing. The most important of these is the need to undertake transplantation soon after the discovery of relapse.

It is likely that the results of marrow transplantation of patients with AML are heavily influenced by the induction regimen used to procure and maintain remission. The optimal initial induction regimen may be different for patients with potential donors than for those who have no possibility of transplantation. The design of treatment for patients with suitable marrow donors should begin with the selection of this initial induction regimen.

The possibilities for studying strategies for the incorporation of transplantation into the treatment of patients with AML are limited mainly by the number of patients available for study. The full testing of design strategies which start at the time of diagnosis will probably require an international cooperative study. Cooperative studies even within one country contain so much experimental noise that it is difficult to believe that we shall soon see productive international studies addressing complex problems. However, it is clear that even a small improvement in relapse-free survival after initial induction will add great urgency

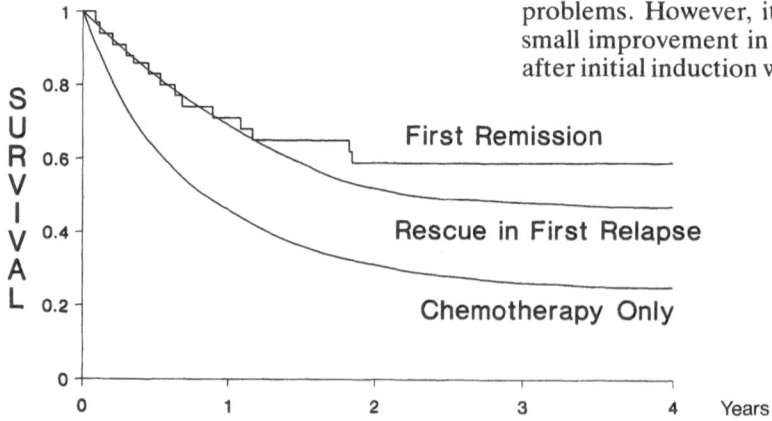

Fig. 9. The probability of relapse-free survival for patients with AML. The First Remission patients were transplanted between April 1985 and July 1990. The Chemotherapy Only curve was constructed from the statistics of the AML Coop Group Study (BMFT) [11], and the statistics for the Rescue in first Relapse curve was calculated from the Chemotherapy only curve with modification for the effects of rescue using a regimen of CY + 15.75 Gy TBI + MTX

to the need to determine the best timing for intervention by marrow transplantation.

References

1. Clift RA, Buckner CD, Thomas ED et al. (1987) The Treatment of acute non-lymphoblastic leukemia by allogeneic marrow transplantation. Bone Marrow Transplant 2: 243–258
2. Gale RP, Horowitz MM, Biggs JC et al. (1989) Transplant or chemotherapy in acute myelogenous leukaemia. Lancet i: 1119–1122
3. Geller RB, Saral R, Piantadosi S et al. (1989) Allogeneic bone marrow transplantation after high-dose busulfan and cyclophosphamide in patients with acute nonlymphocytic leukemia. Blood 73: 2209–2218
4. Tutschka PJ, Copelan EA, Klein JP (1987) Bone marrow transplantation for leukemia following a new busulfan and cyclophosphamide regimen. Blood 70: 1382–1388
5. Helenglass G, Powles RL, McElwain TJ et al. (1988) Melphalan and total body irradiation (TBI) versus cyclophosphamide and TBI as conditioning for allogeneic matched sibling bone marrow transplants for acute myeloblastic leukaemia in first remission. Bone Marrow Transplant 3: 21–29
6. Blume KG, Forman SJ, O'Donnell MR et al. (1987) Total body irradiation and high-dose etoposide: A new preparatory regimen for bone marrow transplantation in patients with advanced hematologic malignancies. Blood 69: 1015–1020
7. Maraninchi D, Gluckman E, Blaise D et al. (1987) Impact of T-cell depletion on outcome of allogeneic bone-marrow transplantation for standard-risk leukaemias. Lancet ii: 175–178
8. Champlin R, Ho W, Gajewski J et al. (1990) Selective depletion of CD8+ T lymphocytes for prevention of graft-versus-host disease after allogeneic bone marrow transplantation. Blood 76: 418–423
9. Clift RA, Buckner CD, Appelbaum FR et al. (1990) Allogeneic marrow transplantation in patients with acute myeloid leukemia in first remission. A randomized trial of two irradiation regimens. Blood 76: 1867–1871
10. Appelbaum FR, Clift RA, Buckner CD et al. (1983) Allogeneic marrow transplantation for acute nonlymphoblastic leukemia after first relapse. Blood 61: 949–953
11. Büchner T, Hiddeman W (1990) Treatment strategies in acute myeloid leukemia (AML). Blut 60: 61–67

Possible Effect of Autologous Blood Stem Cell Transplantation on Outcome of Acute Myeloid Leukemia in First Relapse

J. Reiffers, G. Marit, P. Cony-Makhoul, C. Faberes, P. Fernandez, and A. Broustet

Introduction

Despite recent progress in the treatment of acute myelogenous leukemia (AML), most patients who achieve complete remission (CR) relapse within 2 years following induction chemotherapy. In some of these latter patients (40%–70%), especially when the duration of first complete remission has been longer than 18 months, a second complete remission may be obtained using different salvage chemotherapeutic regimens. High-dose cytosine arabinoside (HD ARA-C) either alone or in combination with other drugs such as intercalating agents are commonly used in such situations. Once a second CR is achieved, its duration is usually short and does not exceed 1 year in most patients.

Allogeneic bone marrow transplantation (AlloBMT), when performed in patients with AML in second CR, may produce 25%–40% longterm survivors, which compares favorably with the results of chemotherapy alone [2]. However, this technique, which is only applicable in young patients having an HLA-identical donor, can only be proposed in a minority of patients. Autologous bone marrow transplantation (AutoBMT) is an alternative treatment for these latter patients [3] and can be applied to a larger population of patients. Autologous blood stem cell transplantation (ABSCT) has more recently been introduced and may be used instead of AutoBMT. The main advantage of ABSCT as opposed to ABMT is that ABSCT is associated with rapid engraftment, thus leading to a decrease in toxicity [10]. The aim of this study is to analyze the results of ABSCT in patients with AML in second CR and to evaluate its contribution to the prolongation of survival in the overall population of patients in first relapse.

Patients and Methods

Patients

A total number of 62 patients (male = 33; female = 29) with AML in first relapse (blast cells >20%) were hospitalized to receive a second-line induction chemotherapy. The mean age of patients was 44.5 years (5–73 years). The mean duration of first CR was 21.5 months (1–98 months). The duration of first CR was less than 6 months for 7 patients and less than 18 months in 38 patients. The FAB classification was as follows: M1 = 12, M2 = 12, M3 = 3; M4 = 10, M5 = 17, others = 8. Twelve of these latter 62 patients who achieved a second CR underwent ABSCT and their characteristics are summarized in Table 1.

Induction and Consolidation Chemotherapy

Three different protocols were used. Forty-two patients received HD ARA-C (3 g/m² × 4 doses) and amsacrine (150 mg/m² per day

Department of Hematology and Bone Marrow Transplant Unit, CHR Bordeaux, Hôpital Haut-Levêque, 33604 Pessac, France

Table 1. Patient characteristics (ABSCT)

Patients (male/female)	4/8
Mean age (years)	34.5 ± 14
Duration of first CR (months)	27.5
PBSC collection (CR1/CR2)	4/8
Conditioning regimens	4
Busulfan + melphalan	
Cyclophosphamide	6
(CYC) + TBI	
HD ARA-C + CYC + TBI	2

× 5) as previously described [8]. Once a second CR was achieved the patients received consolidation therapy with the same drugs at lower doses (ARA-C, × 1 g/m² × 2; AMSA, × 100 mg/m² per day × 3).

Thirteen other patients received a combination of mitoxantrone (12 mg/m²/day × 5 and VP-16 (80 mg/m²/day × 5, continuous infusion) [8]. The patients who responded were given consolidation therapy with the same drugs at lower doses.

Finally, seven patients were treated according to the IDARUB-IDARAC protocol [4].

Post Remission Treatment

Twenty-one patients in second complete remission were designated to receive monthly courses of maintenance chemotherapy using 6-thioguanine and ARA-C. The reasons for not transplanting these patients were as follows: age over 60 years, poor performance status, impaired cardiac function, previous transplantation in first CR, early relapse. Three other patients were allocated to receive AlloBMT from an HLA-identical (two cases) or haplo-identical family donor (one patient).

Twelve patients (Table 1) received ABSCT after different conditioning regimens: cyclophosphamide (120 mg/kg) + fractionated TBI (400 rads × 3) alone (six patients) or preceded by HD ARA-C (3 g/m² × 3) (two patients); and busulfan (4 mg/kg per day × 4) combined with melphalan (140 mg/m²) four patients). Following this conditioning regimen, the patients were infused with peripheral blood stem cells collected after induction or consolidation chemotherapy during first (four patients) or second CR (eight patients). No further antileukemic agents were administered after transplantation.

Results

Induction Chemotherapy

Twenty-six patients (58%) achieved a complete remission after 1 or 2 courses of induction chemotherapy, 4 patients died during treatment and 22 patients were non-responsive to chemotherapy. Four of these latter patients underwent ABSCT in resistant relapse but died early either from transplant-related toxicity or from leukemia. The CR rate was not influenced by the age or sex of patients, by the FAB morphology or the initial WBC count. However, the CR rate was significantly higher for patients treated with HD ARA-C + AMSA (28/42; 67%) or IDARUB-IDARAC (5/7; 71%) than for patients who received mitoxantrone + VP 16 (3/13; 23%) ($p < 0.01$). The CR rate was significantly influenced by the length of first remission: the CR rate was 31.5% in patients (15/38) for whom the first CR was less than 18 months and 88% in the other patients (21/24) ($p < 0.0005$).

Outcome

The median duration of second remission for the 36 CR patients was 6 months. The actuarial proportion of patients surviving at 2 years without recurrent leukemia was 21%. The duration of second remission was significantly longer (13 months) for patients in whom the first CR was longer than 18 months than for the other patients (5 months) ($p < 0.03$). It was not influenced by the age or sex of patients or by the type of chemotherapy used for the induction treatment of first relapse. More surprisingly the outcome was not influenced by the treatment administered once a second CR was achieved:

– For the 21 patients given chemotherapy, the median duration of second CR was very short (5 months) but the estimated chance of surviving without disease at 2 years was 31%.

- The three patients who underwent AlloBMT died from either transplant-related toxicity (two cases) or relapse (one case)
- For the 12 patients who underwent ABSCT, one patient died from bleeding before platelet reconstitution [9]. Eight other patients had leukemic relapse, 3–12 months after ABSCT (median = 8 months). Finally only three patients are still alive, in second CR 8, 48 and 50 months after ABSCT. For two of these latter patients, the duration of second CR was longer than the duration of their first remission. The estimated chance of surviving at 2 years was 19% and not statistically different from that observed in the chemotherapy group.

Discussion

We have treated 62 AML patients in first relapse with three different chemotherapeutic regimens. Our results confirm that a high CR rate can be obtained in patients whose first remission duration lasted longer than 18 months [1, 6]. They also confirm that ID or HD ARA-C is able to overcome drug resistance [5]. However as we have previously reported [8], we were unable to reproduce the results of Ho et al. [7] who documented the efficacy of the combination of mitoxantrone and VP 16 as treatment for refractory or relapsed leukemia. The resistance of leukemic cells to these two drugs may be due to the same mechanism (multidrug resistance) and it may be hypothesized that the poor results were due to the expression of the mdr phenotype by the leukemic cells of the majority of patients treated with the combination of mitoxantrone and VP 16.

The median duration of second remission was not different to that usually reported [6]. As reported elsewhere, it was influenced by the length of first remission [1]. The results for the 12 patients who underwent ABSCT did not differ significantly from those usually reported after ABMT [3]. As with ABMT, the results were similar when the hematopoietic stem cells were collected in first or second CR. Thus, as for AML in first CR, ABSCT seems to be as effective as AutoBMT in maintaining remission and its major advantage over ABMT is the reduction in the duration of granulocytopenia [10].

The results of ABSCT, however, do not differ significantly from those obtained from patients given chemotherapy alone as maintenance treatment. Moreover, only 12 of the 36 patients who achieved a second CR underwent ABSCT. Thus, it may be concluded that ABSCT does not significantly modify the outcome of patients in first relapse.

References

1. Amadori S, Meloni G, Petti MC, Papa G, Miniero R, Mandelli F (1989) Phase II trial of intermediate dose ARA-C (IDAC) with sequential Mitoxantrone (MITOX) in acute myelogenous leukemia. Leukemia 3: 112–114
2. Bortin MM, Gale RP, Kay HEM, Rimm AA (1983) For the Advisory Committee of the International Bone Marrow Transplant Registry. Bone marrow transplantation for acute myelogenous leukemia. JAMA 249: 1166–1175
3. Gorin NC, Herve P, Aegerter P, Goldstone A, Linch D, Maraninchi D, Burnett A, Helbig W, Meloni G, Verdonck LF, De Witte T, Rizzoli V, Carella A, Parlier Y, Auvert B, Goldman J (1986) For the Working Party on Autologous Bone Marrow Transplantation of the European Bone Marrow Transplantation Group (EBMTG). Autologous bone marrow transplantation for acute leukemia in remission. Br J Haematol 64: 385–395
4. Harousseau JL, Reiffers J, Hurteloup P, Milpied N, Guy H, Rigal-Huguet F, Facon T, Dufour P, Ifrah N (1989) For the French Study Group of Idarubicin Leukemia. Treatment of relapsed acute myeloid leukemia with idarubicin and intermediate-dose cytarabine. J Clin Oncol 7: 45–49
5. Heinemann V, Jehn U (1990) Rationales of a pharmacologically optimized treatment of acute nonlymphocytic leukemia with cytosine arabinoside. Leukemia 4: 790–796
6. Hiddemann W, Kreutzmann H, Straif K, Ludwig WD, Mertelsmann R, Planker M, Donhuijsen-Ant R, Lengfelder E, Arlin Z, Buchner T (1987) High-dose cytosine arabinoside in combination with mitoxantrone for the treatment of refractory acute myeloid

and lymphoblastic leukemia. Semin Oncol 14 [Suppl 1]: 73–77

7. Ho AD, Lipp T, Ehninger G, Illiger HJ, Meyer P, Freund M, Hustein W (1988) Combination of mitoxantrone and etoposide in refractory acute myelogenous leukemia. An active and well-tolerated regimen. J Clin Oncol 6: 213–217

8. Marit G, Cony P, Duclos F, Puntous M, Broustet A, Reiffers J (1990) Treatment of relapsed or refractory acute leukemia: comparison of two different regimens. Haematol Blood Transfus 33: 614–617

9. Reiffers J, Castaigne S, Tilly H, Lepage E, Leverger G, Henon P, Douay L (1987) Hematopoietic reconstitution after autologous blood stem cell transplantation: a report of 46 cases. Plasma Ther Transfus Technol 8: 360–362

10. Reiffers J, Leverger G, Marit G, Castaigne S, Tilly H, Lepage E, Henon P, Douay L, Troussard X for the France Auto Greffe Group (1989) Haematopoietic reconstitution after autologous blood stem cell transplantation. In: Gale RP, Champlin RE (eds) Bone marrow transplantation: current controversis. Liss, New York, pp 313–320

Therapy of Acute-Phase Chronic Myelogenous Leukemia with Intensive Chemotherapy, Blood Cell Autotransplantation and Cyclosporine A

A. M. Carella

Introduction

Therapy of chronic myelogenous leukemia (CML) is unsatisfactory. The disease is characterized by two phases: a chronic phase lasting approximately 3 years and an acute phase lasting approximately 6 months. All patients with CML in chronic phase survive sufficiently long to progress to acute phase. The annual rate of transformation is approximately 25 %. No therapy convincingly prolongs the duration of the chronic phase. Therapy of acute phase is unsatisfactory with clinical remission rates of 25 %–30 % and a median survival of approximately 6 months [1–3].

In contrast to the usual fatal course of CML, persons receiving allogeneic bone marrow transplants achieve long-term disease-free survival. Results are best in persons receiving allogeneic transplants in chronic phase where 5-year disease-free survival is approximately 50 %. Results of allogeneic transplants in persons in acute phase are inferior with about 15 % 5-year disease-free survival [4].

Autotransplants are also used in persons with CML [4]. Results in acute phase are disappointing with less than 5 % 5-year disease-free survival. Results of autotransplants in chronic phase are somewhat better but there are not yet sufficient data for critical analysis.

Recently we reported that persons with AP-CML treated with idarubicin, intermediate-dose cytarabine and VP-16 may 'achieve clinical remissions. In some instances, blood cells obtained from these persons *immediately* after recovery from marrow aplasia contain large numbers of myeloid progenitor cells which are Ph-negative. We wondered whether such cells could be used for autotransplants in persons in acute phase prepared for transplantation with high-dose therapy and total body radiation.

Considerable data indicate that graft-versus-host disease (GvHD) is associated with a substantial antileukemic effect in animals and humans. Recently, use of cyclosporine A postautotransplant has been shown in rodents and humans to induce a syndrome resembling acute GvHD [5, 6]. Consequently, we wondered whether adding cyclosporine A to the posttransplant therapy of our autotransplant recipients might not decrease the probability of leukemia recurrence. In this report we indicate the results of this approach in eight persons with AP-CML.

Materials and Methods

Patients and Therapy

Eight consecutive patients with AP-CML entered the study between July 1989 and September 1990 (Table 1). Written informed consent was obtained from all subjects. Median age at the time of the autotransplant was 40 years (range, 30–67

Onchematologic and ABMT Unit, Division of Hematology II, Ospedale S. Martino, Via Acerbi 10/22, 16148 Genoa, Italy years). Acute phase was characterized as myeloid in four subjects, erythroid in one, and lymphoid in three by standard criteria, including morphologic studies (generally, the presence of 30% or more blasts in the marrow and blood), cytochemical reactions (peroxidase, specific and nonspecific esterases, Sudan black, and periodic acid-Schiff) and flow cytometry using a battery of monoclonal anti-bodies designed to detect either myeloid or lymphoid antigenic determinants [7].

Initial chemotherapy of acute phase consisted of idarubicin (6–8 mg/m^2 per day for 5 days intravenously), cytarabine (600–800 mg/m^2 per day for 5 days infused intravenously over 2 h), and VP-16 (150 mg/m^2 for 3 days infused intravenously over a period of 2 h). The drugs were given concurrently. Peripheral stem cells were collected following recovery from initial intensive chemotherapy. Leukapheresis was initiated when the WBC reached 0.3–1 × 10^9. Details of blood stem cell collection were reported [8]. Twenty-nine leukapheresis procedures were done in the eight patients (median, three per patient; range, to five on consecutive days. Procedures were completed in all cases. Nucleated cells collected varied between 0.5 and 0.8 × 10^9 kg body weight (median, 0.7 × 10^9). Autologous bone marrow was harvested and treated „in vitro" with the ASTA-Z "adjusted-dose" technique [9] only to be used if peripheral blood stem cells failed to engraft. The patients whose blood stem cell resulted Ph-negative after a single course of initial intensive chemotherapy were considered for an autotransplant (Table 1, subjects 1, 3, 4, 5, and 8). These subjects received VP-16 (800 mg/m^2 per day for two consecutive days, intravenously), cyclophosphamide (60 mg/kg per day for each of two consecutive days) followed by 10 Gy total body irradiation at a dose rate of 5–9 cGy/min. Within 24 h following radiation, the cryopreserved blood cells were defrosted and reinfused intravenously. This is designated day O.

Cyclosporine A at a dose of 1.5 mg/kg per day by continuous intravenous infusion was initiated on day+1 and continued for 4 weeks.

Cytogenetic Analyses

Cytogenetic studies were done on peripheral blood stem cells and on bone marrow using short-term (24–48 h) cultures without the addition of mitogens. Chromosomes were analyzed using G and Q techniques and classified according to ISCN [10]. Patients were studied at diagnosis of acute phase on BM and on peripheral blood stem cell collection after leukapheresis prior to autografting. Subsequently, cytogenetic evaluation was done on BM at 4, 12, 20, 28, 36, and 44 weeks following autografting. At least 10–60 metaphases were examined in all cases on BM and on peripheral blood.

Results

Eight previously untreated patients in AP-CML have so far been treated with this intensive inductive regimen (Table 1). Five (62.5%) out of eight patients achieved peripheral blood stem cell remission with 100% Ph-negative blood cells, disappearance of other cytogenetic abnormalities and negative PCR in one patient. The parallel evaluation of bone marrow demonstrated clinical and cytogenetic remission in two patients (Table 2, subjects 1,8) and a good response in two other patients (Table 2, subjects 3, 4). The five subjects with Ph-negative peripheral blood cells then received high-dose therapy followed by blood stem cell reinfusion. Three out of five subjects remain in clinical and cytogenetical remission 5, 9, and 15 months posttransplant. This is an interesting result, which may perhaps explain the good outcome of these patients, derived from PCR analysis performed on the leukapheresis cells from patient 4 (Table 1). The results of this analysis (the sensitivity of which may be estimated to range between 1 × 10^4 and 1 × 10^5 cells) failed to show the presence of an amplification fragment of 273 bp (base pairs), corresponding to the presence of *Bcr-Abl* hybrid transcripts with a junction between the *"bcr"* region exon 3 and the Abl exon 2, which was the one expected on the basis of a PCR done on the patient cells before treatment.

Table 1. Clinical features and results

Patients	Sex/age	Prior therapy	Duration of chronic phase (months)	Blast cell morphology	Karyotype at acute phase (N metaphases]	PS at APBSC	Recovery data (days) N	P	Results and outcome (months)
1	M/30	BU, HU, VND, PTC	19	Erythroid	46xy, Ph+[10]	1	15	25	A/W Ph-negative (15+)
2	M/67	BU, HU, RhU-alpha INF, VND	24	Myeloid	46xy, Ph+[20]	1	10	30	Died in AP
3	M/39	BU, HU, VND	20	Myeloid	46xy, Ph+[16]	1	14	28	A/W Ph-negative (9+)
4	M/41	VCR+PRED	–	Lymphoid ("d'emblee" at diagnosis)	46xy, [3] 46xy, Ph+[6] 54–70,xy, Ph+Complex [35]	1	18	34	Ph-negative (5+) PCR-negative, relapsed, alive
5	M/47	BU, HU	20	Lymphoid	46xy, Ph+[10] 46xy, Ph+, t (14: 19) (q11; p13) [30]	1	21	40	Ph-negative (7+), relapsed, died
6	M/62	BU, HU	22	Myeloid	46xy, Ph+[20]	1	20	46	Alive in PR
7	F/35	BU, HU, DNR, ARA-C, VCR	31	Myeloid	46xx,t(1;9:22)(q22;q34:q11)[20]	1	40	50	Died in AP
8	F/37	BU, HU, VCR, DNR, PRED	14	Lymphoid	46xx,Ph+[20]	1	12	41	A/W Ph-negative (5+)

Cytogenetic PBSC renormalization and clinical remission; CP, chronic phase; AP, acute phase; BU, busulphan; HU, hydrossiurea; RhU-alpha INF, alpha-interferon; VND, vindesine; PTC, Peptichemio; PRED, prednisolone; DNR, daunorubicin; ARA-C, Cytarabine; VCR, vincristine; A/W, alive and well; CP, chronic phase; PBC, peripheral blood cell; PR, partial remission; PS, performance status; APBSC, autografting peripheral blood stem cells; N, neutrophils > 0.5 × 10⁹; P, platelets > 50 × 10⁹

Table 2. Results of cytogenetic analysis

Patient	% Ph-negative metaphases[a] Before PBSC Autografting	At PBSC Collection PBSC/BM		After PBSC Autografting (weeks) 4	12	20	28	36	44	60
1	0 (0–30)	100 % (10/10)	100 % (20/20)	100 % (10/10)	100 % (20/20)	NE	100 % (40/40)	100 % (40/40)	100 % (40/40)	100 % (50/50)
2	0 (0–50)	0 (0–40)	0 (0–40)	–	–	–	–	–	–	–
3	0 (0–20)	100 % (2/2)	75 (3/4)	NE	100 % (20/20)	100 % (20/20)	NE	100 % (30/30)	–	–
4	0 (0–60)	100 % (38/38)	82 (50/60)	100 % (40/40)	100 % (50/50)	100 % (40/40)	0 % (0/40)			
5	0 (0–50)	100 % (20/20)	NE	100 % (10/10)	100 % (20/20)	100 % (30/30)	0 % (0/30)			
6	0 (0–40)	50 % (10/20)	NE	50 % (10/20)	50 % (10/20)	50 % (20/40)	NE			
7	0 (0–40)	0 (0–30)	0 (0–40)	0 (0–40)	–	–	–			
8	0 (0–50)	100 % (20/20)	100 % (30/30)	100 % (30/30)	NE	100 % (30/30)				

[a] The number of Ph-negative metaphases and the total number of examined on each occasion are specified in parentheses; NE, not examined

Table 3. Therapy of acute phase CML with intensive chemotherapy, blood cell autotransplantation and cyclosporine A: an update of the genoa experience.

No. Patients	28
Blastic Phase (BP)	25
BP "d'emblee"	1
Chronic Phase (CP)	2
Transplant Source	BSC
Age	16–67
BP: duration CP (median)	24 months (14–52)
CP: duration disease	8, 12 months
Early deaths	5 (all BP)
Restore CP in BP patients	13 (My:7; Ly:6)
BSC Ph-negative	9 (32.1%)
CBR (Ph-/PCR-)	3 (LyBP:1; MyBP:1; CP:1)
CR (Ph-)	6
Mosaicism (Ph−/Ph+)	4 (CP:1; MyBP:3)
Alive and well	4 (CP:2; MyBP:1; LyBP:1)

BSC: Blood Stem Cell; CBR: Complete Biological Remission; CR: Complete Remission.

A rash developed in four of five recipients posttransplant at a median of 13 days (range, 9–20 days). GVHD of the skin was confirmed by histological criteria in three patients [11, 12]. The rash resolved within 1–2 weeks. There was no clinical or biochemical evidence of hepatic or gastrointestinal GVHD. All patients tolerated cyclosporine A treatment without serious complications.

Discussion

For patients with CML the only available chance of avoiding fatal blastic transformation is the allogeneic BMT. This procedure is limited by age and the availability of an HLA-matched donor. For the patients without a matched HLA-compatible donor, the outlook is less hopeful. Various methods are being utilized to prevent graft rejection and GvHD when mismatch transplants are performed but transplantation of mismatched marrow still has a high risk of failure and/or complications. Also the idea of possible donation of marrow through banks still remains very difficult. One possibility of helping such patients might come from the development of a better treatment of AP, which is able to induce a Ph-negative remission. It has been known for some years that pluripotential hemopoietic stem cells capable of reconstituting hemopoiesis after "supralethal" myelo-ablative chemoradiotherapy were present in the marrow and blood of untreated CML patients in greatly increased numbers. What was not so obvious until recently is the fact that Ph-negative hemopoietic stem cells persist intact possibly in normal concentrations, in the marrow of CML patients even though their presence is difficult to demonstrate [13]. The induction regimen employed by our team appears promising. The peripheral stem cells collected *immediately* after postchemotherapeutic aplasia were Ph negative in five of eight patients. Moreover, even if only one case has been examined so far, the negative result of the PCR analysis performed on the cells derived from the leukapheresis of patient 4 is remarkable. This procedure is able to detect the presence of residual Ph-positive cells with a sensitivity of at least $1/10^4$–$1/10^5$, and therefore the chemotherapy regimen proposed has the potential to induce a very profound suppression of the Ph-positive clone in least some of the responsive patients. As suggested by a few investigators, the expansion of Ph-chromosome clone in CML might have a proliferative advantage over the proliferation of "putative" normal Ph-negative hemopoietic stem cells, but this proliferative advantage might in certain circumstances be reversible [14–17]. Although in most patients Ph-negative cells cannot be routinely identified, recent analysis of BM in patients undergoing chemotherapy has shown that a Ph-negative chromosomal status can be achieved [16–21] and further work is needed to evaluate the durability of such treatments. This suggests that treating patients before the onset of blastic transformation with high-dosage chemoradiotherapy followed by autografting with hematopoietic blood cells collected at diagnosis or, better, in the postaplastic phase after an intensive chemotherapy protocol, might facilitate the restoration of Ph-negative hematopoiesis.

In the attempt to evaluate whether this theory could have a clinical application, we have treated eight patients with CML in BC and three of them are now Ph-negative alive and well. Further results are needed to prove the efficacy of the above treatment.

Summary

Eight patients with acute-phase chronic myelogenous leukemia (AP-CML) were treated with idarubicin, intermediate-dose cytarabine and etoposide. During recovery from bone marrow aplasia, when WBC reached $0.3–1 \times 10^9$, blood cells were collected by leukapheresis carried out two to five times (median, three) consecutively. In five to eight patients, these peripheral cells were Ph-negative on cytogenetic analysis. Moreover, in one case polymerase chain reaction (PCR) analysis performed to detect the presence of minimal residual disease in the cells collected by leukapheresis was negative, further confirming that this approach may induce a very high degree of suppression of Ph-positive clones.

After complete recovery, these five patients were subsequently treated with high-dose etopopside, cyclophosphamide, and total body radiation (10 Gy, single dose) followed by reinfusion of Ph-negative peripheral blood stem cells. All these patients received cyclosporine A post-auto-transplant in an attempt to induce acute GVHD. Three out of five patients remained in clinical and cytogenetic remission 5–15 months posttransplant. We conclude that Ph-negative peripheral blood stem cells can be recovered from patients with AP-CML and used successfully to restore Ph-negative hemopoiesis after high-dose therapy.

References

1. Canellos GP (1977) The treatment of chronic granulocytic leukemia. Clin Hematol 6: 113–116
2. Sokal JE (1976) Evaluation of survival data for chronic myelocytic leukemia. Am J Hematol 1: 493–496
3. Desforges JF, Miller KB (1986) Blast crisis. Reversing the direction. N Engl J Med 315: 1478–1481
4. Butturini A, Keating A, Goldman J, Gale RP (1990) Autotransplants in chronic myelogenous leukaemia: strategies and results. Lancet i: 1255–1258
5. Jones RJ, Vogelsang GB, Hess AD et al. (1989) Induction of graft versus host disease after autologous bone marrow transplantation. Lancet i: 754–757
6. Talbot DC, Powles RL, Sloane JP et al. (1990) Cyclosporine – induced graft-versus-host-disease following autologous bone marrow transplantation in acute myeloid leukaemia. Bone Marrow Transplant 6: 17–20
7. Lovett EJIII, Schnitzer B, Karen DF et al. (1984) Application of low cytometry to diagnosis pathology. Lab invest 50: 115–140
8. Goldman JM, Catovsky D, Hows J et al. (1979) Cryopreserved peripheral blood cells functioning as autografts in patients with chronic granulocytic leukaemia in transformation. Br Med J i: 1310–1313
9. Rizzoli V, Mangoni L, Carella AM et al. (1989) Drug-mediated marrow purging: maphosphamide in adult acute leukemia in remission. The experience of the Italian study group. Bone Marrow Transplant 4 [Suppl 1]: 190–194
10. Harnden DG, Klinger HP (eds) (1985) An international system for human cytogenetic nomenclature, Karger, Basel. Also in Birth defects, no 1. March of Dimes Birth Defects Foundation, New York, 1985
11. Lerner KG, Kao GF, Storb R (1974) Histopathology of GVHD in human recipients of marrow from HLA matched sibling donors. Transplant Proc 6: 367–371
12. Elliot CJ, Sloane JP, Sanderson KV, Vincent M, Sheperd V, Powles R L (1987) The

histological diagnosis of cutaneous GVHD: relationship of skin changes to marrow purging and other clinical variables. Histopathology 11: 145–155

13. Goldman JM (1990) Options for the management of chronic myeloid leukaemia 1990. Leukemia Lymphoma 3: 159–164

14. Advisory commitee of the International Bone Marrow Transplant registry (1989) Report from the International Bone Marrow Transplant Registry. Bone Marrow Transplant 4: 221–228

15. Frassoni F, Sessarego M, Bacigalupo A, et al. (1988) Competition between recipient and donor cells after bone, marrow transplantation for chronic myeloid leukaemia. Br J Haematol 69: 471–475

16. Goto N, Nishikori M, Arlin Z et al. (1982) Growth characteristics of leukemic and normal hematopoietic cells in Ph+ chronic myelogenous leukemia in vivo and in vitro and effects of intensive treatment with the L-15 protocol. Blood 59: 793–808

17. Coulombel L, Kalousek DK, Eaves CH et al. (1983) Long term marrow culture reveals chromosomally normal hemopoietic progenitor cells in patients with Philadelphia chromsome-positive chronic meylogenous leukemia. N Engl J Med 306: 1493–1498

18. Singer CRJ, Mc Donald GA, Douglas AS (1984). Twentyfive year survival of chronic granulocytic leukemia with spontaneous varyotype conversion. Br J Haematol 57: 309–314

19. Talpaz M, Kantarjian HM, McCredie K et al. (1986) Hematologic remission and cytogenetic improvement induced by recombinant human interferon alpha in chronic myelogenous leukemia. N Engl J Med 314: 1065–1069

20. Barnett MJ, Eaves CJ, Phillips GL et al. (1989) Successful autografting in chronic myelogenous leukemia after maintenance of marrow in culture. Bone Marrow Transplant 4: 345–351

21. Brito-Babapulle F, Bowcok SJ, Marcus RE et al. (1989) Autografting for patients with chronic myeloid leukaemia in chronic phase: peripheral blood stem cell may have a finite capacity for maintaining haemopoiesis. Br J Haematol 73: 76–81

Allogeneic Bone Marrow Transplantation in Patients with Acute Leukemia with More Advanced Disease*

R. Arnold, D. Bunjes, B. Hertenstein, D. Hueske, M. Theobald, M. Weiss, M. Wiesneth, and H. Heimpel

Introduction

After first relapse disease-free survival (DFS) is poor for patients with acute leukemia treated with chemotherapy alone. Chemotherapy studies revealed a long-term disease-free survival below 5 % for patients with acute myeloid leukemia (AML) [1] and with acute lymphoblastic leukemia (ALL/AUL) (D. Hoelzer, personal communication). When a MHC (major histocompatibility complex) compatible bone marrow donor exists, the indication for bone marrow transplantation (BMT) is given. The following data represent the results of BMT in patients with acute leukemia beyond first remission transplanted between 1975 and 1990 at the University of Ulm.

Patients

Forty-four adult patients with acute leukemia were transplanted beyond first remission. The median age was 29 years (15–50 years) for the whole group. For AML patients the median age was 36 years (24–50 years) and for ALL/AUL patients 21 years (15–48 years). There were 25 males and 19 females. Nineteen out of 44 patients had AML and the stage of disease at BMT was as follows: second CR $n=9$; third CR $n=2$;

* This work was supported by Deutsche Krebshilfe, M 71-90-HE7.
Departments of Internal Medicine III and Transfusion Medicine, University of Ulm, Robert-Koch-Str. 8, W-7900 Ulm, FRG

first PR $n=2$; second PR $n=1$, first relapse $n=3$, third relapse $n=1$, refractory disease $n=1$. Twenty-five out of 44 patients had ALL/AUL and the stage of disease at BMT was as follows: second CR $n=12$, third CR $n=1$, fourth CR $n=1$, second PR $n=1$, first relapse $n=2$, second relapse $n=7$, third relapse $n=1$. When remission could be achieved, patients were transplanted as soon as possible. The median time between complete remission (CR) and BMT was 30 days (18–135 days) for AML patients and 44 days (10–106 days) for ALL/AUL patients.

Bone Marrow Transplantation

Conditioning Regimens

Most of the patients received VP-16 (60 mg/kg) and total body irradiation (TBI) ($n=17$) or cyclophosphamide and TBI ($n=15$). In nine patients Ara-C and VP-16 were given in addition to cyclophosphamide and TBI. Three patients received chemoconditioning only (busulfan/cyclophosphamide). The conditioning regimens were not different between AML or ALL/AUL patients.

Bone Marrow Donors

Thirty-five out of 44 patients were transplanted from an HLA-identical, MLC-negative sibling donor. Two patients had an identical twin donor. Seven patients were transplanted from a haploidentical family member (parents $n=5$, sibling $n=1$, cousin $n=1$).

GvHD Prophylaxis

In 42/44 patients prophylaxis for prevention of graft versus host disease (GvHD) was given. Seventeen patients received methotrexate/cyclosporin A, six patients MTX alone, and two patients CSA alone. Seventeen patients received a T-cell-depleted bone marrow transplant.

Results

Twelve of 44 patients remain in complete remission after BMT with a median follow-up of 52 months (3–100 months). Eighteen out of 44 patients relapsed after BMT and are dead. Fourteen out of 44 patients died due to transplant-related death, mainly infections (Table 1). The probability of disease-free survival is 18 % for AML patients (Fig. 1) and 29 % for ALL/AUL patients (Fig. 2).

Table 1. Results of allogeneic BMT in more advanced leukemia

1. AML Patients (n)	19	
Alive in CR	4/19	
Dead	15/19	
Transplant related	5/15	
Relapse	10/15	
Median survival after BMT	107 days	
Time of relapse	median 100 days (40–513 days) after BMT	
2. ALL/AUL patients (n)	25	
Alive in CR	8/25	
Dead	17/25	
Transplant related	9/17	
Relapse	8/18	

Median survival after BMT: 140 days
Time of relapse: median 84 days (11–259 days) after BMT

Analysis of Risk Factors for Relapse After BMT

Duration of First Remission

The duration of first CR was short for the whole group. In AML patients the median

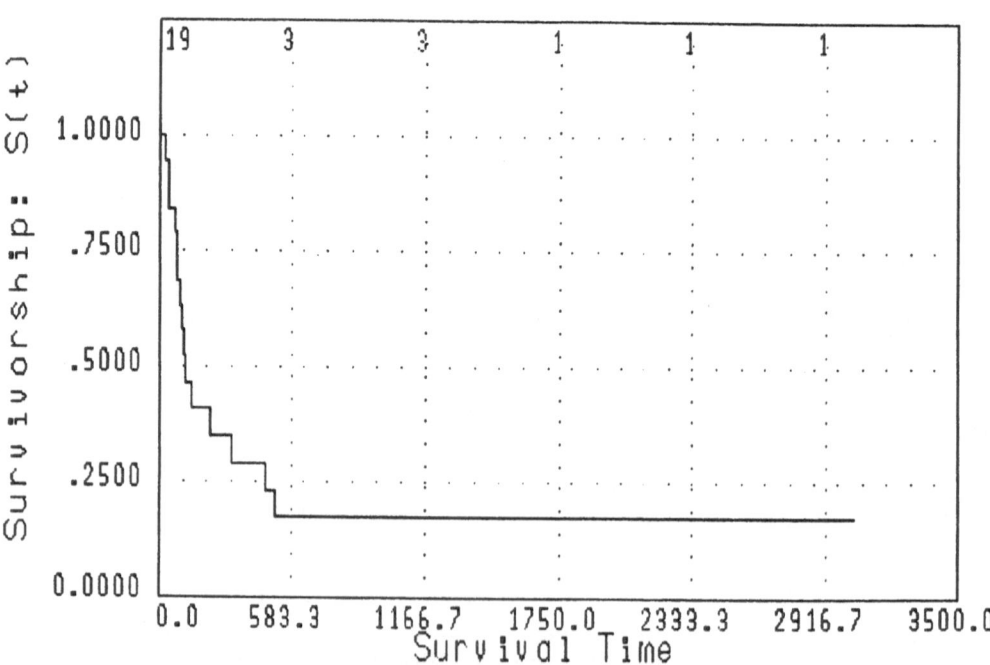

Fig. 1. Probability of disease-free survival for AML patients

530

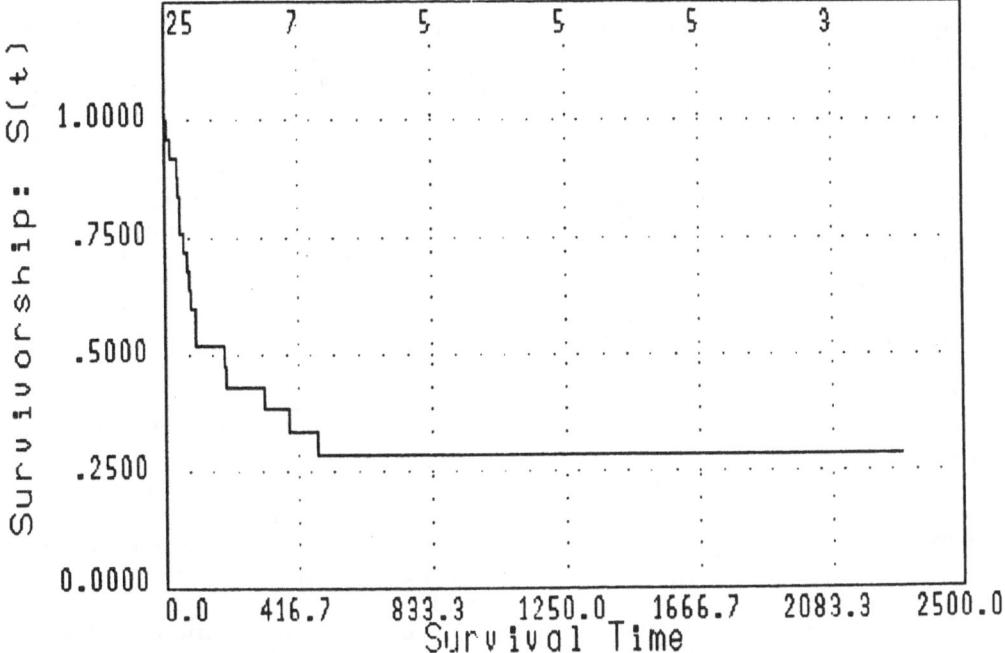

Fig. 2. Probability of disease-free survival for ALL/AUL patients

duration of first CR was 103 days for patients who relapsed after BMT vs. 165 days for patients who remained in remission after BMT. In ALL/AUL patients the median duration of first CR was 166 days for patients who relapsed after BMT vs. 197

Table 2. Outcome of allogeneic BMT (1975–11/1990)

Diagnosis	Total	Alive in CR	BMT-related death	Relapse	DFS
	(*n*)	(*n*)	(*n*)	(*n*)	
AML First CR	46	29	15	2	0.52
ALL/AUL First CR	18	11	6	1	0.55
AML > first CR	19	4	5	10	0.18
Second CR	9	2	4	3	
First relapse/first PR	5	2	0	3	
Third CR	2	0	0	2	
Second PR/third relapse/refr.	3	0	1	2	
ALL/AUL > first CR	25	8	9	8	0.29
Second CR	12	4	6	2	
First relapse	2	1	0	1	
Third CR	1	1	0	0	
Second PR	1	0	1	0	
Second relapse	7	2	1	4	
Fourth CR	1	0	1	0	
Third relapse	1	0	0	1	

531

days for patients who remained in remission after BMT.

Status of Disease at BMT

The stage of leukemia at BMT is important. In AML only patients transplanted in second CR, first PR or first relapse survived in remission after BMT. In ALL/AUL patients a certain proportion of patients transplanted beyond second CR became long-term survivors. The comparison of the results of BMT in more advanced disease with BMT in first CR is depicted in Table 2.

Discussion

Allogeneic BMT can cure a certain proportion of patients with relapse after chemotherapy. In 1991 the IBMTR [2] reported a 5-year probability of disease-free survival of 28% ± 8% for patients with AML ≥ second CR (n=196), 20% ± 6% for patients with AML in relapse (n=357), 33% ± 5% for patients with ALL ≥ second CR (n=515) and 18% ± 6% for patients with ALL in relapse (n=256). Because of the small numbers of patients involved, we have not subdivided AUL and ALL with advanced disease any further. The disease-free survival of our group of 19 AML patients is 18%, of our group of 25 ALL/AUL patients 29%. These results are essentially equivalent to the IBMTR data.

The major causes of treatment failure were transplant-associated mortality (30%) and leukemic relapse (30%–50%). Whereas the procedure-related mortality was similar to that observed in patients grafted in first CR, the incidence of relapse was significantly higher. Our experience, albeit in a limited number of patients, suggests that, in contrast to the IBMTR data, AML beyond first relapse is essentially refractory to current conditioning regimens. This difference could be due to the more intensive induction and reinduction regimens currently being used in the German multicenter chemotherapy trials. In contrast, a certain proportion of ALL beyond first relapse remains sensitive and can be potentially cured by BMT.

These differences may be related to differences in the biology of AML and ALL or could be the result of differences in susceptibility to the effector mechnisms of the graft-versus-leukemia effect, which is probably important for the induction and maintenance of remission after allogeneic BMT.

In summary, bone marrow transplantation is currently the only means of achieving a cure in adults with advanced leukemia. Attempts to reduce the high risk of relapse in these patients by intensifying the conditioning regimens will probably fail due to an increase in procedure-related mortality. We feel that a more effective manipulation of the graft-versus-leukemia effect is currently our best hope for progress in this difficult area.

References

1. Hiddemann W, Büchner T (1990) Treatment strategies in acute myeloid leukaemia (AML). Blut 60: 163–171
2. International Bone Marrow Transplantabion Registry (IBMTR) (1991) January 1991, Statistical Center, Medical College of Wisconsin

Engraftment-Promoting Potential of High-Dose Cytostatic Agents in Allogeneic Bone Marrow Transplantation*

B. Glass, W. Gassmann, L. Uharek, A. Erbersdobler, H. Loeffler, and W. Mueller-Ruchholtz

Introduction

Graft rejection is a serious problem in HLA-mismatched and in T-cell-depleted HLA-identical bone marrow transplantation. Rejection rates of up to 35% have been observed in cases where HLA-identical bone marrow depleted of T lymphocytes was grafted following conventional conditioning with cyclophosphamide and total body irradiation [1].

Cyclophosphamide as well as irradiation are potent immunosuppressants, so that substitutes for either modality may imply an even higher risk of graft rejection. Consequently, substitutes for cyclophosphamide have to be tested for their engraftment-promoting potency in allogeneic bone marrow transplantation. To test the immuno-suppressive engraftment-promoting potential of cyclophosphamide, ifosfamide, ACNU, BCNU, thiotepa, melphalan, and carboplatin, we used a modification of the experimental model of Tutschka and Santos [2], namely the busulfan-treated rat. Busulfan is a myeloablative cytostatic agent which has only limited immunosuppressive potential and does not allow engraftment of allogeneic marrow. Therefore it could be used to test the engraftment-promoting potential of cytostatic agents given in addition to busulfan.

Materials and Methods

The experimental model has been described previously. Briefly, LEW rats received a myeloablative dose of busulfan (35 mg/kg) via a gastric tube 24 h prior to transplantation of 1×10^8 allogeneic bone marrow cells. To avoid GvHR-induced mortality, (CAP $\times$ LEW)F1 marrow was used for grafting. Since preliminary experiments have shown that the preparatory regimens tested would be highly toxic, with a substantial portion of the rats dying even after syngeneic bone marrow transplantation, it proved necessary to determine in each individual rat whether death was due to graft rejection or to toxicity of the preparatory regimen. Consequently, hematocrit, leukocyte counts and differential blood counts were done in each animal twice weekly for the first 3 weeks and on every 10th day until day 100. The day of marrow grafting was termed day 0. Death with granulocyte counts below 500/μl was considered to be caused by graft rejection, death with higher granulocyte counts was considered to be due to other reasons, e.g., toxicity. Death of animals that never achieved a granulocyte count above 500/μl was termed primary rejection. Animals initially reaching this granulocyte count, but dying thereafter in secondary aplasia, were counted as secondary rejections. All rats surviving the 100-day observation period received an allogeneic CAP skin graft to

Second Department of Internal Medicine and Department of Immunology, University of Kiel, Chemnitzstraße 53–57, 2300 Kiel, FRG

* Supported by a grant from Heinz and Gudrun Bauer, Hamburg/FRG, in memoriam of their son Hendrik.

indicate persistence or rejection of the transplanted marrow, since rejection might have been masked by autologous recovery.

Results

Cyclophosphamide

After preparation with 35 mg/kg busulfan, 60 mg/kg cyclophosphamide, and grafting of 1×10^8 marrow cells, the total rejection rate was 59 %. The rate that completely prevented rejection was 120 mg/kg, representing 33 % of the maximum dose applicable in conjunction with busulfan (Table 1).

Ifosfamide

Ifosfamide is a cytostatic agent structurally related to cyclophosphamide. In conventional polychemotherapeutic regimens it is given in doses of 5–10 g/m², equivalent to 120–240 mg/kg (K. Havemann 1987, study protocol). We have tested it in combination with busulfan in doses of 60–1200 mg/kg i.p. on day –2 (doses up to 90 mg/kg), or in divided doses on days –4, –3, and –2. Doses of up to 120 mg/kg did not prevent rejection of the allogeneic marrow. Following 180 mg/kg, the rejection rate was 67 % and no rejections were observed when 240 mg/kg was given in addition to busulfan (Table 1).

ACNU

According to our knowledge, ACNU has been used as a conditioning agent in clinical bone marrow transplantation only in single cases [3]. We have tested ACNU in doses of 7–40 mg/kg given intravenously on day –2. All rats receiving doses up to 10 mg/kg in addition to the lethal dose of busulfan rejected the allogeneic marrow. Following 15 mg/kg, rejection rate was 45 % and no rejections were observed with doses of 20 mg/kg ($n = 10$) or more. The maximum dose applicable in addition to the lethal dose of busulfan prior to allogeneic or syngeneic (data not shown) bone marrow transplantation was 30 mg/kg (Table 2).

BCNU

In clinical autologous bone marrow transplantation, doses of 10–30 mg/kg BCNU are given for conditioning [4]. Following 10 mg/kg BCNU given in addition to the lethal dose of busulfan, the immunosuppressive potential was limited with only one of seven animals transiently accepting the allogeneic bone marrow graft. After 20 mg/kg the rejection rate dropped to 64 "%, and only 2 rejections in 17 animals transplanted were seen when 30 mg/kg BCNU was given in addition to the lethal dose of busulfan (Table 2).

Thiotepa

Thiotepa has been given prior to autologous bone marrow transplantation in doses

Table 1. Rejection rates following allogeneic BMT after conditioning with 35 mg/kg busulfan and a varying dosis of cytostatic agents with high immunosuppressive potency

Dosis (mg/kg)	Rejection rate (%)	n	Toxic death rate (%)
	Cyclophosphamide		
30	100	4	0
60	59	32	9
90	20	21	5
120	0	19	0
180	0	4	0
	Ifosfamide		
60	100	4	0
90	100	4	0
120	100	9	0
180	67	12	0
240	0	10	0
360	0	3	0
480	0	4	0
600	0	4	50
750	0	4	50
900	0	4	25
1200	0	2	100

Table 2. Rejection rates following allogeneic BMT after conditioning with 35 mg/kg busulfan and a varying dosis of cytostatic agents with intermediate immunosuppressive potency

Dosis (mg/kg)	Rejection rate	n	Toxic death rate
	ACNU		
7	100	4	0
10	100	6	0
15	45	11	18
20	0	10	10
30	0	10	60
40	0	2	100
	BCNU		
5	100	4	0
10	100	7	0
20	64	17	35
30	12	17	76
40	17	6	83
80	0	2	100

Table 3. Rejection rates following allogeneic BMT after conditioning with 35 mg/kg busulfan and a varying dosis of cytostatic agents with low immunosuppressive potency

Dosis (mg/kg)	Rejection rate (%)	n	Toxic death rate (%)
	Thiotepa		
5	100	7	0
10	100	7	0
15	0	6	100
20	0	4	100
	Melphalan		
1	100	2	0
2	100	2	0
3	100	4	0
5	100	7	0
7	57	14	36
10	0	4	100
	Carboplatin		
30	100	7	0
40	100	7	0
60	100	8	0
80	71	7	29
120	0	2	100
180	0	2	100

of 3–22 mg/kg [5]. We tested doses of 5–20 mg/kg (i.p., day –2) in conjunction with busulfan before allogeneic bone marrow transplantation. The maximum tolerable dose in this setting was 10 mg/kg but it did not prevent rejection in all seven rats transplanted (Table 3). Toxic effects of thiotepa on the transplanted marrow were excluded. Five syngeneic controls injected with 10 mg/kg thiotepa on day –1 showed rapid and lasting engraftment.

Melphalan

In the clilnical setting, melphalan doses of 100–260 mg/m², equivalent to 2.5–4 mg/kg, have been used with or without total body irradiation prior to marrow transplantation [6]. In the animal model described here, rejection of allogeneic marrow could not be prevented by doses of up to 5 mg/kg melphalan, given i.v. on day –2 in addition to busulfan. The maximum tolerable dose was 7 mg/kg (Table 3). To make sure that rejection or primary graft failure was not mediated by toxic effects of the

drug on the incoming marrow, melphalan was given to syngeneic controls on day –1, instead of day –2, as in the allogeneic situation. Both rats receiving 5 mg/kg and all four receiving 7 mg/kg melphalan on day –1 with busulfan and 1×10^8 syngeneic marrow cells showed rapid and lasting engraftment and survived the full observation period.

Carboplatin

Pilot studies with syngeneic marrow transplants showed that doses up to 80 mg/kg given in addition to the lethal dose of busulfan can be administered as a preparatory agent prior to syngeneic transplantation [7, 8]. Even the highest doses of carboplatin given in addition to a lethal dose of busulfan were not sufficiently immunosup-

535

pressive to allow engraftment of the allogeneic bone marrow (Table 3).

Discussion

Our previously published experiments revealed that cytarabine and etoposide, if added to lethal doses of busulfan, are clearly inferior to cyclophosphamide in their ability to promote the engraftment of allogeneic bone marrow [9, 10]. The experiments described here show that melphalan, thiotepa and carboplatin should be used with caution as substitutes for cyclophosphamide in preparation for transplantation of T-cell-depleted or HLA-mismatched bone marrow. Their potential for preventing rejection of allogeneic bone marrow was clearly inferior to that of cyclophosphamide. BCNU, and especially ACNU, gave much better results. The most potent immunosuppression was provided by ifosfamide, which proved equivalent to cyclophosphamide in equitoxic doses. Accordingly, these latter three drugs might be suitable candidates for conditioning of recipients of allogeneic bone marrow who bear an increased risk of rejection.

References

1. Patterson J, Prentice HG, Brenner MK, Gilmore M, Janossy G, Ivory K, Skeggs D, Morgan H, Lord J, Blacklock HA, Hoffbrand AV, Apperley JF, Goldman JM, Burnett A, Gribben A, Alcorn M, Pearson C, Mcvickers I, Hann IM, Reid C, Wardle D, Gravett PJ, Bacigalupo A, Robertson AG (1986) Graft rejection following HLS matched T-lymphocyte depleted bone marrow transplantation. BR J Haematol 63: 221–230
2. Tutschka PJ, Santos GW (1975) Bone marrow transplantation in the busulfan-treated rat. Transplantation 20: 101–106
3. Harada M, Yoshida T, Funada H, Hattori K-I for the Kanazawa University Bone Marrow Transplant Team (1984) Clinical trial of intensive therapy and autologous bone marrow transplantation in the treatment of malignant diseases. Jpn J Clin Oncol 14 [Suppl 1]: 543–552
4. Carella AM, Congiu AM, Gaozza E, Ricci P, Visani G, Meloni G, Cimino G, Mangoni L, Coser P, Cetto GL, Cimino R, Alessandrio EP, Brusamolino E, Santini G, Tura S, Mandelli F, Rizzoli V, Bernasconi C, Marmont AM (1988) High-dose chemotherapy with autologous bone marrow transplantation in 50 advanced Hodgkin's disease patients: an Italian study group report. J Clin Oncol 6: 1411–1416
5. Lazarus HM, Reed MD, Spitzer TR, Rabaa MS, Blumer JL (1987) High-dose iv thiotepa and cryopreserved autologous bone marrow transplantation for therapy of refractory cancer. Cancer Treat Rep 71: 689–695
6. Powles RL, Milliken S, Helenglass G, Treleavan J, Pinkerton R, Zuiable A, Nandi A, Aboud H, Millar J (1989) The use of melphalan in conjunction with total body irradiation as treatment for acute leukaemia. Transplant Proc 21: 2955–2957
7. Nichols CR, Tricot G, Williams SD, van Besien K, Loehrer PJ, Roth BJ, Akard L, Hoffman R, Goulet R, Wolff SN, Gianonne L, Greer J, Einhorn LH, Jansen J (1989) Dose-intensive chemotherapy in refractory germ cell cancer – a phase I/II trial of high-dose carboplatin and etoposide with autologous bone marrow transplantation. J Clin Oncol 7: 932–939
8. Shea TC, Flaherty M, Elias A, Eder JP, Antman K, Begg C, Schnipper L, Frei EIII, Henner WD (1989) A phase I clinical and pharmacokinetic study of carboplatin and autologous bone marrow support. J Clin Oncol 7: 651–661
9. Gassmann W, Uharek L, Wottge HU, Schmitz N, Loeffler H, Mueller-Ruchholtz W (1988) Comparison of cyclophosphamide, cytarabine, and etoposide as immunosuppressive agents before allogeneic bone marrow transplantation. Blood 72: 1574–1579
10. Schmitz N, Gassmann W, Rister M, Johannson W, Suttorp M, Brix F, Holthuis JJ, Heit W, Hertenstein B, Schaub J, Loeffler H (1988) Fractionated total body irradiation and high-dose VP 16–213 followed by allogeneic bone marrow transplantation in advanced leukemias. Blood 72: 1567–1573

Impact of Total Body Irradiation and Marrow Transplantation in Early and Advanced Leukemia*

F. Frassoni

Introduction and Background

The treatment of leukemia, as for other neoplastic diseases, faces the problem that chemotherapy does not act selectively on neoplastic cells and does not spare their normal counterparts. However, a high proportion of acute leukemias are sensitive to a given "induction treatment" and enter so-called complete remission (CR) [1].

How does remission occur? Once chemotherapy (CT) is administered the marrow of the patient is monitored to see whether marrow aplasia has been achieved: this mainly because the aplasia signifies that the vast majority of blasts have disappeared. It is therefore assumed that marrow aplasia is a necessary factor although not sufficient to achieve CR [2]. If remission is going to be achieved after approximately 20 days the marrow is populated by maturing cells of various hemopoietic lineages. The question is then: what are these cells and where do they originate? It has generally been accepted that the marrow of CR originates from residual normal bone marrow (NBM) cells. It can be concluded that after CT, when marrow aplasia is achieved, the normal bone marrow has a proliferative advantage as compared to the leukemic cells: without this property we would never had

the possibility to put a patient into CR. In recent years the concept of heterogeneity of the cell composition within a tumor has been expanding. In addition, new available techniques have revealed that in some cases part or the majority of the "normally" maturing cells are "clonal" with the leukemic cells. This has ended with a new definition of "clonal remission" [3]. This has a tremendous impact on the management of leukemia. (1) Some cells belonging to the leukemic clone can mature as well as the normal cells do. (2) Many of the situations which we define as remission are not true remissions. Therefore the statement, after CT and marrow aplasia the NBM has a growth advantage (temporary) over leukemic cells, should be motified to: not only do NBM cells have a growth advantage but also those leukemic cells which are similar to normal ones, i.e., those subclones that can mature. This is the hypothesis [4]. It is noteworthy that in chronic myeloid leukemia (CML) the possibility of inducing lasting CR is very unlikely [5]: this probably because the CML cells in CP are very similar to the normal ones [4]. Therefore the achievement of complete remission is dependent upon the following:

1. leukemic cells should be sensitive to a given drug combination,
2. marrow aplasia should be achieved,
3. normal bone marrow cells must be present in the system in a sufficient number and quality in order to regrow faster than leukemic cells.

The CR lasts for a given period but in the great majority of cases relapse occurs. At

* This work was supported by the Associazione Italiana per la Ricerca sul Cancro (A.I.R.C.) Milano – Italia.

Centro Trapianti Midollo Osseo, Divisione Ematologia, Ospedale San Martino, Genova, Italy

this stage the induction of a new CR might still be possible but the length of a new CR is shorter than the first one, and subsequently the disease becomes resistant and CR is no longer achieved [1]. In addition there are leukemias which are refractory to the induction treatment. The first question is why resistance occurs? Namely why are there leukemias which are chemosensitive and others which are chemoresistant? Is it the leukemic cell itself that is more or less sensitive to a given chemotherapeutic agent or is it the environment which is different, or both? For example, myelodysplastic syndromes are unlikely to enter CR because it is assumed that there are no more normal bone marrow cells spared.

Bone marrow transplantation (BMT) provides a situation in which the marrow aplasia is obtained by a more aggressive treatment of the host marrow without taking into consideration the residual NBM because a healthy NBM is provided by the donor. There is no question that the TBI and BMT greatly modify the environment. CR is very difficult to achieve in CML although there is evidence that some Ph-negative cells exist in many patients [2, 6, 7]. However, after allogeneic BMT a long-lasting remisson (cure) can be obtained. An extremely important observation has emerged from autologous BMT for CML [8]. Using the chronic phase (CP) cryopreserved cells (which were 100% Ph positive) a transient take of Ph-negative cells has been obtained. This suggests that the few Ph-negative cells (which were so diluted as to be undetectable by cytogenetics) have found a favorable microenvironnement and have repopulated the marrow faster than the Ph-positive cells [4].

There is no doubt that after allogeneic BMT the chance of remaining in CR is by far more probable than after any other treatment. This is due to the fact that, in terms of leukemic cell killing, the conditioning regimen used in BMT is superior to any other consolidation or intensification chemotherapy schedule. It should be pointed out that there is a constellation of data indicating that a consistent number of residual host cells (including leukemic and nonleukemic cells) remain alive after the BMT-conditioning regimen. In fact one of

reduced risk of relapse is the graft-versus-the factors found to be associated with the host activity [9, 10, 11].

It intriguing that the pheneotype of leukemia (at least in AML) turns out to be relevant as far as relapse is concerned. If the cells which sustain leukemia are pluripotent stem cells, the phenotypic expression of the majority of the cells we observe at the onset or at relapse (representing a progeny of the stem cells) should be irrelevant to the treatment response. But this is not the case: at least in the IBMTR data M4 and M5 have a higher chance of relapsing than M1, M2, and M3. So far there has not been a ready explanation for this fact [12].

Data concerning an analysis of patients grafted in the bone marrow transplant center in Genoa from 1982 to 1990 are presented. The analysis will focus on the effect of a protocol of TBI which has been used either for early or advanced disease in AML and CML. Furthermore the effect of the variations of the TBI dose within the same TBI schedule will be discussed.

Patients and Methods

All patients entered in this study received non-T-cell-depleted allograft from their HLA-identical siblings in the bone marrow transplant center of Genoa. Acute myeloid leukemia in first remission and chronic myeloid leukemia in chronic phase were considered early disease (ED); any other phase was considered advanced disease (AD).

Conditioning

Both 97 acute myeloid leukemia (AML) patients ($n=84$ first CR and $n=13$ in advanced disease) and 62 CML patients ($n=43$ in first CP and $n19$ in advanced disease) were conditioned with the same protocol: 60 mg/kg per day on day -7, -6, followed by fractionated total body irradiation (TBI) of 330 cGy on each of three consecutive days (-3, -2, -1) using a single source of cobalt -60 for a total scheduled dose of 990 cGy. The TBI was delivered with the patient in the lateral position, half a dose per side with a horizontal beam at 3m source-axis distance. A lead shield was used to reduce overdosage to the eyes, mouth and lungs. The lungs were shielded to receive the same dose of the prescription point.

Total Body Irradiation Dose

A retrospective analysis of the total received dose of TBI, carried out by dosimetric recordings, indicated that 70 patients (30 AML in first CR and 8 in AD; 19 CML in first CP and 13 in AD) received less than 990 cGY and 72 patients (36 AML in first CR and 5 in AD; 16 CML in first CP and 15 in AD) received more than 990 cGy. This difference between the two series of doses in cGy is significant ($p=0.0001$). The variation of the total dose was $\pm$ 18% (range 820–1185 cGy). Because of the uncertain measurements, the data were recorded without considering possible corrections for the dose. A retrospective evaluation of the measurement revealed the correlation reported in these results: this suggests that the measurements were reliable. The median TBI dose for patients receiving more than 990 cGy was 1038 cGy (1042 cGy for AML and 1019 cGy for CML) while the median TBI dose for patients receiving less than 990 cGy was 915 cGy (909 cGy for AML and 923 cGy for CML). There was no correlation between TBI dose and time of relapse after BMT. The distribution of age, sex, diagnosis and FAB classification for AML was no different in patients receiving more or less than 990 cGy. Patients receiving T-cell-depleted grafts were excluded from this analysis.

Results and Discussion

Effect of Diseases Status

The actuarial relapse incidence at 8 years was 31% for patients ($n=127$) grafted in early disease and 54% for patients ($n=32$) grafted in advanced disease ($p=0.001$). For CML patients the actuarial relapse incidence was 13% and 44% at 3 years and 28% and 63% ($p=0.001$) at 8 years for patients grafted in chronic phase or in advanced disease respectively. For AML patients the actuarial relapse incidence was 34% and 38% for patients grafted in first remission or in advanced disease respectively.

Effect of TBI Dose

Early Disease. The actuarial probability of relapse for patients (30 AML+19 CML) receiving <1000 cGy was 56% while for patients (36 AML, 16 CML) receiving >1000 cGy it was 12% at 8 years ($p=0.004$). In AML in first CR only, the probability of relapse at 8 years was 20% and 50% respectively ($p=0.01$) for patients receiving more and less than 1000 cGy. For CML in first CP only, the probability of relapse at 8 years was 52% and 0% respectively for patients receiving less and more than 1000 cGy ($p=0.001$).

Advanced disease. The actuarial probability of relapse for patients (8 AML+13 CML) receiving less than 1000 cGy was 69% while for patients (5 AML+15 CML) receiving more than 1000 cGy it was 37% at 8 years.

Early+Advanced Disease. The actuarial probability of relapse was 21% and 53% for patients receiving more ($n=67$ patients) and less ($n=62$ patients) than 1000 cGy respectively ($p=0.0003$). For the two groups of patients the actuarial survival at 8 years was 60% and 36% respectively ($p=0.03$). From these data it comes out clearly that the transplant-related mortality was higher in patients receiving higher doses of TBI. This indicates that even small variations in the dose of TBI, within a TBI schedule which is among the mildest used, can produce detrimental effects on tissues other than bone marrow.

Allogeneic Effect of NBM

There is no doubt that donor bone marrow obstructs the regrowth of host marrow and consequently counteracts the possible proliferation of leukemic cells. This is best

539

supported by the higher relapse rate in allografts performed with T-cell depletion [13] and data concerning the incidence of mixed chimerism [14]. The presence of acute and chronic GvHD seems to be correlated with reduced risk of relapse [9, 10]. However, data concerning the patients included in this study show a reduced risk of relapse associated only with severe chronic GvHD: this holds true either for early and advanced disease ($p=0.001$).

It is of interest to note that this analysis, although carried out in a limited number of patients, comes from a single center and that all patients have been treated with the same schedule. It must be pointed out that in all studies the concept of eradication is not absolute but applies only in the operational situation where an allogeneic marrow is infused after chemoradiotherapy. Moreover, to some extent, this applies also to chemotherapy: to obtain a complete remission normal bone marrow is needed as stated earlier on in this paper.

Conclusions

1. The impact of BMT on relapse incidence is greatly affected by the disease status: this is mainly observed in CML. However, other studies have shown a more important role of the disease stage also for AML [13].
2. Total body irradiation dose has a major effect on both early and on advanced disease. This suggests that the resistance acquired with the progression of the disease can be, in part, overcome with the appropriate TBI dose. However, as the disease advances, it becomes more resistant to TBI and BMT than to chemotherapy. How can we put these data together. One can speculate that at the onset of the disease the majority of leukemias have few cells with a high proliferative potential. At the time of relapse (namely at any given opportunity to proliferate) the number of leukemic cells with a high proliferative potentiality is increased. In this way the number of cells that have to be knocked down by chemo- and radiotherapy is increased.
3. Chronic myeloid leukemia is a peculiar

disease: it is not easily treated with an acute leukemia like treatment but after TBI and non-T-depleted BMT the incidence of relapse is very limited. In this case the two approaches (chemotherapy vs. TBI and BMT) have a totally different impact on the disease. However with T-cell depletion the relapse rate is very high. Once the CML becomes AD the relapse rate after BMT increses dramatically.

4. It is clear from this analysis that increasing the dose of TBI is associated with a reduced incidence of relapse. This indicates that with a higher TBI dose one can kill a higher number of target leukemic cells: this besides the allogeneic graft-versus-leukemia effect. In fact the TBI dose came out to be the most important factor for the prevention of relapse in a multivariate analysis [16, 17]. In addition a direct correlation was found between TBI dose and the incidence/severity of chronic graft-versus-host disease which also correlated inversely with the recurrence of leukemia [16]. This raises several questions about the significance of the correlation between graft-versus-host disease and prevention of relapse [15].
5. While few relapses occurred in patients receiving more than 990 cGy, a more complex situation was observed in patients receiving less than 990 cGy [16]. It was therefore interesting to analyze in detail why some patients receiving less than 990 cGy relapsed and some did not. Indeed a dose effect was still seen in patients receiving less than 990 cGy in CML but not in AML. This may reflect a heterogeneity among the radiosensitivity of various acute myelogenous leukemias. It is also possible that some AML patients could have already been cured by previous chemotherapy before BMT. The impact of allogeneic bone marrow transplant on leukemias reproduced to some extent the features of chemotherapy but in many aspects BMT is totally different. From the data presented one can conclude that increasing the dose of TBI a good proportion of leukemias can be controlled in either early or advanced disease [16]. However, what are the

consequences of increasing the dose of TBI? It has recently been reported [18] that increasing the dose of TBI from 1200 cGy to 1575 cGy has a beneficial effect on relapse rate but a detrimental effect on survival. In contrast with this report [18], the observed variations in the TBI dose, within our protocol, did not have major effects on the transplant-related mortality but only on survival [15]: indeed a higher dose correlated not only with lower relapse rate but also with a better survival, 60 % vs. 36 %.

It should be noted that a fractionated TBI consisting of 330×3 cGy represents a dose which is radiobiologically lower than the dose reported in the study by Clift et al. [18]. It is likely that our TBI protocol (330 cGy $\times 3$) represents a threshold dose: small variations have major effects on the hemopoietic but not on other tissues [15]. Indeed in our protocol the incidence of interstitial pneumonitis is 5 %. We are aware that this regimen is possibly associated with a higher incidence of relapse which can be avoided by giving a correct dose of at least 990 cGy. This prospective study is ongoing and, although the follow-up is short, results are promising both in terms of relapse and survival.

References

1. Rohatiner ZS, Lister TA (1990) The treatment of acute myelogenous leukemia. In: Henderson ES, Lister TA (eds) Leukemia. Saunders, Philadelphia, p 485
2. Frassoni F, Repetto M, Prodestà M et al. (1986) Competitive survival/proliferation of normal and Ph1 positive haematopoietic cells. Br J Haematol 63: 135–141
3. Fearon ER, Burke PJ, Shiffer CA et al. (1986) Differentiation of leukemic cells to polymorphonuclear leukocytes in patients with acute nonlymphocytic leukemia. N Engl J Med 315: 15–24
4. Frassoni F, Sessarego M, Bacigalupo A et al. (1988) Competition between recipient and donor cells after bone marrow transplantation for chronic myeloid leukaemia. Br J Haematol 69: 471–475
5. Cunninghan I, Gee T, Dowling M et al. (1979) Results of treatment of Ph+ chronic myelogenous leukemia: with an intensive

6. Coloumbel L, Kalousek DK, Eaves CJ et al. (1983) Long-term culture reveals chromosomally norma hemopoietic progenitors cells in patients with Philadelphia-chromosome positive chronic myelogenous leukemia. N Engl J Med 304: 700–704
7. Turhan AG, Humphries RK, Eaves CJ et al. (1990) Detection of breakpoint cluster region-negative and nonclonal hematopoiesis in vitro and vivo after transplantation of cells selected in cultures of chronic myeloid leukemia marrow. Blood 76: 2404–2410
8. Goldman JM (1991) Use of autologous stem cells in support of the intensive treatment of chronic myeloid leukemia, vol 13. In: Deisseroth AB, Arlinghaus RB (eds) Dekker, New York, p 455
9. Sullivan KM, Weiden PL, Storb R et al. (1989) Influence of acute and chronic graft-versus-host disease on relapse and survival after bone marrow transplantation from HLA-identical siblings as treatment of acute and chronic leukemia. Blood 73: 1720–1728
10. Horowitz MM, Gale RP, Sondel PM et al. (1990) Graft-versus-leukemia reactions after marrow transplantation. Blood 75: 555–562
11. Marmont AM, Horowitz MM, Gale PR et al. (1991) T-cell depletion of HLA-identical transplants in leukemia. To be published
12. International Bone Marrow Transplant Registry (1989) Transplant or chemotherapy in acute myelogenous leukaemia? Lancet i: 1119–1121
13. Clift RA, Buckner CD, Thomas ED et al. (1987) The treatment of acute non-lymphoblastic leukemia by allogeneic marrow transplantation. Bone Marrow Transplant 2: 243–258
14. Goldman JM, Gale RP, Horowitz MM et al. (1988) Bone marrow transplantation for chronic myelogenous leukemia in chronic phase. Increased risk of relapse associated with T-cell depletion. Ann Intern Med 108: 806–814
15. Frassoni F, Sessarego M, Strada P et al. (1990) Mixed chimerism after marrow transplantation for leukaemia: correlation with dose of total body irradiation and graft-verus-host disease. Bone Marrow Transplant 5: 235–240
16. Frassoni F, Scarpati D, Bacigalupo A et al. (1989) The effect of total body irradiation dose and chronic GvHD on leukaemic relapse incidence after allogeneic bone marrow transplantation. Br J Haematol 73: 211–216

treatment regimen (L-5 protocol). Blood 53: 375–394

17. Scarpati D, Frassoni F, Vitale V et al. (1989) Total body irradiation in acute myeloid leukemia and chronic myelogenous leukemia: influence of dose and dose-rate on leukemia relapse. Int J Radiat Oncol Biol Phys 17: 547–552

18. Clift RA, Buckner CD, Appelbaum FR et al. (1990) Allogeneic marrow transplantation in patients with acute leukemia in first remission: a randomized trial of two irradiation regimens. Blood 76: 1867–1871

High-Dose ARA-C, Cyclophosphamide and Etoposide with Noncryopreserved Autologous Bone Marrow Transplantation in Acute Myeloid Leukemia in Remission: A Pilot Study

H. Köppler, K. H. Pflüger, M. Wolf, M. Klausmann, and K. Havemann

Introduction

Conventional chemotherapy regimens produce 60 %–70 % complete remissions (CR) in patients with acute myeloid leukemia (AML). Long-term survival, however, is poor due to a high relapse rate. In most trials the long-term disease-free survival is in the range of 10 %–20 % [1–5]. Strategies to stabilize remission include maintenance therapy, early or late intensification or ablative forms of therapy with allogeneic or autologous bone marrow transplantation. While maintenance therapy gives a statistically significant but only small advantage in disease-free survival [1, 2], the role of intensification with conventional chemotherapy as double induction or late intensification has not been clearly established. Initial results show an increased number of disease-free survivors [6–8]. Increased long-term survival has been achieved with ablative therapies and allogenic bone marrow transplantation resulting in 5-year disease-free survival between 40 % and 50 % [9, 10]. This approach, however, is limited to patients <45 years with an HLA-identical related donor.

Recently similar results have been achieved in studies using ablative therapies with autologous bone marrow as a source for hematopoietic reconstitution [11–16]. Results of these studies, however, are difficult to interpret because of different conditioning regimens, timing of transplant and the use of purging procedures. We report the results of a prospective phase I–II trial in which 16 consecutive patients who achieved CR with a standardized induction and consolidation regimen were treated with escalating doses of ara-C, cyclophosphamide and etoposide combined with autologous noncryopreserved bone marrow transplantation.

Patients and Methods

Patients

Sixteen consecutive patients aged <65 years with AML who had achieved CR after one or two cycles of the TAD 9 regimen [1] were consolidated with the same regimen and then treated with high-dose chemotherapy and ABMT. Median time from CR to ABMT was 2 months (range 1–5 months). Median age was 45 years (range 25–63 years). Age, sex, FAB classification, prior chemotherapy and time from CR to ABMT are shown in Table 1. Additionally four patients with AML in second or subsequent CR were treated with high-dose chemotherapy and ABMT.

Bone Morrow Procurement and Reinfusion

The technique of bone marrow harvesting has been described elsewhere [17]. The heparinized whole bone marrow was stored in bone marrow collection containers with 10 % $CPDA_1$ (Bone Marrow Collection Kit,

Department of Hematology, Philipps University, 3550 Marburg, FRG

Table 1. Patient characteristica

Pa-tient	Age/sex	FAB	Status	Cycles to CR	Induction/Consolidation	Interval CR → ABMT months	Number of ABMTs	CR duration after ABMT (months)
1	25/M	4	CR1	1	TAD × 2	4	1	11
2	43/F	5	CR1	1	TAD × 2	1	1	8
3	49/F	5	CR1	1	TAD × 2	1	1	36+
4	41/M	4	CR1	1	TAD × 2	2	2	30+
5	63/F	5	CR1	2	TAD × 2. AD × 1	1	1	10
6	51/M	1	CR1	2	TAD × 3	2	2	8
7	47/M	4	CR1	2	TAD × 2. AD × 1	5	1	8
8	55/F	4	CR1	1	TAD × 2	1	2	24+
9	55/F	5	CR1	2	TAD × 3	5	1	3
10	33/M	5	CR1	2	TAD × 3	5	1	5
11	40/F	2	CR1	1	TAD × 2	1	1	5
12	54/M	1	CR1	1	TAD × 2	1	2	15+
13	23/F	4	CR1	2	TAD × 3	2	1	2
14	40/M	1	CR1	2	TAD × 3	2	2	4+
15	52/M	2	CR1	2	TAD × 3	3	1	4+
16	33/F	4	CR1	2	TAD × 3	3	1	3+
17	56/F	2	CR2	1	TAD × 2	2	1	0
18	22/F	5	CR2	1	VP16 / Mitox × 2	5	2	24+
19	44/F	5	CR2	1	TAD × 2	2	2	27+
20	41/F	2	CR3	2	HAM. Acla.. VP16	1	1	1

Baxter, Fenwal Division) for 48–72 h at 4 °C. Before reinfusion over a central line on day 0, the marrow was filtered through the three steel filters of the Bone Marrow Collection Kit to remove particles and aggregates. Previous studies have shown that liquid storage at 4 °C results in stem cell survival as determined by measuring CFU-GM, BFU-E, CFU-E and CFU-GEMM of 70 %–100 % after 72 h [18, 19].

High-Dose Chemotherapy

Patients 1–3 were treated with cytosine arabinoside 1000 mg/m² q 12 h × 5, cyclophosphamide 60 mg/kg day –2, etoposide 800 mg/m² days –2, –1. Patients 4–6 were treated with cytosine arabinoside 1000 mg/m² 912 h × 6, cyclophosphamide 60 mg/kg day –2, etoposide 700 mg/m² days –3, –2, –1. Patients 7–20 were treated with cytosine arabinoside 1000 mg/m² q 12 h × 6, cyclophosphamide 60 mg/kg days –3, –2, etoposide 700 mg/m² days –3, –2, –1. Cytosine arabinoside and cyclophosphamide

were infused over 60 min and etoposide over 30 min.

Statistical Analysis

Survival probabilities were calculated according to the actuarial method of Kaplan and Meier [20].

Results

Hematopoietic Reconstitution and Toxicity

Sixteen patients in first CR and four patients in second or subsequent CR were treated with ACE and noncyropreserved bone marrow transplantation. Seven of 20 patients received a double transplantation with the same regimen. A median number of 1.5 × 10⁸ nucleated cells per kilogram body weight (range 1.0–3.1 × 10⁸ kg) were reinfused. Eighteen evaluable patients had a full hematopoietic reconstitution. Median time to achieve 500 neutrophils/µl was 18 days (range 12–26 days). Median time to achieve an unsupported platelet count of 20 000/µl was 15 days (range 10–22 days). One patient in second CR (No. 17) died on day +7 from progressive cardiac failure. One patient in third CR died from intracerebral hemorrhage on day + 45 after having reconstituted neutrophils (1500/l) but still being transfusion dependent on platelets. No difference in terms of reconstitution was observed between patients in the three escalative steps or between first and second transplantation. Toxicity of the procedure is shown in Table 2. Besides patient No. 17, another patient in second CR suffered from cardiac failure after transplantation. No other severe or life-threatening toxicity was observed.

Outcome

Nine of 16 patients treated in first CR relapsed with a median of 8 months (range 2–11 months) after ABMT. Seven patients remain in CR 3+, 4+, 4+, 15+, 24+, 30+, 36+ months after ABMT. The projected disease-free survival at 36 months is 32 % (Fig. 1). Two of four patients in second CR remain in CR 24+ and 27+ months after ABMT.

Discussion

The best postremission therapy for patients with AML is a continuing controversial issue. The few prospective studies comparing allogeneic bone marrow transplantation (BMT) versus autologous bone marrow transplantation versus conventional chemotherapy suggest that allogeneic bone marrow transplantation achieves the best relapse-free survival [21–24]. This approach however is limited to patients <45 years with an HLA-identical-related donor. The majority of patients depend on alternative treatment modalities. Recently intensive chemotherapy +/– TBI with ABMT has produced relapse-free survival rates up to 60 % at 3 years [11–16, 25–28]. Analysis of these data, however, reveals that results are

Table 2. Toxicity

Side effects	Patients with Who grade	
	3	4
Nausea/vomiting	20/20	–
Mucositis	5/20	2/20
Diarrhea	5/20	–
Hemorrhagic cystitis	1/20	–
Cardiac failure	1/20	1/20

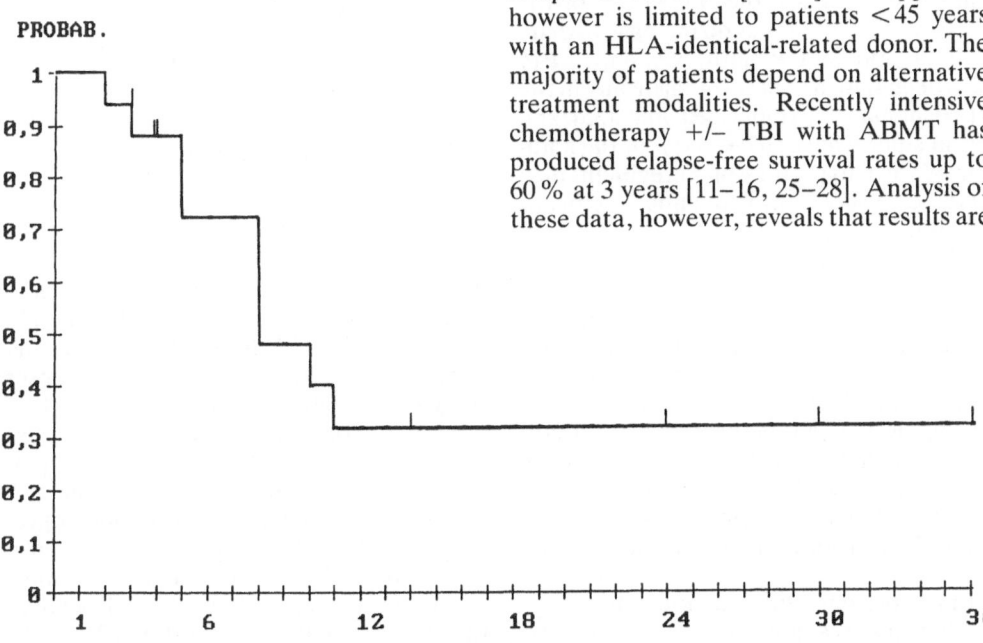

Fig. 1. Relapse-free survival of 16 patients transplanted in first remission. The projected relapse-free survival is 32 % at 36 months

strongly related to timing of transplantation [29] and patients transplanted within 6 months after CR have relapse rates of up to 70%. The high relapse rates in patients receiving allogeneic T-cell-depleted or syngeneic marrow indicate that the major antileukemic effect of allgeneic BMT is mediated by graft versus leukemia events and that the standard conditioning cyclophosphamide + TBI is not sufficient in this aspect. More effective antileukemic treatment is needed.

The aim of the present study has been to investigate a new preparative regimen with intermediate-dose cytosine arabinoside (ara-C), high-dose cyclophosphamide (Cy) and etoposide (VP16). The rationale for combining ara-C, VP16 and Cy was derived from preclinical in vitro data and clinical observations with high-dose Cy and VP16. Ara-C is one of the major antileukemic agents with a characteristic steep dose response curve in vitro [30, 31]. Studies in relapsed or refractory AML produce high response rates with high-dose ara-C [32, 33]. Recent data, however, indicate that, due to the limited intracellular conversion to ara-C, monophosphate doses above 1 g/m do not increase the conversion of the active derivates [34] but do increase toxicity without apparent benefit. Cy and VP16 have been shown to act synergistically in the HL60 human leukemia cell line [35] and recent studies have suggested that the addition of VP16 to pretransplant regimens may increase the antileukemic efficacy [36–38].

The use of liquid-stored bone marrow for hematopoetic reconstitution was safe and all evaluable patients had a rapid engraftment. One patient in third CR died 45 days after ABMT from intracerebral hemorrhage. At this time she had a reconstituted myelopoiesis (2500 neutrophil/μl) but still needed platelet support. Bone marrow aspiration showed an active myelopoiesis but no megakaryocytes, suggesting a delayed reconstitution or an autoimmune process.

In the present study the nonhematological toxicity was low and not treatment-limiting in any escalation step. This was also true for patients undergoing a double transplantion with the same regimen. In contrast to protocols with single short-term VP-16 infusions [37, 39] or continuous infusions [38] no severe mucositis, liver dysfunction, pulmonary toxicity or neurotoxicity was observed with the 3-day intermediate-dose short-term infusions. Two patients in second CR suffered from cardiac failure which was fatal in one patient 7 days after first ABMT. The second patient who presented with cardiac failure WHO grade 3, 4 weeks after second ABMT, is alive and well but is dependent on treatment with captopril. Both patients had a high cumulative anthracycline dose and had already been at risk for cardiomyopathy.

Though the number of patients in our study is small, the relapse-free survival for patients in first remission in this in all respects unselected patient group is promising and in the range reported in other prospective trials with unselected patients [21, 22]. As reported by other groups [40] patients undergoing double transplantation seem to benefit from this approach as compared to patients with a single transplantion. The small numbers, however, preclude any final conclusion. We conclude that high-dose ACE with noncryopreserved bone marrow transplantation is a safe procedure. The lack of toxicity and the preliminary follow-up data suggest a useful efficacy, making this straightforward to perform approach suitable for comparative studies with conventional chemotherapy.

Summary

Twenty patients with acute myeloid leukemia (AML) in remission (CR), (16 patients in first CR, four patients in second CR) were treated with escalating high doses of cytosine arabinoside (1000 mg/m^2 q12 h × 5–6), cyclophosphamide (60–120 mg/kg) and etoposide (1600–2100 mg/m^2) combined with an autologous bone marrow transplantation (ABMT) with noncryopreserved marrow. Seven patients received a double transplantation with the same protocol within 6 weeks of first ABMT. Median time between CR and ABMT was 2 months (range 1–5 months). All evaluable patients showed a rapid and full hematopoietic reconstitution. Nonhematological toxicity was low for patients in first CR with moderate nausea/vomiting, mild mucositis and diarrhea. Two patients with heavy anthracycline pretreatment in second CR suffered from cardiac failure, which was fatal in one patient 7 days after ABMT. One patient in third CR died on day +45 from intracerebral hemorrhage having reconstituted neutrophils but not platelets.

Seven of 16 patients transplanted in first CR remain in CR with a median of 18 months (range 3–36 months). Two patients in second CR are free of disease 24+ and 27+ months after ABMT. We conclude that high-dose ACE with noncryopreserved ABMT is a safe procedure with low toxicity and preliminary data suggest a useful efficacy.

References

1. Büchner T, Urbanitz D, Hiddemann W et al. (1985) Intensified induction and consolidation with or without maintenance chemotherapy for acute myeloid leukemia (AML): two multicenter studies of the German AML cooperative group. J Clin Oncol 3: 1583–1589
2. Rees JKH, Gray RG, Swirsky D, Hayhoe FGJ (1986) Principal results of the medical research council's 8th acute myeloid leukaemia trial. Lancet i: 1236–1241
3. Zittoun R, Jehn U, Fiere D et al. (1989) Alternating v repeated postremission treatment in adult acute myelogenous leukemia: a randomized phase III study (AML6) of the EORTC leukemia cooperative group. Blood 73: 896–906
4. Geller RB, Burke PJ, Karp JE et al. (1989) A two-step sequential treatment for acute myelocytic leukemia. Blood 74: 1499–1506
5. Brincker H, Christensen BE (1990) Long-term survival and late relapses in acute leukaemia in adults. Br J Haematol 74: 156–160
6. Mayer RJ, Weinstein JH, Coral FS et al. (1982) The role of intensive postinduction chemotherapy in the management of patients with acute myelogenous leukemia. Cancer Treat Rep 66: 1455–1462
7. Glucksberg H, Cheever MA, Farewell VT et al. (1983) Intensification therapy for acute nonlymphoblastic leukemia in adults. Cancer 52: 198–205
8. Champlin R, Gajewski J, Nimer S et al. (1990) Postremission chemotherapy for adults with acute myelogenous leukemia:
9. Clift RA, Buckner CD, Thomas ED et al. (1987) The treatment of acute non-lymphoblastic leukemia by allogeneic bone marrow transplantation. Bone Marrow Transplant 2: 243–258
10. European Group for Bone Marrow Transplantation (1988) Allogeneic bone marrow transplantation for leukaemia in Europe. Lancet i: 1379–1388
11. Goldstone AH, Anderson CC, Linch DC et al. (1986) Autologous bone marrow transplantation following high-dose chemotherapy for the treatment of adult patients with acute myeloid leukaemia. Br J Haematol 64: 529–537
12. Gorin NC, Herve P, Aegerter P et al. (1986) Autologous bone marrow transplantation for acute leukaemia in remission. Br J Haematol 64: 385–395
13. Calm IY. Herve P, Flesch M et al. (1986) Autologous bone marrow transplantation (ABMT) for acute leukaemia in complete remission: a pilot study of 33 cases. Br J Haematol 63: 457–470
14. Burnett AK. Watkins R, Maharaj D et al. (1984) Transplantation of unpurged autologous bone marrow in acute myeloid leukaemia in first remission. Lancet ii: 1068–1070
15. Löwenberg B, Abels J, Van Bekkum DW et al. (1984) transplantation of non purified autologous bone marrow in patients with AML in first remission. Cancer 54: 2840–2843
16. Stewart P, Buckner CD, Bensinger W et al. (1985) Autologous marrow transplantation in patients with acute non lymphocytic leukemia in first remission Exp Hematol 13: 267–272
17. Robinson WA, Hartmann DW, Mangalik A, Morton N, Joshi J (1981) Autologous non frozen bone marrow transplantation after intensive chemotherapy: a pilot study. Acta Haematol 66: 145–151
18. Mangalik A, Robinson WA, Drebing C, Hartmann D, Joshi JH (1979) Liquid storage of bone marrow. Exp Hematol 7 [Suppl 5]: 76–94
19. Lasky LC, MC Cullough J, Zanjani ED (1986) Liquid storage of unseparated human bone marrow. Transfusion 26: 331–334
20. Kaplan EL, Meier P (1958) Nonparametric estimation from incomplete observations. J Am Stat Assoc 53: 457–481
21. Löwenberg B, Verdonck LJ, Dekker AW et al. (1990) Autologous bone marrow transplantation in acute myeloid leukemia in first

improved survival with high-dose cytoarabine and daunorubicin consolidation treatment. J Clin Oncol 8: 1199–1206

remission: results of a Dutch prospective study. J Clin Oncol 8: 287–294

22. Reiffers J, Gaspard MH, Manraninchi D et al. (1989) Comparison of allogeneic or autologous bone marrow transplantation and chemotherapy in patients with acute myeloid leukaemia in first remission: a prospective controlled trial. Br J Haematol 72: 57–63

23. Zander AR, Keating M, Dicke K et al. (1988) A comparison of marrow transplantation with chemotherapy for adults with acute leukemia of poor prognosis in first remission. J Clin Oncol 6: 1548–1557

24. Conde E, Iriondo A, Rayon C et al. (1988) Allogeneic bone marrow transplantation versus intensification chemotherapy for acute myelogenous leukaemia in first remission: a prospective controlled trial. Br J Haematol 68: 219–226

25. Körbling M, Hunstein W, Fiedner TM et al. (1989) Disease-free survival after autologous bone marrow transplantation in patients with acute myelogenous leukemia. Blood 74: 1898–1904

26. Beelen DW, Quabeck K, Graeven U et al. (1989) Acute toxicity and first clinical results of intensive postinduction therapy using a modified busulfan and cyclophosphamide regimen with autologous bone marrow rescue in first remission of acute myeloid leukemia. Blood 74: 1507–1516

27. Meloni G, De Fabritiis P, Carella AM et al. (1990) Autologous bone marrow transplantation in patients with AML in first complete remission. Results of two different conditioning regimens after the same induction and consolidation therapy. Bone Marrow Transplant 5: 29–32

28. Spinolo JA, Dicke KA, Horwitz LJ et al. (1990) Double intensification with amsarine/high-dose ara-C and high dose chemotherapy with autologous bone marrow transplantation produces durable remissions in acute myelogenous leukemia. Bone Marrow Transplant 5: 111–118

29. Gorin NC, Aegerter P, Auvert B et al. (1990) Autologous bone marrow transplantation for acute myelocytic leukemia in first remission: a European survey of the role of marrow purging. Blood 75: 1606–1614

30. McCullough EA, Buick RN, Curtis JE et al. (1981) The heritable nature of clonal characteristics in acute myeloblastic leukemia. Blood 58: 105–109

31. Cappizi TL, Yang JL, Rathmell JP et al. (1985) Dose related pharmacologic effects of high-dose ara-C and its self potentiation. Semin Oncol 12 [Suppl 2]: 65–75

32. Rudnick SA, Cadman EL, Capizzi RL et al. (1979) High-dose cytosine arabinoside (HDARAC) in refractory acute leukemia. Cancer 44: 1189–1193

33. Herzig RH, Wolff SN, Lazarus HM et al. (1983) High-dose cytosine arabinoside therapy for refractory leukemia. Blood 62: 361–369

34. Plunkett W, Liliemark JO, Adams TS et al. (1987) Saturation of 1-B-D-arabinofuranosylcytosine 5'-triphosphate in the leukemic cells from bone marrow and peripheral blood of patients receiving 1-B-D arabinofuranosylcytosine therapy. Cancer Res 47: 3005–3011

35. Chang TT, Glulati SC, Chou TC et al. (1985) Synergistic effect of 4-hydroperoxycyclophosphamide and etoposide on a human promyelocytic leukemia cell line (HL-60) demonstrated by computer analysis. Cancer Res 45: 2434–2439

36. Zander AR, Culbert S, Jagannath et al. (1987) High dose cyclophosphamide, BCNU and VP-16 (CVB) as a conditioning regimen for allogeneic bone marrow transplantation for patients with acute leukemia. Cancer 59: 1083–1086

37. Schmitz N, Gassmann W, Rister M et al. (1988) Fractionated total-body irradiation and high-dose VP16–213 followed by allogeneic bone marrow transplantation in advanced leukemias. Blood 72: 1567–1573

38. Bostrom B, Weisdorf DJ, Kim T, Kersey JH, Ramsay NKC (1990) Bone marrow transplantation for advanced acute leukemia: a pilot study of high-energy total body irradiation cyclophosphamide and continuous infusion etoposide. Bone Marrow Transplant 5: 83–89

39. Blume KG, Forman SJ, O'Donnenn MR et al. (1987) Total-body irradiation and high-dose etoposide: a new preparatory regimen for bone marrow transplantation in patients with advanced hematologic malignancies. Blood 69: 1015–1020

40. Gribben JG, Goldstone AH, Linch DC, Mc Millan AK, Richards JDM (1989) Double autologous bone marrow transplantation in acute myeloid leukemia. Bone Marrow transplant 4: [Suppl 1]: 209–211

Autologous Bone Marrow Transplantation in Patients with Acute Lymphoblastic Leukemia in Second or Subsequent Complete Remission

R. Haas[1], B. Dörken[1], E. Ogniben[1], S. Hohaus[1], B. Witt[1], G. Kvalheim[2], and W. Hunstein[1]

Introduction

With intensive conventional chemotherapy a complete remission (CR) can be achieved in more than 90 % of children and 70 % of adults with ALL [1]. The long-term disease-free survival for patients with ALL depends on certain prognostic factors [2]. As it has been shown by several investigators, high-risk patients can be defined on the basis of initial white blood count, age, the immunological phenotype of blast cells, the time to achieve CR after the induction phase of chemotherapy and by the presence of a Philadelphia chromosome. With respect to the therapeutic benefit of bone marrow transplantation (BMT) in high-risk ALL, the data of the International Bone Marrow Transplant Registry demonstrate that for allogeneic BMT the 5-year probability of disease-free survival (DFS) is 50 % in first complete remission (CR) versus 32 % in second CR [3]. Kersey et al. [4] reported a series of patients with high-risk ALL who were transplanted either in first or second CR. These patients demonstrated an overall disease-free survival of 20 % at 5 years post-BMT.

It was the purpose of our study to evaluate the therapeutic efficacy of ABMT in patients with ALL in second or subsequent CR. In nine patients the BMT was performed with mafosfamide purged bone

marrow (chemoseparation), whereas in the remaining nine patients the autograft was purged with monoclonal antibodies and immunomagnetic beads to remove residual tumor cells. All patients received the same pretransplant conditioning regimen. We compared the kinetics of hematopoietic reconstitution after ABMT, disease-free survival and relapse rate for these two patient groups.

Material and Methods

Patients

After informed consent was obtained, a total of 18 patients with ALL were included in this bone marrow transplantation protocol. All BMTs were performed either in second or subsequent CR following intensive conventional chemotherapy. In group I four patients were transplanted in third or higher CR compared to only two patients in group II. In nine patients (group I) the bone marrow was purged with mafosfamide, whereas the remaining nine patients received bone marrow treated with monoclonal antibodies and immunomagnetic beads. The patient characteristics are summarized in Table 1.

Bone Marrow Harvesting, Purging and Cryopreservation

The bone marrow was harvested by multiple aspirations from the posterior iliac crest. For the purging procedure with mafosfamide, a stable substitute of the

---

[1] Department of Internal Medicine V, University of Heidelberg, Hospitalstr. 3, 6900 Heidelberg, FRG
[2] The Norwegian Radium Hospital, Oslo, Norway

Table 1. Patient characteristics prior to ABMT

Group I (BM purged with mafosfamide)

Patient	Age/sex	Diagnosis	Date of initial diagnosis	No. of relapses	Duration of last CR prior to ABMT (days)
1	13/f	ALL[a]	09/75	2	216
2	31/m	c-ALL	07/83	2	73
3	20/m	T-ALL	10/82	1	416
4	22/m	c-ALL	11/84	1	211
5	23/f	O-ALL	10/86	1	136
6	26/m	c-ALL	02/82	2	96
7	48/m	ALL[a]	12/80	1	480
8	21/f	O-ALL	02/90	1	45
9	44/f	c-ALL	09/89	2	53

Group II (BM purged with moAb and immunomagnetic beads)

1	17/m	c-ALL	10/86	1	40
2	19/m	c-ALL	06/81	1	126
3	16/f	O-ALL	06/87	1	99
4	26/f	pre-B-ALL	01/76	1	247
5	15/m	c-ALL	11/88	1	32
6	24/f	ALL[a]	02/74	3	42
7	19/f	c-ALL	12/87	1	78
8	22/m	T-ALL	08/89	1	124
9	29/m	c-ALL	01/86	2	44

m, male; f, female; Immunophenotypes not done BM, bone marrow; moAb, monoclonal antibodies

activated primary metabolite of cyclophosphamide, the cell suspension was treated as previously described [5]. For the immunoseparation, the cell suspension was incubated with a cocktail of 3 monoclonal antibodies according to the immunophenotype of the leukemic blast cells (CD19, CD20, CD10 or CD2, CD5, CD7). After an incubation period of 30 min the cells were carefully washed and incubated with immunomagnetic beads (Dynabead M450, sheep-anti-mouse, IgGl, Fc). Thereafter, the cells bound to the monoclonal antibody/immunomagnetic beads were removed in a strong magnetic field and the remaining cells were collected from the blood bag in a constant flow rate of 40 ml/min by a peristaltic pump.

The cells were transferred into freezing bags (Delmed, Canton, MA) and frozen to −100 °C using a computer controlled cryopreservation device (Cryoson-BV-6; Cryoson Deutschland GmbH, FRG). The cells were transferred into the liquid phase of nitrogen and stored at −196 °C.

Pretransplant Conditioning Regimen

For all patients the myeloablative conditioning regimen consisted of TBI superfractionated over 4 days at doses of 1.2 Gy 3 ×/day to a total of 14.4 Gy (lungs 9.0 Gy) followed by 50 mg/kg body weight (bw) cyclophosphamide on each of 4 consecutive days (total dose: 200 mg/kg bw).

Results

Hematopoietic Reconstitution

The purging with mafosfamide caused a median reduction in the number of CFU-GM to 11.2 % (range: 1.6 %–58.7 %.) The median number of CFU-GM/kg bw infused into the patients following the treatment with mafosfamide was 1.1×10^3 (range: 0.2–13.2); see Table 2. The median number of TNC transfused/kg bw was 7.1×10^7 (range: 3.4–15.2). Due to one early death 10 days after ABMT eight patients could be

Table 2. Hematologic reconstitution and clinical status after ABMT

Patient No.	No. of cells infused		Time to reach			Status posttransplant (update: 31. Jan 91)	
	TNC x 10⁷/kg	CFU-GM x 10³/kg	WBC 1.0/nl (days)	PMN 0.5/nl (days)	Platelet 20.0/nl (days)	DFS (days)	Survival (days)
(BM purged with mafosfamide)							
1	15.2	13.2	16	18	23	206	268
2	10.3	0.3	n.r.	n.r.	n.r.	10	10
3	10.1	0.7	31	32	35	175	327
4	10.3	1.1	26	39	114	365	736
5	3.9	0.6	36	36	38	242	268
6	5.4	1.6	32	25	n.r.	89	122
7	5.7	2.7	28	39	29	135	135
8	7.1	0.2	27	26	45	55	67
9	3.4	1.3	52	53	67	76	76
Median	7.1	1.1	29.5	34	38		
Range	3.4–15.2	0.2–13.2	16–52	18–53	23–114		
(BM purged with moAb and immunomagnetic beads)							
1	6.6	0.4	57	54	48	1089+	1089+
2	2.5	3.7	23	33	44	1033+	1033+
3	7.3	cont.	30	37	55	816+	816+
4	8.6	5.7	24	40	36	606+	606+
5	6.8	9.9	54	49	63	501+	501+
6	10.1	15.7	32	32	34	448+	448+
7	17.1	17.5	29	41	35	273+	273+
8	5.9	2.2	n.r.	n.r.	n.r.	222	222
9	3.7	6.7	45	47	46	46	46+
Median	6.8	6.2	31	40.5	45		
Range	2.4–17	0.3–17.4	23–57	32–54	34–63		

TNC, total nucleated cells; CFU-GM, colony-forming unit granulocyte-macrophage; WBC, white blood count; PMN, polymorphonuclear count; DFS, disease-free survival; n.r., not reached; cont., contaminated; BM, bone marrow; moAb, monoclonal antibodies

evaluated for hematological recovery. All of them had a stable trilineage engraftment with subsequent hematopoietic reconstitution. A WBC of 1.0/nl was reached within 16–52 days (median: 29.5) and a PMN count of 0.5/nl within 18–53 days (median: 34). A stable platelet count of > 20/nl was observed after a median time of 38 days (range: 23–114). Reticulocytes appeared after 7–68 days (median: 13.5). For the patients autografted with bone marrow purged with monoclonal antibodies and immunomagnetic beads the median recovery of CFU-GM was 63% (range: 2.1%–310%). The median number of transplanted CFU-GM was 6.2 × 10³/kg bw (range: 0.3–17.4). With respect to the number of TNC the recovery after the immunoseparation was 73.2% (median, range:

36.4%–91.1%) and the total number of TNC/kg bw transfused was 6.8 × 10⁷ (median, range: 2.4–17). All patients demonstrated a stable trilineage engraftment with the following reconstitutional pattern: WBC >1.0/nl after 31 days (median, range: 23–57), PMN >0.5/nl after 40.5 days (median, range: 32–54) and stable platelet count of >20/nl after 45 days (median, range: 34–63). Reticulocytes appeared after 4–25 days (median: 6).

Early and Late Toxicity

Four of the 18 patients died of transplantation-related complications. In one patient a fatal gram-positive septicemia occurred 10 days after ABMT. The other patient died 76

551

days after BMT of acute respiratory distress syndrome. In this patient a postmortem lung biopsy demonstrated an interstitial pneumonitis, but no CMV or other viral infection could be documented. Another patient with delayed hematological recovery of cerebral hemorrhage due to thrombocytopenia 222 days after BMT. The fourth patient died of an encephalitis on day 135 post-transplantation.

In almost all patients a transient supraventricular tachycardia developed starting after high-dose cyclophosphamide which lasted approximately 2–3 weeks after ABMT. Furthermore, all patients developed fever within the first days after ABMT which dissolved in most of the patients after empirical administration of antibiotics. In case of antibiotics resistant fever amphotericin B was administered systemically.

Disease-Free Survival and Relapse Rate

In patient group I, three patients (No. 2, 7 and 9) died of transplantation related complications. The remaining six patients relapsed after a median time of 190.5 days (range: 55–365). The overall survival for the whole group of patients showed a median of 135 days (range 10–736). In patient group II, only one late treatment-related death (pat. No. 8) was observed 222 days after ABMT and one patient (No. 9) autografted in third CR relapsed 46 days after ABMT. The remaining seven patients are in unmaintained complete remission, with a median follow-up of 606 days (range: 273–1089) (Fig. 1).

Discussion

High-dose consolidation such as myeloablative chemo- and/or radiotherapy followed by ABMT provides a treatment modality for patients with high risk ALL [6]. It is still controversial whether purging for the removal of residual tumor cells from the autograft has an impact on disease-free survival and the rate of relapses [7]. Basically, two different purging procedures are available: chemoseparation with the in vitro active cyclophosphamide-derived mafosfamide and immunological targeting of tumor cells using specific monoclonal anti-

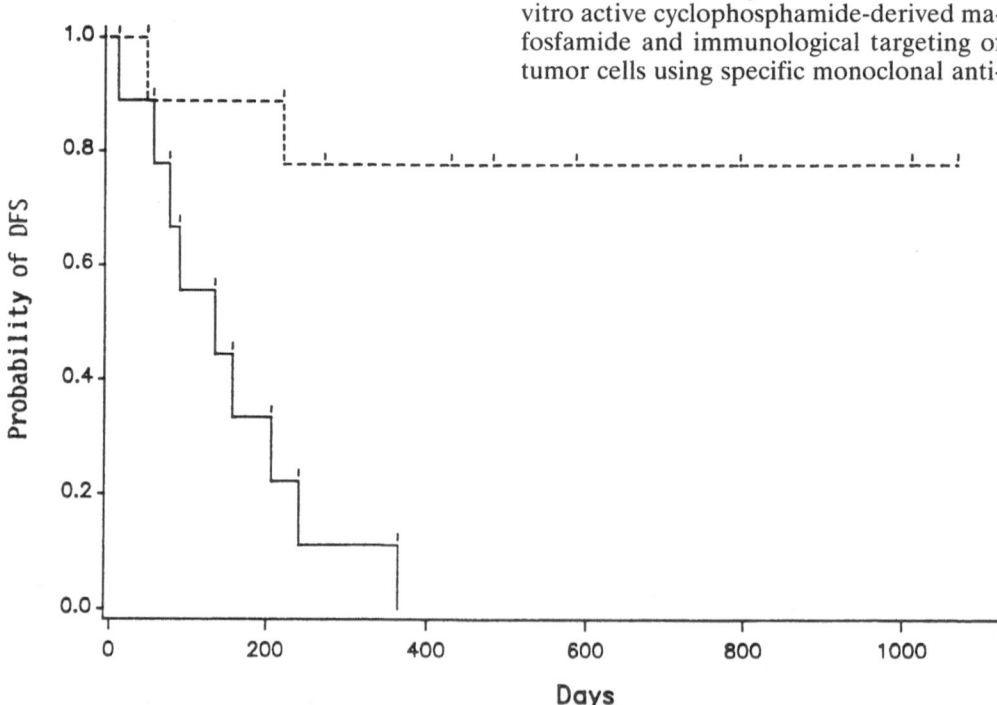

Fig. 1. Disease-free survival of patient group I (BM purged with mafosfamide, –) versus patient group II (BM purged with moAb and immunomagnetic beads, ----)

bodies. Among the different immunological purging procedures the use of immunomagnetic beads provides a standardized and most efficient technique for the removal of tumor cells [8].

In a preclinical study we have shown that the immunoseparation with a panel of B-cell antibodies and magnetic beads does not affect hemopoiesis as assessed by CFU-GM growth [8]. Based on these in vitro results we initiated an autologous BMT protocol with immunomagnetic bone marrow purging for patients with ALL in second or subsequent remission. Since January 1988 nine patients were autografted according to this ex vivo purging method. All patients demonstrated a stable trilineage engraftment. Although the median number of CFU-GM/kg bw transfused was substantially lower in the patient group I (mafosfamide purging) there was no difference between the two groups with respect to the kinetics of hematological reconstitution. One patient died of treatment-related late toxicity. Only one patient developed a relapse on day 46 after ABMT, whereas the remaining seven patients are in unmaintained complete remission after a median follow-up of 606 days (range: 273–1089). We compared these results to a group of nine patients with ALL in second or subsequent CR who were transplanted with bone marrow purged with mafosfamide. The patient groups are comparable with respect to sex and age distribution and prior conventional chemotherapy. However, four patients of group I were transplanted in third CR versus two patients in group II. Three patients died of transplantation related early or late toxicity and the remaining six patients relapsed after a median time of 190.5 days after ABMT.

In conclusion, our data suggest that ABMT with bone marrow purged by monoclonal antibodies and immunomagnetic beads offers a promising therapeutic alternative for high-risk ALL patients. The therapeutic value of this purging procedure has to be carefully assessed by molecular biological studies for the detection of minimal residual disease.

Summary

We evaluated the therapeutic efficacy of autologous bone marrow transplantation (ABMT) using bone marrow purged with either mafosfamide (group I) or with monoclonal antibodies (moAbs) and immunomagnetic beads (group II). A total of 18 patients with ALL in second or subsequent remission were autografted (9 patients in each group). Eight patients were female, ten patients were male. Their median age was 22 years (range: 13–48). The bone marrow was harvested after a median remission duration of 48 days (range: 5–383). The median duration of the last CR prior to ABMT was 97.5 days (range: 32–480). The myeloablative conditioning regimen consisted of TBI (14.4 Gy) and cyclophosphamide (200 mg/kg bw). Of the 18 patients, 16 patients are evaluable for hematological reconstitution. A WBC of 1.0/nl was reached on day 31 (median; range: 16–57), PMN count of 0.5/nl on day 38 (median; range: 18–54), and a platelet count of 20/nl on day 44 (median; range: 23–114). In group I, three patients died of transplantation-related complications, whereas the remaining six patients relapsed after 190.5 days (median, range: 55–365). In contrast, in patient group II one death was observed due to transplantation-related late toxicity and one patient relapsed 46 days after ABMT. Seven patients are in unmaintained CR, with a median follow-up of 606 days (range: 273–1089). Our data demonstrate that bone marrow purged with moAbs and immunomagnetic beads can be safely used as autograft following a myeloablative conditioning regimen. Furthermore, the high rate of disease-free survival in patient group II suggests a beneficial role of immunomagnetic bone marrow purging compared to the chemoseparation with mafosfamide.

References

1. Hoelzer D, Thiel E et al. (1984) Intensified therapy in acute lymphoblastic and acute undifferentiated leukemia in adults. Blood 64: 38–47

2. Clarkson B, Ellis S et al. (1985) Acute lymphoblastic leukemia in adults. Semin Oncol 3: 271–282

3. International Bone Marrow Transplantat Registry (IBMTR) (1991) January, 1991, Statistical Center, Medical College of Wisconsin

4. Kersey JH, Weisdorf D et al. (1987) Comparison of autologous and allogeneic bone marrow transplantation for treatment of high-risk refractory acute lymphoblastic leukemia. N Engl J Med 317: 461–467

5. Körbling M, Hunstein W et al. (1989) Disease-free survival after autologous bone marrow transplantation in patients with acute myelogenous leukemia. Blood 74: 1898–1904

6. Simonsson B, Burnett AK et al. (1989) Autologous bone marrow transplantation with monoclonal antibody purged marrow for high risk acute lymphoblastic leukemia. Leukemia 3: 631–636

7. Dicke KA, Spinolo JA (1989) High dose therapy and autologous bone marrow transplant (ABMT) in acute leukemia: is purging necessary? Bone Marrow Transplant 4: 184–186

8. Kiesel S, Haas R et al. (1987) Removal of cells from a malignant B-cell line from bone marrow with immunomagnetic beads and with complement and immunoglobulin switch variant mediated cytolysis. Leuk Res 11: 1119–1125

Two Murine Leukemia Models for the Investigation of New Treatment Strategies in Bone Marrow Transplantation

L. Uharek, W. Gassmann, B. Glass, B. Focks, H. Bolouri, H. Loeffler, and W. Mueller-Ruchholtz

Introduction

Leukemic relapse is still the major cause of death after bone marrow transplantation in hematological malignancies [1]. Recent clinical data have indicated that the relapse risk is markedly influenced by certain properties of the bone marrow graft. In particular, it has been demonstrated that GvH reactivity, T-cell depletion, and natural killer cell activity can affect leukemic relapse rates [2–4]. Whereas the clinical significance of graft-versus-leukemia activity is now commonly accepted [5], the underlying mechanisms remain obscure [6]. Since it is impossible to analyze complex interactions of host, leukemia, and marrow graft in the clinical setting, we have started to develop preclinical models for the investigation of factors influencing leukemic relapse after bone marrow transplantation. Here we report our results obtained with the B-cell leukemia cell line A-20 and the myelomonocytic cell line WEHI-3.

Materials and Methods

Cell Lines. A20 is a B-cell neoplasia that has occurred spontaneously in a more than 15-month-old Balb/c mouse [7]. WEHI-3 is a chemically induced myelomonocytic leukemia cell line of Balb/c origin [8]. No viral antigens have been detected on both cell lines; both express H-2^d MHC class I sur-

face antigens. Cell lines were maintained in culture in RPMI 1640 and 5 % FCS at 37 °C, 5 % SO$_2$.

Experimental Animals. Mice used in this study were obtained from our own breeding facilities (Dept. of Immunology, University of Kiel, FRG). Female Balb/c mice (H-2^d), 8–14 weeks of age and weighting 20–26 g, were used for in vivo transfer of leukemia cells and as bone marrow recipients. Bone marrow donors were Balb/c mice, aged 10–20 weeks and of either sex. All animals were kept in conventional cages (five to ten animals in each cage) and received unsterilized food and water ad libitum. For 6 weeks posttransplant, the drinkung water contained cotrimoxazol. Experimental animals were inspected daily for survival.

Leukemia Cell Inoculation. After several weeks in culture, the tumor cells were maintained in Balb/c mice for two to five intravenous passages. Thereafter, spleen cells of mice with marked splenomegaly (>0.3 g) were pooled and stored in liquid nitrogen. This procedure was used, since it guaranteed a reliable transfer of highly malignant cells, in contrast to preliminary inoculation trials with cultured cells. To investigate the therapeutic effect of syngeneic BMT, Balb/c mice were injected with 10^6 stored spleen cells derived from animals inoculated with A-20 or WEHI-3, as described above. The cells were washed twice prior to injection in a constant volume (0.3 ml) of RPMI 1640. Leukemia cell suspensions contained less than 20 % trypan blue stained "nonviable" cells.

Tumor Diagnosis. Experimental animals were examined daily. Total body, spleen and

Department of Immunology and Department of Internal Medicine II, University of Kiel, Brunswikerstr. 4, 2300 Kiel, FRG

liver weights were determined after death. Cytological investigations of spleen, liver and blood smears were performed in a number of cases. Death due to leukemia was defined as death with macroscopic evidence of tumor, liver weight >1.5 g, and spleen weight >0.15 g. The follow-up period was 100 days, if not stated otherwise.

Total Body Irradiation. Five to ten mice each were placed in plastic boxes ($20 \times 20 \times 2.5$ cm) and irradiated with a ^{137}Cs source (gamma cell, Atomic Energy of Canada, Ottawa, Canada). Immediately prior to marrow grafting, mice received a single dose of TBI through opposing portals delivering approximately 1.2 Gy/min.

Bone Marrow Preparation. Donor animals were killed by cervical dislocation under ether anesthesia. Marrow was rinsed from femurs, tibias and humeri with 0.3 ml of a 50% normal mouse serum in RPMI 1640. Cells were triturated with a Pasteur pipette, washed once and resuspended in RPMI 1640. Nucleated cells were counted and injected intravenously in a constant volume of 0.3 ml. Marrow suspensions contained 5–10% trypan blue stained "nonviable" cells. The day of marrow grafting was termed day 0.

Statistics. The percentage of animals with "freedom from leukemia" was estimated and documented in accordance to the method of Kaplan and Meier. Experimental groups were compared using the Cox-Mantle test.

Results

Survival and Tumor Growth Characteristics After Injection of Leukemia Cells Obtained from Different Sources. The median survival time for recipients of 10^6 untreated, cell culture derived WEHI-3 leukemia cells was 18.5 days. Overall mortality was 93% for these animals (Table 1). Even higher doses of cultured cells were not completely lethal (data not shown). When spleen cells of tumor-bearing animals were transferred, 10^6 cells invariably resulted in death due to leukemia with a median survival time of 14 days. There was no difference in survival time between groups that had received cells from first, second, third, or fourth in vivo

passage. Interestingly, a tendency towards higher spleen weights at the time of death was observed with increasing numbers of passages. Transfer of bone marrow cells from animals previously inoculated with WEHI-3 or A-20 leukemia cells was invariably lethal, suggesting the potential usefulness of this model for the development of new purging techniques. Whereas storage in liquid nitrogen markedly reduced the malignancy of cultured cells (as indicated by a mortality rate of only 40%), there was no significant difference in mortality and survival time between recipients of either frozen or unmanipulated spleen cells from leukemia bearing animals. Similar results were observed for A-20 (data not shown).

After injection of either WEHI-3 or A-20 cells, all animals died with obvious hepatosplenomegaly. In contrast to untreated Balb/c mice, none of these animals had a spleen weight of less than 0.15 g and a liver weight of less than 1.5 g. We therefore used these two parameters for leukemia diagnosis (see also "Methods"). In a number of animals with WEHI-3 or A-20 leukemia, a marked leukocytosis with a high percentage of peripheral blast-like cells was detected at a terminal stage of the disease. Other animals, however, developed no persistent leukocytosis or suffered from pancytopenia. Thus, the peripheral blood count proved to be no valid indicator for leukemic cell growth. Cytological and histological investigations of the liver were performed in a number of cases and showed diffuse perivascular infiltration with WEHI-3 blasts or characteristic tumor nodules in case of A-20. Leukemia cells were the predominant ($>90\%$) cell population in all spleens studied.

Survival After Injection of Increasing Doses of A-20 and WEHI-3 Leukemia Cells. To determine the influence of leukemia cell dose on survival time and mortality rate, we transferred 10^4, 10^5, or 10^6 spleen cells of tumor-bearing animals. As shown in Fig. 1, the survival time depended on the number of leukemia cells transferred: for 10^4, 10^5, or 10^6 cells the median survival times were 24, 21, or 16 days in the case of A-20, and 25, 21, or 15 days in the case of WEHI-3. The overall mortality remained 100% for all cell doses tested. All animals

Table 1. Influence of the tumor inoculum source on mortality, liver and spleen weight after injection of WEHI-3 leukemia cells

Source	n	Median survival time days	Percentage mortality	Liver weight absolute (g)	Relative (%)	Spleen weight Absolute (g)	Relative (%)	Time of death (days)
Cell culture untreated cells	29	18.5 (13, >99)	93	2.53 (0.73)	10.18 (2.8)	0.38 (0.12)	1.51 (0.48)	13, 13, 14, 14, 14, 14, 15, 15, 17, 17, 17, 18, 18, 18, 19, 20, 20, 20, 20, 23, 23, 26, 28, 30, 33, 33, 48, 99, 99
Cell culture frozen cells	10	<100 (22, <99)	40	n.d.	n.d.	n.d.	n.d.	22, 22, 29, 29, 99, 99, 99, 99, 99
Untreated spleen cells from first in vivo passage	21	14 (11, 22)	100	2.38 (0.69)	10.41 (2.38)	0.44 (0.16)	1.93 (0.61	11, 12, 12, 12, 12, 14, 14, 14, 14, 14, 14, 14, 15, 16, 19, 19, 21, 21, 21, 21, 22
Untreated spleen cells from second in vivo passage	12	14.5 (13, 17)	100	1.84 (0.3)	9.37 (2.02)	0.34 (0.11)	1.73 (0.58)	13, 14, 14, 14, 14, 15, 15, 15, 15, 16, 16, 17
Untreated spleen cells from third in vivo passage	12	16 (14, 18)	100	1.9 (0.6)	8.49 (3.24)	0.62 (0.28)	2.88 (1.67)	14, 15, 15, 15, 15, 15, 17,, 17, 18, 18, 18, 18
Untreated spleen cells from fourth in vivo passage	12	13.5 (12, 19)	100	2.47 (0.31)	9.81 1.33	0.78 (0.15)	3.10 (0.67)	12, 13, 13, 13, 13, 13, 14, 14, 14, 16, 16, 16, 19
Frozen spleen cells from second or third in vivo passage	11	16 (13, 21)	100	2.56 (0.42)	10.22 (2.08)	0.85 (0.34)	3.35 (1.33)	13, 14, 14, 15, 15, 17, 19, 19, 19, 19, 20, 21
Untreated marrow cells from second in vivo passage	6	14 (12, 18)	100	1.99 (0.55)	8.32 (1.27)	0.37 (0.13)	1.60 (0.62)	12, 12, 14, 14, 17, 18

died due to leukemia. In subsequent experiments 10^6 cells were transferred, if not stated otherwise.

Effect of Prior Immunization with Irradiated Leukemia Cells on Survival After Injection of A-20 and WEHI-3. To test the immunogenicity of both leukemia cell lines in syngeneic hosts we injected 10^6 highly irradiated (80 Gy) leukemia cells prior to injection of 10^6 vital tumor cells. As indicated in Fig. 2, repeated (day -7 and -21) systemic exposure to irradiated A-20 or WEHI-3 cells was shown to exert no influence on subsequent proliferation of vital tumor cells, as indicated by nearly similar survival curves as compared to controls. These data strongly argue against the induction of classical immune reactivity directed against both leukemia cell lines in syngeneic hosts.

Leukemic Relapse Rates After Injection of A-20 Followed by Syngeneic BMT at Day 2, 5, or 10. Animals reveived 10^6 in vivo passaged leukemia cells at different times prior to irradiation with 7.5 Gy and bone marrow rescue with 10^7 syngeneic cells in order to determine the optimal interval between leukemia cell injection and BMT. Syngeneic BMT at day 10 or 5 resulted in a small but statistically significant ($p < 0.05$)

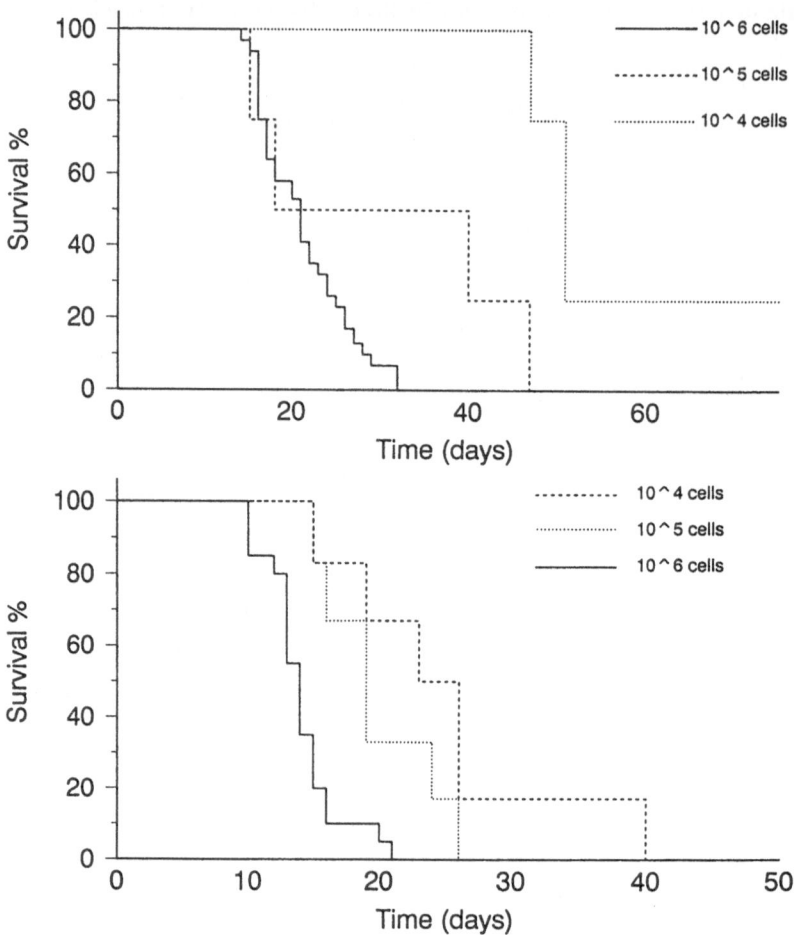

Fig. 1. Survival of Balb/c mice after injection of escalating doses of frozen A-20 *(top)* or WEHI-3 *(bottom)* leukemia cells (for details see text)

prolongation of the median survival time but was without influence on long-term survival rates (Fig. 3). All animals died due to leukemic relapse between day 20 and 45 after leukemia cell injection. When BMT was performed at day 2, the median survival time increased from 21 to 32 days. In addition, long-lasting (>100 days) freedom from relapse was observed in 20% of these animals.

Leukemic Relapse Rates After Injection of WEHI-3 Followed by Syngeneic BMT at Day 2, 5, or 10. When animals were treated with 7.5 Gy and syngeneic BMT at a late stage of the disease (10 days after WEHI-3 cell inoculation), all mice died due to

leukemic relapse (Fig. 4). The median survival time was only moderately increased from 14.5 to 23 days (p <0.05). Syngeneic BMT performed at day 5 after tumor cell inoculation resulted in a median survival time of 42 days and a disease-free survival rate of 45%. No recurrence of the leukemia was observed in mice that had been treated with BMT at a very early stage of the disease (2 days after tumor cell inoculation). All these animals survived more than 100 days. In a small number of cases (*n*=4), secondary recipients received 10^6 spleen cells of long-term survivors. None of these animals showed any evidence for subsequent growth of WEHI-3 leukemia cells.

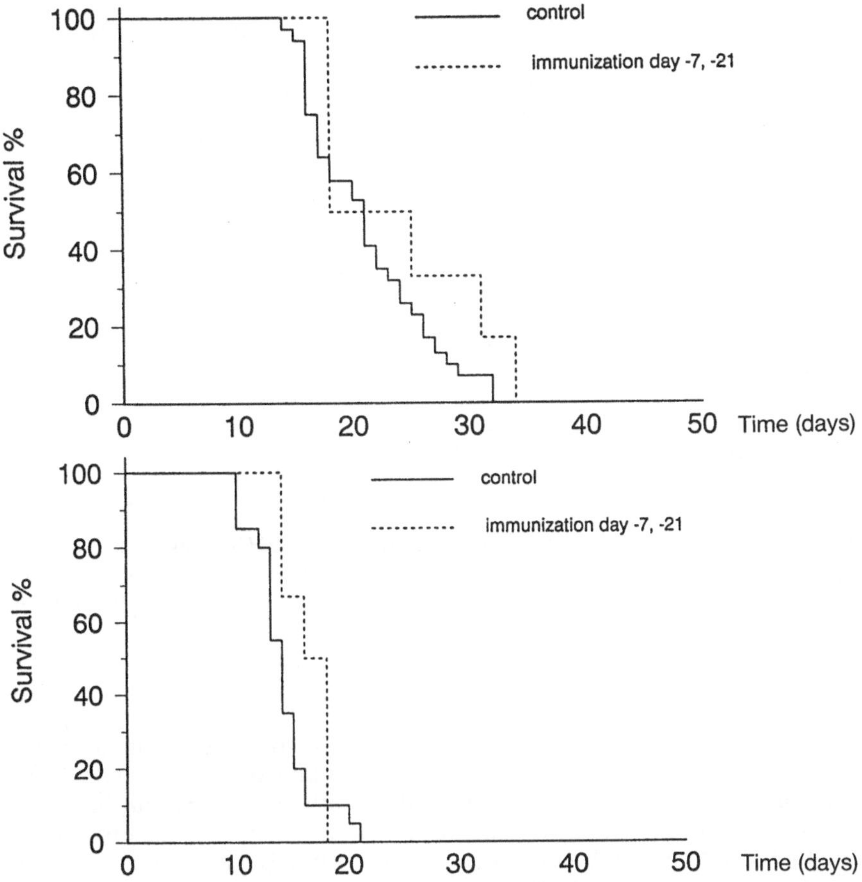

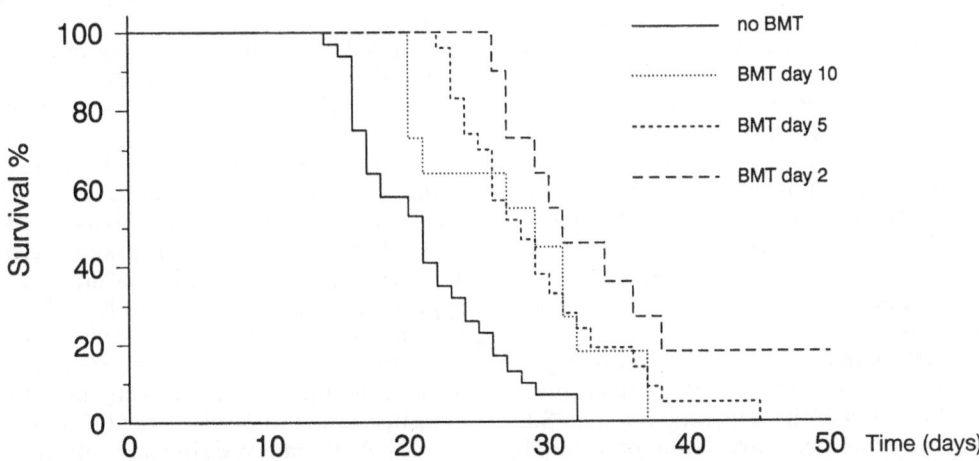

Fig. 2. Effect or prior immunization with irradiated A-20 (top) or WEHI-3 (bottom) leukemia cells on survival rates after injection of 10^6 vital leukemia cells. Balb/c mice received 10^6 irradiated (80 Gy) leukemia cells 21 and 7 days before tumor cell inoculation

Fig. 3. Freedom from leukemia after injection of 10^6 A-20 leukemia cells and syngeneic bone marrow transplantation at different times after tumors inoculation. At day 2, 5, or 10 after leukemia cell injection, Balb/c mice received a lethal dose (7.5 Gy) of total body irradiation prior to injection of 10^7 syngeneic bone marrow cells

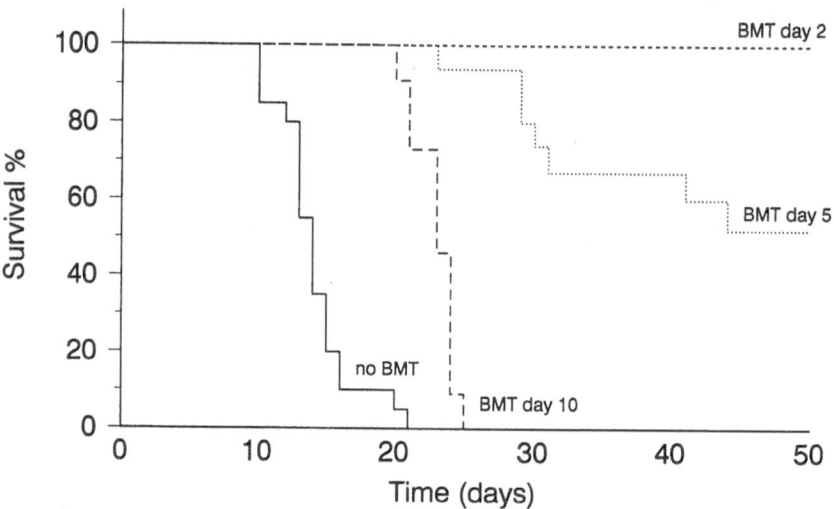

Fig. 4. Freedom from leukenia after injection of 10⁶ WEHI-3 leukemia cells and syngeneic bone marrow transplantation at different times after tumor inoculation. At day 2, 5, or 10 after leukemia cell injection, Balb/c mice received at lethal dose (7.5 Gy) of total body irradiation prior to injection of 10⁷ syngeneic bone marrow cells

Discussion

The preclinical models described in this study were developed to investigate new treatment strategies in bone marrow transplantation. In particular, they were designed to allow the investigation of graft-versus-leukemia (GvL) effects. In the clinical situation, marked differences have been observed between lymphatic and myelocytic neoplasms in terms of susceptibility towards antileukemic effects of allogeneic bone marrow grafts [5, 9, 10]. Thus, it would be inappropriate to generalize findings obtained with a single leukemia model. According to the data presented here, the B-cell leukemia A-20 [7] and the myelomonocytic leukemia WEHI-3 [8], fulfill a number of criteria fundamental for their application in the context of preclinical BMT.

First, both cell lines were shown to grow in vivo, resulting in death due to continuous proliferation of the leukemic cell line. Similar observations have been reported by others [11–13]. The direct transfer of cultured cells, however, was hampered by the fact that even cell doses of ashigh as 10⁷ were not able to ensure 100 % mortality. In vivo passaged cells, usually splenocytes of tumor-bearing animals, have been used by others [11, 13], but have the disadvantage of a relatively heterogeneous cell population. Nevertheless, we could demonstrate that their malignancy is significantly higher as compared to cultured cells but is not further enhanced by continuous in vivo passage (Table 1). To standardize the inoculum, we have pooled large numbers of spleen cells from tumor-bearing mice and stored them in liquid nitrogen. As few as 10⁴ of these cells were shown to be lethal (Fig. 1).

Second, both cell lines were shown to be nonimmunogenic in syngeneic hosts. In man, classical immune reactivity is not evocable against autologous leukemia cells. To get close to the situation in humans, it appears essential to work with leukemia cells not expressing immunogenic surface structures, e.g., viral antigens. In contrast to several other leukemia cell lines that have been used to investigate GvL effects, [14–17] A-20 and WEHI-3 are not virally induced.

Third, markedly enlarged spleen and liver weight provide a genuine and simple post-mortem criterion for the diagnosis of leukemia as the cause of death after injection of A-20 or WEHI-3. In several other studies, comparable criteria have not been established and survival time was the major parameter analyzed [18–20]. In the context of experimental bone marrow transplantation, death of an animal per se does not provide sufficient information, since causes other than recurrence of leukemia are known to influence survival rates, e. g., GvH disease or graft rejection. Regrowth of leukemic cells in secondary recipients which has been used in a number of other studies [21] to demonstrate or exclude the presence of leukemic cells is not a feasible criterion to study larger number of animals but might provide additional information about minimal residual disease. Unfortunately, leukocyte counts are not invariably elevated and thus allow no continuous monitoring of leukemic cell growth in case of A-20 or WEHI-3.

Fourth, bone marrow transplantation improves the median survival time and can be performed safely without any increment in treatment-related toxicity due to leukemia-related factors, e. g., tumor-lysis syndrome. It is an important feature of the WEHI-3 model that the leukemic relapse rate can be modified over a wide range (100 %–0 %) by varying the time interval between leukemia cell inoculation and bone marrow transplantation (Fig. 4). It is therefore possible to define optimal conditions for the investigation of different factors influencing the risk of relapse in a positive or negative direction. In contrast to WEHI-3, A-20 represents a higher malignant hematological neoplasia that is difficult to treat with radiotherapy, even at an early stage of the disease (Fig. 3).

We have now started a series of experiments to examine the antileukemic effect of allogeneic as compared to syngeneic bone marrow transplantation. Preliminary data are encouraging and indicate that GVHR is not a prerequisite for GvL activity of allogeneic grafts. Thus it may become possible to enhance the antileukemic effect of allogeneic bone marrow grafts without a concomitant increase in GvHR-induced mortality.

Summary

We have developd two murine models for bone marow transplantation in hematological malignancies. A-20 (B cell) and WEHI-3 (myelomonocytic) are murine leukemia cell lines of Balb/c (H-2^d) origin. After several weeks in culture, tumor cells were maintained in Balb/c mice for two to five intravenous passages. Thereafter, spleen cells of tumor-bearing mice were pooled and stored in liquid nitrogen. After injection of in vivo passaged leukemia cells into Balb/c mice, 10^6, 10^5, and 10^4 cells invariably lead to hepatosplenomegaly and death with a median survival time (MST) of 16, 21, or 24 days (A-20) and 15, 21, or 25 days (WEHI-3). Prior immunization with irradiated A-20 or WEHI-3 cells did not affect MST. For transplantation experiments, the follow-up period was 100 days and relapse was defined as death with spleen weight >0.15 g. Lethal irradiation (7.5 Gy) followed by syngeneic BMT at day 10, 5, or 2 after inoculation of 10^6 tumor cells resulted in prolonged survival times: 26, 27, or 32 days for A-20 and 23, 42, or >100 days for WEHI-3. After syngeneic BMT at day 5, relapse rates of 100 % (A-20) and 55 % (WEHI-3) were observed. Our data indicate that these two models can be used to investigate factors that are supposed to influence leukemic relapse after bone marrow transplantation.

References

1. Bortin MM, Horowitz MM, Gale RP (1989) Current status of bone marrow transplantation in humans: report from the international bone marrow transplant registry. Nat Immun Cell Growth Regul 7: 334
2. Weiden PL et al. (1979) Antileukemic effect of graft-versus-host disease in human recipients of allogeneic-marrow grafts. N Engl J Med 300: 1068
3. Mitsuyasu RT, Champlin RE, Gale RP, Ho WG, Lenarsky C, Winston D, Selch M, Elashoff R, Giorgi JV, Wells J, Terasaki P, Billing R, Feig S (1986) Treatment of donor bone marrow with monoclonal anti T-cell antibody and complement for the prevention of graft-versus-host disease. A prospective, randomized, double blind trial. Ann Intern Med 105: 20

4. Prentice HG, Hermans J, Zwaan FE (1988) Relapse risk in allogeneic BMT with T cell depletion of donor marrow. Bone Marrow Transplant [Suppl] 3: 30

5. Horowitz MM, Gale RP, Sondel PM, Goldman JM, Kersey J, Kolb H-J, Rimm AA, Ringdén O, Rozman C, Speck B, Truitt RL, Zwaan FE, Bortin MM (1990) Graft-versus-leukemia reactions after bone marrow transplantation. Blood 75: 555

6. Butturini A, Gale RP (1989) How can we cure leukaemia. Br J Haematol 72: 479

7. Kim KJ, Kannellopoulus-Langevin C, Mervin RM, Sachs DH, Asofsky R (1979) Establishment and characterization of Balb/c lymphoma lines with B cell properties. J Immunol 122: 549

8. Ralph P, Nakoinz I (1977) Direct toxic effects of immunopotentiators on monocytic, myelomonocytic, and histiocytic or macrophage tumor cells in culture. Cancer Res 37: 546

9. Butturini A, Bortin MM Gale RP (1987) Graft-versus-leukemia following bone marrow transplantation. Bone Marrow Transplant 2: 233

10. Sullivan KM, Weiden PL, Storb R, Witherspoon RP, Fefer A, Fisher L, Buckner CD, Anasetti C, Appelbaum FR, Badger C, Beatty P, Bensinger W, Berenson R, Bigelow C, Cheever MA, Clift R, Deeg HJ, Doney K, Greenberg P, Hansen JA, Hill R, Loughran T, Martin P, Neiman P (1989) Influence of acute and chronic graft-versus-host disease on relapse and survival after bone marrow transplantation from HLA-identical siblings as treatment of acute and chronic leukemia. Blood 73: 1720

11. Berdel WE, Okamoto S, Danhauser-Riedl S, Hong CI, Winton EF, West CR, Rastetter J, Vogler WR (1989) Therapeutic activity of 1-ß-D-arabinofuranosylcytosine conjugates of lipids in WEHI-3B leukemia in mice. Exp Hematol 17: 364

12. Gamba-Vitalo C, Carman MD, Sartorelli AC (1989) Development of neomycin-resistant WEHI-3B D$^+$ murine cells as an in vivo model of acute nonlymphocytic leukemia. Exp Hematol 17: 130

13. Ratech H, Kim J, Asofsky R, Thorbecke RJ, Hirschhorn R (1984) Effects of deoxycoformycin in mice. II. Differences between the drug sensitivities and purine metabolizing enzymes of transplantable lymphomas of varying immunologic phenotypes. J Immunol 132: 3077

14. OKunewick JP, Meredith RF, Brozovich BJ, Seeman PR, Schieb AL (1979) Rauscher leukeimia as a model for studies of marrow transplantation therapy: results using syngeneic, allogeneic and hybrid donors. Int J Cancer 24: 438

15. Floersheim GL (1981) Treatment of Moloney lymphoma with lethal doses of dimethylmyleran combined with injections of haemopoietic cells. Lancet i: 233

16. Iorio AM, Neri M, Zei T, Romeo G, Rossi GB, Bonmassar E (1989) Natural resistance mice against Friend leukemia cells. II. Studies with in vivo passaged interferon-sensitive and interferon-resistant cell clones. Cell Immunol 118: 425

17. Pierpaoli W (1985) Growth of transplantable melanoma and leukaemia and prevention of virus-induced leukaemia in long lived radiation chimeras constructed with unmanipulated bone marrow. Clin Exp Immunol 59: 210

18. Bitran JD, Williams SF, Moormeier J, Mick R (1990) High-dose combination chemotherapy with thiotepa and autologous hematopoietic stem cell reinfusion in the treatment of patients with relapsed refractory lymphomas. Semin Oncol 17 [Suppl 3]: 39

19. Sykes M, Sachs DH (1989) Genetic analysis of the anti-leukemic effect of mixed allogeneic bone marrow transplantation. Transplant Proc 21: 3022

20. Truitt RL, Shih CC, LeFever AV (1986) Manipulation of graft-versus-host disease for a graft-versus-leukemia effect after allogeneic bone marrow transplantation in AKR mice with spontaneous leukemia/lymphoma. Transplantation 41: 301

21. Weiss L (1983) Suppression and elimination of BCL1 leukemia by allogeneic bone marrow transplantation. J Immunol 130: 2452

Immunomagnetic Removal of Malignant Cells from Human Bone Marrow Prior to Autologous Bone Marrow Transplantation

J. Zingsem, T. Zeiler, V. Weisbach, K. Stahlhut, R. Zimmermann, S. Serke, W. Siegert, and R. Eckstein

Introduction

Autologous bone marrow transplantation (ABMT) following myeloablative chemo-radiotherapy is an alternative to conventional chemotherapy for poor prognosis lymphoid malignancies in patients without HLA- and MLR-identical donor for allogenous bone marrow transplantation [1]. However, the patient's bone marrow (BM) might be infiltrated by tumor cells even in clinically complete remission. Many transplantation centers are investigating different techniques to remove these tumor cells from the BM prior to the marrow reinfusion, therefore. Monoclonal antibodies directed against tumor associated antigens are being used either in the presence of complement or bound to toxins or inert particles as magnetic microspheres [2, 3]. We report here purging results in the BM of the last 27 out of 33 patients suffering from

Blutbank Abteilung Innere Medizin und Poliklinik, Universitätsklinikum Rudolf Virchow, Standort Charlottenburg, Freie Universität, Berlin, FRG

C-ALL, B-ALL, Burkitt's lymphoma, T-ALL or T-cell-lymphoma (Fig. 1).

Materials and Methods

Bone Marrow Processing

Under general anesthesia, BM was harvested from the posterior and anterior iliac crests and collected in RPMI 1640 with preservative-free heparin. The cells were filtered through stainless steel mesh before they were concentrated with a blood cell separator (Haemonetics V50, Cobe 2997 or Cobe Spectra). The hemolytic plasma was rejected and the red blood cells were retransfused to the patient. As the obtained BM-cell concentrates contained more than 80% mononuclear cells, no further centrifugation procedure has been done.

Monoclonal Antibodies and Immunobeads

Immunobeads are monodisperse, magnetizable polymer particles with a diameter of

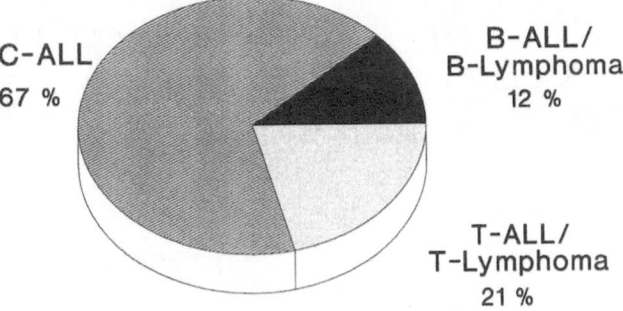

Fig. 1. Bone marrow purging: distribution of patients

Table 1. Composition of Moab cocktail

Subtype	Moab specificity	Clone [5]	source
C-ALL	Anti-CD10	ALB1	Immunotech, France
	Anti-CD10	ALB2	Immunotech, France
	Anti-CD19	CLB-B4	Jannsen, Belgium
	Anti CD24	ALB9	Immunotech, France
B-ALL/	Anti-CD19	CLB-B4	Jannsen, Belgium
Burkitt's lymphoma	Anti-CD10	ALB2	Immunotech, France
	Anti-CD10	ALB1	Immunotech, France
	Anti-CD24	ALB9	Immunotech, France
T-ALL/	Anti-CD2	6F10-3	Immunotech, France
T-lymphoma	Anti-CD3	X35-3	Immunotech, France
	Anti-CD5	BL1a	Immunotech, France
	Anti-CD7	8H8-1	Immunotech, France

4.5 μm and a surface area of 3–5 m²/g (Dynabeads M-450, Dynal, Norway) [4]. They are coated with approximately 5 μg affinity-purified sheep-anti-mouse IgG/mg beads (SAM beads).

A cocktail of target cell specific monoclonal antibodies (MoAb) was coupled to the SAM beads in a ratio of 3.3 μg MoAb cocktail/mg SAM beads by incubation overnight at 4 °C. Depending on the patient's lymphoma or ALL subtype, the MoAb cocktail was composed as shown in Table 1.

In addition to these individually coated beads, Dynabeads M-450 Pan-B (anti-CD19, clone AB1) and Dynabeads M-450 Pan-T (anti-CD2, clone ITI4C1) were used.

Before use, the beads were washed three times in phosphate-buffered salt solution (Seromed, FRG).

Treatment of Bone Marrow Cells with Beads

In a first step, BM cells were incubated with MoAb-conjugated beads at a bead/cell ratio of two beads per mononuclear cell for 30 min at 4 °C in Baxter transfusion bags on a flat bottom agitator. Subsequently, the blood bag with the BM cells was placed upside down in a magnetic cell separation unit (Dynal, Norway) as schematically shown in Fig. 2.

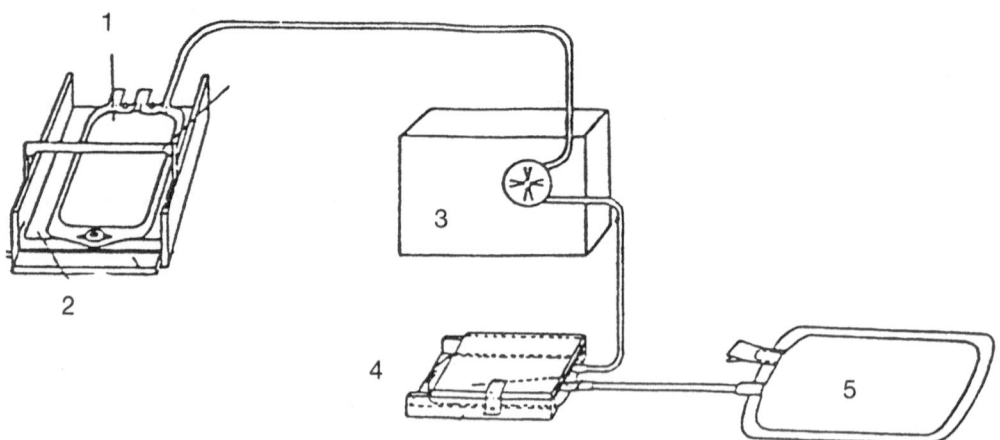

Fig. 2. Magnetic cell separation unit. 1 = blood bag containing BM with beads, 2 = magnetic cell separation unit, 3 = peristaltic pump, 4 = magnetic trap, 5 = collection bag

While stepwise reducing the distance between the bag and the magnets, the magnetic field strength in the bag was increased from 10 % to 100 % of the maximal field strength. The cell suspension was then sucked out of the bag to an attached 600-ml collection bag using a peristaltic pump (Watson Marlow 503S) while the bead-cell rosettes and the excess beads were fixed in the blood bag. To remove beads that might have left the bag, a 150-ml bag in a magnetic trap was inserted between the pump and collection bag. In the following second purging cycle the bead/cell ratio was one bead per mononuclear cell, the incubation and separation remaining as described for cycle 1.

After the second purging cycle, the cell suspension was concentrated by centrifuging when necessary, resuspended and mixed with freezing medium to a final concentration of 10 % DMSO in 700 ml Gambro hemofreeze bags (Gambro, FRG). The purged BM was then cooled to $-100\,°C$ in a Planar freezing machine (Planar, UK) and subsequently stored under liquid nitrogen.

Quality Control

Samples from the initial BM-cell suspension as well as after each step of the procedure were taken for white cell counts and cytomorphologic smears, bacteriological controls, viability tests (trypan blue), immunological phenotyping and stem cell tests (CFU-GM).

Results

Unspecific Cell Losses

The mean MNC and CFU-GM reduction during the complete procedure is shown in Table 2.

This results in a 0.61 log MNC and a 0.56 log CFU-GM reduction.

Efficacy of Tumor Cell Depletion

The initial BM contamination with tumor type related antigen positive cells ranged from less than 0.03 % to 70 %. The tumor

Table 2. Mean MNC and CFU-GM reduction

Tumor type	MNC $\times$ 10^8/kg		CFU $\times$ 10^4/kg	
	Initial	Purged	Initial	Purged
B	3.2	0.8	23.5	4.7
C	3.1	0.8	24.4	7.9
T	3.0	0.8	12.6	5.4

Table 3. Tumor cell reduction achieved

	Log	reduction	for antigen		
Tumor type	CD2	CD5	CD7	CD10	CD19
B	nd	nd	nd	nd	1.8 (1.3–2.6)
C	nd	nd	nd	1.6 (1.0–2.8)	1.7 (1.2–2.8)
T	2.4 (0.9–3.4)	2.0 (0.9–3.5)	2.2 (0.8–3.4)	nd	nd

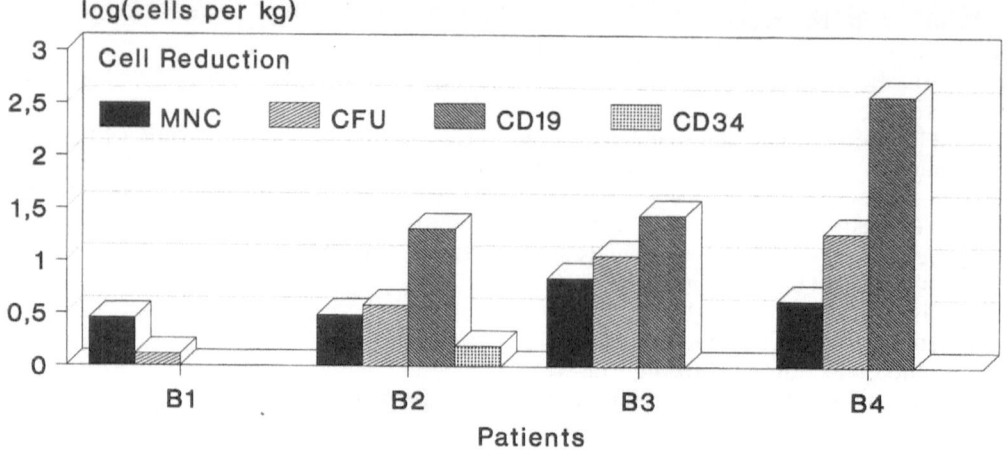

Fig. 3. Bone marrow purging: B-ALL/B lymphoma

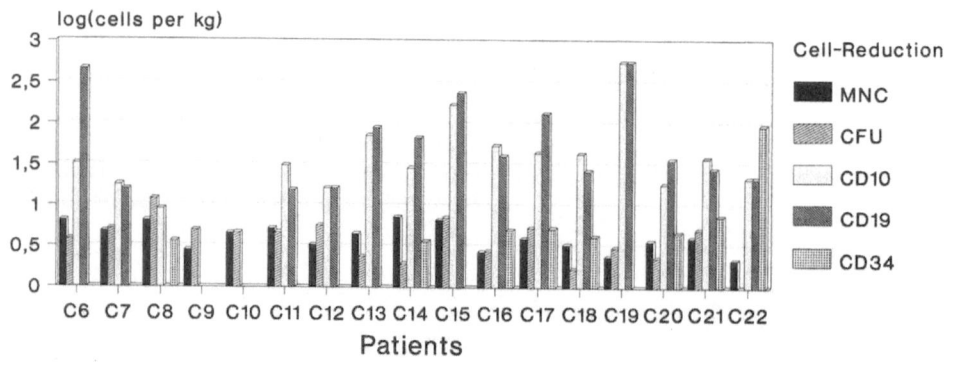

Fig. 4. Bone marrow purging: C-ALL

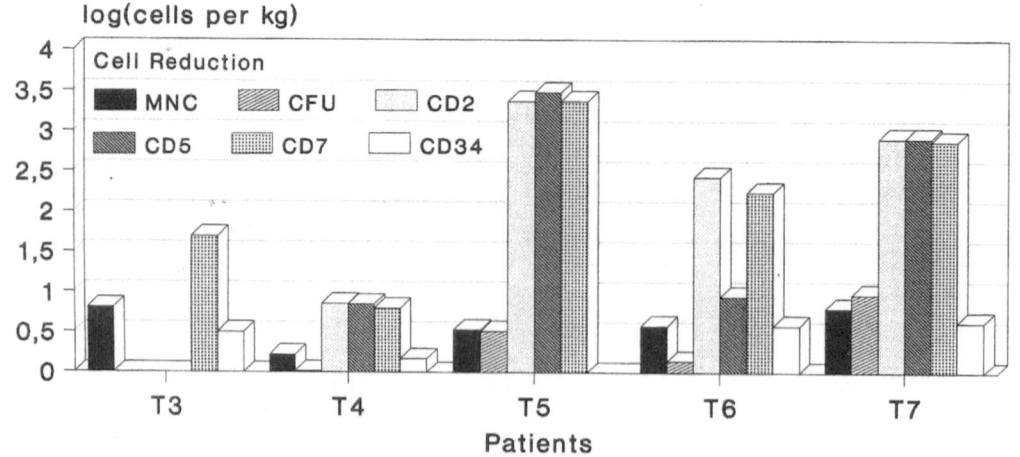

Fig. 5. Bone marrow purging: T-ALL/T lymphoma

cell reduction that could be achieved is shown in Table 3.

Specific data for each purging procedure are shown in Figs. 3–5.

Discussion

In comparison with laboratory experiments showing a 4–5 log tumor cell depletion, the purging of not artificially contaminated bone marrow seems to be less effective. This is especially caused by the limits of cell detection techniques (FACS) that usually enable a detection of less than 3 positive out of 10000 cells (0.03 %) only. However, ex vivo purging of bone marrow prior to ABMT using MoAbs and SAM beads allows satisfactory tumor cell reduction by sufficient stem cell recovery.

References

1. Dicke KA, Zander A, Spitzer G et al. (1979) Autologous bone marrow transplantation: adult acute leukaemia in relapse. Lancet i: 514–517
2. Kemshead JT, Health L, Gibson FM et al. (1986) Magnetic microspheres and monoclonal antibodies for the depletion of neuroblastoma cells from bone marrow. Experience, improvements and observations. Br J Cancer 54: 771–778
3. Bast RC jr, DeFabritiis P, Lipton J et al. (1986) Elimination of malignant clonogenic cells from human bone marrow using multiple monoclonal antibodies and complement. Cancer Res 46: 449–503
4. Ugelstad J, Mork PC (1980) Swelling of oligomer-polymer particles. New methods of preparation of emulsions and polymer dispersions. Adv Colloid Interface 13: 101–140
5. Boucheix CI, Perrot JY, Mirshahi M et al. (1985) A new set of monoclonal antibodies against acute lymphoblastic leukemia. Leuk Res 9: 597–604

High-Dose VP-16 (HD VP-16) and Fractionated Total Body Irradiation (F-TBI) Followed by Autologous Bone Marrow Transplantation (ABMT) in Children with Relapsed or High-Risk Acute Lymphoblastic Leukemia (ALL)

R. Schwerdtfeger[1], H. Schmid[2], J. Zingsem[1], J. Beck[3], C. Bender-Götze[4], R. Dopfer[5], H. Peters[6], G. Hentze[2], and W. Siegert[1]

Introduction

In spite of the increasing knowledge of risk factors in childhood ALL [1] and risk-adapted chemotherapy [2], the prognosis of high-risk ALL remains extremely poor. High-risk factors include abnormal cytogenetics, no response to conventional chemotherapy (CC), relapse within 18 months of diagnosis, relapsed T-ALL and multiple relapses. By CC continuous complete remission (CCR) is achieved in less than 10 % of patients (pts.). Allogeneic bone marrow transplantation in CR2 ALL leads to leukemia-free survival in about 30 % of pts. [3]. In children without a suitable marrow donor the same or an even more aggressive antileukemic treatment and autologous BMT may offer a chance for long-lasting CR or even cure. Stimulated by early promising results in high-risk ALL in CR1 and CR2 [4, 5], we started a clinical study using a new and well-tolerated conditioning regimen and ABMT. The regimen, which was introduced by BLUME for allogeneic BMT, consisted of HD VP-16 and F-TBI [6]. So far, 23 children in first, second, or subsequent remission have entered the study.

Patients and Methods

Between December 1987 and October 1990, 23 children (17 males and 6 females),

median age 3 11/12 (range, 1 4/12 to 13 2/12) with high-risk ALL received ABMT after HD VP-16 and F-TBI. At the time of transplantation 12 pts. were in second, 7 in third, and 2 in fourth remission. The two patients who were transplanted in first remission were Ph1 positive (Pat. #1) and unresponsive to conventional chemotherapy, respectively (Pat. #20). Nine pts. had relapsed within 24 months of diagnosis. For pts. transplanted in CR 2 the median duration of first remission was 18 months (range, 9–26), for those transplanted in CR 3 the median duration of second remission was 40 months (range, 16–68). The median time from last relapse until AMBT was 152 days /range, 63–419).

Relapse

Analysis of the sites of relapse before ABMT showed that 13 pts. had BM relapse only, 5 pts. had CNS relapse only, and 1 pt. had isolated testicular relpase. Two children suffered from recurrent BM and CNS disease (Table 1).

Bone Marrow Harvest

All but three pts. underwent bone marrow harvest at a median of 69 days (range, 1–217) after achieving CR. In three pts. bone marrow was harvested during the preceding CR.

UKRV [1]Med. Klinik and Kinderklinik[2] Berlin; Univ.-Kinderkliniken [3]Erlangen [4]München und [5]Tübingen (FRG); [6]St. Anna-Kinderspital, Wien (Austria)

Table 1. Patient characteristics

Pat.	Sex	Age (yrs) at diagnosis	Date of diagnosis	Pheno-type	Status	Duration of Remission (mths) 1st	2nd	3rd	Site of last relapse	Purged	Date of ABMT	Day after ABMT	Status
1	F	3	Jul-89	p-B-ALL	CR1	–	–	–	–	Yes	Feb-90	+364	A&W
2	M	10	Oct-86	p-B-ALL	CR2	9	–	–	CNS	Yes	May-88	115	R, D
3	M	4	Mar-88	B-ALL	CR2	26	–	–	BM	Yes	Oct-90	+142	A&W
4	M	4	Jun-86	c-ALL	CR2	21	–	–	BM	Yes	Jul-88	212	R, D
5	M	6	Nov-85	c-ALL	CR2	26	–	–	BM/ CNS	No	Mar-89	+702	A&W
6	M	1	Sep-86	c-ALL	CR2	15	–	–	CNS	No	Jul-88	150	R, D
7	M	13	Nov-87	c-ALL	CR2	18	–	–	BM	Yes	Oct-89	144	R, D
8	M	1	Jul-86	c-ALL	CR2	17	–	–	BM	Yes	Apr-88	65	R, D
9	F	4	Jul-86	c-ALL	CR2	11	–	–	BM	Yes	Dec-87	101	R, D
10	M	2	Feb-88	c-ALL	CR2	18	–	–	BM/ CNS	Yes	Feb-90	14	I, D
11	F	11	Mar-88	c-ALL	CR2	24	–	–	BM	Yes	Oct-90	+114	A&W
12	M	2	Jan-83	c-ALL	CR3	34	40	–	BM	Yes	Apr-89	156	R, D
13	M	3	Oct-84	c-ALL	CR3	24	27	–	BM	Yes	May-89	105	R, D
14	M	2	Jan-81	c-ALL	CR3	42	51	–	T	Yes	Jan-89	+752	A&W
15	M	3	Aug-83	c-ALL	CR3	31	22	–	BM	Yes	May-88	99	R, D
16	M	3	Jun-81	c-ALL	CR3	28	68	–	BM	Yes	Jan-90	26	I, D
17	F	4	Mar-86	c-ALL	CR3	33	16	–	BM	Yes	Jun-90	146	R, D
18	F	5	Jul-77	c-ALL	CR3	106	45	–	BM	Yes	Jul-90	+205	A&W
19	M	2	Jun-82	c-ALL	CR4	39	17	8	CNS	Yes	Feb-90	94	R, D
20	F	2	May-87	T-ALL	CR1	–	–	–	–	Yes	Dec-87	41	I, D
21	M	10	Dec-86	T-ALL	CR2	13	–	–	BM	No	May-88	43	R, D
22	M	4	Sep-86	T-ALL	CR2	26	–	–	CNS	Yes	Apr-89	+688	A&W
23	M	3	Dec-82	T-ALL	CR4	18	–	–	CNS	No	Dec-88	132	R, D

Abbreviations: F, female; M, male, p-B, prae-B; AMBT, autologous bone marrow transplantation; BM, bone marrow; CNS, central nervous system; T, testes; A&W, alive and well; R, relapse; I, infection; D, died

Purging

In vitro BM purging was performed in 19 transplants. A cocktail of monoclonal antibodies attached to magnetic beads [7, 8] based on disease lineage was used in 15,4-hydroxycyclophosphamide in two and a combination of both in the remaining two transplants.

Patient Treatment

First-line chemotherapy was performed according to BFM protocols [1] in 19 pts. Different protocols were used in four pts. Leukemic relapse was treated according to BFM-relapse protocols [2]. All pts. received fractionated total body irradiation, i.e., 12 Gy in six divided doses of 200 cGy each on day −6, −5 and −4 with lung shielding at 9–10 Gy. VP-16 (60 mg/kg) was infused over 4 h on day −3. Autologous BM was rapidly thawed and reinfused immediately by intravenous bolus.

Results

Data were analyzed as of 17th February 1991. The probability of event-free survival (EFS) at 2 years after ABMT was 25 % (Fig. 1). Of the 23 pts., 13 relapsed and died, 3 died from infection early in the course of

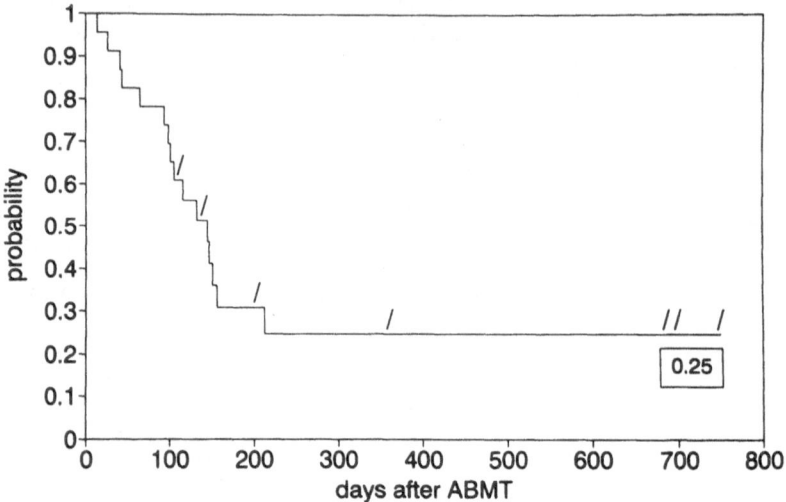

Fig. 1. Event-free survival: all patients (n=23)

ABMT and 7 remained in CCR at a median of 364 days (range, 114–752) (Table 1).

Survivors

One out of the seven surviving pts. was transplanted in first CR, four in second CR and two in third CR. Among the surviving children there was one with pre-B-ALL (PH1+), one with B-ALL, and five with c-ALL.

Relapses

Thirteen pts. (57%) relapsed at a median of 132 days (range, 43–212). Relapse occurred in 7 out of 12 pts. grafted in second CR, in 4 out of 7 grafted in third CR and in both pts. grafted in fourth CR. BM was the site of relapse in 12 pts., CNS in 1 pt. Duration of first remission was a prognostic factor for pts. transplanted in second CR. All pts. with an initial remission duration of 24 months or longer are alive and disease free whereas no pt. with an initial remission duration of less than 24 months survived. This difference is statistically significant (p = 0,0005, chi-square test).

Transplantation-Related Death

Three pts. transplanted in first, second, and third remission died from infectious complications at day 14 (legionella pneumonia), day 26 (aspergillus pneumonia) and day 41 (disseminated aspergillosis).

Discussion

Our group of pts. represents a cohort of typical ALL pts. with very poor prognosis if treated by conventinal chemotherapy. In order to improve treatment results ABMT was performed in 23 children. With high-dose chemoradiotherapy followed by ABMT, 30% of pts. are currently disease free and the probability of EFS is 25% at 2 years. This is an accordance with results reported by Sallan et al. [9], Kersey et al. [10], and Rizzoli et al. [11]. Like Sallan et al. [9] we found that the duration of the initial remission was a highly significant prognostic factor for long-term EFS after ABMT.

Relapse after ABMT was the major problem with an actual rate of 57% and a probability of 71% at 2 years. Our data do not allow any conclusion as to the role of bone marrow purging for prevention of relapse since most pts. received purged marrow. But there is a accumulating evidence that relapse arises rather from refractory disease in vivo than from reinfused BM. HD VP-16 and F-TBI is apparently not sufficient in eradicating residual leukemic cells in CR pts. Since regimen toxicity was low except for severe stomatitis a more aggressive combined chemoradiotherapy before ABMT may lead to an increase in EFS. A deficient immune system due to HD VP-16, F-TBI and ABMT [12, 13] may be a factor contributing to relapse. The early occurrence of relapse after ABMT supports this suggestion. Therefore, a post-transplant immunostimulating or -modulating therapy using cytokines such as IL-2 and interferon may improve EFS following ABMT. If long-term EFS could be increased to more than 30 % ABMT would offer a promising alternative to allogeneic BMT, particularly if one considers morbidity and mortality due to graft versus host disease.

References

1. Riehm H, Feickert HJ, Schrappe M, Henze G, Schellong G (1987) Therapy results in five ALL-BFM studies since 1970: Implications of risk factors for prognosis. In: Büchner T, Schellong G, Hiddemann W, Urbanitz D, Ritter I (eds) Acute leukemias. Berlin Heidelberg New York, pp 139–146 (Hämatologie und Bluttransfusion, vol 30)
2. Henze G, Fengler R, Hartmann R, Niethammer D, Schellong G, Riehm H (1990) BFM group treatment results in relapsed childhood acute lymphoblastic leukemia. In: Büchner T, Schellong G, Hiddemann W, Ritter I (eds) Acute leukemias II. Springer, Berlin Heidelberg New York, pp 619–626 (Hämatologie und Bluttransfusion, vol 33)
3. Gale RP, Horowitz MM, Bortin MM, (for the International Bone Marrow Transplantation Registry) (1989) IBMTR analysis of bone marrow transplants in akute leukaemia. Bone Marrow Transplant 4, Suppl. 3: 83–84
4. Gorin NC, Herve P, Aegerter P, Goldstone A, Linch D, Maraninchi D, Burnett A, Goldman J (1986) Autologous bone marrow transplantation for acute leukaemia in remission. Br J Haematol 64: 385–395
5. Cahn JY, Herve P,, Flesch M, Plouvier E, Noir A, Racadot E, Montcuquet P, Behar C

(1986) Autologous bone marrow transplantation (ABMT) for acute leukaemia in complete remission: a pilot study of 33 cases. Br J Haematol 63: 457–470
6. Blume KG, Forman SJ, O'Donnell MR, Doroshow JH, Krance RA, Nademanee AP, Snyder DS, Schmidt GM (1987) Total body irradiation and high-dose etoposide: a new preparatory regimen for bone marrow transplantation in patients with advanced hematologic malignancies. Blood 69: 1015–1020
7. Kemshead JT, Heath L, Gibson FM, Katz F, Richmond F,, Treleaven J, Ugelstad J (1986) Magnetic microspheres and monoclonal antibodies for the depletion of neuroblastoma cells from bone marrow: experiences, improvements and observations. Br J Cancer 54: 771–778
8. Kvalheim G, Sörensen O, Fodstad Ö, Funderud S, Kiesel S, Dörken B, Nustad K, Jakobsen E, Ugelstad J, Pihl A (1988) Immunomagnetic removal of B-lymphoma cells from human bone marrow: a procedure for clinical use. Bone Marrow Transplant 3: 31–41
9. Sallan SE, Niemeyer CM, Billett AL, Lipton JM, Tarbell NJ, Gelber RD, Murray C, Pittinger TP, Wolfe LC, Bast RC Jr, Ritz J (1989) Autologous bone marrow transplantation for acute lymphoblastic leukemia. J Clin Oncol 7: 1594–1601
10. Kersey JH, Weisdorf D, Nesbit ME, Le Bien TW, Woods WG, McGlave PB, Kim T, Vallera DA (1987) Comparison of autologous and allogeneic bone marrow transplantation for treatment of high-risk refractory acute lymphoblastic leukemia. N Engl J Med 317: 461–467
11. Rizzoli V, Carella AM, Carlo-Stella C, Mangoni L (1990) Autologous marrow transplantation in acute lymphoblastic leukemia: control of residual disease with mafosfamide and induction of syngenic GvHD with Cyclosporine. Bone Marrow Transplant 6 [Suppl 1]: 76–78
12. Anderson KC, Ritz J, Takvorian T, Coral F, Daley H, Gorgone BC, Freedman AS, Canellos GP (1987) Hematologic engraftment and immune reconstitution post transplantation with anti-B1 purged autologous bone marrow. Blood 69: 597–604
13. Welte K, Kolitz JE, Merluzzi VJ, Flomenberg N, Engert A, Miller GA, Holloway K, Sykora KW, Venuta S, O'Reilly RJ, Oettgen HF, Mertelsmann R, Bradley E (1985) The role of interleukin-2 in human immunodeficiency states. In: Sorg C, Schimpl A (eds) Cellular and molecular biology of lymphokines. Academic Press, Orlando, pp 755–759

Understanding the Mechanisms of Cure in Acute Myeloblastic Leukaemia: Towards a Modern Immunotherapy

H. G. Prentice

Introduction: Mechanisms of Cure Revealed by Bone Marrow Transplantation Studies

The published literature suggests that less than 25 % of patients with de novo acute myeloblastic leukaemia (AML), treated by intensive chemotherapy, are cured by this approach [1, 2]. Modest improvements have been claimed for treatment on high-dose cytosine arabinoside (HD-Ara-C) containing combinations [3] and in younger patients on the VAPA protocol [4]. As a rule more than 60 % experience disease recurrence [5, 2].

Although considerable unique morbidity and mortality associated with allogeneic bone marrow transplantation (BMT) restricts the cure rate to 45 %–50 %, this is the only method proven to have a major impact on the disease. International (IBMTR) and European (EBMTR) Marrow Transplant Registry data show a relapse rate (RR) of approximately 20 % for transplants in first complete remission (CR) [6, 7].

In contrast some studies in which the delicate donor/recipient immune balance has been disturbed by T lymphocyte depletion show loss of the anti-leukaemic benefit of BMT and have returned the relapse risk to 60 % [8–10]. At these centres the conditioning regimen was identical to that used prior to the introduction of T-cell depletion suggesting that the difference in RR is

Bone Marrow Transplant Programme, Royal Free Hospital School of Medicine, London, UK

largely due to the loss of the anti-leukaemic activity of the donor-derived immune system (the graft-versus-leukaemia or GvL effect) [11] and that the leukaemia ablative effects of the conditioning regimen make only a modest contribution to cure. Understanding of these phenomena has resulted in a resurgence of interest in immunotherapy which might mimic the GvL effects of allogeneic bone marrow transplantation.

Evidence for the Relative Contributions of the Conditioning Regimen and GvL in the Cure of AML

Recent studies suggest that the anti-leukaemic effect of the conditioning regimen may be modest. First, several studies have failed to show any benefit from increased intensity of conditioning. Second, three groups have reported a substantial increase in relapse risk when donor bone marrow is depleted of T lymphocytes despite the use of unaltered conditioning regimens. The Royal Marsden Hospital [8] reported an RR of 30 % using conventional (non-T-depleted) donor marrow. This increased to 60 % with T-lymphocyte-depleted marrow. Atkinson et al. [9] showed in increase in RR from 37 % to 62 % with T-cell depletion. These findings were confirmed by Maraninchi et al. [10]. For each group the RR for patients receiving T-lymphocyte-depleted bone marrow approached that observed for patients treated with chemotherapy alone. The observations are similar to those made by the Seattle BMT group when they intro-

572

duced the "short methotrexate (MTX) plus cyclosporin A" combination into their standard protocol for BMT in AML. This resulted in a substantial increase in the risk of leukaemia relapse [12]. Although this effect was reversed by redressing the immune imbalance by increasing the total dose of radiotherapy to 1575 cGy, survival was unaffected because of increased toxicity of the conditioning regimen. The most reasonable explanation for this observation is a return of the advantage to the donor-derived immune system rather than a dramatic increse in antileukaemia effect by the modest increment in the radiation dose.

Our inability to identify a relationship between the intensity of conditioning and cure rates suggests that the anti-leukaemic contribution of the conditioning regimen is indeed modest.

Although the studies detailed above indicate that T-cell depletion of donor marrow can be associated with an increse in the RR following allogeneic BMT, this finding is restricted to centres which failed to anticipate the effect of loss of immunosuppressive effect of donor-derived T lymphocytes. Data from the Royal Free Hospital [13], The Glasgow Royal Infirmary [14], Wisconsin [15] and Dutch groups [16] and others show no increase or even a slight reduction in relapse risk with T-cell-depleted BMT. This disparity is probably not attributable to the method (antibody/elutriation, etc.) of T-cell depletion, which is very varied, but to a combination of the *extent* of T-cell depletion and the degree of host immunosuppression by the conditioning regimen.

Effectors of Graft-Versus-Leukaemia

Both preclinical and clinical data (above) support a substantial role for T cells (? CTLs). Our own studies show that the immune reconstitution after either allogeneic or autologous (ABMT) bone marrow transplant is characterised by an environment hostile to residual leukaemic cells [17]. This anti-leukaemic activity has two main components. The first is cell mediated and characterised by the appearance in the circulation of mononuclear cells with large granular lymphocyte (LGL) morphology

able to lyse targets which are relatively resistant to killing by lymphocytes in normal individuals. Since no extraneous lymphokine is applied, we have termed these cells "activated killer" (AK) cells in contrast to "lymphokine activated killer" (LAK) cells.

The phenotype of these AK cells is either CD3-CD16+ (i.e., NK derived) or CD3+CD16-. In vitro, these cells kill leukaemic cell lines and may contribute in vivo to the eradication of minimal residual leukaemia [18]. The increased number and activity of these cells returns to baseline by about 3 months after BMT. Additionally both populations secrete cytokines which have synergistic inhibitory activity against leukaemic cells in culture which we have identified as γ-interferon (γINF) and tumour necrosis factor (TNF) [19]. Neither the cells nor their secondary cytokines are detected after treatment of leukaemia by combination chemotherapy [17, 20] although Kiyohara et al. [21] have found increased NK activity 1 month after certain chemotherapy combinations in patients with urological neoplasms.

Interleukin 2 Treatment of Patients with Residual Leukaemia and New Immunomodulatory Drugs

Following our observation that AK cells briefly exposed to the cytokine IL2 could further substantially augment the lysis of AML blasts and inhibit clonogenic leukaemic growth [22], we embarked on a phase I/II study of the administration of IL2 in 22 patients with a range of haematological malignancies. IL2 was given by intravenous infusion to 14 patients with AML recovering after chemotherapy with or without autologous BMT in either first or second CR. The patients were aged between 18 and 67 years (median 33 years) and received one to two infusions of IL2 over 3–5 days with a maximum daily dose of 3 × 10^6 Cetus units/m^2 per day. Two initial patients were treated in a phase I trial with escalating doses of IL2 given over a 6 h infusion. These patients treated for 11 and 12 days developed severe toxicity with high fever, prostration and cardiovascular collapse. Modification of the protocol with continuous infusions (CI) permitted the administration of equivalent or greater total doses over a shorter period without severe toxicity. Although fever, malaise, nausea and vomiting and hypotension remained common, no patient required admission to an intensive care facility [23]. Lymphokine activated killer (LAK) cells appeared in the peripheral blood during the infusions. These cells, when incubated with myeloid leukaemic blasts, significantly inhibited the growth of leukaemia colonies and also produced high levels of both TNF and γINF [20, 24]. IL2 also increased the peripheral blood neutrophil count and our studies show evidence that this may be due to the secondary production of GM-CSF.

A review of the European experience of IL2 usage in haematological malignancies shows that more than 100 patients have been treated. The most frequent indication has been AML. The most pertinent information concerns patients treated at the two extremes of their disease – chemotherapy resistant and/or relapsed disease and those in first CR. Thirty-eight patients have been treated by IL2 alone for relapsed and/or refractory AML. Six achieved complete remission (+ five partial remissions), these remissions lasting 3–30+ months [25]. Twenty-three patients have had IL2 in first CR (four had preceding MDS). Of the 19 primary cases, 8 had an ABMT prior to IL2 and 7 remain in CR from 1–32+ months (1 died from the treatment). Of those having chemotherapy alone 7 of 11 remain in CR. Four of four with prior MDS relapsed (one had an ABMT). Very few patients treated beyond first CR remain free of disease. Rapid relapse in two cases of M5 AML [26] and laboratory data for IL2 receptor expression in some cases of AML (26, 27) must caution us against undue optimism – although Foa has published encouraging contradictory observations [28].

Preliminary studies with IL2 show that first: toxicity can be manageable; second, patients beyond first CR (however pretreated) are generally not cured, nor are those with a preexisting MDS; third, patients in first CR who have an ABMT prior to IL2 may represent the best prospect for cure by this immunotherapeutic approach. Logic suggests this approach since the disease is likely to be at its nadir at this point and the immune environment may be ideal since it is already primed [17].

Linomide (Pharmacia – Leo) is an orally active drug with a long half-life which when taken in once or twice weekly dosing is apparently able to mimic all of the biological effects of IL2. Early phase I/II studies show only modest toxicity. Randomised studies are now underway in AML after ABMT (placebo controlled).

The outcome of current parallel randomised studies examining the role of IL2 and Linomide are urgently awaited. Immunotherapy is a promising but *weak* modality of therapy and benefit is most likely to be detected in patients with minimal residual disease (MRD). Since ABMT can "prime" the biological effectors we would recommend that such trials be done in patients in first CR having ABMT after best current chemotherapy [29].

Acknowledgements. I wish to express my gratitude to Professors Franco Mandelli, Robin Foa, Dominique Maraninchi, John Barrett, Drs. Didier Blaise, Tony Goldstone, Seah Lim, Adrian Newland, Donald MacDonald and the Eurocetus and Roussell Study Groups for their laudable help in providing much presently unpublished data and to Malcolm Brenner, David Gottlieb, Mike Hamon and many other members of our medical, technical and nursing staff on the bone marrow transplant team at the Royal Free Hospital who have helped in this programme.

References

1. Rees JKH, Gray RG et al. (1986) Lancet ii: 1236–1241
2. Preisler HD, Anderson K, Cuttner J et al. (1987) Br J Haematol 71: 189–194
3. Wolff SN, Herzig AW, Phillips GL et al. (1987) Semin Oncol 14: 12–17
4. Weinstein JH, Mayer RJ, Rosenthal DS et al. (1983) Blood 62: 315–319
5. Garson OM, Hagemeijer A, Sakurai M et al. (1989) Cancer Genet Cytogenet 40: 187–202
6. International Bone Marrow Transplant Registry (1989) Lancet i: 1119–1122

7. Gratwohl A, Hermans J, Barrett AJ et al. (1988) Lancet i: 1379–1382
8. Pollard, CM, Powles RL, Miller JL (1986) Lancet ii: 1343–1344
9. Atkinson K, Biggs J, Dodds A et al. (1988) Aust NZ J Med 18: 587–593
10. Maraninchi D, Gluckman E, Blaise D (1986) Lancet ii: 175–178
11. Weiden PL, Fluornoy N, Thomas ED et al. (1979) N Engl J Med 300: 1068–1073
12. Clift RA, Buckner CD, Appelbaum FR et al. (1990) Blood 76: 1867–1871
13. Prentice HG, Gottlieb DJ et al. (1990) Proceedings of the 3rd International Symposium on Minimal Residual Diseases in Acute Leukaemia. (in press)
14. Burnett AK, Hann IM, Robertson AG et al. (1988) Leukaemia 2: 300–303
15. Ash RC, Jasper D, Lawton CG et al. (1989) Blood 74(1): 163 (abstr)
16. Schattenberg A, De Witte T, Bar B et al. (1989) Bone Marrow Tansplant 4 [Suppl 1]: 111
17. Reittie JE, Gottlieb DJ, Heslop HE et al. (1989) Blood 73: 1351–1358
18. Hercend T, Reinherz ELK, Meuer SC et al. (1983) Nature 301: 158–160
19. Price G, Brenner MK, Prentice HG et al. (1989) Br J Cancer 71: 189–194
20. Heslop HE, Gottlieb DJ, Reittie JE et al. (1989) Br J Haematol 72: 122–126
21. Kiyohara T, Taniguchi K, Kubota S et al. (1988) J Exp Med 168: 2355–2360
22. Leger O, Drexler HG, Reittie JE, et al. (1987) Br J Haematol 67: 273–279
23. Gottlieb DJ, Brenner MK, Heslop HE et al. (1989) Br J Cancer 60: 610–615
24. Gottlieb DJ, Prentice HG, Heslop HE et al. (1988) Blood 74: 2335–2342
25. Foa R, Fierro MT, Tosti S et al. (1990) Leuk Lymph 1: 113–117
26. MacDonald D, Jiang YZ, Swirsky D et al. (1991) Br J Haematol 77: 43–49
27. Carron JA, Cawley JC (1989) Br J Haematol 73: 168
28. Foa R, Caretto P, Fierro NT (1990) Br J Haematol 75: 34–40
29. Geller RB, Saral R, Karp JE et al. (1990) Leukemia 4: 313–315

Interleukin 2 Treatment in the Management of Acute Leukemia Patients*

R. Foa[1], G. Meloni[2], A. Guarini[1], M. Vignetti[2], A. Gillio Tos[1], S. Tosti[2], A. Novarino[1], F. Gavosto[1], and F. Mandelli[2]

Introduction

The possibility of successful employment of an immunotherapeutic approach to the treatment of solid tumor patients has been boosted by the encouraging results obtained starting from the mid-1980s using interleukin 2 G (IL2) usually in association with ex vivo generated lymphokine-activated killer (LAK) cells [1–3]. Though the real impact of this innovative treatment modality still needs to be fully appreciated, a proportion of complete and, more often, partial remissions have been obtained in cancer patients with advanced and resistant disease, particularly renal cell carcinoma and melanoma.

Immunotherapy with IL2/LAK cells is potentially applicable to all neoplastic patients, since the cytotoxic effectors of the lytic activity are present in all body tissues. In view of the lack of available information for acute leukemias and of the necessity of pursuing new therapeutic modalities for this category of patients, different groups including our own have extensively investigated in the preclinical setting the potential applicability of an IL2-mediated approach

[4–9]. The results obtained indicated that both acute myeloid leukemia (AML) and acute lymphoid leukemia (ALL) blasts can be lysed by LAK cells and that few leukemic cells may be eliminated by normal LAK effectors. Furthermore, patients in complete remission (CR) often display a good LAK activity, also against autologous blasts, and a satisfactory LAK function may be generated in bone marrow and peripheral blood samples containing a variable, often high, proportion of leukemic cells. Finally, using as a model immunosuppressed nude mice, it was possible to demonstrate that normal LAK cells, as well as IL2 alone, were capable of blocking the growth of human leukemic cell lines and primary blasts.

Clinical Applications

The above summarized data have represented the necessary background towards the clinical exploitation of immunotherapy in the management of acute leukemia patients. Our experience in vivo was initiated at the beginning of 1988 through a collaborative project between our Institution and the chair of Hematology in Rome. In view of the lack of definitive evidence that the combined use of IL2 and LAK cells was truly superor to IL2 alone, we elected to employ in our patients only IL2 (by Glaxo Imb, Geneva, Switzerland) and opted for a daily continuous infusion protocol. Based on the toxicity observed in the first patients treated, we thereafter used a daily escalating protocol aimed at repeated 5-day cycles

[1] Dipartimento di Scienze Biomediche ed Oncologia Umana, Sezione di Clinica Medica, University of Turin; Via Genova 3, 10126 Turin, Italy
[2] Dipartimento di Biopatologia Umana, Sezione di Ematologia, University of Rome, Rome, Italy
* This work was supported by the Istituto Superiore di Sanita', Rome. AGT has a fellowship from the Associazione Italiana per la Ricerca sul Cancro (AIRC), Milan.

of IL2 with a 2- to 3-day interval between each cycle. The maximum dose reached in the "induction" courses was 1000 Mg/m^2 per day. When applicable, "maintenance" cycles were administered with 5-day monthly low-dose courses of IL2 given i.v. over a 6-h period on an outpatient basis.

In view of the lack of information on the toxicity, hematological modifications and clinical effects, several patients with advanced and resitant acute leukemia were enrolled, particularly in the early entries. Thereafter, and on the basis of the results obtained, different categories of patients in different phases of the disease have entered our protocol.

Summarizing the results obtained during this 3-year experience, it is felt that IL2 alone has little effect in patients with a large marrow blastosis. This is probably contributed by a numerical insufficient quantity of evocable cytotoxic effectors due to the heavy blastic contamination, namely at the marrow level. In addition, it should be noted that our group has recently shown that in most acute leukemia patients at diagnosis and in relapse there is a defect of the LAK machinery, often recognizable only in an autologous setting [10], suggesting therefore that in patients with a large tumoral mass it may be difficult to generate LAK cells active specifically against the leukemic population of the host.

It is worth noting that in individual patients who did not respond to IL2 alone, an unexpected response to chemotherapy was thereafter observed, suggestive of a possible synergistic effect between the cytokine and the cytotoxic drugs. We have recently confirmed in vitro this in vivo clinical observation, using a clonogenic system in semisolid media which showed that AML blasts preincubated with IL2 may become significantly more susceptible to the lytic action of Ara-C [11].

The situation appeared quite different when patients with small, but detectable reistant disease were enrolled. So far, seven patients with 8%–15% resistant bone marrow blasts have been treated with IL2 alone. Of the five AMLs, three have obtained a complete remission (CR) with two to four cycles of IL2. One patient persists in fourth CR 38 months later,

another remained in third remission for 4 months and the last for 9 months before relapsing. It should be noted that the latter obtained a fourth CR with low-dose Ara-C and is currently again on a maintenance protocol with IL2. Of the two ALLs, one obtained a short-lived CR. The detailed clinicohematological information on the AML cases treated with IL2 and hereby discussed are reported in Foa et al. [12, 13].

The side effects in the treated patients were, using the daily escalating protocol, acceptable and in line with those described for other patient categories. None of the patients ever required intensive case treatment. The "maintenance" cycles were of overall easy administration in the outpatients department and, as expected, the side effects of lesser severity. In terms of clinical modifications, most patients experienced, after the IL2 "induction" courses, a more or less evident splenohepatomegaly. Hematologically, under IL2 infusion a neutrophilia with eosinophilia was noted. After stopping IL2, an increase in WBC count was recorded coupled to a lymphocytosis with large granular lymphocytes, often with prominent polar protrusions rich in azurophilic granules (Fig. 1).

Prolonged "induction" treatment is frequently followed by a moderate anemia and by a moderate to severe thrombocytopenia. The latter in some cases necessitates supportive treatment. Recent data by our group [14] suggest that the IL2-generated LAK cells are capable of playing a marked inhibitory effect on the in vitro growth of autologous bone marrow megakaryocytic progenitor cells. This effect appears to be largely mediated by tumor necrosis factor (TNF) alpha.

Another clinical setting in which the administration of IL2 bears a relevant potential application is after an autologous bone marrow transplantation, in an attempt to boost the cytotoxic compartment, which has been suggested to be amplified following this procedure [15]. The results so far reported suggest that this approach is feasible and that the LAK compartment may be amplified [16] and personal data); it should, however, be noted that relatively high doses of IL2 could be administrered only at

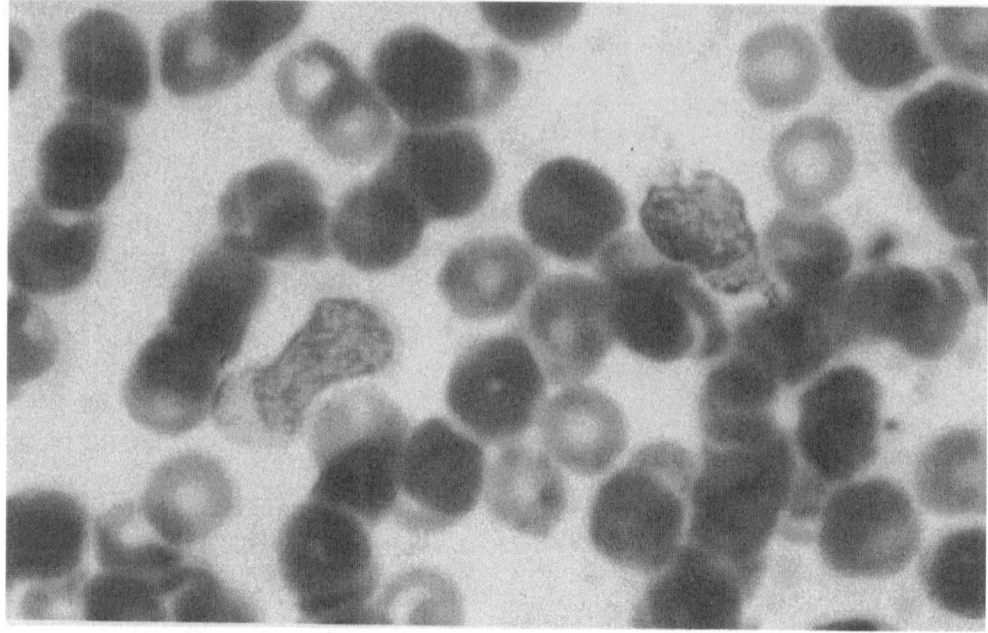

Fig. 1. Granular lymphocytes with marked polar protrusions following in vivo cycles of recombinant IL2

approximately 2 months from grafting, when a satisfactory hemopoietic recovery has been achieved. Whilst this may be acceptable for some disorders, for others – for example ALL – a scheme contemplating the early infusion of IL2, possibly associated with LAK cells, may prove to be preferable.

Finally, some preliminary data have suggested that IL2 in combination with chemotherapy may be an option for the lymphoid blast crisis of chronic myeloid leukemia [17].

Biological Modifications

The immunological monitoring of the treated patients has documented several modifications of both peripheral blood and bone marrow lymphocytes [18]. At the phenotypic level, while no major difference in the distribution of circulating CD3, CD4 and CD8 lymphocytes could be documented after two cycles of IL2, in patients who underwent four cycles a significant increase of CD3+ and CD8+ cells was seen. The presence of CD25+ cells, as well as an increase of CD16+ lymphocytes, was

recorded both in the blood and in the marrow. Functionally, an amplification of the natural killer (NK) compartment was observed, particularly in patients with more limited disease, as well as an increase of LAK effectors both in the blood and in the marrow. Furthermore, we could document that the administration of IL2 is followed by the in vivo generation of "spontaneous" LAK cells, and, of relevance in view of the disease under study, that this event occurs also in bone marrow lymphocytes. An example of the amplification of the cytotoxic compartment after treatment with IL2 is shown in Fig. 2.

Similarly to what was observed in other tumors, also in acute leukemia patients the administration of IL2 is followed by an in vivo release of TNF alpha and of interferon gamma, as documented by the increased levels detected in the serum.

Considerations and Future Perspectives

Taken together, the results so far obtained with recombinant IL2 in acute leukemia allow us to consider a role for this innova-

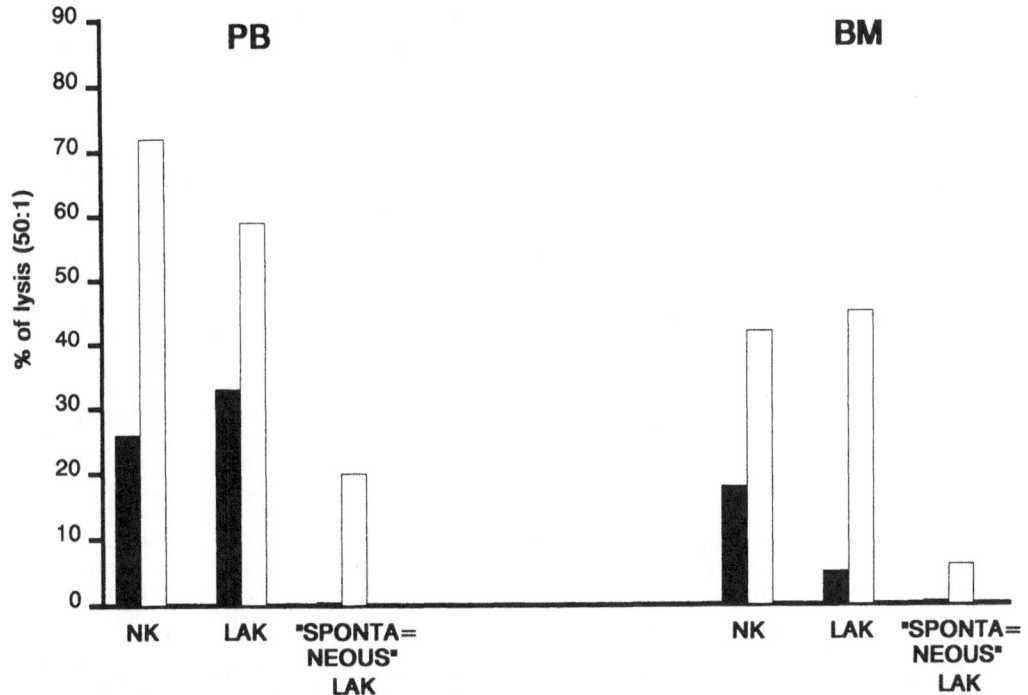

Fig. 2. Modification of the NK, LAK and "spontaneous" LAK activity in peripheral blood and bone marrow lymphocytes of a representative leukemic patient following in vivo administration of IL2

tive therapeutic modality in the management of these patients and also allow us to suggest some considerations with regard to patient selection, as guidelines for future studies.

It seems quite convincingly shown that IL2 alone has little effect in patients with a large tumoral mass, and for such situations a combined approach between IL2 and chemotherapy will need to be carefully investigated. This approach may also benefit from in vitro preclinical evaluations. The possible role of IL2 + LAK may also deserve some consideration.

The potential role of IL2 alone in patients with limited, but detectable resistant disease obviously requires further confirmation, particularly in AML. In this regard, the search for additional biological informations, for instance susceptibility of the blasts to autologous LAK effectors, will represent a major goal in terms of predictive tests for patient selection.

It is clear that the encouraging results obtained in the latter category of patients indicate that studies in AML in remission

are warranted. These will be probably directed, initially, to pilot studies in first CR, as a baseline for a possible randomized trial, and to multicenter randomized studies for AML patients in second CR.

The role for IL2, with or without LAK cells, following a bone marrow autograft still awaits data to support not only the feasibility of this approach, but also its clinical impact. Furthermore, the validity of the two administration modalities above suggested (early and late IL2 infusion) will need to be defined, before drawing any firm conclusion on the potential efficacy of IL2 treatment after autotransplanting.

In conclusion, it is realistic to state that the clinical results so far obtained are in agreement with earlier laboratory data and suggest the potential activity of IL2 in the management of acute leukemia patients, particularly with limited or minimal residual disease. The ongoing trials and the search for response predictive factors should allow us in the relatively near future to define more targeted protocols of IL2 treatment for acute leukemia patients.

References

1. Rosenberg SA, Lotze MT, Muul LM, Leitman S, Chang AE, Ettinghausen SE, Matory YL, Skibber JM, Shiloni E, Vetto JT. Seipp CA, Simpson C, Reichert CM (1985) Observations on the systemic administration of autologous lymphokine-activated killer cells and recombinant interleukin-2 to patients with metastatic cancer. N Engl J Med 313: 1485–1492

2. Rosenberg SA, Lotze MT, Muul LM, Chang AE, Avis FP, Leitman S, Linehan WM, Robertson CN, Lee RE. Rubin JT. Seipp CA, Simpson CG, White DE (1987) A progress report on the treatment of 157 patients with advanced cancer using lymphokine-activated killer cells and interleukin-2 or high dose interleukin-2 alone. N Engl J Med 316: 889–897

3. West WH, Tauer KW, Yannelli JR. Marshall GD, Orr DW, Thurman GB. Oldham RK (1987) Constant-infusion recombinant interleukin-2 in adoptive immunotherapy of advanced cancer. N Engl J Med 316: 898–905

4. Oshimi K, Oshimi Y, Akutsu M. Takei Y, Saito H, Okada M, Mizoguchi H (1986) Cytotoxicity of interleukin 2-activated lymphocytes for leukemia and lymphoma cells. Blood 68: 938–948

5. Lotzova E, Savary CA, Herberman RB (1987) Induction of NK cell activity against fresh human leukemia in culture with interleukin 2. J Immunol 138: 2718–2727

6. Fierro MT, Xin-Sheng L, Lusso P, Bonferroni M, Matera L, Cesano A. Arione R. Forni G, Foa R (1988) In vitro and in vivo susceptibility of human leukemic cells to lymphokine activated killer activity. Leukemia 2: 50–54

7. Adler A, Chervenick PA, Whiteside TL, Lotzova E, Herberman RB (1988) Interleukin 2 induction of lymphokine-activated killer (LAK) activity in the peripheral blood and bone marrow of acute leukemia patients. I. Feasibility of LAK generation in adult patients with active disease and in remission. Blood 71: 709–716

8. Lista P, Fierro MT, Xin-Sheng L, Bonferroni M, Brizzi MF, Porcu P, Pegoraro L, Foa R (1989) Lymphokine-activated killer (LAK) cells inhibit the clonogenic growth of human leukemic stem cells. Eur J Hematol 42: 425–430

9. Foa R, Caretto P, Fierro MT, Bonferroni M, Cardona S, Guarini A, Lista P, Pegoraro L, Mandelli F, Forni G, Gavosto F (1990) Interleukin 2 does not promote the in vitro and in vivo proliferation and growth of human acute leukaemia cells of myeloid and lymphoid origin. Br J Haematol 75: 34–40

10. Foa R, Fierro MT, Cesano A, Guarini A, Bonferroni M, Raspadori D, Miniero R, Lauria F, Gavosto F (1991) Defective lymphokine – activated killer cell generation and activity in acute leukemia patients with active disease. Blood 78: 1041–1046

11. Lista P, Brizzi MF, Resegotti L, Allione B, Pegoraro L, Foa R (1992) Interleukin 2 may improve the therapeutic effect of Ara-C in acute myeloid leukaemia. Br J Cancer: (in press)

12. Foa R, Fierro MT, Tosti S, Meloni G, Gavosto F. Mandelli F (1990) Induction and persistence of complete remission in a resistant acute myeloid leukemia patient after treatment with recombinant interleukin-2. Leuk Lymph 1: 113–117

13. Foa R, Meloni G, Tosti S, Novarino A, Fenu S. Gavosto F, Mandelli F (1991) Treatment of acute myeloid leukaemia patients with recombinant interleukin 2: a pilot study. Br J Haematol 77: 491–496

14. Guarini A, Sanavio F, Novarino A, Gillio Tos A, Aglietta M and Foa R (1991) Thrombocytopenia in acute leukaemia patients treated with IL2: cytolytic effect of LAK cells on megakaryocytic progenitors. Br J Haematol 79: (in press)

15. Reittie JE, Gottlieb D, Heslop HE, Leger O, Drexler HG, Hazlehurst G, Hoffbrand AV, Prentice HG, Brenner MK (1989) Endogenously generated activated killer cells circulate after autologous and allogeneic marrow transplantation but not after chemotherapy. Blood 73: 1351–1358

16. Blaise D, Olive D, Stoppa AM, Viens P, Pourreau C, Lopez M, Attal M, Jasmin C, Monges G, Mawas C, Mannoni P, Palmer P, Franks C, Philip T, Maraninchi D (1990) Hematological and immunologic effects of the systemic administration of recombinant interleukin-2 after autologous bone marrow transplantation. Blood 76: 1092–1097

17. Meloni G, Foa R, Tosti S, Vignetti M, Gavosto F, Mandelli F (1990) IL-2 in the treatment of chronic myeloid leukemia after lymphoid blast crisis: a pilot study. Haematologica 73: 502–505

18. Foa R, Guarini A, Gillio Tos A, Cardona S, Fierro MT, Meloni G, Tosti S, Mandelli F, Gavosto F (1991) Peripheral blood and bone marrow immunophenotypic and functional modifications induced in acute leukemia patients treated with interleukin 2: evidence of in vivo lymphokine activated killer cell generation. Cancer Res 51: 964–968

Assessment of Lymphokine-Activated Killer Activity Against Myeloid Leukemic Blasts and the Myeloid Cell Line K562 by Flow Cytometry

H. S. P. Garritsen[1], G. M. J. Segers-Nolten[1], K. Radoševic[1], B. G. de Grooth[1], M. Kiehl[2], B. Wörmann[2], W. Hiddemann[2], and J. Greve[1]

Introduction

It is well known that recombinant interleukin-2 (rIL-2) and other lymphokines can be used to increase cell mediated cytotoxicity of PBL against non-HLA restricted targets. Futhermore rIL-2 is able to induce cell mediated cytotoxicity of PBL against tumor cells which were first insensitive to cell mediated cytotoxicity. These activated lymphocytes are called lymphokine-activated killer (LAK) cells. It is of great importance to determine the functional capacities of these activated cells for killing specific target cells like leukemic blasts. In this study we determined the functional capacity of activated killer cells from healthy donors for killing blasts from acute myeloid leukemia (AML) patients and compared it with the capacity for killing K562 cells. We use newly developed flow cytometric assays for determination of cytotoxicity [1] and conjugate formation. In this way we obtain information on whether leukemia related defects in the killing mechanism occur and to what extent it is possible to overcome these defects by using specific cytokines.

Materials and Methods

Effector cells were obtained from ten healthy donors. Peripheral blood lymphocytes

were obtained after density separation (density 1.077 g/cm^3), (Percoll, Pharmacia Uppsala, Sweden). The effector cells were cultured for 3 days ($1 \times 10^6/ml$) either with or without rIL-2 (500 U/ml) to generate LAK cells. Bone marrow aspirates before treatment from four AML patients were used to obtain mononuclear target cells. Mononuclear cells were separated by Ficoll-Hypaque gradient centrifugation. All aspirates contained over 90 % leukemic blasts. Cell were stored in liquid nitrogen for 2–3 months. The blasts were thawed 2 days prior to the experiments. Before the assay, cells were checked for viability (viability test using ethidium bromide and acridine orange staining [2]). Preparations with more than 70 % viable cells were used as targets. K562, an NK sensitive cell line [3], was also used as target. Both types of targets were kept in suspension culture at 37 °C, in a 5 % CO_2 incubator.

Staining Procedures

F-18 staining of target cells was performed at a cell concentration of $10^6/ml$ using an F-18 concentration of 0.010–0.025 µg/ml. The staining procedure was performed as described [1]. For determination of conjugate formation effector cells were stained with F-18 using the same procedure. Tetramethylrhodamine isothiocyanate (TRITC) of cells was performed using a 1.3-mM stock solution of TRITC (Serva, Heidelberg, FRG) in ethanol. Twenty microliters of the stock solution was added to 1 ml of the target cell suspension (cell concentra-

[1] University of Twente, Department of Applied Physics, Cell Characterization Group PO Box 217, 7500 AE Enschede, The Netherlands
[2] Department of Internal Medicine A, Westfälische Wilhelms University, Münster, FRG

tion 10^6/ml). Target cells were incubated in the dark, at 37°C, in 5% CO_2 for 1 h. Subsequently incubation cells were washed twice with excess volume of cold medium and resuspended at a final concentration of 2.10^5/ml.

Flow Cytometer

Experiments were performed with a home-built flow cytometer equipped with a 100-mW air-cooled argon ion laser tuned to 488 nm and operating at a power output of 50 mW. The instrument has been described in detail elsewhere [4]. For measuring the F-18 fluorescence a six-cavity filter 530-nm DF 50-nm (Omega) was used, for PI fluorescence and TRITC fluorescence an RG 610–4 mm was used.

Flow Cytometric Cytotoxicity Assay

A flow cytometric cytotoxicity test was used as described in [1]. Basically this test determines the number of live target cells (N_l) and the total number of target cells, alive or dead (N_t) in the test sample and in a control sample. In this test target cells are flow cytometrically identified by F-18 mem-brane labeling. Dead target cells are characterized by F-18 labeling and simultaneous propidium iodide (PI) uptake. Cytotoxicity is then defined as:

$$\frac{N_{l_c} - N_{l_{test}}}{N_{l_c}} \cdot 100\%$$

Each sample was made in triplicate. Three effector: target ratios were tested: 12.5:1, 25:1 and 37.5:1.

Flow Cytometric Measurement of Conjugate Formation

Target cells and effector cells were stained with TRITC and F-18 respectively. Effector cells (PBL) were resuspended at the concentration of 5.10^6/ml and 0.1 ml of each effector cell suspension was mixed with 0.1 mgl target cell (K562) suspension (2.10^5/ml). Each sample was made in triplicate. Control samples consisted of target cells in medium only. Samples were incubated at 37°C for 0, 1, 2, 3 and 4 h. The double fluorescent positive particles were sorted on a cell sorter to verify that they were conjugates. Fluorescence microscopy was used to verify that the stains used (F-18 and TRITC) did not influence conjugate formation and cytotoxicity.

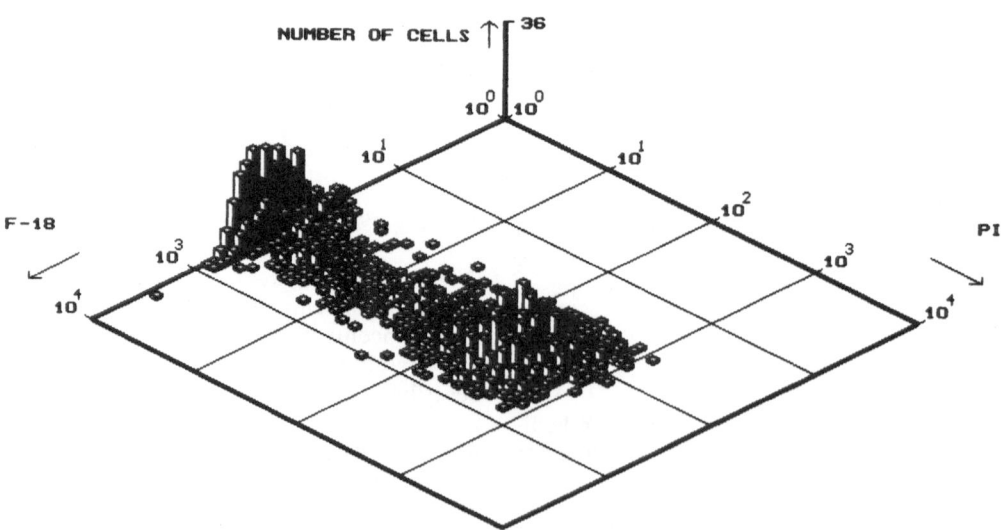

Fig. 1. Flow cytometric cytotoxicity assay using F-18 and PI. rIL-2 stimulated lymphocytes were incubated for 4 h with F-18 labeled K562 cells (ratio 37:1). Only F-18 positive cells are displayed. In this plot the number of cells is plotted versus F-18 fluorescence intensity and PI fluorescence intensity (note the log scale)

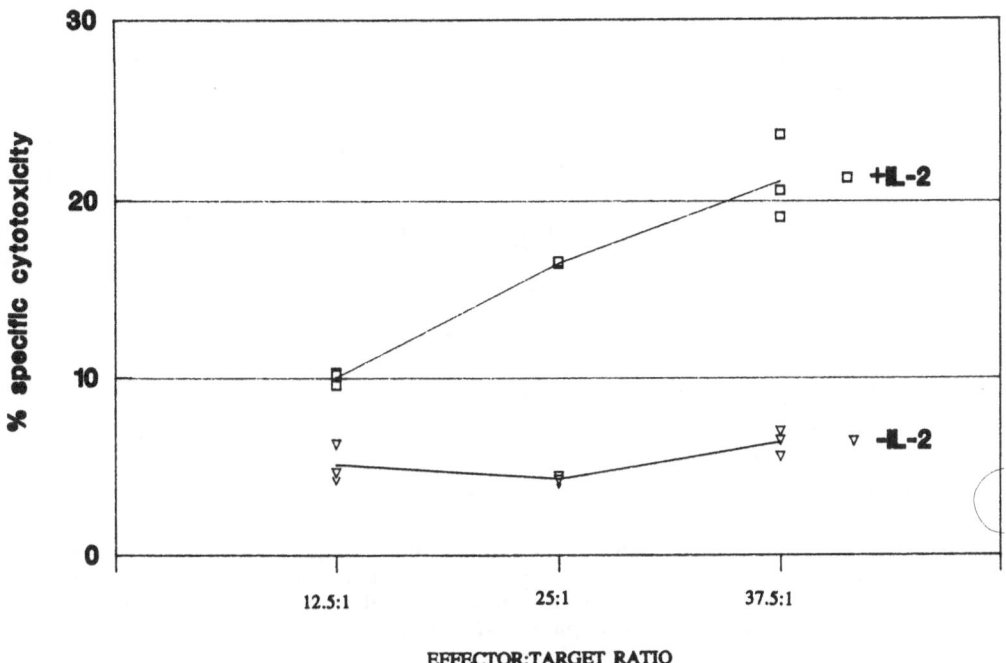

Fig. 2. Cytotoxicity of activated lymphocytes from one healthy donor against allogeneic blasts of one AML patient donor at different effector to target ratios. Each marker (square or triangle) represents one measurement

Results

Cytotoxicity

We determined the cytotoxicity of lymphocytes isolated from the blood of healthy donors against K562 and allogeneic leukemia blasts. For this determination we used the flow cytometric method described previously. Figure 1 gives an example of a flow cytometric plot obtained in such a test. It shows the number of target cells as a function of F-18 fluorescence (which identifies target cells) and P1 fluorescence (which identifies dead cells). The influence of culturing lymphocytes with or without 500 U/ml rIL-2 on the cytotoxicity is shown in Fig. 2. In this case we used leukemic blasts from one AML patient as target cells. Clearly the cytotoxicity is much higher and the influence of the effector/target cell ratio is greater after culturing with rIL-2. That the cytotoxicity against K562 is strongly dependent on the individual healthy donor

is shown in Fig. 3. From Fig. 4 it becomes clear that similar effects are present for cytotoxicity against allogeneic leukemic blasts.

Conjugate Formation

Using the flow cytometer we also studied the conjugate formation. The principle of the determination is illustrated in the dotplot of Fig. 5. In this particular case we used an effector/target cell ratio of 25:1 and studied the conjugate formation between rIL-2 stimulated lymphocytes and K562. In the dotplot separate clusters are obtained: unconjugated lymphocytes (F18 positive, TRITC negative); unconjugated K562 (TRITC positive, F18 negative); conjugates (TRITC and F18 positive). To check whether this last category of cells were really conjugates we sorted this population and studied the sample by means of fluorescence microscopy. Figures 6 shows the

583

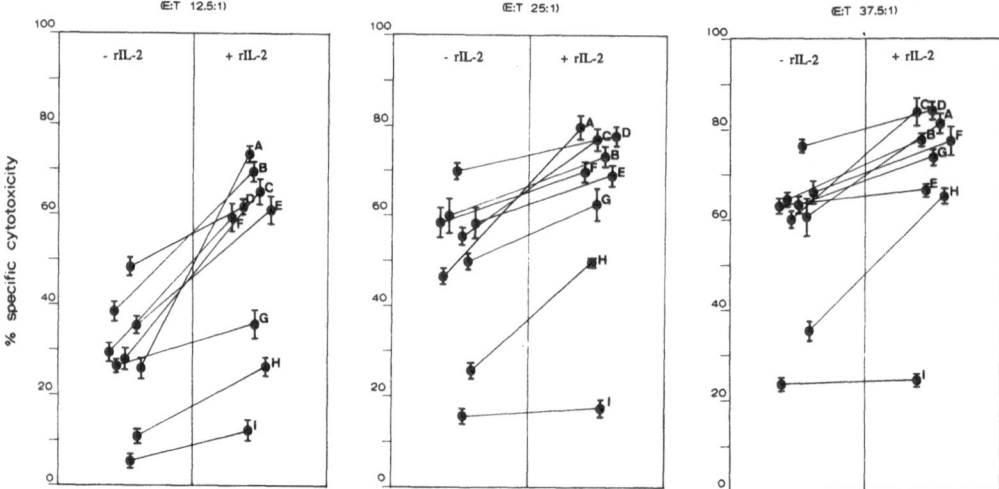

Fig. 3. Cytotoxicity against K562 with lymphocytes from nine different healthy donors (A–I). Each point represents mean and standard error of the results obtained from three measurements. The results obtained with and without rIL-2 stimulation of lymphocytes at the same E:T ratio are interconnected by a *solid line*. Measurement prints were put on arbitrary positions along the horizontal axis

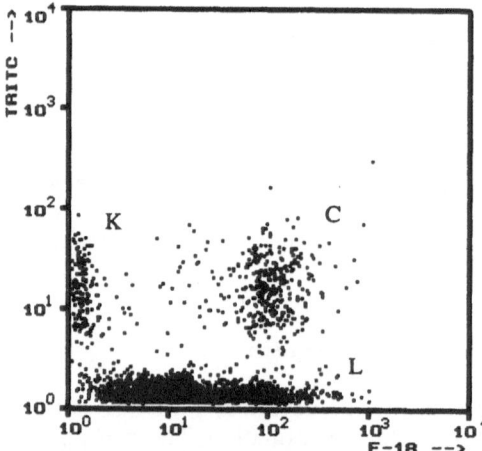

Fig. 5. Dotplot showing conjugate formation between F-18 labeled lymphocytes and TRITC labeled K562. Three clusters of events are observed: A cluster only positive for F-18, which are unconjugated lymphocytes (*L*); cluster positive only for TRITC, which are unconjugated K562 (*K*) and a cluster positive for TRITC and F-18 which are conjugates (*C*)

results of such a measurement (85 % conjugates, 15 % single K562). Figures 6 and 7 show the simultaneous measurements of conjugate formation (Fig. 6) and cell

mediated cytotoxicity (Fig. 7) using K562 as target cells after 0, 1, 2, 3 and 4 h of incubation. rIL-2 stimulated lymphocytes of two donors were used at an E:T ratio of 25:1. It is clear that stimulation with rIL-2 increases both conjugate formation and cytotoxicity.

Influence of the Fluorochromes TRITC and F-18 on Conjugate Formation

Tables 1 and 2 show that F-18 and TRITC singly or in combination do not significantly influence conjugate formation or viability of the target cells as assessed by fluorescence microscopy.

Discussion

The flow cytometric method presented in this paper to measure cell mediated cytotoxicity is a good replacement for the ^{51}Cr release assay and can be used with target cells which display a relatively low uptake of ^{51}Cr and a relatively high spontaneous leakage. Even after 4 h of incubation at 37 °C, in 5 % CO_2 the separation between target and effector cells was no problem. Against the NK-sensitive cell line K562 the

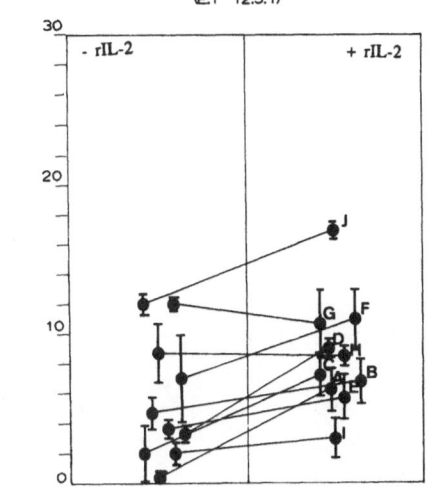

(E:T 12.5:1)

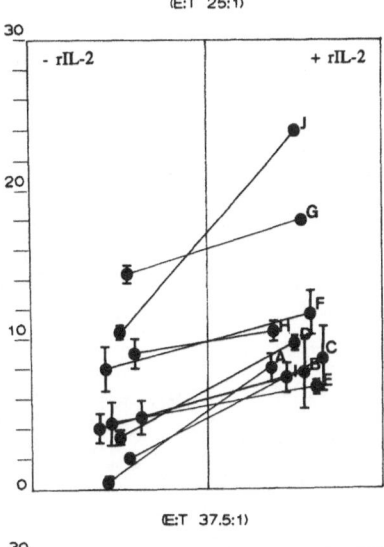

(E:T 25:1)

(E:T 37.5:1)

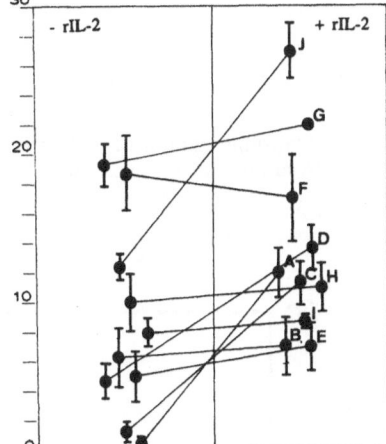

Fig. 4. Flow cytotoxicity of lymphocytes from ten different donors (*A–J*) against allogeneic leukemic blasts from one AML patient. Each *point* represents mean and standard error of the results obtained from three measurements with lymphocytes from a single donor. The results obtained with and without rIL-2 stimulation at the same E:T are interconnected by a *solid line*. *Right panels* give the results with rIL-2 stimulation

majority of healthy donors display a considerable (40%–70%) specific cytotoxicity (E:T 25:1), although there exist donors with a rather low cytotoxicity. Coculturing for 3 days with 500 U/ml rIL-2 increases specific cytotoxicity, especially in the low E:T ratios. The ability of NK and LAK cells from normal donors to lyse cultured allogeneic leukemic blasts is also assessed. NK activity against cultured leukemic blasts was low (0%–10% specific cytotoxicity) for most donors at all E:T ratios tested. Only three of ten donors in the highest E:T ratio were able to display more than 10% specific cytotoxicity, indicating that leukemic blasts usually escape NK-mediated lysis. The sti-

mulation of LAK cells revealed an increse in the specific cytotoxicity against leukemic blasts. Seven out of ten donors in the highest E:T ratio were able to display more than 10% specific cytotoxicity. In view of the short generation time of the LAK cells (3 days) and the applied concentration of rIL-2 (500 U/ml) this is remarkable. However, successful LAK activation and lysis of leukemic blasts occurred with some but not with all donors.

Labeling effectors with F-18 and K562 targets with TRITC provided information about the kinetics of conjugate formation. It is shown that rIL-2 stimulated lymphocytes display different conjugate formation

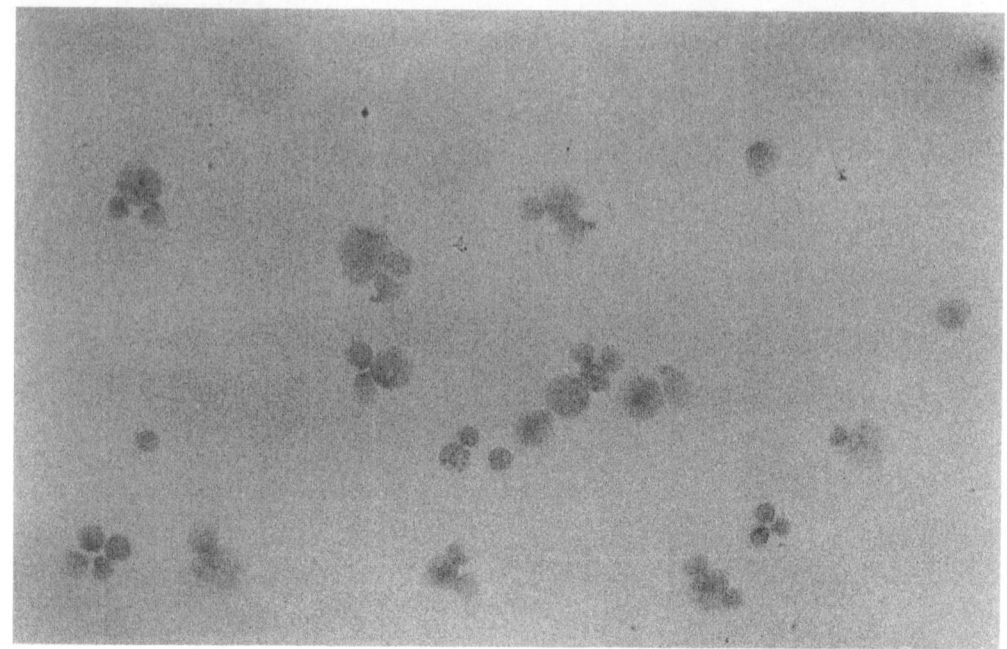

Fig. 6. Photomicrograph of cells obtained after sorting, selecting the double positive fluorescent events from Fig. 5. Cells were diretly sorted on a microscopic slide and stained with May-Grünwald Giemsa

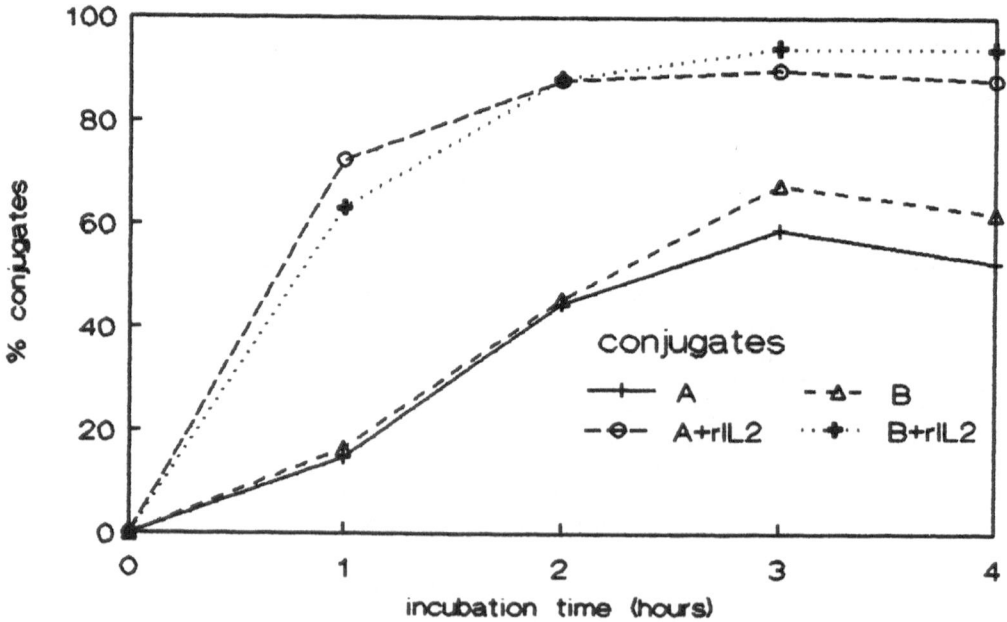

Fig. 7. Conjugate formation of lymphocytes of two donors (*A* and *B*) with K562. Lymphocytes were preincubated with (*A*+, *B*+) or without (*A*−, *B*−) rI-2. *Markers* represent the mean of triplicate measurements

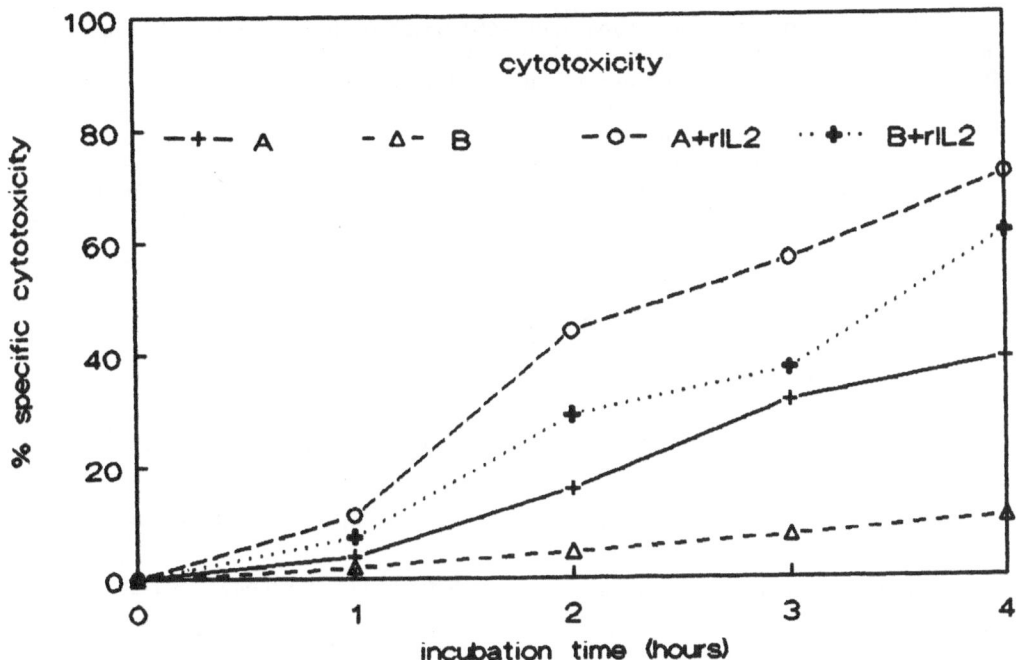

Fig. 8. Cell mediated cytotoxicity of lymphocytes of two donors (*A* and *B*) against K562. Lymphocytes were preincubated with (*A+*, *B+*) or without (*A–*, *B–*) rIL-2. *Markers* represent the mean of triplicate measurements

Table 1. Conjugate formation and viability of K652 tested by fluorescence microscopy with a combination of ethidium bromide and acridine orange. K562 with rIL-2 stimulated lymphocytes as effector cells (E:T) = 25:1). Results of triplicates are displayed as mean +/–standard error

	Single K562 cells			K562 cells in conjugates	
	Viable	Death		Viable	Death
$\dfrac{-}{-}$	21.5 ± 0.7	20.5 ± 0.7	$\dfrac{-}{-}$	47.5 ± 2.5	8 ± 3.6
$\dfrac{+}{-}$	20.5 ± 3.5	23 ± 8.5	$\dfrac{+}{-}$	45 ± 8.5	11.5 ± 3.5
$\dfrac{-}{+}$	22.5 ± 3.5	24.5 ± 7.8	$\dfrac{-}{+}$	43.5 ± 3.5	9.5 ± 0.7
$\dfrac{+}{+}$	22.3 ± 4	21.3 ± 7.5	$\dfrac{+}{+}$	44.7 ± 6.4	11.7 ± 3.5

$\dfrac{-}{-}$ K652 + lymphocytes unstained $\dfrac{-}{+}$ K562 unstained + lymphocytes F-18

$\dfrac{+}{-}$ K562 TRITC + lymphocytes unstained $\dfrac{+}{+}$ K562 TRITC + lymphocytes F-18

587

Table 2. Conjugate formation and viability of K652 tested by fluorescence microscopy with a combination of ethidium bromide and acridine orange. K562 with unstimulated lymphocytes as effector cells (E:T = 25:1). Results of triplicates are displayes as mean +/−standard error

	Single K562 cells			K562 cells in conjugates	
	Viable	Death		Viable	Death
−/−	36 ± 5.6	19 ± 4	−/−	29.7 ± 4	15.3 ± 4.6
+/−	35 ± 5.7	13 ± 5.7	+/−	42 ± 12.7	10 ± 4
−/+	34.5 ± 3.5	17 ± 4.2	−/+	35 ± 1.4	13.5 ± 0.7
+/+	31.6 ± 6.5	30.3 ± 16.3	+/+	22.3 ± 8.9	15.7 ± 5.6

−/− K652 + lymphocytes unstained   −/+ K562 unstained + lymphocytes F-18

+/− K562 TRITC + lymphocytes unstained   +/+ K562 TRITC + lymphocytes F-18

kinetics even when correlated with the percentge of killing. To prove that the conjugate formation took place, we sorted the double positive events and scored them after May-Grünwald Giemsa staining. The results shown in Figures 6 show that the double positive events are indeed conjugates. Also lymphocytes containing membrane-debris (from K562?) were visible, suggesting that a conjugate was possibly disrupted by sorting. The high number of conjugates in the cytospin preparations (85%) in our view justifies the conclusion that TRITC and F-18 double positive events are indeed conjugates. F-18 and TRITC used singly or in combination do not significantly influence conjugate formation or viability of the target cells as assessed by fluorescence microscopy.

Our aim is to evaluate LAK cell activity against autologous leukemic blasts, to be able to investigate aspects of the killing mechanism in leukemia. Conventional radioactive methods [5] gave frequent problems with high spontaneous release while flow cytometric alternatives using internal dyes [6–9] also showed high leakage during the 4 h of incubation. The methods presented in this paper offer the possibility to investigate the cell mediated cytotoxicity at a very detailed level, where killing, conjugate formation and for example immunophenotype of effector cells involved in killing can be revealed. This is of great importance in the study of acute myeloid leukemia where multiple defects in the killing mechanism of effector cells have been reported [10–12].

Conclusions

The flow cytometric method presented here can be used to assess cell mediated cytotoxicity of lymphocytes against myeloid leukemic blasts. By labeling effector cells with F-18 and target cells with TRITC it is now also possible to study conjugate formation with a flow cytometer. Differences in cell mediated cytotoxicity against K562 and allogeneic leukemic blasts were found between rIL-2 stimulated and unstimulated lymphocytes of the same donor.

References

1. Radoševic K, Garritsen HSP, van Graft M, de Grooth GB, Greve J (1990) A simple and sensitive flow cytometric assay for the determination of the cytotoxic activity of human natural killer cells. J Immunol Methods 135: 81–89

2. Parks DR, Bryan VM, Oi VM, Oi VT, Herzenberg LA (1968) Antigen specific identification and cloning of hybridomas with a fluorescence activated cell sorter (FACS). Proc Natl Acad Sci USA 76: 1962–1967

3. Lozzio CB, Lozzio BB (1975) Human chronic myelogenous leukemia cell line with positive Philadelphia chromosome. Blood 45: 321–334

4. Terstappen LWMM, de Grooth BG, Nolten GMJ, ten Napel, van Berkel W, Greve J (1986) Physical discrimination between human lymphocyte subpopulations by means of light scattering, revealing two populations of T8 positive cells. Cytometry 7: 178–184

5. Brunner KT, Mauel J, Cerottini JC, Chapuis B (1968) Quantitative assay of the lytic action of immune lymphoid cells on Cr 51-labeled allogenic target cells in vitro; inhibition by isoantibody and by drugs. Immunology 14: 181–189

6. McGinnes K, Chapman G, Marks R, Penny R (1986) A fluorescence NK assay using flow cytometry. J Immunol Methods 86: 7–16

7. Papa S, Vitale M, Mariani AR, Roda P, Facchini A, Manzoli FA (1988) Natural killer function in flow cytometry. I Evaluation of NK lytic activity on K562 cell line. J Immunol Methods 107: 73–79

8. Shi TX, Tong MJ, Bohman R (1987) The application of low cytometry in the study of natural killer cell cytotoxicity. Clin Immunol Immunopathol 45: 356–365

9. Kolber MA, Quinones RR, Gress RE, Henkart PA (1988) Measurement of cytotoxicity by target cell release and retention of the fluorescent dye bis-carboxyethyl-carboxy-fluorescein (BCECF). J Immuno Methods 180: 225–264

10. Teichmann JV, Ludwig WD, Seibt-Jung H, Thiel E (1990) Lymphokine-activated killer (LAK) cells against human leukemia – Augmentation of LAK-cell cytotoxicity by combinations of lymphokines or cytokines. In: Büchner T, Schellong G, Hiddemann W, Ritter J (eds) Acute leukemias II. Springer, Berlin Heidelberg New York (Haematology and blood transfusion, vol 33)

11. Tratkiewicz JA, Szer J, Boyd RL (1990) Lymphokine-activated killer cytotoxicity against leukemic blast cells. Clin Exp Immunol 80: 94–99

12. Lotzová E, Savary CA, Keating MJ (1982) Studies on the mechanism of defective natural killing in leukemia-diseased patients. Exp Hematol 10: 83–89

Effect of Cyclosporine on the Frequency of LAK Precursor Cells In Vivo and In Vitro*

D. Bunjes[1], M. Theobald[1], B. Hertenstein[1], M. Weiss[1], M. Wiesneth[2], R. Arnold[1], and H. Heimpel[1]

Introduction

A considerable part of the therapeutic efficacy of allogeneic bone marrow transplantation (BMT) has been attributed to the so-called graft-versus-leukemia effect (GvL) [1]. Lymphokine-activated killer cells (LAK) have been suggested as possible effector cells. Previous studies had demonstrated a very rapid regeneration of LAK cells after T-depleted BMT [2, 3]. The most effective conventional GvHD prophylaxis regimen currently available, cyclosporine plus methotrexate (CSA/MTX), has not been evaluated with respect to its effect on LAK regeneration after BMT. Such an investigation might be of considerable interest because there is some evidence that CSA/MTX and CSA alone are associated with an increased risk of relapse in patients with acute leukemias.

We have therefore employed a limiting dilution assay to evaluate the early regeneration of LAK precursor cells after allogeneic BMT. In addition, the in vitro effects of CSA were investigated in the same system.

Patients

Patient characteristics are summarized in Table 1.

Methods

Cells

Peripheral blood mononuclear cells (PBMNC) were obtained from healthy bone marrow donors and patients after BMT by centrifugation of either diluted peripheral blood or buffy coat cells over Ficoll-Hypaque ($d = 1.077$) and then cryopreserved. Patients were sampled 30 days and 60 days after BMT. Leu11b$^+$ cells and Leu4$^+$ cells were obtained by sorting PBMNC with an EPICS V cell sorter after labeling with the monoclonal antibodies Leu-11b-FITC and Leu-4-PE (Becton-Dickinson Inc.). The puritiy of the cell populations exceeded 95 % as determined by reanalysis.

Limiting Dilution Culture

Microcultures were performed in round-bottom microtiter plates. Sixteen replicate cultures were set up with cell numbers ranging from 40 to 40960 cells/well. Each culture contained 1×10^4 irradiated (40 Gy) autologous PBMNC as feeder cells, the culture medium consisting of RPMI 1640 supplemented with 10 % FCS, 100 U/ml recombinant human interleukin-2 (Sandoz) and antibiotics. The culture period was 7 days.

[1] Department of Internal Medicine III and [2]Department of Transfusion Medicine, University of Ulm, Robert-Koch-Str. 8, W-7900 Ulm , FRG
* This work was supported by the SFB 322.

Table 1. Patient characteristics

UPN	Diagnosis	Ages (years)	Conditioning	GvHD	Outcome
120	AML 1st CR	21	TBI/CTX	None	CCR
143	AML 1st CR	28	TBI/CTX	None	Isolated CNS relapse
140	AML in PR	29	TBI/VP16	None	Relapse
152	ALL 1st CR	39	TBI/CTX	None	CCR
154	ALL 1st CR	32	TBI/CTX	aGvHD II°	CCR
159	ALL 1st CR	37	Busulfan/CTX (200)	None	CCR
164	AML 1st CR	28	TBI/CTX	cGvHD	CCR
174	ALL 2nd CR	19	TBI/VP16	None	Relapse
122	CM: CP	38	TBI/CTX/DNR	None	Relapse
139	CML 2nd CP	37	TBI/VP16	None	Relapse
161	CML CP	36	TBI/CTX/DNR	aGvHD II°/cGvHD	CCR
172	CML CP	54	TBI/CTX/DNR	cGvHD	Relapse
199	CML CP	34	TBI/CTX/DNR	cGvHD	CCR
201	CML CP	45	TBI/CTX/DNR	cGvHD	CCR
205	CML CP	26	TBI/CTX/DNR	aGvHD II°/cGvHD	CCR

TBI, total body irradiation 6×2 Gy; CTX, cyclophosphamide 120 mg/kg; VP16, etoposide 60 mg/kg; busulfan, 16 mg/kg; DNR, daunorubicin 60 mg/m²

Cytotoxicity Assay

After 7 days, each microculture was split into three and the cytolytic activity was assessed in a 4-h ^{51}Cr release assay using labeled Daudi, K562 and autologous PHA-blasts as targets. Specific lysis was defined as

$$\frac{\text{experimental } ^{51}\text{CR release} - \text{spontaneous } ^{51}\text{CR release}}{\text{maximum } ^{51}\text{Cr release} - \text{spontaneous } ^{51}\text{Cr}} \times 100.$$

Proliferation Assay

Proliferation was assessed by measuring [³H]thymidine incorporation during the last 18 h in culture.

Statistical Analysis

The frequencies of LAK precursor cells (LAK-p) were determined by Poisson analysis. Individual cultures were scored as positive if their specific ^{51}Cr release exceeded the mean of spontaneous ^{51}Cr release by at least three standard deviations. The values for the frequencies, the 95% confidence limits of the frequencies, and the probability of single hit kinetics were calculated by likelihood maximization and chi-squared minimization as described by Taswell. Only experiments with a $p > 0.05$ were considered valid.

Results

LAK-p in PBMNC of Healthy Volunteers

As illustrated in Fig. 1, the cells expanded in our culture system fulfil the criteria of LAK cells in that they kill the NK-resistant Daudi cells without significantly lysing autologous PBMNC. The LAK-p frequencies of healthy volunteers showed a wide range (1/300–1/100000) with the majority of values clustering between 1/2000 and 1/30000. Figures 2 and 3 show that the majority of LAK-p reside in the CD16

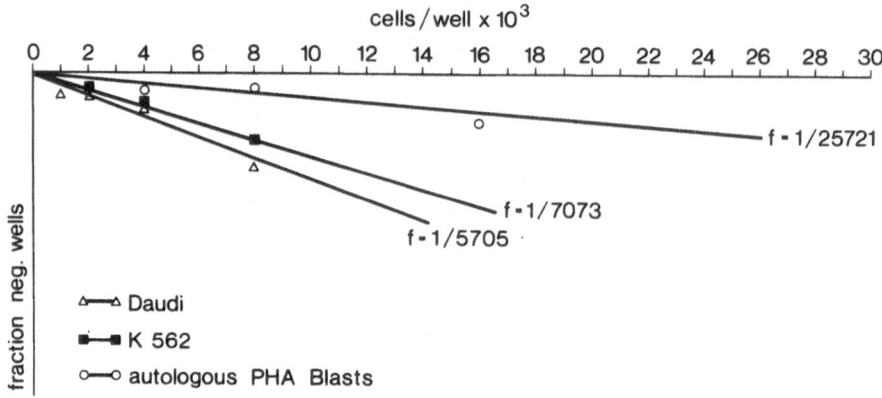

Fig. 1. LAK-p in PBMNC

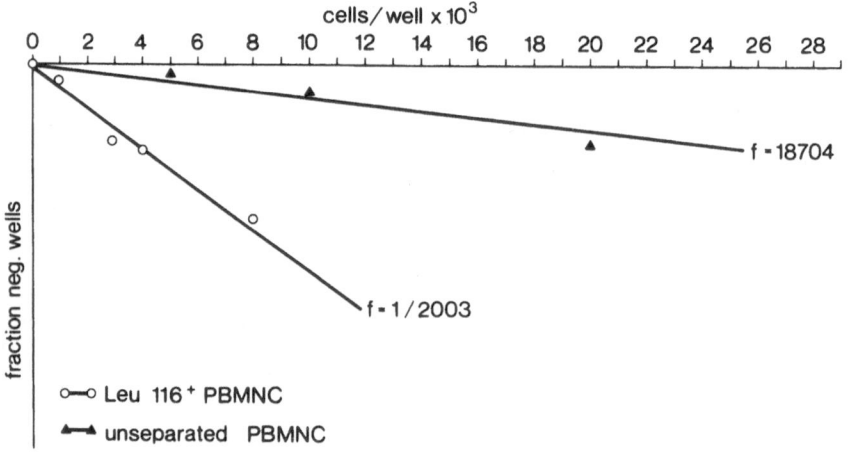

Fig. 2. LAK-p in Leu 11b⁺ PBMNC

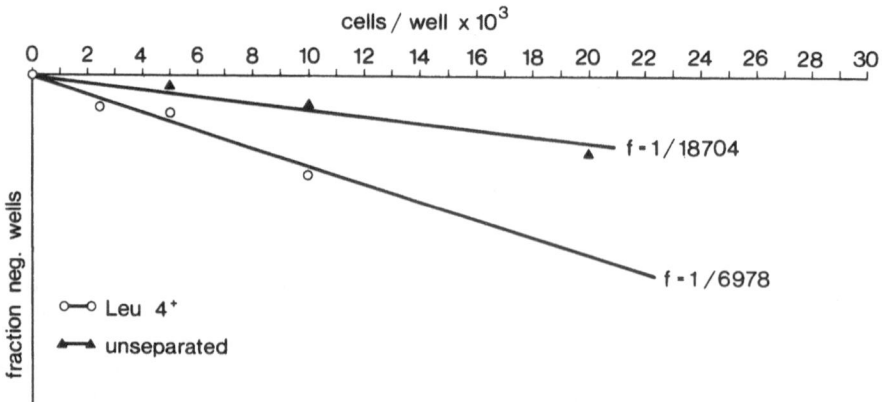

Fig. 3. LAK-p in Leu4⁺ PBMNC

Table 2. Results

UPN	Donor	Day 30 post-BMT	Day 60 post-BMT
120	1/3317	1/309 756	1/12 309
140	0	1/20 323	1/4624
143	1/3258	1/56 880	1/12 309
152	1/3651	1/30 132	1/10 285
154	1/15 603	1/187 453	0
159	1/100 742	1/97 495	1/309 756
164	1/6481	1/25 981	1/12 487
174	1/28 001	1/50 680	1/65 427
122	1/22 512	1/125 980	1/96 203
139	1/29 440	0	0
161	1/2557	1/8857	1/3007
172	1/11 572	0	1/70 974
199	1/5705	0	0
201	1/417	1/11 316	1/2338
205	1/33 568	1/50 521	1/175 934

positive (Leu11b⁺) NK cell population with CD3 positive (Leu4⁺) T cells making a smaller contribution.

LAK-p Regeneration After Allogeneic BMT

Patients were investigated 1 and 2 months after allogeneic BMT with CSA/MTX as GvHD prophylaxis. The marrow donor pre-BMT served as the normal control. The results are summarized in Table 2. Clearly, LAK-p regeneration is delayed and incomplete with the majority of patients achieving no more than 25 % –50 % of normal values.

Effects of CSA on LAK-p In Vitro

Figure 4 shows the effect of CSA on the IL-2 induced proliferation of PBMNC. There is a clear dose-dependent reduction of proliferation. There was no IL-2 inducible cytolytic activity detectable even in a CSA concentration as low as 100 ng/ml.

Discussion

We have investigated LAK regeneration after BMT using a limiting dilution assay (LDA) because previous experience had shown that LDA is more sensitive than bulk culture in detecting impaired regeneration

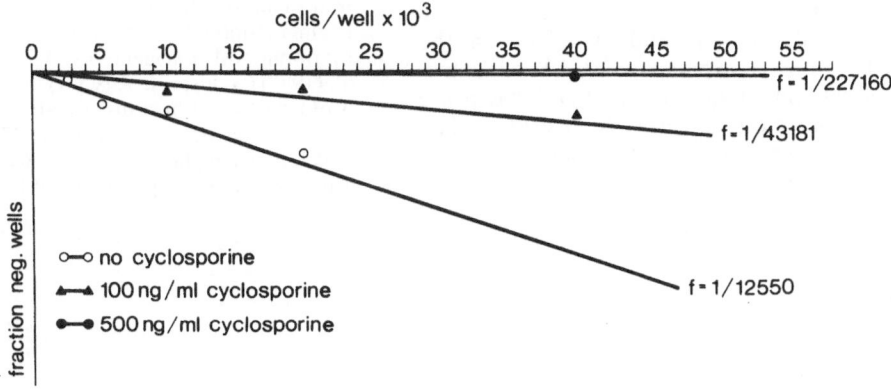

Fig. 4. Influence of cyclosporine on IL-2 induced proliferation

of cytotoxic T cell precursors after BMT [4]. In our culture system, the majority of LAK-p in normal peripheral blood were demonstrated to be in the $CD16^+$ NK cell population as previously reported by Ortaldo et al. [5]. The wide range of LAK-p values observed in healthy volunteers was not unexpected because of the wide variation of $CD16^+$ PBMNC observed by others [6].

Regeneration of LAK-p in patients with CSA/MTX as GvHD prophylaxis was delayed and incomplete. These results are in complete contrast to those reported for patients with T cell depletion as GvHD prophylaxis [2, 3]. This is probably not simply due to the more sensitive LDA we used, because bulk cultures performed in parallel in three of the patients produced similar results and no endogenous activation could be detected (data not shown). This delay could be the result of a direct CSA effect or could be de to the higher incidence of GvHD in this group of patients compared with patients receiving T cell depleted grafts. The numbers are too small at present to discriminate between these possibilities but our in vitro results clearly suggest that CSA has a direct effect on LAK-p. A further interesting point to emerge from these studies is the suggestion that LAK-p regeneration after BMT correlated with LAK-p frequency of the marrow donor. Similar observations have been reported by Hauch et al. [7]. We have been unable to correlate LAK-p reconstitution with the risk of relapse in patients with acute leukemias or CML, but a trend may emerge with larger numbers of patients.

Our in vitro studies show that CSA has a profound, dose-dependent effect on the activation and expansion of LAK-p in vitro. In fact, our data suggest that LAK-p are probably more sensitive than CTL-p. The mechanism of this effect is unclear but may be related to an effect of CSA on IL-2 receptor expression. Interestingly, Marmont et al. have recently reported a randomized trial in which the risk of relapse in patients with acute leukemia correlated with the dose of CSA used in GvHD prophylaxis [8]. Overall, these studies suggest that CSA impedes LAK regeneration after allogeneic BMT and that this may have an impact on the risk of relapse after allogeneic BMT.

References

1. Gale RP, Horowitz MM et al. (1990) Graft-versus leukaemia in bone marrow transplantation. Bone Marrow Transplant 6 [Suppl 1]: 94–97
2. Reittie JE, Gottlieb D, Heslop HE et al. (1989) Endogenously generated activated killer cells circulate after autologous and allogeneic bone marrow transplantation but not after chemotherapy. Blood 73: 1351–1358
3. Keever CA, Welte K, Small T et al. (1987) IL-2 activated killer cells in patients following transplants of soybean lectin-separated and E-rosette-depleted bone marrow. Blood 70: 1893–1903
4. Rozans MK, Smith BR, Burakoff et al. (1986) Long-lasting deficit of functional T-cell precursors in human bone marrow transplant recipients revealed by limiting dilution methods. J Immunol 136: 4040–4048
5. Ortaldo JR, Mason A, Overton R (1986) Lymphokine activated killer cells: analysis of progenitors and effectors. J Exp Med 164: 1193–1205
6. Trinchieri G (1989) Biology of natural killer cells. Adv Immunol 47: 187–376
7. Hauch M, Gazzola MV, Small T et al. (1990) Antileukaemic potential of Interleukin-2 activated natural killer cells after bone marrow transplantation for chronic myelogeneous leukaemia. Blood 75: 2250–2262
8. Marmont AM, Bacigalupo A, Van Lint MT et al. (1990) Cyclosporin A (CyA) for prophylaxis of graft versus host disease after allogeneic bone marrow transplantation (BMT for acute leukaemia: a higher relapse rate with 5 mg vs. 1 mg/kg. Blood 77 [Suppl 1]: 551a

Adoptive Immunotherapy in Human and Canine Chimeras*

H. J. Kolb, K. Beißer, E. Holler, J. Mittermüller, C. Clemm, M. Schumm,
G. Ledderose, W. Wilmanns, and S. Thierfelder

Bone marrow transplantation is an effective method for treatment of acute and chronic leukemia. Allogeneic transplants are superior to autologous and syngeneic transplants in the prevention of recurrence of leukemia. Unfortunately the occurrence of graft-versus-host disease (GVHD) is associated with a high risk of treatment-related complications. Some evidence of a graft-versus-leukemia (GVL) reaction separable from a graft-versus-host reaction has been reported [1], but neither the target antigens nor the effector cells have been well defined. Immune reactivity against histocompatibility antigens expressed by hemopoietic progenitor cells and clonogenic leukemia cells may be sufficient for a strong antileukemic effect. We treated patients with hematologic relapse of chronic myelogenous leukemia (CML) after marrow transplantation by transfusion of viable peripheral blood lymphocytes from their marrow donor and interferon-α (IFN-α) [2]. The effect of donor lymphocyte transfusions was further investigated in mixed DLA-identical canine chimeras at various times after transplantation. The aim of the study was the evaluation of an effect on residual hemopoietic cells of the host as compared to the development of GVHD.

Materials and Methods

Patients were prepared for bone marrow transplantation by either the combination of total body irradiation (4 Gy on each of 3 successive days) and cyclophosphamide (50 mg/kg on each of 4 successive days) or busulfan (16 mg/kg within 4 days) and cyclophosphamide (as above). GVHD prophylaxis consisted of cyclosporin A as continuous infusion for 28 days and orally thereafter and short course of methotrexate. Two patients with relapse had been given syngeneic marrow, eight allogeneic marrow from HLA-identical siblings. Buffy coat was prepared from the marrow donor by a continuous flow cell separator (Fa. Cobe, model 5000). Between 250 ml and 365 ml were collected per session, and between three and five sessions were performed within 5–9 days. Chimerism was studied by cytogenetic analyses and determination of polymorphic isoenzymes in blood and marrow cells. Dogs were transplanted with marrow from DLA-identical littermates of the opposite sex following conditioning treatment with total body irradiation in a single dose of 10 Gy. The marrow was treated with absorbed rabbit antithymocyte globulin for GVHD prophylaxis. Buffy coat was prepared by centrifugation of heparinized blood collected from an arteriovenous shunt.

---
* Supported by the Wilhelm Sander Foundation.

Medizinische Klinik III, Klinikum Großhadern, Universität München, Institut für Immunologie, und Institut für Klinische Hämatologie der Gesellschaft für Strahlen- und Umweltforschung, Marchioninistr. 15, Munich, FRG

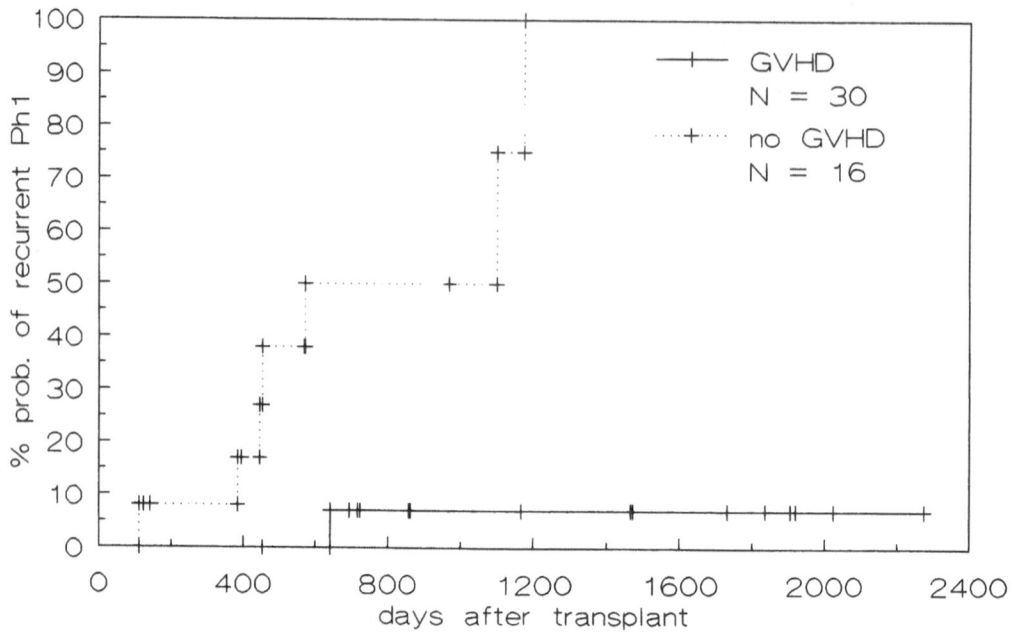

Fig. 1. Recurrence of PH1 after BMT for CML in CP (AG-KMT Munich 2/1991)

Table 1. Recurrence of CML after transplantation and outcome of treatment

UPN	Relapse	Treatment	GVHD	Response	Duration (months)
162	Cytogenetic	DIT	0	CCR	4
165	Cytogenetic	DIT	II–III	CCR	>38
238	Cytogenetic	IFN-α	De novo cGVHD	CCR	>4
105	Chronic	Chemotherapy	–	–	–
		IFN-α + DBC	II–III	CCR	>25
139	Chronic	IFN-α + DBC	II–III	CCR	>13
162	Chronic	IFN-α + DBC	0	CCR	>17
100 (twin)	Chronic	Chemotherapy	–	–	–
		second BMT (different donor)	cGVHD	CCR	>38
079	Transformed phase	Chemotherapy	–	–	–
(twin) 110	Transformed phase	Chemotherapy	–	–	–
145	Transformed phase	Chemotherapy	–	–	–
		Second BMT (same donor)	cGVHD	CCR	35
213	Tansformed phase	(Chemotherapy)	–	–	–

DIT, discontinuation of immunosuppresive therapy; DBC, danor buffy coat; CCR, complete cytogenetic remission

596

Results

Patients

Ten patients had some form of recurrence of CML. The cumulative incidence of patients with Philadelphia-positive cells after transplantation is significantly higher ($p = 0.001$) in patients without acute GVHD of grade II or more and without chronic GVHD (Fig. 1). Three patients showed only cytogenetic evidence of CML recurrence, in four the disease relapsed in chronic phase and in four it relapsed in transformed phase (Table 1). In transformed phase chemotherapy was unsuccessful, a patient was given a transplant a second time from the same donor following preparation with busulfan and VP-16 (60 mg/kg i.v.) and had a complete cytogenetic response for 35 months. Patients with cytogenetic recurrence only responded to the discontinuation of immu-nosuppressive therapy and IFN-α. In UPN 162 a hematologic relapse terminated the cytogenetic response. In contrast to the other patients she did not develop clinical signs of GVHD. UPN 100 had been transplanted with marrow of her syngeneic twin sister. She was prepared with busulfan and cyclophosphamide and given a marrow transplant from her allogeneic, HLA-identical twin sister. She developed chronic GVHD and is still in complete cytogenetic remission.

Three patients were treated with IFN-α without cytogenetic response (Table 2). They were transfused with $4.4–7.4 \times 10^8$/kg viable mononuclear cells. These patients have been in complete cytogenetic remission for between 13 and 25 months. Two patients developed acute GVHD, one patient did not. Chimerism and cytogenetic response is shown for UPN 105 (Table 3). This patient developed a subclone charac-

Table 2. Summary of clinical data

	UPN 105	UPN 139	UPN 162
Age/sex	22, male	39, female	30, female
Stage of disease	CP	CP	CP
Donor	Brother	Brother	Brother
GVHD	0	0	0
Recurrence	CP, 3 yrs	CP, 3 yrs 3 mos	2 yrs 2 mos
Duration of IFN-α treatment	4 mos	2.5 mos	3 mos
Response	No	No	Hematology yes Cytogenetics no
Donor buffy coat Transformation	4.4×10^8/kg	7.4×10^8/kg	5.1×10^8/kg
GVHD	II skin, liver	II skin, oral mucosa (encephalitis)	0
Treatment	Prednisone cyclosporine, azathioprine	Prednisone cyclosporine, azathioprine	None
Result	GVHD resolved, hematologic remission at 27 months	GVHD and encephalitis resolved hematologic remission at 15 mos	Hematologic remission at 17 mos
Last cytogenetics	Ph-negative at 24 months	Ph-negative at 13 mos	Ph-negative at 17 mos

Table 3. Response of leukemia and chimerism in UPN 105

Time (weeks post-transplant)	Clinical condition	Treatment	Blood MNC	PMN	RBC	Marrow MNC	Karyotypes
49	Remission	None	D	D	–	D	46 XY (20)
121	Remission	None	D	D	D	D	46 XY (16)
166	Hematologic relapse	None	M	R	M	–	46 XY Phl+ (2) 46 XY Phl– (14)
170	Remission	IFN-α	M	R	M	–	–
177	Remission	IFN-α	M	R	M	M	46 XY Phl+ (18)
183	Remission	IFN-α + buffy coat	–	–	R	–	46 XY Phl+ 14q+ (1)14
187	Remission	IFN-α discontuation	M	R	M	R	46 XY Phl+ 14q+ (15)
191	GVHD	–	M	R	–	M	46 XY Phl+ (12) 46 XY Phl– (6)
193	GVHD	CSA, predisone azathioprine	D	M	–	–	46 XY Phl– (13)
199	GVHD	CSA	D	D	D	–	46 XY Phl– (16)
208	GVHD decreased	CSA discontinued	D	D	D	D	46 XY Phl– (12)
230	Remission	None	–	–	–	–	46 Phl– (10)
236	Remission	None	–	–	–	–	46 XY Phl– (10)
244	Remission	None	D	D	D	–	46 XY Phl– (10)
275	Remission	None	D	D	D	–	46 XY Phl– (9)
287	Remission	None	–	–	–	–	46 XY Phl– (10)

terized by 14q+, his polymorphonuclear cells were of the recipient type, and red cells and mononuclear blood cells were mixed until the disease disappeared.

Dogs

In DLA-identical chimeras the GVHD prophylaxis with "in vitro" treatment of marrow with ATG was successful, nine dogs not given buffy coat transfusions surviving without GVHD (Table 4). Persistent mixed chimerism was found in two of three dogs given 2×10^8/kg mononuclear marrow cells, a dog given 1.5×10^8/kg and three of five dogs given $1,0 \times 10^8$/kg. Dogs transfused with buffy coat of their marrow donor on days 1 and 2, or 21 and 22, developed severe GVHD and died. After transfusion at later times (days 61 and 62, 2 years and 4.5 years) they did not develop GVHD. Nevertheless transfused dogs showed an increase of donor type mitoses as compared to their contemporary controls and their own pretransfusion values (Table 5).

Discussion

The beneficial effect of buffy coat transfusions on the hematologic relapse of our patients cannot be explained easily, since these patients had not developed GVHD prior to and UPN 162 did not develop GVHD even after buffy coat transfusions.

Table 4. Graft versus host disease and survival after DLA-identical marrow transplantation

Buffy coat transfusion	Number of Dogs			Survival time (months)
	Studied	GvHD	Alive	
–	9	0	9	>71, >54, >57, >55, >34, >32, >24, >13
Days 1 + 2	2	2	0	51 days, 83 days
Days 21 + 22	2	2	0	56 days, 72 days
Days 61 + 62	3	0	3	>12, >9, >7
2 years	1	0	1	>5
4.5 years	1	0	1	>5

Table 5. Effect of donor buffy coat transfusions on chimerism

Donor	Host		Day 20		Day 50		Day 100	1 year	2 years
96N	98N		–/5		70/25		100/95	85/95	75/90
96N	101N	BC d1+2	100/100		–/100		GVHD+		
116N	112N		–/17		–/0		0/0	0/0	0/0[a]
116N	114N		–/0		–/10		0/0	0/0	0/0[b]
116N	111N	BC d1+2	–/95		75/100		GVHD+		
110N	107N		–/20		11/12		100/100	50/90	20/55
110N	106N		–/33	BC d21+22	–/–		GVHD+		
200N	196N		–/0	BC d21+22	100/100		GVHD+		
170N	176N		73/25		0/15		55/80	71/80	
170N	175N		100/5		83/25	BC d61+62	100/90	–/100	
220N	217N		–/0		100/50	BC d61+62	93/100		
231N	228N		33/0		65/10	BC d61+62	89/90		
		Before BC		d50		d100 after BC			
N975	N970	–/75 (4.5 yrs)		63/90		100/95			
110N	107N	20/55 (2yrs)		22/80		25/82			

[a] 112N donor skin grafted 20 months post-BMT is tolerated for more than 7 months

[b] 114N donor skin graft was rejected after 17 days

It is possible that transfused T lymphocytes reacted against minor histocompatibility antigens present on hemopoietic cells and not present on other tissue. Minor histocompatibility antigens on hemopoietic progenitors detected by cytotoxic T cells have been described [3]. The expression of these antigens may be reinforced by the treatment with IFN-α. On the other hand, activation of helper T cells [4] producing IFN-γ, IL-2 and other cytokines may equally well be responsible for clinical signs of GVHD as well as for the response of leukemic cells. One patient responded without GVHD. This indicates that an antileukemic effect may be obtained without clinical GVHD.

This finding is confirmed by our studies in dogs where the degree of chimerism increased without significant GVHD. In contrast to human chimeras canine chimeras did not develop GVHD more than 2 months after transplantation. Several explanations are possible: the dogs were not treated with IFN-α, they had received a different method of GVHD prophylaxis, and their residual hemopoiesis was not leukemic. The latter explanation appears most plausible, since GVHD was also seen in patients treated with IFN-α only and patients whose prophylactic cyclosporine had been discontinued. It is known that CML cells produce a high amount of tumor necrosis factor α (TNFα) and are thus potent stimulators of allogeneic T cells.

References

1. Horowitz MM, Gale RP, Sondel P et al. (1990) Graft-versus-leukemia reactions after bone marrow transplantation. Blood 75: 555–562
2. Kolb HJ, Mittermüller J, Clemm C et al. (1990) Donor leukocyte transfusions for treatment of recurrent chronic myelogenous leukemia in marrow transplant patients. Blood 76: 2462–2465
3. Voogt PJ, Goulmy E, Veenhof WFJ et al. (1988) Cellularly defined minor histocompatibility antigens are differentially expressed on human hematopoietic progenitor cells. J Exp Med 168: 2337–2347
4. Van Els CACM, Bakker A, Zwinderman AH et al. (1990) Effector mechanism in graft-versus-host disease in response to minor histocompatibility antigens. II Evidence of a possible involvement of proliferative T-cells. Transplantation 50: 67–71

Interleukin-2 in the Treatment of Acute Myelocytic Leukemias: In Vitro Data and Presentation of a Clinical Concept*

L. Bergmann, P. S. Mitrou, and D. Hoelzer

Introduction

The relapse-free survical and overall survival in patients with acute myelocytic leukemia (AML) especially in first relapse is still unsatisfactory despite strategies such as intensification of chemotherapy (e.g., HDAra-C) and/or bone marrow transplantation (BMT) [1]. For elimination of minimal residual disease predominantly after allogeneic or autologous BMT the induction of graft versus leukemia (GvL) may be important for long-term disease-free survival [2, 3]. Both the activation of cytotoxic cells and the secretion of cytotoxic cytokines such as TNF-α are considered to play a major role in the eradication of residual blasts [4].

Therefore, therapeutic approaches are of interest, which may induce or stimulate the GvL reaction. In this context the administration of interleukin-2 (Il-2) may be of interest, as this cytokine activates autologous cytotoxic lymphocytes (LAK) and induces high secretion of cytokines such as TNF-α, Il-6 and IFN-γ [5, 6]. Additionally, in vitro trials suggest that LAK cells reacting with blasts can be induced by Il-2 [7].

We conducted a clinical phase II trial for AML patients in first relapse with an induction chemotherapy with iHDAra-C/VP-16 and Il-2 as consolidation therapy for patients with and without autologous BMT in second remission. In vitro results and the clinical concept were reported.

Patients and Methods

Patients and Therapy

In a clinical phase II trial patients in first relapse of AML and aged 18–75 years were included. Patients with an allogeneic bone marrow donor or secondary AMLs after myelodysplastic syndrome or myeloproliferative disease were excluded.

For induction therapy patients receive 600 mg/m^2 cytosin-arabinoside (Ara-C) as 2 h infusion every 12 h on day 1–4 and 100 mg/m^2 etoposide (VP-16) on day 1–7 as 1 h infusion. In total, three cycles of this chemotherapy were applied (Fig. 1). Starting 4–6 weeks after the last cycle of iHDAra-C/VP-16, four cycles of rIl-2 (EuroCetus, Frankfurt, FRG) are adjusted every 6 weeks consisting of 1.5 × 10^6 U/m^2 rIl-2 (Cetus units) as 1 h infusion on days 1–5 and 7–13. Patients undergoing autologous BMT also receive four cycles of rIl-2 as indicated in Fig. 1 b.

Up to now eight patients have been entered into the clinical trial. Five patients are too early for evaluation, and one patient underwent autologous BMT. The other two patients had a CR after chemotherapy and were relapse free for 11 and 15+ months. In total, ten therapy cycles with Il-2 have been applied so far.

* This work was supported by the grant 0 1 GA8802 from the Bundesministerium für Forschung und Technologie (BMFT).

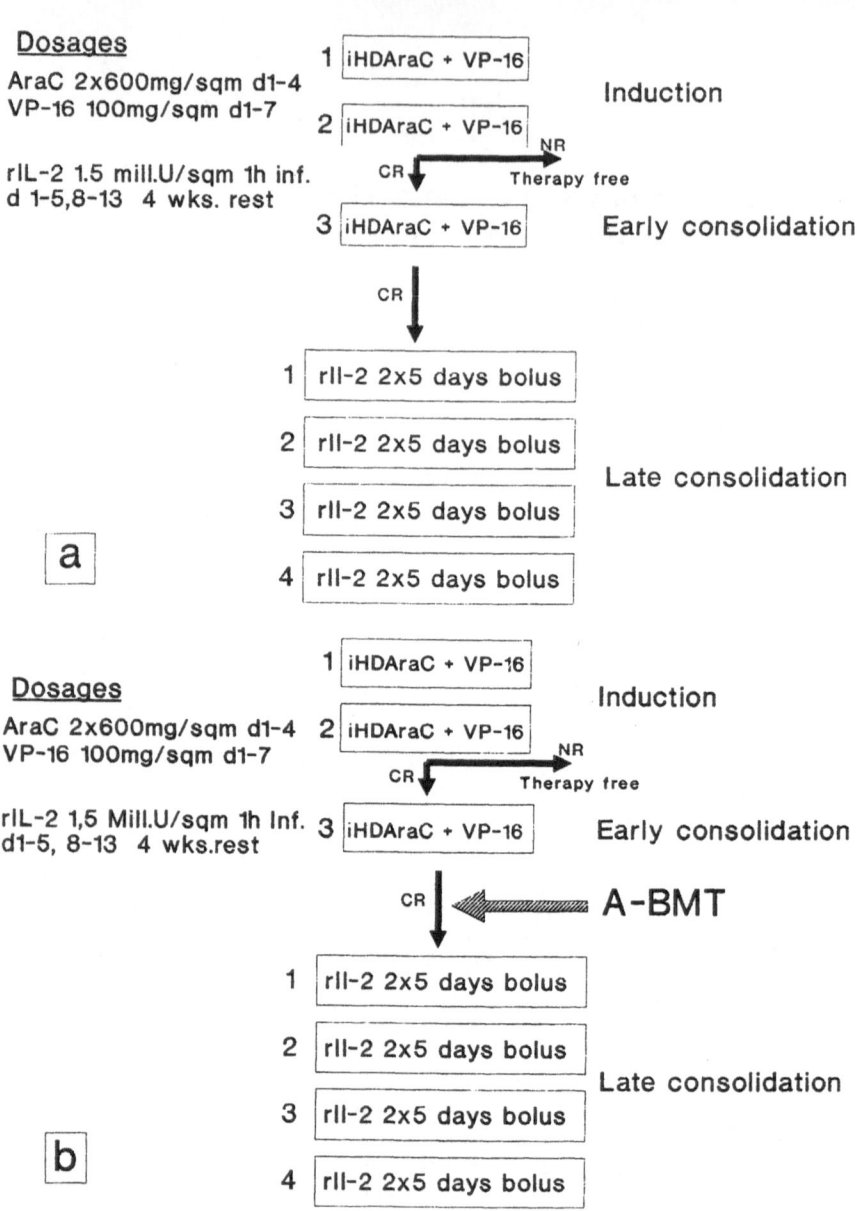

Dosages

AraC 2x600mg/sqm d1-4
VP-16 100mg/sqm d1-7

rIL-2 1.5 mill.U/sqm 1h inf.
d 1-5,8-13 4 wks. rest

1 | iHDAraC + VP-16   Induction
2 | iHDAraC + VP-16
CR ↓   NR
       Therapy free
3 | iHDAraC + VP-16   Early consolidation
CR ↓

1 | rIl-2 2x5 days bolus
2 | rIl-2 2x5 days bolus
3 | rIl-2 2x5 days bolus   Late consolidation
4 | rIl-2 2x5 days bolus

a

Dosages

AraC 2x600mg/sqm d1-4
VP-16 100mg/sqm d1-7

rIL-2 1,5 Mill.U/sqm 1h Inf.
d1-5, 8-13 4 wks.rest

1 | iHDAraC + VP-16   Induction
2 | iHDAraC + VP-16
CR ↓   NR
       Therapy free
3 | iHDAraC + VP-16   Early consolidation
CR ↓ ⟵ A-BMT

1 | rIl-2 2x5 days bolus
2 | rIl-2 2x5 days bolus
3 | rIl-2 2x5 days bolus   Late consolidation
4 | rIl-2 2x5 days bolus

b

Fig. 1 a, b. Therapy schedule for patients with AML in first relapse receiving induction chemotherapy with iHDAra-C/VP-16 and rIl-2 (EuroCetus, Frankfurt, FRG) as late consolidation without (**a**) and with autologous bone marrow transplantation (A-BMT) (**b**). rIl-2 is administered as 1 h infusion on days 1–5 and 8–13. This cycle is repeated after a rest of 4 weeks

Methods

Surface Marker Studies

Phenotypic characterization of MNC and blast of peripheral blood or cell cultures was performed by flow cytometric analyses (FACScan, Becton-Dickinson, Heidelberg) using FITC or PE-labeled monoclonal antibodies.

In Vitro Cultures

For in vitro investigation, heparinized peripheral blood or bone marrow aspiration of patients with AML on first diagnosis or in relapse were used. The mononuclear cells (MNC) including the blast population were separated by Ficoll-Hypaque sedimentation as described elsewhere [7]. The blast-enriched MNC contained at least 70 % blast cells.

To investigate the influence of various cytokines on the proliferation of blasts, they were cultured in the presence of rIl-2, rIl-3, rGM-CSF or rIFN-α at a cell concentration of 50000 cells/well for 72 h. Twenty-four hours prior to harvesting, [³H]thymidine was added and the uptake was counted in a β-counter. The stimulation index (SI) was calculated as the ratio of cytokine-induced stimulation and spontaneous proliferation.

For induction of autologous cytotoxic cells, blasts containing MNC were incubated in culture dishes using supplemented RPMI 1640 (+10 % fetal calf serum) with or without the addition of 500 U/ml rIl-2 (EuroCetus, Frankfurt, FRG) for up to several weeks. During this time, surface marker studies and the measurement of cytokines in the supernatants were performed.

Cytotoxic Assays and Cytokine Levels

Activity of NK and LAK was tested against K562 and Daudi cells using the ⁵¹Cr releases assay as described elsewhere [7]. In the serum of AML patients in the acute phase and in the culture supernatants of blasts the levels of TNF-α, Il-6 and IFN-γ were measured using an ELISA (Medgenix, Brussels, Belgium) [7].

Results

We tested a possible stimulating effect of Il-2 and other cytokines on the proliferation

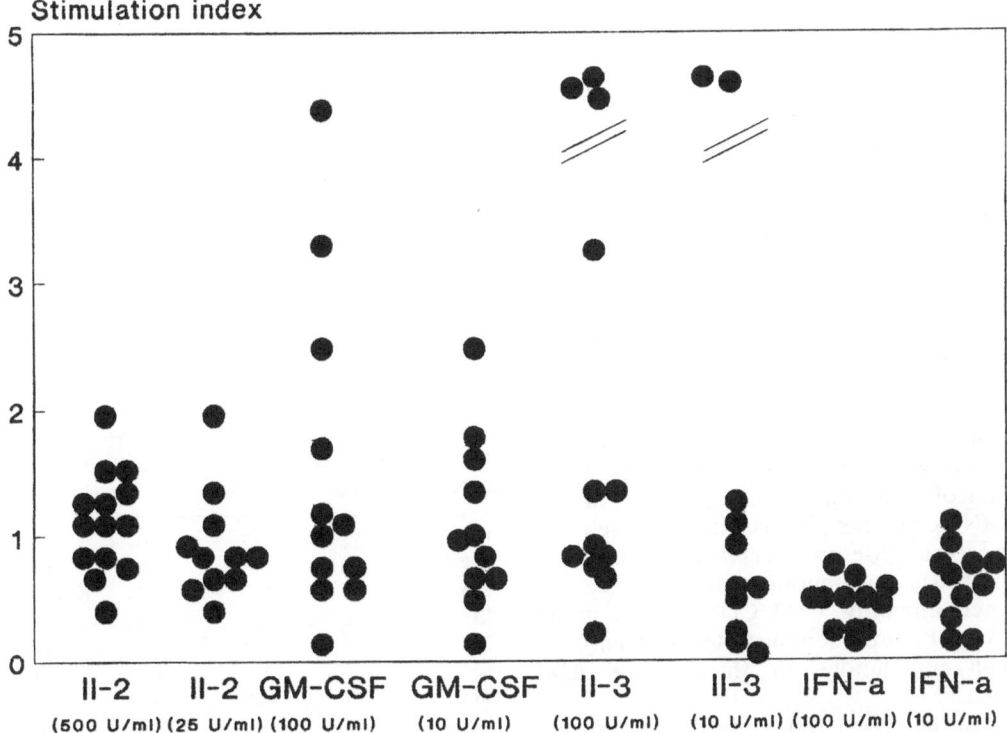

Fig. 2. Stimulation of MNC with >70 % AML blasts by various amounts of recombinant Il-2, Il-3, GM-CSF and IFN-α. The proliferation was measured by ³H thymidine uptake and the stimulation index (SI) was calculated as the proportion of cytokine-induced proliferation and spontaneous proliferation

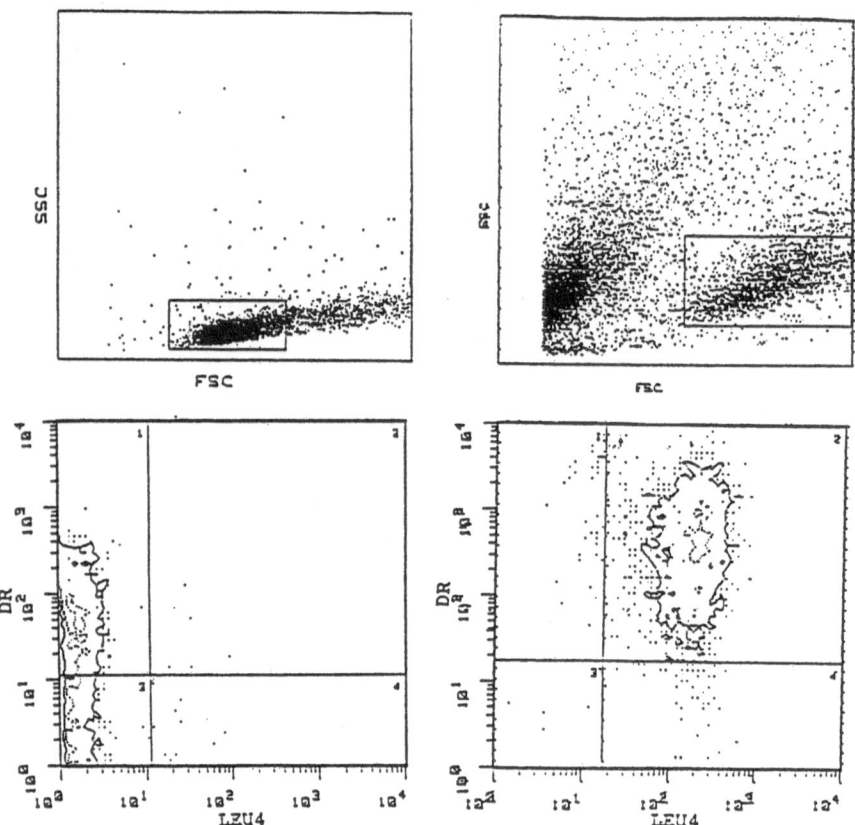

Fig. 3 a, b. Phenotypic characterization of cultures with AML blasts of aⁿ M2 (**a**) and M4 (**b**) leukemia before and after addition of Il-2 using flow cytometric analysis

of blast. So far, only a slight increase of the stimulation index by Il-2 was observed, whereas some patients revealed a very high proliferation by incubation of blasts with GM-CSF or Il-3. In most cases IFN-α had nor or an inhibitory effect on the proliferation of blasts (Fig. 2). Long-term cultures of MNC containing blasts with Il-2 resulted in nearly all cases in a decrease or elimination of blasts concomitant with an increase of predominantly CD3⁺CD4⁺DR⁺ lymphocytes. Figure 3 demonstrates the changes of cell populations in the culture AML blasts.

In the supernatants of AML blasts with and without Il-2, remarkable amounts of Il-6 and TNF-α were found. Whereas in most cases the Il-6 secretion could not be enhanced by the addition of Il-2, the TNF-α

Table 1. In vitro production of Il-6 and TNF-α in cultures of mononuclear cells containing >70% blasts with and without addition of 500 U/ml rIl-2

Patients (FAB)	Il-6 (pg/ml) −Il-2	+Il-2	TNF-α (pg/ml) −Il-2	+Il-2
M4	22	27	210	27
M2	1633	2241	6	558
M5	152	152	302	424
M2	5992	6658	94	546
M4	4793	5323	500	624
M4	880	314	<20	70
M3	1780	866	40	186
M7	48	84	<20	70
M4	1662	1764	<20	1964
M2	64	72	50	<20
M4	262	266	38	116
M4	9912	9448	2952	11476

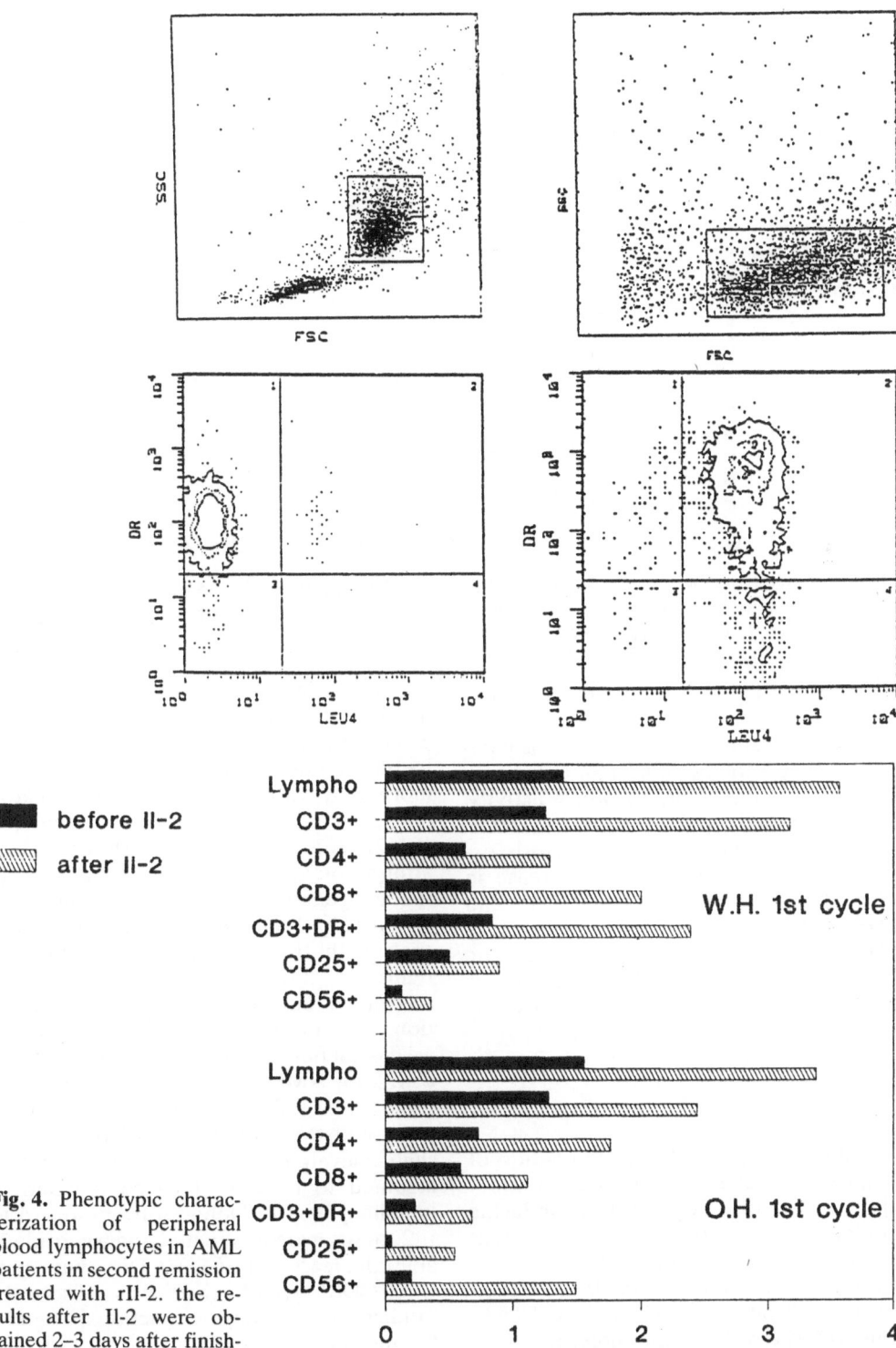

Fig. 4. Phenotypic characterization of peripheral blood lymphocytes in AML patients in second remission treated with rIl-2. the results after Il-2 were obtained 2–3 days after finishing Il-2 administration

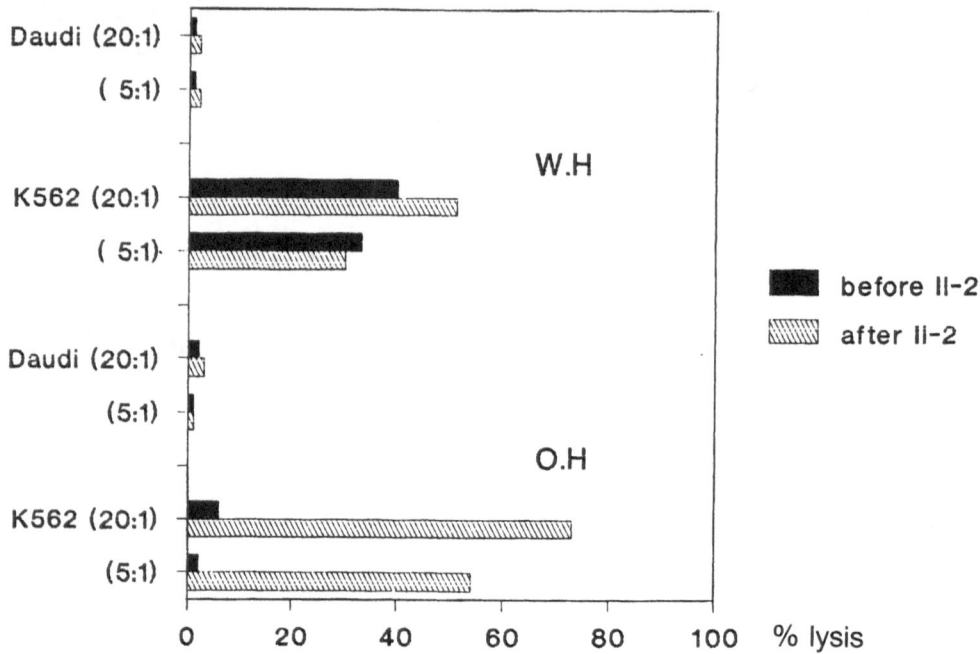

Fig. 5. Acitivity of NK and LAK of peripheral blood lymphocytes in AML patients in second remission treated with rIl-2. The results after Il-2 were obtained 2–3 days after finishing Il-2 administration. *E:T,* effector: target cell ratio

levels were higher in cultures with Il-2 (Table 1).

Patients treated with rIl-2 for consolidation therapy were monitored for changes in lymphocyte subsets and cytotoxic activity. After intermediate high-dose Il-2 bolus infusions a remarkable lymphocytosis occurred, whereby an excessive increase in CD3+ lymphocytes including CD4+ and CD8+ cells was found. The increase in CD56+ cells was moderate (Fig. 4). Testing the cytotoxic acitivity, only an increase of NK but no increase of LAK activity was found (Fig. 5).

Discussion

An intersting approach for elimination of minimal residual disease may be the stimulation of antileukemic potential by inducing autologous LAK cells with Il-2. Various clinical trials with Il-2 predominantly after autologous BMT are ongoing [8, 9]. Additionally, Il-2 induces high secretion of TNF-α and IFN-γ especially after bolus infusions [6]. These cytokines are considered to play a

major role in eradicating minimal residual disease after BMT [5]. It was shown that principally LAK cells in AML patients can be induced despite previous intensive chemotherapy without compromising hematopoietic stem cells in most in vitro models [9, 10–12]. Additionally the synthesis of Il-2 after autologous BMT is impaired, so that the exogenous addition of Il-2 may be useful [13]. Preliminary results of clinical trials with Il-2 in AML patients in first remission, however, did not lead to an advantage and suggest a possible stimulation of M5 blasts by Il-2 [14]. In our hands, we did not find an evident stimulatory effect of Il-2 on AML blasts in vitro, whereas in some cases Il-3 and GM-CSF extensively promoted the proliferation of blasts. The slight elevated SI in cultures with rIl-2 is assumed to be caused by contaminating lymphocytes. In all long-term cultures with Il-2, blasts were eliminated and a considerable increase of CD3+CD4+ but not CD3+CD8+ lymphocytes was observed. Studies investigating the functional properties including possible cytotoxic activities of these CD4+ cells are ongoing. An interesting point is that Il-2 enhanced the TNF-α but not the initially high Il-6 secretion of blast-containing MNC in vitro. This is important as Il-6 may act as a growth factor for blasts.

We think that clinical trials with Il-2 for consolidation therapy in AML with or without autologous BMT may be a promising tool for induction of GvL. A benefit of relapse-free survival will have to be demonstrated. Our scheme with bolus infusions of Il-2 using intermediate high doses (1.5 million U/m²) is high enough to induce LAK cells and remarkable amounts of TNF-α, which exceed that of continuous infusions [15]. The toxicity is moderate, so that the schedule can even be performed with outside patients. The study is ongoing as a multicenter study (South German Hemoblastosis Group; SHG) and at present it is too early for clinical evaluations.

Acknowledgments. The authors thank Mrs. S. Christ, Mrs. S. Fuck, and Mrs. B. Würz for skillful technical assistance.

References

1. Wiernik PH (1990) Leukemias and myeloma. In: Pinedo HM, Longo DL, Chabner BA (eds) Cancer chemotherapy and biological response modifiers. Elsevier, New York, pp 321–342
2. McMillian AK, Goldstone AH, Linch DC, Gribben JG, Patterson KG, Richards JDM, Franklin I, Boughton BJ, Milligan DW, Leyland M, Hutchison RM, Newland AC (1990) High-dose chemotherapy and autologous bone marrow transplantation in acute myelocytic leukemia. Blood 67: 480–488
3. Slavin S, Ackerstein A, Naparsteck E, Or R, Weiss L (1990) The graft versus leukemia (GvL) phenomenon: is GvL separable from GVHD? Bone Marrow Transplant 6: 155–161
4. Skórski T, Kawalec M, Kawiak J (1990) Successful adoptive immunotherapy of minimal residual disease after chemotherapy and transplantation of bone marrow purged of leukemia with mafosfamide. Cancer Immunol Immunother 32: 71–74
5. Duncombe AS, Meager A, Prentice HG, Grundy JE, Heslop HE, Hoffbrand AV, Brenner MK (1990) γ-Interferon and tumor

necrosis factor production after bone marrow transplantation is augmented by exposure to marrow fibroblasts infected with cytomegalovirus. Blood 76: 1046–1053
6. Bergmann L (1990) The clinical significance of interleukin-2. Onkology 13: 416–422
7. Bergmann L, Weidmann E, Bungert B, Hechler P, Mitrou PS (1990) Influence of various cytokines on the induction of lymphocyte activated killer (LAK) cells. Nat Immun Cell Growth Regul 9: 265–273
8. Bolonesi B, Petersen FB, Appelbaum F, Treisman J, Lindgren C, Benz L, Buckner CD, Fefer A (1990) Phase Ib trial of interleukin-2 after autologous marrow transplantation for hematological malignancies. Proc Am Soc Clin Oncol 9: 17 (abstr 59)
9. Hauch M, Gazzola MV, Small T, Bordognon C, Barnett L, Cunningham I, Castro-Malaspinia H, O'Reilly RJ, Keever CA (1990) Anti-leukemia potential of interleukin-2 activated natural killer cells after bone marrow transplantation for chronic myelogenous leukemia. Blood 75: 2250–2262
10. Teichmann JV, Ludwig W-D, Seibt-Jung H, Thiel E (1990) Induction of lymphokine activated killer cells against human leukemic cells in vitro. Blut 59: 21–24
11. van den Brink MR, Voogt PJ,, Marjit WAF, von Luxemburg-Heys, von Rood JJ, Brand A (1989) Lymphokine-activated killer cells selectively kill tumor cells in bone marrow without compromising bone marrow stem cell function in vitro. Blood 74: 354–360
12. Savary CA, Lotzova E (1990) Inhibition of human bone marrow and myeloid progenitors by interleukin-2 activated lymphocytes. Exp Hematol 18: 1083–1089
13. Cayeux S, Meuer S, Pezzutto A, Körbling M, Haas R, Schulz R, Dörken B (1989) T-cell ontogeny after autologous bone marrow transplantation: failure to synthesize interleukin-2 (Il-2) and lack of CD2- and CD3-mediated proliferation by both CD4⁺ and CD8⁺ cells even in the presence of exogenous Il-2. Blood 74: 2270–2277
14. MacDonald D, Jiang Y, Gordow AA, Mahendra P, Oskam R, Palmer PA, Franks CR, Barret J (1990) Recombinant interleukin-2 for acute myeloid leukemia in first complete remission: a pilot study. Leuk 14: 967–973
15. Bergmann L, Hechler P, Weidmann E, Franks CR, Mitrou PS (1990) Daily alternating scheme of bolus recombinant interleukin-2 i.v. and interferon-alpha s.c. in advanced renal cell cancer – a phase II study. Cancer Res Clin Oncol 116 [Suppl]: 145

Idarubicin: New Aspects
in the Treatment of Acute Leukemias

State of the Art and Future Prospects of the Treatment of Acute Myeloid Leukemia

T. Büchner

Introduction

Major clinical trials published during the 1980s failed to demonstrate a substantial therapeutic progress in chemotherapy for patients with AML. In particular, it remained unanswered whether more chemotherapy – in terms of its intensity as well as duration – produces more cures. Bone marrow transplantation has not been adequately compared to chemotherapy on the basis of comparable groups. Chemotherapy may be modulated by hemopoietic growth factors in both its myelotoxicity and its antileukemic activity as from first clinical results. We discuss here major results from the above therapeutic approaches and their role in AML management.

Prolonged Maintenance

A prolonged maintenance strategy designed by Cancer and Acute Leukemia Group B used monthly myelosuppressive chemotherapy courses for 3–5 years resulting in 19 % CCR after 5 years [11]. Subsequently, the role of similar type maintenance has been addressed in several trials [9, 13, 16] but has not clearly been substantiated. Those later trials, however, used less intensive [9, 13, 16] or less frequent [13] maintenance courses. The AMLCG 1981 trial addressed the question whether the effect of the original CALGB type mainte-

nance [11] can be reproduced or even improved when given after the more intensive TAD induction and a TAD consolidation course. Patients of 16 years and over with no upper age limit suffering from newly diagnosed AML received for induction one course of TAD (Fig. 1) and in the case of persisting bone marrow blasts a second identical course. After attaining CR patients were randomized to receive one consolidation course by TAD again and no further treatment or subsequent maintenance by monthly courses of AD, AT or AC (Fig. 1) for 3 years. Median remission duration was 15 months in patients randomized to maintenance treatment and 7 months in the no-maintenance group ($p = 0.0001$). After 5–8 years CCR is 23 % versus 7 % [3]. Thus, the long-term effect of the same type of maintenance achieved by the CALGB [11] was more than confirmed by us when using a more intensive induction and consolidation treatment. As shown in Fig. 2 also patients of 60 years and over similarly benefited from prolonged maintenance [3]. By a metaanalysis of ten multicenter trials (Fig. 3) the superiority of treatment arms containing CALGB type maintenance over treatment arms without comparable maintenance is again confirmed.

Intensified Consolidation

As a new concept intensified consolidation using high-dose Ara-C combined with anthracyclines and not followed by prolonged maintenance has been investigated in some nonrandomized trials [6, 8, 10, 15]

Department of Medicine, Hematology/Oncology, University of Münster, Münster, FRG

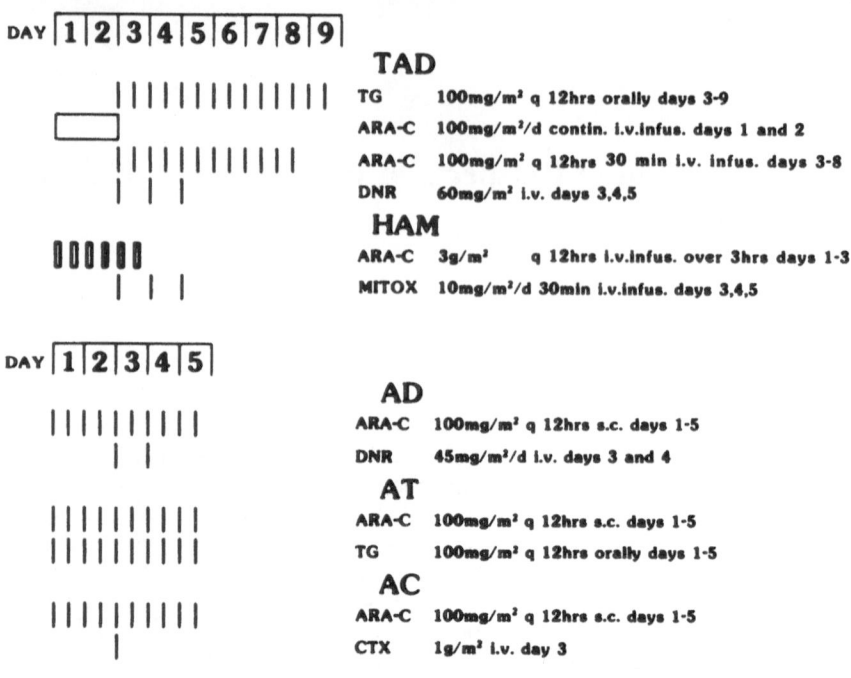

DAY 1 2 3 4 5 6 7 8 9

TAD

| | | | | | | | | | | | | |
TG   100mg/m² q 12hrs orally days 3-9
ARA-C   100mg/m²/d contin. i.v.infus. days 1 and 2
| | | | | | | | | | | | |
ARA-C   100mg/m² q 12hrs 30 min i.v. infus. days 3-8
| | |
DNR   60mg/m² i.v. days 3,4,5

HAM

||||||
ARA-C   3g/m²   q 12hrs i.v.infus. over 3hrs days 1-3
| | |
MITOX   10mg/m²/d 30min i.v.infus. days 3,4,5

DAY 1 2 3 4 5

AD

| | | | | | | | | |
ARA-C   100mg/m² q 12hrs s.c. days 1-5
| |
DNR   45mg/m²/d i.v. days 3 and 4

AT

| | | | | | | | | |
ARA-C   100mg/m² q 12hrs s.c. days 1-5
| | | | | | | | | |
TG   100mg/m² q 12hrs orally days 1-5

AC

| | | | | | | | | |
ARA-C   100mg/m² q 12hrs s.c. days 1-5
|
CTX   1g/m² i.v. day 3

TG = 6-thioguanine, ARA-C = cytosine arabinoside, DNR = daunorubicin, MITOX = mitoxantrone, CTX = cytoxan

Fig. 1. Chemotherapeutic regimens applied in the 1981 trial and/or in the 1985 trial

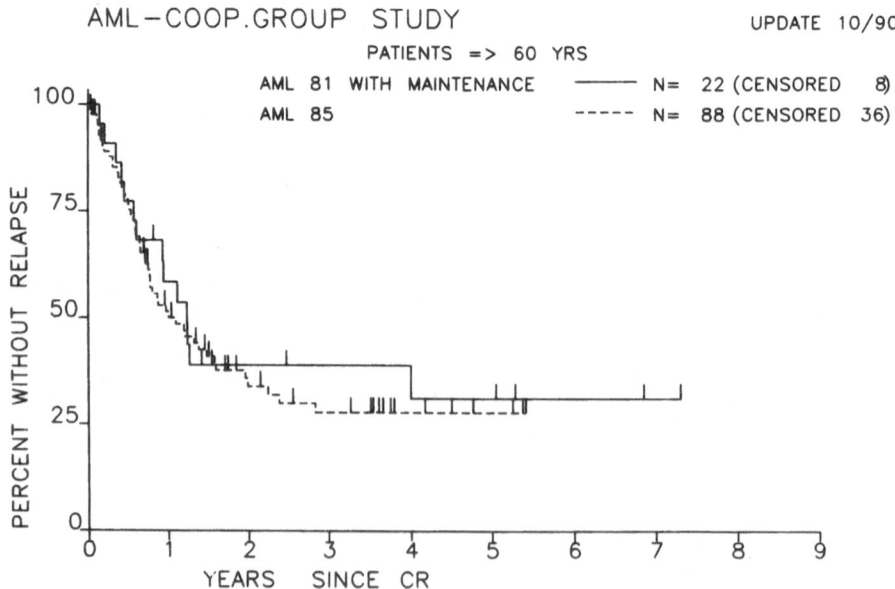

AML – COOP.GROUP STUDY   UPDATE 10/90

PATIENTS => 60 YRS

AML 81 WITH MAINTENANCE ——— N= 22 (CENSORED 8)
AML 85   - - - - N= 88 (CENSORED 36)

Fig. 2. Remission duration in patients of 60 years and over receiving induction, consolidation and maintenance in the 1981 trial and the 1985 trial

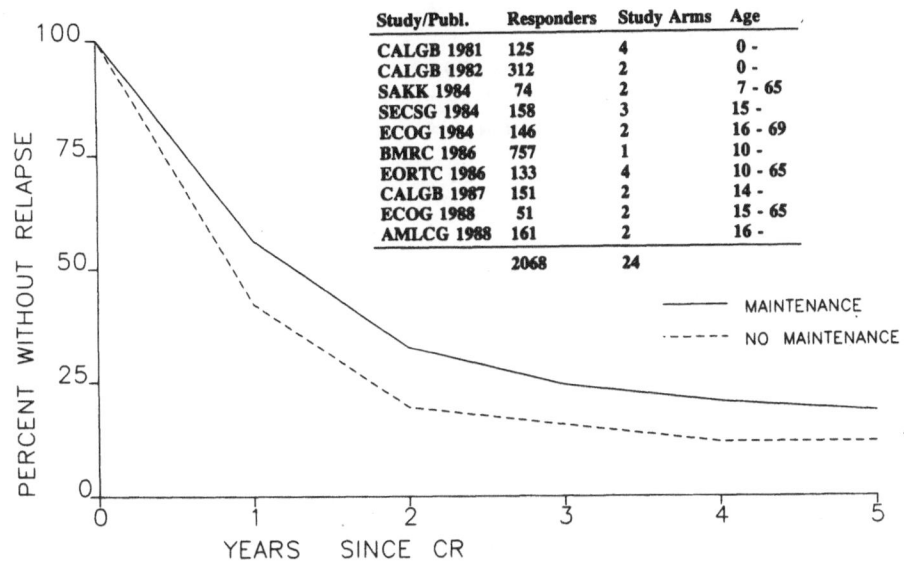

Fig. 3. Metaanalysis of remission duration from multicenter trials on chemotherapy in AML. The average probability of ongoing remission of all treatment arms containing a CALGB type maintenance is compared to the average of all study arms without CALGB type maintenance. The studies listed correspond to the following references: CALGB 1981 [11], CALGB 1982 [16], SAKK 1984 [13], SECSG 1984 [14], ECOG 1984 [4],, BMRC 1986 [12], EORTC 1986 [7], CALGB 1987 [9], ECOG 1988 [5]

where it produced long-term remission rates similar to those from maintenance regimens [6, 8]. In selected patient populations superior results were even obtained [10, 15].

Very Early Intensification

In an attempt to further improve present chemotherapy the AMLCG 1985 trial addressed the question whether a very early intensification by a response nonadapted two-course induction adds to the cure rate produced by maintenance. Patients uniformly received consolidation and maintenance as above. But differently from the 1981 trial, patients under 60 years of age all received two induction courses with the second course starting on day 21 of treatment regardless of the response in bone marrow after the first course. The two courses of double induction consisted randomly of either TAD/TAD or TAD/HAM (Fig. 1). Patients of 60 years and over received a second TAD induction course only if blasts persisted in the bone marrow

after the first course similarly to the 1981 trial. Compared to those in the 1981 trial CR rates in the younger age group are 69% versus 65% and in the over 60s 46% versus 42%. Remission duration of all younger patients in the 1985 trial is compared to that in the same age group of the maintenance arm in the 1985 trial in Fig. 4. Median remission duration is 20 versus 15 months and 5-years CCR is 34% versus 23% [3]. When comparing the two randomized arms in the 1985 trial there is a nonsignificant trend of both remission rate and remission duration in favor of TAD/HAM double induction. Figure 2 compares remission duration in the older age group of the 1985 trial to that of the maintenance arm in the 1981 trial. Figure 5 compares remission duration in patients of all ages in the 1981 and 1985 trials to that published from other randomized multicenter trials comparable in patient selection [3]. Thus, the favorable long-term result from prolonged maintenance in our 1981 trial could be further improved in our 1985 trial by further intensifying chemotherapy in its initial phase. Very early intensification by double induc-

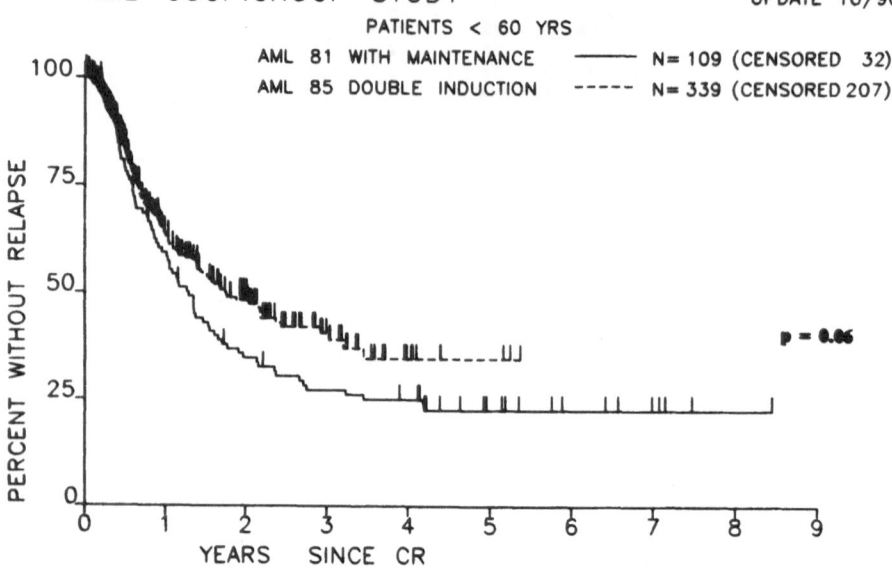

AML—COOP.GROUP STUDY   UPDATE 10/90
PATIENTS < 60 YRS
AML 81 WITH MAINTENANCE   ————— N= 109 (CENSORED 32)
AML 85 DOUBLE INDUCTION   ----- N= 339 (CENSORED 207)

Fig. 4. Remission duration in patients under the age of 60 years receiving induction, consolidation and maintenance in the 1981 trial and double induction, consolidation and maintenance in the 1985 trial

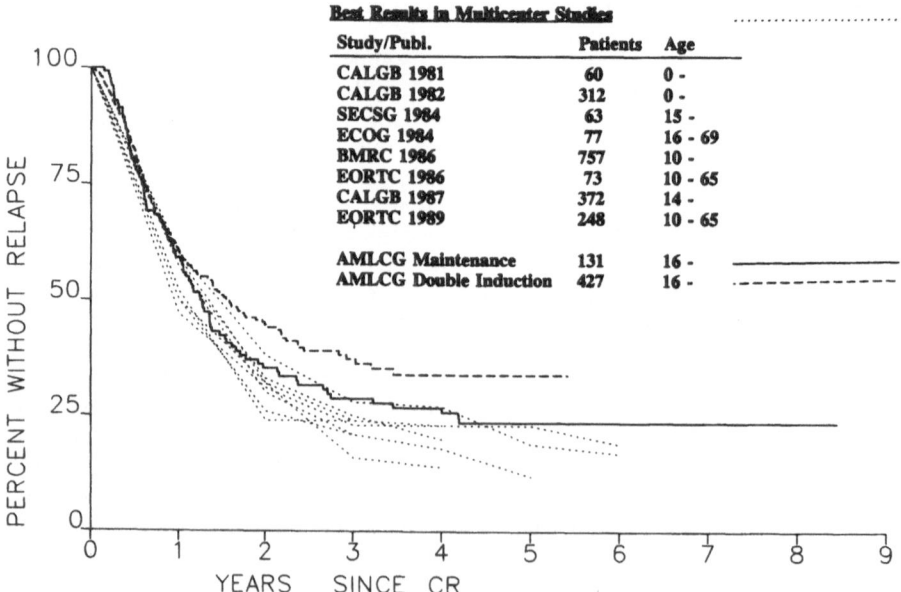

Best Results in Multicenter Studies		
Study/Publ.	Patients	Age
CALGB 1981	60	0 -
CALGB 1982	312	0 -
SECSG 1984	63	15 -
ECOG 1984	77	16 - 69
BMRC 1986	757	10 -
EORTC 1986	73	10 - 65
CALGB 1987	372	14 -
EORTC 1989	248	10 - 65
AMLCG Maintenance	131	16 -
AMLCG Double Induction	427	16 -

Fig. 5. Remission duration in patients at all ages in the 1981 trial and the 1985 trial compared to best results in other randomized trials comparable in patient selection. The studies correspond to the following references: CALGB 1981 [11], CALGB 1982 [16], SECSG 1984 [14], ECOG 1984 [4], BMRC 1986 [12], EORTC 1986 [7], CALGB 1987 [9]

tion followed by consolidation and maintenance as before increased the long-term remission rate to 34 % in patients under 60 years of age. Also in the entire group of unselected patients at all ages this age-adapted very early intensified/prolonged maintenance protocol of our 1985 trial improved the 5-year CCR rate to as much as 34 %. Thus, chemotherapy for AML seems not to be at the limits of its curative potential.

Bone Marrow Transplantation

In the AMLCG 1985 trial allogeneic bone marrow transplantation is offered to every patient of up to 45 years with a compatible donor. For comparison of relapse free survival a prospective matched-pair system is used. At the time of transplantation a control patient in the chemotherapy group matched for age and remission duration already achieved is allocated to each transplant patient. The 30 allogeneic transplant patients compared to their 30 matched controls show a median relapse free survival of 47 versus 26 months and a 3 years relapse free survival of 65 % versus 49 % (n.s.). In the 1985 trial autologous bone marrow transplantation is optional at special centers. In order to circumvent the problems of randomization between chemotherapy and autologous bone marrow transplantation the same prospective matched-pair system is used as in allogeneic bone marrow transplantation. The 20 patients receiving autologous bone marrow transplantation when compared to their matched controls show a median relapse free survival of 15 versus 20 months and a 3 years relapse free survival of 39 % versus 33 % (n.s.). A higher number of patients and another 2–3 years of follow-up will further substantiate the role of bone marrow transplantation in first remission.

Hemopoietic Growth Factors

Further improvements in chemotherapy seem possible when reducing myelotoxicity by hemopoietic growth factors. Data of a first study on GM-CSF following chemo-

therapy in high-risk AML [2] are presented separately (T. Büchner et al., this volume). They show a significant reduction in both neutrophil recovery time and early mortality and a low risk of promoting disease progression. The data lead to the present randomized study on GM-CSF priming and long-term administration in standard risk AML. GM-CSF starts 24 h prior to chemotherapy and is continued until recovery of blood neutrophils. This regimen applies to all induction courses, the consolidation course and the two first maintenance courses. After entering 25 patients preliminary data show consistant priming effects in an increase of blood blasts by factor 1.15 to 6.5 (median 2.0) and evidence of differentiation in the immunophenotype of bone marrow blasts. The tolerability appears acceptable and early relapses have not been observed in the GM-CSF group, so far.

Conclusions

There is clear evidence that more chemotherapy – in terms of its intensity as well as duration – produces more cures in AML. In a metaanalysis of remission duration in ten multicenter trials there is a marked trend in favor of treatment arms with prolonged maintenance. Maintenance proved especially effective when given after TAD induction and consolidation producing 23 % long-term remissions. The addition of very early intensification to this strategy by age-adapted double induction resulted in as much as 34 % long-term remissions in unselected patients at all ages. Allogeneic bone marrow transplantation may further improve on this cure rate demonstrable after a longer follow-up of transplant patients and matched controls. Patients receiving autologous bone marrow transplantation show a relapse free survival almost identical to that in the matched controls when projected to 3 years. GM-CSF appears to effectively reduce neutrophil recovery time and may facilitate more intensive chemotherapy. A possible enhancement of antileukemic effects by GM-CSF priming requires longer follow-up to be objectivated.

References

1. Büchner T, Urbanitz D, Hiddemann W et al (1985) Intensified induction and consolidation with or without maintenance chemotherapy for acute myeloid leukemia (AML): two multicenter studies of the German AML Cooperative group. J Clin Oncol 3: 1583–1589
2. Büchner T, Hiddemann W, Koenigsmann M et al (1991) Recominant human granulocyte-macrophage colony-stimulating factor following chemotherapy in patients with acute mayloid leukemia at higher age or after relapse. Blood 78: 1190–1197
3. Büchner T, Hiddemann W, Löffler H et al (1991) Improved cure rate by very early intensification combined with prolonged maintenance chemotherapy in patients with acute mayloid leukemia (AML): data from AMLCG. Semin Hematol 28, Suppl 4: 76–79
4. Cassileth PA,, Begg CB, Bennett JM et al (1984) A randomized study of the efficacy of consolidation therapy in adult acute nonlymphocytic leukemia. Blood 63: 843–847
5. Cassileth PA, Harrington DP, Hines JD et al (1988) Maintenance chemotherapy prolongs remission duration in adult acute nonlymphocytic leukemia. J Clin Oncol 6 (4): 583–587
6. Champlin R, Gajewski J, Nimer S et al (1990) Postremission chemotherapy for adults with acute myelogenous leukemia: improved survival with high-dose cytarabine and daunorubicin consolidation treatment. J Clin Oncol 8: 1199–1206
7. Hayat M, Jehn U, Willemze R et al (1986) A randomized comparison of maintenance treatment with androgens, immunotherapy and chemotherapy in adult acute myelogenous leukemia. Cancer 58: 617–623
8. Kurrle E, Ehninger G, Fackler-Schwalbe E et al (1990) Consolidation therapy with high-dose cytosine arabinoside: experiences of a prospective study in acute myeloid leukemia. In Büchner T, Schellong G, Hiddemann W, Ritter J (eds) Acute leukemias II. Springer, Berlin Heidelberg New York, pp 209–215 (Hämatologie und Bluttransfusion, Vol 33)
9. Preisler H, Davis RB, Kirshner J et al. (1987) Comparison of three remission induction regimens and two postinduction strategies for the treatment of acute nonlymphocytic leukemia: a Cancer and Leukemia Group B study. Blood 69: 1441–1449
10. Preisler HD, Raza A, Early A et al. (1987) Intensive remission consolidation therapy in the treatment of acute nonlymphocytic leukemia. J Clin Oncol 5: 722–730
11. Rai KR, Holland JF,, Glidewell OJ et al. (1981) Treatment of acute myelocytic leukemia: a study by Cancer and Leukemia Group B. Blood 58: 1203–1212
12. Rees JKH, Swirsky D, Gray RG, Hayhoe FGJ (1986) Principal results of the Medical Research Council's 8th Acute Myeloid Leukemia Trial. Lancet ii: 1236–1241
13. Sauter C, Fopp M, Imbach P et al. (1984) Acute myelogenous leukaemia: maintenance chemotherapy after early consolidation treatment does not prolong survival. Lancet i: 379–382
14. Vogler WR, Winton EF, Gordon DS et al. (1984) A randomized comparison of postremission therapy in acute myelogenous leukemia: a Southeastern Cancer Study Group Trial. Blood 63: 1039–1045
15. Wolff SN, Marion J, Stein RS et al. (1985) High-dose cytosine arabinoside and daunorubicin as consolidation therapy for acute nonlymphocytic leukemia in first remission: a pilot study. Blood 65: 1407–1411
16. Yates J, Glidewell O, Wiernik P et al. (1982) Cytosine arabinoside with daunorubicin or adriamycin for therapy of acute myelocytic leukemia: a CALGB study. Blood 60: 454–462
17. Zittoun R, Jehn U, Fière D et al. (1989) Alternating v repeated postremission treatment in adult acute myelogenous leukemia: a randomized phase III study (AML6) of the EORTC leukemia Cooperative Group. Blood 73: 896–906

Idarubicin Pharmacokinetics

E. Schleyer, S. Budeus, J. Reinhardt, C. Rolff, T. Büchner, and W. Hiddemann

Introduction

Idarubicin is one of the most recently introduced agents which has gained increasing interest andd is beginning to be widely administered both for the first and second line treatment of AML as well as in breast cancer [1, 2]. In order to provide the basis for its clinical use the pharmacokinetics of this agent have been the topic of many investigations [3–5]. This paper gives an overview of the available literature on the pharmacokinetics of idarubicin and its main metabolite idarubicinol after intravenous and oral administration and demonstrates the results from our own pharmacokinetic studies on the pharmacokinetics of idarubicin after repeated oral administration. In order to obtain an overwiew of the pharmacokinetics of idarubicin the following key determinants must be evaluated.
1. Determination of terminal half-life, metabolic pathways, methods of elimination, area-under-curve concentration and peak plasma concentration related to the given dosis.
2. The kinetic characteristics in the case of multiple dosing, evaluating for example a change from first-order to zero-order kinetics.
3. Interindividual variations of kinetic parameters and a relation to therapeutic response and toxicity.
4. Intraindividual variations in the case of multiple dosing. While these questions must be addressed for the intravenous administration of idarubicin, its administration via the oral route requires additional information about:
1. Bioavailability of idarubicin
2. Differences in drug metabolism between intravenous and oral administration, for example due to a first-pass effect
3. Differences in plasma kinetics after oral and intravenous administration

These questions are addressed in the present paper on the basis of previously published data and the results of our own investigations.

Patients, Material and Methods

Patients

Pharmacokinetic investigations were performed in six patients with acute myeloid leukemia (AML) at third relapse. Treatment consisted of a combination of low-dose cytosine arabinoside (AraC) with idarubicin (LAI). Ara-C was given at $10 \, mg/m^2$ per 12 h s.c. on days 1–14 while idarubicin was given at $20 \, mg/m^2$ per day orally on days 3, 4 and 5 (LAI protocol).

Pharmacokinetic Analyses

Measurements of idarubicin and its metabolite idarubicinol were performed with an isocratic reversed-phase HPLC system and fluorescence detection with an excitation wavelength of 480 nm and an emission

Department of Internal Medicine, University of Münster, Domagkstr. 3, 4400 Münster, FRG wavelength of 560 nm. Plasma idarubicin and idarubicinol were concentrated by extraction on Supelco C 18 columns (Supelco, Bad Homburg FRG). The sensitivity of this assay is about 100 pg/ml plasma for both idarubicin and idarubicinol. Quantification was performed with the external standard method using a computerized integration of peak areas (RAMONA, Nuclear interface, Münster, FRG). Analysis of measured data was based on the TOPFIT program, providing an optimized adaption of coefficient of variation between the observed and calculated respective data [6].

Results

Figure 1 shows time/concentration curves of idarubicin and idarubicinol after an intravenous bolus injection from a paper by Smith and coworkers [7]. Its demonstrates that the maximum concentration of idarubicin is reached immediately after a 15 mg/m^2 intravenous bolus injection and is in the microgram concentration range. The plasma concentrations decline rapidly because of a short distribution phase. The curve fits best a three-compartment pharmacokinetic model with a second distribution phase revealing a half-life of approximately 4 h. The terminal elimination phase starts at 10 h with a half-life of about 25 h. The only detectable metabolite idarubicinol reveals a different pharmacokinetic behavior. Its peak plasma concentration is not reached before approximately 8 h after the i.v. injection. Its terminal half-life is twice as long as for the mother substance. According to the differences in pharmacokinetics idarubicinol plasma levels exceed idarubicin plasma concentrations after 5 h and remain higher for an extended period. Since the cytotoxic activity of idarubicinol is compared to idarubicin it is conceivable that the cytotoxic effects after i.v. injection are largely mediated by idarubicinol.

This fact makes idarubicin a different drug from other anthracyclines or other anthracycline derivates. Although similar plasma concentration curves are found for daunorubicin and daunorubicinol, the metabolite has only minor cytotoxic activity and does not contribute to the cytotoxic effects [3]. The second major differences from other anthracyclines is the applicability of idarubicin via the oral route. Figure 2 depicts the concentration/time curves of idarubicin and idarubicinol from one patient during treatment with idarubicin 20 mg/m^2 per day on three consecutive

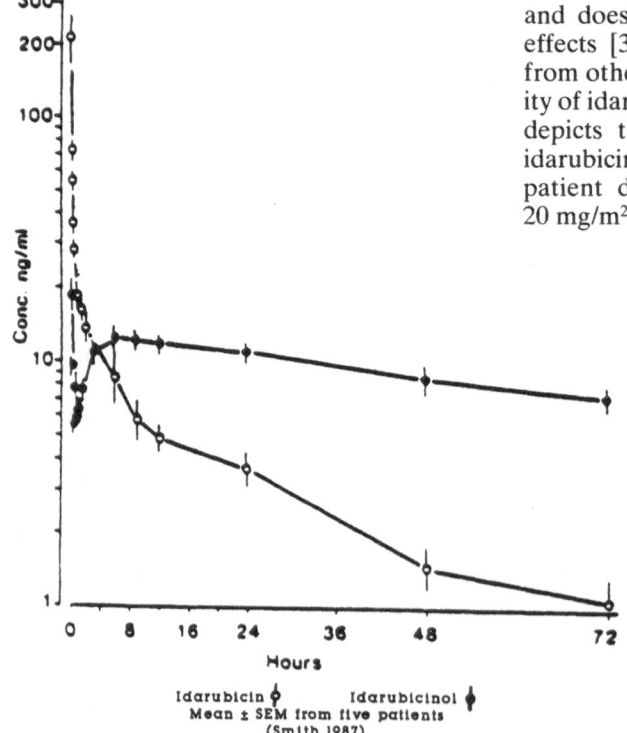

Fig. 1. Plasma concentration curves of idarubicin and idarubicinol after 15 mg/m^2 bolus injection (Smith et al. [7]

618

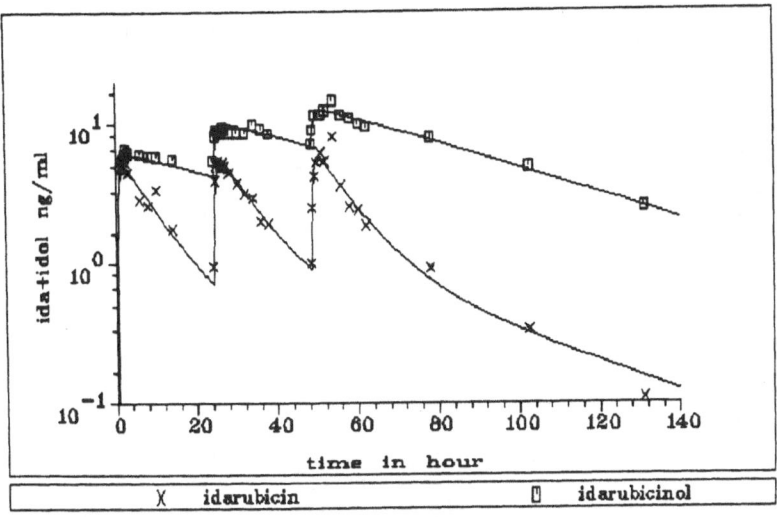

Fig. 2. Plasma concentration curves of idarubicin and idarubicinol from patient No. 3 after oral administration of idarubicin 20 mg/m² per day on three consecutive days

days. While plasma levels of idarubicinol exceed idarubicin plasma concentrations not earlier than 8 h after intravenous injection, they are higher shortly after oral uptake. These data suggest a first-pass effect by the liver after oral administration. Pharmacokinetics of the oral formulation are otherwise identical to the intravenous administration and fit best a three-compartment model. Basically the kinetic behavior is as described in Fig. 1. The terminal half-life of idarubicinol is twice as long as for idarubicin. This diagram demonstrates a constant absorption of the drug over the 3 days as indicated by the reproducible AUCs and the linear increase of the plasma levels of both substances. Table 1 shows additional data from the available literature on the pharmacokinetics of idarubicin after both i.v. and oral administration [5, 7–10]. The upper part lists the most relevant kinetic data after intravenous administration from several studies. As mentioned before the terminal half-life of idarubicinol is about twice that of idarubicin, the AUC three to six times higher. Both idarubicin and idarubicinol are most probably mainly excreted via the gut – the renal clearance is about 12% only. The lower part of the table demonstrates the same kinetic parameters after oral administration of different

doses. Results on the bioavailibility differ greatly and range from 8% to 50% in different studies and individual patients as illustrated for example by Smith and coworkers [7].

The ratio of the AUCs for idarubicinol over idarubicin is constantly higher after oral administration while comparable results are obtained for the dose-independent parameters such as terminal half-life. The comparison of the AUCs after intravenous administration to oral administration leads to an average of bioavailibility between 20% and 30%. Nearly the same result is reflected by the ratio of drug eliminated via the kidneys after intravenous and oral administration. These data allow the following conclusions:

1. The pharmacokinetics of idarubicin and idarubicinol follow a three-compartment model independent of their method of administration, terminal half-life and elimination rates are similar after i.v. and oral administration.
2. Idarubicin has a biovailibility of about 30% with a great variability between different patients from 8% to 50%.
3. After oral administration a higher idarubicinol/idarubicin ratio can be found due to a first-pass effect by the liver. These data emphasize that the oral route

Table 1. Pharmacokinetic overview of idarubicin and idarubicinol

Author	Terminal $t_{1/2}$ Ida	Terminal $t_{1/2}$ Idol	AUC idarubicin 15 mg/m²	AUC idarubicinol 15 mg/m²	Ratio AUC ida/idol	Renal clearance ida idol	Bioavali-billity (%)
Intravenous route							
Tamassia et al. [5]	12 h	69 h	173 ng h/ml	1037 ng h/ml	1: 6.0	3.3% 12.8%	
Smith et al. [7]	35 h	52 h	330 ng h/ml	697 ng h/ml	1: 4.7	2.8% 8.7%	
Speth et al. [8]	15 h	47 h	260 ng h/ml	860 ng h/ml	1: 3.3	– –	
Lu et al. [10]	27 h	66 h	–	–		5.2% 8.8%	
Oral route							
Tamassia et al. [5]	5 h	36 h	92 (45 mg/m²)	920 (45 mg/m²)	1:10.0	0.6% 4.7%	30
Smith et al. [7]	20 h	40 h	82 (15 mg/m²)	331 (15 mg/m²)	1: 4.0	0.6% 3.6%	8.9–38.9
Pannuti et al. [9]	24 h	59 h	46 (10 mg/m²)	306 (10 mg/m²)	1: 6.7	1.5% 9.2%	–
Lu et al. [10]	27 h	38 h	–	–	–	2.4% 7.7%	28–49.4
Schleyer (own data)	31 h	57 h	51 (20 mg/m²)	273 (20 mg/m²)	1: 5.4	–	–
Mean i.v.	22 h	59 h	254 (15 mg/m²)	865/15 (mg/m²)	1: 4.7	3.8% 10.1%	–
Mean oral	21 h	46 h	55 (15 mg/m²)	323 (15 mg/m²)	1: 9.0	1.3% 6.3%	31

should be explored in more detail but seems attractive especially because of the higher idarubicinol/idarubicin ratio translating into a higher AUC for idarubicinol as compared to the i. v. injection. The further exploration of the oral formulation should address the following topics.

1. Confirmation of published data about the kinetics of oral idarubicin
2. Evaluation of intraindividual variations in absorption amount and rate
3. Assessment of a possible therapeutic benefit from adapting drug doese to bioavailability in individual patients

Figure 3 shows the concentration/time curves for idarubicin and idarbucicinol from six patients. The AUCs for both substances show great interindividual variation, but are reproducible in individual patients. This is depicted in more detail in Table 2, which describes the kinetics parameters for the six individual patients. AUC and absorption rate were calculated for every single dose. The results indicate that AUC and absorption rate are constant for idarubicin over the three consecutive doses in every single patient.. AUC values range from 27 to 71 ngh/ml and the absorption rate has a half-life of 0.6–5.1 h. Table 2 again demonstrates a considerable difference in AUCs, reflecting variations in bioavailability between different patients. On a single patient basis, however, it can be shown that the amount and rate of drug absorption remain constant. Table 3 shows the pharmacokinetic parameters for idarubicinol as calculated from the measured data illustrated by Fig. 3. AUCs could not be calculated for every single dose due to the long half-life of idarubicinol.

Table 2. Idarubicin pharmacokinetics; LAI protocol (20 mg/m² per day oral administration)

Patient Given dose	AUC 1 (ng h/ml)	AUC 2	AUC 3	AUC from all data	$t_{1/2abs.}$ h	× VC	Day 1	2	3	$t_{1/2\,y}$ (h)	Clearance$_{total}$ (ml/min)	C_{max} (ng/ml)
1: 3×40 mg	25.1	28.4	26.5	27.5	4.16	25%	3.1	5.1	3.9	24.2	7395	1.37
2: 2×35+30 mg	29.2	33.7	27.1	32.5	1.03	31%	0.8	1.4	0.9	44.4	5382	1.70
3: 3×35 mg	67.3	65.8	72.5	71.4	0.68	16%	0.6	0.6	0.8	21.2	2454	5.01
4: 2×35 mg	55.3	58.7	–	57.7	0.61	42%	0.9	0.4	–	51.4	3030	2.15
5: 1×40 mg	–	–	–	63.0	0.61	42%	–	–	–	18.3	3174	4.29
6: 1×40 mg	–	–	–	52.4	0.68	16%	0.6	0.6	0.8	27.9	3816	3.01
Average	–	–	–	50.8	1.81	–	–	–	–	31.2	4209	2.92
VC				31%	68%					39%	40%	58%

Vc, variance coefficient; c_{max}, peale concentration of idarubicin; $t_{1/2\,y}$, terminal half-life
Dose-dependent data were calculated assuming a bioavailability of 30%

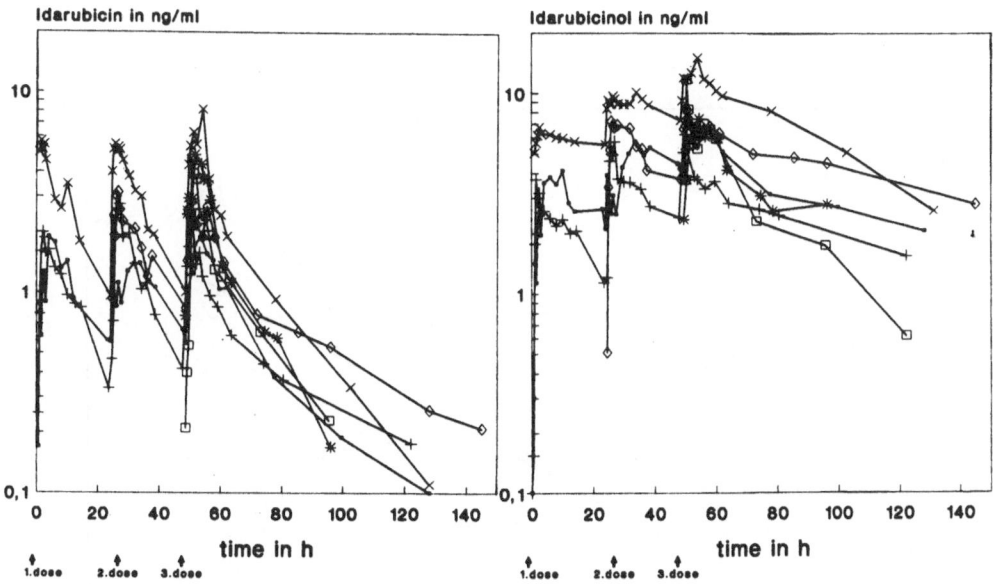

Fig. 3. Plasma concentration curve of idarubicin and idarubicinol after oral administration of 20 mg/m² per day on three consecutive days for all analyzed patients

Assuming that the AUC of idarubicin is related to its cytotoxic activity, these data may pose the question of how to correct for the interindividual differences in absorption and how to achieve comparable plasma concentrations and comparable AUCs between the individual patients. From a practical standpoint this should be possible without the requirement of multiple determination of idarubicin plasma level during

Table 3. Idarubicinol pharmacokinetics; LAI protocol (20 mg/m² per day idarubicin oral administration

Patient Dosis	$t_{1/2\alpha}$ (h)	$t_{1/2\beta}$ (h)	$t_{1/2\gamma}$ (h)	AUC (ng h/ml)	Clearance$_{total}$ (ml/min)	V_{ss} (l)	C_{max} (ng)	Ratio AUC ida/idol
1: 3×40 mg	0.44	5.15	69.17	213	941	4488	3.35	1:7,7
2: 2×35 mg+30 mg	0.76	7.52	55.37	151	1163	5112	3.32	1:4.7
5: 1×40 mg	0.44	2.29	50.21	288	693	2592	7.00	1:4.5
6: 1×40 mg	0.44	6.88	59.92	278	718	2850	7.82	1:5.3
4: 2×35 mg	0.76	13.4	72.00	406	432	2562	5.49	1:7.0
3: 3×35 mg	0.21	4.43	36.8	345	507	1407	6.08	1:4.8
Average	0.51	6.61	57.25	273	742	3169	5.51	1:5.5
VC	38%	53%	21%	29%	34%	40%	31%	22%

$t_{1/2\alpha}$, first distribution half-life; $t_{1/2\beta}$, second distribution half-life; $t_{1/2\gamma}$, terminal half-life; V_{ss}, distribution volume at steady state
Dose-dependent data were calculated assuming a bioavailability of 30%

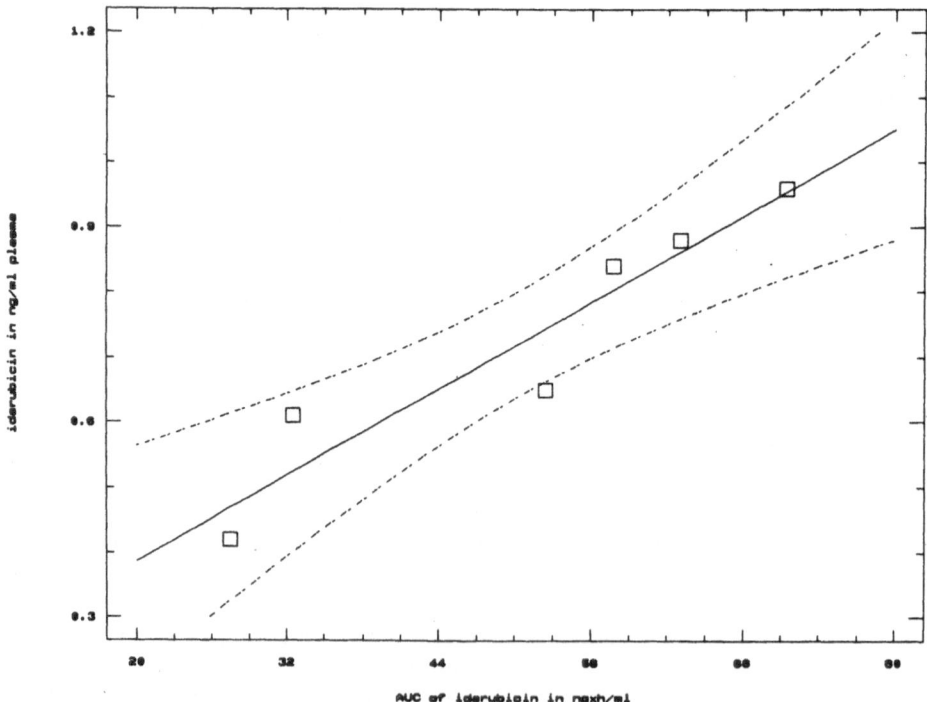

Fig. 4. Regression curve of idarubicin concentration 24 h after 20 mg/m² oral administration versus AUC

the first idarubicin administration to calculate the AUC. Figure 4 indicates that such an approach can be achieved by measuring only the idarubicin plasma concentration 24 h after the first dose. The 24-h plasma concentration is significantly correlated with the AUC and thus allows a respective calculation. The correlation coefficient of this regression is 95 %.

On this basis a dose correction may be possible by a single drug concentration measurement. Hence, a drug-targeted therapy is feasible and may be explored in future studies.

Discussion

The pharmacokinetic of idarubicin and its main metabolite idarubicinol are well defined by available data. Basically all investigators describe the same kinetic behavior of the two substances with numerical variations which are probably due to differences in the methods of analysis and kinetic calculations. The oral route seems to be an attractive method of administration, taking advantage of the first-pass effect in the liver and the transformation of idarubicin into the similarly active but more slowly eliminated idarubicinol. In order to fully explore the possibilities and limitations of oral administration additional data on the bioavailability and the impact of differences between individual patients on treatment outcome are warranted and should be provided by future studies. Preliminary data by Elbeak and coworkers indicate a relation between bioavailibility and white blood cell count [2]. In summary the current data demonstrate:

1. Pharmacokinetics of idarubicin and its main metabolite idarubicinol are well defined by available data.
2. Plasma pharmacokinetics are linear in the dose range tested [1].
3. Dose-independent pharmacokinetic parameters are similar for intravenous and oral administration.
4. Idarubicin bioavailibility is variable among individual patients but constant during multiple dosing in one patient.
5. The idarubicin plasma AUC strongly correlates with the 24-h plasma concentration after oral administration and therefore possibly allows an individualized targeting of drug administration.

Summary

Idarbucin is a new anthracycline analog which lacks the methoxy group in the C4 position of the aglycon moiety. Compared with daunorubicin, idarubicin was found to exert a five to eight times higher antineoplastic activity against a variety of experimental tumor systems. Clinical studies also demonstrated a lower cardiotoxicity. In contrast to other anthracyclines, idarubicin can be administered via the intravenous and oral route. Pharmacokinetics have been evaluated for both methods of administration and were found equivalent for the following dose-independent parameter: The plasma concentration time curve follows a three-compartment model with a terminal half-life of about 25 h. In the therapeutic dose range the kinetics are linear with a proportional increase in the AUC. The distribution volume of about 2000 l indicates a strong tissue binding. The bioavailability of idarubicin amounts to an average of 30 %. One major method of elimination is the hepatic transformation of idarubicin to idarubicinol. The terminal half-life of this metabolite is about 60 h. In vitro studies showed a similar antineoplastic activity of idarubicin and idarubicinol. Due to the first-pass effect after oral administration the ratio of the AUCs of idarbucinol/idarubicin is about twice as high after oral as after i.v. administration. Similar prolonged high plasma levels of idarubicinol can otherwise only be achieved by continuous i.v. infusion. Our own studies on the pharmacokinetics of repeated oral administrations of idarubicin show a reproducible intraindividual rate of drug absorption with substantial interindividual differences.

References

1. Robert J, Rigal-Huguet F, Harousseau JL, Pris J, Huet S, Reiffers J, Hurtelopu P, Tamassia V (1987) Pharmacokinetics of Ida-

rubicin after daily intravenous administration in leukemic patients. Leuk Res 11: 961–964

2. Elbaek K, Ebbehoej E, Jakobsen A, Juul P, Rasmusen S, Bastholt L, Dalmark M. Steiness E (1989) Pharmacokinetics of oral Idarubicin in breast cancer patients with reference to antitumor activity and side effects. Clin Pharmacol Ther 5: 627–634

3. Broggini M, Sommacampagna B, Paolini A, Ersilia D, Grazia D (1986) Comparative metabolism of daunorubicin and 4-demethosydaunorubicin in mice and rabbits. Cancer Treat Rep 6: 697–702

4. Zhini G, Vicario GP, Lazzati M, Armacone F (1986) Disposition and metabolism of (14-C) 4-demethoxydaunorubicin HCL (Idarubicin) and (14-C) daunorubicin HCL in the rat. Cancer Chemother Pharmacol 16: 107–115

5. Tamassia V, Pacciarini MA, Moro E, Piazza E, Vago G, Libretti A (1987) Pharmacokinetic study of intravenous and oral Idarubicin in cancer patients. Int J Clin Pharmacol Res 5: 419–426

6. Heinzel G, Hammer R, Wolf M, Koss FW, Bozler G (1977) Modellentwicklung in der Pharmakokinetik. Drug Res 27: 904–911

7. Smith DB, Margison JM, Lucas SB, Wilkinson PM, Howel A (1987) Clinical pharmacology of oral and intravenous 4-demethosydaunorubicin. Cancer Chemother Pharmacol 19: 138–142

8. Speth P., van de Loo F, Linssen P, Wessels H, Haanen C (1986) Plasma and human leukemic cell pharmacokinetics of oral and intravenous 4-demethoxydaunorubicin. Clin Pharmacol Ther 12: 643–649

9. Pannuti F, Camaggi CM, Strocchi E, Comparsi R, Angelelli B, Pacciarini MA (1986) Low dose oral administration of 4-demethoxydaunorubicin (Idarubicin) in advanced cancer patients. Cancer Chemother Pharmacol 16: 295–299

10. Lu K, Savaraj N, Kavanagh L, Feun LG, Burgess M, Bodey GP, Loo TL (1986) Cancer Chemother Pharmacol 17: 143–148

Toxicity Profile of Idarubicin: Experiences with Oral and Intravenous Idarubicin in the Treatment of Leukemia

J. L. Harousseau, B. Pignon, J. Reiffers, F. Rigal-Huguet, J. Y. Cahn, and P. Y. Le Prise on behalf of the French Idarubicin Study Group

Idarubicin (IDR) is a new potent antileukemic agent and the only anthracycline derivative in current use that can be administered orally. We review here the French experience with oral and IV IDR.

Oral Idarubicin

Up to now, oral IDR has only been used in France in the treatment of de novo acute myeloid leukemia (AML) in elderly patients (over 65 years of age). Two consecutive pilot studies have been conducted. In the first [1], IDR was given as a single agent at a dose of 30 mg/m² per day for three consecutive days with a second course at day 14 if the marrow remained blastic. Twenty patients were enrolled in this study. The results of this first study were encouraging with eight complete remissions (CR) (40%). However, the hematologic toxicity was high and all but one patient were entirely nursed in hospital. Thus, in

the second study [2], the therapeutic protocol was a combination of IDR (20 mg/m² per day, days 1–3) and low-dose cytarabine (LD ARA-C) (10 mg/m² subcutaneously every 12 h, days 1–10). A second course was administered at day 20 if the marrow remained blastic (with 2 days of IDR and 5 days of LD ARA-C). Thirty-two patients received this regimen. The clinical characteristics of the patients treated in both trials are shown in Table 1.

In the first study, eight patients (40%) achieved CR (six after one single course), five patients died and there were seven failures. In the second study, 13 patients (40.5%) achieved CR (12 after a single course), 4 patients died and there were 2 partial remissions and 13 failures.

Severe myelosuppression was noted after one course in 16 out of 19 noncytopenic patients in study 1 and in 22 out of 28 patients in study 2. Only one CR was obtained without neutropenia. The median durations of neutropenia ($<0.5 . 10^9/l$) were respectively 19 and 18 days. As a consequence of this hematologic toxicity, the treatment was entirely done in hospital for

---

* Hotel Dieu, 44035 Nantes Cedex, France

Table 1. Treatment of AML in elderly patients: clinical characteristics

	Study 1: oral IDR as single agent	Study 2: oral IDR plus LD ARA-C
No. of patients	20	32
Age (median)	65–79 (72)	67–82 (76)
Performance status ⩾ 2 WHO	6/20	15/32
Initial WBC count (median) (10⁹/l)	1–168 (12)	0.7–200 (7.7)
Initial platelet count (median) (10⁹/l)	8–230 (33)	5–316 (62)
FAB classification M1–M3 + M6 /M4–M5	14/6	20/11

Table 2. Oral IDR in the treatment of AML in elderly patients: nonhematologic toxicity

Percentage WHO grade	Study 1: oral IDR as single agent			Study 2: oral IDR plus LD ARA-C		
	0–1	2	3–4	0–1	2	3–4
Nausea vomiting	45	25	30	86	10	4
Diarrhea	70	25	5	93	7	–
Mucositis	65	25	10	93	7	–
Hepatic toxicity	90	5	5	76	21	3
Cardiac toxicity	80	20	–	90	10	–

19/20 patients in study 1, and for 27/32 patients in study 2. Of the six patients treated partly at home, three were subsequently admitted to hospital in an emergency for septic complications of aplasia. The extrahematologic toxicity is shown in Table 2. Minor or transient cardiac abnormalities were noted in seven cases but with no case of congestive heart failure.

These results are encouraging and could be favorably compared to those obtained in the same age category with LD ARA-C [3–5] or combination chemotherapy [6]. However, it is difficult to draw any firm conclusion from these two small pilot studies and prospective trials are warranted to define the exact role of oral IDR in the management of AML in the elderly. It should be emphasized that in both trials hematologic toxicity was a limiting factor for treatment on an outpatient basis.

Intravenous Idarubicin

In France, i. v. IDR is administered on five instead of three consecutive days. According to the results of a phase I/II study, the daily dosage used is 8 mg/m² [7].

Idarubicin and Intermediate-Dose Cytarabine in Relapsed AML [8]

High-dose ARA-C (HD ARA-C) is an effective but toxic treatment for relapsed AML. In order to reduce the incidence of severe complications noted with HD ARA-C containing regimens, we used a combination of i. v. IDR at optimal dosage (8 mg/m² per day, days 1–5) and cytarabine at inter-

mediate-dose (ID ARA-C) (1 g/m² by 2 h infusion every 12 h for six doses). Thirty-five patients aged 23–78 years (median 56) with AML in first relapse received this protocol. Of the 35 patients, 21 (60%) achieved CR, 4 had a partial remission, 4 died in aplasia and 6 were nonresponders. The median duration of aplasia was 23 days (15–38). The nonhematologic toxicity was moderate. The main side effect was mucositis (ten patients including six grade 3–4 WHO). Diarrhea, skin toxicity and hepatic disturbances which are side effects of HD ARA-C therapy were rare and mild. No conjunctivitis and, in spite of the age of the patients (25 >50 years), no cerebellar toxicity was recorded. Four patients suffered minor cardiac events.

As a result of this good extra hematologic tolerancce, the CR rate was not affected by age and even in patients >60 years it was 58%. The only factor influencing the CR rate was the duration of the first CR: 35% for patients relapsing before the median duration of first CR (16 months) versus 83% for patients relapsing after 16 months (p = 0.003). This IDR/ID ARA-C protocol is safe and effective in relapsed AML and is currently proposed in frontline therapy of AML.

Phase III Randomized Protocol in Adult AML

The French group GOELAM has initiated in 1987 a randomized study for the treatment of AML in adults. For patients aged 15–50 years the main objective of this protocol is the comparison of autologous bone marrow transplantation and high-dose chemotherapy as postremission consolidation treatment. For the whole group of patients (15–65 years), the induction treatment is randomized between a combination of ARA-C (200 mg/m^2 continuous infusion seven consecutive days) and zorubicine (Rubidazone) (200 mg/m^2 i. v. per day, days 1–4) or IDR (8 mg/m^2 i. v. per day, days 1–5). Zorubicine (ZRB) is a potent antileukemic anthracycline used in France and gives, in combination with conventional doses of ARA-C, a high CR rate in adult AML [9]. Up to October 1990, 380 patients were included and 317 are evaluable for induction therapy (151 in the IDR arm, 166 in the ZRB arm). Both groups were comparable regarding the initial clinical and hematologic characteristics. The overall CR rate is 75 % with no significant difference between the IDR arm (77.5 %) and the ZRB arm (73 %). The CR rates are strictly comparable for patients <50 years (77.3 % versus 77.7 % respectively). However, in the group of patients >50 years, there is a trend in favor of the IDR arm (78 % versus 67 %, $p = 0.15$). In the IDR arm the CR rate is the same for patients over or under the age of 50. The median duration of neutropenia was slightly longer in the IDR arm (26 days versus 24 days, $p = 0.002$) but this did not induce a higher toxic death rate (7.3 % versus 7.8 %). The nonhematologic toxicity was comparable in both arms (Table 3). The only significant differences concerned nausea and vomiting, and mucositis, which were more frequent in the ZRB arm. Twenty-one cardiac events were recorded, 8 (5.3 %) in the IDR arm and 13 (7.8 %) in the ZRB arm. However, only four patients experienced severe cardiac toxicity (three

congestive heart failures, one coronary insufficiency), all four in the ZRB arm.

Thus in combination with ARA-C, IDR gives a high CR rate and appears at least as effective as ZRB in adult AML. It could even be more effective in patients >50 years of age, which could partly be explained by a better tolerance.

These preliminary results have to be confirmed by further analysis of this still ongoing trial.

Table 3. Goelam study: nonhematologic toxicity, percentage of toxicities ≥grade 2 WHO

Toxicity	IDR	ZRB	p value
Nausea vomiting	57	69.5	0.02
Mucositis	38.5	49	0.03
Diarrhea	34.5	45	0.13
Hepatic toxicity	30.5	34	0.43
Renal toxicity	3.5	7	0.30

References

1. Harousseau JL, Rigal-Huguet F, Hurteloup P et al. (1989) Treatment of acute myeloid leukemia in elderly patients with oral idarubicin as a single agent. Eur J Haematol 42: 182–185
2. Harousseau JL, Huguet F, Reiffers J et al. (1991) Oral idarubicin and low dose cytarabine as the initial treatment of acute myeloid leukemia in elderly patients. Leuk Lymph (in press)
3. Seban C, Archimbaud E, Coiffier B et al. (1988) Treatment of acute myeloid leukemia in elderly patients. A retrospective study. Cancer 61: 227–231
4. Powell BL, Capizzi RL, Muss HB et al. (1989) Low dose ARA-C therapy for acute myelogenous leukemia in elderly patients. Leukemia 3: 23–28
5. Tilly H, Castaigne S, Bordessoule D et al. (1990) Low dose cytarabine versus intensive chemotherapy in the treatment of acute non lymphocytic leukemia in the elderly. J Clin Oncol 8: 272–279
6. Champlin RE, Gajewski JL,, Golde DW et al. (1989) Treatment of acute myelogenous leukemia in the elderly. Semin Oncol 16: 51–56
7. Harousseau JL,, Hurteloup P, Reiffers J et al. (1987) Idarubicin in the treatment of relapsed or refractory acute myeloid leukemia. Cancer Treat Rep 71: 991–992
8. Harousseau JL, Reiffers J, Hurteloup P et al. (1990) Treatment of relapsed acute myeloid leukemia with idarubicin and intermediate dose cytarabine. J Clin Oncol 7: 45–49
9. Marty M, Lepage E, Guy H et al. (1987) Remission induction and maintenance modalities in acute myeloid leukemia: a multicenter randomized study. In: Büchner T, Schellong G, Hiddemann W, Urbanitz D, Ritter J (eds) Acute leukemias. Prognostic factors and treatment strategies. Springer, Berlin Heidelberg New York, pp 50–56 (Hämatologie und Bluttransfusion, vol 30)

Prospective Study Comparing Idarubicin and Daunorubicin in Elderly Patients with Acute Myeloid Leukemia

J. Reiffers, F. Rigal-Huguet, A. M. Stoppa, M. Michallet, G. Marit, M. Attal, J. A. Gastaut, B. Corront, G. Lepeu, M. Routy, P. Cony-Makhoul, J. Pris, D. Hollard, D. Maraninchi, M. Mercier, and P. Hurteloup for the BGMT Group

Introduction

There is general agreement about the use of a combination of cytosine arabinoside (Ara-C) and anthracycline as induction chemotherapy for patients with acute myeloid leukemia (AML). Cytosine arabinoside is usually given as a continuous infusion (100–200 mg/m^2 per day) for 7–10 days. Daunorubicin (DNR) is the most commonly used anthracycline and is usually infused for 3 days (45–60 mg/m^2 per day). Using such a combination, complete remission (CR) is achieved in 65%–80% of young adult patients but the CR rate is lower in elderly patients, varying from 40% to 70% [6]. This latter lower CR rate is due to a high proportion of patients who fail to enter remission either because they die during induction treatment (infection, cardial dysfunction, etc.) or their leukemic cells are not sensitive to chemotherapy [6]. In order to increase the CR rate in elderly patients, several therapeutic strategies have been proposed. Hematopoietic growth factors such as GM-CSF or G-CSF may shorten the duration of granulocytopenia following chemotherapy and decrease the number of early deaths [3]. New intercalating agents may be used instead of DNR for both increasing the antileukemic efficacy and decreasing the mortality due to cardiac toxicity. Idarubicin (IDA) (4-demethoxy-daunorubicin) has been recently introduced as treatment for AML patients. Its safety

Department of Hematology,
Hôpital Haut-Levêque,
33604 Pessal, France

and antileukemic activity have been reported in some phase I – phase II studies where IDA was used either alone [7] or in combination with Ara-C [1, 5, 8]. The preliminary results from some ongoing prospective studies indicate that IDA is at least as efficient as DNR for adult patients with AML [2, 10, 12, 13]. We report herein a prospective study comparing IDA and DNR in AML patients aged between 55 and 75 years. Our preliminary results are similar to those reported elsewhere in adult patients and confirm that IDA is at least as effective as DNR.

Patients and Methods

Patients

Between April 1987 and September 1990, 216 patients aged between 55 and 75 years were entered into the protocol BGMT 87 designed to prospectively compare the efficacy and toxicity of IDA and DNR in elderly AML patients. Two hundred and six patients who fulfilled the following criteria were eligible: diagnosis of AML according to the FAB criteria, no assessable preleukemic phase, and normal left ventricular ejection fraction (LVEF). They were randomized to receive either IDA or DNR. One hundred and ninety-seven patients (IDA = 98; DNR = 99) were evaluable for the comparison of the two anthracyclines. The main characteristics of these 197 patients (age, sex, FAB morphology, initial WBC count) did not differ significantly for the different therapeutic arms (Table 1).

Table 1. Characteristics of the 197 evaluable patients

	IDA (n = 98)	DNR (n = 99)
Age (median)	65 (56–75)	65 (56–75)
Sex (M/F)	49/49	50/49
M_1–M_3/ M_4–M_5/others	54/36/8	59/28/12
Initial WBC (/mm³)	9.95 (0.3–260)	5 (0.4–520)

BGMT 87 Study Design

Induction chemotherapy

The patients were given Ara-C (100 mg/m² per day, continuous infusion, 7 days) combined with either IDA (8 mg/m² per day, i. v., 5 days) or DNR (50 mg/m² per day, i. v., 3 days). The patients who did not achieve a complete remission were given a second course of identical chemotherapy. The results of induction chemotherapy were analyzed according to Preisler's criteria [11].

Maintenance Treatment

When complete remission (CR) was achieved after one or two courses of chemotherapy, the patients received consolidation therapy with Ara-C (50 mg/m² per 12 h, subcutaneously, 5 days) combined with either IDA (8 mg/m² per day, i. v., 3 days) or DNR (30 mg/m² per day, i. v., 3 days). After consolidation, the patients received five courses of Ara-C (50 mg/m² per 12 h, s. c., 5 days) and either IDA (10 mg/m²) or DNR (40 mg/m²) administered 1, 3, 6, 9 and 13 months after consolidation and continuous maintenancce chemotherapy (± stonalozolol) consisting of alternating 10-day courses of 6-mercaptopurine (70 mg/m² per day) and methotrexate (15 mg/m² per day, three times for 10 days).

Results

Induction Chemotherapy

A complete remission (CR) was achieved in 129 patients (65.5%) after one (112 patients) or two courses (17 patients) of induction chemotherapy. The CR rate was not influenced by the age or sex of patients, the FAB morphology or the initial WBC count. The patients treated with IDA had a higher CR rate (68/98; 69.4%) than the patients treated with DNR (61/99; 61.6%) but the difference did not reach statistical significance ($p = 0.3$). However, in patients between 55 and 65 years of age, the CR rate was significantly higher with IDA (36/43; 83%) than with DNR (28/52; 52%) ($p < 0.004$). For the patients who entered CR, the median duration of severe granulocytopenia (polymorphonuclear cells <500 mm³) was 24 days in both groups. The reasons for not achieving CR were more often drug resistance in the DNR group (26/38) than in the IDA group (11/30), and the percentage of patients who died during the treatment was higher in the IDA group (19/30) than in the DNR group (12/38). These differences were not statistically significant. There was no difference in the extrahematological toxicity between patients who received IDA and those who received DNR. The three patients who developed severe congestive heart failure leading to the interruption of chemotherapy received DNR.

Outcome

The actuarial median survival of the entire patient population studies was 9 months and was similar in the DNR and IDA groups. The only prognostic factor for the duration of survival was the age of patients since the median survival of patients over the age of 65 years was shorter (7 months) than for the patients between 55 and 65 years (13 months) ($p < 0.003$). Among the 129 patients entering CR after induction chemotherapy, a leukemic relapse occurred in 71 patients. While the follow-up was similar in both groups, the number of patients who relapsed was higher (38/61 = 62%) in the DNR group than in the IDA group (33/68:48.5%) ($p=0.1$). The median duration of remission was longer in the IDA group (19.5 months) than in the DNR group (13 months). The actuarial proportion of long-term survivors was not statistically different in both groups (IDA = 40 %; DNR = 20 %).

Discussion

Idarubicin has been demonstrated to be effective in patients with AML. In refractory of relapsed AML,, a CR rate was obtained in 19/96 patients treated with IDA alone administered either over 3 days (8–15 mg/m^2 per day) or for five consecutive days (7–8 mg/m^2 per day) (for review, see [5]). When IDA was combined with Ara-C either as a continuous infusion or as intermediate dose, the response rate seemed to be higher in both refractory and relapsed AML than that observed after IDA alone [5, 8]. In one of these studies, IDA was administered over 5 days (8 mg/m^2) and was demonstrated to be effective and well tolerated in elderly patients [8]. Thus, this latter schedule was chosen for IDA in the ongoing BGMT phase III study and compared to the standard regimen for DNR. We observed an overall CR rate of 65.5 %, which compares favorably with that usually reported in elderly patients [6]. The CR rate obtained in the 97 patients treated with Ara-C and IDA (69.4 %) was similar to that recently reported in two studies from Italy using IDA combined with Ara-C and VP-16 [4, 9]. Four other studies from Italy and the United States have prospectively compared the efficacy and toxicity of IDA and DNR. In the three studies performed in adult patients with AML, the overall CR rate was higher after IDA (99/135; 73 %) than after DNR but the difference was not statistically significant in one of these studies [13], borderline in the ECOG study [12] and significant in the New York study [2] (Table 2). In the cooperative Italian study performed in elderly AML patients, there was no difference in the CR rate between patients receiving IDA or DNR. However, in this study, IDA seemed to be more effective than DNR as the proportion of patients who achieved CR after one course of chemotherapy was significantly higher after IDA (30 %) than after DNR (20 %) (p=0.02). Moreover the proportion of patients who exhibited drug resistance was less in the IDA group (17/125) than in the DNR group (89/125) (p=0.001). Thus, all these studies indicate that IDA is at least as effective and probably superior to DNR as induction treatment in AML patients. Our own results confirm the efficacy of IDA when administered to elderly patients. As in other studies, they also confirm that the extrahematological toxicity was mild.

Since the follow-up of patients achieving CR is still insufficient in our study, it is not possible to draw any conclusion regarding the comparative efficacy of IDA and DNR

Table 2. Results of prospective studies comparing IDA and DNR in AML

	Age of patients (median; range)	Induction regimen IDA	DNR	Response rate IDA	DNR	P
Petti et al. [10] (n = 245)	62.5 (55–78)	12 mg/m^2 ×3	45 mg/m^2 ×3	50/124 (40 %)	49/125 (39.2 %)	N.S
Vogler et al. [12] (n = 95)	– (15–?)	12 mg/m^2 ×3	45 mg/m^2 ×3	29/39 (74 %)	26/46 (57 %)	0.09
Wiernik et al. [13] (n = 102)	55 (18–?)	13 mg/m^2 ×3	45 mg/m^2 ×3	34/51 (67 %)	27/51 (53 %)	N.S
Berman et al. [2] (n = 86)	38 (17–60)	12 mg/m^2 ×3	50 mg/m^2 ×3	36/45 (80 %)	24/41 (58 %)	0.03
BGMT study (n = 197)	65 (55–75)	8 mg/m^2 ×5	50 mg/m^2 ×3	69/98 (69.5 %)	61/99 (61 %)	N.S

for prolonging survival. However, the percentage of patients who had a leukemic relapse was higher in the DNR group than in the IDA group. Such a finding was also reported in Vogler's Study [12], where the percentage of relapse was higher after DNR (44 %) than after IDA (22 %). A significant prolongation of survival was also reported in patients treated with IDA in two other studies [13]. We feel that identical results will be found in our BGMT study when we have a sufficient follow-up.

References

1. Berman E, Raymond V, Daghestani A, Arlin ZA, Gee TS, Kempin S, Hancock C, Williams L, Stevens YW, Clarkson BD, Young C (1989) 4-Demethoxydaunorubicin (Idarubicin) in combination with 1-b-D-arabinofuranosyl-cytosine in the treatment of relapsed or refractory acute leukemia. Cancer Res 49: 477–481
2. Berman E, Raymond V, Gee T, Kempin SJ, Gulati S, Andreeff M, Kolitz J, Gabrilove J, Heller G, Young CW, Clarkson BD (1989) Idarubicin in acute leukemia: results of studies at Memorial Sloan-Kettering cancer center. Semin Oncol 16 [Suppl 2]: 30–34
3. Buechner T, Hiddeman W, Koenigsmann M, Zuehlsdorf M, Woermann B, Boeckmann A, Aguion Freire E, Innig G, Maschmeyer G, Ludwig W, Sauerland C, Schulz G (1990) Recombinant human GM-CSF following chemotherapy in high-risk AML. Bone Marrow Transplantation 6 [Supp 1], 131–133
4. Carella AM, Martinengo M, Santini G, Gaozza E, Damasio E, Giordano D, Nati S, Congiu A, Cerri R, Risso M, Ganzina F, Marmont AM (1987) Idarubicin in combination with etoposide and cytarabine in adult untreated acute non lymphoblastic leukemia. Eur J Cancer Clin Oncol 23: 1673–1678
5. Carella AM, Berman E, Maraone MP, Ganzina F (1990) Idarubicin in the treatment of acute leukemias. An overview of preclinical and clinical studies. Haematologica 75: 159–169
6. Champlin RE, Gajewski JL, Golde DW (1989) Treatment of acute myelogenous leukemia in the elderly. Semin Oncol 16: 51–56
7. Harousseau JL, Hurteloup P, Reiffers J (1987) Idarubicin in the treatment of relapsed or refractory acute myeloid leukemia. Cancer Treat Rep 69: 1447–1448
8. Harousseau JL, Reiffers J, Hurteloup P, Milpied N, Guy H, Rigal-Huguet F, Facon T, Dufour P, Ifrah N for the French Study Group of Idarubicin in leukemia (1989) Treatment of relapsed acute myeloid leukemia with Idarubicin and intermediate-dose cytarabine. J Clin Oncol 7: 45–49
9. Lambertenghi-Deliliers G, Annaloro C, Cortelezzi A, Cortellaro M, Volpe AD, Maiolo AT, Mozzana R, Pogliani E, Pozzoli E, Polli EE (1989) Idarubicin plus cytarabine as first-line treatment of acute nonlymphoblastic leukemia. Semin Oncol 16: 16–20
10. Petti MC, Mandelli F (1989) Idarubicin in acute leukemias: experience of the Italian cooperative group GIMEMA. Semin Oncol 16: 10–15
11. Preisler HD, Reese PA,, Marinello MJ, Pothier L (1983) Adverse effects of aneuploidy on the outcome of remission induction therapy for acute nonlymphocytic leukaemia: analysis of types of treatment failure. Br J Haematol 53: 459–466
12. Vogler WR, Velez-Garcia E, Omura G, Raney M (1989) A phase-three trial comparing Daunorubicin or Idarubicin combined with Cytosine Arabinoside in acute myelogenous leukemia. Semin Oncol 16 [Suppl 2]: 21–24
13. Wiernik PH, Case CD, Periman PO, Arlin ZA, Weitberg AB, Ritch PS, Todd MB (1989) A multicenter trial of Cytarabine plus Idarubicin or Daunorubicin as induction therapy for adult nonlymphocytic leukemia. Semin Oncol 16 [Suppl 2]: 25–29

Novantrone: Current Status and Future Trends in the Treatment of Leukemias and Lymphomas

New Aspects in the Pharmacokinetics and Metabolism of Mitoxantrone*

G. Ehninger, J. Blanz, K. Mewes, B. Proksch, I. Kumbier, U. Schuler, and K. P. Zeller

Anthracenediones are an important group of naturally occurring quinones found in plants and animals. Many have been used as dyes and laxatives since ancient times. Surprisingly an American National Cancer Institute screening of some 1500 naturally occurring quinones revealed their relative lack of antitumor activity.

In 1973 ametantrone (1,4-bis-[[2-[(2-hydroxyethyl)amino]ethyl]amino]-9, 10-anthraquinone) (Fig. 1), a molecule originally developed to be used as a ballpoint pen ink, showed good antitumor activity [1].Two groups, K. C. Murdock and colleagues (Lederle Laboratories, Pearl River, NY) and R. K. Y. Zee-Cheng and colleagues (Drug Development Laboratory, Mid-American Cancer Center, Kansas City, KS) tested structural variations to develop more active compounds. Among these compounds, the most active was mitoxantrone [2–6].

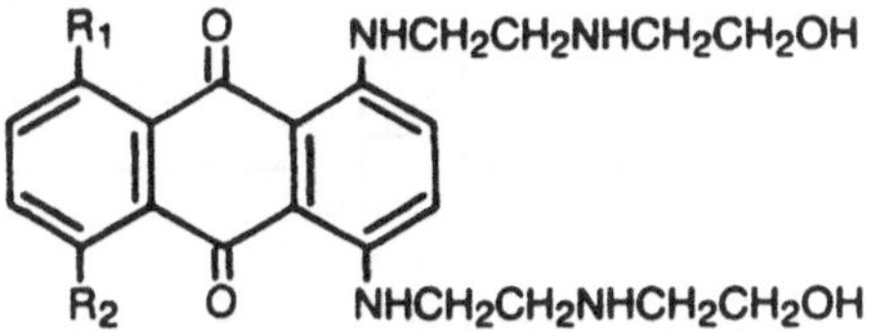

Fig. 1. Structure of mitoxantrone and ametantrone

Medizinische Universitätsklinik und Institut für Organische Chemie der Universität, Tübingen, FRG

* Dedicated to Professor Dr. Dr. H. D.Waller on the occasion of his 65th birthday.

Mitoxantrone, a cytotoxic anthracenedione derivative, has shown clinically beneficial activity in breast cancer, lymphoma and leukemia [7]. Several different mechanisms of action have been suggested to account for this. In addition to intercalation, biological effects such as electrostatic interactions with DNA, DNA-protein crosslinks,, immunosuppressive activities, inhibition of topoisomerase II, prostaglandin biosynthesis, and calcium release have been described [1, 8–24].

Various methods for drug monitoring in biological fluids and tissues are available. Of these the highest sensitivity was achieved using high-performance liquid chromatography (HPLC) with electrochemical detection, radioimmunoassay, and enzyme-linked immunosorbent assay.

A very long terminal half-life of mitoxantrone elimination was reported by our group in patients who were treated with mitoxantrone 14 mg/m^2 and cyclophosphamide 600 mg/m^2 [25, 26]. Serum and urine concentrations were measured by an HPLC method with a limit of sensitivity of 0.2 ng/ml in urine and 1 ng/ml in serum.The pharmacokinetic parameters were estimated using both urinary and serum values. The combined data were best described by an open three-compartment model (Fig. 2). The rapid distribution phase with a half-life of 0.14 h was likely to represent the plasma equilibrium, binding to endothelium, and penetration into the formed elements of blood. The estimated β half-life was 3.1 h and was interpreted to be associated with a redistribution of the drug from the formed elements and surfaces into the tissues. The

635

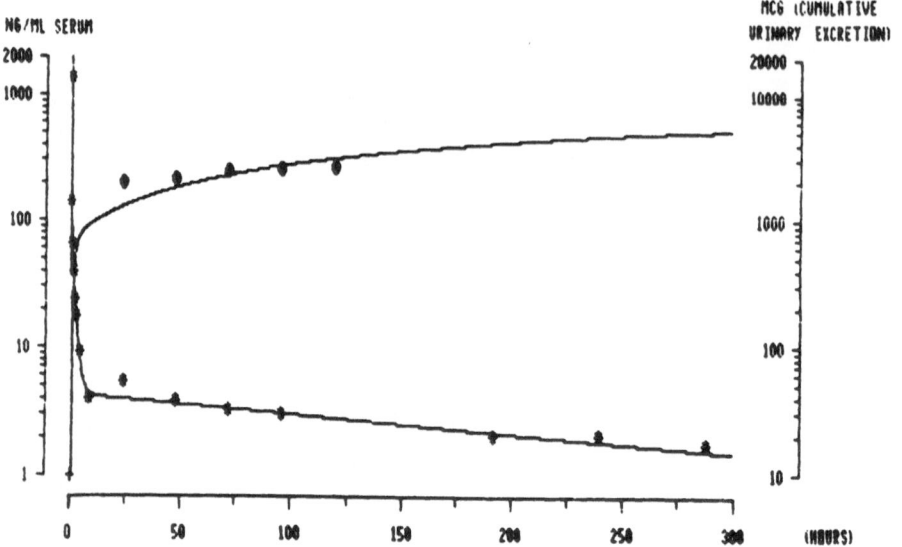

Fig. 2. Plasma concentration versus time curve and urinary excretion of mitoxantrone [26]

terminal half-life was 215 h (range, 125–346 h). The volume of distribution was 2248 l/m²; a total body clearance of 217 ml/min/m² and a renal clearance of 15 ml/min/m² was observed.

Four metabolites were separated in urine and three in serum. The two major metabolites cochromatographed with the synthesized monocarboxylic and dicarboxylic acids of mitoxantrone. Within 48 h, 4.4% of the administered dose was excreted in urine as mitoxantrone and 0.8% as metabolites (Fig. 3).

Data derived from mitoxantrone measurements by use of an radioimmunoassay are

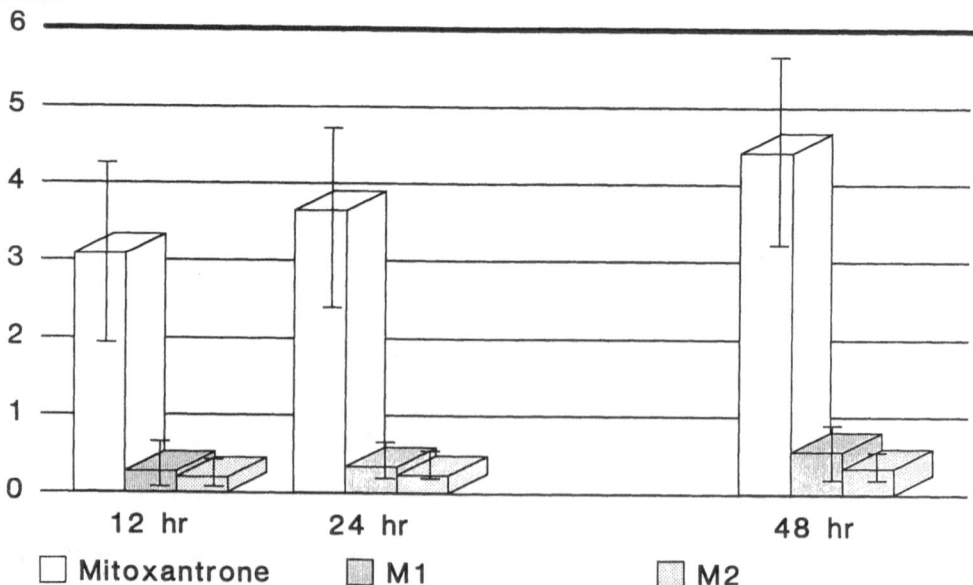

Fig. 3. Urinary excretion of mitoxantrone and two major metabolites

included in one report [27]. Serum samples were obtained from six patients through 3 weeks after treatment. Concentrations of 290–1000 pg/ml were present in serum after 21 days. A terminal half-life of 12.4 ± 3.1 days was calculated.

All pharmacokinetic studies reported a short $t_{1/2\alpha}$ between 4.1 and 10.7 min, with the distribution phase being between 0.3 and 3.1 h. In contrast, the values of the terminal half-life are quite variable ranging from 8.9 h to 9 days [28–35]. Differences might be attributed to assay sensitivity, number and weighting of data points beyond 24 h and coadministered drugs.

Taken together, we may suggest the following consensus: mitoxantrone exhibits a rapid initial distribution phase followed by a relatively slow elimination phase. The results suggest a deep tissue compartment with a slow release. The very large volume of distribution shown by all studies suggests that much of the mitoxantrone is sequestered in the tissues.

All tissue measurements showed that mitoxantrone persists in human tissues for prolonged periods. In autopsy studies, relatively high tissue concentrations have been measured in liver, bone marrow, heart, lung, spleen, and kidney [36, 37]. Concentrations of drug in tissues in which a tumor was located generally did not correlate with concentration of drug in the tumor itself. Exceptions to this were liver and brain.

Pharmacokinetic data of a 21-day continuous infusion of mitoxantrone were reported by a Dutch group. Mitoxantrone at doses of 0.3 mg/m² per day to 1.3 mg/m² per day for 3 weeks was given. Plasma steady-state was reached after 35 h. At the highest dose, steady-state plasma levels of about 3.5 ng/ml were reached. Mitoxantrone could be detected in plasma for at least 5 days after the end of the 21-day infusion period and in leukocytes for at least 14 days. The cellular drug concentration with continuous infusion was about twice as high as with a bolus infusion of an equal myelotoxic dose, expressed as area under the plasma concentration time curve (AUC). It was speculated that, if the same phenomenon takes place in tumor cells, continuous infusion may lead to a higher tumor response rate [38].

Our group reported the results of a study in patients who received mitoxantrone at daily repeated doses [39]. The terminal half-life was 175 h and the volume of distribution in steady state was 3841 l. The urinary excretion of mitoxantrone was unchanged from day 1 through day 5. Therefore the capacity of the tissues to bind mitoxantrone seems to be large.

A clinical study described the administration of mitoxantrone in patients with hepatic dysfunction [40]. In hepatocellular carcinoma patients given 12 mg/m² mitoxantrone, hematologic and other toxic effects were similar in 13 patients with elevated bilirubin compared to 15 with normal bilirubin levels. In contrast, breast cancer patients with elevated bilirubin levels given either 14 or 8 mg/m² mitoxantrone experienced more severe hematologic toxicity than did patients with normal bilirubin levels. The authors suggested that these differences could be explained by the presence of hepatocellular carcinoma cells that retain some variable amount of the usual metabolic capacity. General application rules for patients with impaired liver function cannot be derived from this small study.

Elimination and Metabolism of Mitoxantrone

Investigations with bile-duct cannulated rats,, rabbits, dogs, monkeys, and isolated perfused rat liver [27, 41–44] showed that biliary excretion is the major excretory pathway for mitoxantrone and its metabolites.

Urinary excretion of radioactivity was found to be comparatively low in all species examined. In rabbits, less than 6 % – 8 % of the dose was excreted during a 6-h observation period. In rats and dogs, 6 % or 4.9 % of radioactivity has been found in the same collection time, which increased to 13.6 % of administered dose in rats when the time of collection was extended to 120 h. Following a single i. v. dose of ¹⁴C-labeled mitoxantrone, renal excretion of radioactivity in cancer patients was similar to that in animals.

Some investigators have also examined the collected body fluids by HPLC monitoring light absorption at 658 nm to determine the fraction of radioactivity belonging to the unchanged drug. The significant differences demonstrate that up to 51 % (dogs), 22.5 %–25 % (rabbits) and 40 % (rats) of the total excreted radioactivity has to be attributed to metabolites of mitoxantrone [27, 29, 30, 41, 43, 45]. In an isolated perfused rat liver model three more polar metabolites have been detected after separation via high-performance thin-layer chromatography [44]. HPLC investigations of urine, bile and plasma of patients showed up to four metabolites which were also observed in the urine and bile of rats [41, 46, 47], dogs [43] and rabbits [42]. However, the amount of metabolites detected by light absorption by no means equaled the radioactivity not bound to the parent compound [26].

Few attempts have been made to elucidate the metabolism of mitoxantrone and only two laboratories have reported efforts in chemical structure elucidation of metabolites detected by several investigators [26, 34, 42, 44, 45, 47–50].

Our group was recently able to isolate and characterize several metabolites of mitoxantrone (Blanz et al., unpublished work). The metabolic pathways are shown in Fig. 4. Two metabolites of mitoxantrone have been characterized as the mono- and dicarboxylic acid derivatives resulting from the oxidation of the terminal methylene groups of the side chains. Chicarelli et al. [50] and our group suggested these compounds to be metabolites. Unequivocal proof was provided a few weeks ago. Other metabolic pathways lead to metabolite with a cyclization of the side chain. An intermediate precursor of this metabolite can react with DNA and proteins and shows alkylation activity. In the presence of glutathione the reactive di-imine intermediate reacts to mono- and diglutathione conjugates. In addition mitoxantrone can also bind glucuronic acid (not shown in Fig. 4).

As described above several different mechanisms of action have been suggested to account for the cytotoxic activity of mitoxantrone. In addition to intercalation, biological effects such as electrostatic interactions with DNA, DNA-protein crosslinks, inhibition of topoisomerase II, pros-

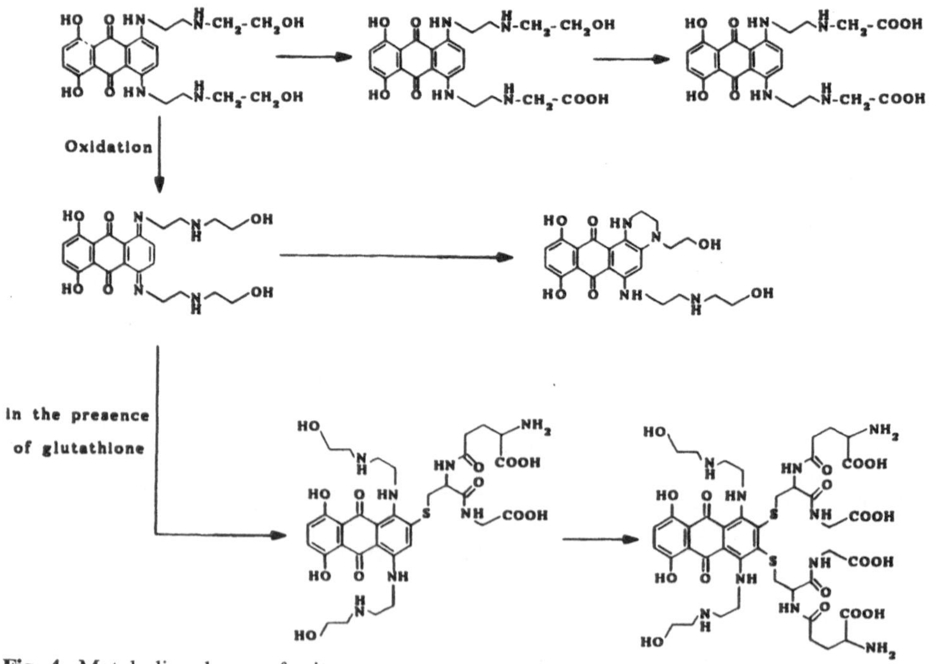

Fig. 4. Metabolic scheme of mitoxantrone

638

taglandin biosynthesis, and calcium release, alkylating properties should now be added.

Perspectives

The efficacy of mitoxantrone is established in breast cancer, leukemia and lymphoma. Further clinical studies should focus on the evaluation of different schedules and application modalities, e. g., locoregional vs. systemic treatment and continuous infusion vs. bolus, to improve activity and further decrease toxicity. The complex and unique pharmacokinetic and metabolic profile should be further investigated in these trials. The influence of disease status with altered conditions of drug elimination should be evaluated. In addition, studies at the cellular level might help to improve our knowledge of drug resistance and drug interactions.

References

1. Johnson RK, Zee-Cheng RKY, Lee WW, Acton EM, Henry DH, Cheng CC (1979) Experimental antitumor activity of aminoanthraquinones. Cancer Treat Rep 63: 425–439
2. Murdock KC, Child RG, Fabio PF,, Angier RB,, Wallace RE, Durr FE, Citarella RV (1979) Antitumor agents. 1. 1,4-Bis((aminoalkyl)amino)-9, 10-anthracenediones. J Med Chem 22: 1024–1030
3. Zee-Cheng RKY, Cheng CC (1982) Structure-activity relationship study of anthraquinones: 1,4-dihydroxy- 5,8-bis ((2-(2-hydroxyethoxy) ethyl)amino)-9, 10-anthracenedione, an analog of an established antineoplastic agent. J Pharm Sci 71: 708–709
4. Cheng CC, Zee-Cheng RKY, Narayanan VL, Ing RB, Paull KD (1981) The collaborative development of a new family of antineoplastic drugs. Trends Pharmacol Sci 2: 223–224
5. Zee-Cheng RKY, Cheng CC (1983) Anthraquinone anticancer agents. Drugs Future 8: 229–249
6. Murdock KC, Wallace RE, White RJ, Durr FE (1985) Discovery and preclinical development of novantrone. Adv Cancer Chemother March 21–24: 3–13
7. Shenkenberg TD, Von Hoff DD (1986) Mitoxantrone: a new anticancer drug with significant clinical activity. Ann Intern Med 105: 67–81
8. Ho AD, Seither E, Ma DD, Prentice HG (1987) Mitozantrone-induced toxicity and DNA strand breaks in leukaemic cells. Br J Haematol 65: 51–55
9. Foye WO, Vajragupta OPA, Sengupta SK (1982) DNA-binding specificity and RNA polymerase inhibitory activity of bis (aminoalkyl) anthraquinones and bis (methylthio) vinylquinone odides. J Pharm Sci 71: 253–257
10. Lown JW, Hanstock CC, Bradley RD, Scraba DG (1984) Interactions of the antitumor agents mitoxantrone and bis-antrene with deoxyribonucleic acids studied by electron microscopy. Mol Pharmacol 25: 178–184
11. Lown JW, Hanstock CC (1985) High field H-NMR analysis of the 1:1 intercalation complex of the antitumor agent mitoxantrone and the DNA duplex [d(CpGpCpG]. J Biomol Struct Dynamics 2: 1097–1106
12. Kapuscinski J, Darzynkiewicz Z, Traganos F, Melamed RR (1981) Interactions of a new antitumoragent, 1,4-dihydroxy-5,8-bis[[2-(2-hydroxyethyl)aminoÄethyl]amino]-9, 10-anthra-cenedione with nucleic acids. Biochem Pharmacol 30: 231–240
13. Alberts DS, Peng YM, Bowden T,, Mackel C, Dalton WS (1986) Mechanisms of action and pharmacokinetic of novantrone in intravenous and intraperitoneal therapy. In: Coltman CA (ed) The current staus of novantrone. Wiley, New York, pp 15–21
14. Cohen LF, Glaubiger DL, Kann HE, Kohn KW (1980) Protein associated DNA single strand breaks and cytotoxicity of dihydroxyanthracenedione (DHAD) in mouse L1210 leukemia cells. Proc Am Assoc Cancer Res 21: 277
15. Su RT (1981) Effect of 1,4-dihydroxy-5,8-bis[[2-(2-hydroxyethyl)amino]-ethylÄamino]-9, 10-anthracenedione (dihydroxyanthraquinone) on the replication of simian virus 40 chromosome. Biochem Biophys Res Commun 103: 249–255
16. Bowden GT, Roberts RA, Alberts DS, Peng YM, Garcia D (1985) Comparative molecular pharmacology in leukemia L1210 cells of the anthracene anticancer drugs mitoxantrone and bisantrene. Cancer Res 45: 4915–4920
17. Crespi MD, Ivanier SE, Genovese J, Baldi A (1986) Mitoxantrone affects topoisomerase activities in human breast cancer cells. Biochem Biophys Res Commun 136: 521–528
18. Frank P, Novak RF (1985) Mitoxantrone and bisantrene inhibition of platelet aggregation and prostaglandin E2 production in vivo. Biochem Pharmacol 34: 3609–3614

19. Bachur NR (1979) Anthracycline antibiotic pharmacology and metabolism The inhibitory effect of 1,4-dihydroxy-5,8-bis[[2-(2-hydroxyethyl)amino]-ethyl]amino]-9, 10-anthracenedione dihydrochloride on dividing and nondividing cells in vitro. Proc Am Assoc Cancer Res 20: 12 (abstr)

20. Doroshow JH (1983) Comparative cardiac oxygen radical production by anthra-cycline antibiotics, mitoxantrone, bisantrene, M-AMSA, and neocarzinostatin. Clin Res 31: 67A (abstr)

21. Frank P, Novak RF (1986) Effects of mitoxantrone and bisantrene on platelet aggregation and prostaglandin/thromboxane biosynthesis in vitro. Anticancer Res 6: 941–947

22. Novak RF, Kharash ED (1985) Mitoxantrone: propensity for free radical formation and lipid peroxidation implications for cardiotoxicity. Invest New Drugs 3: 95–99

23. Tewey KM, Chen GL, Nelson EM, Liu LF (1984) Intercalative antitumor drugs interfere with the breakage-reunion reaction of mammalian DNA topoisomerase II. J Biol Chem 259: 9182–9187

24. Wang BS, Murdock KC, Lumanglas AL, Damiani M,, Silva J, Ruszala-Mallon VM, Durr FE (1987) Relationship of chemical structures of anthraquinones with their effects on the suppression of immune responses. Int J Immunopharmacol 9: 733–739

25. Ehninger G, Proksch B, Heinzel G, Woodward DL (1986) Clinical pharmacology of mitoxantrone. Cancer Treat Rep 70: 1373–1378

26. Ehninger G, Proksch B, Heinzel G, Schiller E, Weible KH, Woodward DL (1985) The pharmacokinetics and metabolism of mitoxantrone in man. Invest New Drugs 3: 109–116

27. Batra VK, Morrison JA, Woodward DL, Siverd NS, Yacobi A (1986) Pharmacokinetics of mitoxantrone in man and laboratory animals. Drug Metab Rev 17: 311–329

28. Savaraj N, Lu K, Manuel V, Burgess M, Umsawasdi T, Benjamin RS, Loo LT (1982) Clinical kinetics of 1,4-dihydroxy-5,8-bis-[[2-[(2-hydroxyethyl)-amino]ethyl]amino]-9, 10-anthracenedione. Clin Pharmacol Ther 31: 312–316

29. Savaraj N, Lu K, Manuel V, Loo LT (1982) Pharmacology of mitoxantrone in cancer patients. Cancer Chemother Pharmacol 8: 113–117

30. Alberts DS, Peng YM, Bowden GT, Dalton WS, Mackel C (1985) Pharmacology of mitoxantrone: mode of action and pharmacokinetics. Invest New Drugs 3: 101–107

31. Alberts DS, Peng YM, Leigh S, Davis TP,, Woodward DL (1985) Disposition of mitoxantrone in cancer patients. Cancer Res 45: 1879–1884

32. Alberts DS, Peng YM, Leigh S, Davis TP, Woodward DL (1983) Disposition of mitoxantrone in patients. Cancer Treat Rev 10 (B): 23–27

33. Alberts PS, Peng YM, Bowden GT, Mackel C, Dalton WS (1989) Mechanism of action and pharmacokinetics of novantrone in intravenous and intraperitoneal therapy. Adv Cancer Chemother 15–21

34. Van Belle SJP, de Planque MM, Smith IE, van Oosterom AT, Schoemaker TJ, Deneve W, McVie JG (1986) Pharmacokinetics of mitoxantrone in humans following single-agent infusion or intra-arterial injection therapy or combined-agent infusion therapy. Cancer Chemother Pharmacol 18: 27–32

35. Larson RA, Daly KM, Choi KE, Han DS, Sinkule JA (1987) A clinical and pharmacokinetic study of mitoxantrone in acute nonlymphocytic leukemia. J Clin Oncol 5: 391–397

36. Stewart DJ, Green RM, Mikhael NZ, Montpetit V, Thibault M, Maroun JA (1986) Human autopsy tissue concentrations of mitoxantrone. Cancer Treat Rep 70: 1255–1261

37. Roboz J, Paciucci PA, Silides D, Greaves J, Holland JF (1984) Detection and quantification of mitoxantrone in human organs. A case report. Cancer Chemother Pharmacol 13: 67–68

38. Greidanus J, de-Vries EG, Mulder NH, Sleijfer DT, Uges DR, Oosterhuis B, Willemse PH (1989) A phase I pharmacokinetic study of 21-day continuous infusion mitoxantrone. J Clin Oncol 7: 790–797

39. Ehninger G, Mjaaland I, Proksch B, Schiller E, Meyer P (1987) Klinische Pharmakologie von Mitoxantron bei Patienten mit Mammakarzinom und Leukämien. Z Antimikrob Antineoplast Chemother 5: 67–70

40. Chlebowski RT, Tong M, Bulcavage L, Woodward DL (1986) Mitoxantrone in hepatic dysfunction: factors influencing toxicity and response. Proc Am Soc Clin Oncol 5: 46–46 (abstr)

41. Chiccarelli FS, Morrison JA, Gautam SR (1984) Biliary pharmacokinetics of C-mitoxantrone in the rat following different intravenous doses and characteristics of drug related material in the bile. Fed Proc 43: 345 (abstr)

42. Richard B, Fabre G, Fabre I, Cano JP (1989) Excretion and metabolism of mitoxantrone in rabbits. Cancer Res 49: 833–837

43. Lu K, Savaraj N, Loo LT (1984) Pharmacological disposition of 1,4-dihydroxy-5,8-bis[[2-(2-hydroxyethyl)amino]ethyl]amino]-9, 10-anthracene-dione dihydrochloride in the dog. Cancer Chemother Pharmacol 13: 63–66

44. Ehninger G, Proksch B, Hartmann F, Gärtner H-V, Wilms K (1984) Mitoxantrone metabolism in the isolated perfused rat liver. Cancer Chemother Pharmacol 12: 50–52

45. Macpherson JS, Smyth JF, Clements JA, Ramsay MW, Warrington PS, Leonard RCF, Wolf CR (1984) Pharmacokinetics and metabolism of mitoxantrone. Br J Cancer 50: 252–253

46. Avramis V (1982) Pharmacokinetics of dihydroxyanthracenedione (DHAD) and its metabolites in rats. Pharmacologist 24: 241 (abstr)

47. Wolf CR, Macpherson JS, Smyth JF (1986) Evidence for the metabolism of mitoxantrone by microsomal glutathione transferases and 3-methylcholanthrene-inducible glucuronosyl transferases. Biochem Pharmacol 35: 1577–1581

48. Ehninger G, Proksch B, Schiller E (1985) Detection and separation of mitoxantrone and its metabolites in plasma and urine by HPLC. J Chromato 342: 119–127

49. Smyth JF, Macpherson JS, Warrington PS, Leonard RCF, Wolf CR (1986) The clinical pharmacology of mitoxantrone. Cancer Chemother Pharmacol 17: 149–152

50. Chiccarelli FS,, Morrison JA, Cosulich DB, Perkinson NA, Ridge DN, Sum FW, Murdock KC, Woodward DL, Arnold ET (1986) Identification of human urinary mitoxantrone metabolites. Cancer Res 46: 4858–4861

Mitoxantrone in the Treatment of Acute Leukemias

M. J. Keating

Introduction

In the late 1960s the introduction of cytosine arabinoside (ara-C) transformed acute myelogenous leukemia (AML) from an incurable to a potentially curable disease. Around the same time clinical research discovered the activity of the anthracycline antibiotic, daunorubicin (DNR), in acute leukemia. Subsequently DNR plus ara-C has provided the backbone of most clinical trials alone or together with other agents such as thioguanine. Cardiac toxicity is dose limiting with DNR at high cumulative doses. Other anthracyclines such as doxorubicin, rubidazone, and idarubicin have been developed with attempts to increase the responsiveness of the leukemia and to decrease the cardiac toxicity. Results of early clinical trials suggest that idarubicin at the dose and schedule studied has a higher response rate than DNR in combination with ara-C. Other agents have been developed which have significant activity in acute myelogenous leukemia. These agents include amsacrine, VP-16, and the topic of this report which will be mitoxantrone.

Mitoxantrone is an anthracenedione with structural similarities to doxorubicin but without the amino sugar moiety at C_9 on the parent anthracycline molecule. A variety of clinical trials with mitoxantrone in patients with relapsed and refractory acute leukemia have shown activity similar to that seen with anthracyclines [1–3]. A variety of combination protocols have been conducted which have resulted in responses in refractory patients and comparative studies have been undertaken in previously untreated patients [4].

The MD Anderson Cancer Center has conducted a variety of studies with mitoxantrone in refractory acute leukemia. In 1983, Estey et al. reported on the use of mitoxantrone in 41 adult patients with refractory acute leukemia [1]. The starting dose was 4 mg/m² per day for 5 days and eventually the dose was escalated to 12 mg/m² per day for 5 days. Higher doses of 12 mg/m² per day for 5 days were associated with dose-limiting mucositis, abnormal liver function tests, and delayed recovery of normal blood counts. One complete remission was noted in ten patients at doses of less than 6 mg/m². Two of 23 patients receiving 6–8 mg/m² achieved a complete remission with only 1 CR among 22 patients receiving higher doses. The antileukemic effect was greater at the higher doses as was the incidence of death during induction. This phase I–II trial formed the basis for subsequent studies in refractory acute leukemia.

Relapse and Refractory AML

Management of patients with AML that have relapsed after a previous remission or have proved refractory to initial remission induction therapy is suboptimal. A variety of analyses have been conducted and have noted that the probability of achieving a

University of Texas MD Anderson Cancer Center, 1515 Holcombe Blvd., Box 38, Houston, Texas 77030, USA

complete remission on salvage therapy is of the order of 20 % – 30 % in patients who are refractory to remission induction therapy and is similar in frequency in patients whose initial remission duration is less than 6 or 12 months [5, 6]. Patients whose initial remission duration is longer than 12 months have a higher response rate of the order of 50 % and, if the initial remission duration was greater than 18 months, the patients have a probability of CR approximating that of frontline induction therapy [5, 6]. The use of chemotherapy regimens in second and subsequent salvage therapy is associated with the response rate of approximately 10 % [6]. Other important prognostic factors include the karyotype of the leukemia, normality of organ function, and the age of the patient [6].

Extensive clinical trials have been conducted with the use of high-dose ara-C and more recently intermediate-dose ara-C in refractory and relapsed AML. Patients who receive high-dose ara-C at a dose of 3 g/m^2 every 12 h for 9–12 doses have response rates variably reported from 25 % to greater than 50 % [7, 8]. We elected to combine mitoxantrone at a dose of 5 mg/m^2 per day for 5 days with ara-C 3 g/m^2 over 2 h every 12 h for six doses in the management of refractory AML [9]. Forty-four patients were treated. Twenty-seven of the patients were less than 50 years of age and 28 received mitoxantrone plus high-dose ara-C as their first salvage therapy. The initial remission duration was less than 1 year in 25 of 44 patients. The overall complete remission rate was 16/44 (36 %) patients. The median survival was 16 weeks. There was a strong association of survival with response with a median survival of responders of approximately 1 year. Patients who were refractory to remission induction and survived therapy with mitoxantrone plus high-dose ara-C had a median survival of 12 weeks. Thirteen of the 16 CR patients achieved complete remission in 1 course. Fourteen patients died during remission induction, 11 in the first course. Fourteen patients were refractory to the combination. Response was more commonly seen in patients under the age of 50 and in patients with APL (Table 1). Patients with impaired performance status had lower response

rates than patients whose performance status was 0–1 (Zubrod scale). Eleven of 28 (40 %) patients receiving mitoxantrone plus high-dose ara-C as first salvage therapy, achieved a complete remission versus 5 of 16 (32 %) who achieved a remission with second or greater salvage therapy. There was a strong association of duration of first remission with response with the CR rate being 4 of 25 (16 %) if the patients were primary refractory or had an initial CR duration of less than 1 year versus 12 of 19 (63 %) if the initial CR duration was longer than 1 year (Table 2). The CR rate according to karyotype was 2/4 (50 %) with translocation 8;21, 3/6 (50 %) with translocation 15;17 and 3/6 (50 %) with inversion of chromosome 16. Five (42 %) of 12 diploid patients achieved CR versus 1/12 (8 %) patients with other abnormalities (Table 3).

Table 1. Mitoxantrone + high-dose ara-C in AML: prognostic factors

Characteristic	Value	CR/total (%)
Age (years)	<50	13/27 (48)
	≥50	3/17 (18)
Morphology	AML	9/25 (36)
	APL	5/8 (63)
	AMOL	0/2 (–)
	AMML	2/8 (25)
	AEL	0/1 (–)
Performance Status (Zubrod)	0–1	14/32 (44)
	2	2/8 (25)
	3–4	0/4 (–)

Table 2. Mitoxantrone + high-dose ara-C: response rate according to salvage attempt and duration of initial CR in AML

First CR duration	Salvage attempt	
	First	≥ Second
<1 year	4/16 (25 %)	0/9 (–)
≥1 year	7/12 (58 %)	5/7 (71 %)

Table 3. Mitoxantrone + high-dose ara-C: clinical outcome by karyotype

Karyotype	Patient No.	% CR	% Died	% Resistant
inv16	6	50 \	17 \	33 \
t(15;17)	6	50 50	50 50	– 25
t(8;21)	4	50 /	– /	50 /
Diploid	12	42	33	25
Other Abnormalities	12	8	25	67
Insufficient metaphases	4	50	50	–

In previous studies using high-dose ara-C alone in AML, the CR rate was 11 of 45 (24 %). The incidence of resistance to high-dose ara-C was 15 of 45 patients (33 %) versus 14 of 44 patients (32 %) for the combination of mitoxantrone plus high-dose ara-C. The major toxicity (moderate-severe grade) of the regimen was vomiting in 16 % of patients, diarrhea in 21 %, and stomatitis in 16 %. Fourteen percent of patients experienced cerebellar neurotoxicity. Febrile episodes occurred in 96 % of patients with hyperbilirubinemia greater than 2 mg % in 37 % of patients and creatinine elevation greater than 1.4 mg/m^2 in 32 % of patients. Recovery from the effects of myelosuppression was delayed in a number of patients so that dose escalation was not increased. The other reason for not increasing dose was the observation that 14 out of 44 (32 %) patients died during the remission induction phase.

Mitoxantrone Plus High-Dose ara-C in CML Blast Crisis

Twenty-seven patients in the blastic phase of CML received similar combination chemotherapy to the AML group [10]. The patients' median age was 42 years with a range of 19–61 years and 26 of them had Philadelphia chromosome positive disease. Seven patients (26 %) achieved a complete remission and one had a partial remission for an overall response rate of 30 %. Eight patients died during remission induction, 11 patients had resistant disease. The median survival was 14 weeks for the total population. The complete remission patients had a median survival of 24 weeks. There was no

Table 4. Prognostic factors for response to mitoxantrone + HD ara-C in CML blast crisis

Characteristic	Value	CR/total (%)
Morphology	Myeloid	2/12 (17 %)
	Undifferentiated	5/13 (38 %)
	Lymphoid	0/2 (–)
Age (years)	<50	5/21 (24 %)
	≥50	2/6 (33 %)
Karyotype	Ph only	6/18 (33 %)
	ph+others	1/8 (13 %)

influence of age on response rate with 5/21 (24 %) patients under the age of 50 achieving a CR versus 2/6 (33 %) patients older than 50 years of age (Table 4). Twelve patients had myeloid blast crisis and 2 (17 %) achieved a CR versus 5/13 (38 %) with undifferentiated blast crisis and 0 of 2 lymphoid blast crisis. The duration of chronic phase was not associated with response. Four of 12 patients with an initial chronic phase of less than 12 months achieved a CR. Eighteen patients had Philadelphia chromosome as the only abnormality at the time of blast crisis and 6 out of 18 (33 %) achieved a complete remission. Only one of eight (13 %) with additional karyotypic abnormalities responded. There was no impact of hemoglobin level or platelet count on response. The incidence of nonmyelosuppressive toxicity was similar to that seen in AML. Severe mucositis and diarrhea was seen in 4 % of patients and hepatic dysfunction with a bilirubin level of >5 mg % in 19 % of patients. Severe cerebellar toxicity occurred in 4 % of patients. While mitoxantrone plus high-dose ara-C had a significant effect in getting patients into complete remission, this did not translate into a meaningful survival of the complete responders. The conclusion from this study was that additional therapeutic initiatives need to be undertaken.

Mitoxantrone Plus High-Dose ara-C in the Treatment of Refractory Acute Lymphocytic Leukemia

Mitoxantrone plus high-dose ara-C plus vincristine 2 mg on day 1 and prednisone 100 mg/day for 5 days was administered to 25 patients with refractory or relapsed acute lymphocytic leukemia [11]. Four of the patients were more than 40 years of age and 92 % had more than 50 % marrow blasts. Ten patients received the combination as their first salvage therapy, seven for their second, and eight for their third or greater salvage attempt (Table 5). Eleven patients (44 %) achieved a complete remission, nine (36 %) died during remission induction attempts and five (20 %) were resistant to therapy. Seven patients had an initial first CR duration of 0–26 weeks and only one out of seven (14 %) responded. No other features were strongly associated with response. Eighteen of the 25 patients had documented infections which were bacterial in 32 %, fungal in 4 %, viral in 4 %, both bacterial and fungal in 8 %, and multiple bacterial infections in 24 % of patients.

Formerly we had published the results of high-dose ara-C as a single agent together with vincristine and prednisone in 30 patients with ALL [12]. Eight out of 30 (27 %) patients achieved a complete remission. A compilation of other studies gives a response rate of 13 of 43 patients for high-dose ara-C regimens (30 %). Mitoxan-trone plus ara-C appeared to be an effective regimen for a number of patients with refractory ALL. In an ongoing study, mitoxantrone plus high-dose ara-C in the same schedule is followed 1 day after discontinuation of chemotherapy with GM-CSF 120 mg/m^2 per day by subcutaneous or short intravenous infusion. So far 23 patients have been treated. Nine out of 23 (39 %) have achieved a complete remission. Only three patients have died during remission induction. However, 11 patients had resistant disease. The decrease in early mortality was associated with an improved early survival but no improvement in long-term survival. There was a shortening by 4 days of the time-to-recovery of 500 granulocytes when mitoxantrone plus high-dose ara-C was compared with and without GM-CSF. In neither the study without GM-CSF nor with GM-CSF was there an association of 5 salvage attempt with a higher remission rate. In the study without GM-CSF, four of ten patients receiving treatment as their first salvage achieved a CR versus four of seven for second salvage and three of eight for third or greater salvage. In the study with GM-CSF, 5 of 13 first salvage patients responded versus 3 of 4 for second salvage and 1 of 6 third or greater salvage. Continued exploration of GM-CSF is occurring to establish whether dose intensity can be increased.

Mitoxantrone Plus Etoposide

Ho et al. [13] have reported a high response rate using mitoxantrone plus VP-16 in poor-risk first-relapse patients, patients relapsing on maintenance therapy, second or subsequent relapses, and patients with secondary AML. In that study 26 of 61 (43 %) patients

Table 5. Results of mitoxantrone + HD ara-C in ALL by salvage attempt

| | Salvage attempt | | | |
	S$_1$	S$_2$	≥S$_3$	Overall
Total	10	7	8	25
CR	4 (40)	4 (57)	3 (38)	11 (44)
Died	3 (30)	3 (42)	3 (38)	9 (36)
Resistant	3 (30)	0	2 (25)	5 (20)

Table 6. Influence of karyotype on response to mitoxantrone + VP-16 in refractory AML

Karyotype	S_1	Salvage attempt $\geq S_2$	Overall
t(8;21), t(15;17)	2/2 (100%)	1/6 (17%)	3/8 (38%)
Diploid	4/10 (40%)	1/11 (9%)	5/21 (24%)
+8/−5/−7	0/4	0/4	0/8
Miscellaneous	0/2	1/8 (13%)	1/10 (10%)

achieved a complete remission. The dose of mitoxantrone in their study was 10 mg/m^2 per day intravenously and etoposide 100 mg/m^2 per day as a short infusion both on days 1–5. We have conducted a study with mitoxantrone 7.5 mg/m^2 intravenously for 5 days and VP-16 in high-dose of 2 g/m^2 over 4 days either as a daily infusion or divided into 2 daily doses (Table 6) [14]. Twenty-one patients received this schedule. Seven patients received mitoxantrone at 6 mg/m^2 per day for 5 days and VP-16 at 1500 mg/m^2 over 3 days. A total of 47 patients have received this combination. Twenty-seven patients were less than 50 years of age and 24 had initial CR duration of less than 6 months. Ten of these 24 were refractory to initial remission induction therapy. Eighteen patients received the combination as their first salvage therapy, 7 during the second salvage, and 12 as their third or greater salvage regimen. The response for first salvage was 6 out of 18 (33%). Seven out of 18 patients died during the treatment with 28% of patients being resistant. Three (18%) patients receiving treatment as their second salvage attempt achieved a CR with 41% of patients dying during salvage therapy. None of the 12 patients who received the combination as their third or greater salvage responded. Six of 27 patients less than 50 years of age responded versus 3 of 20 older patients. Patients whose first CR duration was less than 6 months had a CR rate of 4 of 24 (17%) versus 4/14 (29%) for those whose initial CR duration was 26–51 weeks and only 2/9 (22%) with longer remissions responded. Karyotype was associated with response. Patients with t(8;21) and t(15;17) had a CR rate of three of eight (38%). Both patients with t(8;21) receiving treatment as their first salvage responded.

Diploid patients had a response rate of 5 of 21 (24%). None of the patients with trisomy of chromosome #8 or loss or deletion of either chromosome #5 or #7 responded (none of eight). Of those with miscellaneous other abnormalities only one out of ten patients responded.

Discussion

These studies suggest that mitoxantrone can be incorporated into successful combinations for salvage therapy in a variety of refractory or relapse leukemias. The impression persists that the response to salvage therapy is determined more by the biology of the leukemia, in particular the duration of the initial complete remission and the karyotype of the cells rather than the particular regimen which is being used. Whenever duration of initial CR is analyzed, patients who receive any regimen appear to have a higher response rate if their initial CR duration is longer than 12 months or if they have relapsed off treatment. In addition, patients with inv16, t(8;21), and t(15;17) appear to have higher response rates whereas those who are diploid have intermediate response rates and a very low CR rate in salvage therapy as found for patients with loss of deletion of chromosome #5 or #7, trisomy of chromosome #8, or miscellaneous other abnormalities. The results which were obtained with mitoxantrone and VP-16 were not as satisfactory as those obtained by Ho, where 7 of 21 primary resistant patients responded and 9 of 20 poor risk, high and first relapse patients responded [13]. In addition, 4 out of 11 patients with second relapse achieved a CR and 6 out of 9 patients with secondary

AML responded in that study. The nonhematologic toxicity which was reported by Ho was lower than we had seen with mitoxantrone and high-dose VP-16. In our study, obviously, the VP-16 dose is much higher and the mitoxantrone dose somewhat lower. Thus dose escalation of the VP-16 did not translate into an improved CR rate.

Mitoxantrone appears to have added in our historical experience to high-dose ara-C in the management of refractory AML. The dosage which we have used in salvage therapy (5 mg/m^2 per day for 5 days) is much lower than in other reported studies [15, 16]. It may well be that the mitoxantrone dose should be escalated and the ara-C dosage decreased to once a day rather than twice a day. Others such as Vredenburgh have treated relapsed or refractory AML with 14 mg/m^2 mitoxantrone daily for 3 days and have achieved a 47% complete remission rate [2]. Amadori has used 6 mg/m^2 per day for 6 days with once a day intermediate dose ara-C for 6 days and achieved a complete remission rate of 69% [17]. Hiddemann et al. [15] have used high doses of mitoxantrone also and have achieved a complete remission rate of 54%. Thus the question of dose intensity must be addressed. Overall, the results suggest that mitoxantrone is a useful addition to our therapeutic armamentarium but the majority of patients are still refractory to salvage therapy attempts.

References

1. Estey EH, Keating MJ, McCredie KB, Bodey GP, Freireich EJ (1983) Phase II trial of mitoxantrone in refractory acute leukemia. Cancer Treat Rep 67: 389–390
2. Paciucci PA, Cuttner J, Holland JF (1984) Mitoxantrone as a single agent and in combination chemotherapy in patients with refractory acute leukemia. Semin Oncol [Suppl 1] 11: 36–40
3. Arlin ZA, Silver RT, Cassileth P et al. (1985) Further evaluation of mitoxantrone in acute leukemia. In: Coltman CA Jr (ed) The current status of novantrone. Wiley, New York, pp 91–94
4. Arlin Z, Case DC Jr, Moore J, Wiernik P, Feldman E, Saletan S, Desai P, Sia L, Cartwright K, and the Lederle Cooperative Group (1990) Randomized multicenter trial of cytosine arabinoside with mitoxantrone or daunorubicin in previously untreated adult patients with acute nonlymphocytic leukemia. Leukemia 4: 177–183
5. Hiddeman W, Büchner T (1990) Treatment strategies in acute myeloid leukemia. Blut 60: 163–171
6. Keating MJ, Kantarjian H, Smith TL, Estey E, Walters R, Andersson B, Beran M, McCredie KB, Freireich EJ (1989) Response to salvage therapy and survival after relapse in acute myelogenous leukemia. J Clin Oncol 7: 1071–1080
7. Early AP, Preisler HD, Solcum H et al. (1982) A pilot study of high dose 1-β-D-arabinofuranosylcytosine for acute leukemia and refractory lymphoma: clinical response and pharmacology. Cancer Res 42: 1587–1594
8. Herzig RH, Wolff SN, Lazarus HM, Phillips GL, Karanes C, Herzig GP (1983) High-dose cytosine arabinoside therapy for refractory leukemia. Blood 62: 361–369
9. Walters RS, Kantarjian HM, Keating MJ, Plunkett WK, Estey EH, Andersson B, Beran M, McCredie KB, Freireich EJ (1988) Mitoxantrone and high-dose cytosine arabinoside in refractory acute myelogenous leukemia. Cancer 62: 677–682
10. Kantarjian HM, Walters RS, Keating MJ, Talpaz M, Andersson B, Beran M, McCredie KB, Freireich EJ (1988) Treatment of the blastic phase of chronic myelogenous leukemia with mitoxantrone and high-dose cytosine arabinoside. Cancer 62: 672–676
11. Kantarjian HM, Walters RL, Keating MJ, Estey EH, O'Brien S, Schachner J, McCredie KB, Freireich EJ (1990) Mitoxantrone and high-dose cytosine arabinoside for the treatment of refractory acute lymphocytic leukemia. Cancer 65: 5–8
12. Kantarjian HM, Estey EH, Plunkett W et al. (1986) Phase I–II clinical and pharmacologic studies of high-dose cytosine arabinoside in refractory leukemia. Am J Med 81: 387–394
13. Ho AD, Lipp T, Ehninger G, Illiger H-J, Meyer P, Freund M, Hunstein W (1988) Combination of mitoxantrone and etoposide in refractory acute myelogenous leukemia – an active and well-tolerated regimen. J Clin Oncol 6: 213–217
14. O'Brien S, Witt R,, Talpaz M, Kantarjian H (1991) Extramedullary blast crisis in a patient with Philadelphia chromosome-positive chronic myelogenous leukemia in complete cytogenetic remission. Cancer 67: 1946–1949
15. Hiddemann W, Kreutzmann H, Straif K, Ludwig WD, Mertelsmann R, Planker M,

Donhuijsen-Ant R, Lengfelder E, Arlin Z, Büchner T (1987) High-dose cytosine arabinoside in combination with mitoxantrone for the treatment of refractory acute myeloid and lymphoblastic leukemia. Semin Oncol 14: 73–77

16. Sanz MA, Borrego MD, Martin-Aragones G, Lorenzo I, Sanz G, Sayas MJ, Jarque I, Pastor E, Rafecas I, (1987) High-dose cyto-

sine arabinoside and mitoxantrone in high-risk acute nonlymphoblastic leukemia. Semin Oncol 14: 18–20

17. Amadori S, Mandelli F, Meloni G, Petti MC, Miniero R, Papa G (1988) Phase II study of intermediate-dose Ara-C and mitoxantrone for acute myelogenous leukemia. New Trends Ther Leuk Lymph 3: 17–21

High-Dose Cytosine Arabinoside and Mitoxantrone (HAM) in the Treatment of Acute Leukemias: Results of Salvage and First Line Treatment

W. Hiddemann[1], C. Aul[2] G. Maschmeyer[3], W. D. Ludwig[4], H. Löffler[5],
N. Nowrousian[6], R. Schönrock-Nabulsi[7], P. Bettelheim[8], A. Heinecke[9],
and T. Büchner[1] for the German AML Cooperative Group

Based on the significant single-agent activity of cytosine arabinoside at high doses (HD-AraC) and mitoxantrone (Mitox) in refractory and relapsed acute myeloid leukemia (AML) and the indication of a sequence-dependent synergistic effect of the two-drug combination by in vitro investigations [1, 2], a series of clinical phase II studies was initiated by the German AML Cooperative Group (AMLCG) in order to assess the antileukemic activity and toxicity of the HD-AraC/Mitox combination (HAM). These studies were primarily restricted to patients with refractory disease as previously defined in detail [3]. In addition, the majority of patients were recruited from the studies on first line therapy of the AMLCG and had thus received a standardized induction and postremission therapy [4, 5].

The *original HAM regimen* consisted in HD-AraC 3 g/m^2 by 3 h infusion q 12 h on days 1–4, Mitox was started at 12 mg/m^2 per day on days 3, 4, and 5 and was escalated to 4 and 5 doses of 10 mg/m^2 per day on days 2–5 and 2–6, respectively [6]. A total of 89 pts. with refractory AML ($n=65$) or ALL ($n=24$) have been treated according to this protocol. Results are summarized in Table 1. They indicate a high antileukemic activity of HAM in refractory acute leukemias which compares favorably with the data of

Table 1. High-dose Ara-C and mitoxantrone (HAM) in refractory AML and ALL

	AML	ALL
n	65	24
CR	35(54%)	12(50%)
PR	2(3%)	1(4%)
NR	12(18%)	5(21%)
ED	16(25%)	6(25%)

other AMLC 6 phase II studies, especially in advanced AML (Table 2). Since side effects were also acceptable, the HAM regimen was subsequently incorporated into the first line treatment of patients younger than 60 years of age with de novo AML [5 7].

Table 2. German AML cooperative group: Phase I/II trials in refractory AML

Regimen	n	CR (%)
HD-AraC 3 g/m^2 × 12	9	1(11%)
AMSA/VP-16	20	0(0%)
Acla/VP-16	31	10(32%)
HD-AraC/Mitox	65	35(54%)

On the basis of the *double induction therapy* HAM was applied as second induction cycle following initial TAD-9 treatment (Fig. 1). The TAD-9/HAM sequence was randomly compared with the TAD-9/TAD-9 combination. At the present time,

Departments of Hematology and Oncology University of Münster[1], Düsseldorf[2], Berlin[4], Kiel[5], Essen[6], Vienna[8], Evangel. Krh. Essen-Werden[3], St. Georg's Krh. Hamburg[7], Department of Biostatistics, University of Münster[9], FRG

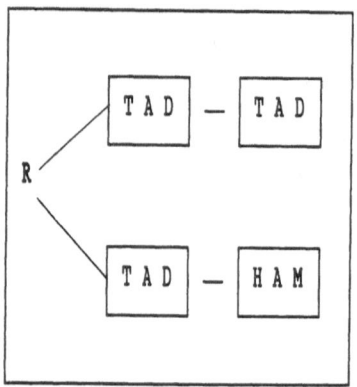

Fig. 1. Acute myeloid leukemia double induction therapy

Table 3. Sequential HAM (S-HAM): Pilot study

Disease	n	CR
AML	10	6
ALL	6	4
Prior HAM therapy	8	6

both sequences appear equally effective with complete remissions of 67 % for TAD-9/TAD-9 and 72 % for TAD-9/HAM [7]. A more detailed analysis of patients experiencing an inadequate clearance of leukemic blasts from the bone marrow after the first TAD-9 cycle indicates, however, that in this subgroup a higher complete remission rate is achieved by applying HAM rather than TAD-9 as the second cycle (58 % versus 46 %). Although this difference is not statistically significant, it strongly suggests that TAD-9 and HAM are not completely cross-resistant and that the TAD/HAM sequence is beneficial, especially in cases with slow initial response. Hence, the most recently initiated trial of the German AMLCG, which is still in its pilot phase, applies a uniform first line regimen using the TAD-9/HAM sequence as the basis to address further questions of postremission treatment and the addition of hematopoietic growth factors.

In parallel to the investigations of HAM in first line treatment, attempts were also

directed to further improvements of salvage therapy. Cell kinetic and pharmacologic data prompted the evaluation of a timed *sequential modification of HAM* (S-HAM) as outlined in Fig. 2. In a first pilot study, 16 patients with advanced AML and ALL at second, third and fourth relapse were treated accordingly and complete remissions were achieved in 10 pts. (62 %) [8]. Remarkably, 8 of the 16 cases had received the original HAM protocol at the preceding relapse and 6 of the 8 cases responded to the S-HAM regimen again (Table 3). These encouraging data provided the means to address further questions such as the most effective and appropriate dose of AraC in relapsed and refractory AML. Hence, using S-HAM as the uniform basis, as prospective randomized trial was initiated by the German AMLCG comparing AraC at doses of 3.0 versus 1.0 g/m² in pts. ≤60 years of age while older cases are assigned to either 1.0 or 0.5 g/m² AraC. With 125 presently evaluable patients similar remission rates were achieved in all treatment groups with an overall response rate of 47 % (Table 4). Reasons for treatment failure, however, were different and suggest a superior antileukemic activity of higher AraC doses which do not translate into an improvement of CR rates due to an enhancced death rate mostly from severe infections. Further

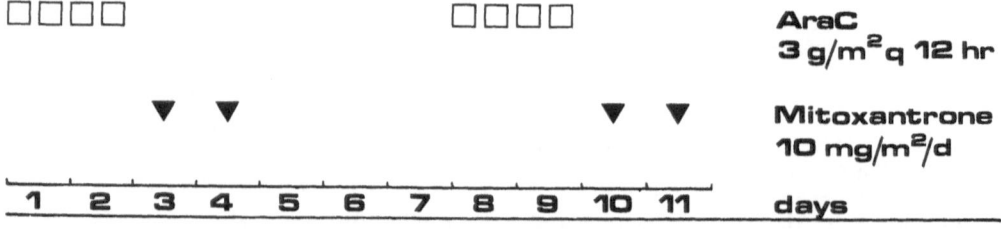

Fig. 2. Sequential HD-AraC and mitoxantrone (S-HAM)

Table 4. Treatment results

	CR	ED	NR + PR	n
Patients <60 years	41(47%)	26(29%)	21(24%)	88
Patients ≤60 years	17(46%)	13(35%)	7(19%)	37
Total	58(47%)	39(31%)	28(22%)	125

results of this trial are given in detail in a separate contribution (9).

Overall, the current data emphazise a significant antileukemic activity of HAM in first and second line treatment of AML, which makes the combination a highly valuable addition substantially contributing to further improvements in AML therapy.

Summary

The significant single-agent activity of high-dose cytosine arabinoside (HD-AraC) and mitoxantrone (Mitox) in relapsed and refractory acute leukemias and the indication of a synergistic antileukemic effect by in vitro investigations led to the clinical application of the two drugs in combination in clinical phase II studies. The original HAM regimen consisted of HD-AraC 3 g/m^2 q 12 h days 1–4 and Mitox 10 mg/m^2 per day days 2–6, and was applied to 89 patients with refractory AML ($n=65$) or ALL ($n=24$). Complete remissions were achieved in 35 of 65 patients with AML (54%) and in 12 of 24 patients with ALL (50%). Pharmacokinetic and cell kinetic data prompted a further modification in a timed sequential application consisting of HD-AraC on days 1+2 and 8+9 and Mitox on days 3+4 andd 10+11 (S-HAM). The encouraging results of a pilot study in 16 patients with advanced refractory AML 10 of whom achieved a CR allowed us to use the S-HAM regimen as the basis to further address the question about the most appropriate dose of ARA-C in relapsed and refractory AML in way of a prospective randomized comparison of 1.0 versus 3.0 g/m^2 AraC in patients <60 years of age while in the older age group 0.5 g/m^2 versus 1.0 g/m^2 AraC are compared. Based on 125 currently evaluable patients no differences in CR rates were observed between the different AraC doses at the present time. The HAM combination was also introduced into the first line treatment of AML as the second course of double induction therapy. The randomized comparison with TAD suggests a higher, though not significant, antileukemic activity especially in patients with slow initial cytoreduction. Hence, the TAD/HAM combination has become the uniform induction treatment used in the current first line trial of the German AML Cooperative Group. In summary, these data indicate a high antileukemic activity of HD-AraC and mitoxantrone in first and second line AML therapy.

References

1. Fountzilas G, Ohnuma T, Okano T, Greenspan EM, Holland JF (1983) Schedule-dependent synergism of cytosine arabinoside (Ara-C) with mitoxantrone in human acute myelogenous leukemia cell line HL 60. Proc Am Soc Clin Oncol 2: 179
2. Krehmeier C, Zühlsdorf M, Büchner T, Hiddemann W (1990) Synergistic cytotoxicity of cytosine arabinoside and mitoxandrone for K562 and CFU-GM. In: Büchner T, Schellong G, Hiddemann W, Ritter J (eds) Acute leukemias II. Prognostic factors and treatment strategies. Springer, Berlin Heidelberg New York, pp 129–132 (Hämatologie und Bluttransfusion, vol 33)
3. Hiddemann W, Martin WR, Sauerland CM, Heinecke A, Büchner T (1990) Definition of refractoriness against conventional chemotherapy in acute myeloid leukemia: a proposal based on the results of retreatment by thioguanine, cytosine arabinoside, and daunorubicin (TAD-9) in 150 patients with relapse after standardized first line therapy. Leukemia 4: 184–188

4. Büchner T, Urbanitz D, Hiddemann W, Rühl H, Ludwig WD, Fischer J, Aul HC et al. (1985) Intensified induction and consolidation with or without maintenance chemotherapy for acute myeloid leukemia (AML): two multicenter studies of the German AML Cooperative Group. J Clin Oncol 3: 1583–1589
5. Büchner T, Hiddemann W, Blasius S et al. (1990) Adult AML: the role of chemotherapy intensity and duration. Two studies of the AML Cooperative Group. In: Büchner T, Schellong G, Hiddemann W, Ritter J (eds) Acute leukemias II. Prognostic factors and treatment strategies. Springer, Berlin Heidelberg New York, pp 261–266 (Hämatologie und Bluttransfusion, vol 33)
6. Hiddemann W, Kreutzmann H, Straif K, Ludwig WD, Mertelsmann R, Donjuijsen-Ant R, Lengfelder E, Arlin Z, Büchner T (1987) High-dose cytosine arabinoside and mitoxantrone: a highly effective regimen in refractory acute myeloid leukemia. Blood 69: 744–749
7. Büchner T, Hiddemann W, Löffler H, Maschmeyer G, Aul C, Nowrousian M, Straif K, Hossfeld D, Heinecke A (1991) Improved cure rate by early intensification combined with prolonged maintenance chemotherapy in patients with acute myeloid leukemia (AML): data from AMLCG. Semin Hemat (in press)
8. Hiddemann W, Büchner T, Essink M, Koch O, Stenzinger W, van de Loo J (1988) High-dose cytosine arabinoside and mitoxantrone: preliminary results of a pilot study with sequential application (S-HAM) indicating a high antileukemic activity in refractory acute leukemias. Onkologie 11: 10–12
9. Hiddemann W, Aul C, Maschmeyer G, Schönrock-Nabulsi R, Ludwig WD et al. (1991) High-dose versus intermediate dose cytosine arabinoside combined with mitoxantrone for the treatment of relapsed and refractory acute myeloid leukemia: results of an age adjusted randomized comparison. In: Hiddemann W, Büchner T, Plunkett W, Keating M, Wörmann B, Andreeff M (eds) Acute leukemias. Pharmacokinetics and Management of Infractory and relapsed disease Springer, Berlin, Heidelberg New York (in press)

Mitoxantrone, Cytosine Arabinoside and VP-16 (MAV) for De Novo Acute Myeloid Leukemia: A Pilot Study

H. Link, M. Freund, H. Diedrich, L. Arseniev, H. Wilke, J. Austein, and H. Poliwoda

Introduction

In several studies it could be shown that mitoxantrone has considerable antileukemic activity [1–3]. In a previous report we showed that the combination of mitoxantrone with cytosine arabinoside and VP-16 is effective in relapsed and refractory acute myeloblastic leukemia (AML) [4]: 21 (58.3 %) of 36 patients achieved a complete hematological remission with a therapy consisting of mitoxantrone (M) 10 mg/m^2 i. v., cytosine arabinoside (A) 100 mg/m^2 continuous infusion and VP-16 (V) 100 mg/m^2 i. v., each for 5 days (MAV protocol). Encouraged by the high antileukemic activity and moderate toxicity, we applied this triple combination in elderly patients with untreated AML. The question was whether the effectiveness of MAV therapy could lead to a high response rate in this group of patients with intermediate risk.

Patients and Treatment Protocol

Eighteen patients with untreated AML and a median age of 58 (49–77) years were entered into the protocol.

Treatment Plan (MAV)

Mitoxantrone (M) 10 mg/m^2 i. v. on days 1–5
Cytosine arabinoside (A) 100 mg/m^2 con-

tinuous infusion on days 1–5 VP-16 (V) 100 mg/m^2 i. v. on days 1–5.

Two cycles were given for remission induction and one for consolidation therapy; one complete remission had been achieved.

Results

Thirteen of 18 (72 %) patients attained a complete remission and three patients died during pancytopenia from bleeding, sepsis or cardiomyopathy. One patient reached a partial remission and one did not respond to therapy. The median duration of remission was 8.25 (1–26+) months; see Fig. 1. The toxicity is summarized in Table 1. In patients surviving the induction therapy, the median duration of granulocytopenia <500/μl was 25 (12–38) days and that of thrombocytopenia <25000/μl 25 (4–38) days.

Discussion

This pilot study showed that the combination of mitoxantrone with ARA-C and VP-16 yielded a remission rate which was in the upper range of the usual conventional chemotherapy. Considering the higher age of this patient population these results look very promising in terms of achieving a complete remission. We therefore recommend testing this combination in comparative clinical trials. Even further improvement might be achieved if the combination of ARA-C and VP-16 were optimized

---

Department of Hematology-Oncology, Konstanty-Gutschow-Str. 8, Medizinische Hochschule Hannover, 3000 Hannover 61, FRG

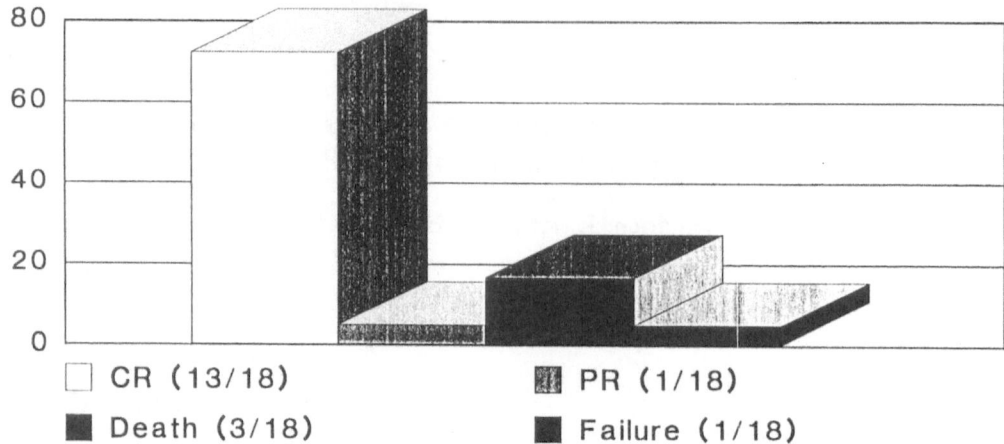

%

☐ CR (13/18) ▨ PR (1/18)

■ Death (3/18) ■ Failure (1/18)

Fig. 1. Results of induction chemotherapy in 18 patients with de novo AML. *CR*, complete remission; *PR*, partial remission; the median duration of remission was 8.25 (1–26+) months

Table 1. Toxicity observed in 28 MAV cycles

WHO grade (%)	1	2	3	4
Bilirubin	32.4	3.6	3.6	
Alkaline phosphatase		3.6	3.6	
ALT	17.4	10.8		
Creatinine	21.6		3.6	
Proteinuria	10.8	21.6		
Hematuria	21.6	21.6		
Hemorrhage	39.6	10.8	3.6	3.6
Nausea	32.4	18	18	
Diarrhea	21.6	36	10.8	
Mucositis	18	25.2	18	
Skin reaction	21.6	21.6		
Local infection		7.2	3.6	
Sepsis			10.8	7.2
Fever of unknown origin	7.6	32.4	25.2	
Congestive heart failure				3.6
Neurological symptoms	10.8	3.6		

according to in-laboratory experiments. In vitro data strongly suggest an inhibitory effect of VP-16 on the uptake of ARA-C by leukemic cells when both drugs are given simultaneously [5]. In our protocol for relapsed and refractory patients we therefore recommend giving ARA-C in the form of a short infusion with a 12-h interval between the applications of ARA-C and of VP-16 in order to further improve the response rate.

Summary

Mitoxantrone is an effective drug against acute myeloid leukemia (AML) and might be valuable in combination with other AML-active drugs such as cytosine arabinoside (ARA-C) and VP-16. In a previous trial we had studied the effectiveness and toxicity of the combination of mitoxantrone (M) 10 mg/m² i.v. for 5 days, cytosine arabinoside (A) 100 mg/m² in the form of a continuous infusion for 5–8 days and VP-16 (V) 100–120 mg/m² i. v. for 5 days (MAV protocol) for relapsed and refractory AML. Out of 36 patients, 21 (58.6%) attained a complete remission (CR) with a median duration of 4.5 (1–12+) months. The median survival of all patients was 5.5 (0.5–15.5+) months. We concluded that the MAV protocol was highly effective against leukemic cells and only moderately toxic. We then applied the 5-day MAV protocol with 100 mg VP-16/m² per day to 18 elderly patients with de novo AML and a median age of 58 (49–77) years. Thirteen of the 18 (72%) patients attained a complete remission and 3 patients died during pancytopenia from bleeding, sepsis or cardiomyopathy. One patient reached a partial remission and one did not respond to therapy. The median duration of remission was 8.25 (1–26+) months. In 28 MAV courses we did not observe any unusual toxicity. In patients surviving the induction therapy, the median duration of granulocytopenia <500/μl was 25 (12–38) days and that of thrombocytopenia <25000/μl 25 (4–38) days. We conclude that MAV therapy is a highly active antileukemic combination with acceptable toxicity and deserves further clinical evaluation in patients with AML.

References

1. Ho AD, Lipp T, Ehninger G, Illinger HJ, Meyer P, Freund M, Hunstein W (1988) J Clin Oncol 6: 213–217
2. Brito-Babapulle F, Catovsky D, Slocombe G et al. (1987) Cancer Treat Rep 71: 161–164
3. Prentice HG, Robbins G, Ma DDF, Ho AD (1984) Semin Oncol 11: 32–35
4. Link H, Freund M, Diedrich H, Wilke H, Austein J, Henke M, Wandt H, Fachler E, Hoffmann R, Poliwoda H (1990) In: Büchner T, Schellong G, Hiddemann W, Ritter J (eds) Acute leukemias II. Prognostic factors and treatment strategies. Springer, Berlin Heidelberg New York, pp 322–326 (Haematology and Blood Transfusion, vol 33)
5. Ehninger G,, Proksch B, Wanner T, Schmidt H, Jaschonek K, Hiddemann W (1990) Blood 76 [Suppl 1] 266 a (abstr)

Role of Mitoxantrone, High-Dose Cytosine Arabinoside, and Recombinant Human GM-CSF in Aggressive Non-Hodgkin's Lymphoma

A. D. Ho[1, 10], F. Del Valle[2], R. Haas[1], M. Engelhard[3], W. Hiddemann[4], H. Rückle[5], G. Schlimok[6], E. Thiel[7], R. Andreesen[8], W. Fiedler[9], and W. Hunstein[1]

Introduction

The activity of mitoxantrone in patients with pretreated aggressive non-Hodgkin's lymphoma (NHL) has been demonstrated in several phase II studies [1–3]. In a previous phase II trial, the present authors investigated the efficacy of mitoxantrone combined with cytarabine (Ara-C) in conventional doses for patients with refractory disease [4], but the response rates did not seem to have improved as compared with mitoxantrone alone. Encouraging results have been reported on the use of high-dose Ara-C alone in relapsed NHL [5–7]. In patients with refractory acute leukemia, the combination of high-dose Ara-C and mitoxantrone has been shown to be active [8, 9].

We have initiated a series of studies with this combination for refractory NHL.

The results in our first trial were encouraging but showed that myelosuppression was the dose-limiting toxicity whereas non-hematological toxicities were mild [10]. At the same time, as rhGM-CSF was available for clinical trials, we have investigated the efficacy and toxicity of NOAC in combination with the growth factor in patients with refractory NHL. As rhGM-CSF was supplied to some of the participating centers, patients treated with rhGM-CSF are reported and compared to those treated in the same period with rhGM-CSF in a nonrandomized fashion.

Materials and Methods

Patients

Adult patients (15–70 years of age) with advanced NHL (stages II–IV) who had refractory disease were eligible for the study if they had normal liver and kidney functions and did not have active infections or signs of cardiac insufficiency. The working formulation was used for defining disease groups of NHL [11].

The following criteria were used to define refractory disease: (1) primary resistance (i.e., maximally stable disease or less after at least two cycles) to regimens such as CHOP [12]/IMVP-16 [13], COP-BLAM/-IMVP-16 [14, 15], ProMACE/MOPP [16], MACOP-B [17], M-BACOD [18]; (2) early relapse (within 6 months) of first remission;

[1] Department of Internal Medicine, University of Heidelberg, Heidelberg, FRG
[2] Städtische Kliniken Oldenburg, Oldenburg, FRG
[3] Department of Internal Medicine, University of Essen, Essen, FRG
[4] Department of Internal Medicine, University of Münster, Münster, FRG
[5] Department of Internal Medicine, University of Würzburg, Würzburg, FRG
[6] Zentralklinikum Augsburg, Augsburg, FRG
[7] Department of Internal Medicine, Klinikum Steglitz, University of Berlin, Berlin, FRG
[8] Department of Internal Medicine, University of Freiburg, Freiburg, FRG
[9] Department of Oncology and Hematology, University of Hamburg, Hamburg, FRG
[10] Northeastern Ontario Regional Cancer Centre, 41 Ramsey Lake Road, Sudbury, Ontario P3E 5J2, Canada

(3) resistance, i.e., less than stable disease after at least two cycles of second-line regimen (IMVP16, ProMACe or M-BACOD, etc.) upon relapse in patients who have previously achieved CR with CHOP or equivalent as first-line therapy; and (4) second or higher relapses. In addition, there had to be measurable disease.

Regimen

In the first trial, mitoxantrone was administered at a dosage of 10 mg/m^2 per day on days 2 and 3 as rapid intravenous infusion (in 15 min) and Ara-C at 3 g/m^2 per 12 h on day 1 (two doses). If at least a partial response (PR) was achieved with the first course, a second course was administered in the 4th week. The treatment, however, was postponed until the drug-induced myelo-suppression had recovered (i.e., platelet count >100/nl and neutrophil count >3.0/nl). If recovery was not achieved after the 5th week and the patient showed at least a partial response, another course was attempted with both drugs reduced in dose by 50%. Patients with lower platelet and neutrophil counts after the end of the 6th week were taken off study. Nonresponsive patients (stable disease or less after the first course) were also taken off study.

In the second study, mitoxantrone was given at the same dosage, whereas the dose of Ara-C was escalated to 3 g/m^2/12 h on days 1 and 2 (four doses). Of nine treatment centers participating in the trial, rhGM-CSF was made available to five by the supplier (Behringwerke AG, Marburg, FRG). In these patients, rhGM-CSF was administered at a concentration of 250 µg/m^2 per 24 h as a continuous infusion and was started at day 6 until the neutrophil count was more than 3.0/nl for three consecutive days [19].

Response and toxicity were evaluated at the end of each course. Dependent upon drug-related toxicity, patients entering into complete remission (CR) were to be given one to two courses of NOAC with or without rhGM-CSF at the same dosage as a consolidation therapy. Patients who achieved only a partial remission (PR) after two cycles were taken off study and fol-

lowed without further treatment. Toxicity was assessed by World Health Organization (WHO) criteria [20].

Complete remission (CR) was defined as disappearance of all signs and symptoms of disease for at least 4 weeks. Bone marrow and peripheral blood counts must be within normal range. Partial remission (PR) was defined as a reduction of measurable tumor parameters by at least 50% for more than 4 weeks. Bone marrow involvement or lymphoma cells in peripheral blood must have decreased by more than 75%. Response less than PR but not fulfilling the criteria for progressive disease (PD) was classified as stable disease (SD). PD was defined as an increase of measurable tumor parameters by at least 25%. Patients who achieved SD or PD were grouped together as nonresponders (NR).

Time to treatment failure (TTF) was defined as time from study enrolment until relapse, disease progression, treatment-related death, withdrawal or date last known alive. Survival was defined as time from enrolment until death or date last known alive.

The study protocol was approved by the Protocol Review Committee of the Medical Faculty of the University of Heidelberg and the local Ethics Commissions. Informed consent was obtained before therapy.

Statistical Analysis

Differences in duration of severe neutropenia and thrombocytopenia, in incidence of side effects and response rates between patients treated with NOAC and rhGM-CSF, and those treated with NOAC chemotherapy alone were analyzed by means of the Wilcoxon-Mann-Whitney U-test.

Results

In the first trial with two doses of Ara-C at 3 g/m^2 per 12 h for day 1 and mitoxantrone at 10 mg/m^2 per hour for days 2 and 3, 34 patients were enrolled and 31 patients were evaluable for response and toxicity. Three patients were considered ineligible, two had Hodgkin's disease and in another patient the disease was not measurable. Of the 31 evaluable patients, 18 had high-grade NHL and 13 intermediate- or low-grade NHL. A CR was achieved in 6 of the 18 patients with high-grade NHL and in 1 of the 13 with intermediate or low-grade NHL. Two of the patients with high-grade NHL and five of those with intermediate or low-grade NHL attained a PR. The median TTF for patients with CR was 7.0 months with a range from 4.0 to 17.0 months.

Myelosuppression was the major toxic side effect of this regimen: the median duration of severe neutropenia ($<0.5/nl$) after each course was 9 days (range: 0–27 days) and that of severe thrombocytopenia ($<20/nl$) was 5 days (range 0–35 days). Infections as a consequence of neutropenia occurred in 45.5 % of the treatment courses and fever of unidentified origin (FUO) in 42.3 % of courses. Two patients died from disease progression within 6 weeks after initiation of therapy. No other serious nonhematologic side effects were observed.

In the second study with escalation of Ara-C to four doses of 3 g/m^2 per 12 h each on days 1 and 2, 42 patients were enrolled but three were considered to be ineligible: two because of pretreatment with mitoxantrone or high-dose Ara-C and one because of AIDS complex. Two further patients were excluded because of protocol violation. Of the 37 patients evaluable for response and toxicity, 23 received rhGM-CSF in addition and 14 did not. A CR was achieved in 9 and a PR in 6 of 23 patients treated with chemotherapy and rhGM-CSF. Two of 14 patients treated with chemotherapy alone attained a CR and 4 others a PR. The median TTF for patients with CR was 6.0 months (range 2.0–10.0+months). The median survival of the 23 patients treated with rhGM-CSF in addition was 130 days and was significantly higher than that of 95 days in patients treated with chemotherapy alone ($p=0.036$, log rank test).

The major toxicity was again myelosuppression. The median duration of severe neutropenia ($<0.5/nl$) in patients treated with rhGM-CSF in addition was 8.0 days with a range from 4 to 20 days, and that of severe ($<20.0/nl$) thrombocytopenia 3.0 days (range 2–38 days). In patients who received chemotherapy alone, the median duration of neutropenia was 13.0 days (range 2–27 days) and that of thrombocytopenia 7.0 days (range 0–22 days). Only the difference in duration of neutropenia was statistically significant ($p=0.0058$). The major nonhematologic side effects were mucositis, infections and FUO. In relation to treatment with rhGM-CSF,, mucositis was observed in 17 % of patients receiving chemotherapy with rhGM-CSF whereas it was present in 57 % of patients with chemotherapy alone ($p=0.0078$). Infections were documented in 25 % of patients treated with rhGM-CSF versus 57 % of patients without rhGM-CSF ($p=0.0547$, n.s.). There was also no difference in incidences of FUO between the two groups.

Discussion

Our studies have shown that the combination of mitoxantrone and high-dose Ara-C is active in the treatment of NHL refractory to second- or third-generation regimens or sequential regimens. Furthermore, we have demonstrated that the additional administration of rhGM-CSF has reduced myelotoxicity and mucositis, and has caused no adverse effects on tumor response. The complete and overall response rates seem to be even higher in patients who received rhGM-CSF.

With mitoxantrone alone, response rates (CR+PR) of 20 % – 35 % have been achieved in relapsed and refractory NHL (1–3). Mitoxantrone has since been combined with etoposide and ifosfamide as salvage therapy [21], or with prednimustine [22] as primary and salvage therapy in patients with aggressive NHL. An overall response rate of up to 78 % has been reported with these combinations, but the criteria for patient entry in these studies are not comparable to our studies reported here.

Although the results of our trials did not appear to be superior to those of other salvage regimens reported in the literature, these patients were more heavily pretreated and most of these patients had disease that was primarily refractory to two or more different regimens before entry into the trials and all had progressive disease before treatment.

As rhGM-CSF was first introduced into our regimen, the main concern was whether the application of hematopoietic growth factors might have any adverse effects on response rates and response duration. Despite all the limitations of a nonrandomized trial and disparity between the two groups, our pilot study indicates that the response rate might be higher in those patients treated with rhGM-CSF in addition to chemotherapy. Based on the preliminary results from these sequential trials, we are concurrently conducting a placebo-controlled, randomized trial using NOAC with rhGM-CSF in patients with refractory NHL.

A number of risk factors for relapse in patients with aggressive NHL have recently been defined [23, 24]. It seems that patients with elevated LDH, bulky tumor mass, extranodal sites, or poor performance status have a poor prognosis and that such patients should be treated with more intensive chemotherapy followed by autologous stem cell transplantation. In another ongoing trial, the regimen NOAC combined with rhGM-CSF is used as a consolidation regimen and at the same time for enhancement of peripheral stem cell yield for autologous stem cell transplantation. The aim of this study is to improve the duration of CR and incrase the cure rate by consolidating the responders to primary regimens with mitoxantrone and high-dose Ara-C and subsequent autologous stem cell transplantation for patients with poor prognostic factors.

Summary

Mitoxantrone (Novantrone, NO) and high-dose cytarabine (Ara-C, AC) have each been shown to be active in non-Hodgkin's lymphoma (NHL). This is a report on our past experience with these two agents and on the use of recombinant human granulocyte-macrophage colony-stimulating factor (rhGM-CSF) for aggressive NHL. The first study combined high-dose cytarabine (3 g/m^2 per 12 h as a 3 h infusion on day 1) with mitoxantrone (10 mg/m^2 per day on days 2 and 3). Of 31 patients with relapsed and refractory NHL, 7 achieved complete remission (CR) and 7 partial remission (PR). In the second study the dosage of cytarabine was escalated to 3 g/m^2 per 12 h on days 1 and 2 (four doses) while mitoxantrone remained at 10 mg/m^2 per day on days 2 and 3. RhGM-CSF was administered at 250 $\mu g/m^2$ per day as a continiuous i. v. infusion from day 6 until the neutrophils were >3.0/nl for three consecutive days. Twenty-three patients from 5 centers were treated with NOAC + rhGM-CSF while 14 patients from 4 other centers received NOAC alone. A CR was achieved in 9 of 23 patients who received rhGM-CSF in addition and in 2 of 14 patients treated with NOAC alone. With rhGM-CSF the median duration of severe neutropenia (<0.5/nl) after chemotherapy was 8 days versus a median of 13 days without rhGM-CSF ($p=0.0058$). The rates of infection and mucositis were 25 % and 17 % respectively with rhGM-CSF compared to 57 % ($p = 0.0547$) and 57 % ($p = 0.0078$) without rhGM-CSF. Concurrently, a double-blind controlled study is being conducted comparing the treatment outcome of patients with refractory disease treated with NOAC and rhGM-CSF versus patients treated with NOAC and placebo. In another trial for patients with defined poor risks, the same regimen combined with rhGM-CSF is used as an induction or consolidation regimen and simultaneously for stimulation of peripheral stem cells for autologous transplantation.

References

1. Coltmann CA Jr, McDaniel TM, Balcerzak SP et al. (1982) Mitoxantrone hydrochloride in lymphoma. Cancer Treat Rev 10: 73–76
2. Gams RA, Steinberg J, Posner L (1984) Mitoxantrone in malignant lymphoma. Sem in Oncol 1 [Suppl] 47–49
3. Shenkenberg TD, Von Hoff DD (1986) Mitoxantrone: a new anticancer drug with significant clinical activity. Ann Intern Med 105: 67–81
4. Ho AD, Dörken B, Hunstein W (1985) Mitoxantrone Monotherapie und in Kombination mit Cytosin-Arabinosid bei refraktären Hodgkin und Non-Hodgkin-Lymphomen. Cancer Res Clin Oncol 111: 105
5. Kantarjian H, Barlogie B, Plunkett W et al. (1983) High dose cytosine arabinoside in

non-Hodgkin's lymphoma. J Clin Oncol 1: 689–694

6. Shipp MA, Takvorian RC, Canellos GP (1984) High-dose cytosine arabinoside: active agent in treatment of non-Hodgkin's lymphoma. Am J Med 77: 845–850

7. Adelstein DJ, Lazarus HM, Hines JD et al. (1985) High-dose cytosine arabinoside in previously treated patients with poor prognosis non-Hodgkin's lymphoma. Cancer 56: 1493–1496

8. Hiddemann W, Kreutzmann H, Straif K, Ludwig WD, Mertelsmann R, Donjuijsen-Ant R, Lengfelder E, Arlin Z, Büchner T (1987) High-dose cytosine-arabinoside and mitoxantrone. A highly effective regimen in refractory adult acute myeloid leukemia. Blood 69: 744–749

9. Hiddemann W, Büchner T, Heil G, Schumacher K, Diedrich H, Maschmeyer G, Ho AD, Planker M, Gerith-Stolzenburg S, Donjuijsen-Ant R, Lengfelder E, Hoelzer D (1990) Treatment of refractory acute lymphoblastic leukemia in adults with high dose cytosine arabinoside and mitoxantrone (HAM). Leukemia 4: 637–640

10. Ho AD, Del Valle F, Rückle H, Schwammborn J, Schlimok G, Hiddemann W, Meusers P, Dörken B, Hunstein W (1989) Mitoxantrone and high-dose cytarabine as salvage therapy for refractory non-Hodgkin's lymphoma. Cancer 664: 1388–1392

11. The non-Hodgkin's Lymphoma Pathologic Classification Project (1982) National Cancer Institute sponsored study of classifications of non-Hodgkin's lymphomas: summary and description of a working formulation for clinical usage. Cancer 49: 2112–2123

12. Armitage JO, Dick FR, Corder MP et al. (1982) Predicting therapeutic outcome in patients with diffuse histiocytic lymphoma treated with cyclophosphamide, adriamycin, vincristine, and prednisone (CHOP). Cancer 50: 1695–1702

13. Cabanillas F, Hagemeister FB, Bodey GP, Freireich EJ (1982) IMVP-16: An effective regimen of patients with lymphoma who have relapses after initial combination chemotherapy. Blood 60: 693–697

14. Laurence J, Coleman M, Allen SL, Silver RT, Pasmantier M (1982) Combination chemotherapy of advanced diffuse histiocytic lymphoma with six-drug COP-BLAM regimen. Ann Intern Med 97: 190–195

15. Thiel E, Gerhartz HH, Brittinger G (1988) Response-adapted COP-BLAM/IMVP-16 chemotherapy for advanced stage aggressive non-Hodgkin's lymphoma. Proc Am Soc Clin Oncol 7: 244

16. Fisher RI, DeVita VT Jr., Hubbard SM et al. (1983) Diffuse aggressive lymphomas: increased survival after alternating flexible sequences of ProMACE and MOPP chemotherapy. Ann Intern Med 98: 304–309

17. Klimo P, Connors JM (1985) MACOP-B chemotherapy for the treatment of diffuse large-cell lymphoma. Ann Intern Med 102: 596–602

18. Skarin AT, Canellos GP, Rosenthal DS et al. (1983) Improved prognosis of diffuse histiocytic and undifferentiated lymphoma by use of high-dose methotrexate alternating with standard agents (M-BACOD). J Clin Oncol 1: 91–97

19. Ho AD, Del Valle F, Engelhard M, Hiddemann W, Rückle H, Schlimok G, Haas R, Thiel E, Andreesen R, Fiedler W, Frisch J, Schulz G, Hunstein W (1990) Mitoxantrone/high-dose Ara-C and recombinant human GM-CSF in the treatment of refractory non-Hodgkin's lymphoma. Cancer 66: 423–430

20. Miller AB, Hoogstraten B, Staquet M et al. (1981) Reporting results of cancer treatment. Cancer 47: 207–214

21. Heinz R, Dittrich CH, Ludwig H et al. (1986) Results of a new combination chemotherapy (etoposide-ifosphamide-mitoxantrone) in advanced NHL. Cancer Res Clin Oncol 111:[Suppl] 38

22. Landys KE (1988) Mitoxantrone in combination with stereocyte (NOSTE) in treatment of unfavorable non-Hodgkin's lymphoma. Invest New Drugs 6: 105–113

23. Coiffier B, Gisselbrecht C, Vose J, Tilly H, Herbrecht R, Bosly A, Armitage JO (1991) Prognostic factors in aggressive malignant lymphomas: description and validation of a prognostic index that could identify patients requiring a more intensive therapy. J Clin Oncol 9: 211–219

24. Hoskins PJ, Ng V, Spinelli J, Klimo P, Connors JM (1991) Prognostic variables in patients with diffuse large-cell lymphoma treated with MACOP-B. J Clin Oncol 9: 220–226

Treatment of Low-Malignant Non-Hodgkin's Lymphoma by Cytoreductive Chemotherapy with Prednimustine/Mitoxantrone (PmM) Followed by Interferon-α2b Maintenance

M. Unterhalt[1], P. Koch[1], M. Nahler[1], R. Herrmann[2], and W. Hiddemann[1]

Introduction

The prognosis of patients with low-grade malignant non-Hodgkin's lymphomas in advanced stages III and IV has not significantly changed within the past 15 years. The median survival after diagnosis is 6–10 years [2, 6, 10]. While patients in stages I and II, in some cases also in stage III, can be cured by radiotherapy [9], only palliative treatment concepts are available for patients with advanced disease. Although low-grade non-Hodgkin's lymphomas respond to different forms of cytostatic therapy in the vast majority, a significant prolongation of survival has not been demonstrated. In 1988, Landys et al. [7] reported on a high antilymphoma activity of the combination of prednismustine and mitoxantrone with a low incidence of therapy-associated side effects.

Several groups have demonstrated a significant antilymphoma activity of interferon-α also in patients resistant to conventional cytostatic therapy [3, 8, 11]. Based on experimental data and preliminary clinical observations, the application of interferon-α seems to be more promising in patients with a lower tumor load after initial chemotherapy has significantly reduced the number of lymphoma cells [1]. Based on these data, a phase II study was initiated for patients with advanced low-malignant non-Hodgkin's lymphoma using prednimustine and mitoxantrone for initial cytoreductive therapy and interferon-α as maintenance therapy [4].

Patients and Methods

The initial cytoreductive therapy in this study consisted of a combination of 100 mg/m^2 per day prednimustine, given on days 1–5 p. o. and the intravenous administration of mitoxantrone 8 mg/m^2 per day on days 1 and 2. This therapy was repeated after a minimum of 4 and a maximum of 6 weeks. Inclusion criteria for the study were B symptoms, hematopoietic insufficiency, objective progression of the lymphoma or bulky disease. After every two cycles of therapy the treatment success was reevaluated. In patients with progression of the lymphoma the therapy was discontinued. Patients who achieved a complete remission after four cycles of therapy received two further cycles as consolidation. The other patients also received two additional cycles of chemotherapy. If they achieved at least a partial remission, i. e., at least 50 % reduction of the initial lymphoma mass, two further cycles of PmM were applied as consolidation. This group of patients received a total of eight cycles. In patients with posttherapeutic cytopenia with less than 1 500 neutrophils/µl or less than 75 000 platelets/µl the dose of prednimustine and mitoxantrone was reduced by 25 % in the subsequent cycles [4].

A total of 19 patients have been treated in the pilot study. The median age was 59

Department of Internal Medicine, University of Münster, Albert-Schweitzer-Str. 33, 4400 Münster, FRG
Department of Internal Medicine, University of Berlin, FRG

661

years. Eight patients were female, 11 male. The histological diagnosis according to the Kiel classification was centroblastic-centro-cytic in 13 cases, centrocytic in 3 cases. The remaining three patients were diagnosed as lymphoplasmocytoid immunocytomas. Two of the 19 patients had not received prior therapy. Seventeen patients had received at least one course of chemotherapy with drugs not tested in the pilot study. Five of the 17 patients had received radiotherapy.

Results

A total of 137 therapy cycles were eva-luated. The most significant side effect was myelosuppression with an incidence of leu-kocytopenia of WHO grade III or IV in 29 %. The rate of severe infections was 9 %. A significant thrombocytopenia of WHO grade III and IV occurred in only 5 % of cycles. Dose reduction was necessary in 48 % of all courses.

Two of the 19 patients achieved a com-plete remission after only 2 cycles. One patient achieved complete remission after four, another patient after six cycles. So the total rate of complete remissions was four patients. Nine patients had a reduction of the initial lymphoma manifestations of at least 50 %, defined as partial remission. Two patients had no change, while four patients showed progression of lymphoma under therapy. The 13 patients with a signif-icant response to the initial chemotherapy received 2 further courses of consolidation followed by maintenance therapy with 5 million IU interferon-α s.c. 3 × per week. The median remission duration of these patients was 14.5+ months. In comparison with the preceding chemotherapies in these patients maintenance therapy with interfe-ron-α shows a tendency toward a longer remission duration. The results of this pilot study are the basis for the current, multi-center study in patients with centroblastic-centrocytic lymphoma and centrocytic lymphoma at advanced stages III and IV. The goal of this study is a randomized comparison of the currently described PmM regimen with standard COP chemo-therapy. COP consists of 400 mg/m^2 per day cyclophosphamide i.v. on days 1–5,

1.4 mg/m^2 vincristine with a maximum of 2 mg/dose on day 1 and 100 mg/m^2 per day prednisone p.o. on days 1–5. Inclusion criteria were identical to those of the pilot study. Patients were randomized by the study center in Münster into one of the two therapy arms. As in the pilot study, all patients received a minimum of six and a maximum of eight cycles, depending on the results after four cycles of therapy. Therapy was discontinued in patients with progres-sion of the disease. Patients who achieved a complete or at least a partial remission, under initial COP or PmM therapy, were randomized for maintenance therapy with interferon-α versus observation only. As of February 1991, 141 patients from 55 centers have entered the study. The histological diagnoses were centroblastic-centrocytic lymphoma in 100 patients and centrocytic lymphoma in 37 patients. Four patients with different histological diagnoses were excluded.

Patient recruitment has increased steadi-ly after the start of the study in May 1988. Eighty-nine patients of the 141 patients entered the study after June 1989 and have been randomized between COP and PmM. Before this date each center treated with either PmM or COP. Only the randomized patients form the basis of the comparative evaluation of the two chemotherapy proto-cols. Seventy-eight of the 141 patients were male, 63 were female. As expected, patients with centrocytic lymphoma showed a preponderance of male patients while in the group of cb-cc lymphomas a slightly higher number of female patients was registered. The median age was 53 years. Analysis of therapy-related toxicity was performed on the basis of 187 treatment courses with COP and 241 treatment courses with PmM (Table 1). The most significant side effect of the two initial chemotherapies in this group of not pre-viously treated patients was myelosuppres-sion, most notably granulocytopenia. There was no significant difference in hematotox-icity between the two therapy arms. How-ever, differences have been noted in cardio-toxicity which was more pronounced in patients receiving PmM, while neurotoxici-ty and alopecia were more frequently observed in patients receiving COP. The

Table 1. COP vs. PmM: side effects

WHO toxicity	COP					PmM				
	I (%)	II (%)	III (%)	IV (%)	N	I (%)	II (%)	III (%)	IV (%)	N
Hemoglobin	22.0	3.3	2.1	0.8	241	12.9	5.0	1.1	0.0	280
Leukocytes	10.0	17.1	30.8	11.7	240	8.8	21.9	27.9	8.8	283
Granulocytes	7.5	13.4	21.4	12.3	187	12.0	13.7	19.5	14.9	241
Thrombocytes	4.8	0.9	0.9	0.4	231	8.9	5.0	1.8	0.7	280
Bleeding	0.0	0.0	0.4	0.0	235	1.4	0.7	0.0	0.0	289
Nausea/vomiting	18.9	4.5	2.5	1.6	243	24.7	5.8	3.4	0.0	291
Mucositis	3.0	0.4	0.0	0.0	237	5.6	1.4	0.0	0.0	287
Obstipation	3.8	0.8	0.0	0.0	237	1.1	1.1	0.0	0.0	285
Diarrhea	5.9	2.1	0.8	0.0	236	1.4	0.3	0.0	0.0	287
Fever	2.9	3.8	0.4	0.0	238	2.4	1.7	0.0	0.0	288
Alopecia	22.0	30.9	26.3	0.0	236	15.5	8.3	0.0	0.0	278
Infection	3.8	5.0	0.8	0.4	238	5.9	2.8	0.3	0.3	290
Cardiac dysfunction	0.8	0.0	0.0	0.0	236	4.5	1.0	3.1	0.0	289
Neurotoxicity	19.3	0.8	0.4	0.0	238	2.4	1.0	0.0	0.0	287

Table 2. Response after induction therapy with COP (35) or PmM (49)

N	CR 4	CR 6	PR	NC	PD	Dead	Excl.
84	21	13	31	5	5	4	5
	25.0%	15.5%	36.9%	6.0%	6.0%	4.8%	6.0%

combined analysis of treatment response for both treatment arms shows a complete remission after 4 cycles in 21 of the 84 patients (Table 2). An additional 13 patients achieved CR after 6 cycles. Thirty-one patients achieved partial remissions after six cycles. Five patients had no change and five patients progressed under therapy. During the course of therapy four patients died. Five patients were excluded due to protocol violation. After the consolidation therapy patients in CR or PR are randomized between interferon-α maintenance and no further therapy. So far, 63 patients have been randomized.

Conclusion

Stimulated by the results of Landys on PmM [7] and reports on a beneficial effect by interferon-α [1, 3, 8, 11], we initiated a pilot study in 1987, which confirmed the excellent therapeutic results. This was the basis for the current study randomizing PmM versus COP in induction therapy and randomizing interferon-α versus no therapy in patients with CR or PR. Preliminary analysis shows a comparable toxicity in both induction treatment arms. Definitive evaluation requires the recruitment of additional patients and longer observation times.

Summary

In a clinical phase II study the antilymphoma activity of the recently introduced combination of prednimustine and mitoxantrone (PmM) was evaluated in 19 patients with advanced low-malignant non-Hodgkin's lymphomas after failure or relapse after standard chemotherapy. The PmM regimen consisted of prednimustine 100 mg/m^2 per day orally days 1–5 and mitoxantrone 8 mg/m^2 per day i. v. days 1 and 2 and was repeated every 4–6 weeks to a maximum of six cycles. Patients achieving a complete or partial remission (PR or CR) received two additional courses for consolidation followed by interferon-α2b 5 × 10^6 units s. c. three times weekly until progression or relapse. Thirteen of the 19 patients (68 %) responded with four CRs and nine PRs. PmM side effects consisted mainly of neutropenia requiring dose reduction in 48 % of treatment cycles. All 13 responding patients subsequently received IFN-α2b maintenance treatment. At the present time remission duration ranges from 4.5+ – 17.5+ months with a median of 14.5 months. In comparison to unmaintained first remission preceding the PmM/IFN trial a tendency towards a longer period of freedom from progression was apparent in the 13 patients receiving IFN maintenance treatment during their second PR or CR. These data provided the basis for a currently ongoing multicenter study randomly comparing initial chemotherapy by PmM versus COP in patients with advanced CB-CC and CC-non-Hodgkin's lymphomas followed by a second randomization in CR and PR patients for maintenance with IFN-α versus observation, only. The PmM regimen is applied as indicated above. The COP regimen consists of cyclophosphamide 400 mg/m^2 per day i. v. days 1–5, vincristine 1.4 mg/m^2 (max. 2 mg) i. v. day 1 and prednisone 100 mg/m^2 per day orally days 1–5. At the present time 141 patients have been enrolled into this ongoing study, 84 of whom are currently evaluable for response and toxicity. CR was achieved in 34 cases (40 %) while an additional 31 cases (37 %) obtained a PR. Side effects were mild to moderate with neutropenia occurring in 33 % of treatment courses. Further accrural of patients and longer observation times are needed to confirm these promising results and to disclose the comparative analysis of PmM vs. COP and IFN maintenance versus observation only.

Reference

1. Balkwill FR (1985) Antitumor effects of interferons in animals, In: Finter NB, Oldham RK (eds) Interferon, in vivo and clinical studies, vol. 4. Elsevier, Amsterdam, pp 23–45
2. Brittinger G, Meusers P, Engelhard M (1986) Strategien der Behandlung von Non-Hodgkin-Lymphomen. Internist 27: 485–497
3. Chisesi T, Capnist G, Vespignani M, Cetto G (1987) Interferon alfa-2b and chlorambucil in the treatment of non-Hodgkin's lymphoma. Invest New Drugs 5 [Suppl]: 35–40
4. Hiddemann W, Koch P, Essink M, et al. (1989) Treatment of low-grade non-Hodgkin's lymphoma with prednimustine/mitoxantrone followed by interferon alpha-2b. A clinical phase II study. Contrib Oncol 37: 287–291
5. Horning SJ, Nademanee AP, Chao NJ, Schmidt GM, Hoppe RT, Lipsett JA, Negrin RS, Forman SJ, Blume KG (1990) Regimen-related toxicity and early post-transplant survival in patients undergoing autologous bone marrow transplantation (ABMT) for lymphoma: combined experience of Stanford University and the City of Hope National Medical Center. Proc Am Soc Clin Oncol 9: 271
6. Horning SJ, Rosenberg SA (1984) The natural history of initially untreated low-grade non-Hodgkin's lymphomas. N Engl J Med 311: 1471–1475
7. Landys KE (1988) Mitoxantrone in combination with prednimustine in treatment of unfavorable non-Hodgkin lymphoma. Invest New Drugs 6: 105–113
8. Ozer H, Anderson JR, Peterson BA, Budman DR, Henderson ES, Bloomfield CD, Gottlieb A (1987) Combination trial of subcutaneous interferon alfa-2b and oral cyclophosphamide in favorable histology, non-Hodgkin's lymphoma. Invest New Drugs 5 [Suppl]: 27–33
9. Portlock CS (1983) "Good risk" Non-Hodgkin's lymphomas: approaches to management. Semin Hematol 20: 25–36
10. Portlock CS (1990) Non-Hodgkin's lymphomas. Advances in diagnosis, staging, and management. Cancer 65 [Suppl]: 718–722
11. Rohatiner AZ, Richards MA, Barnett MJ, Stansfeld AG, Lister TA (1987) Chlorambucil and interferon for low grade non-Hodgkin's lymphoma. Br J Cancer 55: 225–226
12. Young RC, Longo DL, Glatstein E, Ihde DC, Jaffe ES, DeVita VT Jr (1988) The treatment of indolent lymphomas: watchful waiting v aggressive combined modality treatment. Semin Hematol 25 [Suppl 2]: 11–16

Subject Index

A

Aclacinomycin A
– in combination with
  – VP16 for relapsed AML   392–393,
    458–461
– multidrug resistance   49–54
Aclarubicin see Aclacinomycin A
Acute myeloid leukemia see AML
Acute myelogenous leukemia see AML
Acute non-lymphocytic leukemia see AML
Adriamycin see Doxorubicin
Adult ALL
– G-CSF in   101–107
– multidrug resistance   4–5
– treatment of relapse   472–480, 481–485
Aldehyde dehydrogenase
– and resistance against cyclophosphamide
  60–64
ALL
– allogeneic bone marrow transplantation
  529–532
– and sarcoidosis   248–250
– autologous bone marrow transplantation
  549–553
– detection of minimal residual disease
  – by immunophenotype   228–232
  – by PCR   171–177, 178–183
– renal failure in   503–507
– response to
  – Il 3   148–151
  – Il 7   148–151
ALL trans retinoic acid
– mechanism of response   187–188
Allogeneic bone marrow transplantation
– engraftment-promoting potential of high-
  dose AraC   533–536
– in first remission AML   463–465, 511–517
– in second and third remission AML
  511–517, 529–532
AML
– abnormal marker expression   196–200
– CNS involvement in childhood AML
  491–496
– consolidation therapy with
  – allogeneic bone marrow transplantation
    463–465, 511–517

– high-dose AraC   425–428, 463–465
– mitoxantrone and etoposide
  439–444
– detection of minimal residual disease
  196–200, 204–207, 228–232
– G-CSF in   101–107
– GM-CSF in   81–96, 97–100, 108–117,
  118–130, 615
– immunotherapy   572–575, 601–607
– induction therapy
  – double induction   611–616
  – with
    – AraC and AMSA   445–448
    – AraC, mitoxantrone and etoposide
      653–655
    – high-dose AraC and mitoxantrone
      430–432
    – idarubicin and AraC   439–444,
      462–465
    – sequential AraC and mitoxantrone
      421–424
– LAK cell activity against   581–589, 601–607
– maintenance therapy   611–616
– multidrug resistance   5–7, 29–31
– prognostic factors for salvage therapy
  379–387, 394
– prognostic relevance of immunophenotype
  222–227
– relapse
  – allogeneic bone marrow transplantation
    511–517, 529–532
  – autologous blood stem cell transplan-
    tation   518–522
  – characterization by immunophenotyping
    208–213
  – consolidation therapy   404–410
  – high-dose AraC plus mitoxantrone
    434–438, 643–646, 649–653
    – in childhood AML   418–420
  – high-dose versus intermediate dose AraC
    plus mitoxantrone   412–416
  – karyotype in   383
– renal failure in   503–507
– response to SCF   73–78
– T-cell receptor gene rearrangement
  198–199, 241–247
– therapy with

M

Macrophage-Colony Stimulating Factor
  see M-CSF
MDS
– erythropoietin production in   163–167
– intensive chemotherapy   466–471
– postremission therapy   469–471
Methotrexate
– DHFR gene amplification   16–17
– impairement of
  – polyglutamation   19–20
  – transport   17–18
– plasma pharmacokinetics
  – and prognosis in childhood ALL
    338–342
– resistance to   16–21
Minimal residual disease
– detection by
  – in situ hybridization   190–194
  – premature chromosome condensation
    185–188
– in
  – ALL
    – detection by
      – immunophenotype   228–232
      – PCR   171–177, 178–183
  – AML
    – detection by
    – DNA aneuploidy   198
    – immunophenotype   196–201
    – PCR   198–199
Mitoxantrone
– and
  – mdr expression   52, 53
– cytotoxic activity on CFU-L   302
– in
  – combination with
    – etoposide for consolidation therapy in
      AML   439–444
    – high-dose AraC and GM-CSF in non-
      Hodgkin's lymphoma   656–660
    – prednimustine in low-grade non-Hodg-
      kin's lymphoma   661–664
  – de novo AML
    – in combination with
      – standard-dose AraC   421–424
      – and VP 16   653–655
  – relapsed AML
    – in combination with
      – continuous infusion AraC
        481–485
      – etoposide   382–383, 393–394,
        437–437, 645–646
        – and intermediate dose AraC
          401–403
      – high-dose AraC   434–436, 643–646,
        649–652
      – in childhood AML   418–420
      – in MDS   466–471

– high-dose versus intermediate dose
  AraC   412–416
– idarubicin   396–399
– intracellular concentration   301–302,
  306–308
– plasma pharmacokinetics   300–303,
  635–639
– therapeutic response in AML   301, 642–647
Multidrug resistance see also p-glycoprotein
– circumvention of   7–8, 33–39, 40–42,
  324–325
– in
  – ALL   4–5, 23–26, 321–326, 332–337
  – AML   5–7, 29–31
– mechanism of   3
– through DNA topoisomerase II   11–14
Myelodysplastic syndromes see MDS
M-CSF
– in vitro response to   132–136

N

Natural Killer cells see NK cells
NK cell activity
– in childhood ALL   152–156

PCR

for detection of minimal residual disease in
  ALL
  – bcr/abl rearrangement   175–176
  – immunoglobulin heavy chain rearrange-
    ment   178–183
  – T-cell receptor gene rearrangements
    171–177
P-glycoprotein   3–8
– and
  – AML   5–7, 29–31
  – anthracycline uptake   33–39
  – response to aclacinomycin A   49–54
  – secondary AML   6
– determination by flow cytometry   33–39
– expression in
  – ALL   4–5, 23–26, 324–326
  – AML   5–7, 29–31
  – CLL   34–39
  – Friend leukemia   56–58
  – HL 60   46
  – secondary AML   6
Platelet transfusion
– in patients with bone marrow aplasia
  501–502
Polymerase chain reaction see PCR
Premature chromosome condensation
– for detection of
  – leukemic cell maturation   186–188
  – minimal residual disease   185–188
Programmed cell death   255–256

669

5q-syndrome
- and loss of GM-CSF gene heterozygosity 238–240
- c-fms in   238–240

S

SAENTA fluoresceins   65–71
SFC
- and other growth factors   73–78
- biologic effects in AML   73–78, 110–113
- receptor expression in AML   73–78
Stem cell factor see SCF

T

T-cell receptor gene rearrangements
- for detection of minimal residual disease 171–177, 198–199

- TCR delta rearrangement in AML 241–247
Teniposide
- and AraC accumulation   262–264
- pharmacokinetics and protein binding 343–350
Topoisomerase II
- and response to aclacinomycin A   49–54
- in HL 60   46, 47
- mechanism of drug resistance by   11–14
Triglycidylurazol
- clinical response   359–367
- pharmacology   359–367

V

Vepesid see Etoposide
Vincristine
- and mdr expression   52, 53
VP16 see Etoposide